# Preventive
# Newborn Health

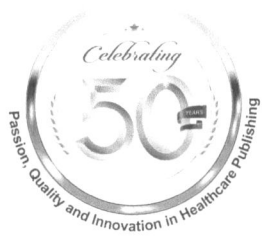

# Preventive
# Newborn Health

*Editor-in-Chief*
**Balaji Govindaswami** MBBS MPH FAAP
Professor of Pediatrics and Associate Chair for Research, Department of Pediatrics
Endowed Chair, Preventative and Addiction Medicine
Professor, Department of Clinical and Translational Sciences
Office of Research and Graduate Education
Marshall University Joan C Edwards School of Medicine
Division Chief, Neonatology; Director - NICU
Hoops Family Children's Hospital at Cabell Huntington Hospital
Huntington, West Virginia, USA

*Associate Editor*
**Robin Daughters Wu**

*Assistant Editor*
**Nisha Bedi Donley**

*Section Editors*
**Glenn Henry DeSandre**
**Kamakshi Devarajan**
**Matthew J Garabedian**
**Priya Jegatheesan**
**Rupalee Patel**
**Audra Pritt**
**Dongli Song**

*Illustrative Editor*
**Albert H Alhatem**

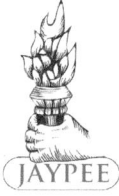

**JAYPEE BROTHERS MEDICAL PUBLISHERS**
*The Health Sciences Publisher*
New Delhi | London

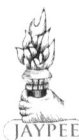 **Jaypee Brothers Medical Publishers (P) Ltd**

**Headquarters**

Jaypee Brothers Medical Publishers (P) Ltd
EMCA House, 23/23-B
Ansari Road, Daryaganj
New Delhi 110 002, India
Landline: +91-11-23272143, +91-11-23272703
+91-11-23282021, +91-11-23245672
Email: jaypee@jaypeebrothers.com

**Corporate Office**

Jaypee Brothers Medical Publishers (P) Ltd
4838/24, Ansari Road, Daryaganj
New Delhi 110 002, India
Phone: +91-11-43574357
Fax: +91-11-43574314
Email: jaypee@jaypeebrothers.com

**Overseas Office**

JP Medical Ltd
83 Victoria Street, London
SW1H 0HW (UK)
Phone: +44 20 3170 8910
Fax: +44 (0)20 3008 6180
Email: info@jpmedpub.com

Website: www.jaypeebrothers.com
Website: www.jaypeedigital.com

© 2021, Jaypee Brothers Medical Publishers

The views and opinions expressed in this book are solely those of the original contributor(s)/author(s) and do not necessarily represent those of editor(s) of the book.

All rights reserved. No part of this publication may be reproduced, stored or transmitted in any form or by any means, electronic, mechanical, photocopying, recording or otherwise, without the prior permission in writing of the publishers.

All brand names and product names used in this book are trade names, service marks, trademarks or registered trademarks of their respective owners. The publisher is not associated with any product or vendor mentioned in this book.

Medical knowledge and practice change constantly. This book is designed to provide accurate, authoritative information about the subject matter in question. However, readers are advised to check the most current information available on procedures included and check information from the manufacturer of each product to be administered, to verify the recommended dose, formula, method and duration of administration, adverse effects and contraindications. It is the responsibility of the practitioner to take all appropriate safety precautions. Neither the publisher nor the author(s)/editor(s) assume any liability for any injury and/or damage to persons or property arising from or related to use of material in this book.

This book is sold on the understanding that the publisher is not engaged in providing professional medical services. If such advice or services are required, the services of a competent medical professional should be sought.

Every effort has been made where necessary to contact holders of copyright to obtain permission to reproduce copyright material. If any have been inadvertently overlooked, the publisher will be pleased to make the necessary arrangements at the first opportunity. The **CD/DVD-ROM** (if any) provided in the sealed envelope with this book is complimentary and free of cost. **Not meant for sale.**

**Inquiries for bulk sales may be solicited at**: jaypee@jaypeebrothers.com

*Preventive Newborn Health*

*First Edition:* **2021**

ISBN: 978-93-5270-473-6

Printed at Repro India Limited

## Dedicated to

माता
*Mother*

पिता
*Father*

गुरू
*Guru*

देवम्
*Divine Grace*

*James Donald Whitaker, Jr*

*In memory of Ira Adams-Chapman*

# Contributors

**Ira Adams-Chapman** MD MPH FAAP
Associate Professor of Pediatrics
Director, Developmental Progress Clinic
Jennings Watkins Scholar in Neuroscience
Emory University School of Medicine
Department of Pediatrics/Division of Neonatology
Children's Healthcare of Atlanta
Atlanta, Georgia, USA

**Albert H Alhatem** MD PhD
Dermatopathology Fellow
Department of Dermatology
Saint Louis University School of Medicine
Saint Louis, Missouri, USA

**Steven M Barlow** PhD
Corwin Moore Professor
Associate Director
Center for Brain, Biology and Behavior
SECD and Biological Systems Engineering
University of Nebraska
Lincoln, Nebraska, USA

**Rebecca Barnett** DO FAAP
Attending Neonatologist
Hoops Family Children's Hospital at
Cabell Huntington
Director, High Risk Infant Follow-up
Marshall Pediatrics
Assistant Professor of Pediatrics
Division of Neonatology
Marshall University Joan C Edwards School of Medicine
Huntington, West Virginia, USA

**Robert M Bernstein** MD
Chief of Staff
Shriners Hospital for Children
Portland, Oregon, USA
Medical Advisory Board
Little People of America
Pediatric Orthopedic Advisory Board
Global Help

**Stephanie D Chao** MD FACS FAAP
Assistant Professor of Surgery
Division of Pediatric Surgery
Stanford University School of Medicine
Stanford, California, USA

**Lily C Chen** MD FAAP
Attending Neonatologist
Saddleback Medical Center
Laguna Hills, California, USA

**John Patrick Cleary** MD FAAP
Associate Clinical Professor
Department of Pediatrics
University of California Irvine
ECMO Director
Associate Director, CVICU
Children's Hospital of Orange County
Regional Director of Neonatology
CHOC Children's Specialists
Orange, California, USA

**Noah Craft** MD PhD
CEO, People Science, Inc.
Los Angeles, California, USA

**Glenn Henry DeSandre** MD FAAP
Attending Neonatologist
Permanente Medicine
Kaiser Permanente Oakland Medical Center
Oakland, California, USA

**Kamakshi Devarajan** MD FAAP
University of California, Irvine
Children's Hospital of Orange County
CHOC Children's Specialists, Orange
Chair of Pediatrics
Director, Neonatal Intensive Care Unit
Saint Francis Medical Center
Lynwood, California, USA

**Nisha Bedi Donley** BA MBA
Los Angeles, California, USA

**Shannon Dralla** MD FACOG
Physician
Department of Obstetrics and Gynecology
The Permanente Medical Group
San Jose and Gilroy, California, USA

**Gregory M Enns** MB ChB
Professor of Pediatrics
Director, Biochemical Genetics Program
Stanford University
Stanford, California, USA

**Christopher Fink** MD MPH FAAP
Clinical Assistant Professor of
Pediatric Gastroenterology
Stanford University School of Medicine
Pediatric Gastroenterologist
Lucile Packard Children's Hospital
Santa Clara Valley Medical Center
San Jose, California, USA

**Susan Flesher** MD FAAP
Associate Professor
Interim Chair, Department of Pediatrics
Director, Pediatric Hospital Medicine Fellowship
Marshall University
Huntington, West Virginia, USA

**Sharyn Frentner** RNC MSN CNS NNP
Clinical Nurse Specialist (Retired)
Neonatal Intensive Care Unit
Santa Clara Valley Medical Center
San Jose, California, USA

**Julie R Fuchs** MD FACS FAAP
Clinical Associate Professor of Surgery
Stanford University School of Medicine
Chief, Pediatric Surgery
Santa Clara Valley Medical Center
San Jose, California, USA

**Matthew J Garabedian** MD MPH FACOG
Chief, Women's Health Subspecialties
Kaiser Permanente
Sacramento and Roseville, California, USA

**Zachary Max Goldstein** MD
Dermatopathologist
Contra Costa Pathology Associates
Pleas-ant Hill, California, USA

**Balaji Govindaswami** MBBS MPH FAAP
Professor of Pediatrics and
Associate Chair for Research
Department of Pediatrics
Endowed Chair, Preventative and Addiction Medicine
Professor, Department of Clinical and
Translational Sciences
Office of Research and Graduate Education
Marshall University Joan C Edwards School of Medicine
Division Chief, Neonatology; Director - NICU
Hoops Family Children's Hospital at
Cabell Huntington Hospital
Huntington, West Virginia, USA

**Stephen Harris** MD FAAP
Clinical Professor (Affiliated) of Pediatrics
Stanford University School of Medicine
Department of Pediatrics
Santa Clara Valley Medical Center
San Jose, California, USA

**Emily Altick Hartford** MD MPH
Assistant Professor of Pediatrics
University of Washington
Seattle Children's Hospital
Formerly at UCLA Center for World Health
Mozambique Partnership Director
Maputo, Mozambique

**Francesca C Ianovich** MD
Resident (PGY-2)
Department of Anesthesiology
University of California San Diego School of Medicine
La Jolla, California, USA

**Priya Jegatheesan** MD FAAP
Clinical Assistant Professor (Affiliated) of Pediatrics
Neonatal and Developmental Medicine
Stanford University School of Medicine
Director, Neonatal Intensive Care Unit
Chief, Division of Neonatology
Santa Clara Valley Medical Center
San Jose, California, USA

**Korinne S Van Keuren** DNP RN CPNP-AC PNP-BC
Director of Advanced Practice Providers
Clinical Assistant Professor of Nursing
University of Virginia Medical Center
Charlottesville, Virginia, USA

**Alganesh G Kifle** RN BSN IBCLC
Volunteer Faculty
Tikur Anbessa Hospital
Vermont Oxford Network, Addis Ababa, Ethiopia
Lactation Program Coordinator (Retired)
Neonatal Intensive Care Unit
Santa Clara Valley Medical Center
San Jose, California, USA

**Rashmi Kirpekar** MD FAAP
Clinical Assistant Professor (Affiliated) of Pediatrics
Stanford University School of Medicine
Chief, Division of Pediatric Nephrology
Santa Clara Valley Medical Center
San Jose, California, USA

**Yueh-Tze Lan** MD FAAP
Clinical Assistant Professor (Affiliated) of Pediatrics
Stanford University School of Medicine
Pediatric Cardiologist
Santa Clara Valley Medical Center
San Jose, California, USA

**Sangeeta Mallik** PhD
Director, NICU Family-Centered Care
Developmental Psychologist and
Early Childhood Researcher
Santa Clara Valley Medical Center
San Jose, California, USA

**Sonya Misra** MBBS MPH FAAP
Clinical Associate Professor (Affiliated) of Pediatrics
Neonatal and Developmental Medicine
Stanford University School of Medicine
Attending Neonatologist
Santa Clara Valley Medical Center
San Jose, California, USA

**Sudha Rani Narasimhan** MD IBCLC FAAP
Clinical Assistant Professor (Affiliated) of Pediatrics
Neonatal and Developmental Medicine
Stanford University School of Medicine
Director, NICU, O'Connor Hospital
Medical Director of Lactation
Director, Well Baby Nursery
Santa Clara Valley Medical Center
San Jose, California, USA

**Elizabeth M Nielsen** CFRE
Chief Executive Officer
Youth on Their Own
Tucson, Arizona
Formerly Chief Development Officer
Valley Medical Center Foundation
San Jose, California, USA

**Matthew JR Nudelman** MD MAS
Pediatric Intern
Marshall Pediatrics
Marshall University Joan C Edwards School of Medicine
Huntington, West Virginia, USA

**Adebola Olarewaju** PhD(c) MS RNC-NIC CPNP
Pediatric Otolaryngology and Head & Neck Surgery
UC Davis Children's Hospital
Sacramento, California, USA

**Rupalee Patel** DNP MS BSN C-PNP RN C-PHN IBCLC
Director, BRIDGE Home Follow-up Program
Director, High Risk Infant Follow-up Clinic
Santa Clara Valley Medical Center
San Jose, California, USA

**Valerie D Phebus** PA-C
Physician Assistant
Envision Physician Services
Joe DiMaggio Children's Hospital
Hollywood, Florida, USA

**Audra Pritt** MD
Associate Professor of Pediatrics
Director, Pediatric Residency Program
Associate Director, PHM Fellowship Program
Director, Pediatric Hospital Division
Marshall University Joan C Edwards School of Medicine
Hoops Family Children's Hospital at
Cabell Huntington Hospital
Huntington, West Virginia, USA

**Dechu P Puliyanda** MD FAAP
Professor of Pediatrics
University of California, Los Angeles David Geffen School of Medicine
Director, Pediatric Nephrology and Transplantation
Cedars-Sinai Medical Center
Los Angeles, California, USA

**Aarti Raghavan** MD FAAP
Director, Neonatal-Perinatal Fellowship Training Program
Director, Master of Science in Patient Safety Leadership
Attending Neonatologist
Assistant Professor of Clinical Pediatrics
Children's Hospital University of Illinois
University of Illinois Hospital and
Health Sciences System
Chicago, Illinois, USA

**Ronald A Roiz** MD CO
Assistant Professor
Division of Pediatric Orthopedics
Department of Orthopedics
Loma Linda University
Loma Linda, California, USA

**Austin O Rosner** PhD
Senior Medical Writer
Vertex Pharmaceuticals
Boston, Massachusetts, USA

**Joseph Schulman** MD MS FAAP
Director
NICU Quality Measurement and Improvement
Associate Medical Director, Medical Policy and
Operations Branch
Integrated Systems of Care Division
California Department of Health Care Services
Sacramento, California, USA

**Christina T Sheridan** MD FAAP
Clinical Assistant Professor (Affiliated) of Pediatrics
Stanford University School of Medicine
Chair of Pediatrics
Pediatric Cardiologist
Santa Clara Valley Medical Center
San Jose, California, USA

**Augusto Sola** MD FAAP
Neonatologist
General Director
Ibero-American Society of Neonatology (SIBEN)
Adjunct Professor of Epidemiology and
Community Health
School of Public Health
New York Medical College
Valhalla, New York, USA

**Antoine Soliman** MD FAAP
Associate Clinical Professor
Department of Pediatrics
University of California
Irvine School of Medicine
Division Chief, Neonatology
Medical Director, Neonatal Intensive Care Unit
Miller Children's and Women's Hospital Long Beach
Long Beach, California, USA

**Dongli Song** MD PhD FAAP
Associate Clinical Professor (Affiliated)
Department of Pediatrics
Neonatal and Developmental Medicine
Stanford University School of Medicine
Eugene H Kim Chair, Newborn Research
Department of Pediatrics
Santa Clara Valley Medical Center
San Jose, California, USA

**John Sum** MD FAAP
Clinical Associate Professor (Affiliated)
Department of Neurology and Neurological Sciences
Stanford University School of Medicine
Chief, Pediatric Neurology
Department of Pediatrics
Santa Clara Valley Medical Center
San Jose, California, USA

**Cherry C Uy** MD FAAP
Clinical Professor
Department of Pediatrics
University of California
Irvine School of Medicine
Attending Neonatologist
Medical Director, NICU
University of California, Irvine Medical Center
Orange, California, USA

**Arwin Valencia** MD FAAP
Attending Neonatologist
Saddleback Medical Center
Laguna Hills, California, USA

**Donna F Wallerstein** MS
Certified Genetic Counselor
Silicon Valley Genetics Center
Santa Clara Valley Medical Center
San Jose, California, USA

**Robert L Wallerstein** MD FAAP
Department of Pediatrics
Division of Medical Genetics
University of California San Francisco
San Francisco, California, USA

**Laishuan Wang** MD PhD
Staff Neonatologist
Department of Neonatology
Children's Hospital of Fudan University
Shanghai, China

**Robin Daughters Wu** BA
Research Associate
Division of Neonatology
Department of Pediatrics
Santa Clara Valley Medical Center
San Jose, California, USA

**Stacy Yadava** MD FACOG
Director of Maternal-Fetal Medicine
Valley Perinatal and Genetics
Stockton, California, USA

**Ki-Young Yoo** MD
Department of Dermatology
Kaiser South Bay Medical Center
Gardena, California, USA

# Foreword

Maternal, perinatal and newborn health should matter to all of us, and should be viewed from both a human rights and public health perspective. We are only beginning to comprehend the interplay of risk and protective factors, such as socioeconomic status, stress, toxic environmental exposures, and social, nutrition and health behaviors that are at play throughout our lifetime. The potential cumulative effects of these influences on health outcomes may be significant. As research continues to demonstrate the important role of early life events in shaping our health trajectory, we must learn and respond.

Through science, we have now been able to establish key links between early life events and the occurrence of many common chronic diseases that usually manifest in adulthood. A mechanism may be that early events are programed into the developing immune, cardiovascular, endocrine and other physiologic systems. For instance, fetal malnutrition can lead to long-term physiologic changes in lipid and carbohydrate metabolism, increasing the risk of obesity in adulthood with consequent diabetes, heart disease, hypertension and arthritis. Animal studies have indicated that epigenetic phenomena may be important mechanisms underlying programing, and that nutritional interventions may need to begin before conception. These new discoveries at the intersection of the biological, behavioral, and social sciences can now explain not only how healthy development happens, but where it may go awry and what we can do about it.

A broad new paradigm is emerging which can potentially address longstanding differences in health across populations. This "life course" approach to conceptualizing healthcare needs and services may be able to better discern the challenges and help improve the health and well-being of all women, children, youth and families in a transgenerational manner. Our efforts must be coordinated both across life stages and across the lifespan. However, we must be clear – the life course approach is not a one-size-fits-all model, but instead a perspective that should be incorporated into future research, programs, policies and partnerships to optimize health outcomes and reduce disparities across populations. If successful, we may be able to uncover early factors that influence infant mortality, including birth defects and preterm birth, leading to reduction in inequities in birth outcomes, and improved reproductive potential. We thus endeavor to improve the health of future generations by introducing a longitudinal, integrated, and ecological approach to implementing maternal and child health programs.

**Rahul Gupta** MD MPH MBA FACP
Chief Medical and Health Officer
Senior Vice-President
March of Dimes
Clinical Professor of Medicine
Georgetown University School of Medicine
Washington DC, USA

# Preface

Every year approximately 140 million babies are born alive on this planet, a large proportion of whom die of preventable causes, including perinatal asphyxial injury, prematurity, infection, and severe birth defects. Maternal risk factors for infant morbidity are pre-existing maternal disease, disorders in pregnancy, and diseases of the placenta, cord and membranes. Recognition and optimum management of these predispositions will lead to better infant outcomes.

In this age of information, it is possible to search vast amounts of literature and data, giving us new perspectives on our experiences and the variation in disease burden in our own communities. Understanding disparities within and between populations may illuminate fundamental genetic disposition or healthcare delivery differences based on socioeconomic determinants of disease.

The impact of the environment and rapid shifts in climate are just beginning to be explored. Effects on our gametes, the early embryo, pregnancy, fetus, developing nervous system, and our entire life cycle are subjects of much-needed exploration. The effects of endocrine disruptive compounds and "forever chemicals" need to be studied with a sense of urgency. The same is true of the myriad new drugs on the market, many seeking to attenuate the way we feel and perhaps altering the way we are, by their effects on the adult central nervous system.

Mental health in general and infant mental health in particular are barely in the infancy of understanding. Sociological determinants of disease, especially adverse childhood experiences, have important consequences for an individual's lifetime, and may negatively impact the next generation. Both genetic code and zip code (i.e. place/circumstances at birth) are critically important to health and well-being; inequities of wealth in any society invariably lead to inequities in health. Addressing disparities in perinatal healthcare delivery will optimize maternal and neonatal outcomes.

It is estimated that the lifetime impairment rate of cognitive processes in our central nervous system is 47%. Thus, even a "perfect" newborn has a 1 in 2 lifetime risk of transient or long-term central nervous system dysfunction. Approaches to enhance neurocognition have critical windows of opportunity in early infant neurodevelopment and throughout childhood and adolescence. Conversely, exposure to the wrong agent at the wrong time can have devastating consequences. Early identification of at-risk infants and intervention programs aimed at enhancing function are essential to reducing long-term societal costs. A commitment to understanding differences in practice variations, both local and global, is fundamental to implementing pathways for minimizing risk of injury, else preventable morbidities often have consequences for a lifetime. Healthcare providers must carefully consider both big data and individual circumstance in order to deliver the most precise care. The instant availability of big data to providers no matter in what part of the world they practice, while fraught with inherent dangers if ill-understood or misapplied, generally holds great promise for the future of clinical practice.

**Balaji Govindaswami**

# Acknowledgments

We would like to thank Mala Arora, editor of World Clinics: Obstetrics & Gynecology, for the inspiration, and Jaypee Brothers Medical Publishers for convincing us that there is a global need to provide transdisciplinary approaches to newborn care.

This book is truly the product of the ultimate devotion and fierce determination of Robin Daughters Wu, Research Associate extraordinaire with our Newborn division of medicine at Santa Clara Valley Medical Center, who has toiled effortlessly and ungrudgingly through a decade of collaboration among authors in different departments, institutions, states, and nations. It is her singular focus and catholic intent that brings this publication to its fruition.

Thank you to the many distinguished authors and faculty who have been incredibly patient and shared their knowledge and gifts with us selflessly, generously, and with private time taken from family and friends. To this group, our gratitude is eternal.

We would like to thank the Santa Clara Valley Medical Center obstetric residents and Stanford pediatric house staff for their questions, for their inquisitive participation, hard work, and feedback, which keep us vigilant. In addition, we thank our students – Sherwin Abdoli, Esther Belogolovsky, Kylie Burdsall, Tatiana Caine, Ashton Easterday, Bella Anderson Enni, Claudia Flores, Erica Flores, Ixtaso Garay, Keshav Goel, Ben Kifle, Melissa Ling, Pooja Rathi Shah, Maricela Vallejo, and so many others for their diligence, conscientious skepticism, and thoughtful work which has supported clinical investigation and made innovative learning fun.

The editorial support team has been ad hoc, extensive, and indispensable at every varied part of this journey. Their contributions to the final product cannot be under-emphasized. That said, any shortcomings, unwitting errors or failure on the part of being true to our stated mission, are mine, and mine alone.

This book would not have been possible without the support of Stacey D Stewart (President and CEO) and the March of Dimes Foundation, Arlington County, Virginia; Jolene Smith (CEO) and FIRST 5 Santa Clara County, San Jose, California; Santa Clara Valley Health and Hospital System, Santa Clara County, California; E Christopher Wilder (President and Executive Director) and the Valley Medical Center (VMC) Foundation, San Jose, California; Jeff Smith, MD, JD, County Executive Officer for the County of Santa Clara, California; Marshall Pediatrics, Huntington, West Virginia; Marshall University Joan C Edwards School of Medicine, Huntington, West Virginia; Hoops Family Children's Hospital at Cabell Huntington Hospital, Huntington, West Virginia; and Kristi Arrowood (Director of Development) and the Mountain Health Network Foundations, Huntington, West Virginia. Net proceeds will be administered through the VMC Foundation in San Jose for the ultimate benefit of disadvantaged women and children in need, anywhere, and with a sense of urgency to those with preventable morbidity and mortality.

The leadership of Dr Rajul Jain and her team at Jaypee Brothers Medical Publishers brought much needed momentum to us, in our eleventh hour. We are very grateful.

Finally, we would like to thank our patients, families, their advocates and caregivers, whose feedback over the years has been an invaluable gift helping to shape future, more civil approaches in healthcare. They remind us that health must be viewed through the eyes of the consumer, as we seek to do unto others as they would prefer to have done unto them, with the overall intent of enhancing "a state of complete physical, mental, and social well-being."

# Contents

## Section 1: Introduction to Newborn Medicine

1. Evidence-based Neonatology in the Age of Information and Big Data — 3
   *Balaji Govindaswami*

2. Historical Understanding and Current Approaches in Neonatology — 12
   *Sharyn Frentner, Robin Daughters Wu, Balaji Govindaswami*

3. Educational Interventions to Improve Newborn Care — 21
   *Emily Altick Hartford*

4. Managing Your Patients' Data with an Electronic Database — 31
   *Joseph Schulman*

5. Quality and Safety — 46
   *Aarti Raghavan*

## Section 2: Healthcare Services Delivery

6. Mental Health and Emotional Well-being in the NICU: Addressing the Next Frontier in Family-integrated Care — 59
   *Sangeeta Mallik*

7. Utilization of Advanced Practice Providers in the Neonatal Intensive Care Unit — 65
   *Valerie D Phebus, Korinne S Van Keuren*

8. Pediatric Hospital Medicine and its Evolution in the United States — 70
   *Susan Flesher*

9. Home Follow-up of the High-risk Infant — 74
   *Rupalee Patel, Adebola Olarewaju*

10. How Charitable Giving can Enhance Newborn Care — 85
    *Elizabeth M Nielsen*

## Section 3: Perinatal

11. Obstetric Contributions to Neonatal Morbidity and Mortality—Overview — 95
    *Francesca C Ianovich, Matthew J Garabedian*

12. Disorders of the Membranes, Placenta, and Cord — 104
    *Shannon Dralla, Matthew J Garabedian*

13. Neonatal Encephalopathy: An Obstetric Perspective — 112
    *Stacy Yadava, Matthew J Garabedian*

## Section 4: Normal Newborn Care

14. Newborn Physical Examination — 121
    *Cherry C Uy*

15. Caring for Families through Pregnancy Loss or Death of an Infant — 129
    *Donna F Wallerstein*

| 16. | Circumcision | 136 |
|---|---|---|
| | *Stephen Harris* | |
| 17. | Couplet Care and Common Nursery Issues | 145 |
| | *Priya Jegatheesan, Sudha Rani Narasimhan, Dongli Song* | |

## Section 5: Disorders of Structure and Function in the Fetus and Neonate

| 18. | Prenatal Diagnosis | 155 |
|---|---|---|
| | *Robert L Wallerstein* | |
| 19. | Birth Defects | 160 |
| | *Robert L Wallerstein* | |
| 20. | Inborn Errors of Metabolism and Newborn Screening | 166 |
| | *Gregory M Enns* | |
| 21. | Common Surgical Conditions of the Neonate | 177 |
| | *Stephanie D Chao, Julie R Fuchs* | |
| 22. | Point-of-Care Testing in Newborn Screening: Hearing Loss and Critical Congenital Heart Disease | 191 |
| | *Rebecca Barnett* | |

## Section 6: Cardiorespiratory Disorders

| 23. | Extracorporeal Membrane Oxygenation in the Neonate | 205 |
|---|---|---|
| | *John Patrick Cleary* | |
| 24. | Assessment and Treatment Options for Neonates with Congenital Heart Disease | 211 |
| | *Christina T Sheridan* | |
| 25. | Pulmonary Hypertension in the Neonatal Intensive Care Unit Setting | 223 |
| | *Yueh-Tze Lan* | |
| 26. | Patent Ductus Arteriosus | 235 |
| | *Priya Jegatheesan, Balaji Govindaswami* | |
| 27. | Common Cardiorespiratory Disorders at Birth | 243 |
| | *Kamakshi Devarajan, Balaji Govindaswami* | |

## Section 7: Fetal and Neonatal Brain Development, and Neurodevelopmental Follow-up

| 28. | Feeding and Brain Development in Preterm Infants: Central Pattern Generation and Suck Dynamics | 255 |
|---|---|---|
| | *Steven M Barlow, Austin O Rosner, Dongli Song* | |
| 29. | Feeding and Brain Development in Preterm Infants: Role of Sensory Stimulation | 264 |
| | *Steven M Barlow, Austin O Rosner, Dongli Song* | |
| 30. | The Gut-Microbiota-Brain Axis: Implications for Neonatal Neurodevelopment | 275 |
| | *Dongli Song, Laishuan Wang* | |
| 31. | Neonatal Seizures | 284 |
| | *John Sum* | |
| 32. | Newborn Populations at Risk for Adverse Neurodevelopmental Outcomes | 292 |
| | *Ira Adams-Chapman* | |
| 33. | Late Preterm Infants, Cerebral Palsy, and Hypoxic-Ischemic Encephalopathy | 305 |
| | *Ira Adams-Chapman* | |

## Section 8: Growth, Lactation and Nutrition

**34. Body Composition and Electrolytes** — 321
*Sonya Misra*

**35. Macronutrients and Micronutrients** — 331
*Sonya Misra*

**36. Stages of Nutritional Support** — 345
*Sonya Misra*

**37. Human Milk Composition and Lactation** — 355
*Sudha Rani Narasimhan, Alganesh G Kifle*

**38. Necrotizing Enterocolitis** — 365
*Arwin Valencia, Antoine Soliman*

## Section 9: Pain and Addiction

**39. Newborn Pain: Recognition and Management** — 377
*Matthew JR Nudelman*

**40. Introduction to Addiction Medicine** — 390
*Balaji Govindaswami*

## Section 10: Other Common Newborn Conditions

**41. Skin Disorders in the Newborn** — 403
*Noah Craft, Zachary Max Goldstein, Ki-Young Yoo*

**42. Common Orthopedic Problems in the Newborn** — 423
*Robert M Bernstein, Ronald A Roiz*

**43. Oxygenation, Oxygen Saturation, Retinopathy of Prematurity and Other Hyperoxia-related Damage in Newborn Infants: A Return to the Basics** — 432
*Augusto Sola, Lily C Chen*

**44. Neonatal Gastrointestinal and Liver Disease** — 441
*Christopher Fink*

**45. Nephrology in the Neonate** — 451
*Dechu P Puliyanda, Rashmi Kirpekar*

*Index* — *465*

Plate 1

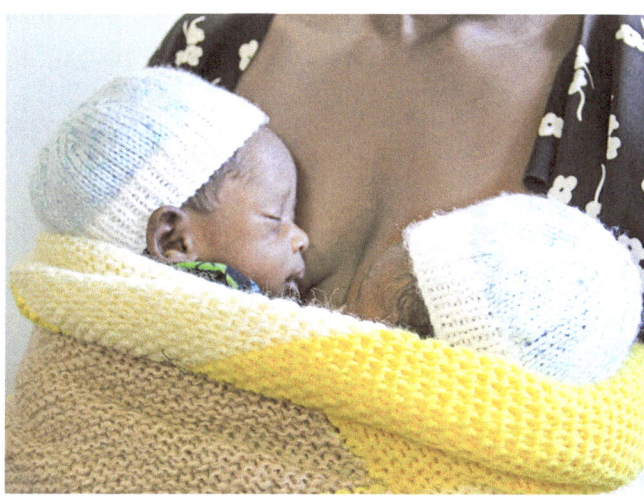

**Fig. 4 (Chapter 2):** Kangaroo care of twins at Queen Elizabeth Hospital, Blantyre, Malawi. The infants have been placed skin-to-skin with their grandmother.

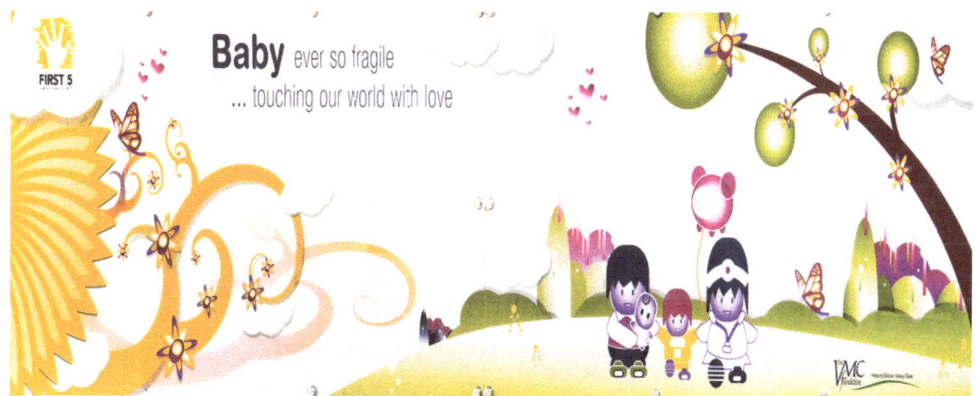

**Box 2 (Chapter 10):** Case Study: FIRST 5.

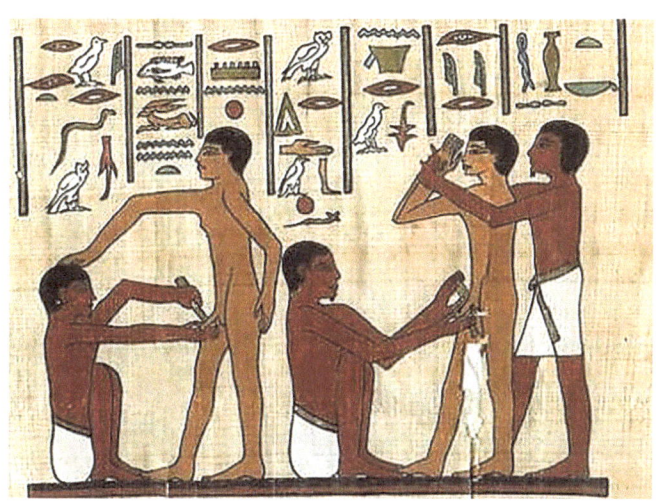

**Fig. 1 (Chapter 16):** Ancient Egyptian depiction of circumcision. *Source:* Anonymous (https://commons.wikimedia.org/wiki/File:Circumcision_Sakkara_3.jpg), Circumcision Sakkara 3 (https://commons.wikimedia.org/wiki/Template:PD-old).

Plate 2

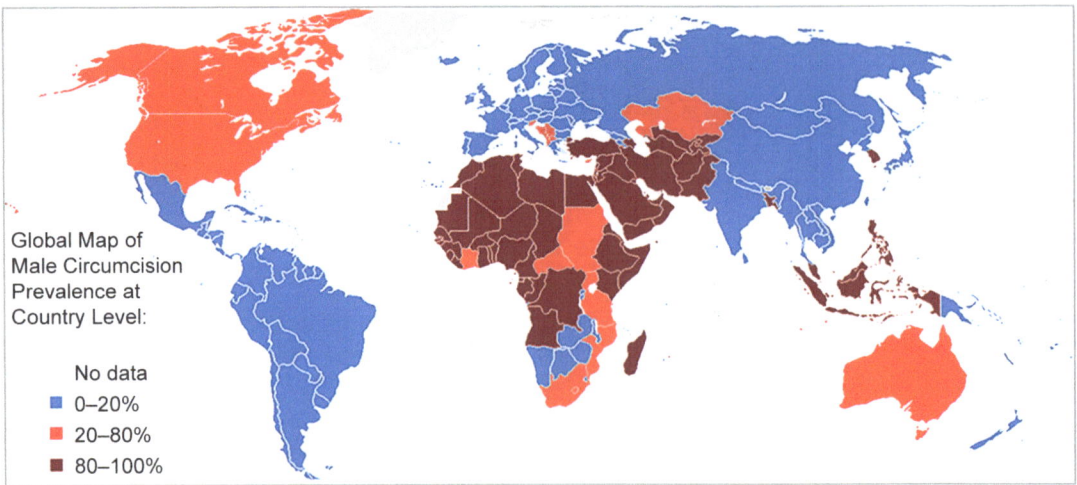

**Fig. 2 (Chapter 16):** Global map of male circumcision.
*Source:* WHO. London School of Hygiene and Tropical Medicine, the World Health Organization and the Joint United Nations Programme on HIV/AIDS (UNAIDS). Geneva: WHO; 2007.

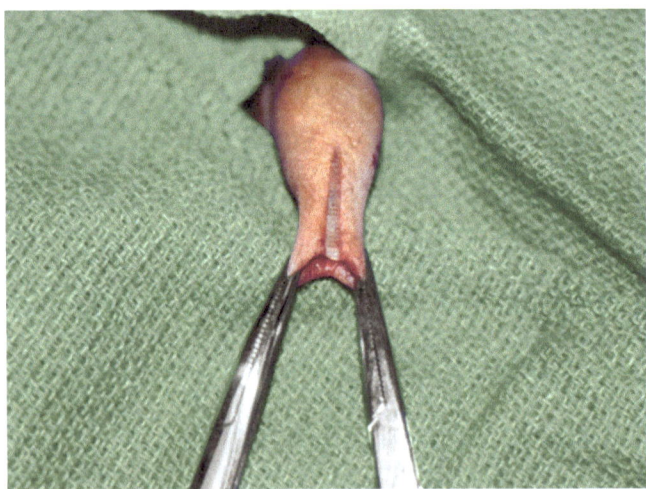

**Fig. 3 (Chapter 16):** Applying hemostats to the foreskin in preparation for circumcision.

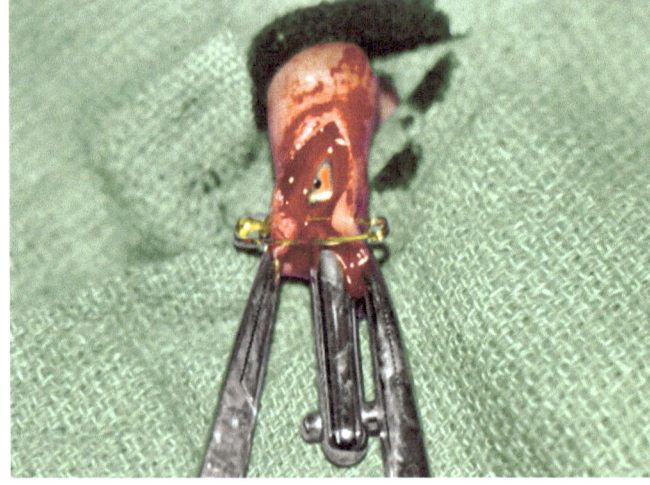

**Fig. 4 (Chapter 16):** An incision is made where the hemostat has created the linear crushed foreskin tissue.

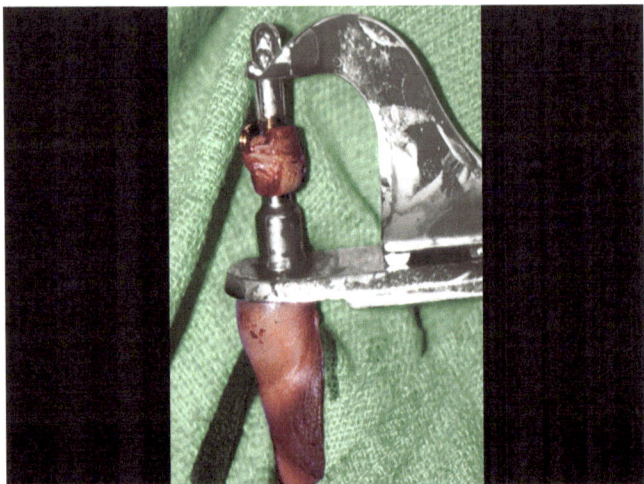

**Fig. 5 (Chapter 16):** Use of the Gomco clamp.

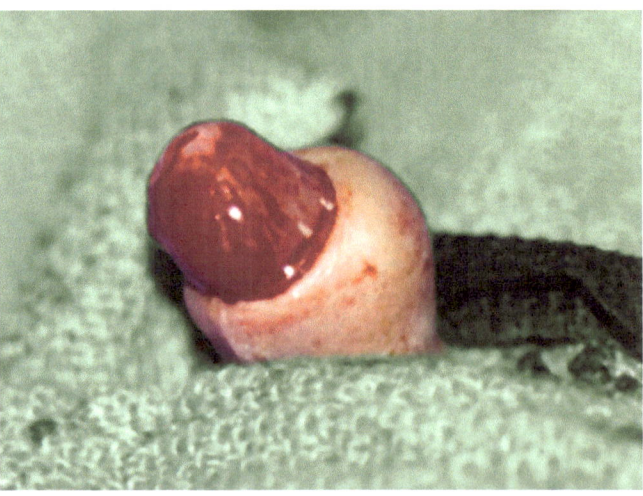

**Fig. 6 (Chapter 16):** The newly cirumcised penis.

## Plate 3

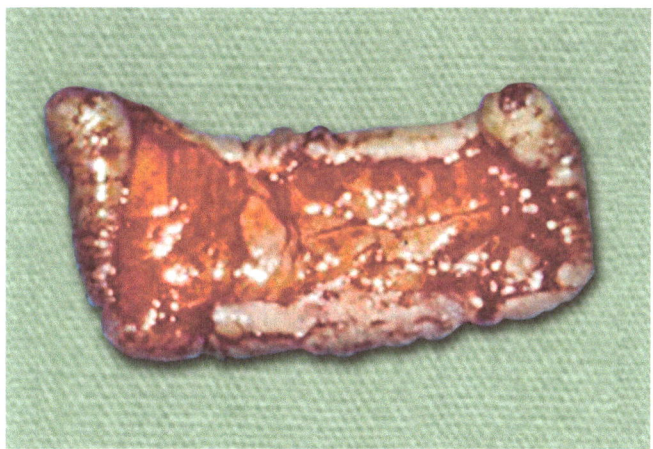

**Fig. 7 (Chapter 16):** The residual foreskin.

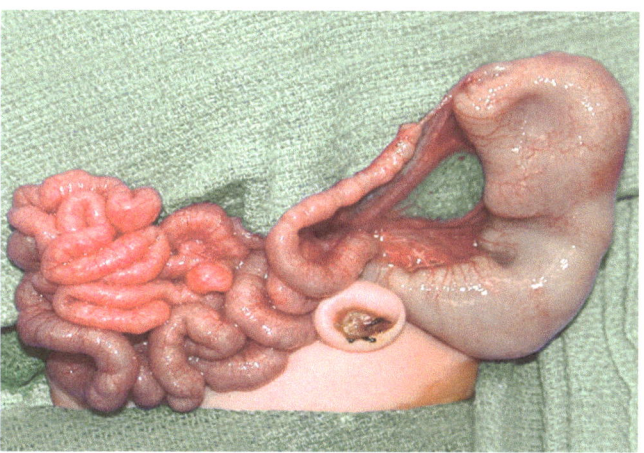

**Fig. 3 (Chapter 21):** Type II intestinal atresia.

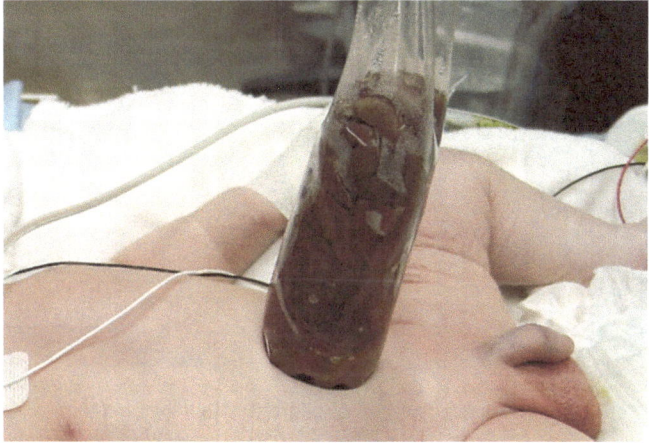

**Fig. 4 (Chapter 21):** Preformed spring-loaded silo used in gastroschisis reduction at bedside.

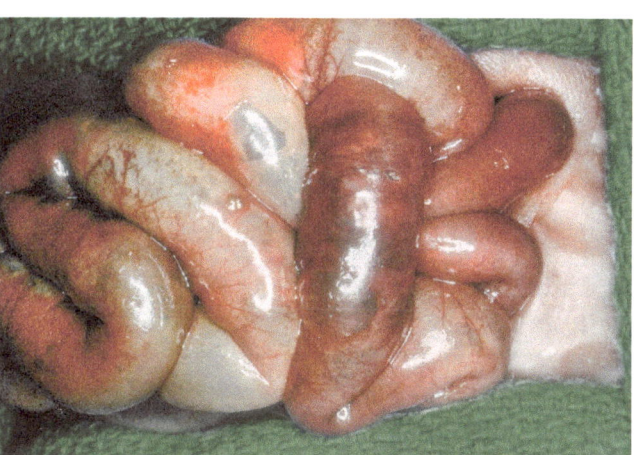

**Fig. 5 (Chapter 21):** Pneumatosis intestinalis.

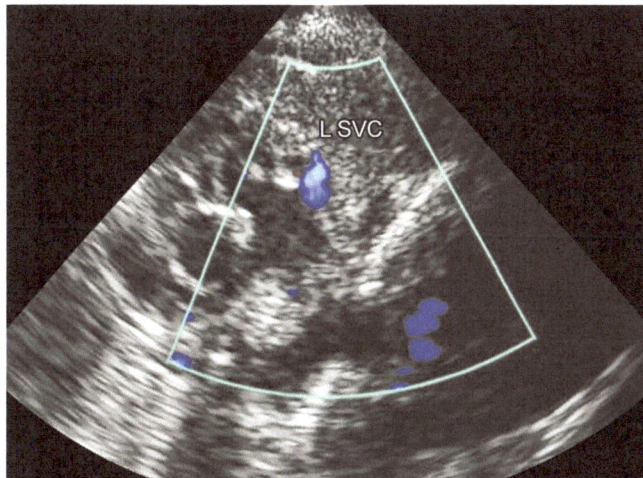

**Fig. 7 (Chapter 24):** High parasternal transverse three-vessel view of fetal chest in two-dimensional (2D), confirming relationship of the great vessels and their relative size to one another. A persistent left superior vena cava (SVC) would be seen as a small circle on the other side of the pulmonary arter (PA).

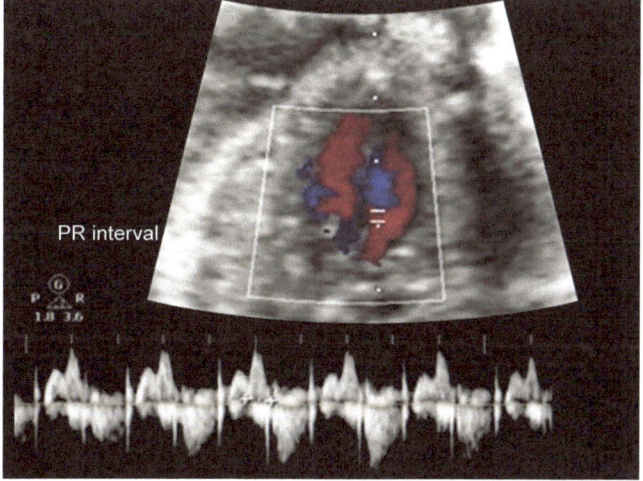

**Fig. 8 (Chapter 24):** Mechanical PR interval in a fetus. Doppler gate is placed at the junction of mitral and aortic valves. The mechanical PR interval (in milliseconds) is measured from beginning of the A wave of mitral valve to the beginning of the left ventricular outflow tract (LVOT) signal.

Plate 4

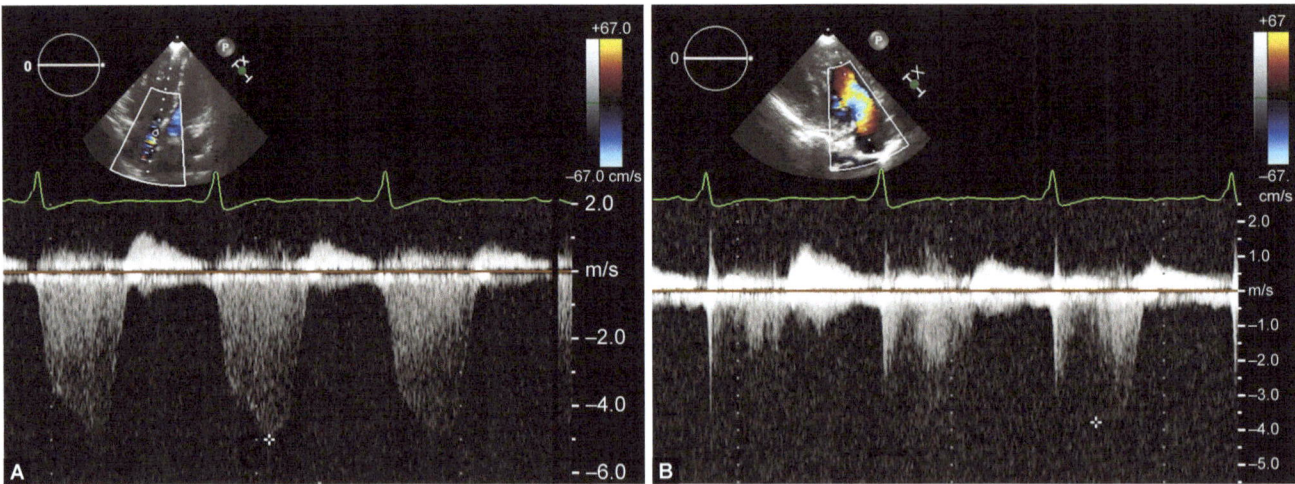

**Figs. 1A and B (Chapter 25):** TR jet peak velocity for estimate of RV systolic pressure. (A) Clear TR jet where peak velocity is clearly visualized with calculated peak gradient of 100 mm Hg; (B) TR jet in the same patient during the same study. TR jet is indistinct and peak velocity could not be determined but was guessed and resulted in calculated peak gradient of 57 mm Hg. (TR: tricuspid regurgitation; RV: right ventricular)

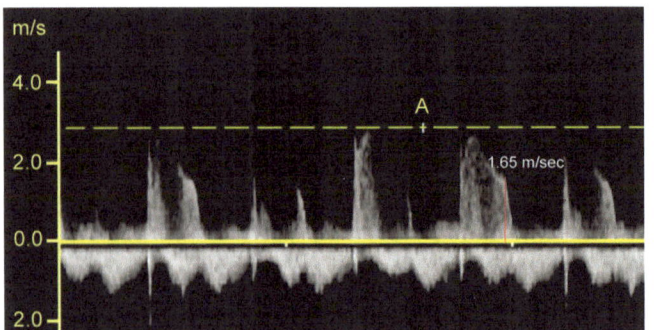

**Fig. 2 (Chapter 25):** Pulmonary insufficiency jet for estimate of PAEDP where PA velocity at end diastole is 1.65 m/s, which predicts PAEDP of 21 mm Hg. (PAEDP: pulmonary arterial end-diastolic pressure; PA: pulmonary artery)

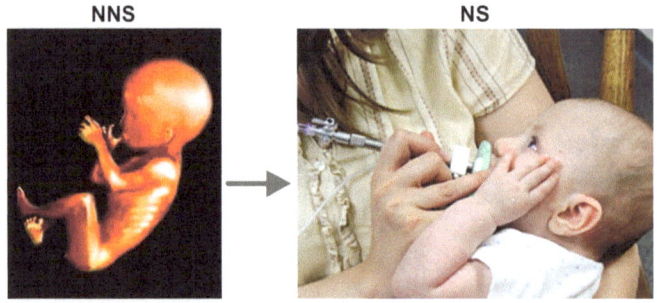

**Fig. 3 (Chapter 28):** Progression from non-nutritive sucking (NNS) to nutritive sucking (NS). (GA: gestational age)
*Source:* Communication Neuroscience Laboratories, Lincoln NE USA.

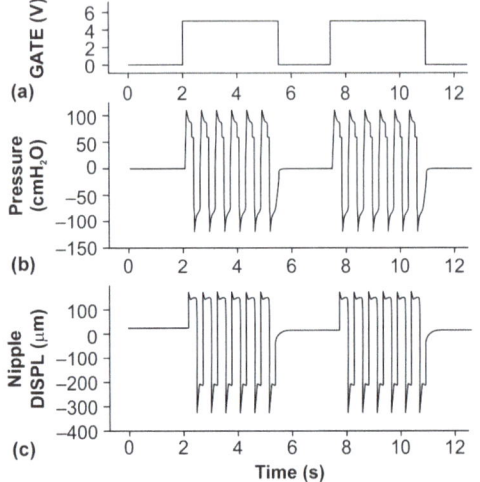
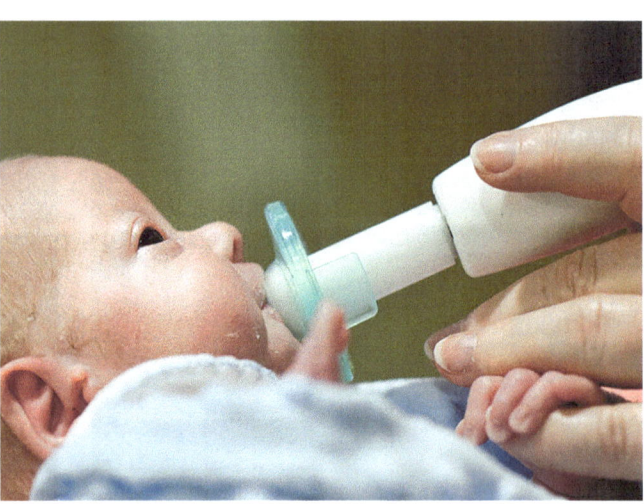

**Fig. 1 (Chapter 29):** Preterm infant receiving pulsed orocutaneous therapy. Synthesized burst-pause stimulus features delivered as frequency-modulated pneumotactile pulse trains through the pacifier nipple (left panel), (a) voltage-controlled gate signal, (b) pressure inside the nipple, and (c) mechanical displacement of the nipple cylinder wall.
*Courtesy:* Innara Health, Inc., Olathe, Kansas USA.

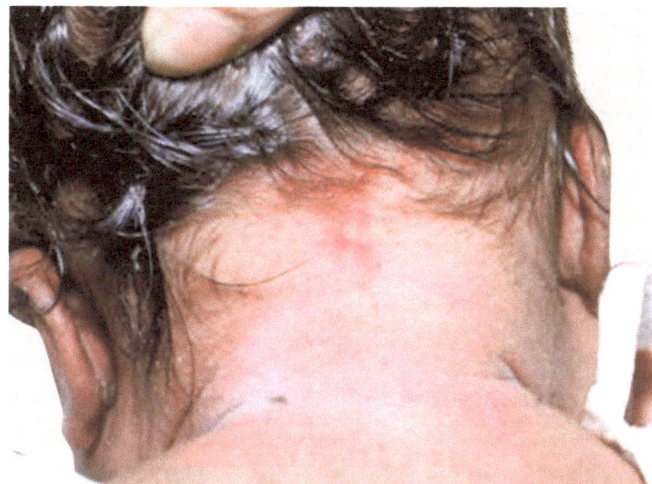

**Fig. 1 (Chapter 41):** Salmon patch.
*Source:* Image appears with permission from VisualDx (www.visualdx.com).

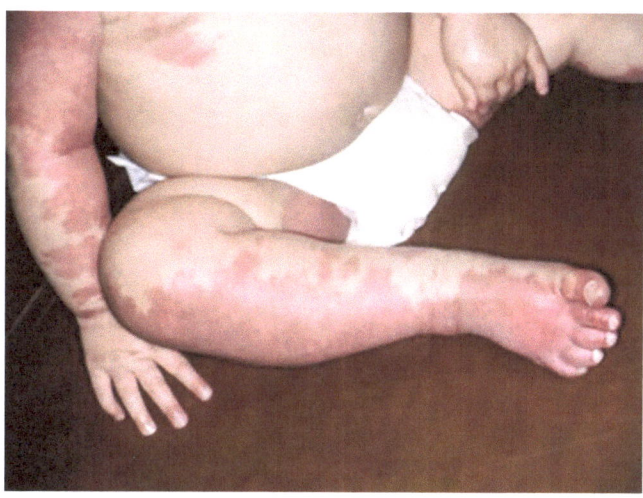

**Fig. 2 (Chapter 41):** Port-wine stain.
*Source:* Image appears with permission from VisualDx (www.visualdx.com).

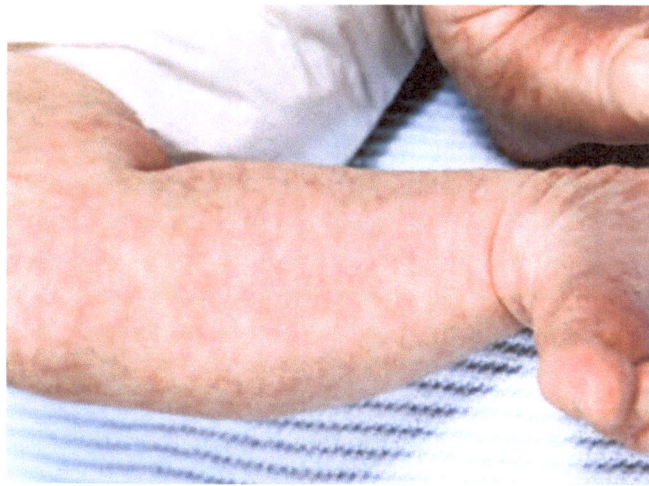

**Fig. 3 (Chapter 41):** Cutis marmorata.
*Source:* Image appears with permission from VisualDx (www.visualdx.com).

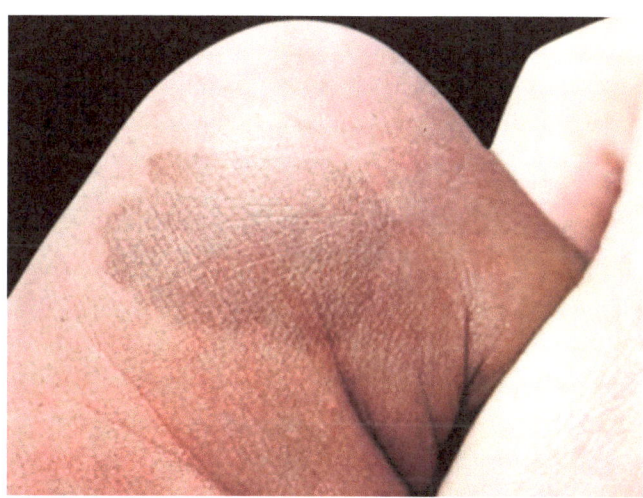

**Fig. 4 (Chapter 41):** Café-au-lait macule.
*Source:* Image appears with permission from VisualDx (www.visualdx.com).

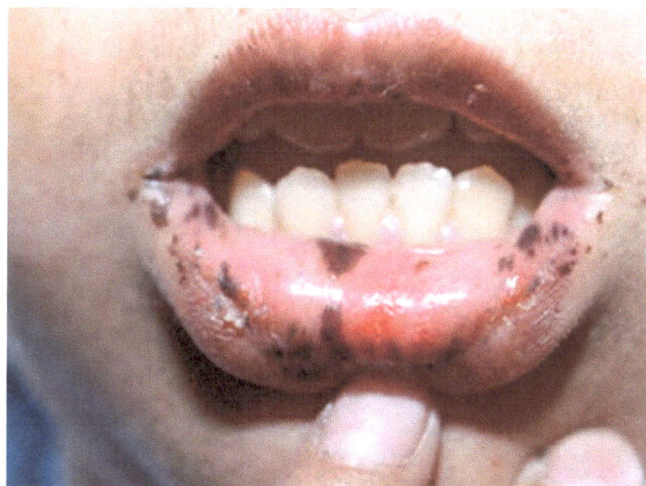

**Fig. 5 (Chapter 41):** Peutz–Jeghers syndrome.
*Source:* Image appears with permission from VisualDx (www.visualdx.com).

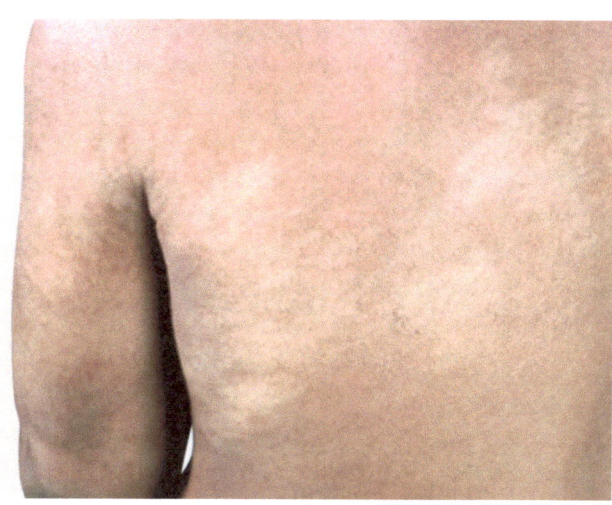

**Fig. 6 (Chapter 41):** Nevus depigmentosus.
*Source:* Image appears with permission from VisualDx (www.visualdx.com).

Plate 6

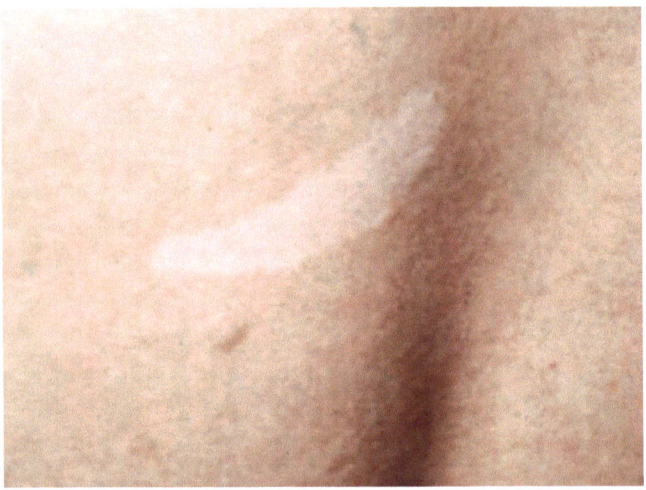

**Fig. 7 (Chapter 41):** Ash leaf macule.
*Source:* Image appears with permission from VisualDx (www.visualdx.com).

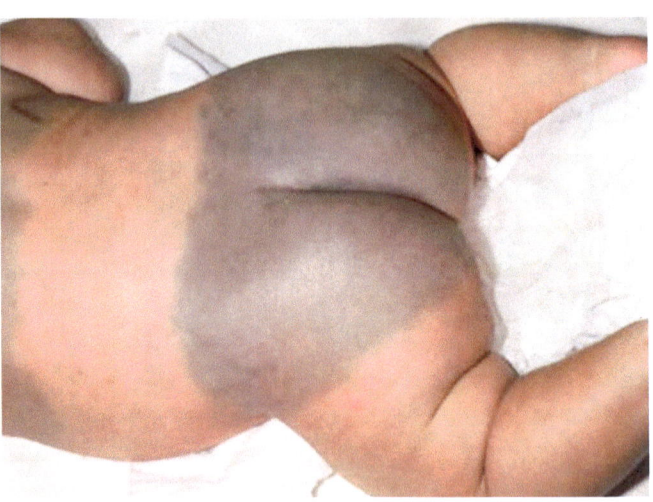

**Fig. 8 (Chapter 41):** Blue-gray spot (Mongolian spot).
*Source:* Image appears with permission from VisualDx (www.visualdx.com).

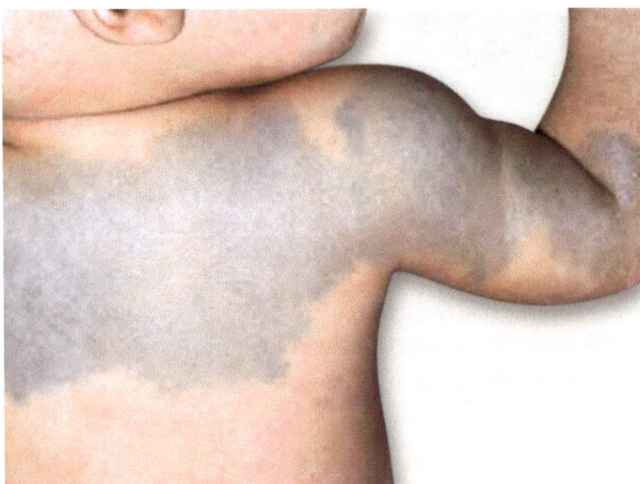

**Fig. 9 (Chapter 41):** Nevus of Ito.
*Source:* Image appears with permission from VisualDx (www.visualdx.com).

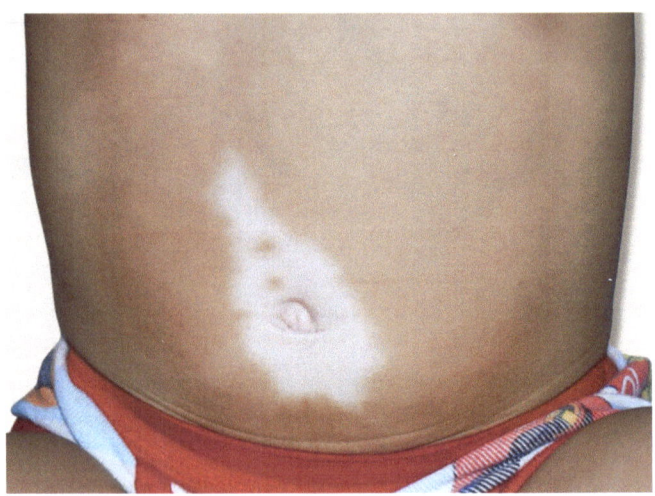

**Fig. 10 (Chapter 41):** Piebaldism.
*Source:* Image appears with permission from Dr Ki-Young Yoo.

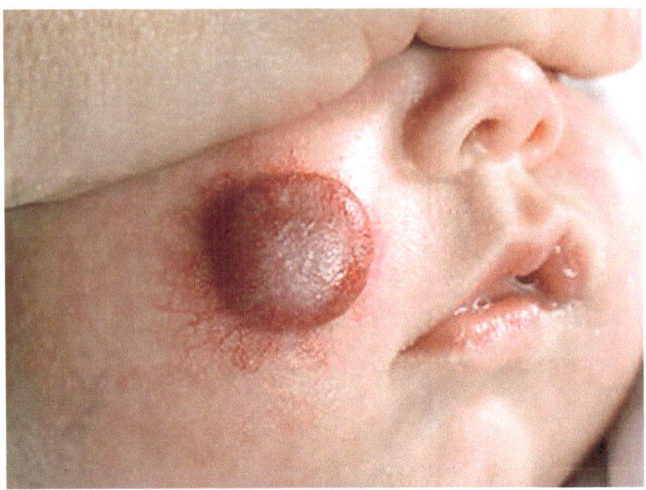

**Fig. 11 (Chapter 41):** Hemangioma, infantile.
*Source:* Image appears with permission from VisualDx (www.visualdx.com).

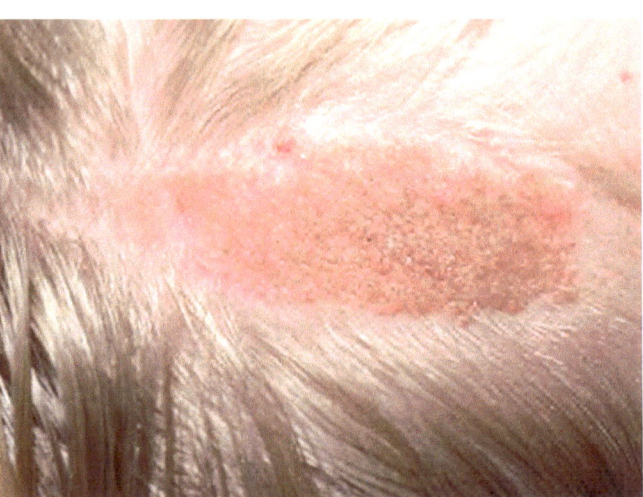

**Fig. 12 (Chapter 41):** Nevus sebaceous.
*Source:* Image appears with permission from VisualDx (www.visualdx.com).

Plate 7

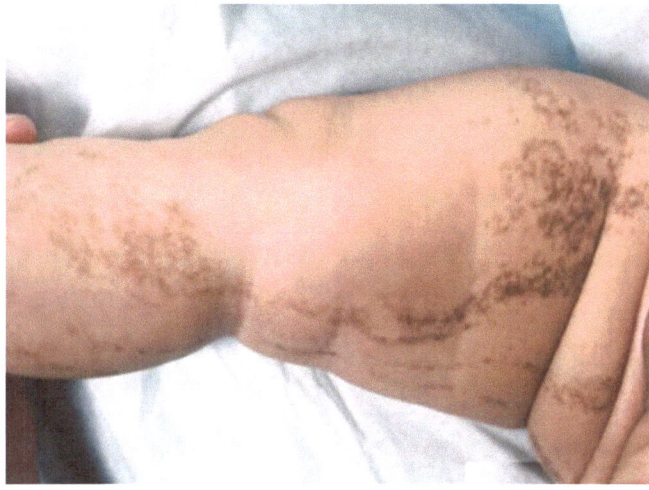

**Fig. 13 (Chapter 41):** Epidermal nevus.
*Source:* Image appears with permission from VisualDx (www.visualdx.com).

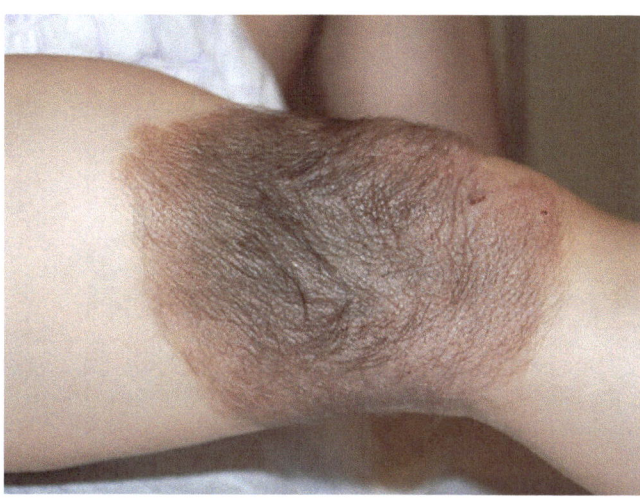

**Fig. 14 (Chapter 41):** Medium congenital nevus.
*Source:* Image appears with permission from Dr Ki-Young Yoo.

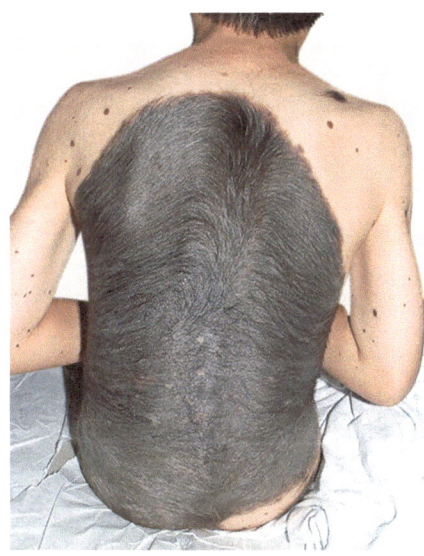

**Fig. 15 (Chapter 41):** Giant congenital nevus.
*Source:* Image appears with permission from Dr Ki-Young Yoo.

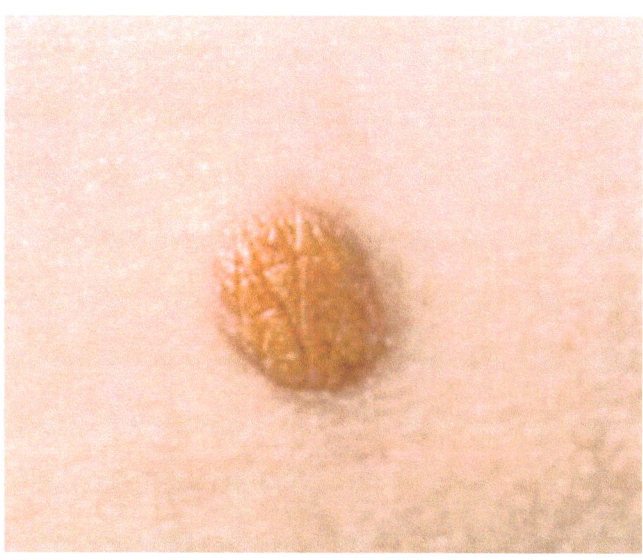

**Fig. 16 (Chapter 41):** Juvenile xanthogranuloma.
*Source:* Image appears with permission from VisualDx (www.visualdx.com).

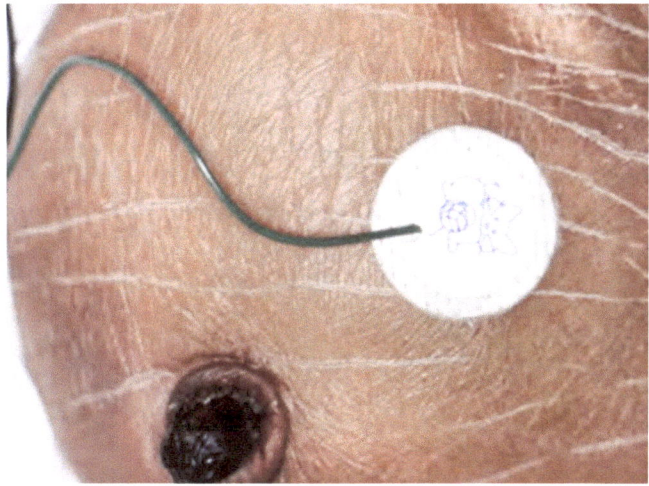

**Fig. 17 (Chapter 41):** Postmaturity desquamation.
*Source:* Image appears with permission from VisualDx (www.visualdx.com).

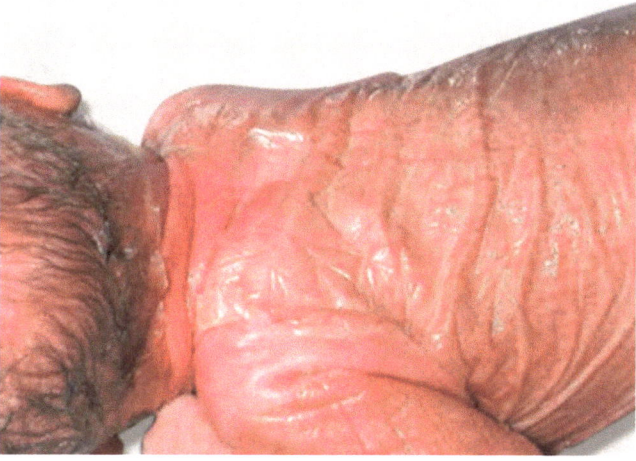

**Fig. 18 (Chapter 41):** Collodion baby.
*Source:* Image appears with permission from VisualDx (www.visualdx.com).

Plate 8

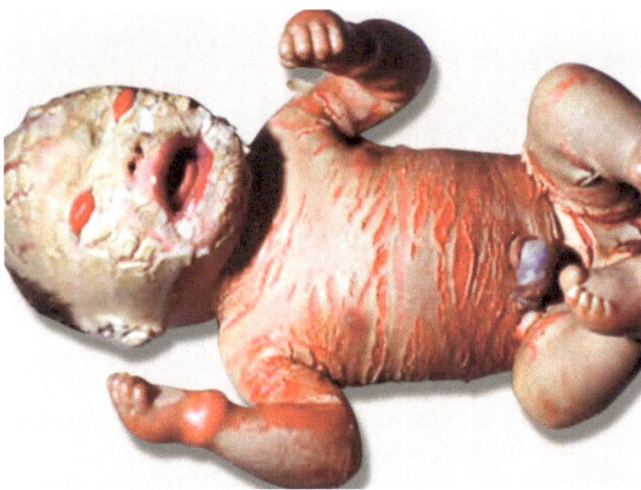

**Fig. 19 (Chapter 41):** Harlequin fetus.
*Source:* Image appears with permission from VisualDx (www.visualdx.com).

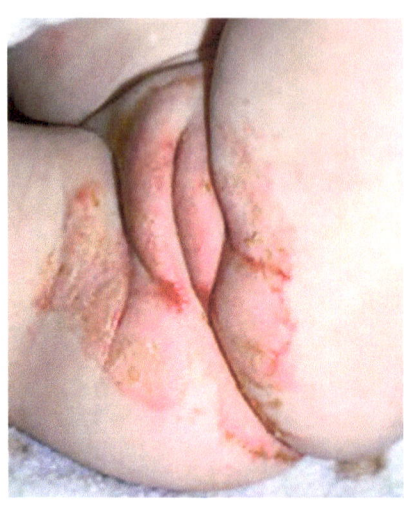

**Fig. 20 (Chapter 41):** Hereditary acrodermatitis enteropathica.
*Source:* Image appears with permission from VisualDx (www.visualdx.com).

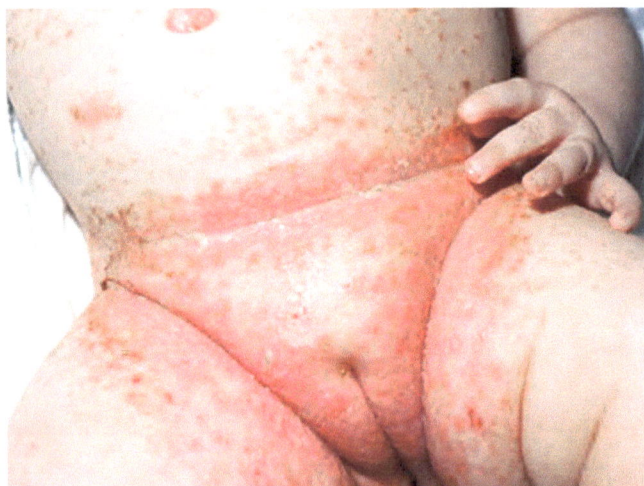

**Fig. 21 (Chapter 41):** Langerhans cell histiocytosis.
*Source:* Image appears with permission from VisualDx (www.visualdx.com).

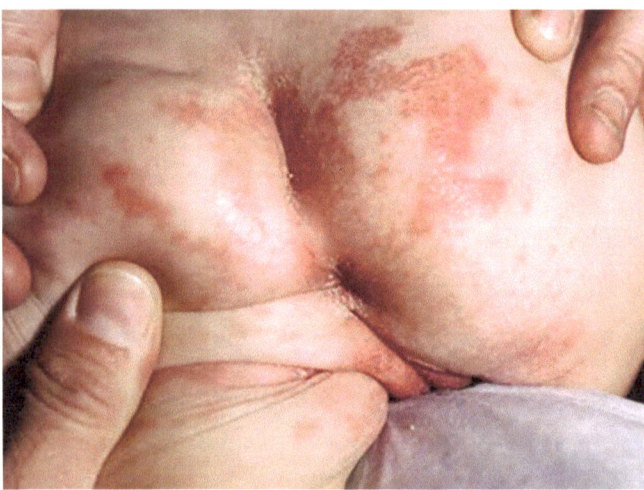

**Fig. 22 (Chapter 41):** Psoriasis.
*Source:* Image appears with permission from VisualDx (www.visualdx.com).

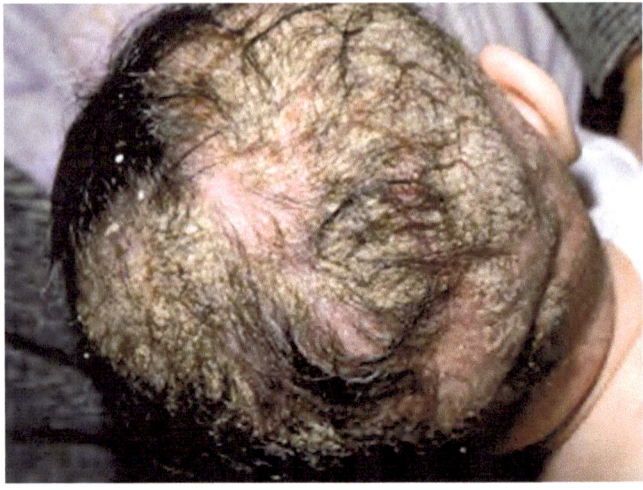

**Fig. 23 (Chapter 41):** Seborrheic dermatitis.
*Source:* Image appears with permission from VisualDx (www.visualdx.com).

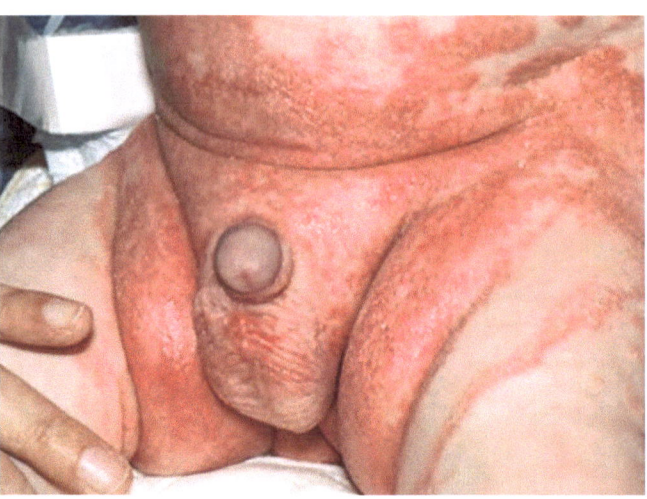

**Fig. 24 (Chapter 41):** Seborrheic dermatitis.
*Source:* Image appears with permission from VisualDx (www.visualdx.com).

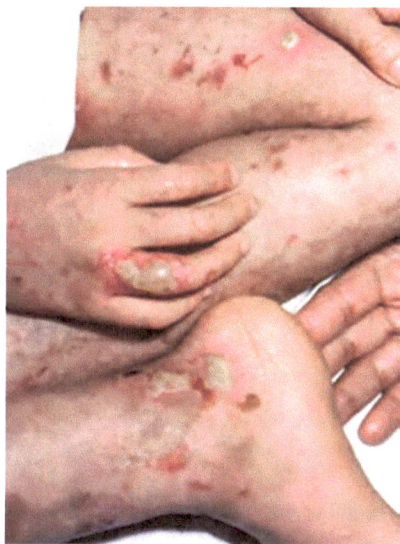

**Fig. 25 (Chapter 41):** Epidermolysis bullosa simplex.
*Source:* Image appears with permission from VisualDx (www.visualdx.com).

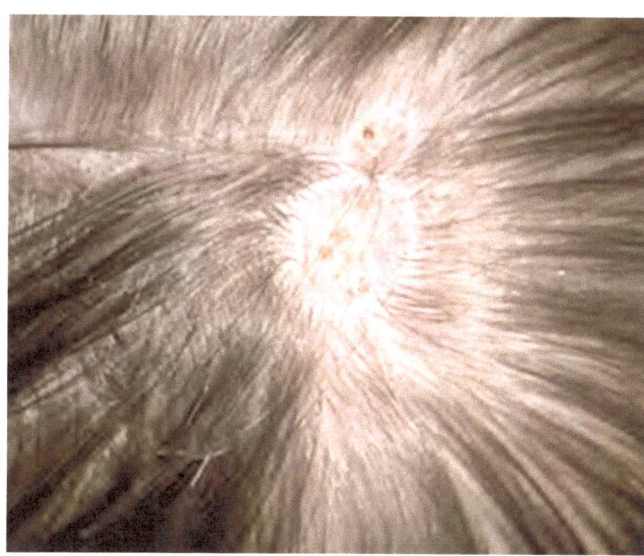

**Fig. 26 (Chapter 41):** Aplasia cutis congenita.
*Source:* Image appears with permission from VisualDx (www.visualdx.com).

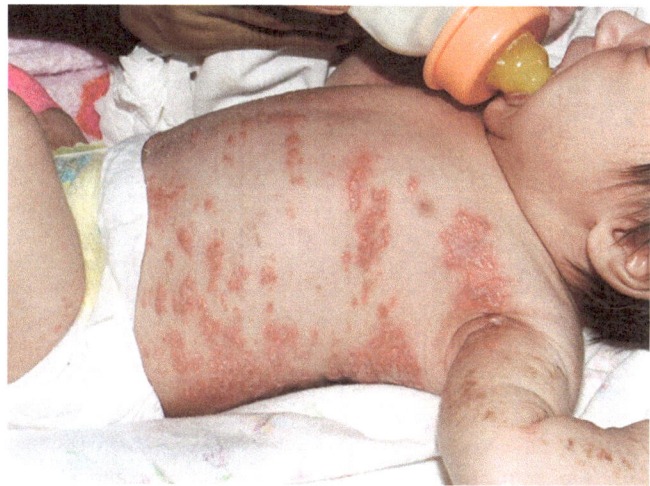

**Fig. 27 (Chapter 41):** Incontinentia pigmenti.
*Source:* Image appears with permission from Dr Ki-Young Yoo.

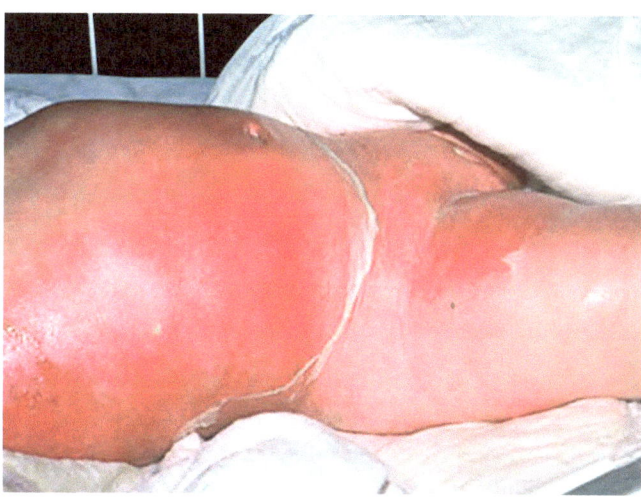

**Fig. 28 (Chapter 41):** Staphylococcal scalded skin syndrome.
*Source:* Image appears with permission from VisualDx (www.visualdx.com).

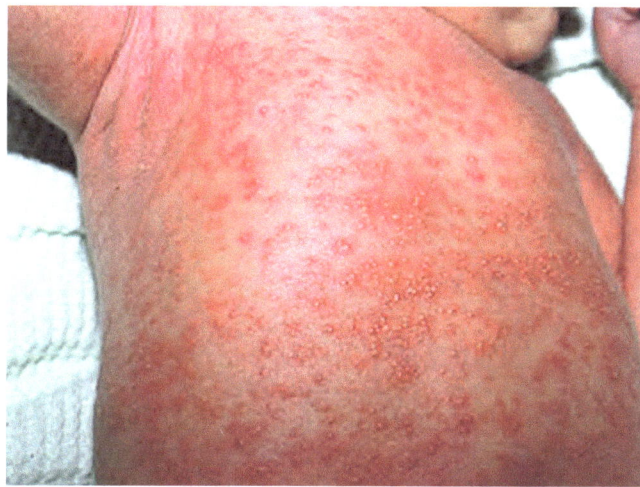

**Fig. 29 (Chapter 41):** Erythema toxicum neonatorum.
*Source:* Image appears with permission from VisualDx (www.visualdx.com).

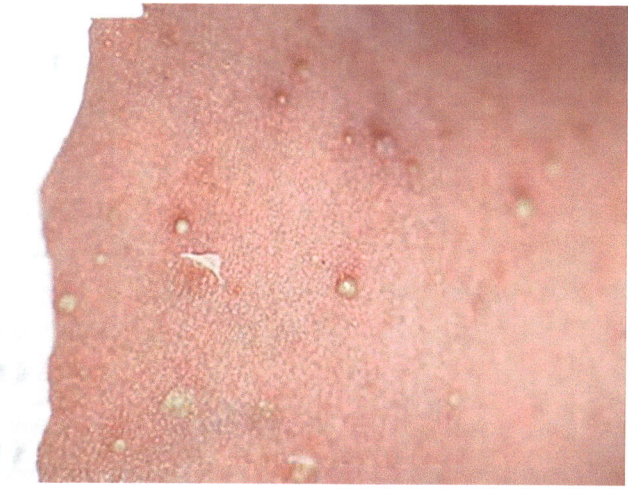

**Fig. 30 (Chapter 41):** Transient neonatal pustular dermatosis.
*Source:* Image appears with permission from VisualDx (www.visualdx.com).

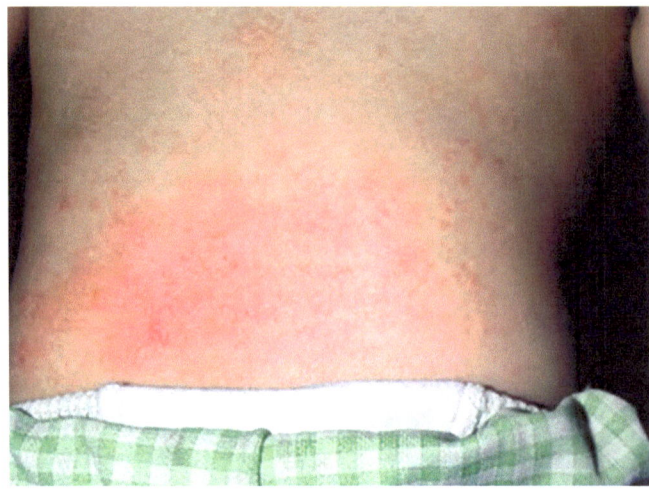
Fig. 31 (Chapter 41): Miliaria rubra.
Source: Image appears with permission from VisualDx (www.visualdx.com).

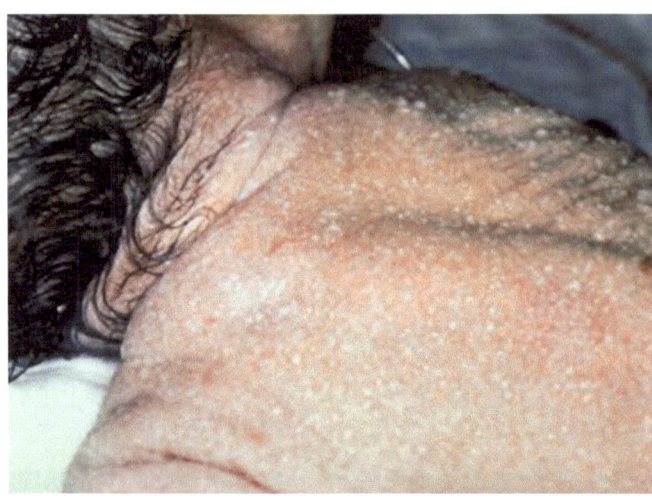
Fig. 32 (Chapter 41): Miliaria crystallina.
Source: Image appears with permission from VisualDx (www.visualdx.com).

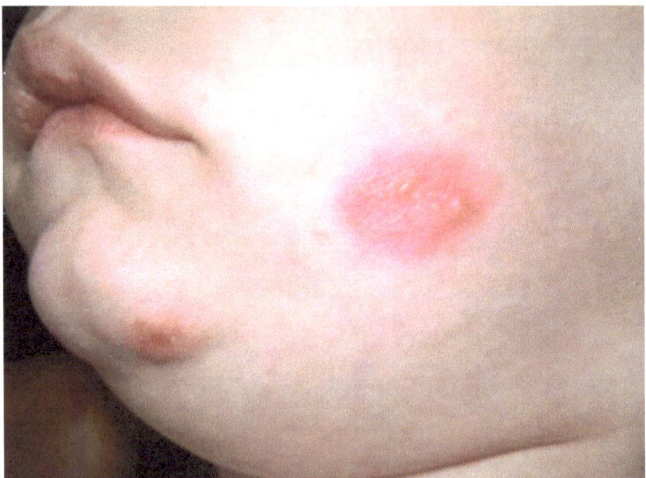
Fig. 33 (Chapter 41): Herpes simplex virus.
Source: Image appears with permission from VisualDx (www.visualdx.com).

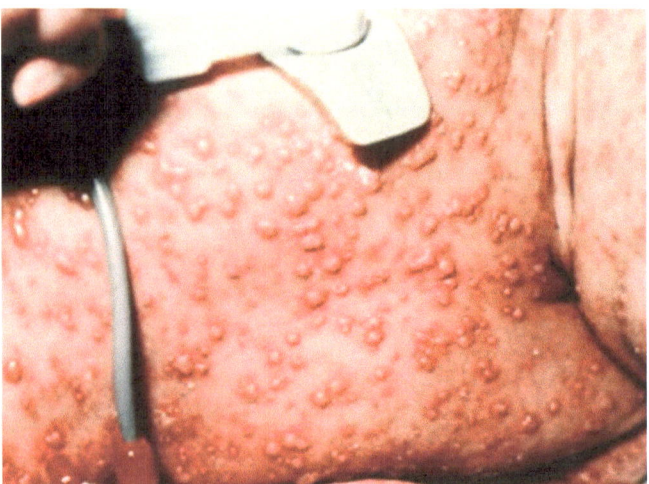
Fig. 34 (Chapter 41): Neonatal varicella (chickenpox).
Source: Image appears with permission from VisualDx (www.visualdx.com).

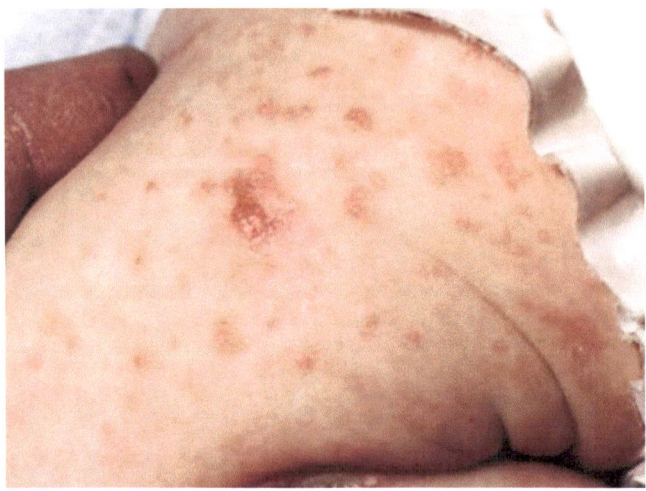
Fig. 35 (Chapter 41): Scabies.
Source: Image appears with permission from VisualDx (www.visualdx.com).

## Plate 11

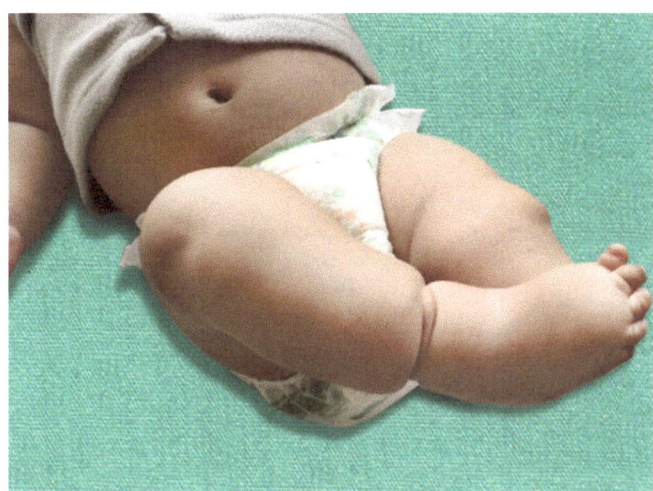

**Fig. 2 (Chapter 42):** Congenital constriction band of the distal tibia.

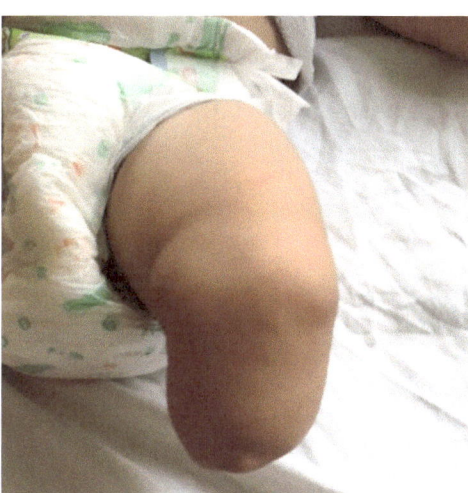

**Fig. 3 (Chapter 42):** Intrauterine transtibial amputation in the same child as the result of congenital constriction band syndrome.

# SECTION 1

# Introduction to Newborn Medicine

- Evidence-based Neonatology in the Age of Information and Big Data
  *Balaji Govindaswami*

- Historical Understanding and Current Approaches in Neonatology
  *Sharyn Frentner, Robin Daughters Wu, Balaji Govindaswami*

- Educational Interventions to Improve Newborn Care
  *Emily Altick Hartford*

- Managing Your Patients' Data with an Electronic Database
  *Joseph Schulman*

- Quality and Safety
  *Aarti Raghavan*

# CHAPTER 1

# Evidence-based Neonatology in the Age of Information and Big Data

*Balaji Govindaswami*

"I honestly beleave it iz better tew know nothing than two know what ain't so." 1874

(Everybody's Friend, or Josh Billing's Encyclopedia and Proverbial Philosophy of Wit and Humor)

## ABSTRACT

Globally, disease burden is borne disproportionately by the poor. Those working in newborn medicine have the opportunity and responsibility to optimize the health of mothers and infants, moving towards health equity even in resource-poor populations. Worldwide implementation of simple public health measures and lifesaving practices at birth can improve newborn outcomes regardless of where they are born.

Information and big data assist in incorporating evidence-based medicine into practice, providing both best practices and best value for the community, families, and infants at birth and beyond. Education of both providers and society at large will ensure that advancements in knowledge and technology are employed to improve empathy and healthcare delivery for families and their newborn infants.

## INTRODUCTION

As we begin the year 2020, much global news is devoted to dramatic climactic shifts, species extinctions, raging fires, and renewed projections of midcentury demographic changes, with rising waters and migratory populations ravaged no longer solely by Malthusian fears of war, famine, and disease. Still, many billion humans are successfully reproducing, with over 120 million live-born babies each year, while enjoying a century of dramatic increase in life expectancy and general quality of life. The probability of death remains greatest most proximate to the moment of birth. How many neonatal deaths are preventable? Equally importantly, how much early morbidity is preventable, avoiding a lifetime of crippling disability due to moderate and severe birth defects, many of which are amenable to repair and/or significant remediation? Inequities in distribution of wealth and resources combined with geopolitical instability have resulted in varied healthcare delivery models with much disparity in healthcare structures, processes, and outcomes. Great global institutions including the United Nations' World Health Organization, myriad nongovernmental institutions (e.g., March of Dimes, Red Cross, and Red Crescent), and numerous academic and professional societies are devoted to the health of women and children, and health of the family and human population at large. How shall we use these resources to our collective human advantage?

For those of us privileged to witness the moment of birth, we have the opportunity not only to ameliorate the burden of death, disease, and disability, but also to promote individual well-being and joy in society. Neonatology, perceived as a pediatric subspecialty in recent decades, has existed through millennia as a tribal role borne largely by peer women birth attendants present in pregnancy and the puerperium. Disease burden in newborns has shifted to various providers in all manner of healthcare systems due to a wide spectrum of heterogeneity in newborn disease, complicated by resurgence of infectious disease (e.g., congenital syphilis in high-risk populations), novel viral diseases (H1N1, ZIKV, and hepatitis C), improved knowledge of rare disease (metabolic, genetic, environmental, or other largely unknown etiology), and novel application of surgical and nonsurgical [e.g., total body cooling (TBC)] technologies. Much disease burden accrues to infants born into disadvantaged populations with substance use and/or mental health and hygiene disorders.

Newborn medicine provides much opportunity for improved global health in this age of information and big data. We "labor" in a time and place, fraught with tedium, inequity, ethical dilemma, uncertainty, and exhaustion, and yet that joyous moment of birth is a daily reminder that every great journey, in personhood, deserves a healthy beginning.

## ART, SCIENCE, AND HUMANITIES

Nowhere in human medicine is the complex interplay between art, science, and humanity more evident than in our nascent field of newborn medicine. Birthing is a normal physiological process, accompanied by the evolution of care to help both mother and child achieve a peaceful and healthy transition and to promote bonding of the mother-child couplet, eventually leading to a more united family and society. A significant proportion of these births are complicated by maternal, fetal, neonatal, or other disease. The increasingly stratified societies of today, with our microclimates of abundance and despair, make it difficult to generate solutions across socioeconomic boundaries and geopolitical axes. The age of information is transformative in that we can learn from experience in different parts of the world and bring it to bear relevance to our local environment and prioritize development of local programs and solutions.

Traditional models have explained natural disease progression[1,2] as it relates to infectious particle burden (**Fig. 1**). Newer paradigms seek to illuminate risk-factor-based contribution to prevalence of other disease, e.g., congenital disorders (**Fig. 2**).[3] Every day new information emerges, providing novel insights into windows of opportunity for intervention,[4] rare/orphan diseases,[5,6] or into fetal and neonatal developmental biology. Encoding of light in the developing retina drives several early physiological processes, including photoentrainment of circadian rhythm, light aversion, and pupillary light reflexes.[7] Dramatic changes in the remarkably stable developmental trajectory in the first week of life are illustrated using extraction of transcriptomic, proteomic, metabolomic, and chemokine signaling, validated across two independent newborn cohorts from West Africa and Australasia.

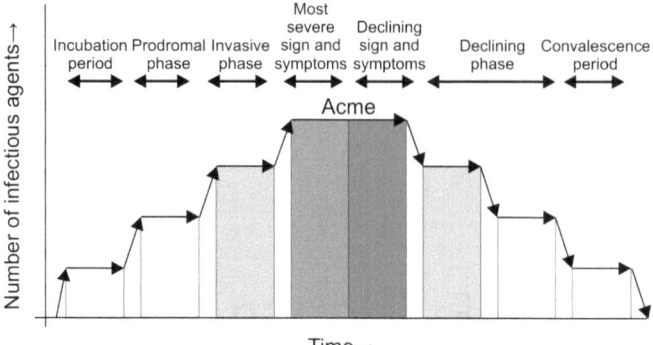

**Fig. 1:** Stages of disease progression.

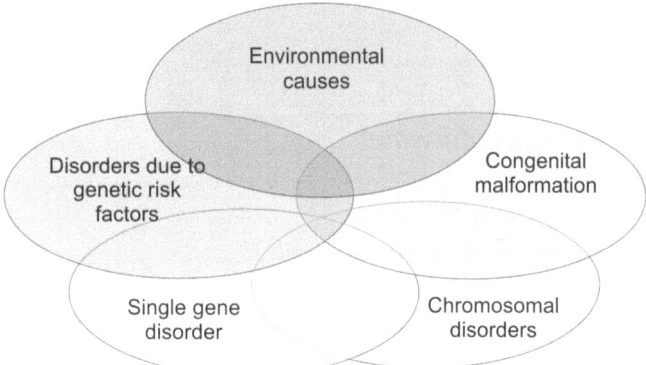

**Fig. 2:** Causes of congenital disorders.[3]
*Source:* Adapted from Modell B, Darlison MW, Lawn JE. Historical overview of development in methods to estimate burden of disease due to congenital disorders. J Community Genet. 2018;9(4):341-5.

Innovative data integration and systems biology approaches provide insight into a dynamic phase key for health and disease.[8] Disruption in maternal proinflammatory cytokines may irreversibly alter infant brain connectivity and future executive function.[9] Furthermore, changes in healthcare service delivery models, diminishing societal inequity, and long predating the moment of birth can alter infant morbidity and mortality patterns.

## ROLE OF HEALTHCARE EDUCATION AND INFORMATICS IN BETTER SERVICE DELIVERY FOR NEWBORNS

We seek to provide tools and experience to educate providers, from the basics of "Helping Babies Breathe" to emphasizing the growing list of advanced practice providers and subspecialist pediatricians engaged in current healthcare delivery for newborns. The role of the general practitioner and family practice in global newborn medicine is vital and cannot be overemphasized. Our future belongs to communities of learners and learning devoted to newborn medicine. Novel definitions and nascent approaches to understanding of palliative and hospice care are requisite for optimal approaches to infants who cannot survive infancy. Furthermore, frameworks for electronically managing infant data have obvious implications for the growing application of informatics to healthcare service delivery improvement.

## PATIENT SAFETY AND QUALITY, INFANT MENTAL HEALTH, FAMILY INTEGRATED CARE, AND HOME FOLLOW-UP

The Institute of Medicine report "To Err is Human" and subsequent iterations by the Institute for Healthcare Improvement have immortalized the principles of quality and safety in US healthcare delivery. Additional paradigms for addressing mental health and emotional well-being with family-integrated care during hospitalization followed by home follow-up for high-risk infants study other vital domains critical to establishing thoughtful systems of integrated care. The importance of charitable giving emphasizes the creative nature of addressing local gap funding vital to optimizing services for high-risk women, infants, and children. The quadruple aim of improved individual healthcare experience, value of care (i.e., better outcomes at lower per capita cost), equitable population health and bringing joy into the healthcare environment are now widely espoused and embraced principles.[10]

## MATERNAL HEALTH AND PRECONCEPTION CARE

Maternal nutrition inclusive of adequate prenatal folate to prevent neural tube defects, prevention of maternal teratogen use (e.g., alcohol) and reducing frequency of smoking, marijuana, and medications and illicit substances known to adversely affect perinatal outcomes are critical to fetomaternal well-being. Maternal disease/disorders in pregnancy and obstetrical contributions to neonatal morbidity and mortality provide key insights into underlying risk to optimal newborn outcomes. The membranes, placenta, and umbilical cord are underappreciated and their disorders have not been optimally studied. Their contribution to perinatal sentinel events (PSE) relevant to neonatal encephalopathy is summarized in Section 3, Perinatal Medicine. Perspectives on PSE relevant to cerebral palsy by the neonatologist[11] and pediatric neurologist[12] are recommended reading. The global importance of preterm birth risk reduction has been reviewed elsewhere.[13]

Opportunities exist for optimizing neonatal care through understanding gaps in study areas between and within different expert clinician groups. Three recent public health examples in neonatal and infant mortality and morbidity reduction come to mind as examples of this transformative process.[14]

1. *Delayed cord clamping (DCC) and its impact on preterm and term brain structure and function:* Prematurity is the leading cause of death in the US, accounting for a third of infant mortality in 2002[15] and globally the leading cause of death in children under age 5.[16] DCC decreases mortality in preterm infants. A study of 18 randomized clinical trials (RCTs) comparing delay of ≥30 seconds (compared to early cord clamping of <30 seconds) in infants born at less than 37 weeks gestation showed reduced hospital mortality, with $I^2 = 0$ indicating no study heterogeneity.[17] In three trials with 996 infants less than 29 weeks gestation, DCC reduced hospital mortality with a number needed to benefit of 20 (95% confidence interval, 11:100, $I^2 = 0$). It has thus been estimated that 300,000–700,000 lives could be saved annually worldwide with implementation of DCC for very preterm infants.[17] Furthermore, in a Canadian retrospective cohort study of 4,680 infants born 2011–2015 at 22–28 weeks gestation, of whom 1,852 received DCC, compared to 2,828 receiving immediate cord clamping (ICC), DCC was associated with reduced risk of severe neurological injury or mortality.[18] Cord milking in the very preterm is unsafe due to fourfold risk of major intraventricular hemorrhage (IVH).[19] Long-term neurodevelopmental benefit has been shown in preterm infants randomized to DCC at ages 1.5 years[20] and 6.5 years.[21] These benefits, attributed to brain structural and functional enhancement (volume and myelination), favor visual motor integration and fine language skill function.

   Studies in term babies also have shown long-term neurodevelopmental benefits associated with DCC. Emerging brain imaging studies indicate that brain myelination at age 4 months is altered favorably in term infants who received ~3 minutes of DCC compared to those receiving <1 minute.[22] Furthermore, long-term neurodevelopmental benefit, particularly in male infants, has been noted as late as age 4 years.[23] In spite of these emerging data, implementation of DCC in high-risk populations is limited even in centers choosing to implement DCC.[24] Optimal duration of "delay"[25] is not currently offered to the majority of the world's newborns at birth. Early implementation experience in DCC in California newborns shows disappointing results even in centers that intend to do so.[24]

2. *Universal saturation screening for critical congenital heart disease (CCHD):* Congenital heart disease is the leading cause of death globally in the first five years of life for infants born with birth defects.[26] In the last two decades, advances in cardiovascular surgery have allowed for definitive care (defined as a

restored circulation with two functioning ventricles) rather than palliative care for many infants with CCHD. In parallel, advances in prenatal diagnosis[27] and newborn saturation[28] have allowed for earlier diagnosis by prenatal detection[14] or by transcutaneous saturation screening in up to 75% of asymptomatic term newborns when prenatal detection rates are <35%.[29] Centers for Disease Control and Prevention (CDC) data[30] from the first US states implementing universal CCHD screening corroborate earlier estimates of reduction in mortality from CCHD[29] in the US. Several nations have attempted to implement early saturation screening to prevent mortality and morbidity from CCHD, but without comprehensive screening, its usefulness is limited. In the People's Republic of China (PRC), universal saturation screening for infants with CCHD is planned for the ~15 million infants expected to be born in the year 2020. Even if and when fully implemented in the PRC, however, the majority of the world's newborns will not yet have benefit of this simple early CCHD detection/intervention. Early experience from California from universal CCHD implementation remains disappointing.[31]

3. *Total body cooling and perinatal asphyxia:* A portion of the world's annual 3 million stillbirths (sometimes miscategorized[32]) may be preventable with simple public health measures such as introduction of birth attendants.[33] Perinatal asphyxia is a primary cause of early neonatal death, affecting 900,000 babies annually worldwide.[34]

While TBC success in the adult and pediatric populations has been limited, investigations ranging from early lamb experiments[35] to human randomized trials[36,37] have established TBC as standard of care for newborn perinatal asphyxia in much of the industrialized world. Standardized registry protocols[38] and collaborative guidelines[39] have facilitated potentially best practice diffusion. Cooling increases survival without increasing disability.[40] While other therapies such as inhaled xenon and high dose erythropoietin (EPO) continue to be studied, it appears that additional high dose EPO benefit may be attenuated by underlying placental pathophysiology.[12] The importance of placental examination in the perinatal asphyxia population cannot be overemphasized.[41] The majority of global newborn citizenry have no access to blood gas analysis at birth, thus providers are unable to ascertain asphyxial definition criteria for these infants, making interventions such as TBC inapplicable. Modified criteria may require consideration until appropriate technology transfer occurs, diminishing further perinatal inequity.

## LEVELS OF EVIDENCE AND GRADING OF RECOMMENDATIONS, ASSESSMENT, DEVELOPMENT, AND EVALUATION

A thoughtful review of incorporating evidence-based medicine into practice is provided here and is recommended reading.[42] Different medical and surgical societies have used mild variations in levels of evidence to guide best practice.[43,44] An illustration is given in **Table 1**.

The EQUATOR (Enhancing the QUality and Transparency Of health Research) network is developing a global initiative to achieve reporting of all health studies to increase value and minimize avoidable waste of human and financial investments in health research (equator-network.org)[46] by providing reporting guidelines for the main study types, in addition to developing other goals and resources. Examples include STROBE (Strengthening The Reporting of OBservational studies in Epidemiology),[47] SQUIRE (Standards for Quality Improvement Reporting Excellence),[48] guideline CONSORT (Consolidated Standards for Reporting Trials),[49] and PRISMA (Preferred Reporting Items for Systematic Reviews and Meta-Analyses).[50]

### Why most published research findings are false?

While Ioannidis meant to be provocative in his sentinel paper with that title,[51] he has brought attention to the fact that using $p < 0.05$ for statistical significance still only means that published studies likely conclude correctly two-thirds of the time and incorrectly one-third of the time if held to a higher degree of statistical certainty (e.g., $p < 0.005$). Uncertainties in the peer-review process[52-55]

**TABLE 1:** Classification of category and strength of evidence.[45]

| | Category of evidence |
|---|---|
| 1A | Meta-analysis of randomized clinical trials (RCTs) |
| 1B | Evidence from ≥1 RCT |
| 2A | Evidence from ≥1 controlled study without randomization |
| 2B | Evidence from ≥1 quasi-experimental study |
| 3 | Evidence from nonexperimental, descriptive, comparative, correlation, and case-control studies |
| 4 | Expert opinions/respected authority/committees |
| | *Strength of recommendation* |
| A | Directly based on Category 1 evidence |
| B | Directly based on Category 2 or extrapolated recommendation from Category 1 evidence |
| C | Directly based on Category 3 or extrapolated recommendation from Category 1 or 2 evidence |
| D | Directly based on Category 4 or extrapolated recommendation from Category 1, 2 or 3 evidence |

*Source:* Modified from Shekelle PG, Woolf SH, Eccles M, et al. Developing clinical guidelines. West J Med. 1999;170(6):348-51.

and the movement toward democratizing knowledge (i.e., open-access publishing) are certain to aid dissemination of knowledge across socioeconomic boundaries.

## PATIENT SAFETY

### Shifting Landscapes: Implications for Research, Education, and Frontline Clinician Practice

A recent paper illustrates how medication side effects may be under-reported and provides a provocative new democratic paradigm for how both providers and patients can contribute in novel ways to reporting adverse effects.[56] Medication error prevention is comprehensively reviewed here and is recommended reading.[57] Providers treatment strategies may fall victim to the "twin traps of overtreatment and therapeutic nihilism"[58] often related to sociocultural bias in our (mis)interpretation of patient's background or our own inadvertent indoctrination. It is important to address these issues in ongoing medical education. Inappropriate management of "conflicts of interest" in US federally funded research is particularly alarming, as revealed recently by ProPublica.[59] This is also an opportune reminder that consumer-based investigation of current health research, conducted in this instance by using publicly available "big data", will necessarily disrupt prior behavioral transgressions and helped clarify future regulation and research practice. Transparency and the necessary disinfectant of sunlight will eventually lead to more clarity in scientific findings, making them less likely to be manipulated by special interests in Big Pharma, establishment investigators and institutions. Ongoing ethics and leadership courses should seek to continually educate providers and institutions based on these rapidly shifting paradigms.

## POTENTIAL OPPORTUNITIES IN FURTHER EXPLORATION OF KNOWLEDGE GAPS

An important part of evaluating newborn well-being at birth must include a visual examination of the placenta, cord, and membranes that have served the infant-mother couplet for months prior to delivery. Current reviews highlight the indications for submission of the placenta for a pathological examination.[60,61] While defined criteria for placental examination have existed for three decades,[62] only a few institutions have >80–85% compliance.[63] Moreover, studies show that the majority of these recommendations are presumably unmeasured or disregarded in the majority of institutions.[64,65] It is concerning that nonmedically indicated examinations (e.g., from surgical deliveries) would result in more placental pathology examinations than those recommended for maternal, fetal/neonatal, or placental indications.[66] Establishing and maintaining placental registries may prove important to a better understanding of newborn health,[67] but historically have been complicated by ethical transgressions in early registry experience.[68]

Since 1997, Denmark has instituted mandatory placental weight examination. An elegant observation of 924,422 liveborn Danish singletons (1997–2011), including 7,569 infants with congenital heart disease, has shown that tetralogy of Fallot, double-outlet right ventricle, and major ventricular septal defects are all associated with deviations in fetal somatic and cerebral growth, possibly related to impaired placental growth.[69] This work exemplifies important contributions to understanding the relationship between congenital heart disease and placental anomalies, and possible implications for fetal growth in infants with heart disease. The association would have been missed, save for the 15 years of data yielded by the Danish approach to universal placental weight examination at birth.

In contrast, cord blood registries, with their better-understood utilitarian ethics, have gained more rapid public, consumer, and institutional support.[70] Their potential; however, has yet to be fully understood, explored, and utilized.

In an era of declining pediatric autopsy, postmortem radiograph[71] and whole exome and genomic sequencing[72] are tools worthy of further study to understand early, obscure causes of neonatal and infant mortality. Obviously, these approaches are currently limited to highly resourced settings and fundamental to exploration of these novel applications are indications;[73-76] ongoing yield, cost and value studies from Europe are forthcoming, and should enhance and refine approaches to infrequent causes of neonatal and infant death.

## REDEFINING NORMAL AND ABNORMAL USING NOVEL NONINVASIVE APPROACHES

The growing role of noninvasive technology in the future of newborn medicine cannot be overemphasized. Applications range from early physiological responses predicting later illness severity in preterm infants[77] to algorithms for predictive monitoring of sepsis in neonatal intensive care unit (ICU).[78] While cerebral near-infrared spectroscopy monitoring for prevention of brain injury in very preterm infants requires further study[79] it appears application in newborns with hypoxic ischemic encephalopathy (HIE) treated with hypothermia may enhance understanding of brain perfusion, in conjunction with other technologies.[80,81] Addition of amplitude-integrated electroencephalography (aEEG) to near-infrared spectroscopy may improve short-term prognostication.[82] Furthermore studies of bilirubin in different race and ethnicity show sufficient variation in "nomograms"[83-85] that when placed in context of gestational age, chronological age, and underlying population genetic risk of red cell membrane or enzyme disorders[86] may lead to novel predictive management algorithms in the future. These select illustrative examples, while far from exhaustive, seek merely to illustrate the range of emerging and future possibilities in newborn care utilizing big data and noninvasive technology.

## CONCLUSION

Societal sociopolitical commitment to universal healthcare coverage, particularly with attention to focused shift of public resources to populations with perinatal inequity and disparity, is fundamental to optimizing care for women and children from the moment of birth. In fact, commitment to societal health with an emphasis on population health education, mental hygiene, and well-being increases the likelihood of more planned pregnancies with greater devotion to optimal preconception care. In an era of "infinite" capital and thus much increased health resource inequity, present-day family variations include both gender binary and nonbinary adults aided by reproductive technology-assisted conception. The modern virtual village supporting this family has a different visual gestalt (genderbread.org), but not dissimilar needs for health equity and education. We need to ask the patient, who are you? and let their answer help inform the optimal treatment strategy. Advancement in technology has made it possible for conception and birthing to occur continents apart, and more recently, uterine transplants and three-parent embryos[87] to prevent lethal congenital mitochondrial disease raise further questions in future reproductive possibilities.

Similarly, awareness of healthcare options for best value in resource-constrained environments needs much critical self-examination in equitable investment of resources; each community must decide for itself what its choices are. Societal priorities may sometimes be fraught with danger prior to birth (e.g., selective prenatal female infanticide) or in childhood (e.g., ritual scarring, piercing, and genital mutilation). Societal education, including that of the growing body of stakeholders in newborn medicine, should seek to keep up with the rapid advancements in knowledge necessary to alter our attitudes and practices. An understanding of the rapidly shifting sands of mental health and substance use in populations is key to serving our newborns and families well. Awareness of preventable mortality and morbidity, investments in family planning, palliative care, and pediatric hospice while embracing missed opportunity for contribution to big data from "minority" populations give the healthcare community much to ponder, plan, and act upon as we embark on the third decade of this new millennium.

The moment of birth represents a triumphant opportunity for hope and joy for the family, community, and our species. Healthcare providers and systems need to build birthing facilities on this concept, providing optimal approaches to couplet care, early optimal bonding and nourishment with a deliberate focus on eliminating unnecessary interventions or needless mother-infant separation at birth or thereafter. High-risk pregnancies managed in regionalized perinatal systems provide opportunity for optimizing outcomes in the minority of situations that require focused devotion of resources and expertise to minimize morbidity and mortality, while providing kindness and supportive palliative care to that very small group unlikely to enjoy pleasure or endure pain, harm, and prolongation of suffering from any measure of care.

## REFERENCES

1. Centers for Disease Control and Prevention (CDC). (2012). Lesson 1: Introduction to Epidemiology. Section 9: Natural History and Spectrum of Disease. [online] Available from: https://www.cdc.gov/csels/dsepd/ss1978/lesson1/section9.html. [Last accessed March, 2019].
2. Jewell NP. Natural history of diseases: Statistical designs and issues. Clin Pharmacol Ther. 2016;100(4):353-61.
3. Modell B, Darlison MW, Lawn JE. Historical overview of development in methods to estimate burden of disease due to congenital disorders. J Community Genet. 2018;9(4):341-5.
4. de Leeuw F, Barkhof F, Scheltens P. Progression of cerebral white matter lesions in Alzheimer's disease: a new window for therapy? J Neurol Neurosurg Psychiatry. 2005;76:1286-8.
5. McGovern MM, Aron A, Brodie SE, et al. Natural history of Type A Niemann-Pick disease. Neurology. 2006;66(2):228-32.
6. Pineda M, Juríčková K, Karimzadeh P, et al. Disease characteristics, prognosis and miglustat treatment effects on disease progression in patients with Niemann-Pick disease Type C: an international, multicenter, retrospective chart review. Orphanet J Rare Dis. 2019;14:32.
7. Caval-Holme F, Feller MB. Gap Junction Coupling Shapes the Encoding of Light in the Developing Retina. Curr Biol. 2019;29(23):4024-35.e5.
8. Lee AH, Shannon CP, Amenyogbe N, et al. Dynamic molecular changes during the first week of human life follow a robust developmental trajectory. Nat Commun. 2019;10(1):1092.
9. Rudolph MD, Graham AM, Feczko E, et al. Maternal IL-6 during pregnancy can be estimated from newborn brain connectivity and predicts future working memory in offspring. Nat Neurosci. 2018;21:765-72.
10. Sikka R, Morath JM, Leape L. The Quadruple Aim: care, health, cost and meaning in work. BMJ Qual Saf. 2015;24:608-10.

11. Wallenstein M, Sunshine P. Neonatal encephalopathy. In: Stevenson D, Benitz W, Sunshine P, Hintz S, Druzin M (Eds). Fetal and Neonatal Brain Injury. Cambridge: Cambridge University Press; 2017. pp. 1-20.
12. Wu YW, Goodman AM, Chang T, et al. Placental pathology and neonatal brain MRI in a randomized trial of erythropoietin for hypoxic-ischemic encephalopathy. Pediatr Res; 2019.
13. Govindaswami B, Jegatheesan P, Nudelman MJR, et al. Prevention of Prematurity: Advances and Opportunities. Clin Perinatol. 2018;45(3):579-95.
14. Levy DJ, Pretorius DH, Rothman A, et al. Improved prenatal detection of congenital heart disease in an integrated health care system. Pediatr Cardiol. 2013;34(3):670-9.
15. Callaghan WM, MacDorman MF, Rasmussen SA, et al. The contribution of preterm birth to infant mortality rates in the United States. Pediatrics. 2006;118(4):1566-73.
16. Chawanpaiboon S, Vogel JP, Moller A, et al. Global, regional, and national estimates of levels of preterm birth in 2014: a systematic review and modelling analysis. Lancet Glob Health. 2019;7(1):e37-e46.
17. Fogarty M, Osborn DA, Askie L, et al. Delayed Versus Early Umbilical Cord Clamping for Preterm Infants: A Systematic Review and Meta-Analysis. Am J Obstet Gynecol. 2017; 300(3):531-43.
18. Lodha A, Shah PS, Soraisham AS, et al. Association of Deferred vs Immediate Cord Clamping With Severe Neurological Injury and Survival in Extremely Low-Gestational-Age Neonates. JAMA Netw Open. 2019;2(3):e191286.
19. Katheria AC, Reister F, Hummler H, et al. LB 1: Premature Infants Receiving Cord Milking or Delayed Cord Clamping: A Randomized Controlled Non-inferiority Trial. Am J Obstet Gynecol. 2019;220:S682.
20. Mercer JS, Erickson-Owens DA, Vohr BR, et al. Effects of Placental Transfusion on Neonatal and 18 Month Outcomes in Preterm Infants: A Randomized Controlled Trial. J Pediatr. 2016;168:50-5.e1.
21. Bolk J, Padilla N, Forsman L, et al. Visual–motor integration and fine motor skills at 6½ years of age and associations with neonatal brain volumes in children born extremely preterm in Sweden: a population-based cohort study. BMJ Open. 2018;8:e020478.
22. Mercer JS, Erickson-Owens DA, Deoni SCL, et al. Effects of delayed cord clamping on 4-month ferritin levels, brain myelin content, and neurodevelopment: a randomized controlled trial. J Pediatr. 2018;203:266-72.e2.
23. Andersson O, Lindquist B, Lindgren M, et al. Effect of Delayed Cord Clamping on Neurodevelopment at 4 Years of Age: A Randomized Clinical Trial. JAMA Pediatr. 2015;169(7):631-8.
24. Tran CL, Parucha JM, Jegatheesan P, et al. Delayed Cord Clamping and Umbilical Cord Milking among Infants in California Neonatal Intensive Care Units. Am J Perinatol. 2020;37(2):151-7.
25. Nudelman MJR, Belogolovsky E, Jegatheesan P, et al. Effect of Delayed Cord Clamping on Umbilical Blood Gas Values in Term Newborns: A Systematic Review. Obstet Gynecol. 2020;135:576-82.
26. March of Dimes. (2006). Global Report on Birth Defects: The Hidden Toll of Dying and Disabled children. [online] Available from https://www.marchofdimes.org/materials/global-report-on-birth-defects-the-hidden-toll-of-dying-and-disabled-children-executive-summary.pdf. [Last accessed March, 2020].
27. Sklansky MS, Berman DP, Pruetz JD, et al. Prenatal Screening for Major Congenital Heart Disease. J Ultrasound Med. 2009;28:889-99.
28. de-Wahl Granelli A, Wennergren M, Sandberg K, et al. Impact of pulse oximetry screening on the detection of duct dependent congenital heart disease: A Swedish prospective screening study in 39, 821 newborns. BMJ. 2009;338:a3037.
29. Govindaswami B, Jegatheesan P, Song D. Oxygen saturation screening for critical congenital heart disease. Neoreviews. 2012;13(12):e724-31.
30. Abouk R, Grosse SD, Ailes EC, et al. Association of US State Implementation of Newborn Screening Policies for Critical Congenital Heart Disease With Early Infant Cardiac Deaths. JAMA. 2017;318(21):2111-8.
31. Siefkes H, Jocson M, Lakshminrusimha S, et al. Hospital reporting of critical congenital heart disease screening. J Investig Med. 2020;68:7.
32. Spector JM, Daga S. Preventing those so-called stillbirths. Bull World Health Organ. 2008;86(4):241-320.
33. Daga SR, Daga AS, Dighole RV, et al. Rural neonatal care: Dahanu experience. Indian Pediatr. 1992;29:189-93.
34. Lawn JE, Manandhar A, Haws RA, et al. Reducing one million child deaths from birth asphyxia: a survey of health systems gaps and priorities. Health Res Policy Syst. 2007;5:4.
35. Gluckman PD, Gunn TR, Johnston BM. The Effect of Cooling on Breathing and Shivering in Unanesthetized Fetal Lambs in Utero. J Physiol. 1983;343:495-506.
36. Shankaran S, Laptook AR, Ehrenkranz RA, et al. Whole-Body Hypothermia for Neonates with Hypoxic-Ischemic Encephalopathy. N Engl J Med. 2005;353:1574-84.
37. Shankaran S, Pappas A, McDonald SA, et al. Childhood Outcomes after Hypothermia for Neonatal Encephalopathy. N Engl J Med. 2012;366:2085-92.
38. Olsen SL, Dejonge M, Kline A, et al. Optimizing therapeutic hypothermia for neonatal encephalopathy. Pediatrics. 2013;131(2):e591-603.
39. Jegatheesan P, Morgan A, Shimotake T, et al. (2015). Early Screening and Identification of Candidates for Neonatal Therapeutic Hypothermia Toolkit. [online] Available from: https://www.cpqcc.org/sites/default/files/FINAL%20HIE%20Toolkit_2-15-15%20California%20Perinatal%20Quality%20Care%20Collaborative.pdf. [Last accessed March, 2020].
40. Jacobs SE, Berg M, Hunt R, et al. Cooling for newborns with hypoxic ischaemic encephalopathy. Cochrane Database Syst Rev. 2013;(1):CD003311.
41. Harteman JC, Nikkels PG, Benders MJ, et al. Placental pathology in full-term infants with hypoxic-ischemic neonatal encephalopathy and association with magnetic resonance imaging pattern of brain injury. J Pediatr. 2013;163(4):968-95.e2.
42. Burns PB, Rohrich RJ, Chung KC. The levels of evidence and their role in evidence-based medicine. Plast Reconstr Surg. 2011;128(1):305-10.
43. Siemieniuk R, Guyatt GH. (2019). What is GRADE? [online] Available from: https://bestpractice.bmj.com/info/toolkit/learn-ebm/what-is-grade/. [Last accessed March, 2020].

44. CEBM. (2016). OECBM Levels of Evidence. [online] Available from: https://www.cebm.net/2016/05/ocebm-levels-of-evidence/. [Last accessed March, 2020].
45. Shekelle PG, Woolf SH, Eccles M, et al. Developing clinical guidelines. West J Med. 1999;170(6):348-51.
46. EQUATOR Network. EQUATOR Network: what we do and how we are organised. [online] Available from: https://www.equator-network.org/about-us/equator-network-what-we-do-and-how-we-are-organised/. [Last accessed March, 2020].
47. von Elm E, Altman DG, Egger M, et al. The Strengthening the Reporting of Observational Studies in Epidemiology (STROBE) statement: guidelines for reporting observational studies. PLoS Med. 2007;4(10):e296.
48. Ogrinc G, Davies L, Goodman D, et al. SQUIRE 2.0 (Standards for QUality Improvement Reporting Excellence): revised publication guidelines from a detailed consensus process. BMJ Qual Saf. 2016;25:986-92.
49. Schulz KF, Altman DG, Moher D. CONSORT 2010 statement: updated guidelines for reporting parallel group randomised trials. PLoS Med. 2010;7(3):e1000251.
50. Moher D, Liberati A, Tetzlaff J, et al. Preferred reporting items for systematic reviews and meta-analyses: the PRISMA statement. PLoS Med. 2009;6(7):e1000097.
51. Ioannidis JPA. Why most published research findings are false. PLoS Med. 2005;2(8):e124.
52. Tancock C. (2018). When reviewing goes wrong: the ugly side of peer review. [online] Available from: https://www.elsevier.com/connect/editors-update/when-reviewing-goes-wrong-the-ugly-side-of-peer-review. [Last accessed March, 2020].
53. Smith R. Peer review: a flawed process at the heart of science and journals. J R Soc Med. 2006;99(4):178-82.
54. Pollett M. (2020). The Evolution and Critical Role of Peer Review in Academic Publishing. [online] Available from: https://www.wiley.com/network/researchers/being-a-peer-reviewer/the-evolution-and-critical-role-of-peer-review-in-academic-publishing-2. [Last accessed March, 2020].
55. Balietti S. (2016). Science is suffering because of peer review's big problems. [online] Available from: https://newrepublic.com/article/135921/science-suffering-peer-reviews-big-problems. [Last accessed March, 2020].
56. Healy D, Mangin D. Clinical judgments, not algorithms, are key to patient safety—an essay by David Healy and Dee Mangin. BMJ. 2019;367:l5777.
57. Antonucci R, Porcella A. Preventing medication errors in neonatology: Is it a dream? World J Clin Pediatr. 2014;3(3):37-44.
58. Mamede S, Schmidt HG. The twin traps of overtreatment and therapeutic nihilism in clinical practice. Med Educ. 2014;48(1):34-43.
59. Armstrong D, Waldman A. (2019). Federally Funded Health Researchers Disclose at Least $188 Million in Conflicts of Interest. Can You Trust Their Findings? [online] Available from: https://www.propublica.org/article/federally-funded-health-researchers-disclose-at-least-188-million-in-conflicts-of-interest-can-you-trust-their-findings?utm_source=pardot&utm_medium=email&utm_campaign=majorinvestigations. [Last accessed March, 2020].
60. Baergen RN. Indications for submission and macroscopic examination of the placenta. APMIS. 2018;126:544-50.
61. Roberts DJ, McKenny A, Barss VA. (2019). The placental pathology report. [online] Available from: https://www.uptodate.com/contents/the-placental-pathology-report. [Last accessed March, 2020].
62. Yetter JF 3rd. Examination of the placenta. Am Fam Physician. 1998;57(5):1045-54.
63. Sills A, Steigman C, Ounpraseuth ST, et al. Pathologic examination of the placenta: recommended versus observed practice in a university hospital. Int J Womens Health. 2013;5:309-12.
64. Curtin WM, Krauss S, Metlay LA, et al. Pathologic examination of the placenta and observed practice. Obstet Gynecol. 2007;109(1):35-41.
65. Al Harazi AH, Frass KA. Low rate of placental pathological examination in a tertiary care hospital in Sana'a, Yemen. East Mediterr Health J. 2011;17(4):277-80.
66. Booth VJ, Nelson KB, Dambrosia JM, et al. What factors influence whether placentas are submitted for pathologic examination? Am J Obstet Gynecol. 1997;176(3):567-71.
67. Terry M. (2018). Modern Tech Teases out Important Role of the Placenta. [online] Available from: https://www.biospace.com/article/modern-tech-teases-out-important-role-of-the-placenta/. [Last accessed March, 2020].
68. Neumeister L. (2006). Up to 700 Women in West Not Told about Placenta Registry. [online] Available from: https://www.insurancejournal.com/news/west/2006/02/13/65318.htm. [Last accessed March, 2020].
69. Matthiesen NB, Henriksen TB, Agergaard P, et al. Congenital Heart Defects and Indices of Placental and Fetal Growth in a Nationwide Study of 924422 Liveborn Infants. Circulation. 2016;134:1546-56.
70. American College of Obstetricians and Gynecologists. (2016). Cord Blood Banking. [online] Available from: https://www.acog.org/Patients/FAQs/Cord-Blood-Banking?IsMobileSet=false. [Last accessed March, 2020].
71. Arthurs OJ, Hutchinson JC, Sebire NJ. Current issues in postmortem imaging of perinatal and forensic childhood deaths. Forensic Sci Med Pathol. 2017;13(1):58-66.
72. European Society of Human Genetics. (2018). Genomic testing for the causes of stillbirth should be considered for routine use. [online] Available from: www.sciencedaily.com/releases/2018/06/180617204419.htm. [Last accessed March, 2020].
73. Bouchireb K, Teychene AM, Rigal O, et al. Post-mortem MRI reveals CP2 deficiency after sudden infant death. Eur J Pediatr. 2010;169(12):1561-3.
74. Methner D, Scherer S, Welch K, et al. Postmortem genetic screening for the identification, verification, and reporting of genetic variants contributing to the sudden death of the young. Genome Res. 2016;26:1170-7.
75. Armes JE, Williams M, Price G, et al. Application of Whole Genome Sequencing Technology in the Investigation of Genetic Causes of Fetal, Perinatal, and Early Infant Death. Pediatr Dev Pathol. 2018;21(1):54-67.
76. Oshima Y, Yamamoto T, Ishikawa T, et al. Postmortem genetic analysis of sudden unexpected death in infancy: neonatal genetic screening may enable the prevention of sudden infant death. J Hum Genet. 2017;62:989-95.
77. Saria S, Rajani AK, Gould J, et al. Integration of early physiological responses predicts later illness severity in preterm infants. Sci Transl Med. 2010;2(48):48-65.

78. Fairchild KD. Predictive monitoring for early detection of sepsis in neonatal ICU patients. Curr Opin Pediatr. 2013;25(2):172-9.
79. Hyttel-Sorensen S, Greisen G, Als-Nielsen B, et al. Cerebral near-infrared spectroscopy monitoring for prevention of brain injury in very preterm infants. Cochrane Database Syst Rev. 2017;(9):CD011506.
80. Dix LML, van Bel F, Lemmers PMA. Monitoring Cerebral Oxygenation in Neonates: An Update. Front Pediatr. 2017;5:46.
81. Wintermark P, Hansen A, Warfield SK, et al. Near-infrared spectroscopy versus magnetic resonance imaging to study brain perfusion in newborns with hypoxic-ischemic encephalopathy treated with hypothermia. Neuroimage. 2014;85:287-93.
82. Goeral K, Urlesberger B, Giordano V, et al. Prediction of Outcome in Neonates with Hypoxic-Ischemic Encephalopathy II: Role of Amplitude-Integrated Electroencephalography and Cerebral Oxygen Saturation Measured by Near-Infrared Spectroscopy. Neonatology. 2017;112:193-202.
83. Olusanya BO, Mabogunje CA, Imosemi DO, et al. Transcutaneous bilirubin nomograms in African neonates. PLoS One. 2017;12(2):e0172058.
84. De Luca D, Jackson GL, Tridente A, et al. Transcutaneous Bilirubin Nomograms: A Systematic Review of Population Differences and Analysis of Bilirubin Kinetics. Arch Pediatr Adolesc Med. 2009;163(11):1054-9.
85. Varughese PM, Rajan N, Mani M, et al. Race specific nomograms: time for change? Int J Contemp Pediatr. 2018;5(2):420-6.
86. Hansen TWR. (2017). Neonatal Jaundice. [online] Available from: https://emedicine.medscape.com/article/974786-overview. [Last accessed March, 2020].
87. Hamzelou J. (2016). Exclusive: World's First Baby Born with new "3 parent" technique. [online] Available from: https://www.newscientist.com/article/2107219-exclusive-worlds-first-baby-born-with-new-3-parent-technique/. [Last accessed March, 2020].

# CHAPTER 2

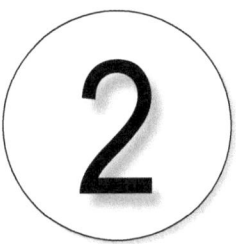

# Historical Understanding and Current Approaches in Neonatology

*Sharyn Frentner, Robin Daughters Wu, Balaji Govindaswami*

*"History will be kind to me, for I intend to write it."*
—Winston Churchill

## ABSTRACT

The practice of caring for newborn infants has evolved significantly over the past century. Highly skilled providers, family-friendly policies, specialized techniques, and equipment tailored to the ill and/or premature infant has made it possible to save lives that in past years could not be saved. This historical perspective should serve to enhance our understanding of current approaches, which surely shall be re-evaluated by a future but different standard of care and practice.

## INTRODUCTION

The term neonatology began being used in the 1960s. The etymology of the word is *neos*: new (Greek) + *natus*: born (Latin) + *logos*: science (Greek) = *new born science*.[1] The neonatal intensive care unit (NICU) of the late 1960s and 70s would be considered primitive by today's standards. There were no infant ventilators, only adult ones that had been modified to attempt to meet infant needs. High-frequency oscillatory ventilation (HFOV), "Jet" ventilation, specialized skin care, "smart pumps," nitric oxide, extracorporeal membrane oxygenation (ECMO), and family-centered care were unknown at the time. This chapter will focus on major shifts in paradigms of neonatal care.

## EVOLUTION

Historically, sick infants were cared for at home, primarily by their mothers and midwives. The first institutional care probably began in the 13th century with the establishment of a foundling hospital by Pope Innocent III.[2] Much later, other hospitals for infants and foundlings were opened in Paris and London—L'Hôpital des Enfants-Trouvés in Paris (1670)[3] and the Foundling Hospital in London (1741).[4] The first children's hospital opened in Paris in 1802 (L'Hôpital des Enfants-Malades).[5] The first American children's hospitals in the US, New York Nursery and Child Hospital, and Children's Hospital of Philadelphia, were founded in 1854 and 1855.[6,7]

Initially, care for the premature newborn was provided by the obstetrician and the parents. There was debate as to which specialty was better prepared to care for premature infants—the obstetrician or the pediatrician?[8] When US birth registries in the early 1900s revealed significantly high infant mortality rates, pediatricians became increasingly involved in improving infant care.

## RESUSCITATION

*"If the child does not breathe immediately upon delivery, which sometimes it will not, especially if it has taken air in the womb; wipe its mouth and press your mouth to the child's, at the same time pinching the nose with your thumb and finger, to prevent the air escaping; inflate the lungs; rubbing it before the fire, by which method I have saved many."* Benjamin Pugh (a London surgeon), 1754.

Although mouth-to-mouth and other forms of resuscitation had been performed for many years, there was no organized assessment or defined procedure for infants until the 1950s. In 1957, Virginia Apgar, an anesthesiologist, devised a systematic scoring system to assess the newborn; in 1958, she suggested that someone apart from the delivering obstetrician or midwife should perform this assessment.[9] The Apgar score became the standard of care. Over the next 30 years, improvements in equipment and procedure were made, including intubation and suctioning for meconium on the perineum. The Neonatal Resuscitation Program (NRP), published in 1988 and now in its seventh edition, has since been taught as standard of care in the United States and around the world.[10]

## Incubator

Caregivers noted early on that survival of a preterm infant depended upon keeping the infant warm. In 1880, ES Tarnier, a Paris Maternity Hospital obstetrician, observing that "the minute and delicate care which these weakly (premature born) infants require, especially in winter, to protect them from the cold is so great that till now most of them have died," invented an incubator that would keep premature infants warm and improve their survival.[11] This incubator revolutionized neonatal care, and precipitated the "incubator baby side shows" **(Fig. 1)**.[12] One of Tarnier's students, Pierre Budin, wrote a number of articles on care of "weaklings," including the importance of thermoregulation and maintenance of a clean environment. At the Berlin Exposition in 1896, Martin Couney, who had studied with Budin, opened an exhibit of premature infants, utilizing the Budin approach. Couney brought his show to the United States in 1901 as part of the Trans-Mississippi Exposition in Omaha. He continued exhibiting the incubator babies at a number of world's fairs and at Coney Island, New York, until 1943.

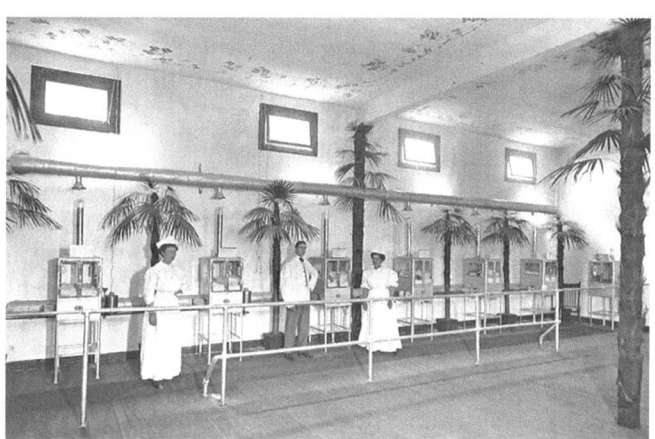

**Fig. 1:** Incubator baby side show.[12]

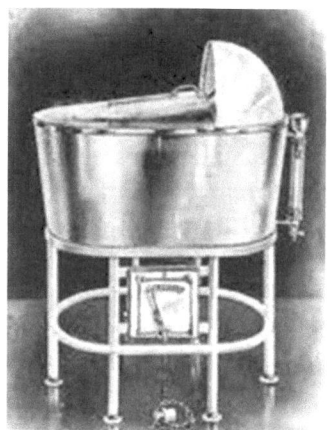

**Fig. 2:** Hess incubator.[13]

Julius Hess, Pediatric Chief at Michael Reese Hospital in Chicago, created the Hess incubator **(Fig. 2)**[13] which provided heat and oxygen to the infant. This incubator was also able to be transported by ambulance.[14] A disadvantage of this incubator was limited visibility of the infant.

By the 1940s, incubators became more modern devices with transparent walls. In the 1970s, overhead warmers and double walls were developed. Continued improvements allow for better access to the infant while maintaining warmth.

## Thermoregulation

Although Budin and colleagues demonstrated the importance of thermoregulation to preterm infant survival, it was not until the 1950s that the benefits of thermoregulation were documented by William Silverman and Richard Day at Columbia Presbyterian Hospital (then Babies' Hospital). They did the first randomized, controlled trials in neonatology, affirming the importance of maintaining a neutral thermal environment.[15] Thermoregulation remains vital to optimal neonatal care.

## Neonatal Intensive Care Unit

In the 1920s, hospitals developed units specifically designed for preterm infant care. One of the earliest was Michael Reese Hospital in Chicago (1922), where Julius Hess wrote the first Textbook of Newborn Care.[16] The first NICUs began to open in the 1960s and were brought to the US public's attention by the death of the president's son in 1963. Patrick Bouvier Kennedy, born at 34½ weeks gestation and weighing 2,112 g, was transported to Boston Children's Hospital, where he died of respiratory distress syndrome, or RDS (then called hyaline membrane disease) at 39 hours of life.[17] His death inspired increased research into treatment of RDS and newborn intensive care practices.

Yale and Vanderbilt Universities[18,19] established their own NICUs in the early 1960s. By 1975, neonatology was designated as a pediatric subspecialty. In the 1970s, regionalization was the norm; ill infants routinely were transported from local hospitals to regional centers, often distant from their families. As more neonatologists, respiratory therapists, and nurses were trained in neonatal care, the ability to care for infants locally improved significantly, with only the most complicated cases requiring transfer to regional centers. Current NICU practice, learned over several decades, includes much improved obstetric/perinatal care and neonatology, aided by explosive growth in innovation and technology.

## Nursing

Florence Nightingale's book *Notes on Nursing*, published in 1860, continues to be relevant today. She challenged nursing practice, both in her work in the Crimea and her efforts later to reform the reputation of nursing from disreputable (exemplified by Dickens' character Sairey Gamp) to what is now a highly respected profession. She transformed the patient experience by improving the environment, personal hygiene, and nutrition, which directly led to such practices as hand-washing and today's decreased noise levels in the NICU. Working to improve patient outcomes, she formulated statistical records, beginning by tracking nosocomial deaths in Scutari, Istanbul (where she was stationed during the Crimean War), and comparing those numbers to battlefield injuries. Her Model Hospital Statistical Form continues to impact quality management today. Using statistical data to guide changes in practice, she promoted care based on evidence. Florence Nightingale also promoted nursing education and mentoring, as she established the Nightingale Training School in 1860 and continued to provide mentoring to former students.[20] Although Nightingale was not a neonatal nurse, she viewed the care of children as particularly demanding.[21]

Nursing has always been an indispensable part of neonatology, from caring for infants in foundling hospitals, to working in sick infant units, and eventually NICUs. No matter who directed treatment—obstetrician, family practitioner, pediatrician or neonatologist—it was the nurse who provided the care. Neonatal nursing has changed dramatically over the years. In the past, a nurse was not allowed to start an IV; that was the doctor's job. In fact, most procedures were performed exclusively by doctors. However, medical residents heeded the experience of the nurse, who was with the patient constantly, and knew when a change was harmless, or cause for concern. As NICUs grew, the nurse's role began to expand. Nurses began to accompany the doctors when transporting a patient; they knew how to set up the IV pump, assist with line insertion, and bag ventilate the infant during the trip to the destination hospital (before the days of transport ventilators). As medical training programs changed, residents spent less time in the NICU, and skilled nurses were needed to attend deliveries, manage patients, and perform procedures.

### Evolution of the Nurse's Role—the Neonatal Nurse Practitioner

In the late 1970s to early 1980s, training programs were established to educate nurses in an advanced practice role. Initially these programs were directed by the hospital, usually in conjunction with a local university. The programs required both didactic and clinical hours. The didactic portion usually lasted about 9 months, followed by an internship in which an attending neonatologist would mentor the nurse in skills and patient care management. Once the internship was complete, the neonatal nurse practitioner (NNP) qualified for certification, which may have been issued from the hospital or from the State Board of Nursing. Later, many Universities began NNP programs at the Masters level. Licensure or certification was dependent on each State Board of Nursing.

National Certification testing became available, at first for clinical nurse specialists/NNPs and later for bedside nurses. Nurses could be credentialed for their knowledge of their specialized field, such as neonatal nursing. These dramatic changes in neonatal nursing over the years were built on the groundwork of Florence Nightingale. It is the ultimate tribute of recognition for the role of nursing in neonatology that the Vermont Oxford Network (VON) has named its reporting process "the Nightingale Network."[22]

## Nutrition

Nutrition is vital to optimal neonatal care. Gavage feedings have been used for preterm infants since the 1800s, using rubber tubes or even a nasal spoon. In the 1970s, feedings were often withheld if the infant had respiratory difficulty or there was concern about infection.

Throughout the US in the 1960s and 1970s, breastfeeding was becoming more popular than it had been in the 1950s. Preterm infant formulas did not exist until the 1980s, when ingredients such as sugar or corn oil were added to term formulas to help boost carbohydrates or fat. Mothers' milk banks made human milk available for infants who did not have their own mother's milk available to them. In the early 1980s, research was begun on fortifiers for human milk to improve infant nutrition with calories and other nutrients. This research continues, with new formulations arriving on the market every day.

As smaller and younger infants arrived in the NICU, IV access for parenteral nutrition became increasingly challenging. In response to this problem, smaller and easier to use IV catheters were designed for use for both peripheral and central access. Glucose solutions were the only parenteral nutrition available until the 1960s. In the late 1960s and early 1970s, Stanley Dudrick pioneered the use of products containing protein, glucose, and other nutrients.[23] By the mid-1970s, intralipids were added to IV solutions, providing phytocholesterols as a source of fat. Present-day practice has substituted plant-based cholesterol with animal-based products, such as SMOF (soybean oil, medium-chain triglycerides, olive oil, and fish oil) and Omegaven (fish oil). These novel lipid formulations are indicated in prolonged use and are less likely to cause liver injury.

Initially, IV pumps were hard to set up and it was difficult to control their flow rate accurately. It was impossible to use IV pumps for blood transfusions as IV flow was controlled by rollers (similar to a Kangaroo pump). Instead, blood was given by gravity, with a nurse counting each drop to determine flow rate. Present-day pumps facilitate much more accurate fluid and drug administration.

## Respiratory Management

Respiratory management is a major concern to those providing neonatal care. Over 50 years ago, cyanotic infants were treated with oxygen; bag and mask ventilation were the only options available if the infant became apneic. Autopsies of premature infants who had difficulty breathing showed the presence of hyaline membranes in their lungs, hence the name "hyaline membrane disease" (now called RDS). In 1959, Mary Ellen Avery determined that preterm infants lacked surfactant, a substance that prevents the lungs from collapsing with each breath.[24] Treatment could be provided with the use of a ventilator, but as infant ventilators were not developed before the mid-1970s, modifications were made to adult ventilators in an attempt to assist preterm infants to breathe without causing additional lung trauma. Some of these ventilators were pressure-driven, while others were volume-controlled. Many were difficult to control; if the pressure or rate was changed, they would often stop working properly, and one nurse would have to bag ventilate the infant while another tended to the machine. Inspiration to expiration or I:E ratios had to be hand-counted. In the early 1970s, the Baby Bird was developed, a ventilator designed for infants. Preterm infants still experienced surfactant deficiency, however, and the pressures required during ventilation often resulted in barotrauma and chronic lung disease (then called bronchopulmonary dysplasia).

Another respiratory device used in the 1970s was a negative pressure isolette.[25] This machine worked like an iron lung; negative pressure on the infant's chest helped to pull out the chest wall, and cycled at a given rate, providing ventilation. The infant's head was placed in the top portion with the padded porthole sleeve, infusing oxygen around the head. The rest of the infant's body was placed in the larger compartment of the isolette. An advantage of this system is that the infant did not require intubation. The disadvantages were: (1) the force of the cycling could move the infant around in the compartment (the device was used only for infants > 1,000 g) and (2) careful attention was required during blood draws to avoid blood being pulled out of the syringe into the chamber.

In 1971, George Gregory designed a continuous positive airway pressure (CPAP) device,[26] which could be used with an endotracheal tube (ETT), nasal prongs, or a hood. While cumbersome, most infants had excellent results with ETT CPAP, which worked in much the same way that modern CPAP devices do. Ventilatory advances in high frequency oscillators and jets came in the 1980s and 1990s.

The definitive treatment of infant respiratory distress was the advent of surfactant use in the early 1990s. The importance of the lecithin to sphingomyelin (L/S) ratio was established in the late 1960s as an indicator of fetal lung maturity; increased L/S and presence of phosphatidylglycerol suggested a lower risk of RDS. Often a shake test[27] was used as a quick determination of lung maturity. The amniotic fluid obtained would be shaken; if it foamed (indicating surfactant presence), there was a probability of lung maturity. Louis Gluck and colleagues looked at the relationship of surfactant and RDS and explored ways to provide surfactant to infants born prior to lung maturity.[28] Although human amniotic fluid was used initially, the first commercially available surfactant was Exosurf,[29] a synthetic product developed at University of California San Francisco (UCSF). Later products include Survanta, Infasurf (bovine) and Curosurf (porcine), all with surface active proteins. Current surfactants include lucinactant, a pentapeptide containing synthetic protein elements.[30,31]

## Retinopathy of Prematurity

Oxygen was used for treatment of apnea and cyanosis as early as 1780, with prolonged use of oxygen supplied directly into the isolette for small, premature infants beginning in the mid-1940s.[32] Retinopathy of prematurity (ROP), an abnormal development of blood vessels in the eye that can lead to blindness, has been associated with oxygen use in preterm infants. A study done in the 1950s to determine if restricting oxygen use would decrease ROP provided confusing findings, leading to the belief that if oxygen concentration remained under 40%, the infant would suffer no eye damage. Some incubators were designed with red flags that would pop up automatically if oxygen concentration rose above 40%. It was later noted that when oxygen was restricted, both the death rate and the rate of brain damage increased. Fortunately, trials in the 1980s and 1990s and the use of pulse oximetry to monitor infant oxygenation have resulted in reduced ROP. Frequency of ophthalmological screening and follow up has also been standardized in subsequent years.

## A BRIEF HISTORY OF NEONATAL SURGERY

A comprehensive review of neonatal surgical history is beyond the scope of this chapter. Neonatal surgery, primarily for congenital defects, has been performed for centuries. It was not until the 20th century that pioneering surgeons devised better techniques with much improved outcomes. A few of the many surgeons who developed new treatments for infants with a variety of surgically correctable defects follow:

- Cameron Haight at the University of Michigan was the first to perform a one-stage repair of esophageal atresia.
- Alfred Blalock and Helen Taussig at Johns Hopkins were the first to develop a technique for correction for Tetralogy of Fallot.
- Benjy Brooks, an innovative pediatric surgeon at the University of Texas-Houston, was the first female pediatric surgeon in Texas.
- More recently, Michael Harrison became the "father of fetal surgery" at University of California at San Francisco, performing different types of surgery on the unborn fetus.

Improved technology, pain management, and optimal anesthesia also have contributed to better infant outcomes. The invention of infant ventilators has made many neonatal surgeries possible. Prior to having the ability to adequately ventilate these infants, surgical intervention was often a major risk. For example, before infant ventilators existed it was not possible to close gastroschisis. Specially-designed IV equipment made parenteral nutrition possible, providing adequate nutrition to infants requiring abdominal surgery for congenital anomalies and/or necrotizing enterocolitis. Modern prenatal diagnostic tools such as ultrasound and magnetic resonance imaging have also led to improved neonatal outcomes through early fetal diagnosis. Currently, interventional radiological, minimally invasive (including robotic) approaches are rapidly replacing traditional open surgery for a variety of medical conditions. Staged surgical procedures and deferring risks of pediatric anesthesia are important studied approaches to optimize long-term surgical and neurodevelopment outcomes.

### Pain Management

There has been a multitude of changes in newborn pain management in the last 50 years. Historically, many in the medical profession claimed that infants did not feel pain and the practice of withholding anesthesia to infants was widespread into the 1980s.[33] Most mothers and nurses knew that infants do feel pain, however, and used nonpharmacologic soothing methods when the infant appeared uncomfortable. Nevertheless, when surgery was performed or procedures were done, no anesthetic or analgesic was provided to the infant. Many doctors who thought pain medication was appropriate were reluctant to administer it because the correct dosage for the smallest infants was unknown. Some surgeons would prescribe a "whiskey nipple" to be provided postoperatively. The procedure was simple; an order was made for bourbon or scotch (dependent on the attending). A small bottle was sent from pharmacy and locked up in the narcotics cabinet. When the nurses decided the infant needed pain management, they would mix a small amount of the whiskey with some glucose water, soak a cotton ball in the mixture and put the wet cotton ball into a nipple. The infant would suck on it and it is hoped, get some relief. There was no dosage written and the procedure would be repeated until the baby seemed to be comfortable.

The current consensus is that infants do indeed feel pain. Just like in the adult world, pain assessment is now one of the five vital signs regularly monitored in healthcare settings. Various scoring methods have been developed to determine if an infant is in pain; usually it is treated appropriately with narcotics and other analgesics. In addition, comfort measures are provided during painful or uncomfortable procedures.

### Transport

Safely transporting a sick infant from one hospital to another for advanced care has always been challenging. A major problem with early transports (**Fig. 3**)[34] was

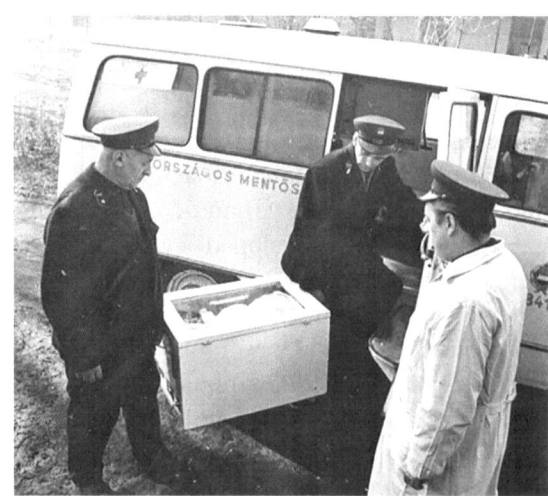

**Fig. 3:** Infant transport in Hungary, 1968.[34]

thermoregulation. It was quite difficult to keep the infant warm during transport, particularly during winter, or when using helicopters, which tended to be quite cold, breezy and noisy. Another issue was the lack of oxygen blenders. The infant could only be transported in room air or 100% oxygen. Transport ventilators did not become available until the mid- to late 1970s, so if the baby needed to be ventilated during transport, a nurse was required to bag by hand the entire way. Many monitors and IV pumps that were available in the NICU were too large to be used in transport.

Most of the improvements in neonatal transport coincide with those made within the NICU itself. The development of sophisticated transport incubators has allowed for better thermoregulation. Smaller monitors and other equipment have made it possible, while on the road or in the air, to provide a similar level of care to that of the NICU.

## Historical Insights from Obstetrics and Perinatology

### Antenatal Steroids to Decrease Neonatal Morbidity and Mortality

Almost a third of the 4 million global deaths in first year of life are attributable to prematurity. In Liggins and Howie's 1972 sentinel paper, a controlled trial of betamethasone therapy for mothers that threatened preterm delivery less than 37 weeks with the hope of reducing infant RDS, showed early neonatal mortality was reduced (3.2% of treated group vs 15% of control group, p = 0.01).[35] RDS reduction benefit was confined to babies less than 32 weeks gestation who had been treated more than 24 hours (11.8% of treated vs 69.6% of controls, p = 0.02). 77% of treated mothers had received betamethasone at least 24 hours prior to delivery. Subsequent surfactant replacement therapy (SRT) trials in the 1980s established further benefit of reduced mortality and morbidity from respiratory distress in the early neonatal period.[36]

### Public Health-based Approaches to Prematurity Prevention

Prevention of premature birth has recently been comprehensively reviewed.[37] Current public health-based approaches seeking to prevent prematurity have incorporated new testing methods and practices, based on studies and observations. In one study, women who had contractions at 24–34 weeks were assessed for preterm birth risk by noting clinical findings and presence of fetal fibronectin. Antenatal steroids (ANS) were administered based on this evidence-based decision model, resulting in standardized management and quick identification of candidates for ANS.[38] Prevention of prematurity with medications includes various 17-hydroxyprogesterone treatment protocols to reduce preterm birth.[37] A meta-analysis suggesting that active women, as compared to those who are relatively inactive, have a 10–14% reduced risk of preterm birth.[39] Emerging evidence from Limerick, Ireland[40] has shown reduced preterm birth in the COVID era. It remains to be seen whether this will be true in other populations and epochs.

### Postpartum Hemorrhage

Active management of the third stage of labor, once used primarily for women who were high risk for post-birth hemorrhage, has become standard of care around the world. However, for mothers with low risk of bleeding, it may not help and could even lead to worse outcomes.[41]

### Cesarean Section

Practice patterns including nonmedically indicated cesarean section (CS) and a reluctance to attempt vaginal birth after CS have resulted in much variation in international and institutional CS rates. It is not known what CS rate is optimal; in aggregate, it is estimated that global rates higher than 10% do not result in improved maternal or neonatal outcomes.[42] A comparative analysis of 40 hospitals found that CS rates for the average nulliparous term singleton vertex (NTSV) delivery varied widely, from 10.3% to 34.2%. It is notable that factors which increased the NTSV CS rate included not only individual variables (e.g., induced labor, higher birth weight, increased maternal age, African American race, hypertension, diabetes) but also institutional variables, such as delivery at hospitals with an obstetric and gynecological residency.[43] Quality improvement initiatives can decrease the NTSV cesarean delivery rate. Any increased incidence of fetal or maternal complications associated with decreased NTSV CS rate should be considered in the context of the risks and benefits of vaginal delivery compared to cesarean delivery.[44]

### Rhesus Isoimmunization Disease

Hemolytic disease of the newborn (HDN) was recorded as early as 1609. It was not until 1954 that fetal hemolysis was proven to be caused by the mother's production of anti-RhD alloimmune antibodies. HDN prevention began in earnest in 1970.[45] Current treatment approaches, including intravenous immune globulin (IVIG) administration in ABO blood type incompatibility in significant hemolytic disease, have decreased exchange transfusions and the duration (e.g., phototherapy) and frequency (e.g., necessity or number of blood transfusions) of other interventions.

## Perinatal Asphyxia

Early observation by Ramji in India showed that mortality was increased in hospitals using oxygen to resuscitate term infants with perinatal asphyxia. Room air is as effective, although possibly not superior to 100% oxygen in infant resuscitation.[46] Subsequent multicenter international trials (RESAIR I and II) led to further validation and confirmation of these observations; resuscitation can be performed on room air just as effectively as oxygen.[47] Institutions vary in their approaches to using oxygen in infant resuscitation, some believing that supplemental $O_2$ is detrimental. Much opportunity exists for further study on this subject.[48-50]

## Total Body Cooling for Neonatal Encephalopathy

Early studies showed in the asphyxiated lamb model that secondary oxygen mediators led to exacerbation of asphyxial injury and that therapeutic hypothermia was neuroprotective.[51] Data from a study of a mixed population of infants with neonatal encephalopathy (NE) suggest that induced cerebral hypothermia may improve neurodevelopmental outcome in infants with less severe NE, but does not improve outcome for those with more severe aEEG changes.[52] Total body cooling has now emerged as standard of care in the prevention of NE.[53]

## Developmental Care

Developmental care for infants was unheard of until fairly recently. If infants had an umbilical artery catheter or umbilical vein catheter in place, they remained on their back with all four extremities restrained. If babies were intubated, small sandbags were often used to keep them from turning their heads and possibly becoming extubated. Parents were not allowed to hold their babies if they had a central line or were on a ventilator.

Later, problems were noted in high-risk follow-up clinics when these children were unable to bring their arms to midline, or had abducted hips. Over time and with the help of such forward-thinking practitioners as Heidelise Als, developmental care has become as much a part of patient care as suctioning or medication administration.[54] In the 1990s, kangaroo care (placing the infant directly on the parent's skin for hours each day) was introduced in many units, which encouraged families to become a part of their infant's care team **(Fig. 4)**.[55] Sibling visitation and family-centered care soon followed.

## Family-centered Care

Family integration with care, an idea which has been present in many realms since the nineteenth century, returned to the forefront in the mid-twentieth century as

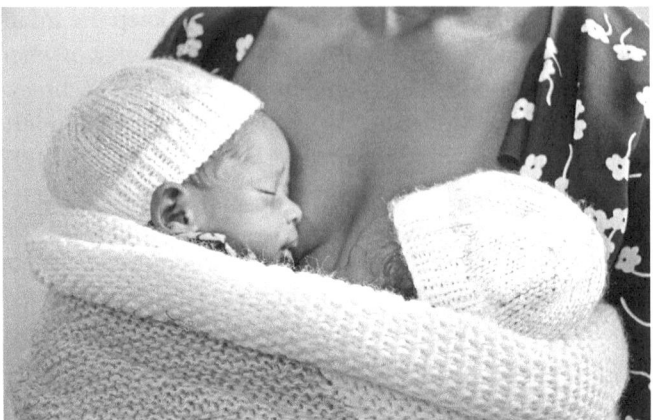

**Fig. 4:** Kangaroo care of twins at Queen Elizabeth Hospital, Blantyre, Malawi. The infants have been placed skin-to-skin with their grandmother[55] (For color version see Plate 1).

the psychologist John Bowlby's work in separation anxiety and grief became popular. In 1955, the Citizens' Committee for Children of New York City was founded in an effort to increase parental access to their hospitalized children. In the UK, the precursor to the British parent advocacy group "Action for Sick Children" formed in 1959 in response to a published report on the conditions in children's hospitals. Worldwide, advocacy groups composed of both parents and healthcare professionals now have input into policy and children's health initiatives.[56] Currently there are many good examples of consumer-led advocacy for improved outcomes for mothers and babies.[57,58] Benchmarking institutions such as the VON and California Perinatal Quality Care Collaborative continually emphasize family integration into quality improvement processes. Numerous benefits arise from family-centered care, including reduced NICU length of stay.[59,60] Current approaches to promote early mother-infant bonding include delayed cord-clamping, early skin-to-skin contact, early administration of colostrum, and exclusive breastfeeding, if, when, and where possible. These approaches have been traditional historical standards of care. Best practice models exist for future building of sustainable family-centered care.[61]

## CONCLUSION

Neonatology is a relatively recent science that has developed rapidly. Although many years ago sick and premature infants were largely cared for at home, now their unique needs are addressed by teams of specialized personnel and their own hospital intensive care environment, the NICU. Advancements in technology, highly skilled providers, and continually evolving standards for the care of premature and ill infants are all factors that have led to improvements in the care of our smallest patients. At the same time, a return to the basic healthy couplet approach for low-risk births and minimizing mother-infant separation is being reintroduced. We live in an era of highly-intensified medical treatment, but intervention is not always clearly indicated. Obstetrics has improved testing and treatment for mothers, preventing many cases of disease and prematurity. As fewer infants need the intensive treatment that the NICU offers, NICU staff can then focus on these children and minimize preventable morbidity. As we begin to address rare and orphan diseases earlier in infancy, there is increasing opportunity for early diagnosis, prevention, and treatment of these conditions in future obstetric and neonatal care.

## REFERENCES

1. Mosby. Mosby's Medical Dictionary, 10th edition. St Louis, Missouri: Mosby Elsevier; 2017.
2. Herlihy D. Women, Family and Society in Medieval Europe: Historical Essays, 1978-1991. New York: Berghahn Books; 1995.
3. Fuchs RG. Abandoned Children: Foundlings and Child Welfare in Nineteenth-Century France. Albany: State University of New York Press, 1984.
4. Pugh G. London's Forgotten Children: Thomas Coram and the Foundling Hospital. Stroud, United Kingdom: The History Press Ltd.; 2007.
5. T.E.C., Jr. L'Hôpital des Enfants-Malades, the world's first children's hospital, founded in Paris in 1802. Pediatrics, May 1981;67(5)670.
6. Christiansen A. Nursery and Child's Hospital Records: 1854-1934, MS 443.20. New-York Historical Society; 2011. Available from: http://dlib.nyu.edu/findingaids/html/nyhs/nursery/bioghist.html [Last accessed July 2020].
7. Children's Hospital of Philadelphia. About the History of Children's Hospital. [online] Available from: https://www.chop.edu/about-us/about [Last accessed July 2020].
8. Baker JP. The incubator and the medical discovery of the premature infant. J Perinatol. 2000;20(5):321-8.
9. Apgar V, Holaday DA, James LS, et al. Evaluation of the newborn infant; second report. J Am Med Assoc. 1958;168:1985-8.
10. Weiner G, Zaichkin J, Kattwinkel J (Eds). Textbook of Neonatal Resuscitation (NRP), 7th edition. Elk Grove Village, IL: American Academy of Pediatrics and American Heart Association; 2016.
11. Silverman WA. Incubator-baby side shows (Dr. Martin A. Couney). Pediatrics. 1979;64(2):127-41.
12. Nowell FH (1909). Baby incubator exhibit interior, Alaska-Yukon-Pacific-Exposition, Seattle, Washington, 1909. University of Washington: Special Collections. [online] Available from: https://commons.wikimedia.org/wiki/File:Baby_Incubator_exhibit_interior,_Alaska-Yukon-Pacific-Exposition,_Seattle,_Washington,_1909_(AYP_977).jpg [Last accessed July 2020].
13. Incubatrice di Hess. Francesco Val/CC BY-SA (https://creativecommons.org/licenses/by-sa/3.0). [online] Available from: https://upload.wikimedia.org/wikipedia/commons/6/6b/Incubatrice_di_Hess.jpg [Last accessed July, 2020].
14. Hess JH. An Electric-Heated Water-Jacketed Infant Incubator and Bed: for use in the care of premature and poorly nourished infants. JAMA. 1915;64(13):1068-9.
15. Silverman WA, Fertig JW, Berger AP. The influence of the thermal environment upon survival of newly born preterm infants. Pediatrics. 1958;22(5):876-86.
16. Hess JH. Premature and Congenitally Diseased infants. Philadelphia: Lea and Febiger; 1922.
17. James SD (2013). JFK Baby Death in 1963 Sparked Medical Race to Save Preemies. ABC News, August 7, 2013. [online] Available from: https://abcnews.go.com/Health/jfk-baby-death-50-years-ago-today-sparked/story?id=19883153 [Last accessed July 2020].
18. National Institutes of Health (1992). Neonatal Intensive Care. A History of Excellence. A Symposium Commemorating National Child Health Day. [online] Available from: http://www.neonatology.org/classics/nic.nih1985.pdf [Last accessed July 2020].
19. Department of Pediatrics, Vanderbilt University School of Medicine. Mildred Stahlman Division of Neonatology: History. [online] Available from: https://www.childrenshospitalvanderbilt.org/program/neonatal-intensive-care-unit-nicu#:~:text=Founded%20in%201961%20by%20Mildred,the%20care%20of%20preterm%20infants. [Last accessed July 2020].
20. Munro CL. The "lady with the lamp" illuminates critical care today. Am J Crit Care. 2010;19(4):315-7.
21. Jolley J. Florence Nightingale and children's nursing. Paediatr Nurs. 2007;19(8):12.
22. Horbar JD, Soll RF, Edwards WH. The Vermont Oxford Network: A Community of Practice. Clin Perinatol. 2010;37(1):29-47.
23. Dudrick SJ, Wilmore DW, Vars HM, et al. Long-term total parenteral nutrition with growth, development, and positive nitrogen balance. Surgery 1968;64(1):134-42.
24. Avery ME, Mead J. Surface properties in relation to atelectasis and hyaline membrane disease. Am J Dis Chil. 1959;97(5, Part 1):517-23.
25. Stern L, Ramos AD, Outerbridge EW, et al. Negative pressure artificial respiration: use in treatment of respiratory failure of the newborn. Can Med Assoc J. 1970;102(6):595-601.
26. Gregory GA, Kitterman JA, Phibbs RH, et al. Treatment of the respiratory distress syndrome with continuous positive airway pressure. N Engl J Med. 1971;268(24):1333-40.
27. Alexander JP. The shake test and the respiratory-distress syndrome. N Engl J Med. 1977;296(21):1236.
28. Gluck L, Kulovich MV, Borer RC, et al. Diagnosis of the respiratory distress syndrome by amniocentesis. Am J Obstet Gynecol. 1971;109:440-5.
29. Phibbs RH, Ballard RA, Clements JA, et al. Initial clinical trial of EXOSURF, a protein-free synthetic surfactant, for the prophylaxis and early treatment of hyaline membrane disease. Pediatrics. 1991;88(1):1-9.
30. Cochrane CG, Revak SD, Merritt TA, et al. The efficacy and safety of KL4-surfactant in preterm infants with respiratory distress syndrome. Am J Respir Crit Care Med. 1996;153(1):404-10.
31. Cochrane CG, Revak SD. Pulmonary surfactant protein B (SP-B): structure-function relationships. Science. 1991;254(5031):566-8.

32. Silverman WA. A Cautionary Tale about Supplemental Oxygen: The Albatross of Neonatal Medicine. Pediatrics. 2004;113(2):394-6.
33. Tara M, Dickerson ML. History and Overview of Neonatal Pain. In: Clinical Handbook of Neonatal Pain Management for Nurses. Springer Publishing Company Connect; 2016. [online] Available from: https://connect.springerpub.com/content/book/978-0-8261-9438-1/part/part01/chapter/ch01 [Last accessed July, 2020].
34. Infant transported in an incubator by ambulance, Hungary, 1968. FOTO:FORTEPAN/Magyar Hírek folyóirat/CC BY-SA (https://creativecommons.org/licenses/by-sa/3.0). [online] Available from: https://commons.wikimedia.org/wiki/File:Ambulance,_incubator_Fortepan_84699.jpg [Last accessed July, 2020].
35. Liggins GC, Howie RN. A controlled trial of antepartum glucocorticoid treatment for prevention of the respiratory distress syndrome in premature infants. Pediatrics. 1972;50(4):515-25.
36. Gyamfi-Bannerman C, Thom EA, Blackwell SC, et al. for the NICHD Maternal-Fetal Medicine Units Network. Antenatal Betamethasone for Women at Risk for Late Preterm Delivery. N Engl J Med. 2016;374:1311-20.
37. Govindaswami B, Nudelman M, Jegatheesan P, et al. Prevention of Prematurity: Advances and Opportunities. Clin Perinatol. 2018;45(3):579-95.
38. Byrne J, Govindaswami B, Jegatheesan P, et al. 480: Perinatal core measure: antenatal steroid performance improvement following a preterm birth risk assessment decision model and perinatal QI toolkit. Am J Obstet Gynecol. 2011;204(1):S193.
39. Aune D, Schlesinger S, Henriksen T, et al. Physical activity and the risk of preterm birth: a systematic review and meta-analysis of epidemiological studies. BJOG. 2017;124(12):1816-26.
40. Philip RK, Purtill H, Reidy E, et al. Reduction in preterm births during the COVID-19 lockdown in Ireland: a natural experiment allowing analysis of data from the prior two decades. medRxiv 2020.06.03.20121442; doi: https://doi.org/10.1101/2020.06.03.20121442.
41. Begley CM, Gyte GML, Devane D, et al. Active versus expectant management for women in the third stage of labour. Cochrane Database Syst Rev. 2019;2:CD007412.
42. World Health Organization (2015). WHO statement on caesarean section rates. [online] Available from: https://apps.who.int/iris/bitstream/handle/10665/161442/WHO_RHR_15.02_eng.pdf;jsessionid=B168854F3403333A3105E79E99D895A6?sequence=1 [Last accessed July, 2020].
43. Coonrod DV, Drachman D, Hobson P, et al. Nulliparous term singleton vertex cesarean delivery rates: institutional and individual level predictors. Am J Obstet Gynecol. 2008;198:694.e1-694.e11.
44. Vadnais MA, Hacker MR, Shah NT, et al. Quality Improvement Initiatives Lead to Reduction in Nulliparous Term Singleton Vertex Cesarean Delivery Rate. Jt Comm J Qual Patient Saf. 2017;43(2):53-61.
45. Sciencedirect (2012). Hemolytic Disease of the Newborn. [online] Available from: https://www.sciencedirect.com/topics/biochemistry-genetics-and-molecular-biology/hemolytic-disease-of-the-newborn [Last accessed July, 2020].
46. Ramji S, Ahuja S, Thirupuram S, et al. Resuscitation of asphyxic newborn infants with room air or 100% oxygen. Pediatr Res.1993;34(6):809-12.
47. Saugstad OD, Rootwelt T, Aalen O. Resuscitation of asphyxiated newborn infants with room air or oxygen: an international controlled trial: the Resair 2 study. Pediatrics. 1998;102(1):e1.
48. Saugstad OD. The role of oxygen in neonatal resuscitation. Clin Perinatol. 2004;31(3):431-43.
49. Uslu S, Bulbul A, Can E, et al. Relationship between oxygen saturation and umbilical cord pH immediately after birth. Pediatr Neonatol. 2012;53:340-5.
50. Saugstad OD. Asphyxia in the Third Millennium: From Virginia Apgar to Metabolomics. In: Selected Lectures of the 13th International Workshop on Neonatology; Cagliari (Italy); October 25-28, 2017. J Pediatr Neonat Individual Med. 2017;6(2):e060235.
51. Gunn AJ, Gunn TR, Gunning MI, et al. Neuroprotection with prolonged head cooling started before postischemic seizures in fetal sheep. Pediatrics. 1998;102(5):1098-106.
52. Gluckman PD, Wyatt J, Azzopardi D, et al. Selective head cooling with mild systemic hypothermia after neonatal encephalopathy: multicentre randomised trial. Lancet. 2005;365(9460):663-70.
53. Shankaran S, Laptook AR, Ehrenkranz RA, et al. Whole body hypothermia for neonates with hypoxic-ishcemic encephalopathy. N Engl J Med. 2005;353:1574-84.
54. Als H, Gilkerson L. The role of relationship-based developmentally supportive newborn intensive care in strengthening outcome of preterm infants. Semin Perinatol. 1997;21(3):178-89.
55. Twin boys strapped to their grandmother's chest in the maternity unit in the Queen Elizabeth hospital in Blantyre, Malawi. Lindsay Mgbor/Department for International Development/CC BY (https://creativecommons.org/licenses/by/2.0). [online]. Available from: https://commons.wikimedia.org/wiki/File:Born_too_soon_and_too_small_-_Ediths_twin_boys_(7497732174).jpg [Last accessed July, 2020].
56. Jolley J, Shields L. The Evolution of Family-Centered Care. J Pediatr Nurs. 2009;24(2):164-70.
57. NEC Society. Building a World Without NEC. [online] Available from: https://necsociety.org/. [Last accessed July, 2020].
58. Redesign Healthcare (2016). About the Instructors. Course: Designing for Safety in Labor and Delivery 2016. [online] Available from: https://www.redesignhealthcare.org/designing-for-safety-in-labor-delivery/about-the-instructor/ [Last accessed July, 2020].
59. Johnson B, Abraham M, Conway J, et al. Partnering with Patients and Families to Design a Patient- and Family-Centered Health Care System. Recommendations and Promising Practices. Bethesda, Maryland: Institute for Family-Centered Care; 2008.
60. Johnston AM, Bullock C, Graham J, et al. Implementation and Case-Study Results of Potentially Better Practices for Family Centered Care: The Family Centered Care Map. Pediatrics. 2006;118;S108.
61. Institute for Patient- and Family-Centered Care. Patient- and Family-Centered Care Defined. [online] Available from: https://www.ipfcc.org/bestpractices/sustainable-partnerships/background/pfcc-defined.html [Last accessed July 2020].

CHAPTER

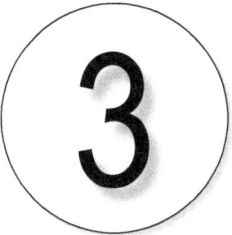

# Educational Interventions to Improve Newborn Care

Emily Altick Hartford

## ABSTRACT

Education for medical personnel is crucial to reducing preventable newborn deaths. Investing in the education of healthcare providers in countries with the highest rates of neonatal mortality has the potential not only to reduce neonatal mortality, but also strengthen staff retention and increase the healthcare workforce. Strong educational partnerships between entities such as governments, academic institutions, medical suppliers, non-governmental organizations (NGOs), and local experts can empower all parties involved. An example of one effective partnership is a "Train the Trainers" course, where a single facilitator can provide materials and support for a class of local experts to go into the community and teach the class to others. Education must not only address birth, but also prenatal and postnatal care, as neonatal outcome is inseparable from maternal health and the health of the family. Educational interventions for newborn health vary according to the setting, and the requirements of each needs to be assessed and education provided across the continuum of care providers. Teaching should go beyond didactic sessions to include hands-on training and mentorship, with focus on supporting implementation, as well as providing necessary supplies and equipment.

To maintain practice standards, the issue of staff turnover needs to be addressed with a careful plan for repeated training and continuing medical education. Key curriculum topics for improving newborn care should address those diagnoses that are responsible for the majority of neonatal mortality: management of prematurity, prevention of birth asphyxia, and prevention and treatment for sepsis. Empowering providers with knowledge in research, administrative techniques and quality improvement should also be a component in an educational program, as these management skills will be necessary in the future.

## WHY IS EDUCATION IMPORTANT?

Despite gains over recent decades, child mortality remains unacceptably high with an estimated 6.6 million deaths among children under 5 years of age worldwide in 2012.[1] Of these deaths, 2.9 million occurred in the neonatal period. Childhood deaths are becoming increasingly concentrated in certain geographical regions such as sub-Saharan Africa and Asia and among newborns less than 28 days of age. Improvements in neonatal mortality still lag behind those made in overall child mortality and represent an ever-increasing proportion of child deaths worldwide. In 2012, 44% of all under-5 mortality could be attributed to neonatal deaths. Another factor that has slowed improvement in neonatal mortality is a lack of funding for programs in newborn health. From 2003 to 2008, the amount of official development assistance for maternal and child health programs nearly doubled, but funds targeted specifically to newborn survival still represented only 0.1% of the total.[2]

In 2014, the World Health Organization (WHO) and UNICEF led the collaborative development of a call to

*This chapter is for the dedicated and inspiring providers in Mozambique who have patiently taught their partners many of these lessons over the years.

action for newborns entitled *Every Newborn: An Action Plan to End Preventable Deaths*. This document outlines the key actions toward achieving a significant reduction in neonatal mortality and stillbirths by 2035.[3] Of the five strategic objectives outlined in this plan **(Fig. 1)**, three are directly related to the education of healthcare workers to increase access to high quality care during labor and birth. It is clear that a major barrier to reducing preventable newborn deaths is the shortage of healthcare workers adequately trained to care for newborns at birth. Neonatal mortality rates across the world correlate with the ratio of providers available for the population.[4] The education of doctors, midwives, nurses, and birth attendants as well as laboratory technicians, pharmacists, administrators, and public health professionals is therefore crucial for ensuring continued and sustainable improvement toward the goal of reducing newborn deaths.

Care provider education also represents the greatest opportunity for sustainable improvement in newborn health around the world. While many interventions can only have limited lasting impact, empowering individuals within a health system to fully understand the challenge before them, to provide high quality care, to work in multi-disciplinary teams, and to continually measure their successes and opportunities to improve can be truly transformative. In the countries with the highest burden of neonatal mortality, there are too few providers, but they also receive minimal investment in their continuing education and opportunities for career development. Therefore, education should be tailored to both pre-service and in-

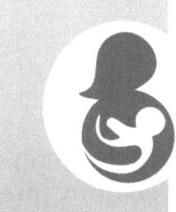

**Strategic objective 1**

**Strengthen and invest in care during labor, birth and the first day and week of life.** A large proportion of maternal and newborn deaths and stillbirths occur within this period, but many deaths and complications can be prevented by ensuring high-quality essential care to every woman and baby during this critical time.

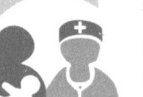

**Strategic objective 2**

**Improve the quality of maternal and newborn care.** Substantial gaps in the quality of care exist across the continuum for women's and children's health. Many women and newborns do not receive quality care even when they have contact with a health system before, during and after pregnancy and childbirth. Introducing high-quality care with high-impact, cost-effective interventions for mother and baby together—delivered, in most cases, by the same health providers with midwifery skills at the same time—is key to improvement.

**Strategic objective 3**

**Reach every woman and newborn to reduce inequalities.** Having access to high-quality health care without suffering financial hardship is a human right. Robust evidence for approaches to ending preventable newborn deaths is available and, if applied, can effectively accelerate the coverage of essential interventions through innovations and in accordance with the principles of universal health coverage.

**Strategic objective 4**

**Harness the power of parents, families and communities.** Engaged community leaders and workers and women's groups are critical for better health outcomes for women and newborns. Education and empowerment of parents, families and communities to demand quality care and improve home care practices are crucial.

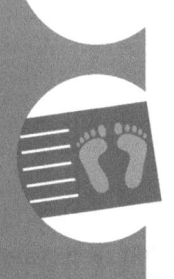

**Strategic objective 5**

**Count every newborn through measurement, program-tracking and accountability.** Measurement enables managers to improve performance and adapt actions as needed. Assessing outcomes and financial flows with standardized indicators improve accountability. There is a need to improve metrics globally and nationally, especially for birth outcomes and quality of care around the time of birth. Every newborn needs to be registered and newborn and maternal deaths and stillbirths need to be counted.

**Fig. 1:** Five strategic objectives outlined in 2014 World Health Organization and UNICEF's action plan.

service healthcare workers—within faculties of medicine and nursing as well as the hospitals and clinics themselves. Investing in existing healthcare workers also has the potential to improve retention, and when combined with scaling up the number of future providers, this will have the greatest impact on increasing the healthcare workforce.

## Partnerships for Education: A Pathway to Success

Creating strong partnerships is foundational to providing the education that is needed for healthcare providers. Countries that partner with one another can develop better techniques for instruction, learn lessons from implementing protocols, and access methods from successful birth providers worldwide. Partnerships among governments, NGOs, and academic institutions can also play a role in supporting education through funding and technical expertise. Academic institutions from high-income countries receive the benefit of establishing a research partner or securing an educational site for their trainees. Both institutions can then participate in educational initiatives, and learnings can benefit both sides. Partnerships may be even more beneficial when they are between countries in the same geographical region and of similar resource level so that practice patterns are more similar to one another. It is crucial that the development of educational priorities and strategies for healthcare providers be led by the local officials in the Ministry of Health to assure relevance, engagement, and sustainability.

Developing educational interventions for newborn health within partnerships require good communication and flexibility. Often priorities will change and each party needs to be ready to adapt and respond appropriately. This is especially true in resource-limited environments where the pressures are greater. Providers are overburdened not only with clinical care but also with administrative and educational responsibilities. Political pressures or new strategies from health authorities may also play a role in changing or developing different priorities quickly. For example, new equipment acquisition might make training staff to use it suddenly become more urgent than another project that had first priority. It is crucial to develop and establish effective and regular communication channels within partnerships in order to navigate all of these situations and achieve the overall result of providing useful educational interventions for staff. Typically this involves a point-person such as a nursery director in a provincial hospital or the district medical officer for a group of rural clinics. It is prudent to plan together to have regular and in-person meetings to assure ongoing effective educational planning.

In the development of educational initiatives, it is critical to include a local provider who is actually practicing in that setting and knows current practice, gaps, and availability of supplies. Ideally it is someone who could help teach as well to assure relevance and increase learner understanding. It is important to consider what supplies are currently available or being procured before the training and develop the material accordingly. Ideally the training would only include what is locally available or familiar to participants.

When partnerships exist between academic institutions in different countries, training exchanges between sites can be a very useful method for empowering providers, increasing knowledge, generating new ideas, sharing important methods, and ultimately improving care. When these exchanges occur within an ongoing collaboration, the benefits increase substantially.

## A Model for Partnerships: Training the Trainers

An important approach to maximize impact when considering global newborn education is employing the "train the trainers" method. This is particularly important where there are few teachers and providers. An experienced facilitator can teach a course in newborn resuscitation, for example, and then multiply his or her efforts by also dedicating time to teaching adult learning methods, course facilitation, and by providing the necessary materials and support for the participants to give the course themselves. Providers can be empowered to become facilitators themselves by practicing teaching some of the material or demonstrating techniques during a course.

In most settings, it will be important to consider the usual hierarchy of the medical system when employing the "train the trainers" method. Careful selection of future facilitators who have had some experience in newborn health, are already managers in their setting, and who have the authority to make changes and monitor outcomes will maximize the likelihood and success of future training. It is also essential to support the process of planning future sessions, provide funds for training materials and participants, and encourage feedback and reports from successful training sessions. It has also been shown that, although skills and knowledge both improve after course participation, practical skills can quickly deteriorate making it necessary to implement an ongoing educational curriculum for providers.[5]

## ▎ THINKING ALONG THE CONTINUUM: ADDRESSING PRENATAL/PERINATAL/POSTNATAL CARE

Education to improve newborn care cannot stop with the newborn alone but must include the entire continuum of maternal and newborn interventions. Eighty percent of newborn deaths can be attributed to just three causes: (1) prematurity, (2) birth asphyxia, and (3) infection.[6] All three of these are inseparable from the maternal counterparts of preterm labor recognition and management, labor progression and fetal position, and infections such as chorioamnionitis. Furthermore, healthy pregnancies, which are more likely to carry to term and produce healthy newborns, receive antenatal care with essential disease screening, nutritional counseling, malaria prophylaxis (where appropriate), and early recognition and management of complications. Birth spacing also improves the health of mothers and infants making access to reproductive health another essential component of comprehensive newborn care. Finally, although the first day of a neonate's life carries the highest risk of mortality,[7] a significant number of deaths also occur in the immediate postnatal period. Careful follow-up of all newborn infants to encourage exclusive breastfeeding and recognize and treat infections is another fundamental part of improving education in newborn care. **Figure 2**[8] shows a continuum of newborn care that encompasses the entire spectrum of maternal and child health, from women of childbearing age through the postnatal and childhood period.

Effective education in any of these areas requires careful coordination with different types of providers across disciplines caring for mothers, infants, and families. The providers and structure of health care will differ by country, and this requires careful analysis. In some settings, there is a single provider responsible for maternal and child health that might be tasked with caring for pregnant mothers, providing skilled delivery care, following newborns, and counseling in reproductive planning. Alternatively, care for mothers and for infants could be provided by different healthcare workers each focused in their specialty or perhaps a birth attendant would provide care during labor but all prenatal and postnatal care would involve different providers. The most important point for successful

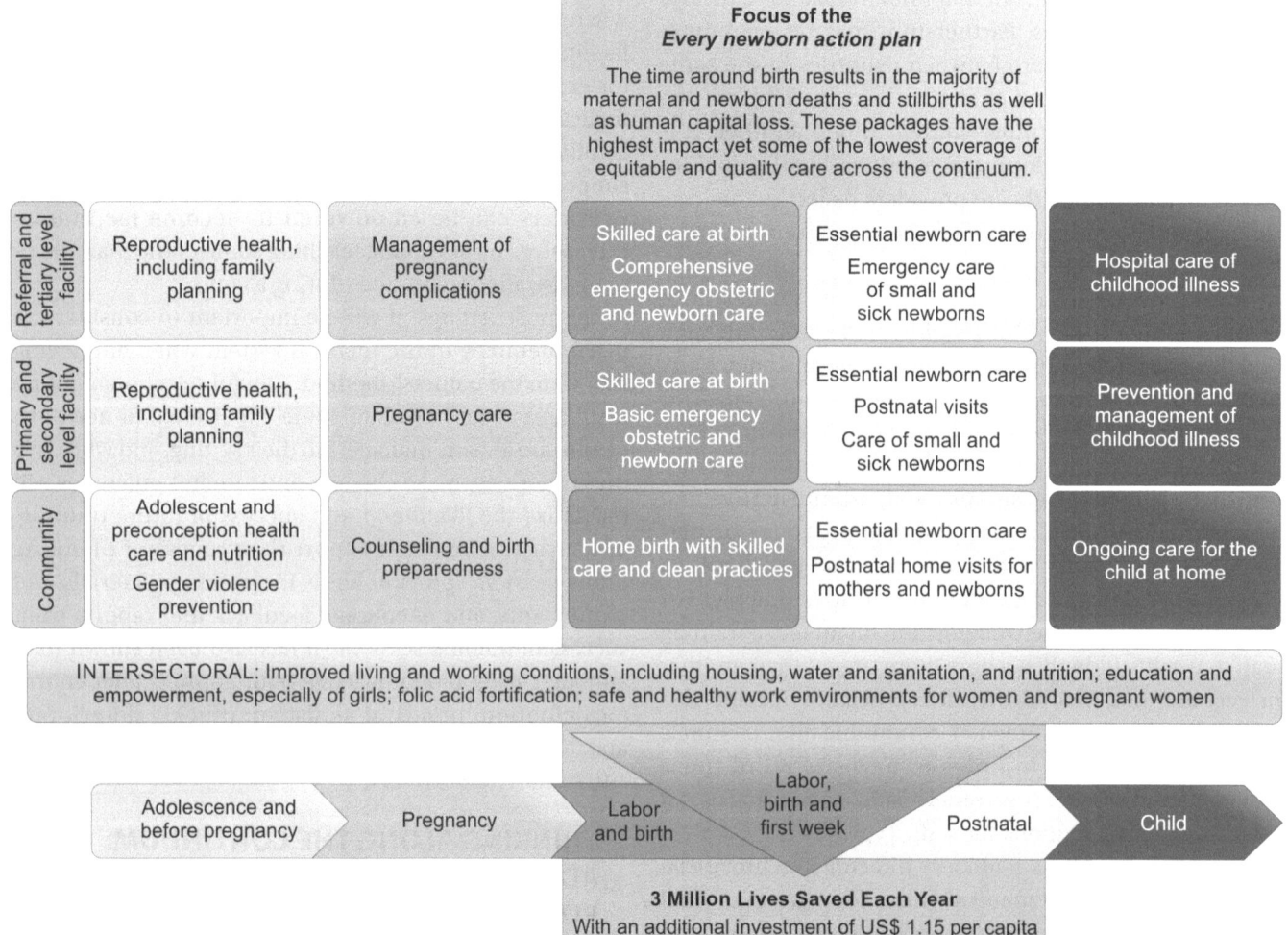

**Fig. 2:** Continuum of newborn care that encompasses the entire spectrum of maternal and child health.
*Source:* Mason E, et al. The Lancet Every Newborn Series. Lancet, 2014.

educational interventions in newborn health is to assess the individual setting and to include all providers involved in this continuum, including doctors, nurses, mid-level providers, midwives, traditional birth attendants, and community health workers. In more rural and underserved areas, this might also include district administrators, public health officials, ambulance drivers, or support staff as they often have a role in supporting the limited number of health care providers to care for mothers and newborns. It may also be beneficial to include practitioners of traditional medicine, community leaders, village chiefs or matriarchs who might have a strong influence on community health-practices. Community education regarding practices that will save newborn lives across the maternal child health continuum will support engagement and understanding and help to ensure success.

## UNDERSTANDING THE PROVIDERS AND THEIR SETTING

All successful educational interventions to improve newborn care should begin with a deep understanding of the providers being taught, their roles, and their previous level of education. Ideally, one would also assess their current practice and the reasons behind it, as well as the resources they have access to and adapt the training accordingly. Without this thorough preparation, providing relevant and actionable training to providers will be difficult, and participants may complete a course feeling confused or frustrated instead of equipped and ready. Coordination with local authorities within the Ministry of Health to understand existing protocols, educational priorities, and supply chain as well as priorities for interventions and future plans will also improve the overall relevance of the material.

An example of how important this process is can be seen in a training, which was prepared to support infection control in a neonatal unit in a major referral hospital in sub-Saharan Africa. Newborns in the unit had a high rate of skin and soft tissue infections resulting in sepsis; the most common site for these infections was in the groin. Nurses were observed frequently drawing blood from a femoral vein with inadequate aseptic technique, and so, a training course was developed regarding drawing blood, aseptic procedural technique, and ideal practice for neonates. After the course, there was little improvement in the rates of skin and soft tissue abscesses in the unit. Upon further investigation, it was discovered that nurses were required to draw at least 5 mL of blood for each laboratory analysis requested by the physicians, and they were unable to achieve such a large amount of blood through different body sites other than the femoral vein. A frequent lack of gloves was also noted as a reason for not following the aseptic procedural technique which all of the nurses understood well. Meetings were held between the leadership in the laboratory and the neonatal unit, and the necessary supplies were procured to carry out analysis with 1–3 mL of blood each. Nurses then received on-the-job clinical mentoring while drawing blood and managing intravenous lines for 1 week. Only after these additional interventions did the problem with groin skin infections resolve almost entirely. The important lesson to learn from this is that providers are almost always doing the best they can with their given resources to provide excellent care to their patients. By overcoming a seemingly insignificant barrier such as the lack of laboratory supplies, this facility made huge improvements. This is a prime example of how combining education with a careful assessment of the provider's environment effectively resolved a care issue.

## Multidisciplinary Approach: Address the Needs of All Types of Providers in Different Settings

Educational interventions for newborn health will vary widely by the type of participants targeted but can be successfully adapted for each setting. Consider the differences, for example, in the topics, course organization, and curriculum for all of the following:

- *Specialists and nurses in a central referral hospital:* Course topics will be highly specialized in neonatology and may include neonatal resuscitation, thermoregulation, intravenous fluids and nutrition, infection control, respiratory support (including mechanical ventilation), perfusion support, management of complications of prematurity, surgical problems in the neonate, and ethics in neonatology.
- *Specialist, generalists, mid-level providers, and nurses at a provincial referral hospital:* Course topics will be relatively specialized in neonatology but may differ from above depending on available resources. They may include neonatal resuscitation, respiratory support [continuous positive airway pressure (CPAP) and oxygen], kangaroo mother care for thermoregulation, treatment of sepsis, and infection control.
- *Generalists, mid-level providers, and nurses at a district hospital:* In these settings, depending on resources available such as oxygen or CPAP in the delivery rooms, neonatal resuscitation may be adapted using *Helping Babies Breathe* (HBB).[9] Additional course topics might include kangaroo mother care, essential newborn care,[10] and recognition and treatment of sepsis.
- *Nurses and support staff at a rural clinic:* In a more rural setting, course topics may include *HBB*, early recognition and risk factors for neonatal sepsis, essential newborn

care, and kangaroo mother care for small or preterm infants. These providers are more likely to also care for mothers so one might highly consider combining educational interventions regarding newborn health with relevant obstetric training as well.
- *Community health workers, birth attendants, traditional healers, and village leadership in the community:* These courses would ideally include essential newborn care and *HBB* with careful attention to the availability of supplies, practicing the required skills and frequent follow-up training and assessments. Many successful training programs for birth attendants or community health workers in sub-Saharan Africa, Asia, and Latin America have recently been described (given later). In addition to overall improvement in provider skills and knowledge, some have also achieved an associated reduction in neonatal mortality by up to 50% when combined with recognition and early treatment of sepsis in the community.[11]
- *Mothers:* Courses could include a variety of important topics including family planning, recognition of illness, kangaroo mother care, and feeding and nutrition. Course material could be provided and taught to community health workers or nurses who would then teach it to mothers in the community itself.

## Going beyond Didactic Educational Sessions

Effective education to improve newborn health must involve hands-on clinical training in addition to didactic sessions. Even with the best course preparation and integration, staff will need support in actually practicing the newly acquired skills in their work environment. An example of this can be seen in newborn resuscitation training in a large referral hospital in sub-Saharan Africa. A 3-day comprehensive course was offered for all nurses and providers in obstetrics and pediatrics that included multiple simulation sessions to practice skills and to integrate the knowledge into various different clinical scenarios. Almost all of the nurses and midwives who care for newborns at this hospital attended the training session and seemed to demonstrate successful knowledge and skills acquisition. However, there was no difference seen in the number of infants successfully resuscitated or in the rates of birth asphyxia in the hospital after the course. When one midwife was alone to care for both the newborn and the mother, the infant was not receiving a timely intervention when needed.

After careful assessment and discussion, an organizational change was made which allowed for a rotating team of two nurses to be dedicated to infant resuscitation and newborn care immediately after birth. Upon starting this new role, these nurses experienced many challenges: the optimal location for their work (near the delivery rooms or the operating rooms), how to maintain supportive care during the transfer of sick infants to the nursery, how to manage their equipment needs to assure they were always ready to attend to a sick newborn, shift and staffing planning, ongoing education, and interactions with the other care providers across the departments of Obstetrics and Pediatrics. A highly experienced team of two perinatal nurse specialists with a combined experience of over 25 years working in delivery rooms was then paired for 2 weeks with these two nurses, attending deliveries and discussing and addressing challenges as needed. The result was impressive because the experienced nurses empowered this newer team with ideas and knowledge, and they acted as a resource for ongoing collaboration and improvements. It was only after this intensive clinical mentoring that infants began to receive immediate resuscitation and post-birth care effectively, and providers noticed dramatic improvements in the rates and severity of birth asphyxia.

Another important factor for effective education in newborn care is the focus on implementation after any given training is completed. Providers should not be given information, only to later face insurmountable barriers to applying this knowledge to practice. It is therefore essential for trainers to not only prepare the course with relevant knowledge but also to follow-up carefully and address challenges and questions as they inevitably arise. Any training course would ideally include several follow-up sessions to meet with staff, review the uses of the information learned in training, and discuss any difficulties or concerns that arise.

Careful consideration must also be given to the provision of necessary supplies and equipment for the successful implementation of newly acquired knowledge. It does not make sense, for example, to train providers in the use of positive pressure ventilation in HBB without first assuring they will have access to a neonatal bag and mask once they acquire the skills. Similarly, teaching nurses how to use lancets to draw smaller volumes of blood from neonates via a "heel stick" will not be useful unless they have access to the lancets and the appropriate tubes. The provision of consumable supplies always brings up an important concern for sustainability. However, this must be balanced with effective education. When possible, training should be combined with sustainable provision of the necessary supplies for a given setting. When this is not possible, educators should at least consider supporting the procurement or provision of a set of supplies in order for providers to continue practicing with the knowledge and skills they have acquired. That knowledge and capability will ultimately be the most sustainable investment even if the supply chain is irregular.

## Addressing Issues of Staff Turnover

Any investment in the education of staff caring for newborns must be followed up carefully, not just for successful implementation and preventing practice deterioration over time, but also to maintain practice in a setting that may have a high turnover of staff. Medical emigration is a known challenge, especially in low-income countries, and often causes frequent staffing changes. In a recent analysis of medical schools across sub-Saharan Africa, for example, there was a reported loss of between 6% and 18% of their faculty to other opportunities or emigration in the 5 years prior.[12] There are also often frequent changes or rotations in nursing staff or new nurses being added to the unit workforce. This requires a careful plan for repeated training and a comprehensive continuing medical education program, headed by an individual responsible for monitoring staffing and providing education in the unit.

## Focus on Key Curriculum Topics for Newborn Health

There is a great deal of existing work in the literature that can help to guide the optimal focus and expected outcomes for newborn education. Topics should focus on the newborn diagnoses (prematurity, asphyxia, and infections) largely responsible for the majority of neonatal mortality.

### Prematurity

Infants who are premature or small for gestational age, represent the largest proportion of neonatal deaths.[6] Improving care for this group requires the prompt recognition and treatment for preterm labor in the mother as well as careful delivery and early postnatal care. Interventions, therefore, might be more complicated as they will require training and coordination for both obstetric and pediatric providers, when they are not the same individual, as well as providing access to the necessary medications and supplies. Priorities for supporting the preterm and low birth weight population in a low-resource setting are antenatal steroid treatment for the mother in preterm labor, thermoregulation through kangaroo mother care, protection from infection, and careful exclusive breastfeeding regimens for the baby. In facilities, interventions may also include intravenous fluids and support for respiratory distress, feeding problems, and temperature.[3]

### Asphyxia

In recent years, there have been many groups studying the impact of educational interventions in resource-limited facilities, with birth attendants who decrease birth asphyxia by providing adequate resuscitation and appropriate care in the early newborn period. A specific curriculum, HBB, was developed in 2010 by the American Academy of Pediatrics to support neonatal resuscitation in resource-limited areas and has since been taught extensively to nurses, doctors, and birth attendants throughout the world.[9] The program emphasizes immediate newborn assessment and action, within the first minute of life, to ensure breathing, color, and reactivity, and it includes positive pressure ventilation with a bag and mask when necessary, without requiring access to oxygen or medications. Comprehensive neonatal resuscitation (NRP) is more often taught in facilities that can provide oxygen, intravenous access, and other aspects of advanced care. The underlying concepts of HBB and NRP, however, are the same. The majority of infants who require intervention at birth will only require what is provided in the HBB educational package, whereas only a small minority would require advanced care such as endotracheal intubation, medications or cardiac massage.[13]

Essential newborn care (ENC)[10] is a course that was developed by the World Health Organization in 2010 for birth attendants caring for newborns within the first week of life in primary health facilities. It includes standard precautions, immediate postdelivery care, infant thermoregulation, cord care, early breastfeeding, basic resuscitation and assessment of breathing, and monitoring for danger signs. The program can also be taught over 4–5 days. ENC has also been taught widely with benefits for neonatal mortality and stillbirths.

The following is a brief summary of the educational interventions for neonatal resuscitation (HBB and NRP) and ENC and their impact in resource-limited settings around the world:

### Educational Outcomes

Although newborn care training is effective to helping providers achieve higher care standards, some studies have shown that providers face a deterioration of skills over time. Furthermore, optimal interval for refresher training is still unknown. As an example, midwives working on a busy labor ward in Ghana were trained in NRP; their exam scores and practical skills significantly improved after training and were retained 9 and 12 months after the training.[5] Ethiopian care providers also demonstrated increased knowledge and skills after receiving training in neonatal resuscitation; their scores improved more with a lower ratio of trainer to trainees. Pretraining differences by the type of healthcare worker (i.e. doctor versus nurse) also disappeared after training.[14] Healthcare workers in Rwanda improved their skills and knowledge immediately after training, but the practical skills deteriorated after only 3 months when they were retested.[15] The authors postulated this was likely due to relatively little practice of attending deliveries in their daily work.

## Patient Outcomes

Many studies have been published in this area, and there is a decrease in perinatal mortality associated with teaching NRP or HBB to birth attendants. However, there is still some discrepancy in the literature regarding the impact on neonatal mortality versus rate of stillbirths.

At primary health clinics in Zambia, a course was taught to midwives on ENC and was associated with a decrease in neonatal mortality by 40% (11.5 per 1,000 to 6.8 per 1,000) at 7 days due to a decrease in deaths from asphyxia and infections. Additional training in NRP decreased mortality further.[16] In another cluster-randomized study in rural Zambia, traditional birth attendants were taught HBB as well as recognition of sepsis. They were taught to give one dose of oral amoxicillin to infants less than 7 days who met sepsis criteria and transfer them to a facility. In the intervention group, they saw an overall significant decrease in neonatal mortality by 45%, a decrease in death from birth asphyxia of 61%, and a decrease in of deaths within the first 2 days of life by 81%. There was no difference in the rate of stillbirths or death from severe infection.[11]

In the large "first breath" trial held in six countries, training of birth attendants in ENC was associated with a decrease in the rates of stillbirths but did not affect neonatal mortality. Subsequent training in HBB also did not decrease mortality. The study concluded that perhaps any benefit of additional resuscitation training in HBB was masked by the improvement after the ENC course. The trial also determined that stillbirths were reduced because minimally responsive infants were resuscitated at birth instead of classified as a stillbirth.[17]

Implementation of a course in HBB taught by local master trainers in Tanzania significantly decreased early neonatal mortality by 48% (13.4/1,000 to 7.1/1,000), fresh stillbirth rate by 24% (19/1,000 to 14.5/1,000), and early perinatal mortality by 33% (32.2 to 21.6 per 1,000).[18]

In another study in India, training of birth attendants in HBB decreased rates of stillbirth and fresh stillbirth but, similar to the First Breath trial, did not change the neonatal mortality rate.[19]

## Review Articles

A meta-analysis evaluating six cluster-randomized trials and seven nonrandomized trials showed a significant decrease in both perinatal and neonatal mortality associated with the training, linkage, and support of traditional birth attendants.[20]

In a systematic review and expert panel on the effect of neonatal resuscitation on mortality, the greatest benefit was found in training birth attendants in facilities, which decreased neonatal mortality by an average of 30%. A smaller benefit (decrease of 10%) was estimated from the available and heterogeneous data on educational interventions for basic resuscitation based in the community.[21]

Training traditional birth attendants in neonatal resuscitation has been described as a highly cost-effective measure.[22]

## Infections

The third most common cause of neonatal mortality worldwide is a severe infection such as sepsis, meningitis, or pneumonia.[6] The risk of infection is often connected to antenatal and intrapartum care for the mother; therefore, education to promote diagnosis and treatment of maternal infections is necessary. Once the newborn has an active infection, however, she will require injectable antibiotics and potentially additional supportive care for treatment. This is another active focus for research and education depending on the setting. In a referral hospital, it might involve implementing early laboratory diagnosis, promoting appropriate antibiotic selection, and improving supportive care. In a community setting, it would also involve promotion of prompt diagnosis but treatment options would certainly differ.

Prevention of infection in the neonatal period in any setting should also include education regarding hygiene, careful cord care, and early exclusive breastfeeding. In facility-based education, infection control is an important investment for training with great potential for impact to decrease mortality. Infants in the hospital are at risk for acquiring an infection after birth, but many infections can be avoided with careful and rigorous infection control measures including hand hygiene. In many low-resource settings, access to alcohol gel or soap and water can be challenging for providers, and supplies such as procedural gloves and gowns might be even more difficult to acquire. In addition, a shortage of warmers might require neonates to share one unit, complicating efforts to implement standard precautions. It has been shown that implementing a comprehensive low-cost infection control program can significantly reduce neonatal sepsis and sepsis-related mortality.[23] Including an algorithm for sepsis diagnosis and treatment as well as nursing interventions has also been associated with a decrease in antimicrobial therapy and drug resistance among pathogens.[24]

According to the available evidence on the impact of educational interventions in low-resource settings, the current priorities for training are neonatal resuscitation (HBB or NRP depending on setting); essential newborn care; antenatal steroids for the mother in preterm labor; kangaroo mother care; exclusive breastfeeding; recognition and treatment of intrapartum infections; prompt diagnosis and treatment of sepsis; and infection control.

## EMPOWERING PROVIDERS WITH KNOWLEDGE IN RESEARCH, ADMINISTRATIVE TECHNIQUES AND QUALITY IMPROVEMENT

In addition to addressing the core medical topics likely to improve newborn care, educational interventions must also cover other topics for local providers in order to empower them with administrative skills, research knowledge, and training in quality improvement. Decreasing neonatal mortality and improving newborn care will require a generation of medical providers adept at these management skills, and improving the quality of both newborn and maternal care has been identified as one of the five major strategic objectives in the Every Newborn Action Plan.[8] Providing education in these topics will differ by setting and provider type, but it is important to consider in any educational program.

One potential model for strengthening capacity in these areas is to establish ongoing collaboration between individuals within a partnership. A neonatologist from an institution in a high-resource country could partner directly with another in a low-resource country to offer guidance and support. With regular travel, training, and observation in the two units, the pair can then develop plans to for their respective settings, write collaborative research protocols, and identify areas for quality improvement measures. Ideally this team could be multidisciplinary, involving both nurses and physicians. It is critical that the travel exchanges occur in both directions to learn context and develop relationships. Another option would be to seek out short courses or master's programs that can address administrative, research, or quality improvement skills. These might be especially worth pursuing for certain individuals in leadership within their setting.

## CONCLUSION

Improving newborn survival around the world has become an urgent goal in the field of global medicine as the proportion of child mortality represented by newborn deaths increases. The tools and practices for saving many of these lives are within reach, and the strengthening of local capacity to care for newborns through education is a sustainable investment to improve care. A thoughtful approach is required to avoid pitfalls, develop lasting partnerships, and ultimately improve outcomes.

## REFERENCES

1. UN Inter-agency Group for Child Mortality Estimation (IGME). Levels and trends in child mortality: Report 2013. New York: UNICEF, 2013.
2. Lawn J, Kinney M, Black R, et al. Newborn survival: a multi-country analysis of a decade of change. Health Policy Plan. 2012;27:iii6-iii28.
3. World Health Organization. Every Newborn: an action plan to end preventable deaths. Geneva: WHO. 2014.
4. Dickson K, Simen-Kapeu A, Kinney M, et al. Every newborn: health-systems bottlenecks and strategies to accelerate scale-up in countries. Lancet. 2014;384:438-54.
5. Bookman L, Engemann C, Srofenyoh E, et al. Educational impact of a hospital-based neonatal resuscitation program in Ghana. Resuscitation. 2010;81:1180-2.
6. World Health Organization. Global Health Observatory Data Repository. Geneva: World Health Organization; 2014.
7. Lawn JE, Cousens S, Zupan J. Four million neonatal deaths: When? Where? Why? Lancet. 2005;365:891-900.
8. World Health Organization. (2018). Every Newborn Action Plan. [online] Available from: https://www.who.int/maternal_child_adolescent/newborns/every-newborn/en/. [Last Accessed November, 2019].
9. Little G, Keenan W, Niermeyer S, et al. Neonatal nursing and helping babies breathe: An effective intervention to decrease global neonatal mortality. Newborn Infant Nurs Rev. 2011;11:82-7.
10. World Health Organization. Essential Newborn Care Course 2010. [online] Available from: http://www.who.int/maternal_child_adolescent/documents/newborncare_course/en/. [Last Accessed November, 2019].
11. Gill C, Phiri-Mazala G, Guerina N, et al. Effect of training traditional birth attendants on neonatal mortality (Lufwanyama Neonatal Survival Project): randomised controlled study. BMJ. 2011;342:d346.
12. Mullan F, Frehywot S, Omaswa F, et al. Medical schools in sub-Saharan Africa. Lancet. 2011;377:1113-21.
13. Wall S, Lee A, Carlo W, et al. Reducing Intrapartum-Related Neonatal Deaths in Low- and Middle-Income Countries – What Works? Seminars in Perinatology. 2011;34:395-407.
14. Hoban R, Bucher S, Neuman I, et al. "Helping babies breathe" training in sub-Saharan Africa: Educational impact and learner impressions. J Trop Pediatr. 2013;59(3):1806.
15. Musafili A, Essen B, Baribwira C, et al. Evaluating helping babies breathe: training for healthcare workers at hospitals in Rwanda. Foundation Acta Pædiatrica. 2013;102:e34-e38.
16. Carlo W, McClure E, Chomba E, et al. Newborn care training of midwives and neonatal and perinatal mortality rates in a developing country. Pediatrics. 2010;126;e1064.
17. Carlo W, Goudar S, Jehan I, et al. Newborn-care training and perinatal mortality in developing countries. N Engl J Med. 2010;362:614-23.

18. Msemo G, Massawe A, Mmbando D, et al. Newborn mortality and fresh stillbirth rates in tanzania after helping babies breathe training. Pediatrics. 2013;131;e353.
19. Goudar S, Somannavar M, Clark R, et al. Stillbirth and newborn mortality in India after helping babies breathe training. Pediatrics. 2013;131;e344.
20. Wilson A, Gallos I, Plana N, et al. Effectiveness of strategies incorporating training and support of traditional birth attendants on perinatal and maternal mortality: Meta-analysis. BMJ. 2011;343:d7102.
21. Lee A, Cousens S, Wall S, et al. Neonatal resuscitation and immediate newborn assessment and stimulation for the prevention of neonatal deaths: A systematic review, meta-analysis and Delphi estimation of mortality effect. BMC Public Health. 2011;11(Suppl 3):S12.
22. Sabin L, Knapp A, MacLeod W, et al. Costs and cost-effectiveness of training traditional birth attendants to reduce neonatal mortality in the Lufwanyama Neonatal Survival Study (LUNESP). PLoS ONE. 2012;7(4):e35560.
23. Darmstadt G, Ahmed A, Saha S, et al. Infection control practices reduce nosocomial infections and mortality in preterm infants in Bangladesh. J Perinatol. 2005;25:331-5.
24. Landre C, Ka A, Peigne V, et al. Efficacy of an infection control programme in reducing nosocomial bloodstream infections in a Senegalese neonatal unit. J Hosp Infect. 2011;79:161-5.

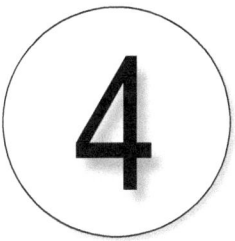

CHAPTER 4

# Managing Your Patients' Data with an Electronic Database

*Joseph Schulman*

## ABSTRACT

This chapter describes how to think about organizing, storing, and retrieving patient information by means of an electronic database—implemented as an electronic medical record system; and how to evaluate the success of the endeavor. Such NICU systems leverage human cognition, speed workflow, and improve patient safety and clinical outcomes in relation to the degree they succeed in capturing the pertinent knowledge and work processes consistent with optimal information management and human factors. Since both the knowledge of basic science underpinning neonatal care and of how to apply it to patients continually advances, the cognitive tool for managing the information of the NICU is a work always in progress.

## INTRODUCTION

The aim of this chapter is to provide an overview of essential concepts for organizing, storing, and retrieving information about patients in a neonatal intensive care unit (NICU), and for reflecting on the success of attempts at implementing those ideas. The following discussion derives, with permission, from previous overviews[1,2] and sources providing greater detail.[3,4]

The daily work of the NICU is too complicated and demanding for a provider to rely on rummaging through a traditional paper-based patient chart to answer a particular question. Such records may not provide much guidance in finding exactly where the required information may lie, nor can they reliably answer a specific question that may arise.

A central aim of patient information management is to ensure that one retrieves the required information quickly; ideally, in the first place one looks for it. But that is far from all that a NICU patient information system should aim to achieve.

In conducting the daily work of the NICU, we often deal with overwhelming amounts of information. To some extent, we recognized this information overload long ago, when we set up paper-based information systems—the traditional medical chart. But, a paper-based system is inadequate.[5,6] In order to recall a laboratory value or remember to check on an X-ray, we may jot the information down on an index card or the back of an envelope. Even better, so we do not lose it, we might write it on the leg of our scrub pants. The problem becomes much larger when we try to learn from past experience. Systematic review of previous patients is labor intensive. Provider notes in paper-based charts commonly are free-form and free-text. That is, there are no strict rules about precisely what must appear in each note; the user can write anything at all (within a size limit). People newly introduced to computers tend to like free-text entry because they believe this "gets all the data into the computer". Unfortunately, typical database query programs cannot reliably search this kind of data. Nor can one be certain that what was entered in free text amounts to an accurate, apropos, clear, coherent, and complete description of the notion to be captured. This potential variability and inconsistency can crucially limit accurate and robust inference and new learning. As a result, chart reviews cannot be counted on to inform unbiased and unconfounded learning from experience; relevant factors may be omitted.

Then, there is the issue of workflow. It takes much time to meticulously work through large amounts of information, filter what is pertinent, reflect on it, draw inferences, devise a plan, implement it, and document everything. Even today, many medical providers need a tool that can speed up their workflow and give them greater mastery over the data with which they work.

A computer-based information system is potentially such a tool. Several vendors of electronic medical records now offer a tool for the NICU. For readers who work in institutions that provide such products, this chapter aims to provide a framework for understanding and evaluating such a tool's performance. However, only a fraction of neonatologists currently can take advantage of such tools, so this chapter's aims are broader still—to provide an overview of electronic database design and implementation sufficient to guide readers who wish to create their own NICU tool.

## HOW WE KNOW: TACIT, IMPLICIT, AND EXPLICIT

A tool that leverages a NICU provider's mastery of patient information may require profound advances in several key areas of work: how an organization's members collect, manage, and interpret data; how they learn from their experience; and how they share the learning. These advances may require fundamental changes in how providers think about their work and their patients, namely, changing from tacit or implicit thinking to explicit ways of thinking.

Tacit knowledge tends to be hard to communicate to another person, either through speech or writing it down. Examples of tacit knowledge include how to ride a bicycle, how to play the piano, and how to be a neonatologist. Although one can read a textbook on any of these skills, the explicit knowledge communicated will fall short of all that must be known to achieve authentic competence. Explicit knowledge can be written down, communicated, and understood by another person. For example, identifying that a neonate has a serum sodium concentration of 123 mEq/L and is therefore hyponatremic, is explicit knowledge. Implicit thinking and knowledge entail unspecified elements and algorithms; in certain settings, some may consider this to be intuitive thinking. For example, an NICU may have an implicit policy for screening visitors who may have a communicable illness. That is, staff may know that they need to ask visitors about this concern, but no written document exists that explicitly articulates exactly who asks a visitor exactly what questions, or exactly when.

Unless a NICU process is written down—explicitly mapped or meticulously described in words, it may well be implicit. Consider, for example, the process of intubating a neonate. There are many details that might be specified, including the particular staff involved, exactly what each one does (consider precisely in how much detail this should be done), the supplies and medications to be made available, and exactly how the endotracheal (ET) tube is placed. Again, consider precisely how much detail could be specified, from opening the neonate's mouth, to positioning the tongue, to how the laryngoscope is held and moved in response to what is visualized, to exactly how the tube is advanced in response to what is visualized, to how the laryngoscope is withdrawn from the oropharynx, to exactly how the ET tube is secured, and exactly how it is determined that all went as planned. The point is that dozens and dozens of component steps may rush by us in an instant of time. Humans cannot attend to all this detail. If questioned about it after the fact, how can we formulate answers from a blur?

Paper-based patient information systems allow providers to dodge this troubling reality of NICU care, because such systems generally do not force us to engage with the gap between what we attend to and what must be entered into the data storage system, if it is to genuinely serve our needs. Paper-based patient information systems typically allow providers to decide what to include in a progress note. As a result, such systems allow workers to avoid facing the challenge of transforming the imprecise, tacit, and even ad hoc ways of thinking that have underpinned so much of healthcare, into more useful collections of data and information about our work. This is also true of computerized systems that do not facilitate explicitly identifying and mapping all important aspects of daily work. With paper-based or underconceptualized computerized systems, there is no system other than retrospective review to detect omitted pertinent information.

The important point is, it is only when we carefully reflect on our work and the limitations of paper-based and other underconceptualized patient information systems that we may appreciate that we do not have total mastery over what unfolds in the NICU; and that we could do much better than we currently do.

## REPRESENTING THE WORK OF THE NEONATAL INTENSIVE CARE UNIT IN A COMPUTER

A computer is a wonderful tool to keep track of more things than we can in our heads or on paper. But, most computers and the programs they run are not designed to handle tacit knowledge and implicit processes in a way that leverages human competence. If we are to benefit from the things computers can do enormously better than humans can, we must think explicitly about clinical data elements. This entails articulating precise methods for collecting, managing, analyzing, interpreting, and acting on this data in excruciatingly fine-grained detail. Unfortunately, in their desire to gain end-user acceptance, institutional decision makers may replicate in the new computer technology the long-standing tacit and implicit methods, thereby limiting and obscuring the potential otherwise available. This may well represent an innocent misjudgment. Few clinicians are solidly trained in data modeling, database design, and implementation.[7] Optimized information management tools require designers who can straddle the domains of clinical care, information technology, and data analysis.

Often when clinicians imagine a computer managing their patient information, they imagine the computer is doing it the same way the clinicians have always done it; just faster, and with less direct clinician involvement. But, we cannot consider the computer a "black box" that will do our work if only we enter the kind of unspecified free-text as we did in the days of paper-based charting. A computer is unintelligent; it only does what it is programed to do. If you had to tell a layperson exactly what to do with some data so that it was properly processed, could you? Well, that is all we are doing when we use a computerized patient information system—we tell a software application exactly what data/information are important, where to store it, how to manipulate it, how to display it, so that we can tell an accurate, apropos, and reasonably complete story about our patient; one that will also inform learning from experience. That sounds straightforward enough, until one reflects on the precise operational details to carry it off.

To conduct our work with a computer, we must precisely specify as many essential details about our work as possible. We must meaningfully represent our work on a computer and capture the essentials, carefully map conceptual elements to precise software elements, and specifically structure it. Often, more than one representation option is possible, yielding varying degrees of success for the performance of the resulting tool. That tool, in one form or another, is a database software application.

Microsoft® Access can serve very well for readers who wish to create such a tool for their own NICU. This software application is quite adjustable, especially because it allows one to write programing code to customize features and even to create new features. However, it takes a vast amount of cataloging and narrative to communicate all the necessary information. So, readers should temper their expectations about becoming a powerfully competent Access user (power user) simply by reading the present chapter or even a book devoted to the subject.[3] What this chapter can do is describe the components of the task and provide assurance that success can indeed be achieved over time.

At its simplest, a database is a collection of data. The term does not necessarily imply computers or software program applications. The card catalog (increasingly replaced by a computer) in many public libraries is an example of a useful, low-tech database. Importantly, computerized, high-tech databases are not just faster versions of low-tech databases. Computerized databases usually reflect more sophisticated design principles than traditional, low-tech databases.

## If the Database is the Solution, What is the Problem(s)?

One fundamental design principle for developing a useful database is to articulate clear ideas about the problems it is intended to solve and the goals to be achieved by the product of the software development.

The Institute of Medicine proposed explicit aims for patient records:[6]
- Support patient care and improve its quality
- Enhance the productivity of healthcare professionals and reduce the administrative costs associated with healthcare delivery and financing
- Support clinical and health services research
- Be able to accommodate future developments in healthcare technology, policy, management, and finance
- Keep mechanisms in place to ensure patient data confidentiality at all times.

These are explicit, but broadly articulated. To achieve them, we require aims for the individual components of patient records, described at a fine-grained level of detail. Many clinicians have not thought pointedly about exactly what an admission note, or a progress note, or a discharge summary, should achieve. Further, how many readers can operationally define what they mean by quality of care?

## Ontology

Even if we share a common idea of information and how to explicitly represent it, we may still have problems communicating. The term ontology describes a special kind of framework to represent our shared knowledge. Ontology in our context is how we specify our idea of our work. It includes precisely defining the vocabulary we use in our discourse, and in our databases. On their own, workers in different settings come up with different terms and structures for representing essentially similar information. For example, consider the variety of definitions of chronic lung disease, an entity often represented in a database as a simple "yes" or "no".

The lack of a common ontology has been called the "Tower of Babel" problem.[8] Within different databases, data with the same label may have different meaning. Other times, we may mean the same thing but use different labels. The potential for learning from our aggregate experience is awesome, but it requires that we resolve the inconsistencies among our data tools. Uniform terminology, representation, and data structure are central to achieving the potential of the new information technology.[9] Calibrating all our data models and database applications to one common ontology could produce unimaginable opportunity to do our work better. To learn more about uniform terminology for healthcare records, visit the websites of the standards-development organizations, called Health Level 7[10] and Systematized Nomenclature of Medicine—Clinical Terms.[11]

## Data Modeling

Explicitly structuring the data that constitute our work entails a data model. A data model is an abstraction aimed at broadly representing the ideas and things that constitute an organization's work. It is the framework that specifies what kind of data to keep and how to store them. A data modeler works with information system users much as an architect works with a building's future dwellers.[12] Both architects and data modelers are designers, people who work with problems that have more than one correct solution.[12] One models—maps—the important objects and events of the reality, so they may be "saved" and subsequently "manipulated".

Why provide technical detail on this subject? Well, if you retain an architect to design and oversee construction of your home, would you not want to understand and approve the blueprints? Would you just move in without repeatedly confirming that the design and the product represent your residential needs?

We shall concentrate on a particular type of data model called the relational data model, so named because it is based on the notion of mathematical relations—for our purpose, tables containing $x$ rows and $y$ columns of data. Though tables often are related to each other, that is not why the model is called relational. The relational model specifies a variety of table features. Each of the relations or tables must have a unique name, as must each of the columns or attributes. The values each attribute may have are specified by a domain. This notion of domain introduces meaning to the data contained in an attribute and helps to avoid incorrect relational operations. For example, a domain might dictate that telephone numbers contain only digits and may not be subjected to arithmetical operations. Each row (observation and record) in a table must be unique. Each cell, that is, each intersection of a row and column should contain only one value (jargon: field values should be atomic). In other words, a single cell holds a single answer. Trying to query cells containing multiple answers or free-text may be problematic.

### What is a Query, a Table?

A database query is a question you formally ask of a database. You ask the question operationally, providing a set of instructions for finding a subset of the data in the database. To produce a report, for example, a daily progress note from the data that were entered into a variety of fields, a number of queries must be run. Query results and answers are assembled according to precise instructions specifying exactly where and how they are to appear in the report. Queries yield answers by means of relational operations stemming from mathematical set operations. Queries to a relational database commonly run via a special programing language called structured query language.

The notion of a table is a key concept. A table is a container for storing data that share common attributes. Tables have rows (horizontal divisions) and columns (vertical divisions). Readers who are familiar with Microsoft® Excel's rows and columns are thus familiar with this notion of a table. Each column describes one attribute of the more overarching idea the table is intended to describe. Each row contains one instance of the table's attribute set, one observation of the thing the table describes. Each row is also called a record. Each column is also called a field.

If you had a table for storing several attributes of your patients, i.e. a "patient's table," each row would contain the information for one patient (one record), with each column recording the information for each attribute (field: for example, birth date, birth weight, gestational age, and so on). For reasons beyond the present scope, it is generally not feasible to store all the pertinent information for a patient in the NICU in a single table, so a core challenge is to identify the pertinent tables needed, and the pertinent attributes for each table.

### Relationship Diagram

The logical connection between information in one table (relation) with the information in another table (relation) is called a relationship. When one record in table A can relate to only one record in table B, a one-to-one relationship exists. For example, each patient can have only one set of admission vital signs because a second set would no longer describe the condition at admission. When one record in table A can relate to many records in table B, a one-to-many relationship exists. One mother, for example, can have more than one infant.

Some appreciation of what data modeling is about may be gained by looking at a diagram of a relatively simple NICU data model. **Figure 1** shows the data model for electronic neonatal intensive care unit (eNICU), a software tool for managing patient information in the NICU.[3,13] The figure is very complicated (yes, I also said that this

# CHAPTER 4: Managing Your Patients' Data with an Electronic Database

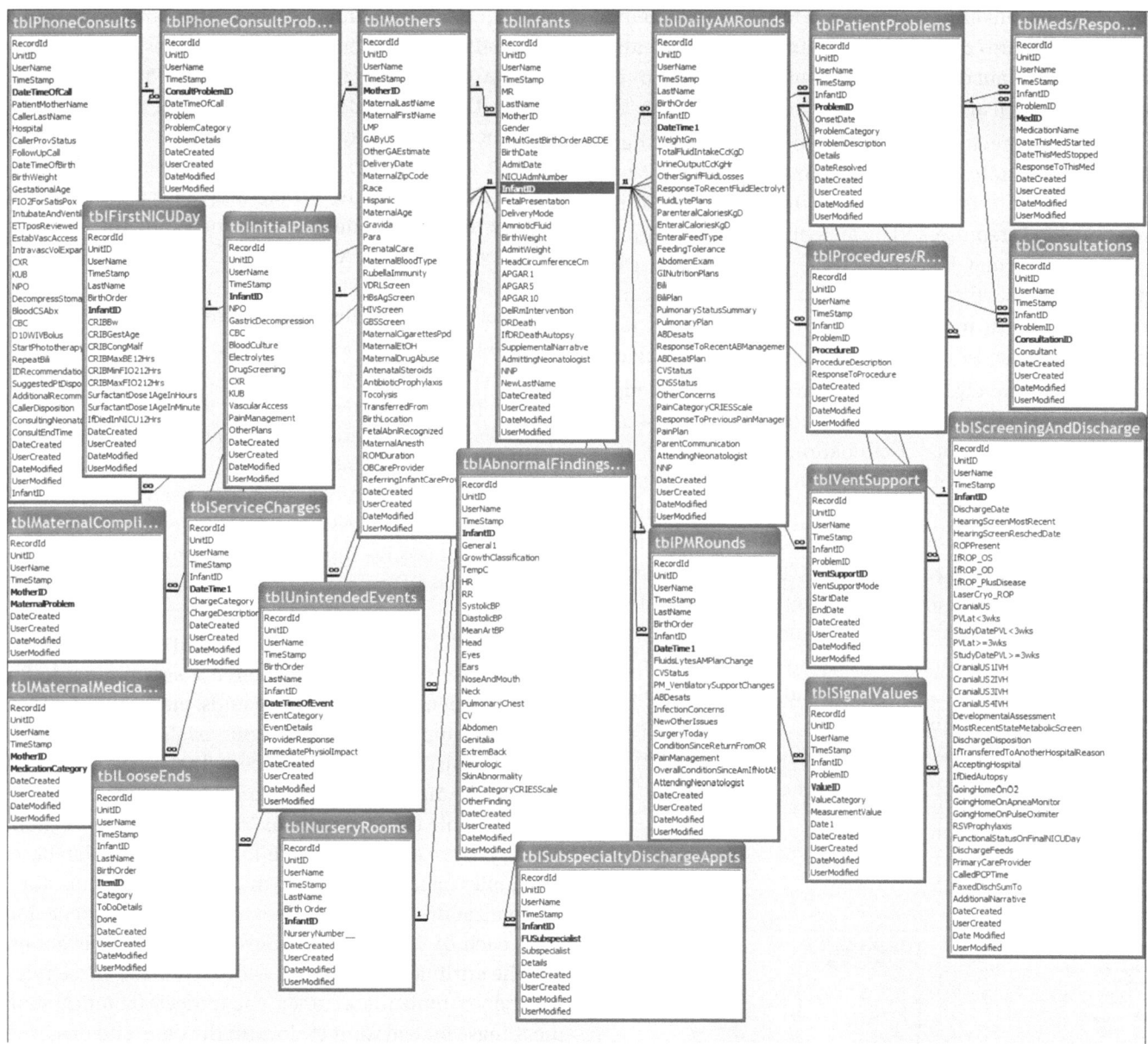

**Fig. 1:** Data model of electronic neonatal intensive care unit. From Schulman[3] with permission.

is a relatively simple NICU data model), but it makes the point that someone ultimately must decide which data elements to include and how to connect them—how they relate. Accepting a data modeler's design without careful reflection on how well the design has mapped the daily work, i.e. the users' (not the modeler's) reality, can result in a disappointing product. Moreover, it is important to note that the disappointment may not be apparent for some time. It may require the accumulation of many records and repetitive querying to discover suboptimal or problematic function.

**Figure 1** uses the convention of naming a table with the prefix "tbl" and "camel caps" instead of a space between words that constitute a name. Relationships between tables are indicated by lines drawn from the primary key field, in bold font, of one table to the foreign key field of the other table. When one or more fields uniquely identify each record in a table, such a field is called a primary key. That is, for each record, the value entered in the primary key field(s) is unique among all records in the table. Without a primary key, records in a database may become confused and database content degraded. A good way to link a record in one table with a record in another table is for each record to share some common attribute value. Thus, if we wish to connect a particular record in a table of infant data with a particular record in another table of maternal data, we would ensure the infant data table includes a field containing the mother's unique identifier—primary key value. Such a linking field is called a foreign key. Together, the linked records describe one instance of a higher entity, the mother/infant dyad in our example, constituted by the various tables in aggregate.

When the relationship is one-to-one, the number 1 appears at each end of the connecting line. When the relationship is one-to-many, the many side of the relationship is represented by the symbol ∞. Occasionally, a relationship may be many-to-many. In **Figure 1**, each patient may have many problems, each of which may be treated with many medications. Similarly, many medications may be used to treat many different problems.

More concretely, consider an infant who experiences multiple episodes of nosocomial infection, each instance treated with the same combination of antibiotics. In a relational database, we cannot directly model the two tables in a many-to-many relationship. Each of the two tables must exist in a many-to-one relationship with a common linking table. In **Figure 1**, tblInfants, tblMeds/Responses, and tblPatientProblems conform to this idea, but this is not readily apparent. **Figure 2** depicts the relationship without the distractions. A many-to-many relationship exists between tblMeds/Responses and tblPatientProblems. That relationship is implemented by using tblInfants as a linking table, in a one-to-many relationship with each of the other two via the InfantID field. At another conceptual level, tblPatientProblems and tblMeds/Responses have a separate one-to-many relationship via the ProblemID field. This relationship models the idea that for each problem, many medications may be used.

One of the tables shown in **Figure 1** is labeled tblSignalValues. Via the ProblemID field, this table is in a many-to-one relationship with the ProblemID field in tblPatientProblems. As just discussed, the latter table is in a many-to-one relationship with tblInfants. The tblSignalValues was designed to store information about particular laboratory studies, those results that signaled meaningful discrimination contributing to establishing a specific patient problem. As such, the model deals with the challenge of ensuring that laboratory information is not merely automatically placed in the patient record without assurance that the information has been processed by the appropriate professional, filtered, and incorporated in decision-making. Thus, the model connects particular laboratory results and specific medications with a particular problem.

The eNICU data model describes, but does not explain. Exactly how did I decide I needed a separate table for infants, patient problems, loose ends, etc.? Truth be told, the scheme did not emerge from one exhilarating epiphany. It is the result of a reiterative process. That process reflected guidelines ranging from simple rules, such as provide a separate table for each class of "real world" objects about which you are trying to store information in the database, to complex ones, such as those that concern normalization. Normalization amounts to a set of design rules specifying what each of the multiple tables in a database is about, and the attributes that belong with each table. These rules generally optimize data storage and retrieval by anticipating the things you will want to do with the data, and ensuring that you will be able to carry them out. By this means, normalization enables reliable queries, i.e. queries that reliably provide the correct answer to a question every time you ask the question. This is a crucial point—if one runs the same query 100 times in an improperly conceived database application, the same result may not appear all 100 times.

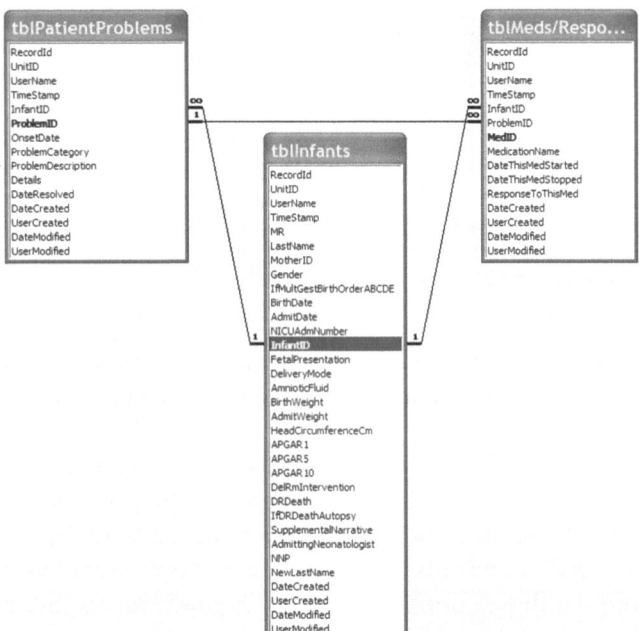

**Fig. 2:** Relationship diagram: tblInfants is the common linking table for the many-to-many relationship between tblPatientProblems and tblMeds/Responses. Each listed attribute represents a table column. The one side of a relationship is denoted by the number 1 at the end of the connecting line. The many side of the relationship is denoted by the symbol ∞. From Schulman[3] with permission.

### A Cognitive Tool for Clarity and Focus

One aspect of the data model in **Figure 1** merits special consideration: the many fields and associated categories that may pertain to an infant. Readers may well ask, "Does the fact that a computer does a better processing job using explicit methods necessarily make it the preferred cognitive tool for a human being in the NICU who is accustomed to tacit thinking?" In 1964, Marshall McLuhan noted that "when International Business Machines Corporation

(IBM) discovered that it was not in the business of making office equipment or business machines, but that it was in the business of processing information, then it began to navigate with clear vision."[14]

Neonatal care providers perform many procedures, but at the core, they must usefully and accurately categorize a patient. The medications provided, the fluid intake, the nutritional support, the respiratory support, the placement of a vascular catheter or a chest tube, and even what we say to the parents, all derive from recognizing that a neonate's profile places that infant in particular categories, and categorical particulars inform what is done for that neonate. Examples of such particulars include elevated $pCO_2$, free water excess, hyponatremia, and growth restriction. Database fields that are not concerned with such categorization still generally support the process. For example, such fields describe what is to be, or was, done for a patient as a result of being in a particular category, or identify the patient; or describe when something happened, or describe a patient exposure or characteristic relevant to establishing a category, or an outcome. Thus, free-text fields provide no advantage in conceptualizing the work of the NICU unless they serve to describe rare situations or other dimensions of neonatal care that have not yet submitted to explicit representation by data modeling.

## Steps in Designing a Patient Database[3]

### Step 1

State what the database is to achieve. For example, "This NICU database will maintain a core data set that attending neonatologists, neonatal nurse practitioners, and residents use in day-to-day patient record documentation and for NICU evaluation".

### Step 2

Specify exactly what you want to accomplish with the data.
a. List specific tasks the database will support, for example:
   i. Produce admission notes
   ii. Produce daily progress notes
   iii. Automatic attending sign-out summary
   iv. Report service charges
   v. Produce discharge summaries
   vi. Satisfy organizational chart audit requirements
   vii. Populate the fields required for other database projects
   viii. Support NICU-level evaluation.
b. It should be appreciated that all above-mentioned points (i-viii), each require specification of fine-grained detail.

### Step 3

Describe the current reality.
a. At present, how do we collect data (forms, index cards, software application interfaces, etc.)?
   i. Collect samples of each way you currently record data:
      - For each, describe how it is used and for what purpose.
b. How do we currently present the information?
   i. Collect sample chart notes, etc.
c. What information do users seem to need that they do not currently have?
   i. Why do we need it?
   ii. How do we know we need it?
   iii. What will be different if we had it?
   iv. What activities or documents rely on it?

### Step 4

Make a list of all fields and calculations gathered from Step 3 (a and b):
a. This is a preliminary field list; it contains current fundamental data requirements of the NICU and is the starting point for the design of the new database.
b. Identify apparent duplicate fields:
   i. Do they represent the same attribute of the same entity?
      - If so, drop all but one
      - If not, rename all but one so each uniquely describes a particular dimension of the entity.
c. Also look for fields with different names that actually describe the same attribute. Drop all but one.
d. Place every calculated field (a field derived from other fields) on a separate calculated field list.

### Step 5

Ask for feedback on the list by all users. To encourage participation, schedule meetings by mutual assent and provide an appealing environment, e.g. offering refreshments.

### Step 6

Create the structures to contain the data.
a. Tables:
   i. Consider which fields appear to belong together:
      - Associate each field from the field list in step 4 with an appropriate table.
   ii. Review each table to ensure that it:
      - Represents only one thing, or entity (object, event, or classification)
      - Contains no duplicate fields.

iii. Describe in writing what each table represents and exactly how it contributes to what the database is to achieve. Return to this description days or weeks later and assure yourself what you wrote is clear and coherent. Next, ask for a coworker's opinion of it.
iv. Edit the table names:
   - Use unique, descriptive, and plural names that make sense to all users.
b. *Fields (attributes):* Assure yourself that each field is indeed an attribute of the object, event, or classification the table represents; relocate or delete fields as you think appropriate. Edit the fields. Use unique, descriptive, and singular names that make sense to all users. Check that each field is designed to contain only a single (atomic) value. Remodel a multivalued field as a discrete table. Designate the primary and foreign keys to link the original table to the new table. Identify each field that serves to link two tables; check that it appears in both tables, albeit under different respective field names.

*Step 7*

Create a table on paper using "dummy" (fabricated) data and look for anomalies.

*Step 8*

Continue to refine the table structures:
a. Aim for redundant data only in linked fields.
b. Aim for duplicate fields only in linked fields.

*Step 9*

Designate keys for each table:
a. Start by identifying all candidate keys.
b. Next, select one primary key per table:
   i. Designate the remaining candidate keys as alternate keys.

## Normalization: Objectives and Strategy

Several of the above database design guidelines endeavor to structure the data to conform to a branch of mathematical set theory called normalization theory. Normalization is a process applied to a set of relations so that:
- Queries that logically may be asked of a set of relations indeed can be asked and will be answered correctly
- Relations store a minimum of redundant data.

An informally determined set of relations (tables) that is not normalized may be incapable of handling all possible queries. Further, such a set of relations may take up more storage space than necessary and therefore, the application will perform slower, increasingly so as the number of patient records grows. As previously mentioned, it may even provide inaccurate query results! Thus, arbitrarily constructed databases, though they may contain the data elements individually deemed appropriate for representing the daily work, when interrogated may function ever more slowly, yield misleading or wrong answers, or at times fail.

Normalization assures the functionality of a database design and provides a nonarbitrary method for determining the appropriate tables. Absent normalization, the patient information management system sooner or later will fail as a tool to facilitate the work of the NICU. Normalization entails applying a series of tests to a group of tables. You apply the tests at successively more detailed levels of scrutiny. Each level imposes greater restrictions on the tables, ensuring greater resistance to problems with data management. Normalizing to three levels usually provides satisfactory performance results. Four more levels may be applied, but these deal with situations that most people are exceedingly unlikely to create, even accidentally.[15,16]

## Implementation of a Database Design

Arcane and intimidating as the preceding overview of database design may be to an individual new to information technology, it covers only foundational aspects of a computerized patient information management system. A selected database design must then be implemented as a software application by which workers can achieve their information management goals. Implementation of a database design is achieved within a general database software platform such as Microsoft® Access, or within a more specific electronic medical record software platform developed by commercial vendors such as Epic, Cerner, and GE, to mention a few.

Implementation entails actually programing into existence the components of the database software application, beginning with the designed relations, the tables. So-called forms are a means for entering data into tables, and also for viewing data already in tables. Forms enable users to add to, or examine what is already in one or more tables without putting at direct risk what already resides in the base tables. Queries pull the required data from the fields in tables. Queries amount to asking questions operationally, by providing a set of instructions for finding a subset of the data in a database. Reports configure and display the results of the various queries to produce products such as admission notes, progress notes, hand-off updates, and discharge summaries.

**Figure 3** illustrates a discharge note constructed by the eNICU software for a fictional patient. It reflects data stored in the model described in **Figure 1**, and is an example of but one of several possible reports that are constituted by results from particular queries that run automatically when requested for a particular patient.

# eNICU: Discharge Note

| | | |
|---|---|---|
| MR 123123 | LMP 35 | Last Name: New Last Name    Female |
| Infant ID: 1231231    GA | U/S | Birth Date 9/25/2002 |
| AMC Adm No 1 | Other est. | Admit Date 9/25/2002 |
| | | Discharge Date 9/30/2002 |

*Amniotic Fluid* clear   *APGAR 1, 5, 10*   **Supplemental narrative at admission:**
*Fetal Presentation* transverse   6 7 8   Concern for GI perforation.
*Delivery Mode* Caesarian   *Birth Weight* 1475
*DelRm Interventio* BMV   *Admit Weight* 1410
   *HC (cm)* 30

## Maternal Information

*OB Care Provider* Dexter, S.
*Referring Infant Care Provider*

| | | | | |
|---|---|---|---|---|
| *Delivery Date* 9/25/2002 | *Transferred From* Bassett (Cooperstown) | | *Birth Location* AMCH | |
| *Last Name* Test3 | *Age* 19 | *Gravida* 2 | *Para* 0010 | *Prenatal Care* Y |
| *First Name* Jane | *Race* White | *Hispanic* N | | |
| *LMP* 1/23/2002 | *Smokes? (ppd)* 2 | | | |
| *GA by U/S* | *Alcohol use?* N | | | |
| *Other GA test.* | *Illicit drug use?* N | | | |
| *Fetal Abnl Recognized* N | *Anesthesia* spinal/epidural | | | |

**Prenatal Screening**

| Blood type | Rubella | VDRL |
|---|---|---|
| AB+ | immune | negative |
| **HBsAg** | **HIV** | **GBS** |
| negative | negative | unknown |

## Maternal Problem    Medication Category

Asthma      *Tocolysis* N
Depression (meds)   antidepressant   *Antenatal steroids?* incomplete (<1 or >7 days PTD
Poor maternal weight gain   bronchodilator   *ROM Duration* 1-12 hours
      *Abx prophylaxis?* none

## Problems/Interventions

| 1. Category | Description | Details | Onset | Resolved |
|---|---|---|---|---|
| CNS | Neuromuscular tone: low | | 9/25/2002 | 9/27/2002 |

*Ventilatory support associated with this problem*

| | Start Date | End Date |
|---|---|---|
| conventional mech ventilation | 9/25/2002 | 9/26/2002 |
| HFOV | 9/26/2002 | 9/26/2002 |
| NCPAP | 9/26/2002 | 9/27/2002 |
| oxyhood | 9/27/2002 | 9/28/2002 |

*Procedures associated with this problem*      *Consultants for this problem*
9/25/2002 10:28:21 AM    LP        Subseq status unrelated      Neurology

---

2. | Category | Description | Details | | Onset | Resolved |
   |---|---|---|---|---|---|
   | INFECTION | sepsis < 72 HRS: suspected | | | 9/25/2002 | 9/28/2002 |

   *Medications associated with this problem*

   | | Started | Response | Stopped |
   |---|---|---|---|
   | Ampicillin | 9/25/2002 | improved | 9/27/2002 |
   | Gentamicin | 9/25/2002 | improved | |

   *Signal values related to this problem*
   WBC      37    9/25/2002

*Procedures associated with this problem*      *Consultants for this problem*
9/25/2002 10:40:38 AM    LP        No detectable effect      ID

---

3. | Category | Description | Details | Onset | Resolved |
   |---|---|---|---|---|
   | PULMONARY | RDS | | 9/25/2002 | 9/30/2002 |

   *Medications associated with this problem*

   | | Started | Response | Stopped |
   |---|---|---|---|
   | O2 | 9/25/2002 | improved | 9/28/2002 |

   *Signal values related to this problem*
   pCO2      96    9/25/2002

*Procedures associated with this problem*
9/25/2002 10:37:22 AM   Endotracheal intubation      improved

4. | Category | Description | Details | Onset | Resolved |
   |---|---|---|---|---|
   | PULMONARY | O2 requirement | | 9/25/2002 | 9/30/2002 |

   *Signal values related to this problem*
   pO2      32    9/25/2002

5. | Category | Description | Details | | Onset | Resolved
SURGICAL | jejunal atresia | | | 9/25/2002 | 9/30/2002

*Procedures associated with this problem*
9/25/2002 11:03:11 AM    jejunostomy                    Improved

## Screening and Discharge Information    *Discharge Date*   9/30/2002

*HearingScreen (most recent)* Passed        *If Screen Re-scheduled, Date:*

*ROP present?* Yes   *If ROP_OS:* Stg 2, Zn 1    *If ROP_OD:* Stg 2, Zn 2   *Plus Disease?* O.S. and O.D
*Laser Cryo_ROP:* O.S. and O.D.

*Cranial US:*   *IVH stage on cranial U/S*   *PVLat<3wks:* N      *Study Date PVL<3wks:*
  Y            #1   0
               #2   1              *PVLat>= 3wks:* Y    *Study Date PVL>= 3wks:* 10/30/2002
               #3   1       *Developmental Assessment* Normal
               #4   1       *Functional status* Normal newborn

*Most recent metabolic screen* Normal           *If died, autopsy*

*Discharge Disposition* Home                    *If transferred, reason*                 *AcceptingHospital:*

*Discharge equip/supplies:*   O2  Y    *Pulse Oximiter:*  Y     *Apnea monitor*   Y

*DischargeFeeds:*  Breast milk + HMF        *RSV Prophylaxis:*  Indicated:<32 wks

*Primary care provider* Tomiak          *Discussed:* 9/30/2002 10:00:00 AM    *Faxed copy to:*  (518) 262-5421

*Pre-discharge exam unremarkable except as noted below:*

## Pertinent Findings on Discharge PE and Supplemental Narrative
Normal exam for age

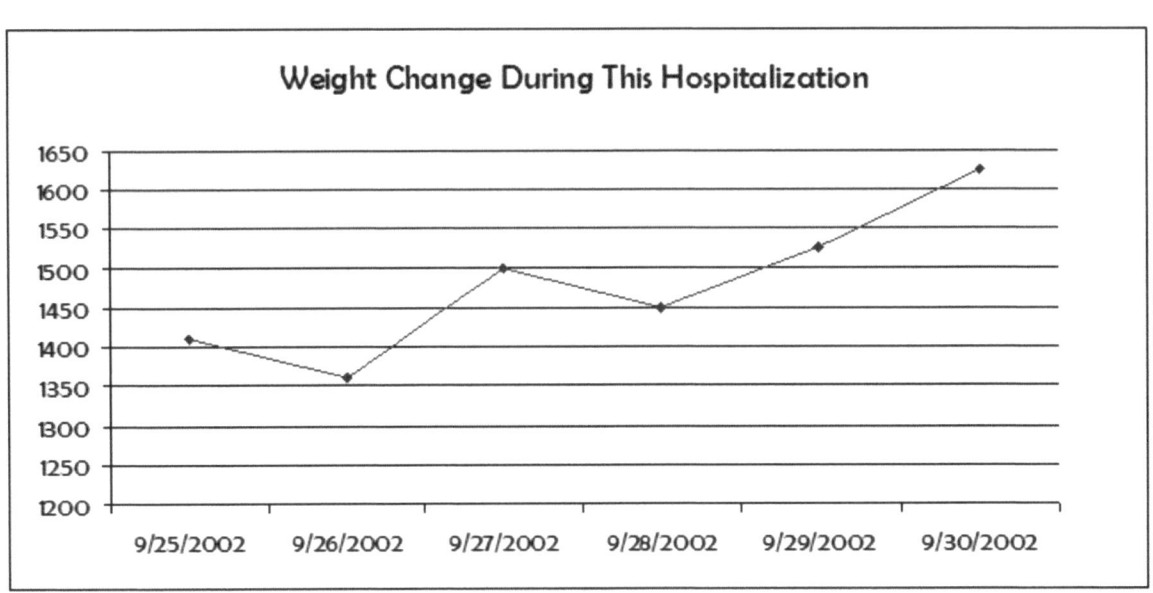

**Fig. 3:** Database software application report: a discharge summary for a fictional patient. From Schulman[3] with permission.

## Backup and Recovery

In data management, to "backup" means to make sure your work can continue to go forward, i.e. to make a copy of your data.[17] You want to ensure that should a problem develop with your stored data, it will not mean you have lost those data. Databases at the scale of a hospital system may experience special problems that are beyond the present scope.

There are a variety of ways for things to go wrong with data. Bad things can happen to the place where you store data. Although unlikely, disasters hit buildings or rooms in a building, destroying the computers within them and the data they contain. In many countries, electric power is reliable, especially within hospitals. But electric power failure can make a hard drive crash, so you want to protect against surges and power failure. Computer data storage devices will fail. Not can fail; will fail. The question is simply when failure will occur. Engineers rate data storage devices such as hard drives by "mean time between failure" rates.[17] The point is, you will experience a disaster with your stored data at some time. Preparation cuts a disaster down to an inconvenience.

Software or data corruption can happen in myriad ways. The operating system that runs a computer tends to become less reliable over time, as users install more and more programs. The operating system is also a common target of computer viruses. Bits of data may vanish or become misplaced from the operating system, or an application file, or a document file as a result of or as an effect of an application freeze. Particularly at risk is a database application that was not correctly set up to handle record locking issues.[17] If you store a database on a network server and the server develops problems, the database can become corrupted.

Routinely backing up is an essential part of maintaining a database. However, backed up files, safely stored in some secure and remote location, have no value unless you can use them to undo a data catastrophe. Try out the recovery tool for your system regularly, so when you really need it to work, deploying it will be routine.

## Security: Encryption

People who should not have access to your database may try to invade. They are far less likely to succeed if you implement some specific safeguards. A secured Access database contains safeguards that make it so time-consuming or expensive for an unauthorized user to enter that it is not worth the effort for an amateur hacker. However, it is important to note that news stories all too frequently report system penetration at large organizations despite deliberate professional efforts to protect stored data.

To encrypt a message is to disguise it. The method by which a message is disguised is called a cipher. Disguised messages are termed ciphertext. Undisguised messages are termed plaintext. The process of changing plaintext to ciphertext is called encryption. Decryption is the process of removing the disguise. Modular mathematics and prime numbers underpin data encryption and decryption. To refresh your memory of modular (modulo functions) math, arithmetical operations based on 12-hour clock time involve mod 12. If we start at 12 o'clock and add 13 hours, we do not arrive at 25 o'clock, but we arrive at 1 o'clock.

Essentially, encryption algorithms convert letters and numbers to other numbers. Decryption algorithms apply a mathematical inverse operation that brings you back to where you started. If very large prime numbers are used in these algorithms, then it can take a very long time, even for extremely powerful computers, to break the cipher. The larger the number of bits in the algorithm, the harder it is for a "black hat," an unauthorized person who tries to intercept data, to figure out what your data says. If you administer a patient information database, one of your duties should include writing a database security policy and making it known to all users. An example of such a policy appears in Schulman.[3]

## IS THE TOOL A SUCCESS?

For each iteration of implementing a NICU information technology system, workers must determine exactly what the desirable features should be, how to minimize work disruption during the implementation, and how to evaluate the consequences of replacing the previous technology. This raises the question of exactly what to measure to determine these ambitions. **Box 1**[4] provides some guidance and insight to the complexity of the task.

## CONCLUSION

### A Neonatal Intensive Care Unit Information Management Tool is always a Work in Progress

An NICU patient information management system is an important cognitive tool for providing neonatal intensive care. For optimal service, it is a tool for which: we must precisely specify as many essential details about our work as possible; we must carefully map the conceptual elements to particular software elements, and specifically structure this mapping; we must calibrate the tool to factors that include the workflow, the available knowledge at the time, the institutional culture, and regulatory requirements. These calibration factors change over time and interact with each other in exceedingly complex and often unpredictable ways.

Therefore, do not expect to spend a few weeks, or a few months, or even a few years developing a product and think the task is finished. Providers certainly understand that the work of basic science research, clinical research, or quality improvement is never finished. For many of the

**BOX 1:** Conceptual framework for probing clinicians' experience using a patient information management system.

*Dimension of IT tool use: Work flow*
- Data entry:
  - Do we impose perceived additional work tasks?
  - Is information displayed in a visual format that facilitates the task?
  - Fonts
  - Background color
  - Content structure.
- Data retrieval:
  - Individual patients
  - Aggregates of patients.
- How soon after creation is a record available?
- *Interruptions:* when distracted by a competing task, do users lose track of thoughts and where they were in the record by the time they return to it, or does the tool remember for them?
- System response time; down time
- Ease of system access
- *Feature navigation:* Ease, and possibility to toggle between features
- *Juxtaposition error:* Is a data element so close to something else on the screen that the wrong option may easily be clicked or an item read in error?
- Have users devised workarounds? That is, have users devised strategies and tactics enabling them to live with the system despite demands they deem unrealistic, inefficient, or harmful?
- To what extent does this tool promote entering information only once, but enable presenting it in varied contexts?

*Dimension of IT tool use: Cognitive enhancement/impedance*
- Does this tool overwhelm users (cause cognitive overload) by overemphasizing structured and complete information entry alerts and reminders?
  - If so, please provide detailed explanation.
- Does this tool cleave information that belongs together, forcing users to switch between different screens, so that users feel deprived of the overview desired?
  - If so, please provide detailed explanation.
- Standard phrases:
  - Are readability and information value of reports diminished by overuse of standard phrases?
  - Does the availability of these standard phrases discourage users' composing thoughts and crafting meaning?
  - As users read a narrative, is understanding sometimes confounded by uncertainty whether a sentence or clause represents thoughtful word use—a spot-on description; or merely a conveniently available selection—a more or less apropos description?
- Have others overused cut and paste or copy and paste text manipulation?
- Redundant information
- Inaccurate information
- Are data provided as abstract cues, or do they contain sufficient context to establish their referential function?[1]
- Do users feel that they function more as data entry workers or as knowledge workers?
- Do users feel that their identity as a professional has changed by using this tool? If so, how?
- To what extent does this tool draw out users' intellect in working with the data and aid their creating meaning from it?[1]

*Dimension of IT tool use: Communication*
- To what extent do users think that another professional reviewing their entry will grasp the essence of what they intended to communicate?
- Do users think that entering their contribution to the patient record replaces their previous means of initiating and communicating their plans?
- Have users noticed a change in the amount of direct interaction among physicians, nurses, and pharmacy? If so, in what direction?
- Is this perceived to be in their patients' and their interests?
- Has overall reliance on the computer system as a source of answers to clinical questions increased, decreased, or stayed the same?

*Dimension of IT tool use: Work/tool interaction*
- Does the tool seem to speed or slow the daily work?
- Does the tool seem to make users feel smarter or dumber?
- Does the tool seem to force users to change the way they think?
  - About the patient?
  - About the work?
  - If so, is the change good or bad?
- What do users need that they are not getting?
- What are users getting that they do not need?
  - For each of the above, exactly how has the user determined this?

(IT: Information technology)
From Schulman[4] with permission.

same reasons that these are never-ending endeavors, so too is it reasonable to consider the cognitive tool for managing the information of the NICU, a never-ending endeavor.

Consider how many versions a software program like Microsoft® Word has gone through so that it can better meet user needs. So, we should not expect that the first

NICU information management product will be the last tool we need. Rather, version 1.0 begins to lay a foundation for what should be an ongoing and reiterative effort to better calibrate the information tool to the work and the work to the information tool.

## REFERENCES

1. Schulman J. Managing NICU patient information with computers requires re-conceptualizing NICU care-Part 1. Neonatology Today. 2007;2(12):1-14.
2. Schulman J. Managing NICU patient information with computers requires re-conceptualizing NICU care-Part 2. Neonatology Today. 2008;3(1):1-13.
3. Schulman J. Managing Your Patients' Data in the Neonatal and Pediatric ICU: an Introduction to Databases and Statistical Analysis. Oxford: Blackwell Publishing Ltd; 2006.
4. Schulman J, Kuperman GJ, Kharbanda A, et al. Discovering how to think about a hospital patient information system by struggling to evaluate it: a committee's journal. J Am Med Inform Assn. 2007;14(5):537-41.
5. Committee on Quality of Health Care in America IoM. Crossing the quality chasm: A New Health System for the 21st Century. Washington, DC: National Academy Press; 2001.
6. Dick RS, Steen EB, Detmer DE (Eds). The Computer-Based Patient Record: An Essential Technology for Health Care. Revised ed. Washington, DC: National Academy Press; 1997.
7. Smith R. Doctors are not scientists. BMJ. 2004;328:7454.
8. Smith B. Ontology. In: Florida L (Ed). The Blackwell Guide to the Philosophy of Computing and Information. Oxford: Blackwell Publishing Ltd; 2004. pp. 155-66.
9. Brailer DJ. Translating ideals for health information technology into practice. Health Aff (Millwood). 2004;Suppl Web Exclusives:W4-318-20.
10. Health Level 7 (HL7). [online] Available from: http://www.hl7.org/about/index.cfm [Last Accessed September, 2019].
11. Systematized Nomenclature of Medicine—Clinical Terms (SNOMED-CT). [online] Available from: http://www.ihtsdo.org/ [Last Accessed September, 2019].
12. Simsion GC. Data Modeling Essentials, 2nd edition. Scottsdale: The Coriolis Group, LLC; 2001.
13. Schulman J. NICU Notes: A Palm OS® and Windows® Database Software Product and Process to Facilitate Patient Care in the Newborn Intensive Care Unit. AMIA Annu Symp Proc. 2003;2003:999.
14. von Baeyer HC. Information: The New Language of Science. Cambridge, MA: Harvard University Press; 2004. p. 36.
15. Chapter 6. Connolly TM, Begg CE. Database Systems: A Practical Approach to Design, Implementation, and Management, 2nd edition. Harlow: Addison Wesley Longman Limited; 1999. p. 49, 77.
16. Chapters 24 and 25. Whitehorn M, Marklyn B. Inside Relational Databases, 2nd edition. London: Springer-Verlag London Limited; 2001.
17. Cougias DJ, Heiberger EL, Koop K. The Backup Book: Disaster Recovery from Desktop to Data Center, 3rd edition. Lecanto, FL: Schaser-Vartan Books; 2003.

# CHAPTER 5

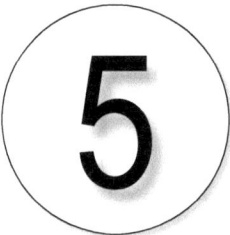

# Quality and Safety

*Aarti Raghavan*

## ■ ABSTRACT

Quality and safety programs are integral to health care in the United States today. A conceptual model such as Donabedian's triad of structure, process and outcome provides a useful framework for quality improvement (QI). Improvement methods such as Lean, Six Sigma or the Institute for Healthcare Improvement (IHI) Model for Improvement can help providers identify areas for improvement, implement changes, and evaluate the effect of these changes. They may also draw from multiple sources of data such as existing hospital-based reportable metrics, or develop simple data gathering tools to reduce the data burden. Use of a mission statement and a SMART (Specific, Measurable, Achievable, Relevant, Time-Bound) aim will keep the team focused on the specific area of improvement. Balance measures will ensure that the "side effects" of changes are monitored, and Plan-Do-Study-Act (PDSA) cycles will ensure that process-related and human factor engineering issues are addressed prior to widespread changes. As with QI, development of a patient safety program involves establishment of leadership that is invested in promoting a culture of improvement and safety rather than assigning individual blame. Multidisciplinary involvement is necessary for success. Although adverse events and healthcare errors vary, evidence suggests that establishing system improvements using solutions from information technology to engaging patients can reduce error. Hardwiring these systems is one of the hallmarks of high reliability organizations.

## ■ INTRODUCTION

The Institute of Medicine's (IOM) sentinel paper "To Err is Human" highlights quality and safety by raising concerns of avoidable deaths due to medical error.[1] Since then, patient safety issues have received significant attention from the scientific community and regulatory agencies.[2,3] As a result, standardization of blood transfusion processes ensued to prevent errors.[4,5] Thereafter, human error recognition led to the Accreditation Council for Graduate Medical Education (ACGME) regulating duty hours of trainees.[6,7] Sharing of common quality and safety metrics has created accountability from the healthcare provider to regulators, payers and the public. Accordingly, the American Board of Pediatrics now requires participation in QI to maintain physician certification. This chapter will focus on definitions, methods, and evidence behind the methods. The IOM defines QI as the "extent to which a change improves a healthcare outcome."[7] The IOM's paper "Crossing the Quality Chasm" includes safety (avoiding preventable injuries and reducing errors), effectiveness (using evidence-based practice), timeliness (reducing wait times and improving workflow), efficiency (reducing overall waste), equity (providing consistent unbiased care) and patient-centeredness (offering respectful and responsive care).[8]

Donabedian's triad model approaches QI through a scaffold of structure (work environment, leadership, organizational culture and information technology), process (what the staff does) and outcomes (results of staff activities).[9] The need for realistic evaluation and contextual relevance in quality processes has been highlighted. Program effectiveness depends on several interrelated variables. This is represented by "Context + Mechanism = Outcome."[10] Although an intervention may not be relevant to an entire group, it may be of value to specific situations. Evidence-based practice, when placed in local context, results in measureable performance improvement.[11] This is dependent on knowledge of local institutional culture, benefits, methods of intervention and the possible side effects of interventions.

Complexity theory states that unlike machines and engineering systems, healthcare systems are deeply interwoven, multidimensional fluid systems where rigid approaches to improvement in one area may have detrimental effects on others.[12] Thus, the ideal framework for improvement in healthcare would be bound by evidence-based principles in local context accounting for unique situations.

## METHODS IN QUALITY IMPROVEMENT

### Lean

Lean is a QI method focused on reducing waste related to processes easily applicable to health care. The most common areas of waste include overproduction, wait times, inventory, transportation, equipment defects, and staffing. This QI method focuses largely on patients and families and promotes value to the patient experience by reducing unnecessary processes.[13]

### Six Sigma

Six Sigma is a QI method using a data-driven approach for eliminating defects (driving toward six standard deviations between the mean and the nearest specification limit) and reducing variation to ensure no more than 3.4 defects per million opportunities.[14] A Six Sigma defect is defined as anything outside of customer specifications. Process sigma can be calculated using a Six Sigma calculator.

Two Six Sigma sub-methodologies are commonly used. The Six Sigma DMAIC process (define, measure, analyze, improve, control) is a system for existing processes falling below specification and looking for incremental improvement. The Six Sigma DMADV process (define, measure, analyze, design, verify) is an improvement system used to develop new processes or products at Six Sigma quality levels. Since this method is heavily based on statistical tools and data, specific training is requisite.

### IHI Model for Improvement

One of the simplest and most popular methods for QI is PDSA.[15] Its ease of use has resulted in its adaptation by the IHI as their standard format for QI. This method consists of: (1) problem identification, (2) aim development, (3) identification of specific interventions that will result in improvement (evidence-based, potentially better practices), (4) trial of the new interventions by the team on a small scale to tease out process related obstacles (PDSA cycles).

## DEVELOPING A QUALITY AND SAFETY IMPROVEMENT STRATEGY

### Culture of Safety

The success of QI and patient safety is rooted in the ability to maintain honesty built on a blame-free culture with an institutional and leadership focus on improvement rather than blame assignment. Institutional culture and behavior are often role-modeled by leadership and management styles.

### Sources of Data

The emergence of technology and health information systems has moved health care from paucity of data to multiple sources of data, which reflect team performance.

### Data for Evaluation

Many sources of data exist for QI leadership to reflect on institutional performance. While many providers may argue to the uniqueness of their own institution and patient population, large databases often account for such differences using risk adjusters. This narrows the focus to comparisons with similar cohorts of patients. For example, the Vermont Oxford Network (VON) provides clinical outcome measures to all participating institutions. Teams review their own data online and compare them to benchmarked data of other centers in the VON system. The easily accessible databases enable institutions to identify areas for improvement.

The success of QI depends upon pinpointing which areas need to change. As QI is very labor-intensive, accurate identification of improvement opportunities conserves resources and limits staff fatigue. When possible, these performance metrics should be benchmarked to national/regional standards. It is the responsibility of QI leadership to select appropriate areas for improvement.

### Development of a QI Team

Quality improvement is a multifactorial process and is therefore dependent on understanding processes and factors affecting outcome. The team composition for QI must be multidisciplinary and can be dynamic depending on the project and composed of representatives from any aspect of care that touches processes that affect outcome.

Ideally, teams should consist of 5–7 individuals. Larger teams may be difficult to manage and smaller teams may not have enough multidisciplinary representation.[16] Overall, the team should represent elements of executive leadership, day-to-day leadership and technical expertise. Executive leadership representation should include at least one individual who has authority to effect change at the institution. The day-to-day leader, who serves as the project champion, ideally has expertise in QI methodology and is invested in the outcome. This provides momentum to the project and takes it past discussion and on to action.[17] Individuals with technical expertise are those who participate actively in the care process that is being reviewed and can highlight system-related issues that obstruct QI.

## Development of a SMART Aim

Following identification of a problem, it is important for a goal to be directed at a specific patient population, for it to have clearly quantifiable/measurable outcomes, to be achievable, realistic and time-bound. For example, if NICU Central Line-Associated Blood Stream Infections (CLABSI) are identified as problematic, the QI project would be to "Reduce the rate of CLABSI in the NICU from 4.7/1,000 central line days to 2.2/1,000 central line days in 6 months through consistent use of the CLABSI bundle."

## Determining Measures and Process of Measurement

Data metrics can be evaluated based on outcome, process and balance measures:

- Outcome measures represent the end point of the healthcare delivery system and are often the most obvious to patients.
- A process measure is made of elements of the workflow system that affect the outcome.
- Balance measures are similar to a side effect profile and represent positive and negative effects of interventions. For example, nosocomial infection rates, particularly CLABSI, are a commonly used metric for healthcare quality. Appropriate hand hygiene and use of a "CLABSI bundle" (grouped elements of maintenance care for a central line) proved to reduce CLABSI. An element of this bundle is removing central lines when they are no longer needed. However, this may result in premature removal of the central catheter. Recognizing the negative outcome related to the positive change in this case represents a balance measure.

In contrast to clinical research, where blinding and randomization are considered the highest standard, QI data are unblinded and focused on measurement of specific outcomes and changes in practices over brief intervals of time without controlling for variables. The focus of QI is to identify the effects of process changes and alter local practices accordingly. Unlike clinical research, it is essential for data to be available as close to real time as possible to facilitate rapid trials of new processes. Ideally, the project would be developed using existing data within the system to reduce the burden of data collection. Whenever data is collected for QI, it is essential to have an "operational definition" of the metric measured to ensure standardization. In the above example, both CLABSI and bundle compliance must be clearly defined to prevent measurement bias.

Unlike clinical research, data in QI is meant to be a mere representation of the whole institutional population. Since the purpose of measurement is sampling, it is not required to collect data on every patient present. Fundamentally, the method of sampling used is dependent on whether within a known population of size $n$ there is a fixed probability of selecting any single element. For this method to be truly objective, statistical methods must be used to ensure random selection. Examples of probability sampling include systematic sampling, simple random sampling, stratified random sampling and stratified proportional random sampling. Nonprobability sampling, on the other hand, is used when the intent is not to generalize the findings to a larger population than the one sampled. This form of sampling is useful in representing the local population where change is to be affected. The limitation of this method is that since selection of sample is not based on statistical methods, the reliability of the sample to be a representation cannot be proven. Examples of nonprobability sampling include convenience sampling, quota sampling and judgment sampling. The choice of sampling method is dependent on the goal of the QI and detailed study of sampling methods is a requisite skill for a quality expert. Further details on sampling are beyond the scope of this chapter.

## Identifying Appropriate Interventions

Multiple methods may guide the QI team toward choosing areas for change. One common starting point is to develop a process map, a diagrammatic depiction of workflow or process. This piece of the QI puzzle that relies most on the team members with technical expertise. A process map serves to identify key areas where process alterations could affect outcome.

## Tools to Examine Different Elements of Process Change

Subsequent to process map creation, multiple tools exist to sort through different elements that could affect change.

These tools provide a system for institutional leadership to identify areas for improvement.

## Key Driver Diagram

The key driver diagram is a depiction of the process showing the sequence of events leading up to the final outcome. This diagram begins with information from the process map, and guides the direction of data gathering. Once the data are gathered, the diagram lists all factors that may have contributed to the occurrence of the event, thereby facilitating solution identification. In this process, multiple areas for change may be recognized. If a single factor is identified, attempts must be made to confirm that the processes of data collection were comprehensive. **Flowchart 1** represents a key driver diagram to improve hand-washing compliance.

## Brainstorming Maps (Flowchart 2)

In brainstorming sessions, all team members present ideas without initial judgment regarding feasibility. Ideas may be presented in a "round-robin" fashion using a white board or a flip chart. The initial discussion presents all possible ideas for change, following which the group explores the pros and cons of each idea. This method is most useful for a group with varied experience with limited exposure to QI methods.

## Fishbone/Ishikawa Diagram

The fishbone is a cause/effect diagram representing a systematic analysis of factors that may affect a given outcome. The diagram **(Fig. 1)** is pictured with the outcome on one end of an arrow and contributing factors pointing towards the main arrow for teams to explore all possible areas for improvement.

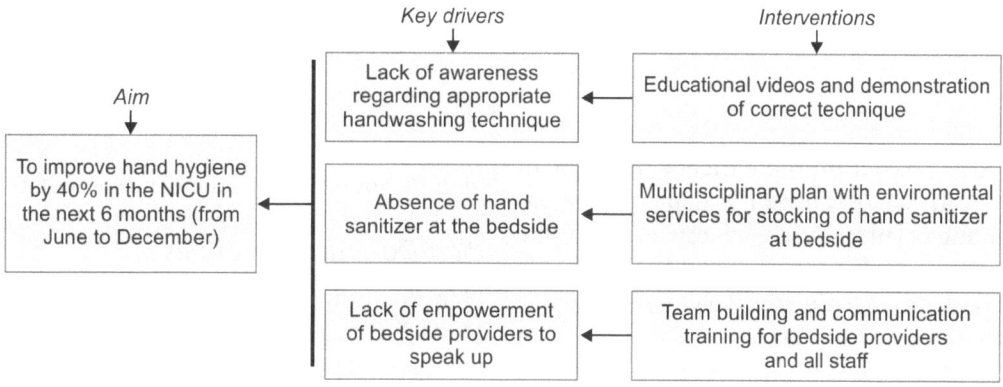

Flowchart 1: Key driver diagram for improving compliance with hand hygiene.

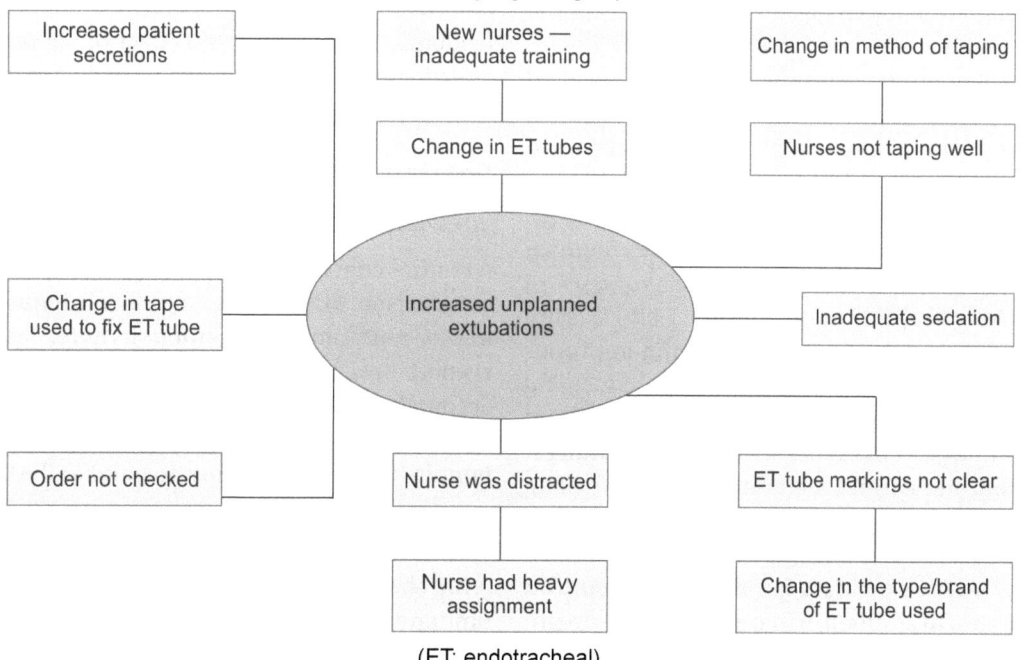

Flowchart 2: Brainstorming regarding unplanned extubations.

(ET: endotracheal).

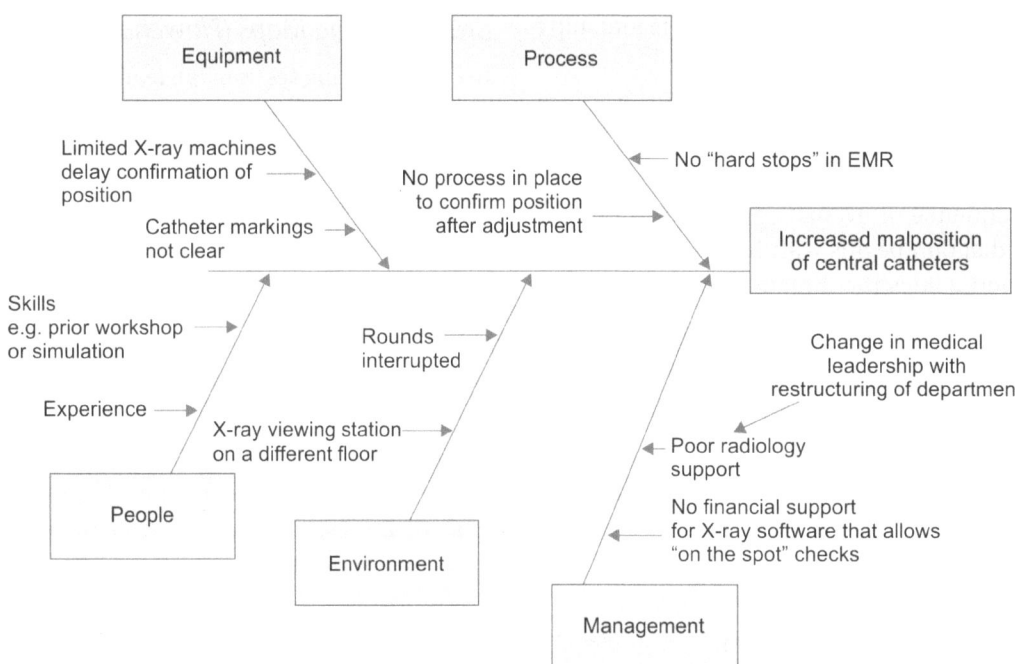

**Fig. 1:** Fishbone diagram regarding malposition of catheters (EMR: electronic medical record).

## Pareto Chart

The Pareto chart is based on the concept that 80% of problems stem from 20% of causes. It is depicted as a bar graph (representing occurrence of each cause) and a line graph representing cumulative totals, and helps identify the few critical rather than many trivial elements that may contribute to an outcome. The focus of this method is on a high yield area of change and appropriate utilization of resources, but it is a data-heavy process since occurrence of each variable needs to be known to analyze the graph.

In identifying areas for change, it is important for the provider to be familiar with two types of change.[18]
1. First Order Change represents changes at the individual level. This type of change typically focuses on individual effort; while easier to implement, it is often subject to significant operator variability and short-lived.
2. The more lasting type of change is Second Order Change, which involves improvement of an entire system, resulting in a new paradigm eliminating suboptimal processes.

Second order change is more sustained albeit more difficult to implement. In a project involving improper dressing material used for central catheters, re-educating and encouraging nurses to use the correct material for dressing change represents a first order change. Removing all but the correct material from the stocking system provides the nurses with only one correct option, representing second order change. Introduction of new processes may stress providers familiar and reliant on previous processes. In addition, while a new process might seem like an excellent idea to a few in the constraints of a conference room, it may not be feasible in reality. It is thus imperative to first test new processes on a smaller scale to identify potential barriers to implementation.

## Plan-Do-Study-Act Cycles

Plan-do-study-act (PDSA) cycles are the keys to the IHI Model for Improvement. This aspect of QI focuses on trialing new processes in small, rapid cycles. The "Plan" stage of this process identifies specific intervention, targets population, and predicts likely outcomes. "Do" implements change and measures effect. "Study" evaluates intervention, receives feedback, and analyzes the effect of the new intervention on outcome. "Act" determines what the next cycle of change should be.

## Sharing Data with the Team Members

### Shewhart/Control Charts

A control chart is a graphical representation of an event in comparison to the upper and lower limits of acceptable norms, represented by continuous lines.[19] The frequency of events between upper and lower control limits is considered acceptable. It is typical to trend format compliance with a prescribed behavior, such as the use of a maintenance bundle for central catheters to reduce CLABSI.[20,21]

### Run Chart

A run chart is a simple depiction of measures plotted against time and is understandable to those with limited knowledge of statistics. It can help identify variations and trends in events, and followed prospectively may identify potential cause-effect relationships between changes in processes and outcomes.[22]

## Value of Collaboration

Although improving outcomes in one's own neonatal intensive care unit (NICU) is worthwhile, collaboration encourages teams to stay accountable to maternal-infant couplet health at a regional level. Collaboration facilitates continuity of care and standardized practice across communities ensuring optimal outcomes for mother and infant regardless of time and place of birth. A national or regional collaborative also provides extensive tools and training in QI methods to providers. Extensive datasets generated through such collaboratives also allow individual institutions to evaluate their own practice and outcomes while providing resources for optimal practice. Hospital outcomes are influenced by demographics, socioeconomic influences, regulatory/insurance profiles, and other factors. Large collaboratives also provide institutions with benchmarks from comparable cohorts of patients and facilitates risk adjustment.

The VON is an international nonprofit established in the 1980s with a goal to promote quality and safety of care to high-risk infants. It allows comparison of each NICU with similar NICUs at a national level by performing multivariate risk adjustment for level of complexity. However, it may not adjust for demographic/socioeconomic risk factors of interest. Data are entered through a confidential system, guided by operational definitions for each outcome, promoting report standardization. The regression model is used to calculate an expected number of cases for each outcome either using standardized mortality or morbidity ratio (observed/expected, O:E) or the difference between observed versus expected (O-E). Statistical methods are used to determine confidence intervals and adjustments are made for noise variation and chance.[23] Reports are generated real time, then quarterly and annually, inclusive of adjusted and unadjusted data.

The California Perinatal Quality Care Collaborative (CPQCC) was initiated in the 1990s in response to payer activity related to quality reporting. The initiative was undertaken with five major stakeholders – the California Association of Neonatologists (CAN), the State of California Maternal-Child Health Branch, California Children's Services (a major payer of NICU care in California), David and Lucile Packard Foundation, and the VON. Over the first year of the initiative, these stakeholders met frequently to develop the mission and goal of the organization. They also evaluated risks and benefits of a collaborative, met individually with other stakeholders and set up meetings between collaborators who may have encountered challenges working together. This facilitated a productive meeting of the executive committee, which further refined the mission, philosophy and goal of the group. In QI the mission statement serves as a compass, to remind the group of the agreed-upon higher goal especially in the face of impasse. The CPQCC is led by its executive steering committee, which is made up of the project Principal Investigator, administrative, data and QI directors. This group oversees the functioning of three arms—data, QI and research. Since the goal of this group was to encompass all NICUs in all regions of the state, the executive committee representatives included representatives from these areas. One of the first goals selected was to increase the rate of antenatal steroids administered to mothers at risk for preterm birth, since this was identified as having the largest impact on outcome. A perinatal QI panel was developed under the QI arm to oversee development of toolkits, conduct training, etc. A data release subcommittee was developed when the executive committee realized the need to promote transparency with data while providing protection to participating hospitals as they developed changes. One of the greatest successes of the CPQCC is its ability to reduce data burden by incorporating its data collection methods into those of VON. The CPQCC data collection system allows participants to collect CPQCC specific data and scan them into a computer, which then generates data tapes that are sent to VON. This allows VON to retain national reports and CPQCC to generate California-specific reports. Regional collaboratives also encourage QI research by exploiting the strengths of local experts and relationships. Successful studies from CPQCC include analysis of "small baby" admission hypothermia and its relationship to morbidity/mortality.[24]

## Patient Safety

Adverse events occur in at least 1 of 10 admissions, and may be as high as 1 in 3-8. While patient safety has made significant progress since the IOM's sentinel paper "To Err is Human," it is still fraught with challenges. Distinguishing preventable adverse events from natural consequences of complex disease or treatment may be the most difficult. Further clarification regarding some overlapping terms is essential to the understanding of patient safety. These terms are defined here:

- Patient safety is defined as freedom from accidental injury.[1]
- Medical errors are those due to failure of the planned action to be completed as intended, or using a wrong plan of action to achieve that goal.
- Adverse events are injuries and harm resulting from a medical intervention, or lack thereof.[1,2]
- "Near misses" are errors that do not result in patient harm, due to chance or timely interventions.[1]

While medical errors, medication errors and adverse events often receive significant attention from the healthcare team, near misses are perhaps a more valuable tool to identify areas for improvement before an adverse event occurs.

## Common Methods to Measure Adverse Events

A common method to measure adverse events is self-reporting. This system is used more often by nurses than physicians, introducing a reporting bias. Having more interdisciplinary team members trained in such reporting is encouraged by agencies such as the University Health Consortium "public safety net" system. Self-reporting is also influenced by the culture of unit-based safety.[25] Another commonly used method is the Agency of Healthcare Research and Quality's (AHRQ) Safety Indicators. AHRQ cautions that this may merely provide clues to patient safety concerns since it is dependent on administrative rather than clinical data. Review of charts requires less knowledge of patient safety methods; however, it is labor-intensive. It is also influenced by individual charting skills and potentially highlights those who chart in detail while missing those who make charting errors. The global trigger tool has come into favor more recently. It raises a flag for tracking when a particular action triggers a certain response. This method also can be labor-intensive, and studies on efficacy have yielded mixed results. Some demonstrate no improvement in patient safety using this tool,[26] while others evaluating patient safety found that global trigger tools were more sensitive and specific (94.9% and 100%) than AHRQ indicators (5.8%, 98.5%) and voluntary error reporting (0, 100%) respectively.[27]

## Basic Principles

Reason's Swiss Cheese Model provides an excellent conceptual framework for understanding patient safety, rather than focus on individual behavior. Improving safety must focus on shrinking the holes in multiple layers of institutional culture. This analogy comes into play as holes represent opportunities for error and solid sections represent layers of protection.[28]

## Types of Errors

### Medication Errors

Medication errors may be defined as "any preventable event that may cause or lead to inappropriate medication use or patient harm while the medication is in the control of the healthcare professional, patient, or consumer."[2] It is estimated that at least 5% of hospital patients experience an adverse drug event at some point and another 5–10% experience a near miss.[29,30] Nearly 1/20 ambulatory patients experiences a potentially preventable error. Standardization of high-risk abbreviations as mandated by The Joint Commission (TJC) is one approach to preventing error. Institutions may mandate their own inviolable agreements, for example: all high-risk medications requiring long-term use need to be approved daily. Employing the "five rights" method of medication administration used by nursing (right patient, right time, right dose, right route, and right drug) is another strategy. "Double-check methods" such as for blood transfusions where two providers must check the blood product prior to transfusion are dependent on vigilance to prevent the process from becoming a mere redundancy. Nurses are often interrupted during medication preparation and must benefit from a "no-interruption zone" to reduce error.[31] Unit dosing, removing medications from certain settings, use of clinical pharmacists, and medication reconciliation are other methods proven to reduce medication errors.[32-34]

### Surgical Errors

While surgical and anesthetic errors receive media attention, more adverse events occur in the NICU during non-surgical bedside procedures. Across all age groups (excluding neonates) studies show 6% of thoracentesis result in pneumothorax.[35] Bedside procedure risk for wrong site and wrong patient errors have been somewhat mitigated by TJC-mandated protocol and have shown better results when nurse presence is mandated and procedural kits used.[36,37] Use of adjunct technologies such as bedside ultrasound for thoracentesis, and use of peripheral intravenous central catheters instead of subclavian or jugular punctures has further reduced errors.[38] Dedicated procedure services with specific individuals trained for high-risk procedures and performing at high volumes reduce adverse events and improve patient satisfaction.[39-41]

### Diagnostic Errors

A diagnostic error is a missed, wrong, or delayed diagnosis, detected by later definitive tests, clinical findings, histopathology, or autopsy results.[42]

### Human Factors and Patient Safety

The impact of human factors on patient safety is perhaps the most difficult to evaluate. Typically these errors occur when a human factor interacts with the healthcare environment, resulting in a preventable error. An example of human factors adversely affecting outcome is the 1984 case of a fatigued resident contributing to a patient fatality. This led to introducing time limits to resident work-weeks to mitigate chronic fatigue, as well as requirements for on-site supervision.

Alarm fatigue as seen in NICUs can be reduced by involving nurses in equipment selection and policy implementation. Human factor engineering focuses on developing equipment with an emphasis on utility, heuristic analysis, and general principles such as visibility of system status, user control and freedom, standardization, flexibility, and efficiency.

### Transition and Handoff Errors

Risk of handoff error can be patient-related (patient moves from one location to another) or provider-related (shift change). Some best practices shown to reduce errors in person-to-person handoffs are: use of standardized formats such as ANTICipate (Administrative, New information/clinical update, Tasks, Illness, and Contingency plans), computerized sign out systems, readbacks, use of a daily goal card, and use of a whiteboard in the patient's room.[43,44] The benefits of optimal transfers extend to transition of care from inpatient units to outpatient services. Approximately 20% of Medicaid patients are readmitted within one month of discharge.[45] Some of the best practices to prevent readmissions include: discharge summary to patient prior to discharge, robust and detailed discharge instructions, follow-up by phone call or any other medium, and postdischarge clinic visits for high-risk patients.[46]

### Teamwork and Communication Errors

The fluid nature of healthcare teams (different individuals working together on a daily basis) increases the risk of communication errors. The authority gradient of an institution may disempower the bedside provider from speaking up when safety is threatened. This authority barrier can be reduced by simple introductions at the beginning of a procedure. Holding standardized briefings and debriefings in one hospital operating room led to improved communications.[47] The use of standardized formats such as SBAR (Situation, Background, Assessment, Recommendations) and CUS (I am Concerned, I am Uncomfortable, this is a Safety issue) improves situational awareness of all individuals on a team.[48] It is imperative not to overuse these terms to facilitate intended impact.

### Healthcare-associated Infections

Healthcare-associated infections such as ventilator-associated pneumonias, CLABSI, and catheter-associated urinary tract infections are examples where standardization of procedures based on potentially better practices with the use of bundles and checklists have resulted in reduction of adverse events.[20,21,49]

## ■ SOLUTIONS

### Root Cause Analysis (RCA)

Once a sentinel or adverse event is identified, it is important to identify contributing factors to prevent recurrence. RCA is a method of investigating latent errors that encourages detailed analysis. The *Five-Why method* is one of the most commonly employed methods in an RCA. Simple to use, the method consists of asking why something happened five times so a minimum of five layers of the system are investigated. Other methods such as fishbone diagrams and Pareto charts may also be used to aid in RCA. Successful RCA requires strong leadership with knowledge of the process, an interdisciplinary approach, the involvement of frontline providers and a clear focus on the process rather than individual blame. Although the goal is to identify system issues that can be improved, individual accountability must be identified and its absence can be addressed in a different forum. While RCA is labor-intensive, time consuming and therefore potentially expensive, its value lies in QI, which cannot be measured. Use of RCAs improve workplace culture from a blame environment to an investigational one.[50]

### Role of IT

Information technology (IT) can significantly contribute to improvement in patient safety by improving communication, dispensing knowledge more easily, prompting for key information, assisting with calculations, providing cross check mechanisms, and providing decision support. An example of successful IT implementation is use of the electronic health record (EHR), use of computerized provider order entry (CPOE), bar coding for medication errors (BCMA) and smart pumps for IV infusions.[51-55] Although these methods have improved patient safety, it is important to remember that each has challenges: structured versus unstructured data of EHR, risk of error with CPOE, time waste with BCMA.

### Education and Training

Teaching hospitals experience yet another challenge with improving patient safety—balance between autonomy and oversight of the trainee. Closer supervision as outlined by regulatory bodies, supported with simulation programs, and conscious training in patient safety should address this issue.

### Patient Engagement and Role in Safety

Language barriers and low health literacy may contribute to safety risk, thus engaging patients in the process of protecting their own safety can improve outcomes. Engaging patients in a hospital hand hygiene campaign did not compromise their relationship with providers while they identified errors that were missed by other methods.[56]

### Organizing a Safety Program

Creating a culture of safety and accountability is critical to the success of any patient safety program. Regardless of methods used, a foundation of honesty and a goal of improvement are imperative. A safety program is often headed by a Patient Safety Officer (PSO) whose role may (but does not have to) overlap with that of Chief Medical or Nursing Officer. The personal qualities of this individual are as important as their qualifications since they will model the culture of safety that the institution develops. An interest in safety, specific training in methods, collegiality, and excellent negotiation skills to collaborate with interdisciplinary teams are desirable qualities. Typically, this individual manages the incident reporting system which can be categorized by domain. In larger institutions, each of these categories may have a different manager (for example, CLABSI, surgical site infections). These domain managers along with the PSO and other key stakeholders make up the Patient Safety Committee. Depending on severity, a report may initiate a baseline inquiry or analysis by a frontline manager, while others may lead to a full RCA with system changes. Aside from supervising the category managers, the PSO is also responsible for managing culture surveys, developing strategies for improvement and developing safety priorities for the institution. It is important for the PSO to engage with frontline personnel by leadership rounds (which may include C-suite officers) or by designating executives with single units for which they are responsible.

## CONCLUSION

Although quality and safety are addressed independently in this chapter, the two concepts are intertwined. Patients have a right to receive care that is high in both quality and safety. As adverse events are commonly self-reported and transparency is dependent on institutional culture, differential payment is likely to affect quality rather than safety. Due to insurance hiding the true cost of care, it is challenging for patients to evaluate the care received. Value based purchasing or nonpayment for errors is an early indicator that reimbursement cuts may be in the direction of cost, rather than performance incentives, further limiting a patient's understanding of the system. In the future, value of health care will be directly woven into the equation of quality and safety. While appearing to be a step in the right direction, it remains to be seen how this will benefit the patient with a right to choose, unless transparency is encouraged.

## REFERENCES

1. Institute of Medicine (US) Committee on Quality of Health Care in America. In: Kohn LT, Corrigan JM, Donaldson MS (Eds). Err Is Human: Building a Safer Health System. Washington DC: National Academies Press (US); 2000.
2. US Federal Drug Administration. Medication Errors. [online] Available from: http://www.fda.gov/Drugs/DrugSafety/MedicationErrors/default.htm. [Last Accessed November, 2019].
3. US Federal Drug Administration. Mandatory Reporting Requirements: Manufacturers, Importers and Device User Facilities. [online] Available from: http://www.fda.gov/MedicalDevices/DeviceRegulationandGuidance/PostmarketRequirements/ReportingAdverseEvents/default.htm. [Last Accessed November, 2019].
4. Biological products: reporting of biological product deviations in manufacturing. Food and Drug Administration, HHS. Final rule. Fed Regist. 2000;65(216):66621-35.
5. Sazama K. Current good manufacturing practices for transfusion medicine. Transfus Med Rev. 1996;10(4):286-95.
6. Pastores SM, O'Connor MF, Kleinpell RM, et al. The Accreditation Council for Graduate Medical Education resident duty hour new standards: History, changes, and impact on staffing of intensive care units. Crit Care Med. 2011;39(11):2540-9.
7. Ulmer C, Miller Wolman D, Johns MM. Institute of Medicine (US) Committee on Optimizing Graduate Medical Trainee (Resident) Hours and Work Schedule to Improve Patient Safety. Resident Duty Hours: Enhancing Sleep, Supervision, and Safety. Washington DC: National Academies Press; 2009.
8. Institute of Medicine (US) Committee on Quality of Health Care in America. Crossing the Quality Chasm: A New Health System for the 21st Century. Washington DC: National Academies Press; 2001.
9. Donabedian A. Evaluating the quality of medical care. 1966. Milbank Q. 2005;83(4):691-729.
10. Pawson R, Tilley N. Realistic Evaluation. Thousand Oaks: Sage, 1997.
11. Batalden PB, Davidoff F. What is "quality improvement" and how can it transform healthcare? Qual Saf Health Care. 2007;16(1):2-3.
12. Plesk P. Redesigning healthcare with insights from the science of complex adaptive systems. Appendix B in Committee on Quality Health Care in America, Institute of Medicine. Natl Acad Press. 2001:309-22.
13. Almorsy L, Khalifa M. Lean Six Sigma in health care: improving utilization and reducing waste. Stud Health Technol Inform. 2016;226:194-7.
14. Trusko B. Improving Healthcare Quality and Cost with Six Sigma. New Jersey: FT Press; 2007.
15. Langley GL. The Improvement Guide : A Practical Approach to to Enhancing Organizational Performance, 2nd edition. San Franciso: Jossey- Bass; 2007.
16. Harkins S. Social loafing: allocating effort or taking it easy. J Exp Soc Psychol. 1980;16(5):457-65.
17. Damschroder LJ, Banaszak-Holl J, Kowalski CP, et al. The role of the champion in infection prevention: results from a multisite qualitative study. Qual Saf Health Care. 2009;18(6):434-40.
18. University of Washington School of Social Work. First Order and Second Order Change. [online] Available from: http://socialwork.uw.edu/programs/henrymaier/quotes/first-order-and-second-order-change. [Last Accessed November, 2019].
19. NHS Scotland. Shewhart Control Charts. [online] Available from: http://www.qihub.scot.nhs.uk/knowledge-centre/quality-improvement-tools/shewhart-control-charts.aspx. [Last Accessed November, 2019].

20. Pronovost P, Needham D, Berenholtz S, et al. An intervention to decrease catheter-related bloodstream infections in the ICU. N Engl J Med. 2006;355(26):2725-32.
21. Pronovost PJ, Goeschel CA, Colantuoni E, et al. Sustaining reductions in catheter related bloodstream infections in Michigan intensive care units: observational study. BMJ. 2010;340:c309.
22. Anhøj J. Diagnostic value of run chart analysis: using likelihood ratios to compare run chart rules on simulated data series. PloS One. 2015;10(3):e0121349.
23. Simpson JM, Evans N, Gibberd RW, et al. Analysing differences in clinical outcomes between hospitals. Qual Saf Health Care. 2003;12(4):257-62.
24. Gould JB. The role of regional collaboratives: the California Perinatal Quality Care Collaborative model. Clin Perinatol. 2010;37(1):71-86.
25. US Department of Health and Human Services, Agency for Healthcare Research and Quality. Comprehensive Unit-based Safety Program. [online] Available from: https://www.ahrq.gov/professionals/quality-patient-safety/cusp/index.html. [Last Accessed November, 2019].
26. Landrigan CP, Parry GJ, Bones CB, et al. Temporal trends in rates of patient harm resulting from medical care. N Engl J Med. 2010;363(22):2124-34.
27. Classen DC, Resar R, Griffin F, et al. "Global trigger tool" shows that adverse events in hospitals may be ten times greater than previously measured. Health Aff Proj Hope. 2011;30(4):581-9.
28. Reason, J. Education and debate - human error: models and management. BMJ. 2000;320:768-70.
29. Bates DW, Cullen DJ, Laird N, et al. Incidence of adverse drug events and potential adverse drug events. Implications for prevention. ADE Prevention Study Group. JAMA. 1995;274(1):29-34.
30. Gandhi TK, Weingart SN, Borus J, et al. Adverse drug events in ambulatory care. N Engl J Med. 2003;348(16):1556-64.
31. Anthony K, Wiencek C, Bauer C, et al. No interruptions please: impact of a No Interruption Zone on medication safety in intensive care units. Crit Care Nurse. 2010;30(3):21-9.
32. Leape LL, Cullen DJ, Clapp MD, et al. Pharmacist participation on physician rounds and adverse drug events in the intensive care unit. JAMA. 1999;282(3):267-70.
33. Kucukarslan SN, Peters M, Mlynarek M, et al. Pharmacists on rounding teams reduce preventable adverse drug events in hospital general medicine units. Arch Intern Med. 2003;163(17):2014-8.
34. Bladh L, Ottosson E, Karlsson J, et al. Effects of a clinical pharmacist service on health-related quality of life and prescribing of drugs: A randomised controlled trial. BMJ Qual Saf. 2011;20(9):738-46.
35. Gordon CE, Feller-Kopman D, Balk EM, et al. Pneumothorax following thoracentesis: A systematic review and meta-analysis. Arch Intern Med. 2010;170(4):332-9.
36. Joint Commission. Approved: Revised Universal Protocol for 2010. Jt Comm Perspect Jt Comm Accreditation Healthc Organ. 2009;29(10):3.
37. Norton E. Implementing the universal protocol hospital-wide. AORN J. 2007;85(6):1187-97.
38. McGee DC, Gould MK. Preventing complications of central venous catheterization. N Engl J Med. 2003;348(12):1123-33.
39. Mourad M, Auerbach AD, Maselli J, et al. Patient satisfaction with a hospitalist procedure service: Is bedside procedure teaching reassuring to patients? J Hosp Med. 2011;6(4):219-24.
40. Smith CC, Gordon CE, Feller-Kopman D, et al. Creation of an innovative inpatient medical procedure service and a method to evaluate house staff competency. J Gen Intern Med. 2004;19(5 Pt 2):510-13.
41. Lucas BP, Asbury JK, Wang Y, et al. Impact of a bedside procedure service on general medicine inpatients: A firm-based trial. J Hosp Med. 2007;2(3):143-9.
42. Graber M. Diagnostic errors in medicine: a case of neglect. Jt Comm J Qual Patient Saf Jt Comm Resour. 2005;31(2):106-13.
43. Pronovost P, Berenholtz S, Dorman T, et al. Improving communication in the ICU using daily goals. J Crit Care. 2003;18(2):71.
44. Sehgal NL, Green A, Vidyarthi AR, et al. Patient whiteboards as a communication tool in the hospital setting: A survey of practices and recommendations. J Hosp Med. 2010;5(4):234-9.
45. Jencks SF, Williams MV, Coleman EA. Rehospitalizations among patients in the Medicare fee-for-service program. N Engl J Med. 2009;360(14):1418-28.
46. Jack BW, Chetty VK, Anthony D, et al. A reengineered hospital discharge program to decrease rehospitalization: a randomized trial. Ann Intern Med. 2009;150(3):178-87.
47. Leonard M, Graham S, Bonacum D. The human factor: The critical importance of effective teamwork and communication in providing safe care. Qual Saf Health Care. 2004;13(Suppl 1):i85-i90.
48. Berenholtz SM, Schumacher K, Hayanga AJ, et al. Implementing standardized operating room briefings and debriefings at a large regional medical center. Jt Comm J Qual Patient Saf Jt Comm Resour. 2009;35(8):391-7.
49. Rebmann T, Greene LR. Preventing catheter-associated urinary tract infections: An executive summary of the Association for Professionals in Infection Control and Epidemiology, Inc, Elimination Guide. Am J Infect Control. 2010;38(8):644-6.
50. Bowie P, Skinner J, de Wet C. Training health care professionals in root cause analysis: a cross-sectional study of post-training experiences, benefits and attitudes. BMC Health Serv Res. 2013;13:50.
51. Bates DW, Leape LL, Cullen DJ, et al. Effect of computerized physician order entry and a team intervention on prevention of serious medication errors. JAMA. 1998;280(15):1311-6.
52. Bates DW, Teich JM, Lee J, et al. The impact of computerized physician order entry on medication error prevention. J Am Med Inform Assoc JAMIA. 1999;6(4):313-21.
53. Poon EG, Cina JL, Churchill W, et al. Medication dispensing errors and potential adverse drug events before and after implementing bar code technology in the pharmacy. Ann Intern Med. 2006;145(6):426-34.
54. Keohane CA, Hayes J, Saniuk C, et al. Intravenous medication safety and smart infusion systems: Lessons learned and future opportunities. J Infus Nurs Off Publ Infus Nurses Soc. 2005;28(5):321-8.
55. Larsen GY, Parker HB, Cash J, et al. Standard drug concentrations and smart-pump technology reduce continuous-medication-infusion errors in pediatric patients. Pediatrics. 2005;116(1):e21-e25.
56. Bittle MJ, LaMarche S. Engaging the patient as observer to promote hand hygiene compliance in ambulatory care. Jt Comm J Qual Patient Saf Jt Comm Resour. 2009;35(10):519-25.

# SECTION 2

# Healthcare Services Delivery

- Mental Health and Emotional Well-being in the NICU: Addressing the Next Frontier in Family-integrated Care
  *Sangeeta Mallik*

- Utilization of Advanced Practice Providers in the Neonatal Intensive Care Unit
  *Valerie D Phebus, Korinne S Van Keuren*

- Pediatric Hospital Medicine and its Evolution in the United States
  *Susan Flesher*

- Home Follow-up of the High-risk Infant
  *Rupalee Patel, Adebola Olarewaju*

- How Charitable Giving can Enhance Newborn Care
  *Elizabeth M Nielsen*

CHAPTER

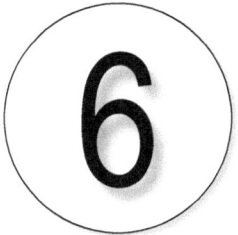

# Mental Health and Emotional Well-being in the NICU: Addressing the Next Frontier in Family-integrated Care

*Sangeeta Mallik*

## ABSTRACT

The birth of an infant if complicated and involving hospitalization can be emotionally and psychologically distressing for families. This chapter highlights the importance of expanding the frontier of family-integrated care in the neonatal intensive care unit (NICU) by supporting mental health and emotional well-being of NICU parents, infants, and staff.

## INTRODUCTION

The birth of an infant can be an amazing and fulfilling experience for parents. However, becoming a parent in an environment that is medicalized can be stressful, even in uncomplicated deliveries, especially for new parents that are relatively unfamiliar with newborn care.[1] If the birth of an infant is complicated, the impact on the family can be even more intense. Many studies have highlighted higher levels of emotional distress in parents during neonatal intensive care unit (NICU) hospitalization and thereafter.[2-6] Furthermore, research on postpartum depression highlights the fact that parental mood disorders do have an impact on child outcomes.[7-9] The National Perinatal Association (NPA) has requested all NICUs to have a psychologist as an essential member of staff.[10] Currently few NICUs have psychologists on staff, although when a family has difficulty, a unit might call for a psychological or psychiatric consult from another department in the hospital. This chapter highlights the importance of expanding the frontier of NICU family-integrated care practices by supporting the mental health and emotional well-being of parents, infants, and staff while in the NICU.[11]

## PARENTAL STRESS AND THE NICU EXPERIENCE

The NICU experience can lead to significant distress in both parents and infants. In fact, studies have found that mothers and fathers with infants in the NICU display a higher percentage of clinical symptomology compared to control parents.[12] Feelings of distress in parents can consist of disappointment, fear about their infant's survival, and the anxiety that accompanies separation and a reduced ability to interact with their infant.[13] Thus, it is no surprise that research findings highlight the fact that parents of preterm and low birth weight infants show elevated levels of distress when compared to parents of healthy infants.[14-16] It is interesting to note that an infant's length of stay in the NICU is predictive of frequency of parental stress, with longer length of stay associated with greater frequency of stress.[17]

What happens to parental stress long-term following birth of an infant in the NICU? Research has shown that individual patterns of maternal distress following the birth of a preterm infant do not consistently decline over time; namely, that different groups of mothers can have varying patterns of distress 24 months following birth of a preterm infant.[18] Some researchers have found that many parents report clinically significant levels of depression 6-months post discharge, and these symptoms remain elevated at 9-months and 27-months post-NICU discharge.[19] Given that parental distress changes over the course of the NICU stay as well as the fact that many of these parents may experience high levels of distress that continues even after their child is discharged home, it is important to address emotional well-being of parents during their child's NICU stay to provide the family with a healthier start post discharge.

## Impact of Parental Stress on Infant Health and Development

The parent-infant dyad is one in which there is a reciprocity of interaction; when parents experience significant stress or psychopathology, it may lead to problematic parent-infant interactions that have a negative impact on the infant's cognitive, behavioral, and social-emotional development.[20] When a parent is distressed, it may affect the parent's ability to adequately care for the infant's needs.[21] In addition, conditions like maternal postpartum depression have been linked to a variety of negative infant outcomes, including avoidant attachment, behavioral and emotional difficulties, and cognitive delay.[22] Anxiety and depression in caregivers can be detrimental to the initiation and maintenance of dyadic relationships important for early infant attachment and development.[23] Caregivers with anxiety and depression may have great difficulty interacting with and being responsive to cues from their preterm infants,[20] may be less sensitive and responsive, and may touch and speak less to their infants.[24,25] Such caregivers also struggle to provide the necessary support, sensitivity, contingent responsiveness, and verbal interactions that promote cognitive development in very low birth weight infants.[25] These less-than-optimal interactions have an impact on the infants. For example, infants of depressed mothers exhibit poor affect regulation, even after depressive symptoms have resolved,[26] while infants of anxious mothers were found to exhibit less mature regulatory behaviors and have high cortisol reactivity compared to those of non-anxious mothers.[27]

Thus, distress that parents experience in the NICU and beyond can impact their thinking and interactions long-term, which can lead to a circular loop of less prosocial behaviors and parent-infant interactions that in turn increase their child's risk for insecure attachment. It is evident that poor parental mental health can lead to poor mental and physical health outcomes in children. For example, highly anxious parents may be less adept at gauging situational demands and fail to behave in a way that supports a child's sense of self confidence, independence and mastery, putting their child at higher risk for developing anxiety as compared to non-anxious parents.[28]

Being in the NICU is stressful to parents. Healthy bonding practices that typically bring the caregiver and child closer like breastfeeding and skin-to-skin care are disrupted. Medical complications of prematurity, emotional exhaustion of the family, and mother-infant separation are further stressors. Early physical closeness and breastfeeding help nurture the intimate mother-infant connection.[29] In fact, skin-to-skin contact has been highlighted as an important intervention to promote breastfeeding, in which oxytocin release is suggested to be an important mediator for the effects of close physical contact on breastfeeding. Moreover, long periods of mother-infant skin-to-skin contact are regarded as an effective way to empower mothers to become familiar with their infants, strengthen their mothering at their own pace and increase feelings of parental competence.[30] When it comes to children who have experienced relational trauma (in foster care or infants up for adoption) such children may not be able to start breastfeeding immediately upon placement with a new caregiver. However, the experience of mothers who have explored breastfeeding with their adopted child is that building trust and attachment with their child, and slowly introducing the idea of breastfeeding, enables the establishment of a breastfeeding relationship.[31]

## Infant Mental Health in the Context of the NICU

Infant and early childhood mental health is defined as the capacity of the child to form close and secure adult and peer connections, to be able to experience, manage, and express a full range of emotions, and explore the environment and learn in the context of family, community, and culture.[32] Infant mental health is associated with healthy social and emotional development, and is linked to the mental wellness of the caregiving relationship between caregiver and child.[33]

It is essential to understand the underpinnings of what supports positive infant mental health as well as maternal health in the context of an NICU and develop expertise in tackling related issues. As mentioned earlier, maternal depression, if left untreated, has the potential to interfere with the quality of the parent-child relationship and can also negatively affect the infant or young child's overall health, development, and learning. Indeed, untreated maternal mental illness is an adverse childhood event (ACE) that can often lead to other adverse events such as child abuse and neglect. Embedding infant mental health education and competency standards in healthcare education professionals' training, coursework, and ongoing professional development is essential as it provides opportunities to build a workforce that understands this area and is prepared to identify situations that may impede children's healthy emotional development.

The field of infant-family and early childhood mental health is an interdisciplinary field of study. Developments in neuroscience, infant mental health, and attachment, as well as prenatal and perinatal psychology and health, indicate that the optimal time to make a lasting positive impact in human development is from the very beginning of life. Research demonstrates that many patterns, such as health or chronic disease, self-regulation, and attachment issues, originate in the prenatal and perinatal periods. It is obvious that best outcomes occur when families are supported in their mental and physical well-being throughout pregnancy, birth, infancy, and early childhood. Infant-family and early childhood mental health services thus emphasize the importance of early caregiving relationships on brain development, attachment, and emotional regulation and can mitigate effects of risk and stress, thereby helping families develop resilience to tackle adversity.

In order to offer effective intervention and support, each provider of service interacting with infants, young children, and their families in the NICU must understand the basic concepts of development and mental health principles of infants and young children. Providers have an equally important professional role to support families in their ability to protect, nurture, and guide their children. Experts in the field of mental health, and particularly infant-family and early childhood mental health, have endeavored for some years to articulate the specialized coursework and skills necessary to build providers' skills and competencies that qualify them as adept in delivering services to infants and young children within the context of their families.[32]

Providers in the NICU that wish to be certified in infant mental health need to be trained in a core set of topics that include the following:[1]

- The importance of responsive and stable caregiving relationships, i.e. understanding the concept of attachment, separation, loss, trauma and grief, etc. in the context of the caregiver/child relationship.
- Understanding early development with special attention to neurological implications.
- The needs (practical and emotional) of culturally diverse families.
- How to identify and access resources to address the complex needs of families in distress and facing challenging circumstances.
- The interdisciplinary nature of the work and the need to collaborate.

Ensuring that staff wanting expertise in the above arenas are appropriately trained and certified is a key responsibility of NICU management. For example, NICU management should ensure that NICU staff gain expertise in identifying signs of postpartum depression in caregivers so that they can guide the provider to appropriate help.

## A MODEL FOR RESILIENCE IN THE NICU: MULTI-TIERED SUPPORT

Given the findings highlighted earlier, it is not surprising that the National Perinatal Association (NPA), with active participation of members of the Neonatology Special Interest Group (Neo-SIG), has called for all NICUs to enlist a psychologist as an essential and core member of the staff.[10] Unfortunately, despite these guidelines, few NICUs have psychologists on staff. Typically, when a family or caregiver experiences distress, an NICU might call for a psychological or psychiatric consult from another department in the hospital.

Family-integrated care should extend a step further in the NICU to address the fact that during the NICU stay, infants, parents, and NICU staff are a closely knit system. Unattended psychological needs of one or more individuals that are part of this system is likely to have a negative impact on all parties concerned, especially the health impacted infant in the NICU. For example, a distressed caregiver in the NICU, as exemplified by the research highlighted earlier in this chapter, is likely to impact her infant negatively and that will in turn have a reciprocal impact on aggravating the caregiver's own psychological distress. In addition, distress and anxiety in NICU staff that remain unaddressed can also potentially affect the quality of family-integrated care disbursed in the NICU.

Keeping these negative circular loops in mind, it is imperative for NICUs to acknowledge the fact that what is needed is a tiered system of care in the NICU addressing mental health and emotional well-being of all parties concerned where families and staff have immediate resources that they can turn to when in distress. In a sense, such a tiered system is likely to build a resilient environment for all parties concerned in the NICU where individuals will feel supported rather than isolated in their unique NICU experiences. Some researchers, in the hope of providing guidance on a tiered model of care in the NICU, have highlighted interventions in the NICU focusing on three areas: (1) the maternal/paternal experience, (2) transition to home, and (3) consultation to staff.[34]

As part of acknowledging the maternal/paternal experience in the NICU, psychologists can focus on the parent-infant dyad by assisting parents with depression, anxiety/panic and any kind of post-traumatic stress disorder (PTSD). This process would involve a model where there is regular contact by the psychologist with parents, taking the effort to listen to their stories in order to provide them with support and empathy as they course through the complexities of their NICU stay, and understanding how well they are able to cope and display resilience through it all. Another key process that has been brought up in the literature is facilitating regular parent NICU support groups, where the underlying goal is to help parents acknowledge their experiences, ambivalence, and help destigmatize depression, help them cope with stress, and help them feel more connected and empowered as parents.[35] The literature also confirms that without mental health professionals on staff, families are burdened and afraid of stigma, and are less likely to follow-up on a mental health referral.[36]

The second area of focus should be helping parents transition back to the home. While many parents might be relieved that their NICU stay has come to an end, it can also be a tremendous source of anxiety in terms of parents feeling anxious about their ability to keep their babies safe and healthy once they return home. Following up on newly discharged families and infants is an essential extension of family-integrated care that should be adopted by NICUs. Indeed, research has clearly shown that high-risk infants that have complex care needs and can benefit from regular follow-up services. For example, home visits provide an opportunity to identify, impact and intervene in, and resolve homecare and healthcare utilization errors.[37] In other words, family-integrated care should not stop once the infant graduates from the NICU, but extend beyond. The reason this is critical is that while some families may manifest symptoms of depression, anxiety and psychological distress during the NICU stay, others may experience symptoms after the baby is discharged, especially when the child is not achieving expected developmental milestones. Parents should be screened following discharge by healthcare home visitors and at developmental follow-up appointments.

The third area of focus in a tiered system of care is the understanding that families form bonds with some NICU staff over the course of their stay. In other words, how families relate to NICU staff is an essential piece that needs to be examined, given that the quality of this interaction impacts the families' overall NICU experience.[38] Once again, if necessary, an NICU psychologist can work with staff and families by facilitating more responsive forms of dialogue between them that will help parents and staff understand each other's intentions and perspectives. The goal is to support both families and staff as they navigate the emotional challenges and distress that may be part of their NICU experience.

It is evident that nurses play a critical role in the NICU for new and anxious mothers and help to maintain the connection between mother and NICU infant during the stay. Research has in fact shown an inverse relationship between depressive symptoms among mothers in the NICU and experiencing support from nurses.[30] Thus, the perception of support from nurses can make a huge impact on the caregivers. Yet, the reality also is that nurses and neonatologists are not immune to the effects of a high-stress environment. In fact, there is a risk that NICU medical staff can suffer from compassion fatigue or burnout without proper psychological support.[31] Three primary factors have been associated with burnout among NICU nurses: (1) elements of the physical and interpersonal work environment (for example, the stress connected with managing distressed families), (2) high workloads of high-maintenance patients and (3) discrepancies between their care-related intentions and their communication skills. In other words, they may have good ideas and intentions with respect to patient care that may not necessarily translate in the way they communicate with the actual patients. A qualified psychologist can help medical staff identify such problems and provide opportunities for growth to medical staff in the NICU.

Bearing in mind the highlighted model of tiered care that is emerging in the medical field, some key recommendations have emerged in the literature to help NICUs equip themselves with the right staffing that can provide the necessary support to parents and staff[10] that include the following:

- NICUs should consider having more NICU mental health professionals (NMHPs) on staff. Having psychologists on the NICU team is a trend that is recently emerging.
- Having one comfortable area for confidential discussions between NICU families and NMHPs like social workers, psychologists and psychiatric staff is important. These staff in turn should have dedicated time to provide verbal therapeutic support to parents and family members.
- NMHPs should educate NICU staff about the importance of the parent–infant dyadic relationship. Furthermore, NMHPs should provide support to staff as well as to families that could include interfacing between staff and families when needed.
- NMHPs should endeavor to create a truly family-integrated culture of understanding and responsiveness for the NICU staff that acknowledges and supports NICU parental/caregiver emotional distress. Within this NICU culture, care for the emotional and educational needs of NICU parents are outcomes that would be just as important as ensuring the health and development of the NICU babies. This shift in perception of family-integrated care is truly important; going beyond episodic health-related events and moving to truly taking care of the infant and family's needs in the context of the NICU, acknowledging the sensitivity of the infant caregiver dyadic experience.
- Ideally there should be a paid parent support coordinator as part of the NICU staff. NMHPs can in turn work closely with the parent support coordinator providing training to recognize parental emotional distress.

- NICUs should also consider having therapeutic parent education groups, which meet on a regular basis.

## SUMMARY

The NICU experience can sometimes have an intense effect on parents, infants as well as staff. NICU parents have a range of emotional responses to the NICU experience that can range from resilience to psychopathology.[18,38] Much of this variability can come from and could be determined by: (1) pre-existing mental health conditions, (2) the severity of the baby's medical condition, and (3) the level of emotional support for parents during the potentially traumatic NICU experience.[39-41] Addressing this third level thoroughly has not historically been considered part of regular family-integrated care in an NICU setting given that NICU care has focused on the medical condition of the baby. Broadening this focus to include the emotional well-being of parents and even staff is indeed the next frontier that NICUs need to universally adopt around the world. Doing so is likely to foster the growth and development of babies by strengthening parent-infant dyadic relationships, promoting the emotional well-being of parents as well as NICU staff and helping the NICU team provide high quality care. Achieving this goal will need to be supported by an NICU environment and culture that values the psychological and emotional well-being of all concerned (parents, infants and staff). This tiered system of care in the NICU will help redefine what it means to provide truly effective albeit compassionate family-integrated care in medical settings.

In conclusion, it is imperative to create a culture to promote comprehensive family support in the NICU as well as prioritize mental health among all parties concerned: doctors, nurses, ancillary staff and families. Families need to feel supported and empowered as this can improve parents' functioning while in the NICU. Once at home, parents that are mentally and emotionally supported can only enhance their connection with their baby. Optimal physical, cognitive and emotional development between caregiver and child occurs only within the context of loving, positive interactions. Providing psychosocial support to all participants in an NICU should not be considered an optional activity, but should be the foundation upon which NICU staff provide excellent medical care.[38] NICU staff that are well supported with respect to mental health issues as well as educated in providing psychosocial support to families can only feel more empowered in ensuring best practices unfold in family-integrated care, ensuring the improved well-being of families in the NICU. This issue is indeed the next frontier in medical care that needs to be embraced by the medical community at large in the near future.

## ACKNOWLEDGMENTS

This chapter would not have been possible without the support of the County of Santa Clara Health System, the VMC Foundation, First 5 Santa Clara County, and the Santa Clara Valley Medical Center (SCVMC) NICU families, providers, nurses, and ancillary staff.

## REFERENCES

1. Steinberg Z, Patterson C. Giving voice to the psychological in the NICU: A relational model. J Infant Child Adol Psychoth. 2017;16(1):25-44.
2. Friedman SH, Kessler A, Yang SN, et al. Delivering perinatal psychiatric services in the neonatal intensive care unit. Acta Paediatr. 2013;102:e392-e397.
3. Penny KA, Freidman SH, Halstead GM. Psychiatric support for mothers in the neonatal intensive care unit. J Perinatol. 2015;35(6):451-7.
4. Holditch-Davis D, Miles MS, Weaver MA, et al. Patterns of distress in African-American mothers of preterm infants. J Dev Behav Pediatr. 2009;30(3):193-205.
5. Brandon D, Tully K, Silva S, et al. Emotional responses of mothers of late-preterm and term infants. J Obstet Gynecol Neonatal Nurs. 2011;40(6):719-31.
6. Voegtline KM, Stifter CA, Family Life Project Investigators. Late-preterm birth, maternal symptomatology, and infant negativity. Infant Behav Dev. 2010;33(4):545-54.
7. Field T. Postpartum depression effects on early interactions, parenting and safety practices: A review. Inf Beh Develop. 2010;33(1):1-6.
8. McManus BM, Poehlmann J. Parent-child interaction, maternal depressive symptoms and preterm infant cognitive function. Inf Beh Develop. 2012;35(3):489-98.
9. Murray L, Arteche A, Fearon P, et al. Maternal postnatal depression and the development of depression in offspring up to 16 years of age. J Am Acad Child Adol Psych. 2011;50(5):460-70.
10. Hynan MT, Steinberg Z, Baker L, et al. Recommendations for mental health professionals in the NICU. J Perinatol. 2015;35(Suppl 1):S14-18.
11. O'Brien K, Bracht M, Robson K, et al. Evaluation of the Family Integrated Care model of neonatal intensive care: A cluster randomized controlled trial in Canada and Australia. BMC Pediatr. 2015;15:210.
12. Carter JD, Mulder RT, Bartram AF, et al. Infants in a neonatal intensive care unit: Parental response. Archiv Disease Child: Fetl Neol Ed. 2005;90(2):F109-13.
13. Miles MS, Funk SG, Kasper MA. The stress response of mothers and fathers of preterm infants. Res Nurs Health. 1992;15(4):261-9.
14. Carter JD, Mulder RT, Darlow BA. Parental stress in the NICU: The influence of personality, psychological, pregnancy and family factors. Behavior. 2007;50:40-50.
15. MacDonald M. Mothers of preterm infants in neonate intensive care. Early Child Dev Care. 2007;177(8):821-38.
16. Treyvaud K, Anderson VA, Lee KJ, et al. Parental mental health and early social-emotional development of children born very preterm. J Ped Psych. 2010;35(7):768-77.

17. Dudek-Shriber L. Parent stress in the neonatal intensive care unit and the influence of parent and infant characteristics. Am J Occup Ther. 2004;58(5):509-20.
18. Holditch-Davis D, Miles MS, Weaver MA, et al. Patterns of distress in African-American mothers of preterm infants. J Dev Behav Ped. 2009;30(3):193-205.
19. Miles MS, Holditch-Davis D, Schwartz TA, et al. Depressive symptoms in mothers of prematurely born infants. J Dev Behav Ped. 2007;28(1):36-44.
20. Forcada-Guex M, Pierrehumbert B, Borghini A, et al. Early dyadic patterns of mother-infant interactions and outcomes of prematurity at 18 months. Pediatrics. 2006;118:107-14.
21. Altman M, Vanpée M, Bendito A, et al. Shorter hospital stays for moderately preterm infants. Acta Paed. 2006; 95(10): 1228-33.
22. Civic D, Holt VL. Maternal depressive symptoms and child behavior problems in a nationally representative normal birthweight sample. Mat Child Health J. 2000;4:215-21.
23. Field T. Postpartum depression effects on early interactions, parenting, and safety practices: A review. Inf Beh Dev. 2010;33:1-6.
24. Zelkowitz P, Papageorgiou A, Bardin C, et al. Persistent maternal anxiety affects the interaction between mothers and their very low birth weight children at 24 months. Early Hum Dev. 2009;85:51-8.
25. Zelkowitz, P, Papageorgiou A. Maternal anxiety: An emerging prognostic factor in neonatology. Acta Paed. 2005;94(12):1704-5.
26. Cohn J, Campbell, S. Influence of maternal depression on infant affect regulation. In: Developmental perspectives on depression. Rochester symposium on developmental psychopathology. Rochester: University of Rochester Press; 1992. pp. 130-30.
27. Feldman R, Granat A, Pariente C, et al. Maternal depression and anxiety across the postpartum year and infant social engagement, fear regulation, and stress reactivity. J Amer Acad Child Adol Psych. 2009;48(9):919-27.
28. Rutherford JL. Impact of parental anxiety on parenting behavior. Dissertation Abs Int. 2004;65:2-9.
29. Flacking R, Lehtonen L, Thomson G, et al. Closeness and separation in neonatal intensive care. Acta Paediatrica (Oslo, Norway 1992). 2012;101(10):1032-7.
30. Zero To Three. The basics of infant and early childhood mental health. [online] Available from: https://www.zerotothree.org/resources/1951-the-basics-of-infant-and- early-childhood-mental-health. [Last Accessed November, 2019].
31. Gribble KD. Mental health, attachment and breastfeeding: implications for adopted children and their mothers. Int Breastfeeding J. 2006;1:5.
32. California Center for Infant-Family and Early Childhood Mental Health. (2016). California Compendium of Training Guidelines, Personnel Competencies, and Professional Endorsement Criteria for Infant-Family and Early Childhood Mental Health. [online] Available at: http://cacenter-ecmh.org/wp/wp-content/uploads/2016/09/compendium-ifecmh-fall-2016.pdf. [Last Accessed November, 2019].
33. Mendez M, Simpson T, Alter A, et al. The Infant Mental Health Workforce: Key to Promoting the Healthy Social and Emotional Development of Children. Farmington, CT: Child Health and Development Institute of Connecticut; 2015.
34. Davis L, Edwards H, Mohay H, et al. The impact of a very premature birth on the psychological health of mothers. Early Hum Dev. 2003;73(1-2):61-70.
35. Braithwaite M. Nurse burnout and stress in the NICU. Adv Neonat Care. 2008; 8(6):343-347.
36. Hall SL, Cross J, Selix NW, et al. Recommendations for enhancing psychosocial support of NICU parents through staff education and support. J Perinatol. 2015;35:S29-S36.
37. Patel R, Olarewaju A, Nudleman M, et al. Homecare and Healthcare Utilization Errors Post Neonatal Intensive Care Unit Discharge. Adv in Neonat Care. 2017;17(4): 258-64.
38. Penny KA, Freidman SH, Halstead GM. Psychiatric support for mothers in the neonatal intensive care unit. J Perinatol. 2015;35(6):451-7.
39. Hynan M, Mounts K, Vanderbilt D. Screening parents of high-risk infants for emotional distress: rationale and recommendations. J Perinatol. 2013;33(10):748-53.
40. Bonanno GA, Westphal M, Anthony D, et al. Resilience to loss and potential trauma. Ann Rev Clin Psychol. 2011;7:511-35.
41. Hall S, Phillips R, Hynan M. Transforming NICU Care to Provide Comprehensive Family Support. Newborn Infant Nurs Rev. 2016;16:10.

CHAPTER

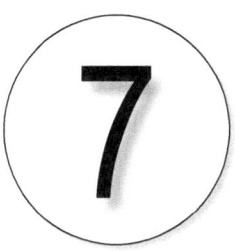

# Utilization of Advanced Practice Providers in the Neonatal Intensive Care Unit

*Valerie D Phebus, Korinne S Van Keuren*

## ABSTRACT

The position of advanced practice provider (APP)—nurse practitioner (NP), nurse anesthetist, nurse midwife, clinical nurse specialist, and physician assistant (PA)—originated in the early 1900s. In the late 1970s–1980s, neonatal prepared NPs and PAs began treating the specific needs of the critically ill infant in the Northern Hemisphere. Since the utilization of APPs, numerous studies have evaluated their role, initially focusing on competency and more recently shifting to quality outcomes and financial incentives.

Over the last 6 years, the number of APPs has grown exponentially. In a recent article published in the New England Journal of Medicine, Auerbach et al. demonstrate that the annual growth of NPs and PAs was 9.6% during the years 2010-2016.[1] The number of APPs is expected to continue to rise through 2030, at an annual rate of 6.8% for NPs and 4.3% for PAs. This expansion of APPs is expected to outpace full-time physician growth, which is anticipated to be slightly higher than 1% per year. This chapter will look at the history, utilization, and outcome studies of APPs.

## HISTORY AND DEVELOPMENT OF ADVANCED PRACTICE PROVIDERS

The role of advanced practice provider (APP) originated in the early 1900s. In the United States, the first formal education program for nurse anesthetists began in 1909; however, nurse anesthetists have been providing anesthesia in combat zones since the Civil War.[2] In the 1920s, nurse midwives worked in the Appalachian Mountains as part of Kentucky's Frontier Nursing service developed by Mary Breckinridge in response to increasing rural rates of maternal and infant mortality.[2]

In 1932, the first nursing certification program was developed in the US. The clinical nurse specialist (CNS) role is more than 50 years old. Dr. Hildegard Peplau of Rutgers University created the first master's degree program in the field. The CNS provides staff and patients with education and serves as a consultant to improve and enhance evidence-based practice and patient outcomes.

In 1965, Dr Loretta Ford and Henry Silver established the first nurse practitioner (NP) certificate program in Colorado. Dr Ford entered nursing as a public health nurse (PHN) as a teacher of patients and families. During this time, she realized she needed to advance her education. In her letter to the Future of Nursing, she discusses how her practice evolved: "I began to examine my practice as a PHN and the needs of children we were serving in homes, schools, well baby clinics, and other clinics, and realized that we, as nurses, could do more to preserve, promote, protect the health and wellness of children, and prevent disease, disability and injury, if we had advanced preparation in their physical, psychological and social growth in their homes, schools, and the community...so the Pediatric Nurse Practitioner model of Advanced Practice in Nursing was born. This model soon gravitated to all other healthcare institutions, hospitals with inpatient neonatal and specialty units, as well as university health services, and all other services."[3]

Similarly, the role of physician assistant (PA) was created in the mid-1960s by Dr Eugene Stead at Duke University to remedy physician shortages in primary care, especially in rural areas. Utilizing Navy corpsmen with a medical background, he created a 2-year intensive curriculum for PAs with an emphasis in general medicine.[4]

In the late 1970s, NPs and PAs began treating the specific needs of critically ill neonates in the US. A neonatal nurse practitioner (NNP) is a registered nurse (RN) with a master's degree, advanced academic training, and experience specific to neonatology. The role developed with the emergence of neonatal intensive care units (NICUs) and need for providers.

## Competencies

### Neonatal Nurse Practitioner

To gain acceptance into an NNP program, one must be licensed as a RN and have at least 2 years of full-time experience working with neonates in a Level III or IV NICU. Generally, programs have 45 class credits and require 600–700 clinical hours.

NNP programs, both traditional and online, offer prospective candidates either a Master's degree or doctorate in nursing. Currently, there are 39 NNP training programs in the US.[5] In order to practice as an NNP, one must complete the national certification exam and participate in specialty-specific continuing education to renew certification. NNPs practice in collaboration with or under the supervision of licensed and credentialed neonatologists. 23 states and the District of Columbia allow NPs to practice autonomously.[6] In the remaining states, NNPs function as part of a healthcare team and may have their own patients; this varies from state to state.[7] The medical staff bylaws of each hospital will further define the NNP's scope of practice at that institution. In a 2007 joint statement, the American Academy of Pediatrics and National Association of Neonatal Nurse Practitioners (NANNP) endorsed NNPs for delivery of expanded neonatal care for patients and families, highlighting their vital role in thoughtful, holistic patient care.[8]

### Physician Assistant

Physician assistants are medically trained professionals who work collaboratively under the supervision of a physician.[9] The PA curriculum, comprised of both didactic and clinical training fashioned after the medical model, is credentialed in the US by the Accreditation Review Commission on Education for the Physician Assistant (ARC-PA). The average PA program is 26 months, with students completing more than 2,000 hours of clinical rotations before graduation.[4] Currently most PA programs result in a Master's of Science degree; by 2020 this will be true of all programs.[10] Certification then requires completion of a national examination every 10 years and ongoing continuing medical education (100 hours) every 2 years.[4] PAs are licensed to practice medicine and authorized to prescribe medication with some variance in scope of practice based on the state of licensure. Since most programs have a general medicine focus, in order to work in neonatology, PAs are hired and given NICU-specific training on the job. Some PAs choose to complete a postgraduate residency for additional expertise. The first neonatal PA program (which required 9 months to complete) was offered from 1981 until the mid-1990s at the University of Southern California Medical Center.[11] For PAs who wish to practice in neonatology, there are three postgraduate residencies in the United States as of 2018. Each offers a 12-month intensive curriculum focused on didactic lectures and clinical training in the field of neonatology.[12]

## Distribution, Utilization, and Evaluation

Both community and academic hospitals may utilize APPs. Data in 2010 revealed that 94% of surveyed NNPs worked in pediatric specialty care (96% in a NICU) with the remaining 6% practicing in primary care (newborn nurseries and hospital wards).[13] Typical duties for APPs in the United States include daily management of infants, including but not limited to physical exams, plans of care, orders, customizing total parenteral nutrition, performing procedures, neonatal resuscitation, transport, admissions, and discharges. Other duties may include palliative care, research, parent and professional education, leadership, and assistance in outpatient NICU developmental care clinics.[14] The neonatal APP (PA or NNP) must understand neonatal anatomy and physiology, have procedural skills, and display critical decision-making ability. This provider should also facilitate clear communication between medical providers and families, and be willing to work as part of a multidisciplinary team.

APPs are not limited to the hospital environment. Position Statement #3058 from the Neonatal Nurse Practitioner Workforce highlights the contribution that neonatal APPs have made with the neonatal population.[8] Using data to demonstrate outcomes has been important to establish the safety of APP care. Some of this data has helped to identify areas where APPs might be able to positively impact care. Brooten, et al. (2002) identified the integral role of the APP and found that very low birth weight (VLBW) infants <1,500 grams were discharged safely 11 days sooner than patients discharged by MD colleagues. This study demonstrates the safe and effective care NNPs provided, as there was no change in the number of readmissions when compared with their physician colleagues.[15]

Due to mandated changes in the infrastructure of US, medical residency programs[16] and the Affordable Care Act, academic hospitals have been forced to reorganize the workforce of the NICU, and many are planning to increase the number of APPs.[17] When medical resident work hours were reduced, Freed et al. surveyed 68% of children's hospitals (n = 114) to determine how they were handling the change.[13] 48% of these institutions increased the number of pediatric NPs, and 42% increased the number of NNPs. In addition, 25% of the surveyed children's hospitals planned to increase the number of PAs over the following 2 years.

Since the employment of APPs, there have been numerous studies to evaluate their role, beginning with a focus on competency and then shifting to quality and financial incentives. Most comparison trials of APPs to residents have demonstrated that they provide as good if not improved care.[11,18-22] Specifically, studies have looked at knowledge, clinical skills, communication, mortality, ventilator days, and length of stay. Additional studies have explored complication rates, quality of care, parent satisfaction, long-term outcomes, and costs. Bissinger and colleagues confirmed the equality of care among practitioners and residents, with a costs savings of $18,240 per patient when care is provided by an APP.[20]

When examining The Office of Technology Assessment study of APPs, Brooten et al. found that APPs are capable of providing 90% of pediatric primary care and 75% of adult care services, and that nurse midwives are 98% as productive as physicians in providing obstetric care.[22] Since APPs are reimbursed at a lower rate, this saves healthcare dollars. APPs order fewer tests and have better patient outcomes in areas such as preventative services, health promotion, quality of life, and patient satisfaction. Patients receiving continued care from APPs had fewer emergency room visits and shorter hospital stays.[23]

Newhouse et al. performed a systematic review of all US randomized control trials (RCTs) and observational studies from 1990-2008 to compare outcomes of two groups: (1) Advanced practice registered nurses (APRNs) and NPs working alone/in teams, and (2) other providers working alone/in teams.[21] The researchers assessed study quality using the Jadad scale (also known as Jadad scoring or the Oxford quality scoring system, used to independently assess the methodological quality of a clinical trial through a three-point questionnaire)[24,25] and additional quality criteria for the observational studies. 107 studies met inclusion criteria [NP: 49; CNS: 22; certified nurse midwife (CNM): 23; certified registered nurse anesthetist (CRNA): 4; and CNS and NP combined: 9]. The researchers also included 20 randomized control studies and 49 observational studies. Results were categorized by the following outcomes for NPs: patient satisfaction, self-reported perceived health, functional status, glucose control, lipid control, blood pressure, erectile dysfunction (ED) or urgent care visits, hospitalization, duration of ventilation, length of stay, and mortality. In all the above categories, there was a high level of evidence to support equivalent levels of care among NPs and MDs, with the exception of duration of mechanical ventilation and length of stay, both found to be equivalent in comparison of NPs and MDs.[21]

Compared with physicians, births assisted by CNMs result in fewer cesarean sections, have comparable rates of low Apgar scores, less epidural usage, less labor augmentation, and comparable rates of low birth weight infants. The studies found that women who deliver using CNMs have higher rates of vaginal birth after cesarean sections, lower third- and fourth-degree perineal lacerations, lower rates of NICU admission, and higher breastfeeding rates.

These studies and comparisons help to demonstrate the cost-effectiveness and high quality of care provided by APRNs. Strictly controlled resident work hours, the reduction of medical providers, and the Affordable Care Act all require healthcare systems to reevaluate the scope and practice of providers in the medical system.

The Federal Trade Commission report in April 2014 estimated that the United States' supply of primary care providers would need to increase by 2.5% in 2014 to accommodate the growing need for these providers. This Federal Trade Commission paper discusses the reports by the Institute of Medicine, National Governors Association, and the US Office of Technology Assessment where NPs were found to perform as well as physicians in primary care with similar health outcomes. As a result, all these agencies have recommended increasing the number of NPs and allowing them to practice to the fullest extent of their education.[6]

## Consensus Model

The APRN consensus model is an effort to standardize licensure, accreditation, certification, and education of APRNs by 2015. Today many states have implemented portions of the model, with variation from state to state.[26,27] Adopting the Consensus model would allow APRNs to swell the ranks of providers and ease the national provider shortage. Centers for Medicare and Medicaid Services (CMS) also have implemented the Graduate Nurse Education Demonstration Project.[28] This project was designed to help increase the base of primary care providers in the country. Much like medical residency programs, CMS chose five hospitals to participate: Hospital of the University of Pennsylvania, Duke University Hospital, Scottsdale Healthcare Medical Center, Rush University Medical Center, and Memorial Hermann-Texas Medical Center Hospital.[28] CMS provided reimbursement for training APRNs at these hospitals, allocating $50 million for fiscal years

2012-2015. The hospitals partnered with academic training programs and payment was linked directly to the increase in advanced practice nursing (APRN or APN) students.[28,29] The evaluation requested by CMS notes the cost for training a NP ranges from $28,000 to $57,000. The cost of training a primary care resident is $157,602.

## Global Use of Advanced Practice Providers

Countries across the world have sought to utilize APPs for reasons similar to the US; a shortage of medical doctors, rising healthcare costs, and need for expert patient care. Globally, APPs may be NPs, PAs, clinical officers, and medical assistants, among other healthcare providers. Nations such as Canada, Australia, New Zealand, the United Kingdom, Ireland, and Finland have well-established advanced nursing practice roles at the graduate or postgraduate level. Taiwan, Hong Kong, Korea, Japan, Singapore, and Thailand also have APNs with required graduate or postgraduate degrees.[30,31] Other countries are evaluating and attempting to utilize a similar role (adapted to their needs).[32] There are challenges to initiating and sustaining APP programs, including differing education and training opportunities, cultural and institutional barriers, and lack of understanding or respect for the role of APP.[33]

Doctorate level nursing programs exist in many Latin American countries, but the role of APN is not yet fully established.[34] Colombia, Chile, Brazil, and Mexico have begun to discuss introducing the APN role into their national healthcare model.[35] Although there is no formal APN program in Israel, many nurses, such as those on kibbutzes, essentially function as NPs. The People's Republic of China has introduced nursing programs designed to train APNs and has recently elevated the status of nursing.[33] Official steps to increase recognition of the APN/APP role will help overcome some of the barriers to sustaining APP programs.

The International Council of Nurses (ICN) was formed in 2000 to facilitate communication worldwide as advanced practice nursing roles have been increasing over the last few decades. The ICN defines APNs as individuals "who have acquired the expert knowledge base, complex decision-making skills, and clinical competencies for expanded practice, the characteristics of which are shaped by the context or country in which they are credentialed to practice. A master's degree is recommended as entry level."[31] Working together with all country members, the ICN is helping to establish international standards for APNs, an important step in promoting their role in healthcare.

Similar to studies performed in the US, studies in Canada and the United Kingdom have shown support by neonatologists of APPs for their contribution to neonatal care.[18] When comparing practitioners with medical doctors, multiple studies found that their outcomes were often of equal quality, if not better.[18] Like North America, the United Kingdom also has had challenges with maintaining appropriate staffing ratios in their neonatal units, and hospitals have had to evaluate and invest in alternative solutions such as advanced NNPs and PAs. For implementation, strategic planning is key from an educational perspective and for recruitment, integration, and sustainability.[32]

## CONCLUSION

Neonatal nurse practitioners and PAs have demonstrated that APPs provide expert and cost-effective care. Studies have supported that APPs enhance quality of care, and enable improved patient outcomes. Originally, an answer to a physician shortage, APPs have impacted the medical ecosystem in a significant way that was not predicted.[13,18-21] It is anticipated that growth for APPs will outpace that of their physician colleagues by 2030.[1,36] Given the current climate in healthcare, utilization of APPs will continue to increase, providing cost-effective quality care to patients in the NICU and beyond.

## REFERENCES

1. Auerbach DI, Staiger DO, Buerhaus PI. Growing Ranks of Advance Practice Clinicians—Implications for the Physician Workforce. N Engl J Med. 2018;378:2358-60.
2. Cronenwett L, Dracup K, Grey M, et al. The doctor of nursing practice: A national workforce perspective. Nursing Outlook. 2011;59:9-17.
3. Institute of Pediatric Nursing. Dr. Loretta Ford's letter to the future of nursing. [online] Available from www.ipedsnursing.org/students/kick-start-your-pediatric-nursing-career/loretta-ford. Last Accessed September, 2019.
4. National Commission on Certification of Physician Assistants. About Us: Purpose and Mission. [online] Available from www.nccpa.net/About. Last Accessed September, 2019.
5. National Association of Neonatal Nurses. APRN Graduate Programs. [online] Available from http://NANN.org/professional-development/graduate-programs. Last Accessed September, 2019.
6. Federal Trade Commission (2014). Policy Perspectives Competition and the Regulation of Advanced Practice Nurses. [online] Available from www.ftc.gov/policy/reports/policy-reports/commission-and-staff-reports?page=4. Last Accessed September, 2019.
7. American Association of Nurse Practitioners. State Practice Environment (interactive map). [online] Available from https://www.aanp.org/legislation-regulation/state-legislation/state-practice-environment. Last Accessed September, 2019.
8. National Association of Neonatal Nurses. Neonatal Nurse Practitioner Workforce Position Statement #3058. NANNP council August 2012; NANN Board of Directors January 2013. [online] Available from http://nann.org/about/position-statements. Last Accessed September, 2019.

9. American Academy of Physician Assistants. What is a PA? [online] Available from https://www.aapa.org/what-is-a-pa/. Last Accessed September, 2019.
10. Accreditation Review Commission on Education for the Physician Assistant, Inc. ARC-PA Standards Degree Deadline Issue. [online] Available from: https://ind01.safelinks.protection.outlook.com/?url=http%3A%2F%2Fwww.arc-pa.org%2Fwp-content%2Fuploads%2F2019%2F07%2FAccredManual-4th-edition.rev6_.19.pdf&data=02%7C01%7Cpm.a%40jaypeebrothers.com%7C268b29f9d00042ca6a3108d78247e14c%7C9e7fa850fd9547b7bda2a51c357d60ae%7C0%7C1%7C637121117546738395&sdata=vNqJwE4eYH3c9%2BL%2Fk4r96KgzBebQ7bL28YHhjNe0maY%3D&reserved=0" http://www.arc-pa.org/wp-content/uploads/2019/07/AccredManual-4th-edition.rev6_.19.pdf
11. Reynolds E, Bricker J. Nonphysician Clinicians in the Neonatal Intensive Care Unit: Meeting the Needs of Our Smallest Patients. Pediatrics. 2007;119:361-9.
12. The Association of Postgraduate PA Programs. Postgraduate PA Program Listings. [online] Available from www.appap.org/post-graduate-pa-programs/programs/. Last Accessed September, 2019.
13. Freed G, Dunham K, Lamarand K, et al. Neonatal Nurse Practitioners: Distribution, Roles, and Scope of Practice. Pediatrics. 2010;126(5):856-60.
14. Vasquez E, Pitts K, Mejia N. A Model Program: Neonatal Nurse Practitioners Providing Community Health Care for High-Risk Infants. Neonatal Network. 2008;27(3):163-9.
15. Brooten D, Naylor M, York R, et al. Lessons learned from testing the Quality Cost Model of Advanced Practice Nursing (APN) Transitional Care. J Nurs Scholars, 2002;34(4):369-75. Available from https://www.ncbi.nlm.nih.gov/pmc/articles/PMC3575196/. Last Accessed September, 2019.
16. Accreditation Council for Graduate Medical Education. Program requirements: Pediatrics. [online] Available from: https://ind01.safelinks.protection.outlook.com/?url=https%3A%2F%2Fwww.acgme.org%2FSpecialties%2FProgram-Requirements-and-FAQs-and-Applications%2Fpfcatid%2F16%2FPediatrics&data=02%7C01%7Cpm.a%40jaypeebrothers.com%7C268b29f9d00042ca6a3108d78247e14c%7C9e7fa850fd9547b7bda2a51c357d60ae%7C0%7C1%7C637121117546748390&sdata=1AL%2BxgwMzYz85LN8TStmlDmHwY99mZB2PmAtQsJTRpQ%3D&reserved=0" https://www.acgme.org/Specialties/Program-Requirements-and-FAQs-and-Applications/pfcatid/16/Pediatrics
17. Freed G, Dunham K, Moran L, et al. Resident Work Hour Changes in Children's Hospitals: Impact on Staffing Patterns and Workforce Needs. Pediatrics. 2012;130:700-4.
18. Fry M. Literature review of the impact of nurse practitioners in critical care services. Nursing in Critical Care. 2011;16(2):58-66.
19. Geiss D, Cavaliere T. Neonatal Nurse Practitioners Provide Quality, Cost-Effective Care. Pediatric Annals. 2003;32:577-83.
20. Bissinger R, Allred C, Arford P, et al. A Cost-Effectiveness Analysis of Neonatal Nurse Practitioners. Nursing Economics. 1997;15:92-9.
21. Newhouse R, Stanik-Hutt J, White K, et al. Advanced Practice Nurse Outcomes 1990-2008: A systematic review. Nursing Economics. 2011;29:1-21.
22. Johnson P. The history of the neonatal nurse practitioner: reflections from "under the looking glass". Neonatal Network. 2002;21:51-60.
23. Brooten D, Youngblut J, Kutcher J, et al. Quality and the nursing workforce: APNs, patient outcomes and health care costs. Nursing Outlook. 2004;(52):45-52.
24. Jadad A, Moore R, Carroll D, et al. Assessing the quality of reports of randomized clinical trials: is blinding necessary? Control Clin Trials. 1996;17(1):1-12.
25. PMID CALC online calculators. Oxford Quality Scoring System. [online] Available from www.pmidcalc.org/8721797/. Last Accessed September, 2019.
26. American Nurses Credentialing Center. APRN State Law and Regulation. Available from https://nursingworld.org/practice-policy/advocacy/state/aprn-state-law-and-regulation/. Last Accessed September, 2019.
27. Phillips S. APRN consensus model implementation and planning. 24th Annual Legislative Update. Nurse Pract. 2012;37:22-24.
28. Centers for Medicare & Medicaid Services. Graduate Nurse Education Demonstration. [online] Available from https://www.cms.gov/newsroom/fact-sheets/graduate-nurse-education-demonstration-0. Last Accessed September, 2019.
29. Aiken L, Dahlerbruch J, Todd B, et al. The Graduate Nurse Education Demonstration—Implications for Medicare Policy. N Engl J Med. 2018;378:2360-3.
30. Delamaire M, Lafortune G. "Nurses in Advanced Roles: A Description and Evaluation of Experiences in 12 Developed Countries", OECD Health Working Papers, No. 54. Paris: OECD Publishing; 2010. Available from http://dx.doi.org/10.1787/5kmbrcfms5g7-en. Last Accessed September, 2019.
31. Sheer B, Wong F. The development of advanced nursing practice globally. J Nurs Scholars. 2008;3:204-11.
32. Smith S, Hall M. Advanced neonatal nurse practitioners in the workforce: a review of evidence to date. Arch Dis Child Fetal Neonatal Ed. 2011;96:F151-5.
33. Kleinpell R, Scanlon A, Hibbert D, et al. Addressing Issues Impacting Advanced Nursing Practice Worldwide. Online J Issues Nurs. 2014;19(2):5. Available from http://ojin.nursingworld.org/MainMenuCategories/ANAMarketplace/ANAPeriodicals/OJIN/TableofContents/Vol-19-2014/No2-May-2014/Advanced-Nursing-Practice-Worldwide.html. Last Accessed September, 2019.
34. Rodriguez J. The challenges of developing the nurse practitioner role in Puerto Rico. INP/APN Network Bulletin 3, September 2004. [online] Available from https://international.aanp.org/Content/Bulletins/Sept04.pdf. Last Accessed September, 2019.
35. Zug K, Cassiani S, Pulcini J, et al. Advanced practice nursing in Latin America and the Caribbean: regulation, education and practice. Rev Lat Am Enfermagem. 2016;24:e2807. Available from https://www.ncbi.nlm.nih.gov/pmc/articles/PMC4990050/. Last Accessed September, 2019.
36. Sullivan Cotter and Associates, Inc. Infographic: 2017 Advanced Practice Clinician Compensation and Pay Practices Survey. [online] Available from https://www.sullivancotter.com/infographic-2017-advanced-practice-clinician-compensation-and-pay-practices-survey/. Last Accessed September, 2019.

# CHAPTER 8

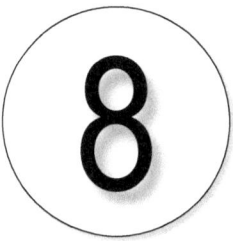

# Pediatric Hospital Medicine and its Evolution in the United States

Susan Flesher

## ABSTRACT

The field of pediatric hospital medicine, the newest subspecialty in pediatrics, is dedicated to providing holistic care for complex hospitalized children. Pediatric hospitalists are increasingly used in hospital settings, as they can focus on ill patients that require more of a doctor's time and attention than patients of yesterday. A number of programs have emerged to teach pediatric hospital medicine (PHM), and certification will soon become available. Addition of PHM positions to hospital staff frees primary care doctors to concentrate on patients outside of the hospital, leading to better results for their patients and less cost. In addition to intensivists (PICU and NICU), nurse practitioners, and physician assistants, PHM promises great contributions to the value of pediatric inpatient medicine.

## HISTORY OF HOSPITAL MEDICINE

The term "hospitalist" was first used in 1996 by Wachter and Goldman[1] to describe the role of a physician who assumes care of patients from primary care doctors when the patient needs hospital care. The hospitalist then has full responsibility for managing care of the hospitalized patient. Once the patient is discharged from the hospital, responsibility is returned to the primary care doctor. Most hospitalists have had their primary training in internal medicine, family practice or pediatrics.[2] One way to view hospitalists is that they are defined by the site where they practice, rather than by a certain organ system. Though recently designated subspecialists, hospitalists are still generalists overseeing all care of the patient, and will consult subspecialists such as gastroenterologists and neurologists while still being the overall decision-maker.[3]

Originally PHM was a very small entity compared to its adult counterpart. The organization and initial growth of pediatric hospital medicine can be traced to the first PHM meeting in 2003.[4] The first three PHM fellowships were started that year in Boston, Washington DC, and Cincinnati. This is a key difference from adult hospitalists, who do not have fellowship training but only tracts in residency programs. As of 2008, internal medicine still dominated the field; 80% of hospitalists were internists, about 10% had subspecialty training, 5% were pediatricians, and 5% family medicine.[5]

The focus on fellowship training has allowed PHM to grow rapidly and has been an impetus for its recognition as a separate pediatric subspecialty. By 2013, the number of PHM fellowships grew to twenty; by 2014 there were thirty-one, and by 2017 there were thirty-four. In November 2015, The American Board of Pediatrics (ABP) voted to establish a recognized 2-year pediatric hospital medicine fellowship. A year later in November 2016, The American Board of Medical Subspecialties (ABMS) granted recognition of the ABP sponsored application to approve subspecialty status and certification for PHM.[6] As of 2019, the ABP has established a procedure for certification in PHM, with the first examination due in November 2019.

The ABP has submitted an application to the Accreditation Council for Graduate Medical Education (ACGME) to request that it will begin a process to accredit

PHM training programs. AGME has distributed proposed program requirements, and PHM fellowships will soon be eligible to apply for accreditation. Residents entering hospital medicine programs before this process is complete are advised to enter programs with faculty that possess appropriate qualifications or are certified in PHM (once certification is available).

Currently, PHM is very solidly established; there are now approximately 4,000–4,500 pediatric hospitalists in the United States.[7] Ninety-eight percent of hospitals associated with academic departments of pediatrics have dedicated PHM services.[8]

## WHY HOSPITAL MEDICINE?

Most hospitalist programs were introduced for efficiency and cost-effectiveness, and to achieve better outcomes at lower costs than a primary care doctor with responsibilities outside the hospital. Hospitalist care was linked to decreased length of stay with greater patient throughput.[9] As previously mentioned, the PHM leadership focus on fellowship training served as a driving force in the rapid growth of PHM, but on a day-to-day, practical level three other factors related to economics and changes in practice influenced this growth, namely, changes in the makeup of inpatient population, changes in outpatient practice, and ongoing healthcare policy.[8]

First, pediatric inpatient populations have developed a higher level of acuity, with more children admitted with medically complex and chronic conditions.[10] Many healthy children with common pediatric conditions that in years past were hospitalized are now managed as outpatients.[8] Successful vaccination use has decreased the incidence of many conditions previously requiring hospitalization. In light of these changes, it is now common to find seriously ill children, such as those with newly diagnosed osteomyelitis, technology-dependent conditions, and multiple comorbidities in the hospital inpatient service, rather than cases of simple dehydration or pneumonia. The increasingly complex hospitalized patients are difficult for outpatient physicians to find time to manage.

At the same time, pediatric outpatient practice has been changing, with increased numbers of visits related to mental health and behavioral issues.[8] Ten years ago, one-fourth of pediatric outpatient visits were for these issues, but now greater than one half of visits to outpatient pediatricians are for mental health and behavioral concerns.[11] Just as current inpatients are requiring more time, outpatients are as well, making it increasingly difficult for the same physician to juggle both types of patient.

While these changes were happening in inpatient and outpatient care, United States health policy also was initiating many advances related to the Affordable Care Act, with overall goals to improve quality, access, and outcomes. These changes have not impacted pediatric medicine to the degree they have adult medicine, but there is more pressure for outpatient pediatricians to see additional patients and to achieve quality benchmarks, and for inpatient physicians to increase efficiency.[12] Where one physician used to see both inpatients and outpatients, these pressures are leading to a division of labor between outpatient physicians and hospitalists to allow each to focus on achieving desired goals in their respective areas. Evidence suggests that patients cared for by hospitalists have decreased length of stay, per-patient costs, and 10% less resource use, as compared to patients cared for by general pediatricians[13-16] This occurs without an adverse effect on 7-day readmissions or mortality. In regard to quality, hospitalists are more likely to follow nationally established guidelines for conditions such as asthma,[17] gastroenteritis,[17] urinary tract infections,[17,18] and bronchiolitis.[17,19,20]

## MAJOR PHM ACCOMPLISHMENTS

Accomplishments in PHM include the establishment of the Pediatric Research in Inpatient Settings Network (PRIS) in 2002. PRIS goals are to "improve the health of hospitalized children, define the national agenda for pediatric research and give better outcomes to hospitalized children."[21] PRIS is a research network with over 120 hospitals and 800 hospitalists participating, and has received over $26 million in research funding over the past 8 years. Compiling data from multiple hospitals, PRIS has had a major impact in changing medical practice. For example, a series of PRIS studies looked at the use of oral versus IV antibiotics in complicated pneumonia,[22] osteomyelitis,[23] and complicated appendicitis.[24] Results showed that early conversion to oral antibiotics for these three diagnoses did not have higher failure rates, and lowered adverse reactions and PICC line complications. The evidence supported a major change in how hospitalists care for ill children, allowing them earlier discharge with no need for a PICC line.

Another major accomplishment of PHM was the establishment in 2008 of the Value in Inpatient Pediatrics (VIP) network. This network is now a part of the American Academy of Pediatrics (AAP) but was initiated as a grass roots organization by a group of concerned pediatric hospitalists. The mission is "to improve the value of care delivered to any pediatric patient in a hospital bed by helping providers implement clinical practice guidelines and other best practices, with a special focus on eliminating harm and waste caused by over utilization."[25] VIP helps hospitalists to implement practice guidelines, particularly when they are practicing in an organization with limited resources available for improvement projects. Projects have included Reducing Excessive Variability in Infant Sepsis Evaluation (REVISE),[26] and the Improving Community-Acquired Pneumonia (ICAP) management project.[27]

As clinical leaders in children's hospitals, pediatric hospitalists and other hospital leaders have created the Children's Hospitals' Solutions for Patient Safety. This is a group of more than 135 children's hospitals who align to achieve safety goals by not letting competition stand in the way of sharing best safety practices. Quality improvement science methods are used to reduce "adverse drug events, catheter-associated urinary tract infections, central line-associated bloodstream infections, injuries from falls and immobility, peripheral intravenous infiltration and extravasations, pressure injuries, surgical site infections, ventilator-associated events, venous thromboembolism, unplanned extubations, *Clostridium difficile* and antimicrobial stewardship, and nephrotoxic acute kidney injury."[28]

Pediatric hospitalists have also joined forces with the Society of Hospital Medicine (SOHM) Choosing Wisely campaign. This campaign has its roots within the National Physicians Alliance and the American Board of Internal Medicine (ABIM). Two examples of areas affected are not routinely treating gastroesophageal reflux in infants with acid suppression and not routinely using bronchodilators in children with bronchiolitis.[29]

## ROLE OF THE PEDIATRIC HOSPITALIST AND THE FUTURE OF PHM

The AAP defines a pediatric hospitalist as "pediatrician who works primarily in hospitals. They care for children in many areas, including the pediatric ward, labor and delivery, the newborn nursery, the emergency department, the neonatal intensive care unit and the pediatric intensive care unit."[30]

The role of the hospitalist continues to expand. In addition to working with primary care physicians, hospitalists often comanage patients with medical and surgical subspecialists (e.g. pediatric neurology, pediatric surgery, and orthopedics), provide inpatient consults and lead rapid-response teams. Particularly in community hospitals and even in a growing number of academic centers, hospitalists provide care in intensive care units under the indirect supervision of neonatologists or pediatric intensivists. They are involved in procedure and sedation teams. A 2017 survey of 220 pediatric hospitalist programs shows the diverse work settings of hospitalists.[31]

While hospitalists may first come to mind as working in pediatric inpatient settings (and many of the major accomplishments of hospitalists have been in the inpatient world), the role of the hospitalist in intensive care settings is expanding. One reason hospitalists have found a niche in the NICU is the decreasing work hours of pediatric residents in that setting. Although further research is needed, pediatric hospitalists likely increase efficiency and decrease costs in the NICU,[32,33] just as they do on inpatient pediatric service and in the wellborn nursery.[34]

This is an exciting time for PHM, with its recognition as a subspecialty complete with an examination for board certification. As PHM fellowships achieve accreditation, the education and scholarly activity of hospitalists will continue to be refined. There is still much work to be done. While the clinical research and quality improvement activities of hospitalists over the past 20 years is impressive, there is still variation in therapies that allows for more streamlining of best practices.[35] The NICU is a particular area for quality and research growth as the majority of hospitalist scholarly work has been in the pediatric inpatient area, perhaps because hospitalists have been in leadership positions in pediatric inpatient units whereas in the NICU they are working under the leadership of neonatologists. This situation should not, however, impede future collaboration.

## REFERENCES

1. Wachter RM, Goldman L. The emerging role of "hospitalists" in the American health care system. N Engl J Med. 1996;335(7):514-17.
2. Lindenauer PK, Pantilat SZ, Katz PP, et al. Hospitalists and the practice of inpatient medicine: results of a survey of the National Association of Inpatient Physicians. Ann Intern Med. 1999;130:342-49.
3. Li JM. Evolution of hospital medicine as a site-of-care specialty. Virtual Mentor. 2008;10(12):829-32.
4. Lye PS, Rauch DA, Ottolini MC, et al. Pediatric hospitalists: report of a leadership conference. Pediatrics. 2006;117(4):1122-30.
5. Society of Hospital Medicine. (2008). 2007-2008 SHM survey: state of the hospital medicine movement. [online] Available from http://www.hospitalmedicine.org/AM/Template.cfm?Section=Survey&Template=/CM/HTMLDisplay.cfm&ContentID=18410. [Last Accessed November, 2019].
6. American Board of Medical Specialties Press Release. (2016). American Board of Medical Specialties officially recognizes pediatric hospital medicine subspecialty certification. [online] Available from https://www.abms.org/news-events/abms-officially-recognizes-pediatric-hospital-medicine-subspecialty-certification/. [Last Accessed November, 2019].
7. Fromme HB, Chen CO, Fine BR, et al. Pediatric hospitalist workload and sustainability in university-based programs: results from a national interview-based survey. J Hosp Med. 2018;13(10):702-5.
8. Barrett DJ, McGuinness GA, Cunha CA, et al. Pediatric hospital medicine: a proposed new subspeciality. Pediatrics. 2017;139(3): e20161823.
9. Bellet PS, Whitaker RC. Evaluation of a pediatric hospitalist service: impact on length of stay and hospital charges. Pediatrics. 2000;105(3 Pt 1):478-84.

10. Berry JG, Hall M, Hall DR, et al. Inpatient growth and resource use in 28 children's hospitals; a longitudinal, multi-institutional study. JAMA Pediatr. 2013;167(2):170-7.
11. Cooper S, Valleley RJ, Polaha J. Running out of time: physician management of behavioral health concerns in rural pediatric primary care. Pediatrics. 2006;118(1):e132-e138.
12. Burwell SM. Setting value-based payment goals – HHS efforts to improve U. S. health care. N Engl J Med. 2015;372(10): 897-99.
13. Srivastava R, Landrigan CP, Ross-Degnan, et al. Impact of a hospitalist system on length of stay and cost for children with common conditions. Pediatrics. 2007;120(2):267-74.
14. Landrigan CP, Conway PH, Edwards S. Pediatric hospitalists: a systematic review of the literature. Pediatrics. 2006;117(5):1736-44.
15. Bekmezian A, Chung PJ, Yazdani S. Staff-only pediatric hospitalist care of patients with medically complex subspecialty conditions in a major teaching hospital. Arch Pediatr Adolesc Med. 2008;162(10):975-80.
16. Mussman GM, Conway PH. Pediatric hospitalist systems versus traditional models of care: effect on quality and outcomes. J Hosp Med. 2012;7(4):350-7.
17. Conway PH, Edwards S, Stucky, et al. Variations in management of common inpatient pediatric illnesses: hospitalists and community pediatricians. Pediatrics. 2006;118(2):441-7.
18. Conway PH, Keren R. Factors associated with variability in outcomes for children hospitalized with urinary tract infection. J Pediatr. 2009;154(6):789-96.
19. McCulloh RJ, Smitherman S, Adelsky S. Hospitalist and nonhospitalist adherence to evidence-based quality metrics for bronchiolitis. Hosp Pediatr. 2012;2(1);19-25.
20. Ralston S, Garber M, Narang S. Decreasing unnecessary utilization in acute bronchiolitis care: results from the value in inpatient pediatrics network. J Hosp Med. 2013;8(1);25-30.
21. PRIS. Available from PRISnetwork.org. [Last Accessed November, 2019].
22. Shah SS, Srivastava R, Wu S. Intravenous versus oral antibiotics for post discharge treatment of complicated pneumonia. Pediatrics. 2016;138(6):1-5.
23. Keren R, Shah SS, Srivastava R. Comparative effectiveness of intravenous vs oral antibiotics for post discharge treatment of acute osteomyelitis in children. JAMA Pediatr. 2015;169(2):120-8.
24. Rangel SJ, Anderson BR, Srivastava R. Intravenous versus oral antibiotics for the prevention of treatment failure in children with complicated appendicitis: has the abandonment of peripherally inserted catheters been justified? Ann Surg. 2017;266(2):361-68.
25. AAP. Value in Inpatient Pediatrics (VIP). [online] Available from https://www.aap.org/en-us/professional-resources/quality-improvement/Pages/Value-in-Inpatient-Pediatrics.aspx. [Last Accessed November, 2019].
26. Biondi EA, McCulloh R, Staggs VS. Reducing variability in the infant sepsis evaluation (REVISE): a national quality initiative. Pediatrics. 2019;144(3): e20182201.
27. Parikh K, Biondi E, Nazif J, et al. A multicenter collaborative to improve care of community acquired pneumonia in hospitalized children. Pediatrics. 2017;139(3):2-9.
28. Children's Hospitals' Solutions for Patient Safety. Results. [online] Available from https://solutionsforpatientsafety.org/our-results/. [Last Accessed November, 2019].
29. Choosing Wisely: An initiative of the ABIM Foundation. Society of Hospital Medicine – Pediatric Hospital Medicine. [online] Available from http://www.choosingwisely.org/wp-content/uploads/2015/02/SHM-Pediatric-Choosing-Wisely-List.pdf. [Last Accessed November, 2019].
30. American Academy of Pediatrics. What is a pediatric hospitalist? [online] Available from www.healthychildren.org/English/family-life/health-management/pediatric-specialists/Pages/What-is-a-Pediatric-Hospitalist.aspx. [Last Accessed November, 2019].
31. American Academy of Pediatrics. Section on Hospital Medicine. Pediatric Hospitalists Programs of North America. [online] Available from https://www.aap.org/en-us/Documents/Ped_Hosp_Prgms_Jan_2017.pdf. [Last Accessed November, 2019].
32. Carlson D, Fentzke K, Dawson J. Pediatric hospitalists fill varied roles in the care of newborns. Pediatr Ann. 2003;32(12):802-10.
33. Hermansen MC. Pediatric practice profile. The Hospitalist. 2005;2005(7).
34. Tieder JS, Migita DS, Cowan CA, et al. Newborn care by pediatric hospitalists in a community hospital. Arch Pediatr Adolesc Med. 2008;162(1):74-8.
35. Landrigan CP, Conway PH, Stucky ER. Variation in pediatric hospitalists use of proven and unproven therapies: a study from the Pediatric Research in Inpatient Settings (PRIS) network. J Hosp Med. 2008;3(4):292-8.

CHAPTER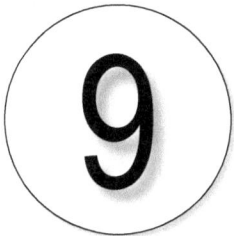

# Home Follow-up of the High-risk Infant

*Rupalee Patel, Adebola Olarewaju*

## ABSTRACT

Globally, infant mortality has declined since 1990, yet 2.9 million infants did not survive the first month of life in 2011. The preterm infant is at high risk for morbidity and mortality through the first year of life and requires intensive follow-up post-hospital discharge. Access to coordinated care, parental empowerment, and establishment of the "medical community" are critical to the well-being of the high-risk infant. International organizations are committed to improving infant survival and recommend home visits by a trained provider for high-risk infants in the hope of decreasing rates of morbidity and mortality. Home visits by advanced practice nurses who bridge inpatient and outpatient infant needs, for example nurse practitioners, can improve health, reduce healthcare costs, improve parent–infant interactions, and can result in optimal growth and development for high-risk infants.

## GLOBAL PERSPECTIVE

The Centers for Disease Control and Prevention, National Center for Health Statistics, has identified that approximately 500,000 premature infants are born in the United States every year.[1] Preterm infants are at an increased risk for morbidity and mortality during the first year of life when compared to healthy term infants. In 2009, the World Health Organization (WHO) and the United Nations International Children's Emergency Fund (UNICEF) published a document addressing how home visits for the newborn child can improve survival rates. While this report looked at newborns in developing countries, the recommendations are very similar to those that have been implemented in developed countries. The WHO and UNICEF recommend home visits for all newborns within the first week of life by trained personnel, in order to assess the infant's and the mother's well-being and to take the necessary steps to decrease infant morbidity and mortality.[2]

## HISTORY

Historically, many industrialized nations have implemented home visitation for the care of preterm and term infants. In most of these countries, home visits are conducted for free, are not income-related, and are often embedded in the maternal-child healthcare systems. Countries that offer extensive home follow-up programs have shown a decrease in infant mortality when compared to those that do not. A home visiting program in Denmark was so successful in decreasing infant mortality that in 1937, the government passed a law requiring that home visits be offered to its citizens. In England, approximately six home visits are performed in the first 5 years of life. France also has healthcare providers who make home visits to the mother–infant dyad. Due to the perceived costs, home-visiting programs in the United States did not begin until the late 19th century.[3] In India and in some African nations, home visitation programs have been developed and implemented to provide care to those mother–infant dyads, who do not have access to a health and hospital system. Furthermore, these programs provide interventions for preventable morbidities such as infection.[4,5]

Overall, when looking at developing countries, most births and neonatal deaths occur at home, especially when families live in areas that are far from healthcare facilities.[6,7] Regardless of whether the mother-infant dyad lives in a developed or developing country, home visitation is an intervention that has the potential to improve access to care, quality of care, and patient outcomes, especially when applied to the premature infant.

## HOME VISITING PROVIDERS

Globally there have been many types of home visiting programs implemented by a variety of different providers for follow-up with the preterm infant. These home visitation delivery providers include and are not limited to paraprofessionals, infant development specialists, medical social workers, nursing students, medical students, public health nurses, midwives, nurse practitioners, and physicians. In areas where there may be a shortage of the "ideal" healthcare provider to conduct home follow-up of the preterm infant, the goal is to identify a provider that can be trained to provide care that targets population-specific needs.

In India as well as in some countries in Africa, home visits are performed by trained village health workers and midwives.[5-7] European countries utilize midwives and nurses to conduct home visits.[3] In the United States, there are currently a variety of home follow-up programs that utilize a range of providers. Some of the most common home visiting providers in the United States are public health nurses, social workers, and infant development specialists.[3,8] However, in the United States, nurse practitioners provide home visits to high-risk infants and high-risk mothers.[9]

## HIGH-RISK INFANTS

According to the American Academy of Pediatrics (AAP 1998), the infants at highest risk for adverse outcomes after Neonatal Intensive Care Unit (NICU) discharge are: (1) Infants born preterm; (2) infants who require technological support; (3) infants primarily at risk because of family issues; and (4) infants whose irreversible conditions will result in death.

Extremely preterm, very low-birth weight, and term infants with complex medical problems are at high risk for neurodevelopmental and medical sequelae.[10] The definition of a "High-risk Infant," for the purpose of this chapter, is based on the California Children's Services medical eligibility criteria (Appendix A). A birth weight of ≤1,500 grams or a gestational age at birth <32 weeks is the most common qualifying criterion. Other criteria include cardiorespiratory depression at birth, prolonged hypoxia, persistent pulmonary hypertension, seizures, or other neurologic abnormalities.[11]

Globally, mothers at highest risk for adverse perinatal outcomes are those living in poverty in a rural or urban setting.[12] Adolescent pregnancy, intellectual disabilities, psychiatric disorders, and lack of prenatal care, all increase the risk of poor maternal and neonatal outcomes. In the United States, studies have shown that mothers at high risk of delivering infants with adverse outcomes tend to be younger, are most likely single, and are less likely to have private insurance, prenatal care, or to have completed high school.[13] Singh and Kogan (2007) reviewed the United States infant mortality statistics that included Very Low-Birth Weight (VLBW) infants between 1969 and 2001 and found that the highest rate of infant mortality occurred with mothers of low socioeconomic status who had not completed high school.[14] These mothers also may have had limited English proficiency, which impacts discharge education learning and comprehension.[15]

The global epidemic of perinatal substance exposure and addiction adversely impacts maternal and neonatal outcomes. In the US, the incidence of Neonatal Abstinence Syndrome (NAS) has increased from 1.20 per 1,000 hospital births to 3.39 per 1,000 hospital births from 2000 to 2009.[16] Infants with NAS typically have mothers who are late to prenatal care and have multiple missed prenatal visits. In many of these cases, child protective agencies have also been involved, and older children are removed from the home. The mothers may have a history of encounters with law enforcement agencies, unstable home environments, and partners who also have issues with substance use. In addition, maternal medical issues and addiction can affect their ability to care for themselves or an infant.

If the home and the family are deemed safe, a qualified healthcare provider should conduct home visits. The home visit allows for assessment of the home environment, assessment of the mother's stability, and compliance with drug treatment programs, if any. The visit also permits assessment of infant feeding, mother-infant bonding, potential neonatal withdrawal symptoms, developmental assessments, comprehensive follow-up, and the ability to make referrals. The provider should have a nonjudgmental approach when working with the mother and infant, and ideally establish a relationship with the family while the infant is inpatient. This approach will increase the likelihood of maintaining contact with the family once the infant is discharged. The rapport built will create a platform of trust between the family and provider, allowing the provider better access to the home. Once the provider establishes this trust, he or she can then follow up on healthcare and developmental needs of the infant, monitor the stability of the home environment, make health and community referrals, monitor maternal health and wellness, and assess mother-infant bonding.

## PARENTAL ANXIETY AND INFANT BONDING

Care of the infant also includes care of the mother. A multidisciplinary team, comprised of representatives from medicine, nursing, and social work, should do an assessment of the home, the family support system and the caregivers while the infant is still inpatient. Parent-infant bonding begins during pregnancy and continues after birth.[17] This bond eventually leads to parent-infant attachment. The initiation of bonding can be affected by parental anxiety, which can begin before or continue post- delivery. Parental concern can be caused by the unexpected delivery of a preterm infant, an infant with an undiagnosed congenital anomaly, or an infant who requires aggressive resuscitation. Anxiety escalates when the infant is separated from the family and admitted to the NICU. The unfamiliar environment of the hospital and the inability to hold their child during the acute phase of the illness hinders parents' natural instincts to take care of their child, which can lead to feelings of inadequacy and interfere with parent–child bonding.[18]

Connections can be maintained through involving caregivers in the infants' daily care at the hospital. While the infant is in the NICU, parents should demonstrate competency in providing care consistently.[19] A teaching plan individualized to each infant and family will aid in parental competence. Anxiety can affect the parent's ability to understand and retain information presented during discharge teaching. Education provided during the home visit reinforces concepts learned at NICU discharge and introduces new concepts based on the infant's stage of development. This plan decreases stress, increases self-efficacy, and enhances positive parent–infant interactions.[20]

Assisting families to have confidence in their abilities to be parents should begin with the NICU admission and continue after discharge through the use of home visits. Studies have shown that 1 month after giving birth, mothers of preterm infants have a greater risk for psychological stress, compared to mothers of term infants.[21] In Switzerland, supporting early positive parent-infant relationships during the first few months of life has shown to be clinically significant.[20] The premature infant's future behavior and development can be impacted by the positive or negative early mother-infant dyad.[19,20] The Durham Connects community-based program and the Home Evidence of Effectiveness study in the United States have been able to demonstrate increased positive parenting behaviors and decreased parental anxiety with home visits.[22]

Parents may continue to feel stressed years beyond the acute phase of their child's illness.[23] Studies have found that up to 6 years after birth, parents still perceive their child as being fragile and vulnerable.[24,25] This may result in ineffective parenting methods, demonstrating a need for provider home visits beyond the first year of life. The high-risk infant potentially will have special health needs through early childhood and beyond, requiring the involvement of specialists, therapists, and social workers. Medication administration, medical supplies, and equipment are a part of the infant's prescribed plan of care. As the infant grows and the needs of the patient and family change, the provider will need to adjust the frequency of home visits, education, and resources provided.

Home visits by a provider can help ease parental anxiety and empower caregivers through reassurance, education, and support. During the home visit and while the patient is enrolled in services, the provider acts as a source of support to caregivers. Support includes linking families to community resources and resources available through the health and hospital system. Providers can also offer reassurance and targeted education to the family, which allows caregivers to have confidence that they are providing the infant optimal care. Furthermore, caregivers can ensure that common deviations in bodily changes and routines are normal. Reassurance can also validate caregiver concerns when they feel that the infant is exhibiting abnormal symptoms. Providers and parents will have confidence in the caregivers' ability to recognize, understand, and respond to the infant's cues. This demonstrates that bonding and attachment has developed between the caregiver and the infant, which preserves the mother-infant dyad.

## DISCHARGE PLANNING

The AAP (2008) has published guidelines on discharge readiness for the NICU graduate. The guidelines include, but are not limited to, assessment of discharge readiness, parental readiness and education, development of a home care plan, communication and follow-up with the primary care provider, and a plan for continued monitoring of growth and development of the infant.[26] The risk of morbidity and mortality of the discharged premature infant or infant with complex medical issues can be minimized by comprehensive discharge planning.

The transition from the hospital to the home requires extensive preparation prior to discharge and intensive follow-up once home. In order to facilitate a smooth transition from the hospital to the home, discharge planning must involve all members of the inpatient and outpatient multidisciplinary teams and must occur soon after admission of the premature infant. The post-hospital discharge home visit is the ideal environment to assess how well the caregivers of the premature infant understand hospital discharge teaching. In circumstances where the premature infant is born at home and there is no access to a health and hospital system, home visitation should take place at birth and teaching should be conducted based on the family's needs and access to care services.

## CARE COORDINATION

Coordination is defined as the organization of patient care activities between the multidisciplinary team members and the patient to facilitate the appropriate delivery of health care services.[27] Organizing care involves coordination of the patients' and caregivers' access to resources, which are needed to carry out all required patient care activities. Care coordination is often guided by the exchange of information among the healthcare providers responsible for different aspects of the patient's care. Poor communication or lack of communication between hospital discharging physicians and primary care providers can contribute to adverse outcomes and the need for readmission.[28-30] It also plays a role in delayed or absent follow-up and failure to order discharge medications.

Care coordination is key to the transition of the high-risk infant from the hospital to the home. A smooth transition from the intensive care unit to the home requires that the families caring for the infants become competent in several key areas, including administering medications, mastering complex feeding regimens, recognizing signs of illness or instability that may indicate the need for medical attention, and navigating the outpatient healthcare system. All these activities are time-consuming to coordinate but are important to ensure successful transition from the hospital to the home and to lessen the risk of preventable morbidities in the high-risk infant. Involving the multidisciplinary team in the coordination of discharge planning provides additional support for caregivers and secures a smooth transition from the hospital to the home. Once the patient has been discharged to home, care coordination facilitated by a healthcare provider becomes an invaluable service. The home visiting provider must serve as a link between the inpatient and the outpatient setting, as well as facilitate care coordination between the patient and primary care provider.

### Family-centered Care

Family-centered care is defined as shared healthcare decision-making between the family and healthcare provider.[31] This definition of family-centered care is crucial to conducting home visits. A clinician who would like to make home visits must not only be aware of the patient's medical needs but also be aware of the family's social, emotional, and financial needs in order to provide a comprehensive home visit. A critical component of family-centered care is involving the family in the patient's activities of daily living from the beginning of admission so that they can start to become comfortable with providing care for their high-risk infant. Empowering caregivers to play an active role in patient care will help to ease the transition from hospital to home. This may potentially create a platform for the home visiting provider to better understand the educational needs of the caregiver and the patient once home.

### Multidisciplinary Team

The saying that "it takes a village to raise a child" is applicable to the home follow-up of the high-risk infant. Whether the infant is born in a developing country or in an industrialized country, it is vital for patient outcomes that care providers play an active role in the patients' care.[3] The multidisciplinary team should begin preparing a plan for home visitation upon the admission of the patient to the NICU. For the inpatient, this team includes the physicians, nurse practitioners, nurses, physical therapists, respiratory therapists, staff nurses, data coordinators, clerical staff, and administrative staff. The home visiting provider should build rapport with all of the providers that make up the multidisciplinary team. It is important for the home visiting provider to open up an avenue of communication with the multidisciplinary team, as well as to create a platform for experts in their fields to serve as consultants and provide specialized guidance once the patient is discharged home.

The home care provider should know the pediatric healthcare providers, pediatric subspecialists, and therapists in the outpatient setting. This enables the home care provider to have access to those directly involved in the patient's care once discharged and can facilitate the prescribed interventions by the various providers in the home. The ultimate goal is for the home provider to build a bridge between the inpatient and outpatient multidisciplinary teams so that open communication can optimize the patient- and family-centered plan of care.

### Home Visits Facilitating the Building of a Medical Community

The AAP believes that the medical care of infants, children, and adolescents ideally should be accessible, continuous, comprehensive, family-centered, coordinated, compassionate, and culturally effective.[32] The academy also recommends that care should be delivered or directed by well-trained healthcare providers who provide primary care and help to manage and facilitate essentially all aspects of pediatric care. The provider should be acquainted with the child and family prior to visitation and should be able to develop a partnership of mutual responsibility and trust with them. These characteristics exemplify the AAP's definition of a "medical home."

Home follow-up facilitates the establishment of a medical home for children with or without special healthcare needs. The medical home provides: (1) comprehensive care from a community-based team, (2) family-centered care, (3) coordination across the continuum of care, (4) establishment of a forum for problem-solving, (5) increased competence of providers, (6) successful transitions of care, and (7) improved satisfaction for the patient, family, and provider.[30,33-35] Galbraith et al. (2003) found that home visits were more likely to be timely than office visits, thus improving parental satisfaction.[36] They also found that home visits may increase newborn follow-up rates post-discharge for mothers who have barriers to care such as lack of childcare, transportation, long waits for office appointments, and maternal postpartum issues.

Recently the term "medical home" has evolved into the term "medical community." In order to cover all aspects of a high-risk infant's care and coordination, a team approach must be implemented.[37] In order to optimize outcomes for high-risk infants, the avenues for communication between all healthcare providers must be maintained even after discharge. Home follow-up programs can help facilitate communication between inpatient and outpatient care teams. The multidisciplinary discharge coordination team is the ideal group to bridge gaps in communication and optimize discharge. This approach can help build a patient's medical home, which involves all providers that are a part of the patient's medical community. In addition, home follow-up provides an opportunity for home health providers to report on the reality of the patient's ability to adhere to prescribed plans of care based on the home environment and financial resources. The high-risk infant has a tremendous need for community support, and efforts to improve comprehensive delivery of patient-centered community-based services such as home follow-up programs are needed.

## Barriers in Access to Care

Marmot (2009) states that the World Health Organization believes, "Social determinants of health are conditions in which people are born, grow, live, work, and age; these circumstances are shaped by the distribution of money, power, and resources at global, national, and local levels".[38] Globally, the highest maternal and child mortality rates are observed among the marginalized and poor who live in remote or rural areas and have limited access to healthcare services. Mortality rates are also high among the urban poor who have poor living conditions and limited social support networks. Additionally, environmental factors such as overcrowding, poor air quality, and poor sanitary conditions can lead to increased disease transmission. In either rural or urban settings, a lack of quality health services, limited knowledge about health services, lack of access to trained professionals, and inadequate public transportation are all contributing factors to mortality rates.[12] Access to and quality of medical care, maternal health, public health practices, and socioeconomic status have also been linked to infant mortality.[39]

The AAP (2010) guidelines for newborn discharge include assessing and addressing barriers to follow up care.[40] Barriers to access to care include language, cultural norms, lack of understanding of the severity of the child's illness, childcare for other children, transportation, and financial constraints.[36] In the United States, an additional barrier is that children with special healthcare needs have higher out-of-pocket expenses than healthy children.[41] Financial burdens may hinder the families' ability to purchase medical supplies and medications, as well as make co-pays for visits. Families may purposely miss follow-up visits if they know that they have not been able to comply with healthcare instructions due to financial constraints.

Having a child with complex medical issues or preterm birth can result in a significant amount of psychological, emotional, and financial stress to parents and families.[42] Financial stress stems from medical costs that increase with every day spent in the hospital. The strain can also come from early or prolonged maternity leave and loss of wages due to work absences. Families may incur additional costs from transportation, parking, food purchases at the hospital, and childcare for other children.[42]

The home visit can help minimize some possible financial strains felt by caregivers, e.g. providers coming into the home alleviate costs related to transportation. For families who do not have a car, they may have difficulties paying for public transportation (buses, taxis, or trains). If there are young children in the home, the caregiver may not be able to manage the older children, the infant, and the infants' medical supplies or equipment while taking public transportation.

Conducting the visit in the infant's home environment alleviates the need for childcare for the other children. Caregivers who cannot afford to pay someone to watch their children often rely on friends and family members for childcare. Unfortunately, friends and family may not always be available, and this can result in missed appointments, which may be critical to the infant's healthcare maintenance. Home visits also can reduce the need for extra visits with specialists outside of the home. Visits with specialists require transportation to the clinic, create a possible need for childcare, and may require payment. The healthcare provider works closely with outpatient providers and is capable of assessing the infant, providing education, and developing a plan of care in conjunction with the specialist.

There are limited data on adverse effects of family disruption, strain on interpersonal relationships, and alteration in the mental health of parents due to the birth of a preterm baby. Studies have found that it is common for these parents to experience post-traumatic stress symptoms.[42-44] In comparison to parents of healthy-term infants, parents of premature infants experience post-traumatic stress symptoms and demonstrate higher rates of ineffective parenting.[20,45] The stress experienced by parents can be alleviated by social support and a good relationship with healthcare providers.[42]

The home visiting provider will assess the caregivers' strengths and identify areas for improvement. Personal and couple strengths are defined as past learning, problem-solving skills, emotional resiliency, and the quality of their relationship.[42] Strengths should be praised and reinforced during the visit, in order to build confidence, empower caregivers, and build a rapport between the provider and the family. Building rapport makes caregivers more receptive to feedback provided in regards to areas that need improvement. The home visiting provider should outline areas for personal growth to parents or caregivers by reinforcing key concepts and appropriate referrals to resources. Typically, an assessment of parents' strengths and weaknesses can most successfully be performed through a home visit, as numerous constraints can exist in clinical practice visits.

A major limitation of clinical practices is the amount of time providers can spend with a patient and their family. Office visits can also be problem-specific, which makes it difficult to coordinate care in the medical home.[46] Medically complex and vulnerable patients can benefit from coordination of care from extended providers. AAP (2010) follow-up guidelines for primary care are applicable to both the office visit and the home visit. They recommend: (1) Assess the general health of the neonate, (2) assess the quality of mother-infant interaction, (3) assess infant behavior, (4) reinforce maternal and family education in regards to infant care and safety, (5) reinforce breastfeeding (if appropriate), (6) review results of outstanding lab tests including the newborn screen, (7) perform any necessary lab tests, (8) verify the plan for healthcare maintenance and the medical home, and (8) assess parental well-being.[40]

## Advanced Practice Nurse

While infant mortality rates have decreased since 1990, as recently as 2011, 2.9 million infants worldwide did not survive the first month of life. This statistic represented 43% of pediatric deaths for children less than 5 years old.[47] The United Nations Millennium Goal 4 is focused on reducing mortality in children under 5 years old by two-thirds from 1990 to 2015. Countries such as Bangladesh have seen a dramatic reduction in infant mortality since introducing interventions such as training community health workers. Infant mortality declined from 100 deaths per 1,000 live births in 1990 to 33 deaths per 1,000 live births in 2012.[48] Surviving birth is only the first challenge in an infant's life. A child is still at risk for morbidity and mortality during the neonatal and infancy stages, and causes for readmission can be related to minor or major health problems. Through implementation of home visits with advanced practice nurses (APNs), minor issues can be managed so that they do not become major problems.

Generally, preterm infants are discharged when their corrected gestational age is at or near 40 weeks' gestation. However, they continue to have greater medical needs than infants born at term. A study by Paul et al. (2006) looked at the readmission rate of 2,540 newborns in the first 10 days of life in Pennsylvania.[49] The researchers found several variables that made readmission more likely: (1) Primi gravida, (2) Mothers over 30 years old, (3) mothers with diabetes or pregnancy-induced hypertension, (4) original hospital length of stay <72 hours, and (5) prematurity. Results showed that the average readmission occurred 62 hours post-NICU discharge. Jaundice was the most common cause of readmission, followed by feeding problems and dehydration. These diagnoses are preventable/manageable in the home by an APN trained in primary care.

A 2004 study by Naylor et al. paired APNs with elderly heart failure patients who had high risk of hospital readmission.[50] The APN conducted the first home visit the day after discharge. Additional visits were conducted at least weekly for 3 months. A year later, results showed 104 readmissions in the intervention group (home visit group) versus 162 among the control group, resulting in an average cost of savings per patient of $4,845.

Advanced practice nurses can perform assessments, diagnose, prescribe medications, make specialty referrals, and connect families to community resources. These skills will be useful to the infant as he or she transitions to primary care. APNs have knowledge of the preexisting medical conditions and the ability to detect and diagnose common medical conditions in the NICU graduate. APNs can be instrumental in the coordination of care and bridge the communication among primary care and specialty providers. They can also perform developmental assessments and follow-up on the infant's developmental needs.

## A Novel Type of Home Follow-up Program

The Institute of Medicine of the United States recommends a wider use of APNs because research studies have demonstrated that APNs such as nurse practitioners are trained to provide expert medical care, and can reduce patient morbidity while reducing healthcare costs.[51] Home visits by providers also create an opportunity to manage the infant's medical needs in the home, providing preventative care that may not be readily available if the family has difficulty accessing a health and hospital system.

Santa Clara Valley Medical Center's Babies Reaching Improved Development and Growth in their Environment (BRIDGE) program was developed in April 2011 in San Jose, California to facilitate the transition of the high-risk infant to the home by providing visits by a Pediatric Nurse Practitioner (PNP). Prior to NICU discharge, the PNP establishes a relationship with the infant's family and works with the inpatient multidisciplinary team. In the home after discharge, the PNP educates caregivers, prescribes needed medications, triages, makes appropriate appointments, and coordinates care with outpatient clinicians. The practitioner also assesses home feeding, medication, equipment use, and healthcare utilization. Based on the frequency of care errors discovered at home visits, caregiver education was modified to prevent the most common errors.[52]

The main goal of the BRIDGE program is to facilitate the creation of a medical community for the patient and family. Additionally, the program focuses on empowering parents and reducing their anxiety about bringing home a medically fragile infant. One crucial aspect of the program is that the advanced practice provider cares for each patient from the first day of admission. The APN attends clinical rounds, and multidisciplinary team rounds and the provider also rounds at the bedside and meets families prior to the infant's discharge. The advanced practice provider assesses the patient and builds a rapport with the family prior to the patient being discharged to solidify a family-centered care approach, as well as to provide continuity of clinical care. Once discharged, a BRIDGE program visit ideally takes place within 2 weeks of the infant returning home.

Since the implementation of the BRIDGE program, challenges and barriers experienced by families of a medically fragile child have become clearer. The program has also demonstrated to the community how the county hospital truly serves the underserved. Although much has been discovered with regard to the needs of families and patients on a day-to-day basis in the home, there is much more that we are still learning. Programs like BRIDGE can assist in building the ideal medical community for the patient. BRIDGE is a cost-effective and home care follow-up program that can minimize length of hospital stay and healthcare utilization errors.

Home visits by providers who bridge inpatient and outpatient infant needs can improve health, reduce healthcare cost, and may result in optimal growth and development for high-risk infants. In 2011, home error identification led to the development and implementation of transitional care interventions targeted toward hospital staff, patient families, and ambulatory caregivers. In 2012 the number of BRIDGE visits per family was increased to enable evaluation of initial interventions and continued education. By 2013, the added family visits resulted in increased error detection, and errors per family also markedly decreased.[52]

## Process of Home Follow-up

The ideal home visit plan can only be developed once a proper assessment is completed of the patient population that is being served, in conjunction with the patient's resources, access to resources, and home environment. Recommendations for developing and implementing a home follow-up program, specifically in developed countries where preterm infants are discharged from a NICU, require additional considerations.

Before a home visit is scheduled, healthcare providers should complete a comprehensive chart review including the patient's past and current medical history, discharge summary, medical social work notes, case manager notes, consults from all specialties, lab results, immunizations, current feeding regimen, medications, equipment, physical therapy recommendations, current contact information, selected pediatrician, pediatric specialty referrals, assigned public health nurse, as well as family history. This information is reviewed so that a highly specialized home visit can cater exactly to the family's needs.

A home visit may take anywhere from 1 hour to 2 hours, depending on the needs of the family and the patient. The visit should include a full-system physical examination, body measurements (weight, length, and head circumference), and vital signs (heart rate, respiratory rate, blood pressure, temperature, and pain score); review of medications, medical equipment, feeding regimen, prescriptions, and referrals, and education including and not limited to anticipatory guidance, healthcare maintenance, and appointment reminders. A home assessment should be performed at the same time as a car seat safety assessment to help parents create the optimally safe home environment for the child. Furthermore, if the child needs a prescription and/or referral, the provider can complete this for the patient at the time of visit.

Upon completion of the home visit, a detailed comprehensive electronic note should be composed and then disseminated to all involved providers, specialists and therapists. This note should be followed up by an e-mail that is sent to all providers that are involved in the patient's care. An e-mail update should also be sent to the discharging NICU provider and primary nurses that were involved with care while in the NICU. The patient and family's needs and medical necessity determine the number of home visits required. Once patients graduate from the BRIDGE program, their families receive an evaluation to provide anonymous feedback regarding their experience and any recommendations for quality improvement.

Advance Practice Nurses monitor, educate, and attenuate home care errors between home visits over time. Collaborating with families and healthcare providers in the inpatient, home, and outpatient environments, APNs have the potential to improve health, reduce healthcare costs, and optimize growth and development for high-risk infants. The BRIDGE program has led to interventions to improve quality of care, opening a path of communication from the home back to the Health and Hospital Systems that can be applied beyond the NICU. The BRIDGE program utilizing APNs can be used as a home care plan model in a variety of healthcare settings.

## Challenges of Home Follow-up

One of the major challenges of home follow-up includes dealing with "difficult" families. These are families who, for instance, may not want home visits but have been ordered to have them as part of their discharge follow-up. They may also not follow discharge education instructions consistently. Or, they may be families who do not return follow-up phone calls, cancel appointments with less than 24-hours notice, or are "no-shows" when the provider arrives at the home. Telephone access may be limited or non-existent; phones may be sometimes disconnected, or there may be no voicemail or text message access. Migrant families (whether due to farm work or lack of stable housing) are difficult to visit, because the "home" address is always in transition. Another challenge to home follow-up is a families' lack of understanding of the child's medical condition and the need for close follow-up. Also, sometimes families do not fully understand the benefits of additional monitoring and care coordination.

## Overall Benefits

Home follow-up programs provide an ideal situation in which the home care provider can assess the patient and customize interventions that will be implemented in the home environment. Home follow-up programs have been proven successful worldwide.[52,56] Reviewed studies suggest that home visiting for preterm infants promotes improved parent-infant interaction. Home follow-up also provides a solution for barriers to patient care, such as lack of access to care and improper healthcare utilization.

Home follow-up programs may also help improve health care utilization follow-up rates by influencing parental behavior through targeted education. These programs may help with reducing disparities among more vulnerable populations by providing education about the importance of closely monitoring the growth and development of high-risk infants to parents of different socio-economic status.[57] Home visits by a trained provider may also help to educate families about available outpatient pediatric services, especially in non-English speaking families.[15]

## Alternatives to Home Visitation

Globally, home visits may not be feasible in some remote locations. The infrastructure of the country may not provide for adequate road maintenance or lighting to reach patients. Access to these families by mobile phone may be hindered by inadequate network service or by inability to purchase a mobile phone and prepaid minutes. A shortage of trained healthcare professionals in developed and developing countries also affects the number of home visits performed. Providers in war-ravaged nations may face serious safety concerns in addition to a lack of medical supplies. In cases where there are insurmountable barriers to the implementation of home visits, there are some alternatives that providers can consider for continued infant care.

### Telemonitoring

Telemonitoring has been trialed in adults with chronic heart failure. These trials have demonstrated variable effectiveness in reducing hospital readmissions.[58] One study was able to demonstrate reduced hospital readmissions and costs when telemonitoring was used in conjunction with nurse follow-up calls with a small sample size.[59]

### Video Interaction Guidance

A study by Tooten et al. (2012) in the Netherlands is looking at Video Interaction Guidance (VIG) to support parent-infant bonding and empower parents while the infant is hospitalized.[17] Edited video feedback will be used to help parents identify their strengths and achieve their goals. Parents enrolled in this study will have 3–5 sessions of VIG. Results of this study are not available at this time. Similar studies by Scheter et al. (2006) and Madigan et al. (2006) saw an increase in positive caregiver behavior after just two sessions.[60,61]

### Utilization of "Apps"

The new age of applications or "apps" on handheld electronic devices (smart phones, tablets, iPads, etc.) may improve access to care in hard-to-reach populations. The ideal "app" would have options such as: (1) Appointment scheduling, (2) appointment reminders, (3) email access to providers, and (4) medication requests and refills. However, financial constraints related to purchasing the device and/or "app" may be a barrier for low-income and at-risk families.

### Community Health Workers

There is currently a shortage of healthcare providers in economically stable countries and in developing countries. Trained healthcare professionals are needed to meet the demands of the population and to provide adequate care. Community health-worker programs in remote populations depend on training and basic toolkits, but frequently have a shortage of supplies, making the programs less effective.[12] These community health programs are now trying to utilize mobile phones to reach remote populations, screen for biomarkers, and improve drug and vaccine delivery.[12]

A systematic review by Prost et al. (2013) found that trained health workers facilitating women's groups in Nepal, Bangladesh, India, and Malawi have helped create a reduction in neonatal and maternal mortality.[47] There was training for the facilitator and the birth attendant; depending upon the facilitator and country, the groups met monthly, biweekly, or 9-13 times per month. These groups practiced participatory learning in regards to health education. The study found that women's groups were a cost-effective intervention and improved maternal and neonatal survival in rural communities.

### National Programs

In 2012, the Nigerian government launched the *Save One Million Lives By 2015* campaign. The interventions included but were not limited to increasing primary care access for women and children, and providing telephone lines for healthcare workers, equipment to prevent maternal-infant transmission of HIV, and bed nets for malaria prevention.[48]

### Healthcare Facilities in Rural Areas

Madhya Pradesh is the second largest state in India and has the highest infant mortality rate in the country.[48] The state government partnered with the United Nations Children's Fund (UNICEF) to build healthcare facilities in remote areas that would link rural communities to district hospitals. One hospital already has been able to save 6,000 children.[48]

## ■ CONCLUSION

There are a variety of home follow-up programs that are geared toward the continued care of high-risk infants in developing and developed countries. Home follow-up providers manage infant health and help educate caregivers, in order to improve preventative care measures that can result in decreased morbidity and mortality. Regardless of the country or population, home follow-up programs have the unique ability to provide access to care for families in need. Whether in neonatology, pediatrics, or adult medicine, a home healthcare program focused on patient follow-up may result in improved quality of care delivery and improved patient outcomes. Extending care into the home post-hospitalization illuminates challenges patients and families face at home due to care transitions. Further study of interventions targeting preterm infants within existing programs may strengthen the impact and cost benefits of home visiting in at-risk populations.

## ■ APPENDIX A

California Children's Services High-Risk Infant Follow-up Eligibility Criteria:
- Birth weight ≤1,500 grams.
- Gestational age at birth ≤32 weeks.
- Birth weight ≥1,500 grams and gestational age at birth ≥ 32 weeks, with one of the following criteria during the NICU stay:
  - Cardiorespiratory depression at birth (defined as pH <7.0 in an umbilical blood sample or a blood gas, obtained within one hour of life) or an Apgar score ≤3 at 5 minutes.
  - A persistently and severely unstable infant manifesting prolonged hypoxia, acidemia, hypoglycemia and/or hypotension requiring pressor support.
  - Persistent apnea which required medication (e.g. caffeine) for the treatment of apnea at discharge.
  - Required oxygen for more than 28 days of hospital stay and had radiographic finding consistent with chronic lung disease (CLD).
  - Infants placed on extracorporeal membrane oxygenation (ECMO).
  - Infants who received inhaled nitric oxide >4 hours for persistent pulmonary hypertension of the newborn (PPHN).
  - History of documented seizure activity.
  - Evidence of intracranial pathology, including but not limited to—intracranial hemorrhage (grade II or worse), periventricular leukomalacia (PVL), cerebral thrombosis, cerebral infarction, developmental central nervous system (CNS) abnormality, or "other

CNS problems associated with adverse neurologic outcome".
- Other problems that could result in a neurologic abnormality, such as history of CNS infection, documented sepsis, bilirubin in excess of usual exchange transfusion level, cardiovascular instability, hypoxic ischemic encephalopathy, etc.

## REFERENCES

1. Hamilton B, Martin J, Sutton P. Center for Disease Control and Prevention, National Center for Health Statistics. Births: preliminary data for 2003. Natl Vital Stat Rep. 2004;53(9):1-17.
2. World Health Organization. (2009). WHO/UNICEF Joint Statement: Home visits for the newborn child: a strategy to improve survival. Geneva: World Health Organization, USAID and Save the Children. [Online]. Available from http://whqlibdoc.who.int/hq/2009/WHO_FCH_CAH_09.02_eng.pdf?ua=1. [Last accessed September 2019].
3. Council on Child and Adolescent Health; American Academy of Pediatrics. The role of home visitation programs in improving health outcomes for children and families. Pediatrics. 1998;101(3):486-9.
4. Bang AT, Bang RA, Baitule SB, et al. Effect of home-based neonatal care and management of sepsis on neonatal mortality: Field trial in rural India. Lancet. 1999;354(194):1955-61.
5. le Roux IM, Tomlinson M, Harwood JM, et al. Outcomes of home visits for pregnant mothers and their infants: a cluster randomized controlled trial. AIDS. 2013;27(9):1461-71.
6. Bang AT, Bang RA, Stoll BJ, et al. Is home-based diagnosis and treatment of neonatal sepsis feasible and effective? Seven years of intervention in the Gadchiroli field trial (1996 to 2003). J Perinatol: Official Journal of the California Perinatal Association. 2005;25Suppl1(S1);S62-71.
7. Bang AT, Baitule SB, Reddy HM, et al. Low birth weight and preterm neonates: Can they be managed at home by mother and a trained village health worker? J Perinatol. 2005;25Suppl1(S1);S72-81.
8. Goyal NK, Teeters A, Ammerman RT. Home visiting and outcomes of preterm infants: A systematic review. Pediatrics. 2013;132(3):502-16.
9. Beal JA, Tiani TB, Saia TA, et al. The role of the neonatal nurse practitioner in post-NICU follow-up. The J Perinat Neonatal Nur. 1999;131(1):78-89.
10. Hintz SR, Kendrick DE, Wilson-Costello DE, et al. Early-childhood neurodevelopmental outcomes are not improving for infants born at <25 weeks' gestational age. Pediatrics. 2011;127(1):62-70.
11. California Perinatal Quality Care Collaborative. (2018). High Risk Infant Follow-up Quality of Care Initiative. Initiative Manual of Definitions. [Online]. Available from https://www.cpqcc.org/sites/default/files/documents/HRIF_QCI_Docs/2018_HRIF-QCI%20Manual%20of%20Defintions%20v01.18_0.pdf. [Last accessed September 2019].
12. Bhutta ZA, Black RE. Global maternal, newborn, and child health—So near and yet so far. N Engl J Med. 2013;369(23):2226-35.
13. De Jesus LC, Pappas A, Shankaran S, et al. Risk factors for post-neonatal intensive care unit discharge mortality among extremely low birth weight infants. J Pediatr. 2012;161(1):70-4.
14. Singh GK, Kogan MD. Persistent socioeconomic disparities in infant, neonatal, and postnatal mortality rates in the United States, 1969-2001. Pediatrics. 2007;119(4):e928-39.
15. Miquel-Verges F, Donohue PK, Boss R. Discharge of infants from NICU to Latino families with limited English proficiency. J Immigr Minor Health. 2011;13(2):309-14.
16. Patrick SW, Schumaker RE, Benneyworth BD, et al. Neonatal abstinence syndrome and associated health care expenditures: United States, 2000-2009. JAMA. 2012;307(18):1934-40.
17. Tooten A, Hoffenkamp HN, Hall RA, et al. The effectiveness of video interaction guidance in parents of premature infants: A multicenter randomized controlled trial. BioMed Central Pediatrics. 2012;12:76.
18. Heringhaus A, Blom MD, Wigert H. Becoming a parent to a child with birth asphyxia—From a traumatic delivery to living with the experience at home. Int Journal Qual Stud Health Well-being. 2013;8:1-13.
19. Smith VC, Stewart J. Discharge planning for high-risk newborns. Up To Date. 2015:1-12.
20. Forcada-Guex M, Pierrehumbert B, Borghini A, et al. Early dyadic patterns of mother-infant interactions and outcomes of prematurity at 18 months. Pediatrics. 2006;118(1):e107-14.
21. Davis L, Edwards H, Mohay H, et al. The impact of very premature birth on the psychological health of mothers. Early Hum Dev. 2003;73(1-2):61-70.
22. Dodge K, Goodman B. (2012). Durham Connects Impact Evaluation Final Report, Pew Center on the States. [online]. Available from https://www.pewtrusts.org/~/media/legacy/uploadedfiles/pcs_assets/2013/durhamconnectsreportpdf.pdf. [Last accessed September 2019].
23. Singer LT, Salvator A, Guo S, et al. Maternal psychological distress and parenting stress after the birth of a very low-birth-weight infant. JAMA. 1999;281(9):799-805.
24. Estroff DB, Yando R, Burke K, et al. Perceptions of preschoolers' vulnerability by mothers who had delivered preterm. J Pediatr Psychol. 1994;19:709-21.
25. De Ocampo AC, Macias MM, Saylor CF, et al. Caretaker perception of child vulnerability predicts behavior problems in NICU graduates. Child Psychiatry Hum Dev. 2003;34:83-96.
26. Committee on Fetus and Newborn; American Academy of Pediatrics. Hospital discharge of the high-risk neonate. Pediatrics. 2008;122(5):1119.
27. McDonald KM, Sundaram V, Bravata DM, et al. Care coordination. In: Shojania KG, McDonald KM, Wachter RM, and Owens DK, eds. Closing the quality gap: A critical analysis of quality improvement strategies. Technical Review 9 (Prepared by Stanford-UCSF Evidence-Based Practice Center under contract No. 290-02-0017). Vol. 7. Rockville, MD: Agency for Healthcare Research and Quality, June 2007. AHRQ Publication No. 04(07)-0051-7.
28. Forster AJ, Clark HD, Menard A, et al. Adverse events among medical patients after discharge from hospital. CMAJ. 2004;170(3):345-9.
29. Forster AJ, Murff HJ, Peterson JF, et al. The incidence and severity of adverse events affecting patients after discharge from the hospital. Ann Intern Med. 2003;138(3):161-7.

30. Kripalani S, LeFevre F, Philips CO, et al. Deficits in communication and information transfer between hospital-based and primary care physicians: Implications for patient safety and continuity of care. JAMA. 2007;297(8):831-41.
31. Kuo DZ, Houtrow AJ, Arango P, et al. Family-centered care: Current applications and future directions in pediatric health care. Matern Child Health J. 2012;16(2):297-305.
32. Medical Home Initiatives for Children with Special Needs Project Advisory Committee; American Academy of Pediatrics. The medical home. Pediatrics. 2002;110(1Pt1):184-6.
33. American Academy of Pediatrics. Ad Hoc Task Force on Definition of the Medical Home. The medical home. Pediatrics. 2002;90:774.
34. Kelly AM, Kratz B, Bielski M, et al. Implementing transitions for youth with complex chronic conditions using the medical home model. Pediatrics. 2002;110(Suppl3):1322-7.
35. Kisker CT, Fethke CC, Tannous R. Shared management of children with cancer. Arch Pediatr Adolesc Med. 1997;151(10):1008-13.
36. Galbraith AA, Egerter SA, Marchi KS, et al. Newborn early discharged revisted: Are California newborns receiving recommended postnatal services? Pediatrics. 2003;111(2):364-71.
37. Hintz SR, Kendrick DE, Vohr BR et al. Community supports after surviving extremely low-birth-weight, extremely preterm birth: special outpatient services in early childhood. Arch Pediatr Adolesc Med. 2008;162(8):748-55.
38. Marmot M. Closing the health gap in a generation: The work of the commission on social determinants of health and its recommendations. Glob Health Promot. 2009;16(Suppl1):23-7.
39. Bryant AS, Worjoloh A, Caughey AB, et al. Racial/ethnic disparities in obstetric outcomes and care: prevalence and determinants. Am J Obstet Gynecol. 2010;202(4):335-43.
40. American Academy of Pediatrics Committee on Fetus and Newborn. Hospital stay for healthy term newborns. Pediatrics. 2010;125:405.
41. Davidoff AJ. Insurance for children with special health care needs: Patterns of coverage and burden on families to provide adequate insurance. Pediatrics. 2004;114(2):394-403.
42. Lasiuk GC, Comeau T, Newburn-Cook C. Unexpected: An interpretive description of parental traumas associated with preterm birth. BMC Pregnancy and Childbirth. 2013;13(Suppl):S13.
43. Holditch-Davis D, Bartlett TR, Blickman AL, et al. Posttraumatic stress symptoms in mothers of premature infants. J Obstet Gynecol Neonatal Nurs. 2003;32(2):161-71.
44. Pierrhumbert B, Nicole A, Muller-Nix C, et al. Parental post-traumatic reactions after premature birth: implications for sleeping and eating problems in the infant. Arch Dis Child Fetal Neonatal Ed. 2003;88(5):F400-4.
45. Wereszczak J, Miles MS, Holditch-Davis D. Maternal recall of the neonatal intensive care unit. Neonatal Netw. 1997;16(4):33-40.
46. McAllister JW, Presler E, Cooley WC. Practice-based care coordination: a medical home essential. Pediatrics. 2007;120(3) e723-33.
47. Prost A, Colburn T, Seward N, et al. Women's groups practising participatory learning and action to improve maternal and newborn health in low-resource settings: a systematic review and meta-analysis. Lancet. 2013;381(9879):1736-46.
48. United Nations. (2016). United Nations Millennium Goal 4.[Online]. Available from https://www.mdgmonitor.org/mdg-4-reduce-child-mortality/. [Last accessed September 2019].
49. Paul IM, Lehman EB, Hollenbeak CS, et al. Preventable newborn readmissions since passage of the Newborns' and Mothers' Health Protection Act. Pediatrics. 2006;118(6):2349-58.
50. Naylor M, Brooten D, Campbell R, Maislin G, McCauley K, et al. Transitional care of older adults hospitalized with heart failure: A randomized, controlled trial. J Am Geriatr Soc. 2004;52(5):675-84.
51. Mager DD, Neal-Boylan L, Kazer MW. Nurse practitioners in home health care: An update. Home Health Care Management & Practice. 2012;24(4):193-7.
52. Patel R, Olarewaju A, Weiss S, et al. A novel home follow-up program for high-risk infants. Pediatric Academic Societies International Conference, Vancouver, Canada. 2014.
53. Barlow A, Mullan B, Neault N, et al. Effect of a paraprofessional home-visiting intervention on American Indian teen mothers' and infants' behavioral risks: A randomized controlled trial. Am J Psychiatry. 2013;170(1):83-93.
54. Khanal S, Sharma J, GC VS, et al. Community health workers can identify and manage possible infections in neonates and young infants: Mini-a model from Nepal. J Health Popul Nutr. 2012;29(3):255-64.
55. LeFevre AE, Shillcutt SD, Waters HR, et al. Economic evaluation of neonatal care packages in a cluster-randomized controlled trial in sylhet, bangladesh. Bull World Health Org. 2013;91(10):736-45.
56. Vimpani G. Home visiting for vulnerable infants in Australia. J Paediatr Child Health. 2000;36(6):537-9.
57. Wang C, Guttmann A, To T, et al. Neighborhood income and health outcomes in infants: How do those with complex chronic conditions fare? Arch Pediatr Adolesc Med. 2009;163(7):608-15.
58. Chaudry SI, Phillips CO, Stewart SS, et al. Telemonitoring for patients with chronic heart failure: A systematic review. J Card Fail. 2007;13(1):56-62.
59. Jerant AF, Azari R, Nesbitt TS. Reducing the cost of frequent hospital readmissions for congestive heart failure: A randomized trial of a home telecare intervention. Med Care. 2001;39(11):1234-45.
60. Schechter DS, Myers MM, Brunelli SA, et al. Traumatized mothers can change their minds about their toddlers: Understanding a novel use of videofeedback supports positive change of maternal attributions. Infant Ment Health J. 2006;27(5):429-47.
61. Madigan S, Hawkind E, Goldberg S, et al. Reduction of disrupted caregiver behavior using modified interaction guidance. Infant Ment Health J. 2006;27:509-27.

CHAPTER

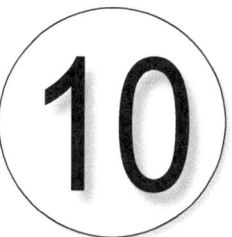

# How Charitable Giving can Enhance Newborn Care

*Elizabeth M Nielsen*

## ABSTRACT

Philanthropy is a proven force for good in global efforts to improve human health. Healthcare institutions can engage charitable organizations and individual philanthropists to build a base of support for research and programs that improve newborn care. By following a defined process for donor research, cultivation, solicitation, and stewardship, healthcare institutions can build or grow a philanthropy program to support under-funded needs within their organizations.

## INTRODUCTION: HOW GLOBAL PHILANTHROPY SUPPORTS MATERNAL AND INFANT HEALTH

Human health can be supported and improved with the help of private funding. Donors are encouraged to support newborn care specifically through a wide range of initiatives taking place both across the world and in their own backyards. Institutional donors and individual philanthropists are important resources for helping healthcare and community organizations achieve improved outcomes in the care of newborns.

## Public Funding

The majority of international aid for newborn health comes from donor countries through international development programs, particularly in supporting efforts to achieve the United Nations Millennium Development Goal 4 (MDG-4) of reducing childhood mortality by two-thirds between 1990 and 2015. This type of global aid architecture primarily addresses goals that are set at the international level.

Through a coordinated and internationally funded effort, countries have achieved promising results. Worldwide between 1990 and 2011, the number of under-5 deaths declined from nearly 12 million to 6.9 million. However, there is still work to do, particularly for neonates whose proportion of under-5 deaths has increased 17% in the same time period.[1] International aid in support of MDG-4 has focused on regions where the majority of under-5 deaths occur, including sub-Saharan Africa and Southern Asia. Interventions have included cultivating government-trained local health educators, providing food subsidies for mothers and babies, and ensuring regular medical visits during and post-pregnancy.

## Public-private Partnerships

Some exciting cross-sector efforts, such as the World Health Organization's Partnership for Maternal, Newborn and Child Health, leverage the expertise and resources of philanthropic, academic, healthcare, and other sectors to adopt aligned strategies and accelerate action by donor and developing countries to achieve MDG-4. Funders include a combination of national governments, international corporate and foundation donors, and high-level individual donors.

## Private Giving

The existing government aid architecture is being challenged by the relatively recent rise in private giving from donors in countries around the world. Over $2.4B in grants was awarded in 2008 by the top 25 private foundations supporting global health efforts.[2] In 2010, Warren Buffet and Bill and Melinda Gates launched the *Giving Pledge* and have inspired dozens of the world's wealthiest families to commit to giving a majority of their wealth to charitable causes, including international health research and programs. At the same time, Peter Singer's advocacy for Effective Altruism continues to gain momentum and growing numbers of individuals are donating significant portions of their income to causes, especially health interventions that have the greatest evidence-supported impact.

Global philanthropy, according to The Philanthropic Initiative, is "the investment of private philanthropic resources without regard to national boundaries. Often, it refers to strategic investments that address issues of world poverty and social injustice."[3] Donors choosing to support causes far from home will often work through an intermediary non-governmental organization (NGO) to steward their gift **(Box 1)**. Well-known NGOs, such as Save the Children, March of Dimes, the Society for Nutrition, Education and Health Action, and many others, support programmatic efforts and research on a range of maternal and newborn health issues, including improvements in prenatal screening and reducing premature birth, birth defects, and infant mortality. Funded through a combination of corporate sponsorships, foundation and government grants, and donations from individuals, NGOs combine and leverage donations from multiple sources to achieve clearly articulated goals.

Private donors also make direct gifts to healthcare institutions whose work they support, most often in or near their own communities. Organizations can develop basic systems for soliciting, accepting, and properly managing donor funds in order to build private support for underfunded initiatives and needs.

Healthcare institutions interested in creating or growing a philanthropy program should first understand how public and private charitable giving currently impacts their organization.

## FOUNDATIONS OF A PHILANTHROPY PROGRAM

Most healthcare providers are not trained fundraisers, yet they can effectively raise philanthropic dollars for a medical institution's research and programs with a basic understanding of the philanthropy landscape and common practices for engaging donors. This practical primer will present information about:
- How to prepare for fundraising by prioritizing needs
- How to research funders and identify strong match potential
- How to approach and cultivate a prospective funder
- How to ask for funding
- How to maintain and strengthen funder relationships.

### Getting Started

Before approaching a funder for a donation, an organization must first determine its greatest needs for funding. Curiously, this step is often overlooked. Most institutions have several priorities and important programs that could benefit from philanthropic support, though often different administrators and providers champion their own unique programs. Ideally, everyone involved with fundraising efforts will have a clear and united understanding of the top needs and priorities for funding, be they equipment, programs, staffing, or research. Competition within an organization for the same charitable funds can leave a donor with the impression of disorganization and unclear leadership. An organization may decide not to seek funds for less pressing programs in the interest of long-term organizational success in meeting top goals.

Identifying funding needs require specificity. Before requesting funding from a donor, an organization must know precisely what goals it aims to achieve and must be able to articulate the potential impact of a donation. When working to raise philanthropic funds, healthcare providers become ambassadors for their institutions and must be ever-ready to communicate a program's benefits to members of the broader community. Every conversation is an opportunity to gain another champion, and having a clear, concise message about goals and impact will help make a strong case for support of your organization.

Another benefit to achieving clarity about goals and priorities for funding is avoiding "mission drift." Once an

---

**BOX 1:** NGO Case Study: SEARCH.

*NGO Case Study: Society for Education, Action and Research in Community Health (SEARCH), Gadchiroli, India*

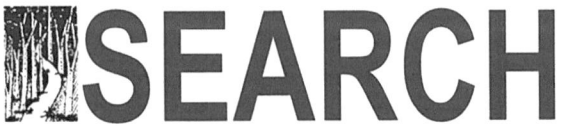

SEARCH works to decrease newborn death rates by training local women as Village Health Workers to attend home deliveries and assist mothers in caring for their newborns. SEARCH provides Home-Based Newborn Care (HBNC) packages to mothers, including health education and home visits during the neonatal period. HBNC packages are being used in 40 villages in rural Maharashtra, India and have decreased the newborn death rate there by 70%.[4]

organization begins to research potential philanthropic partners, it will undoubtedly discover a number of funders with objectives that fall just outside of the institution's main priorities. A healthcare institution may be tempted to adjust its priorities or change a program to better align with these funders' interests. This practice can be extremely detrimental to an organization because it shifts focus and resources away from top priorities—and the organization's core purpose—and instead caters to the desires of a funder. An organization should aim to identify funders with similar priorities for impact, not to refashion its programs in an attempt to be more appealing to a funder.

## Conducting Funder Research

With clearly defined goals for the use of donated funds, an institution can begin searching for philanthropic partners to support its programs and research. Prospect research has become far more accessible in the digital age, though online funder databases are not the only means for identifying prospects. Organizations should consider employing a combination of the following, which are discussed here.

### Online Research

- Unique databases may exist for different countries/regions **(Table 1)**.
- Many online databases require paid registration to access.
- Online databases typically provide access to institutional funders only (not individual donors).

### Researching Like Programs

- Find out who funds other institutions doing similar work in the same area.
- This research can yield information about individual donors with an interest in your work.

### Networking

- Ask contacts at other organizations to make introductions to funders.
- A personal introduction from a trusted source will typically produce a better result than an unknown organization initiating contact with a funder on its own.

Organizations should prioritize funders with the best mission-match potential and avoid casting too broad a net that produces a pipeline of improbable prospects. The goal of prospect research is to develop a strong working list of funders most likely to be interested in an organization's programs and priorities, and to qualify those prospects based on their capacity and inclination to give. This qualification process helps to most efficiently utilize the time of fund developers and healthcare providers in cultivating prospective funders through personal outreach.

**TABLE 1:** Partial List of Available Online Resources for Funder Research.

| Resource | URL/Web Address |
| --- | --- |
| The Foundation Center—Foundation Directory Online (Database) | https://fconline.foundationcenter.org/ |
| The Foundation Center—International Directories of Foundations (List/Links) | http://foundationcenter.org/getstarted/topical/international.html |
| European Foundation Centre—Resources for Grantseekers (Links) | http://www.efc.be/programmes_services/resources/Pages/Advice-for-grantseekers.aspx |
| Grant Select (Database) | http://www.grantselect.com/index.html |
| The Grantsmanship Center—International Funding Resources (Links) | http://www.tgci.com/international-funding-sources |
| The Grantsmanship Center—Grant Domain (Database) | http://www.tgci.com/grantdomain |
| NOZA Search (Database) | http://www.nozasearch.com |

## APPROACHING INSTITUTIONS AND INDIVIDUALS

Once an institution has defined priorities for philanthropic funds and has conducted research to identify funding sources with strong match potential, it can begin a strategy for engaging with potential donors.

Fundraising professionals refer to three stages of donor engagement—cultivation, solicitation, and stewardship. Cultivation is the process of getting a potential donor interested in making a gift to an organization, solicitation involves asking for financial support, and stewardship refers to the ongoing relationship built with a donor once they have made a gift. Successful cultivation, solicitation, and stewardship depend on an understanding of donor motivation so communication can be customized to address a donor's fundamental interests.

Not all donors share the same concerns and motivations, so a one-size-fits-all approach likely will not work. You may find that foundations have a strong interest in specific outcomes of your funded program, with strict methods of evaluation to demonstrate the value of their gift. Individual donors, on the other hand, may want to feel a personal connection to an organization and see the difference their gift makes firsthand or hear stories of inspiring impacts. All outreach should take into account the needs and concerns of each unique donor.

## Institutional Giving

For the purposes of this primer, institutional funders refer to any foundation, corporation, or other organization that makes donations, via grants or sponsorships, to support the work of healthcare institutions.

### How to Approach Institutional Funders

While it is always best to have a mutually known party facilitate an introduction, organizations can initiate new contact with funding institutions by phone or in writing without an introduction. If possible, ask for an in-person meeting to make the communication more personal and establish a face-to-face relationship. Making initial contact with a funder before entering a formal process to request funding is important because it can save organizations time in preparing unnecessary proposals. Funding institutions are typically forthcoming and will inform an organization if it is not a strong candidate for funding. An example of institutional giving is First 5 in Santa Clara County, California (**Box 2**).

### How to Cultivate Institutional Funders

Maintaining contact after an initial phone call or meeting can help an organization remain top-of-mind for a funder. This is especially relevant if a funder has an established timeframe for accepting proposals, as that timeframe may be several months after your initial contact. Keep funders engaged by sending brief emails to share new data or announce other funding partnerships.

### How to Request Funding from Institutional Funders

Nearly all institutional funders have set processes for soliciting and reviewing funding requests. If a formal process is in place, an organization should demonstrate courtesy to the funder by:

- Following the request process as outlined, including respecting deadlines and paying close attention to proposal guidelines or application requirements.
- Keeping the audience in mind. Not everyone reviewing proposals will be a medical professional. Laypeople may not fully comprehend proposals with considerable amounts of medical terminology, so organizations should alter content appropriately.
- Resisting the inclination to simply reuse language from medical publications in proposals to corporate or family foundations. Take the time to revise the language to be more accessible and comprehensible to nonmedical personnel.
- Adhering to the required format for applications/proposals. Follow the required formatting closely so you are not disqualified due to a technical error.

If a funder does not have a required format, follow this narrative outline provided by the Foundation Center:[5] (1) Executive summary/introduction, (2) Description of need, (3) Project description, including implementation and evaluation plans, (4) Project budget, (5) Organization information, and (6) Conclusion.

Remember that a funding proposal is part of a process that starts with research and cultivation. Requesting funding from an institution should be done after careful study of the funder's interests and appropriate contact with the funder's staff or board members.

### How to Steward Institutional Funders

Once funding is secured, an organization should take steps to keep the funder engaged. Many institutional funders will require annual site visits as well as periodic written reports on progress toward established goals. Above and beyond what is required by the funder, an organization should initiate contact to offer gratitude for the donation, share updates from the facility, offer volunteer opportunities, and extend invitations to special events. Assign one person (or a small team) as steward of each funder relationship to ensure consistent communication. In most cases, this will be the same person or team that managed the process of requesting funds. Effective stewardship, along with delivering promised results, can result in recurring donations to an organization from an institutional funder.

---

**BOX 2:** Case Study: FIRST 5. *(For color version see Plate 1)*

*Case Study: FIRST 5 Santa Clara County, California, USA*
FIRST 5 distributes taxes from the sale of tobacco products to programs that support children in their first 5 years of life. Santa Clara Valley Medical Center's neonatal intensive care unit (NICU) established a long-term partnership with FIRST 5 that resulted in concrete enhancements to the treatment of babies, as well as nearly $2M in donated equipment. This funding partnership helped the hospital achieve the elimination of hypothermia in extremely preterm infants, the adoption of therapeutic hypothermia for babies with brain injury, delayed cord clamping for extremely preterm infants as standard practice, and universal screening for critical congenital heart disease.
Ongoing donor stewardship of FIRST 5 included regular reporting on the use of donated funds, annual site visits, NICU tours, meetings with physicians, and permanent recognition of the partnership with the installation of a large donor plaque in the NICU.

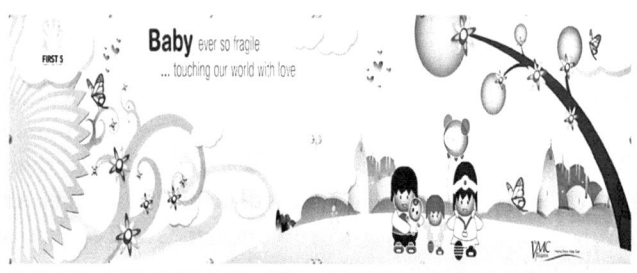

## Individual Giving

While fundraising is a disciplined practice that relies on tested methods, it is fundamentally driven by the motivations and satisfaction of donors, which vary greatly. Because the overwhelming majority of annual philanthropic donations come directly from individuals, not from large institutions, investing the time in building a base of individual supporters can greatly benefit an organization.

### How to Approach Individual Donors

Individual donors make personal, emotional decisions about where to allocate their assets through philanthropic gifts. Therefore, learning about the motivations of individual donor prospects is the most important aspect of this type of donor engagement.

Discovering donor motivation and purposefully segmenting donors accordingly can help organizations tailor their fundraising strategies to best suit each segment, thereby achieving optimal levels of fundraising success. Researchers File and Prince proposed seven distinct segments for donors based on their principal motivation.[6] These segments are:

- *Communitarians:* Those who believe that their personal philanthropy makes good sense and will help the broader community prosper.
- *Devout:* Those who believe that their philanthropy is God's will.
- *Investors:* Those who see financial benefits for themselves as a result of their philanthropy.
- *Socialites:* Those who participate in networks of philanthropy that include regular social events that may affirm status.
- *Altruists:* Those who selflessly give because they believe it is right and that they have a moral imperative to do so.
- *Repayers:* Those who have previously been the recipients of philanthropy and are giving back due to gratitude, a sense of obligation, or loyalty to the organization.
- *Dynasts:* Those who have inherited wealth and carry on a family tradition of philanthropy.

According to File and Prince, "each of these segments represents a distinctive way that a donor group approaches philanthropy, a set of typical attitudes and beliefs about giving."[6] Accordingly, the motivations of these donors will dictate their decisions, and therefore offer key insights to organizations hoping to engage with these individuals.

### How to Cultivate Individual Funders

Approaching fundraising from a donor's point of view helps organizations establish and grow relationships with donors based on what the donor values. For example, for donors who fall into the categories of *altruists and repayers*, fundraising stewards should highlight the good work of the institution with specific stories of patient impact to motivate giving. In contrast, *socialites* may more likely be interested in sponsoring and attending large-scale charity events because philanthropy in the context of a social setting reaffirms social status and provides an opportunity for these donors to mingle with each other. In order to learn a donor's motivation, one must listen attentively and research the donor's other philanthropic interests. Once determined, donor motivation will help inform future cultivation strategies.

For any donor, personal connection to the work of an organization is likely to help create a bond. This can be developed by arranging personalized tours through a hospital or by coordinating a "dinner with the doctors" event so potential donors can hear from medical professionals and researchers about the important work achieved with the help of private funding.

### How to Request Funding from Individual Donors

The process of requesting gifts from individuals can vary greatly and depends entirely on the wishes of the donor. If asked to submit a proposal, the format described in the previous section is applicable. However, expect that soliciting individuals may be a less formal process. Requests for funding may happen in person during a site visit, over the phone, or in a one-page letter. Organizations seeking donations from individuals must remain flexible and responsive to the unique preferences of each donor.

### How to Steward Individual Donors

As with institutional funders, individual donors may request regular reports on the impact of their donation, especially if the gift amount is significant. However, more often, the organization receiving the funds must take the initiative to provide updates about impact.

Maintaining communication with individual donors is crucial to their sustained involvement. As with institutional funders, individual donors should be engaged through regular communication that provides updates on the program or news from the facility. Individual donors should be extended regular opportunities to volunteer or visit the organization. Above all else, organizations should ensure that communication to individual donors does not always contain requests for money. Show individual donors that you value their involvement and partnership in ways that extend beyond their financial resources. As with institutional funders, one person (or a small team) should be assigned as steward of each funder relationship to ensure consistent communication.

> **BOX 3:** Checklist for donor recognition.
> - Thank donors for each gift they make.
> - Keep track of each gift and its purpose.
> - Write a personal message in each thank you letter.
> - Have a formal policy or practice to ensure consistency in managing donor relations.
> - Ensure that every donor is treated equitably and fairly.
> - Send occasional reports to donors on how their funds were used.

Donor recognition is incredibly important when engaging individual donors. For significant gifts, consider semipermanent or permanent recognition via naming opportunities within the facility (e.g., a donor wall in a main lobby, treatment areas named for a donor, etc.). See the Checklist for Donor Recognition, adapted from Fundraising Fundamentals, for guidelines that ensure proper recognition of individual donors **(Box 3)**.[7]

## Crowdfunding

Crowdfunding is a centuries-old technique that has become ever more popular in the digital age. It is the practice of eliciting small donations from a group of individuals, with all donations benefitting a single goal. Crowdfunding is a popular current practice because it can be very effective at raising large amounts of money. A main benefit of crowdfunding is that it can engage donors who do not have significant personal resources, and therefore are not likely to be on an organization's individual donor prospect list. Through crowdfunding, modest donors have the opportunity to participate and be engaged with philanthropic causes in a way never before possible. By showing how small donations add up to have a big impact, organizations are successfully pooling the resources of lower-level donors to achieve major programmatic goals and fund large-scale equipment purchases.

The mechanisms to support crowdfunding campaigns are becoming more accessible around the world, as are the online payment systems that help organizations collect donations. For organizations with a strong social media presence, crowdfunding campaigns are a natural fit because they are easily shared within social networks to increase revenues.

The key to a successful crowdfunding campaign is the thoughtful selection of an achievable goal that can be easily described in an inspirational manner. The purchase of an infant incubator, for example, is easily communicated and the impact can be described through both a concise narrative and moving photographs.

Because donors to crowdfunding campaigns tend to make smaller donations and may not live in an area close to the recipient organization given the wide reach of the Internet, stewardship of these donors typically includes an initial recognition of their gift, and ideally, some level of ongoing communication about an organization's future projects and goals via email.

## ■ THE COSTS OF PHILANTHROPY

Any organization intending to establish or build a philanthropy program should understand the personnel and material costs required for effective donor engagement. The resources required to raise and manage private funds, as well as to maintain funder relationships, are not insignificant. But the benefits of reliable philanthropic support should far outweigh any concern about the costs.

### Personnel Costs

A person or small team of people should be identified to lead philanthropic efforts, including:
- Establishing clear needs and goals for use of charitable gifts.
- Conducting prospect research and identifying funding sources with strong match potential.
- Making contact with donors for initial discussions, meetings, site visits, and tours.
- Coordinating the preparation of funding proposals and formal reports.
- Stewarding donor relationships via personal outreach and regular updates.
- Administration and oversight of donated funds; financial compliance.

The importance of a strong and dedicated team to oversee the fund development process cannot be overstated. Raising philanthropic funds is, at its core, about relationship management. It is necessary to have dedicated individuals to liaise between the funder and the healthcare institution throughout the funding life cycle.

### Nonpersonnel Costs

Keep in mind the other resources required to operate donor engagement efforts, including:
- *Promotional and educational materials:* Brochures and other printed materials about your program and institution.
- *Funding proposals and reports of impact:* Produced in-house or by a design firm.
- *Stationery:* Letterhead, thank you cards, event invitations.
- Donor and financial management software.
- Membership fees to access online research databases.
- Design and installation of any donor recognition plaques within the institution.

Having a realistic understanding of the costs will assist with planning and delegation of responsibilities among staff members. Some healthcare institutions will have resources to contribute directly to fundraising while others may not. Likewise, some healthcare institutions will have professional fund developers on staff (or even a dedicated fundraising organization on-site) while others will divide responsibilities among providers and administrators. Many models can be effective, and anticipating costs from the outset will help build a strong foundation for success.

## CONCLUSION

Charitable giving is the resource that can help healthcare institutions provide better care to people in need. Establishing and growing a philanthropy program requires dedication and effort and can result in new resources to support under-funded research or programmatic and equipment needs.

Engaging institutional and individual donors is a unique process with demands for ethics and accountability. Just as businesses are accountable to shareholders, organizations that receive charitable donations are accountable to their donors. Donors have an investment in the success of the program and deserve to know how their funds were used and how their donations made a difference. By engaging donors as partners in your work, an organization can build a base of champions that will provide long-term energy, passion, and resources that offer sustainability to under-funded programs. Ultimately, these donor contributions can make a major impact on improving health outcomes for people in need, especially newborns and their family members.

## REFERENCES

1. United Nations Children's Fund. Levels and trends in child mortality report 2012. [online] Available from http://www.unicef.org/videoaudio/PDFs/UNICEF_2012_child_mortality_for_web_0904.pdf. [Last Accessed November, 2019].
2. The Foundation Center. Top 25 foundations awarding international grants for global health, circa 2008. [online] Available from http://foundationcenter.org/gpf/health/tables/3-F_Health_Intl_2008.pdf. [Last Accessed November, 2019].
3. The Philanthropic Initiative. Global giving: making a world of difference. [online] Available from http://www.tpi.org/sites/files/pdf/tpi_global_giving_making_a_world_of_difference.pdf. Last Accessed November, 2019].
4. SEARCH. Society for Education, Action, Research and Community Health. [online] Available from http://searchforhealth.ngo/. [Last Accessed November, 2019].
5. Greever JC, McNeill P. The Foundation Center's guide to proposal writing. New York: The Foundation Center; 1997.
6. File K, Prince R. The seven faces of philanthropy: a new approach to cultivating major donors. San Francisco: Jossey-Bass; 1994.
7. Greenfield J. Fundraising fundamentals: a guide to annual giving for professionals and volunteers. San Francisco: John Wiley & Sons, Inc.; 1994.

# SECTION 3

# Perinatal

- Obstetric Contributions to Neonatal Morbidity and Mortality—Overview
  *Francesca C Ianovich, Matthew J Garabedian*

- Disorders of the Membranes, Placenta, and Cord
  *Shannon Dralla, Matthew J Garabedian*

- Neonatal Encephalopathy: An Obstetric Perspective
  *Stacy Yadava, Matthew J Garabedian*

CHAPTER

# Obstetric Contributions to Neonatal Morbidity and Mortality—Overview

Francesca C Ianovich, Matthew J Garabedian

## ABSTRACT

Maternal factors are a significant contributor to neonatal morbidity and mortality. The antenatal condition may dramatically affect the early trajectory of neonatal course. Preterm birth, birth asphyxia, and perinatal infection are obvious factors, but maternal diabetes, hypertension, and obesity are also significant factors. Obstetric interventions are important, but potentially limited, interventions for improving neonatal health. Antenatal corticosteroids (ANS) have been shown to significantly decrease perinatal death, respiratory distress, intraventricular hemorrhage, and necrotizing enterocolitis. Administration of steroids to women at high risk for preterm birth may be the most powerful intervention in the obstetric armamentarium. Antenatal care, addressing maternal nutritional status, management of diabetes, and control of hypertension, as well as access to a skilled birth attendant are feasible and important factors that are thought to improve neonatal outcomes.

## INTRODUCTION

In 2000, the United Nations adopted the Millennium Development Goals (MDGs) to address issues of health, poverty, and well-being worldwide. One of those goals, MDG 4 aims to reduce mortality in children less than 5 years of age by two-thirds between 1990 and 2015. Neonatal mortality accounts for 44% of these under-5 deaths.[1] Though progress has been made toward reducing the under-5 mortality rate (a 47% reduction between 1990 and 2012), the rate of neonatal mortality has only seen a 37% reduction. In 2012, there were 2.9 million neonatal deaths worldwide, compared to 4.6 million neonatal deaths worldwide in 1990.[1] The good news is that progress is being made. We know why maternal and neonatal deaths occur, where they occur, and how they occur, and we have highly effective interventions for preventing them.[2]

Three major causes of neonatal deaths (infections, complications of preterm birth, and intrapartum-related neonatal deaths or "birth asphyxia") account for nearly 80% of all neonatal deaths globally,[3] with prematurity, infection, and asphyxia accounting for 31%, 25%, and 23% of all neonatal deaths, respectively.[4] Developed countries have seen much success in preventing neonatal deaths through implementation of science-driven and highly effective interventions. However, 99% of these deaths now occur in developing countries with unique challenges,[2] which need to make similar interventions to reduce these mortality rates. Up to two-thirds of these deaths are preventable, if mothers and newborns receive known, effective interventions.[2] Key strategies for improving outcomes are providing access to antenatal care and, in particular, the care of a skilled attendant at birth.

## TOP CONTRIBUTORS TO NEONATAL MORBIDITY AND MORTALITY

- *Prematurity*: Preterm birth is the leading cause of neonatal deaths, accounting for almost one-third of worldwide neonatal deaths.[4] Prematurity itself is not only a direct cause of neonatal death, but also is a risk factor for complications such as infection and lifelong disabilities. There are not significant differences among industrialized and developing countries in the incidence of preterm birth; however, a significant gap exists between rich and poor countries in the survival rate of preterm babies.[5] Most preterm births happen spontaneously, yet common causes include multiple pregnancies, infections, and chronic conditions, such as diabetes, high blood pressure, and undernutrition or obesity. However, often no cause is identified.[6] World Health Organization (WHO) guidelines stress the importance of antenatal care to educate mothers about the importance of nutrition and for the screening and management of conditions such as diabetes, high blood pressure, and infections. In the intrapartum period, the WHO recommends the use of tocolytics to slow down labor, administering ANS, using antibiotics for preterm premature rupture of membranes (PPROM), and administering magnesium sulfate for neuroprotection of the newborn.[6] The use of ANS is a missed opportunity with potential to reduce neonatal deaths by up to one-half million per year.[7]

- *Birth asphyxia:* Birth asphyxia is responsible for about 23% of worldwide neonatal deaths.[4] Obstetrical conditions that lead to intrapartum hypoxia include those that (1) primarily impact blood flow through the placenta, such as preeclampsia/eclampsia; (2) separate the placenta from the maternal circulation, such as placental abruption; (3) compress the umbilical cord impeding blood flow; (4) are associated with prolonged labor because contractions themselves decrease fetal oxygenation; and (5) lead to fetal entrapment during delivery, such as a breech presentation or shoulder dystocia.[8] These conditions can be managed and prevented during antenatal care (i.e. detection and management of preeclampsia), and during the intrapartum period (i.e. labor monitoring coupled with access to emergency obstetrical services). Because the most effective interventions for intrapartum-related neonatal deaths are quality antenatal care and skilled attendance at birth with access to emergency obstetrical care, the threat of birth asphyxia is highest in the world's least developed countries where access to such resources is often low. Circumstances common in developing countries increase the prevalence and severity of intrapartum-related hypoxic events—such as delays in problem-recognition/care seeking, inadequate antenatal and intrapartum care, and poor access to health facilities.[8]
- *Infection:* A quarter of the world's neonatal deaths are due to infection.[4] In industrialized countries, the neonatal sepsis rate is one to three per 1,000 live births; in developing countries population-based studies have reported clinical sepsis rates ranging from 49 to 170 per 1,000 live births.[9] This discrepancy highlights the preventable nature of neonatal infections in low-income regions. Risk factors include chorioamnionitis, low birth weight, unhygienic delivery, skin care, cord care, and the environment.[10] In addition to effectively diagnosing and managing cases of neonatal infection, preventative strategies are an integral component to reducing the incidence on neonatal mortality due to infection. These strategies include antenatal visits to educate mothers about clean birth practices and risk factors for infection and supervision by a skilled attendant at birth. Additionally, administering antibiotics to women with PPROM is another intervention with the potential to reduce incidence of all neonatal infections by up to one-third.[11]

## ROLE OF A SKILLED ATTENDANT AT BIRTH

Increasing access to skilled health workers who have the knowledge and ability to deliver effective interventions during the intrapartum period is an integral component of reducing adverse neonatal outcomes and preventing neonatal mortality worldwide. The term "skilled health worker" refers to an accredited health professional (i.e. doctor, nurse, or midwife) who is trained to manage normal pregnancies, child birth, and the immediate postnatal period, and in the identification and management of complications or emergencies.[12] The WHO and UNICEF recommend that a skilled attendant be present during and immediately after birth, regardless of the setting that the birth takes place in.[4] While the percentage of births attended by a skilled health worker has increased globally, certain regions still desperately need increased coverage. In the WHO Africa Region, e.g. fewer than 50% of all births are attended by a skilled worker.[4,13] In general, the low- and middle-income countries that have seen major reductions in neonatal mortality have also had an increase of skilled care during births.[7] Making significant progress toward improving neonatal outcomes and reducing neonatal deaths worldwide will depend upon increased access to skilled health workers who are able to deliver effective interventions.

## WHAT INTERVENTIONS ARE AVAILABLE/ HOW WELL DO THEY WORK?

### Antenatal Corticosteroids

The use of ANS for premature birth is considered one of the most important interventions in obstetric practice.[14]

The most common cause of death and complications among preterm infants is respiratory distress syndrome (RDS), an acute lung disease related to lung immaturity and surfactant deficiency.[15] ANSs help to promote fetal lung maturity in women at risk of preterm delivery, and therefore, reduce the rate of neonatal mortalities and the rate of infants with breathing complications at birth. In the most recent Cochrane review, which included 21 studies and over 4,000 infants, a single course of ANS reduced neonatal deaths by 31% [95% confidence interval (CI) 19-42%, 3,956 infants], RDS by 34% (95% CI 27-41%, 4,038 infants), intraventricular hemorrhage by 46% (95% CI 31-57%, 2,872 infants), necrotizing enterocolitis by 54% (95% CI 26-71%, 1,675 infants), and systemic infection within the first 48 hours of life by 44% (95% CI 15-62%, 1,319 infants). There was also reduction in rates of admission to the neonatal intensive care unit (NICU) and need for respiratory support.[14,16] The Cochrane report concludes that a single course of ANS should be routine for preterm delivery, though further investigation is necessary regarding optimal dosage, the effect in multiple pregnancies, which corticosteroid to use, and to confirm any long-term effects.[16]

Although the effectiveness of ANS was established years ago and is now a common practice in high-income countries, usage rates remain incredibly low in middle- and low-income countries where most of the neonatal deaths occur; this represents a significant missed opportunity for improving survival rates of preterm infants worldwide. There has been some increased use of ANS in middle-income countries such as South Africa and Thailand, although mean coverage in the countries with more than 90% of maternal and neonatal deaths is only around 10%.[15] In a study, assessing the practices of healthcare providers regarding the use of ANS in Latin America, it was noted that barriers to usage could be solved by better providers having better knowledge on the benefits of ANS.[17] This finding reiterates the importance of trained and skilled attendants at birth. The WHO now recommends the administration of ANS (both betamethasone and dexamethasone) as a priority intervention for preterm babies to reduce RDS and considers ANS a priority medicine for reducing mortality among premature babies.[6] In an analysis by Darmstadt et al.[11] administering ANS for preterm labor in low- and middle-income countries is associated with a 40% reduction (25-52% effect range) in neonatal mortality. To date, most trials of ANS have been done in high-income countries and only several have taken place in middle-income countries. Assessing the effectiveness of ANS in lower-level facilities or home births where specialized care tends to be lacking is still needed.[6]

## Antibiotics

Preterm premature rupture of membranes has a strong association with infection of amniotic membranes, thus contributing to preterm birth and other neonatal complications. Antibiotic treatment for PPROM is standard practice in high-income countries in order to reduce the risk of maternal and neonatal infection; however, in low- and middle-income countries many women are not treated with antibiotics for PPROM. Antibiotic treatment for pPROM has been shown to delay labor for up to 48 hours, to reduce neonatal infections, and to reduce abnormal cerebral ultrasounds. Therefore, the WHO now includes antibiotics for PPROM to prevent infection in its priority packages and evidence-based interventions to reduce preterm birth rates.[6] According to an analysis by Darmstadt et al.[11] the administration of antibiotics for PPROM can lead to a 32% reduction (13-47% effect range) in incidence of infection. It has also been suggested that an increase in antibiotic therapy for PPROM will prevent 4% of all preterm neonatal deaths and may reduce sepsis deaths by 8%.[18] The WHO also suggests that screening for and treatment of infections such as asymptomatic bacteriuria and bacterial vaginosis during antenatal care has the potential to reduce preterm births, although it notes inconsistent study results.[6]

## Tocolysis

One of the key interventions to prolong pregnancy and improve neonatal outcomes in cases of preterm labor is the provision of tocolytic agents (i.e. oxytocin antagonists, betamimetics, calcium channel blockers, and magnesium sulfate) to inhibit uterine contractions. The use of tocolytics to slow down labor allows for time to administer ANS and to transfer the mother to a higher-level care facility if necessary. The WHO includes the use of tocolytic agents as part of the priority packages and evidence-based interventions to reduce preterm birth rates.[6]

## Fetal/Labor Monitoring

Carefully monitoring the fetal heart rate pattern can provide useful information about fetal condition during labor. An abnormal fetal heart rate pattern can help to detect many obstetrical conditions associated with birth asphyxia (such as umbilical cord complications, placental abruption, fetal distress, and malposition). Prompt detection of fetal compromise, leading to rapid delivery, can drastically improve outcomes for both mother and newborn.[8] Though further research is necessary, it has been suggested that in low-resource settings a well-trained nurse using a fetoscope or innovative tools, such as hand-held doptone device, may be effective while remaining simple and affordable.[8]

A WHO study in South-East Asia found that partograph use in addition to a labor-management protocol reduced prolonged labor and the need for augmentation; rates of emergency cesarean section and stillbirths also dropped with the partograph use.[19] Darmstadt et al.[11] suggest that labor surveillance (including partograph) for early diagnosis of complications can contribute a 40% reduction in neonatal deaths in low- and middle-income countries.

## Operative Delivery

Once fetal compromise has been detected, often by means of labor and fetal monitoring, rapid delivery usually by cesarean section is paramount for preventing adverse outcomes and mortality. The ability to perform a timely cesarean delivery is a key intervention for reducing neonatal mortalities, again highlighting the importance of a skilled attendant at birth. Darmstadt et al.[11] have suggested that the detection and management of breech (cesarean section) has the potential to reduce perinatal/neonatal death by 71% (14–90% effect range). However, in low-income regions there is often a lack of qualified physicians trained to handle obstetric emergencies. Luckily, there is evidence from Malawi and Mozambique that nonphysician providers can be trained to effectively and safely perform cesarean deliveries, and these providers have the potential to improve emergency obstetric care in low resource regions.[8]

## CONTRIBUTION OF MATERNAL DISEASE

Maternal health and newborn health are intimately linked together. Newborns face a much greater risk of mortality and morbidity when their mothers are ill, malnourished, or receive inadequate care.[20] The major contributors of maternal health on neonatal outcomes include diabetes, hypertension, nutrition (being over/underweight), and HIV/AIDS.

## Diabetes

The global prevalence of diabetes is anticipated to double between 2000 and 2030, with the greatest increase in prevalence in the Middle-East, sub-Saharan Africa, and India.[21] While much of this increase has been attributed to an increasing prevalence of obesity, the global prevalence of diabetes is anticipated to increase, even with stabilization of the prevalence of obesity. Pregestational diabetes has long been known to carry significant risks in pregnancy. When diabetes is recognized in pregnancy, it is considered gestational diabetes mellitus (GDM), or diabetes resulting from a state of insulin resistance created by the pregnant state. Postpartum testing of glucose is recommended for patients with gestational diabetes, as many of these women in fact have previously unrecognized type 2 diabetes mellitus.[22] Additionally, it should be recognized that 15–50% of women with gestational diabetes will develop type 2 diabetes mellitus later in life.

It has been long established that pregnancies conceived during a period of poor glycemic control are subject to a high risk of congenital anomalies, particularly of the heart and neural tube.[23-25] The risk of congenital anomaly correlates with hyperglycemia. With a hemoglobin A1C ≥ 8.6%, the risk of a major congenital anomaly is approximately one-fourth.[26] In these original studies, no excess in congenital anomalies was demonstrated with a hemoglobin A1C ≤ 8.5%.[23,24] More recent work suggests that even in pregnancies of women with pregestational diabetes and a normal hemoglobin A1C, there is an excess risk of congenital heart disease. In a single-institution study of 595 pregestational diabetic women in the United States, Starikov et al. 2013, found that among women with a hemoglobin A1C < 8.5%, there was a 3.9% prevalence of congenital heart disease at the mid-trimester anatomy ultrasound.[27] These authors note that this is roughly five times greater than the < 1% prevalence in the general population, and they argue for congenital heart disease screening with fetal echocardiography in all pregnancies of women with pregestational diabetes.

Diabetes-related complications later in pregnancy are associated with both pregestational and gestational diabetes. Pregestational diabetes is associated with fetal macrosomia and its incumbent risk of neurologic injury, fetal growth restriction, RDS, perinatal asphyxia, hyperbilirubinemia, and metabolic derangement.[28-31] In a single institution study from a teaching hospital in Nigeria, Opara et al. report the most common neonatal morbidities among 47 neonates admitted to the special care nursery to be hypoglycemia (63.8%), neonatal jaundice (57.4%), and respiratory distress disorders (34.0%) among babies of diabetic mothers.[32] While the authors did not account for gestational age at delivery in presenting their results, only 7 of 47 (14.9%) neonates were born before 37 weeks.

Neonatal brachial plexus injury is strongly associated with shoulder dystocia at the time of delivery [odds ratio (OR) 76.1, 95% CI 69–84], and at any given birth weight, the risk of brachial plexus injury is greater among neonates born of diabetic mothers.[33] Gravidas with pregnancies complicated by gestational diabetes and fetal macrosomia are more likely to experience a shoulder dystocia [relative risk (RR) 6.27, 95% CI 2.33–16.88].[34] The risk of shoulder dystocia and brachial plexus injury is greater when the neonate is delivered by operative vaginal delivery.[33,34] There does not appear to be a difference in risk profile for neonates with a proportionate large for gestational age (LGA) birth weight, as compared to those with a disproportionate LGA phenotype, as assessed by Ponderal index.[30]

Fetal growth restriction may arise from maternal vascular disease, particularly in the setting of advanced pregestational diabetes, and results in excessive perinatal mortality.[29] Fetal exposure to a hyperglycemic state leads to excessive production of insulin fetal pancreatic B-cells hyperplasia, possibly leading to insulin resistance, and potentially B-cell failure.[29,31,35] The response of the fetal pancreas to this hyperglycemic milieu is likely the mechanism for transgenerational development of diabetes.[35] These changes in fetal development also increase risk of pediatric impaired glucose tolerance, obesity, and delayed cognitive and motor development.[31]

Gestational diabetes mellitus is also associated with increased risk of short- and long-term effects for both the mothers and their newborns. Immediate adverse maternal outcomes include pregnancy-induced hypertension and need for cesarean delivery. Short-term adverse neonatal outcomes include macrosomia, hypoglycemia, congenital malformation, and perinatal death. For both mothers and newborns, long-term adverse effects are impaired glucose intolerance, an increased risk for development of type 2 diabetes, and obesity.[36] A recent study from India found gestational diabetes to be associated with an increased risk of preterm birth (OR 2.30, 95% CI 1.24-4.27), hypoglycemia (OR 11.97, 95% CI 2.79-51.38), and macrosomia (OR 5.2, 95% CI 1.13-23.99).[37] Additionally, in a review of 25 studies by Wang et al. the adverse outcomes associated with GDM in low- and middle-income countries with highest rates of incidence were cesarean delivery (43.8%, IQR 34.9-65.9%), large for gestational age (17.9%, IQR 12.3-30.5%), newborn jaundice (17.1%, IQR 8.5-22.9%), and macrosomia (17.0%, IQR 8.3-32.5%).[36]

Cardiac and pulmonary disease in the neonates born of mothers with either pregestational or gestational diabetes may be related to structural or functional anomalies. In addition to the increased risk of structural anomalies as described above, poorly-controlled diabetes and hyperinsulinemia may lead to cardiac dysfunction in the fetus and neonate.[38] Fetal hyperinsulinemia is associated with thickening of the fetal intraventricular septum, which may lead to diastolic dysfunction, cardiomegaly, hypertrophic cardiomyopathy, and subaortic stenosis.[28,38] Significant hypertrophic changes may be present in 20–30% of neonates born of diabetic mothers.[38] The resulting cardiac dysfunction may lead to respiratory distress, which may be confused for surfactant deficiency.[39] RDS and surfactant deficiency are more common in neonates of diabetic mothers, as fetal hyperinsulinemia results in abnormalities of glycogen metabolism, leading to a lack of substrates for surfactant production.[31]

While efforts have been made in industrialized countries to improve outcomes of pregnancies complicated by GDM, effective care for women with GDM is less widely available in low- and middle-income countries. The incidence of GDM (along with obesity and type 2 diabetes) has risen in low- and middle-income countries as adoption of the industrialized lifestyle has become more widespread. It is believed that the biggest increases in GDM will arise in India, China, Latin America, and the Middle East.[36] The most effective management of diabetes incorporates glycemic control through diet, exercise, and/or insulin therapy, frequent fetal surveillance using tests of fetal well-being, and/or induction at or before term.[40]

## Hypertension/Preeclampsia

The hypertensive disorders of pregnancy—including pre-existing hypertension, gestational hypertension, and preeclampsia—can lead to serious adverse maternal and fetal outcomes. Hypertension in pregnancy is defined as systolic blood pressure greater than 140 mm Hg or more, or diastolic blood pressure of 90 mm Hg or more on two occasions at least 4 hours apart. This can occur in mothers with chronic hypertension or may arise in a woman that is otherwise normotensive, i.e. gestational hypertension. Preeclampsia is the association of hypertension with significant proteinuria (300 mg of protein in the urine collected over 24 hours or 30 mg/mmol on spot protein: creatinine ratio). Preeclampsia is the most serious of these disorders. The WHO has estimated that preeclampsia is responsible for more than 500,000 fetal and neonatal deaths per year.[41]

An important role of prenatal care is to facilitate the detection of preeclampsia. It is essential to perform blood pressure and urine protein measurements at appropriate intervals during the pregnancy, especially in the third trimester. There are currently new technologies and research tracks with the potential to improve access to accurate, easy to read, community-based blood pressure measurement, and cost-effective urinary protein estimation.[41] Additionally, Doppler ultrasound can provide information about fetoplacental and/or uteroplacental circulatory dynamics. A Cochrane review found a significant 21% reduction in perinatal mortality (RR = 0.71, 95% CI = 0.52–0.98) when Doppler ultrasound was utilized compared to no Doppler use.[40] Several portable machines are available and do not require intensive training or expertise.[41] In high-income countries, significant reductions in the adverse outcomes associated with preeclampsia have been made with widespread use of prenatal care with blood pressure and urine protein measurement and access to hospital care for appropriate induction of labor or cesarean delivery.

Less is known about neonatal outcomes of pregnancies complicated by preeclampsia in low-income countries. It is thought that a substantial reduction in preeclampsia could be made with increased access to antenatal care including blood pressure and proteinuria screening and access to a skilled attendant at birth to perform timely delivery.[42] The major direct contributors to neonatal morbidity and mortality attributable to preeclampsia are preterm delivery and severe hypertension.[43] In a cohort of 171 preeclamptic pregnancies in Uganda, high rates of still birth (13.9%), early neonatal death (8.9%), and birth weight < 2,500 g (45.5%) were observed. In this cohort, the most important predictors of adverse neonatal outcome were birth at ≤ 36 weeks gestational age (OR = 5.97, 95% CI = 2.79–12.7) and severe preeclampsia (OR = 5.17, 95% CI = 2.36–11.3).

The American College of Obstetrician and Gynecologists (ACOG), the Society for Maternal Fetal Medicine (SMFM), and WHO provide guidelines for management of severe preeclampsia presenting in the preterm period.[44-46] These organizations formally recognize that management of this condition requires the balancing of maternal and fetal risks and that iatrogenic preterm delivery may be the best course of action. Additionally, these guidelines provide recommendations for expectant management of severe preeclampsia before 34 weeks gestation, recognizing that there may be neonatal benefit in delaying delivery. These recommendations are mostly drawn from retrospective studies and expert opinion.

A recent Cochrane review draws conclusions that generally support these recommendations.[47] The authors of this review identified four appropriate studies, including 425 pregnancies complicated by preeclampsia between 24 weeks and 34 weeks gestation. A strategy of immediate delivery versus expectant care and delayed delivery was associated with an increased rate of intraventricular hemorrhage (RR = 1.82, 95%, CI = 1.06–3.14), hyaline membrane disease (RR = 2.30, 95% CI = 1.39–3.81), need for ventilation (RR = 1.50, 95% CI = 1.11–2.02), neonatal intensive care admission (RR = 1.35, 95% CI = 1.16–1.58), and experience a longer length of stay in the NICU (mean number of days = 11.14, 95% CI = 1.57–20.72 days). However, given the relative paucity of data, the Cochrane review authors temper their findings, stating that further studies are needed.

In contrast to this Cochrane review, Vigil-de Garcia et al. 2013, demonstrated a lack of benefit from a strategy of delayed delivery in a randomized controlled trial of 267 pregnancies complicated by severe preeclampsia diagnosed between 28 weeks and 34 weeks from 8 Latin American hospitals.[48] In this study, women were randomized to either a strategy of delivery within 24–72 hours, or one of expectant management until 34 weeks gestation. Subjects in both treatment arms received administration of ANS.

The authors found no difference in composite neonatal morbidity comprised of RDS, necrotizing enterocolitis, intraventricular hemorrhage, or neonatal sepsis (immediate delivery 56.4% vs. expectant management 55.6%, RR = 1.01, 95% CI = 0.81–1.26) or any other measure of neonatal morbidity.

The etiology of preeclampsia remains elusive and measures to prevent the development of preeclampsia are limited.[44,46] Administration of low-dose aspirin (60–80 mg daily) appears to offer a reduction in pregnant women who are high risk for developing preeclampsia [RR 0.83, 95% CI = 0.77–0.89; number needed to treat (NNT) 72].[49] Other interventions, such as bed rest, salt restriction, and vitamin C or E supplementation do not seem to reduce the risk of preeclampsia.[44]

## Over/Underweight

Prepregnancy maternal overweight status is associated with a two- to three-fold increase in hypertensive disorders of pregnancy, an approximately 20% risk of gestational diabetes, a two- to three-fold increase in stillbirth, and macrosomia.[50-52] The risk of these complications is related to the severity of excess maternal body mass.[52-54] Additionally, the risk of macrosomia or LGA birth weight is increased in direct proportion to maternal body mass index (BMI).[51,54-56] For example, in a single institution study by Alanis et al. 2010, 1.5% of neonates born to normal weight women were LGA.[56] With increasing maternal BMI, the likelihood of a LGA birth weight neonate increased, to a maximum of 15% among women with a BMI ≥ 50 kg/m$^2$.

Obesity itself does increase the risk of congenital anomaly, particularly of the neural tube (OR 1.2–3.5) and heart (OR 1.18–2.0), which likely contributes in part to the risk of fetal demise.[57] Furthermore, congenital anomalies are less likely to be recognized antenatally in obese women.[57-59] Obesity related risk of both fetal death (OR 2.32, 95% CI 1.64–3.28) and infant death (OR 1.97, 95% CI 1.13–3.45), however, does appear to be independent of the presence of these comorbidities.[60,61] The risk of fetal death appears to occur after 28 weeks gestation, and the strength of association increases with increasing maternal BMI.[62]

Obesity-related neonatal morbidity is also related to an increased risk of preterm delivery.[62] The association with preeclampsia and other obesity-related morbidities leads to an increased risk of indicated or iatrogenic preterm birth. The effect of obesity on spontaneous preterm birth is unclear. Some studies have demonstrated either no change in spontaneous preterm birth or a slight increase in risk (OR 1.2–1.6).[55,62,63] Others, such as Ehrenberg et al. have demonstrated a protective effect, with fewer spontaneous preterm births < 35 weeks among overweight and obese women when compared to normal weight women (8.3% vs. 21.7%, P < 0.01).[64] This protective effect is consistent with the findings of Haeri et al. 2009 (OR 0.29, 95% CI 0.13–0.64).[51] If a protective effect does exist, the mechanism for this is poorly understood. It may be related, however, to alterations in, or hormonal influence over, the oxytocin signally pathway.[65-68]

Prepregnancy maternal underweight status is associated with serious adverse perinatal outcomes including stillbirth, preterm birth, small for gestational age, and low birth weight infants. About one-tenth of newborns in developing countries are born with low birth weight; this can primarily be attributed to maternal poor health and malnutrition.[40] A low birth weight poses increased risks to the newborn, including infection and health problems later in life.

## ANTENATAL CARE

While care during birth—particularly that of a skilled attendant—is absolutely essential to reducing neonatal mortalities and morbidities, care during the antenatal period is also important because it is an opportunity to address other healthcare needs or existing conditions. Continued care during this critical period should address issues such as family planning, immunization against tetanus, identification of conditions detrimental to health during pregnancy, prevention and treatment of human immunodeficiency virus infection, other sexually transmitted infections, and malaria.[40] For example, treating syphilis with penicillin as part of antenatal care has been shown to reduce perinatal mortality by 63% (RR = 0.37, 95% CI = 0.18–0.76). Addressing maternal nutritional status, management of maternal diabetes and hypertension, and identification of pregnancies at heightened risk for preterm birth and neonatal morbidity is paramount to ensuring a healthy neonatal course.

## REFERENCES

1. UNICEF, WHO, World Bank, UN-DESA Population Division. (2013). Levels and Trends in Child Mortality: Report 2013. [online] Available from: https://www.who.int/maternal_child_adolescent/documents/levels_trends_child_mortality_2013/en/ [Last accessed September, 2019].
2. Peterson H, Haidar J, Merialdi M, et al. Preventing maternal and newborn deaths globally: using innovation and science to address challenges in implementing life-saving interventions. Obstet Gynecol. 2012;120(3):636-42.
3. World Health Organization. (2012). Newborns: reducing mortality. [online] Available from: https://www.who.int/news-room/fact-sheets/detail/newborns-reducing-mortality [Last accessed September, 2019].
4. World Health Organization, UNICEF. (2009). Home visits for the newborn child: a strategy to improve survival. [online] Available from: https://www.who.int/maternal_child_adolescent/news_events/news/2009/09_07_08/en/ [Last accessed September, 2019].
5. Belizán JM, Hofmeyr J, Buekens P, et al. Preterm birth, an unresolved issue. Reprod Health. 2013;10(1):58.
6. World Health Organization. (2012). Born Too Soon: The Global Action Report on Preterm Birth. [online] Available from: https://www.who.int/pmnch/media/news/2012/preterm_birth_report/en/ [Last accessed September, 2019].
7. Lawn JE, Kerber K, Enweronu-Laryea C, et al. 3.6 million neonatal deaths—what is progressing and what is not? Semin Perinatol. 2010;34(6):371-86.
8. Wall SN, Lee AC, Carlo W, et al. Reducing intrapartum-related neonatal deaths in low- and middle-income countries: what works? Semin Perinatol. 2010;34(6):395-407.
9. Ganatra HA, Zaidi AK. Neonatal infections in the developing world. Semin Perinatol. 2010;34(6):416-25.
10. Gleason CA, Devaskar SU. Avery's Diseases of the Newborn, 9th edition. Philadelphia: Elsevier Saunders; 2012.
11. Darmstadt GL, Bhutta ZA, Cousens S, et al. Evidence-based, cost-effective interventions: how many newborn babies can we save? Lancet. 2005;365 (9463):977-88.
12. WHO, Department of Reproductive Health and Research. (2008). Proportion of births attended by a skilled health worker: 2008 updates. [online] Available from: https://www.who.int/reproductivehealth/publications/maternal_perinatal_health/2008_skilled_attendants/en/ [Last accessed September, 2019].
13. WHO Media Centre. Millennium Development Goals (MDGs), Fact Sheet N. 290. Geneva: World Health Organization; 2013.
14. Bonanno C, Wapner RJ. Antenatal corticosteroids in the management of preterm birth: are we back where we started? Obstet Gynecol Clin North Am. 2012;39(1):47-63.
15. Mwansa-Kambafwile J, Cousens S, Hansen T, et al. Antenatal steroids in preterm labour for the prevention of neonatal deaths due to complications of preterm birth. Int J Epidemiol. 2010;39:i122-33.
16. Roberts D, Dalziel S. Antenatal corticosteroids for accelerating fetal lung maturation for women at risk of preterm birth. Cochrane Database of Syst Rev. 2006;(3):CD004454.
17. Aleman A, Cafferata ML, Gibbons L, et al. Use of antenatal corticosteroids for preterm birth in Latin America: providers knowledge, attitudes and practices. Reprod Health. 2013;10:4.
18. Cousens S, Blencowe H, Gravett M, et al. Antibiotics for pre-term pre-labour rupture of membranes: prevention of neonatal deaths due to complications of pre-term birth and infection. Int J Epidemiol. 2010;39:i134-43.
19. World Health Organization. Partograph in management of labor. Lancet. 1994;343(8910):1399-404.
20. Tinker A, Ransom E. Healthy mothers and healthy newborns: the vital link. Washington, DC: Population Reference Bureau; 2002.
21. Wild S, Roglic G, Green A, et al. Global prevalence of diabetes: estimates for the year 2000 and projections for 2030. Diabetes Care. 2004;27(5):1047-53.
22. Committee on Practice Bulletins-Obstetrics. Practice Bulletin No. 137: Gestational diabetes mellitus. Obstet Gynecol. 2013;122(2 Pt 1):406-16.
23. Miller E, Hare JW, Cloherty JP, et al. Elevated maternal hemoglobin A1c in early pregnancy and major congenital

anomalies in infants of diabetic mothers. N Engl J Med. 1981;304(22):1331-4.
24. Ylinen K, Aula P, Stenman UH, et al. Risk of minor and major fetal malformations in diabetics with high haemoglobin A1c values in early pregnancy. Br Med J. 1984;289(6441):345-6.
25. Yazdy MM, Liu S, Mitchell AA, et al. Maternal dietary glycemic intake and the risk of neural tube defects. Am J Epidemiol. 2010;171(4):407-14.
26. Kitzmiller JL, Wallerstein R, Correa A, et al. Preconception care for women with diabetes and prevention of major congenital malformations. Birth Defects Res A Clin Mol Teratol. 2010;88(10):791-803.
27. Starikov R, Bohrer J, Goh W, et al. Hemoglobin A1c in pregestational diabetic gravidas and the risk of congenital heart disease in the fetus. Pediatr Cardiol. 2013;34(7):1716-22.
28. Hay WW Jr. Care of the infant of the diabetic mother. Curr Diab Rep. 2012;12(1):4-15.
29. Van Assche FA, Holemans K, Aerts L. Long-term consequences for offspring of diabetes during pregnancy. Br Med Bull. 2001;60:173-82.
30. Persson M, Pasupathy D, Hanson U, et al. Disproportionate body composition and perinatal outcome in large-for-gestational-age infants to mothers with type 1 diabetes. BJOG. 2012;119(5):565-72.
31. Barnes-Powell LL. Infants of diabetic mothers: the effects of hyperglycemia on the fetus and neonate. Neonatal Netw. 2007;26(5):283-90.
32. Opara PI, Jaja T, Onubogu UC. Morbidity and mortality amongst infants of diabetic mothers admitted into a special care baby unit in Port Harcourt, Nigeria. Ital J Pediatr. 2010;36(1):77.
33. Gilbert WM, Nesbitt TS, Danielsen B. Associated factors in 1611 cases of brachial plexus injury. Obstet Gynecol. 1999;93(4):536-40.
34. Athukorala C, Crowther CA, Willson K, et al. Women with gestational diabetes mellitus in the ACHOIS trial: risk factors for shoulder dystocia. Aust N Z J Obstet Gynaecol. 2007;47(1):37-41.
35. Aerts L, Van Assche FA. Animal evidence for the transgenerational development of diabetes mellitus. Int J Biochem Cell Biol. 2006;38(5-6):894-903.
36. Wang Z, Kanguru L, Hussein J, et al. Incidence of adverse outcomes associated with gestational diabetes mellitus in low- and middle-income countries. Int J Gynaecol Obstet. 2013;121(1):14-9.
37. Bhat M, Ramesha KN, Sarma SP, et al. Outcome of gestational diabetes mellitus from a tertiary referral center in South India: a case-control study. J Obstet Gynaecol India. 2012;62(6):644-9.
38. Zielinsky P, Piccoli AL Jr. Myocardial hypertrophy and dysfunction in maternal diabetes. Early Hum Dev. 2012;88(5):273-8.
39. Kjos SL, Walther FJ, Montoro M, et al. Prevalence and etiology of respiratory distress in infants of diabetic mothers: predictive value of fetal lung maturation tests. Am J Obstet Gynecol. 1990;163(3):898-903.
40. Bhutta ZA, Lassi LS, Blanc A, et al. Linkages among reproductive health, maternal health, and perinatal outcomes. Semin Perinatol. 2010;34(6):434-45.
41. von Dadelszen P, Ansermino JM, Dumont G, et al. Improving maternal and perinatal outcomes in the hypertensive disorders of pregnancy: a vision of a community-focused approach. Int J Gynecol Obstet. 2012;119:S30-4.
42. Goldenberg RL, McClure EM, MacGuire ER, et al. Lessons for low-income regions following the reduction in hypertension-related maternal mortality in high-income countries. Int J Gynecol Obstet. 2011;113(2):91-5.
43. Kiondo P, Tumwesigye NM, Wandabwa J, et al. Adverse neonatal outcomes in women with pre-eclampsia in Mulago Hospital, Kampala, Uganda: a cross-sectional study. Pan Afr Med J. 2014;17(Suppl 1):7.
44. American College of Obstetricians and Gynecologists, Task Force on Hypertension in Pregnancy. Hypertension in pregnancy. Report of the American College of Obstetricians and Gynecologists' Task Force on Hypertension in Pregnancy. Obstet Gynecol. 2013;122(5):1122-31.
45. Publications Committee, Society for Maternal-Fetal Medicine, Sibai BM. Evaluation and management of severe preeclampsia before 34 weeks' gestation. Am J Obstet Gynecol. 2011;205(3):191-8.
46. World Health Organization. WHO recommendations for prevention and treatment of pre-eclampsia and eclampsia. Geneva: WHO Publications; 2011.
47. Churchill D, Duley L, Thornton JG, et al. Interventionist versus expectant care for severe pre-eclampsia between 24 and 34 weeks' gestation. Cochrane Database Syst Rev. 2013;7:CD003106.
48. Vigil-De Gracia P, Reyes Tejada O, Calle Miñaca A, et al. Expectant management of severe preeclampsia remote from term: the MEXPRE Latin Study, a randomized, multicenter clinical trial. Am J Obstet Gynecol. 2013;209(5):425 e1-8.
49. Duley L, Henderson-Smart DJ, Meher S, et al. Antiplatelet agents for preventing pre-eclampsia and its complications. Cochrane Database Syst Rev. 2007;(2):CD004659.
50. Lassi ZS, Majeed A, Rashid S, et al. The interconnections between maternal and newborn health—evidence and implications for policy. J Matern Fetal Neonatal Med. 2013;26Suppl 1:3-53.
51. Haeri S, Guichard I, Baker AM, et al. The effect of teenage maternal obesity on perinatal outcomes. Obstet Gynecol. 2009;113(2 Pt 1):300-4.
52. Yogev Y, Catalano PM. Pregnancy and obesity. Obstet Gynecol Clin North Am. 2009;36(2):285-300.
53. Garabedian MJ, Williams CM, Pearce CF, et al. Extreme morbid obesity and labor outcome in nulliparous women at term. Am J Perinatol. 2011;28(9):729-34.
54. Baron CM, Girling LG, Mathieson AL, et al. Obstetrical and neonatal outcomes in obese parturients. J Matern Fetal Neonatal Med. 2010;23(8):906-13.
55. Khashan AS, Kenny LC. The effects of maternal body mass index on pregnancy outcome. Eur J Epidemiol. 2009:24(11):697-705.
56. Alanis MC, Goodnight WH, Hill EG, et al. Maternal super-obesity (body mass index ≥ 50) and adverse pregnancy outcomes. Acta Obstet Gynecol Scand. 2010;89(7):924-30.
57. Racusin D, Stevens B, Campbell G, et al. Obesity and the risk and detection of fetal malformations. Semin Perinatol. 2012;36(3):213-21.

58. Aagaard-Tillery KM, Flint Porter T, Malone FD, et al. Influence of maternal BMI on genetic sonography in the FaSTER trial. Prenat Diagn. 2010;30(1):14-22.
59. Hildebrand E, Gottvall T, Blomberg M. Maternal obesity and detection rate of fetal structural anomalies. Fetal Diagn Ther. 2013;33(4):246-51.
60. Tennant PW, Rankin J, Bell R. Maternal body mass index and the risk of fetal and infant death: a cohort study from the North of England. Hum Reprod. 2011;26(6):1501-11.
61. Chu SY, Kim SY, Lau J, et al. Maternal obesity and risk of stillbirth: a metaanalysis. Am J Obstet Gynecol. 2007;197(3):223-8.
62. Cnattingius S, Bergstrom R, Lipworth L, et al. Prepregnancy weight and the risk of adverse pregnancy outcomes. N Engl J Med. 1998;338(3):147-52.
63. Bhattacharya S, Campbell DM, Liston WA, et al. Effect of Body Mass Index on pregnancy outcomes in nulliparous women delivering singleton babies. BMC Public Health. 2007;7(1):168.
64. Ehrenberg HM, Weiner SJ. Maternal obesity, uterine activity, and the risk of spontaneous preterm birth. Obstet Gynecol. 2009;113(6):1373-4.
65. Garabedian MJ, Hansen WF, McCord LA, et al. Up-regulation of oxytocin receptor expression at term is related to maternal body mass index. Am J Perinatol. 2013;30(6):491-7.
66. Smith RD, Babiychuk EB, Noble K, et al. Increased cholesterol decreases uterine activity: functional effects of cholesterol alteration in pregnant rat myometrium. Am J Physiol Cell Physiol. 2005;288(5):C982-8.
67. Moynihan AT, Hehir MP, Glavey SV, et al. Inhibitory effect of leptin on human uterine contractility in vitro. Am J Obstet Gynecol. 2006;195(2):504-9.
68. Zhang J, Bricker L, Wray S, et al. Poor uterine contractility in obese women. BJOG. 2007;114(3):343-8.

# CHAPTER 12

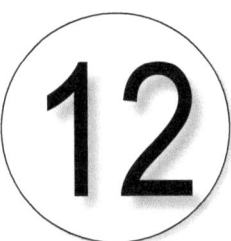

# Disorders of the Membranes, Placenta, and Cord

*Shannon Dralla, Matthew J Garabedian*

## ■ INTRODUCTION

Placental growth is vital to the normal development of the fetus and for the mother to sustain pregnancy. The placenta is a highly regulated interface between mother and fetus, functioning to transport nutrients and immunoglobulins, eliminate fetal waste products, enable gas exchange, and produce steroid hormones and peptides.[1] Pathology of the placenta, membranes, and cord can have a large impact on the health and well-being of both mother and fetus. Abnormalities of the placenta, membranes, and cord may arise from weakening of the membranes or infection [preterm premature rupture of membranes (PPROM)], acute changes in the status of the placenta (abruptio placentae), or may exist from the point of implantation and development of the chorion and amnion [placenta previa, the morbidly adherent placenta (MAP), and vasa previa]. The aim of this chapter is to review the most common disorders and focus on their contributions to neonatal morbidity and mortality.

## ■ DISORDER OF THE MEMBRANES: PRETERM PREMATURE RUPTURE OF MEMBRANES

Preterm premature rupture of membranes is a relatively common condition, representing approximately one quarter of spontaneous preterm births.[2] Currently, the American Congress of Obstetricians and Gynecologists (ACOG) and the Society for Maternal-Fetal Medicine (SMFM) recommend delivery at or beyond 34 weeks in an otherwise uncomplicated pregnancy.[2,3] Intra-amniotic infection and inflammation, in addition to maternal smoking, illicit drug use, low body mass index, low socioeconomic status, and maternal medical conditions may increase the risk of PPROM.[2] The neonatal morbidity associated with PPROM is primarily related to gestational age at delivery. In developing nations, where resources may be limited, the impact of prematurity is a major determinant of outcomes.[4] Decisions about timing of delivery reflect assessment of the risks of prematurity weighed against the risk of infection or other complication with continued pregnancy.[2]

With expectant management, the goal is to safely deliver the neonate at a later gestation to decrease prematurity related risks. The landmark study by Mercer et al. demonstrated that neonatal morbidity was decreased with the use of broad-spectrum antibiotics in cases of PPROM remote from term managed expectantly.[5] In this trial, 610 women were randomized to antibiotics (ampicillin/amoxicillin and erythromycin for 7 days) or placebo. The primary outcome, a composite of fetal or postnatal death, respiratory distress syndrome (RDS), documented sepsis within 72 hours of birth, grade 3 or 4 intraventricular hemorrhage, or stage 2 or 3 enterocolitis, was less common in infants whose mothers received antibiotics than placebo [relative risk (RR) 0.84, 95% confidence interval (CI) 071-0.99]. This result seems to have been driven by a decrease in RDS (RR 0.83, 95% CI 0.69-0.99) and necrotizing colitis (RR 0.83, 0.17-0.95). Improvements in these neonatal outcomes, however, were not seen in women colonized with group B *Streptococcus*. Clinical chorioamnionitis was less common in women receiving antibiotics (23.0% vs 33.9%, P = 0.01) and duration from randomization until delivery was longer (median time to delivery, 6.1 vs 2.9 days, P < 0.01).

Subsequent studies have shown expectant management of PPROM to be associated with longer latencies, less neonatal intensive care unit (NICU) admission, and less neonatal morbidity.[6,7] The occurrence of PPROM at earlier gestational ages is also associated with longer latency.[6,8] There are conflicting data as to whether length of latency is associated with chorioamnionitis and other neonatal morbidity.[6-9] In an observational study of 472 cases of PPROM, elective delivery at 34 weeks without medical complication was associated with less composite neonatal morbidity than a strategy of awaiting spontaneous labor [9% vs 18.8%, P = 0.02, adjusted odds ratio (OR) 0.41, 95% CI 0.19-0.87].[9]

In a 10-year retrospective analysis of PPROM in a Nigerian teaching hospital, early administration of antibiotics was shown to be associated with a decrease in chorioamnionitis (P < 0.0001).[4] Of those neonates with infection, 92% died, in contrast to 35.7% of those without infection (P < 0.0001). These findings support the important role of early administration of antibiotics to improve neonatal survival.

Not all study results agree with the benefit of elective delivery and some question the recommendation for delivery at 34 weeks.[10,11] A Cochrane review, including 690 deliveries, found no clear benefit of early delivery, and insufficient data to guide management in cases of PPROM.[11] This review found no improvement in neonatal sepsis (RR 1.33, 95% CI 0.72-2.47), RDS (RR 0.98, 95% CI 0.74-1.29), or perinatal mortality (RR 0.98, 95% CI 0.41-2.36), but the review did find an increased risk of cesarean delivery (RR 1.51, 95% CI 1.08-2.10). This is consistent with a study of 634 cases of PPROM between 34 and 36 completed weeks, where active management was shown to be associated with an increased risk of oxygen dependence at 24 hours (7.0% vs 1.6%, P = 0.05) and antibiotic usage until 72 hours of life or longer (15.9% vs 5.2%, P = 0.001).[10] However, this review did not find demonstrable increases in the risk of NICU admission (3.2% vs 6.1%, P = 0.28), neonatal infection (3.2% vs 1.7%, P = 0.47), neonatal sepsis (1.6% vs 0%, P = 0.5), or other neonatal morbidities.

Recent data from the Netherlands further questions the recommendation for delivery at 34 weeks in cases of otherwise uncomplicated PPROM.[12,13] The first, dubbed PPROMEXIL, randomized 536 women with PPROM at ≥34 weeks and <37 weeks to immediate delivery or expectant management.[12] Immediate delivery and expectant management had similar rates of proven neonatal sepsis (0.4%, vs 1.1%; RR 0.34, 95% CI 0.04-3.21), RDS (7.8% vs 6.4%; RR 1.25, 95% CI 0.67-2.31), and NICU admission (9.0% vs 5.6%; RR 1.4, 95% CI 0.11-2.74). A meta-analysis, which included this study, showed no statistical difference between immediate delivery and expectant management for neonatal infection (RR 1.06, 95% CI 0.64-1.76), proven neonatal sepsis (RR 0.94, 95% CI 0.43-2.05), and RDS (RR 1.03, 95% CI 0.80-1.33).[12] A strategy of expectant management leads to increased antepartum costs, and on the other hand, the immediate delivery strategy leads to greater intrapartum and postpartum costs.[14] At 6-week postpartum, the net effect seems to be an increase in total costs with immediate delivery, due to an increased need for a higher level and longer duration of neonatal care.[14]

Because of power limitations in the PPROMEXIL trial, a follow-up, PPROMEXIL-II was conducted. With PPROMEXIL-II, an additional 200 subjects were recruited to augment the power of the PPROMEXIL trial.[13] With the additional patients from PPROMEXIL-II, the results from the meta-analysis of key neonatal morbidities was unchanged, without significant differences in neonatal infection (RR 1.02, 95% CI 0.63-1.65), proven neonatal sepsis (RR 0.88, 95% CI 0.42-1.84), or RDS (RR 1.04, 95% CI 0.81-1.33).

## DISORDER OF THE PLACENTA: ABRUPTIO PLACENTAE

Placental abruption (abruptio placentae) is bleeding at the decidual-placental interface that creates partial or total placental detachment. Depending on the amount of separation and acuity of the event, clinically there can be a wide spectrum of outcomes from little to no effect, fetal growth restriction, or massive hemorrhage resulting in stillbirth and maternal death. Abruption may be between the membranes and decidua resulting in vaginal bleeding but less commonly it may be "concealed" with blood collecting behind the placenta with no external bleeding.[15,16] The clinical presentation is commonly painful vaginal bleeding, often also with uterine tenderness, hypertonic contractions, and nonreassuring fetal heath status.[16,17]

Placental abruption occurs in around 1 in 100 births and can lead to hypoxemia, prematurity, and death. In a large Finnish study of over 1 million pregnancies, perinatal mortality with abruption occurred in 119 of 1,000 births and more than double that rate in births before 32 weeks.[16] The risk of prematurity is fourfold higher in abruption as compared to normal pregnancies.[17] Abruptio placentae is an emergency situation for both mother and fetus, often resulting in consumptive coagulopathy for the mother, oxygen and nutrient deprivation to the fetus, and 9-12% perinatal death.[16-18]

Risk factors for abruption include tobacco use, cocaine use, abdominal trauma, polyhydramnios, chronic hypertension, preeclampsia, thrombophilias, intrauterine infections, and advanced maternal age.[15,17] Tobacco and cocaine uses are modifiable risk factors, and management of hypertensive disorders allows for decreased rates of abruption. Predictors of increased risk for perinatal death include tobacco use, prematurity, low birth weight, and male offspring. Tobacco use may increase abruption up to 50%.[15,19,20]

Just as there are broad clinical outcomes and risk factors of abruption, the pathophysiology is also varied.[21,22] Causes such as maternal hypertension, excessive shearing forces during motor vehicle accidents, and premature PPROM may be associated with abruption.[23,24] Diagnosis can be aided by assessing maternal risk factors and ultrasound to look for placental separation and intrauterine growth restriction. Notably, placental abruption is implicated as a risk for sudden infant death syndrome and major congenital anomalies.[25-27]

The management of abruption is early recognition and prompts delivery in near term infants and unstable maternal or fetal status. There are also situations where premature infants with reassuring maternal and fetal status receive conservative management and antenatal steroid administration to improve the sequelae of prematurity and its associated morbidity and mortality.[15] Recognizing the varied presentations and having a high clinical suspicion for abruption will further improve neonatal and maternal outcomes, as seen in multiple retrospective studies.[16,18,22]

## DISORDERS OF THE PLACENTA: PLACENTA PREVIA, ACCRETA, INCRETA, AND PERCRETA

Globally, peripartum hemorrhage is a leading cause of maternal hemorrhage. In developing nations, improvements in medical care are bridging the gaps that persist in the developed world.[28] The management of pregnancy complicated by abnormalities of placental location (placenta previa) or attachment (placenta accreta, increta, or percreta) is driven by attempts to minimize maternal morbidity and mortality.[3,29] Much of this risk comes from antenatal bleeding, and expert opinion argues for the acceptance of some neonatal risk for maternal benefit. Currently, there is no consensus for where the balance lies—ACOG provides no guidelines on timing. The Royal College of Obstetricians and Gynaecologists recommends delivery not occur before 38 weeks in a patient with an asymptomatic placenta previa.[29] The Society for Maternal Fetal Medicine endorses delivery at 36–37 weeks for these patients.[3] A recent analysis of linked vital statistics data supports delivery at the gestational age of 38 weeks being associated with no worse or better neonatal outcomes than delivery at 35, 36, or 37 weeks.[30]

## PLACENTA PREVIA

Placenta previa, occurring in approximately 1:200 pregnancies,[31] is the condition in which the placental disk covers the internal cervical os, either partially (known as a "partial placenta previa") or in entirety ("complete placenta previa").[32] Both conditions result in an increase in maternal morbidity and mortality. A placenta that has its margin within 1 and 2 centimeters of the os, but does not cover the os, is known as a "marginal previa," which also carries risk of maternal morbidity. These disorders of placental location also create an increased risk of neonatal morbidity **(Figs. 1A to D)**.[33] Maternal risk with placenta previa is considerable, with significant risk of antepartum hemorrhage (68%), blood transfusion (15%), and hysterectomy (5%).[34]

One of the strongest risk factors for placenta previa is prior cesarean delivery.[31,35] A history of cesarean delivery is associated with a three-fold increase in likelihood of placenta previa (OR 2.9, 95% CI 2.8–3.0).[31] Additionally, the likelihood of placenta previa increases with the number of prior cesarean deliveries.[31,36] Other risk factors include advanced maternal age, multiparity, prior abortion, and drug use.[31,35,36] In the developing world, the increasing incidence of abnormal placentation may be related to different factors—e.g. in India, increasing utilization of termination procedures has been cited as a contributing factor to a tenfold increase in abnormal placentation.[28]

Placenta previa is also associated with an increase in perinatal morbidity and mortality.[33,37] Neonatal mortality has been demonstrated in pregnancies complicated by placenta previa to be approximately three to four times greater than in pregnancies with normal placentation.[33,38] This risk, however, is influenced by gestational age at birth, and the excess risk attributable to placenta previa may be primarily at 37 weeks or beyond.[33] Older data shows that placenta previa has been associated with an increase in neonatal morbidities such as RDS (OR 4.94, 95% CI 3.45–7.08) and anemia (OR 2.65, 95% CI 1.70–4.15), even after adjusting for gestational age at delivery and other confounders.[37] This is supported by more recent data, demonstrating an association between placenta previa and RDS (OR 3.82, 95% CI 2.91–5.00), prolonged ventilation (OR 3.20, 95% CI 2.50–4.10), and neonatal anemia (OR 6.87, 95% CI 4.43–10.65).[39] Placenta previa may be an independent risk factor for RDS, particularly among neonates born preterm.[39,40] Placenta previa also has been associated, albeit variably, with a risk of fetal growth restriction.[39,41-43] It should

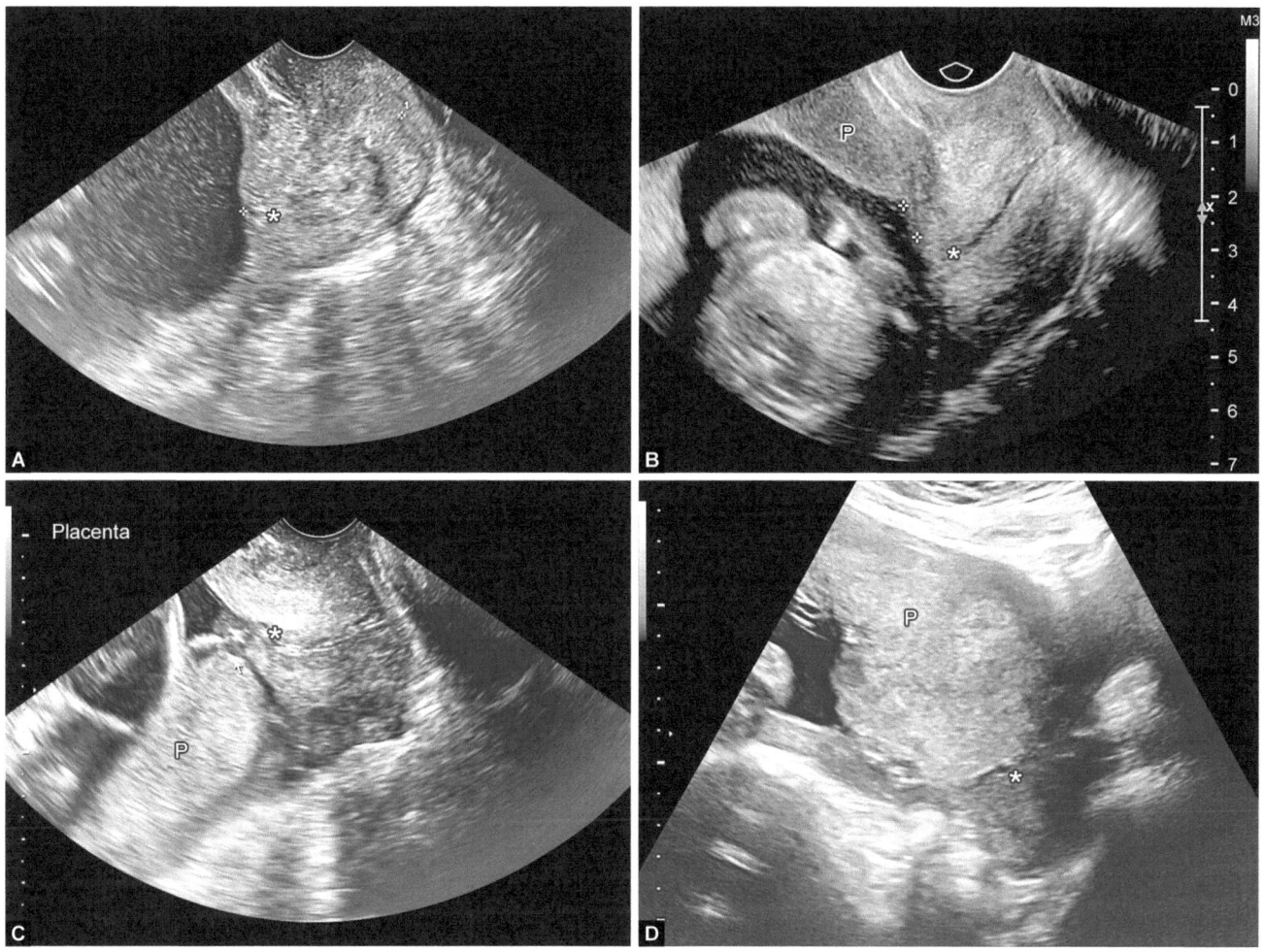

**Figs. 1A to D:** The spectrum of placentation. (A) Normal placentation; (B) marginal placental previa; (C) partial placenta previa; (D) complete placenta previa. Placentation is characterized by the relationship between the placenta (P) and the internal cervical os (*).

be noted, however, that gestational age at delivery remains an important driver of neonatal morbidity and mortality.[30,38]

The diagnosis of placenta previa is made by ultrasound, although patients may present with painless late pregnancy bleeding. Such bleeding should be presumed to be placenta previa until specifically excluded. Many placentas are described as "low-lying," on second trimester ultrasound. Definitive diagnosis should be reserved for third trimester assessment, as more than 90% of such placentas will not persist as true placenta previa by the third trimester.[44-46]

Obstetric management of placenta previa is based upon prevention and treatment of obstetric hemorrhage. The primary maternal risk is that of hemorrhage at the onset of labor. This bleeding may be preceded by "herald" bleeds, but the course of placenta previa is highly variable and difficult to predict.[47] However, these bleeds will frequently prompt hospital admission, administration of antenatal corticosteroids, and close surveillance. The use of tocolytic medications is controversial and likely does not increase short-term morbidity and mortality.[48-50] Tocolytic therapy may lead to significant prolongation and larger birth weights.[49,50]

## MORBIDLY ADHERENT PLACENTA: PLACENTA ACCRETA, INCRETA, AND PERCRETA

Placenta accreta, increta, and percreta are a spectrum of disorders in which abnormal trophoblastic invasion leads to a MAP. Generally, the term placenta accreta is often used to refer to this spectrum of disorders; the term MAP is preferred here to avoid ambiguity of terms. A placenta that is abnormally adherent, without myometrial invasion, is a *placenta accreta*.[51] A *placenta increta* is one that invades the myometrium, but it is contained by the uterine serosa. Extension beyond the uterine serosa with involvement of adjacent tissues (bladder, bowel, and other pelvic structures), defines *placenta percreta*. Of cases of MAP, placenta accreta represents approximately 75% of cases; placenta increta, 18%; and placenta percreta, 7%.[36]

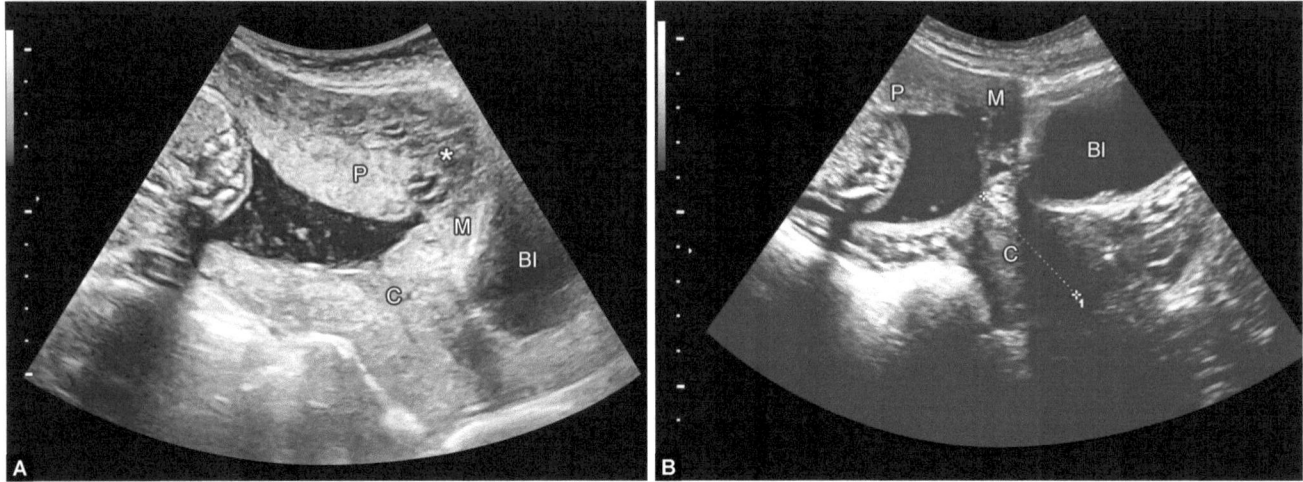

**Figs. 2A and B:** The sonographic appearance of a placenta accreta (A) and normal placenta (B) can be similar. Placenta accreta was confirmed by pathologic examination of hysterectomy specimen in case (A). Placenta accreta is often associated with placenta previa, but may exist in the absence of previa, as demonstrated in (A). In both cases presented, the placenta does not cover the cervix (C). Findings on ultrasound imaging that suggest placenta accreta include loss of a clear distinction between the placenta (P) and myometrium (M), bulging of the interface between the myometrium and bladder (Bl), and abnormal vascularity (*).

Unfortunately, accurate prenatal diagnosis of MAP can be difficult, with neither ultrasound nor magnetic resonance imaging (MRI) having 100% sensitivity or specificity.[52] However, signs such as a loss of distinct border between the placenta and myometrium, a bulge at the border with the bladder, and abnormal vascularity are useful clinical signs **(Figs. 2A and B)**.[53]

Risk factors for MAP are similar to those of placenta previa, with prior uterine surgery and the presence of a placenta previa being the strongest risk factors for MAP.[54] The incidence of MAP has increased over recent decades, likely in association with increasing rates of cesarean delivery.[54-56] The incidence of MAP is approximately 1 in 300-500 pregnancies.[51,54] The combination of multiple prior cesarean deliveries and placenta previa greatly increases the risk of MAP.[57] Among women undergoing a primary cesarean for previa, the risk of MAP is approximately 3%; for women undergoing their third or higher-order cesarean with a concurrent placenta previa, the risk of MAP is >60%.[57] In the absence of a placenta previa, a history of multiple prior cesarean deliveries still confers an increased, although less strikingly so, risk in MAP.

The maternal morbidity associated with MAP is great, with the likelihood of major maternal morbidity of approximately 60%, including a high risk of intensive care admission (>25%), blood transfusion (>80%), surgical injury (cystotomy 15-29%; ureteral injury 2-7%), and pulmonary embolus (2%).[56-58] Maternal mortality may be as high as 6-7%.[51] Data suggests that elective delivery is associated with less maternal and neonatal morbidity than emergent delivery.[55,56,59] Recent decision analysis and expert opinion support scheduled delivery at 34-35 weeks, following administration of antenatal corticosteroids, to be the optimal approach to management of a suspected MAP.[3,60] If no antepartum bleeding or other complications are present, however, delivery in the late-preterm period may be considered.[51] High-quality prospective data supporting these recommendations, however, are lacking.

Neonatal morbidity is increased in pregnancies complicated by MAP, but whether there is an effect of MAP independent than that associated with preterm delivery is unclear.[61] It appears that neonatal morbidity or mortality associated with MAP is similar to that for placenta previa and the most significant differences are those of maternal morbidity and mortality.[58] Antenatal diagnosis of MAP is associated with decreased maternal and neonatal morbidity. There is no difference in NICU admissions noted among infants born following emergent delivery for MAP than those delivering with elective timing (84.6% vs 62.5%, P = 0.17).[59] However, any differences in outcomes may be attributable to a generally earlier gestational age at delivery with antenatal diagnosis (gestational age < 34 weeks 66.7% vs 12.5%, P < 0.001). Current recommendations do not support adjudicating timing of delivery on the results of amniocentesis for lung maturation indexes, as this strategy is not supported by decision analysis.[60] In reality, to see a striking reduction in neonatal morbidity, delivery would need to be delayed until at least 39 weeks gestation, but this strategy would come at the expense of increasing maternal morbidity and mortality. This has been the primary argument to justify iatrogenic prematurity in this population.[53]

## DISORDER OF THE CORD: VELAMENTOUS CORD INSERTION AND VASA PREVIA

A velamentous cord insertion is one in which the umbilical cord inserts into the amniotic membranes and then courses along the membranes to the placenta. This occurs in fewer than 2.5% of pregnancies.[62,63] If these vessels cross or are in close proximity to the uterine cervix, then a vasa previa exists.[64] As the vessels course along the membranes, they are not protected by Wharton's jelly and they are prone to injury.

Risk factors for velamentous cord insertion include multifetal gestation, nulliparity, prior pregnancy termination, obesity, infertility, placenta previa, and maternal smoking.[62,63,65] After adjusting for common risk factors for neonatal morbidity, there remains an association between velamentous cord insertion and preterm birth (OR 2.01, 95% CI 1.53–2.64), NICU admission (OR 1.38, 95% CI 1.06–1.80), and birth weight < 2,500 g (OR 3.39, 95% CI 2.75–5.62).[62] Additionally, velamentous cord insertion is more common with placenta previa (OR 3.71, 95% CI 3.03–4.55), abruptio placentae (OR 2.60, 95% CI 2.12–3.18), and preeclampsia (OR 1.51, 95% CI 1.39–1.65).[63]

With vasa previa, occurring in approximately 1:2,500 pregnancies, there exists the risk of rupture of fetal vessels and fetal exsanguination, a true obstetric emergency.[32] As such, iatrogenic preterm delivery at 34–36 weeks is recommended to avoid labor, and supported by decision analysis.[32,65-67] Unrecognized vasa previa is associated with an approximately 60% risk of perinatal mortality.[32] Screening for vasa previa on second trimester ultrasound can identify cases, which has been shown to lead to a reported 100% neonatal survival rate.[64]

## CONCLUSION

The membranes, placenta, and cord can have significant pathologies that lead to both maternal and neonatal injury and death. The causes of these disorders are varied and often interconnected. With recognition of these pathophysiologic conditions, clinicians can initiate treatments to decrease morbidity and mortality for both mother and infant. Obstetric management of these conditions requires the careful consideration of the maternal-fetal dyad and often requires the consideration of competing risks. Frequently what may decrease maternal risk increases neonatal morbidity.[3] Implementation of evidence based practice finds a rational balance of competing risks, as illustrated clearly by the use of antibiotics in PPROM to decrease neonatal morbidity, counseling tobacco cessation to decreased placental abruption rates, and screening for vasa previa during ultrasound to improve neonatal survival to 100%. Unfortunately, at this point, high quality data do not exist for all obstetric problems, such as timing of delivery of pregnancies complicated by MAP. Until these data exist, careful consideration and personalization of care may be the best approach. Multidisciplinary care teams comprised of neonatology and maternal-fetal medicine should be developed to prevent maternal and fetal morbidity and mortality while striving for increasing healthy family units worldwide.

## REFERENCES

1. Jansson T, Powell TL. Placental nutrient transfer and fetal growth. Nutrition. 2000;16:500-2.
2. Practice bulletins No. 139: premature rupture of membranes. Obstet Gynecol. 2013;122:918-30.
3. Spong CY, Mercer BM, D'Alton M, et al. Timing of indicated late-preterm and early-term birth. Obstet Gynecol. 2011;118:323-33.
4. Obi SN, Ozumba BC. Pre-term premature rupture of fetal membranes: the dilemma of management in a developing nation. J Obstet Gynaecol. 2007;27:37-40.
5. Mercer BM, Miodovnik M, Thurnau GR, et al. Antibiotic therapy for reduction of infant morbidity after preterm premature rupture of the membranes. A randomized controlled trial. National Institute of Child Health and Human Development Maternal-Fetal Medicine Units Network. JAMA. 1997;278:989-95.
6. Nayot D, Penava D, Da Silva O, et al. Neonatal outcomes are associated with latency after preterm premature rupture of membranes. J Perinatol. 2012;32:970-7.
7. Frenette P, Dodds L, Armson BA, et al. Preterm prelabour rupture of membranes: effect of latency on neonatal and maternal outcomes. J Obstet Gynaecol Can. 2013;35:710-7.
8. Aziz N, Cheng YW, Caughey AB. Factors and outcomes associated with longer latency in preterm premature rupture of membranes. J Matern Fetal Neonatal Med. 2008;21:821-5.
9. Pasquier JC, Picaud JC, Rabilloud M, et al. Neonatal outcomes after elective delivery management of preterm premature rupture of the membranes before 34 weeks' gestation (DOMINOS study). Eur J Obstet Gynecol Reprod Biol. 2009;143:18-23.
10. Kayem G, Bernier-Dupreelle A, Goffinet F, et al. Active versus expectant management for preterm prelabor rupture of membranes at 34-36 weeks of completed gestation: comparison of maternal and neonatal outcomes. Acta Obstet Gynecol Scand. 2010;89:776-81.
11. Buchanan SL, Crowther CA, Levett KM, et al. Planned early birth versus expectant management for women with preterm prelabour rupture of membranes prior to 37 weeks' gestation for improving pregnancy outcome. Cochrane Database Syst Rev. 2010;3:CD004735.
12. van der Ham DP, Vijgen SM, Nijhuis JG, et al. Induction of labor versus expectant management in women with preterm prelabor rupture of membranes between 34 and 37 weeks: a randomized controlled trial. PLoS Med. 2012;9:e1001208.
13. van der Ham DP, van der Heyden JL, Opmeer BC, et al. Management of late-preterm premature rupture of membranes: the PPROMEXIL-2 trial. Am J Obstet Gynecol. 2012;207:276.e1-10.

14. Vijgen SM, van der Ham DP, Bijlenga D, et al. Economic analysis comparing induction of labor and expectant management in women with preterm prelabor rupture of membranes between 34 and 37 weeks (PPROMEXIL trial). Acta Obstet Gynecol Scand. 2014;93:374-81.
15. Oyelese Y, Ananth CV. Placental abruption. Obstet Gynecol. 2006;108:1005-16.
16. Tikkanen M, Luukkaala T, Gissler M, et al. Decreasing perinatal mortality in placental abruption. Acta Obstet Gynecol Scand. 2013;92:298-305.
17. Ananth CV, Berkowitz GS, Savitz DA, et al. Placental abruption and adverse perinatal outcomes. JAMA. 1999;282:1646-51.
18. Kayani SI, Walkinshaw SA, Preston C. Pregnancy outcome in severe placental abruption. BJOG. 2003;110:679-83.
19. Kaminsky LM, Ananth CV, Prasad V, et al. The influence of maternal cigarette smoking on placental pathology in pregnancies complicated by abruption. Am J Obstet Gynecol. 2007;197:275.e1-5.
20. Ananth CV, Savitz DA, Luther ER. Maternal cigarette smoking as a risk factor for placental abruption, placenta previa, and uterine bleeding in pregnancy. Am J Epidemiol. 1996;144:881-9.
21. Chang YL, Chang SD, Cheng PJ. Perinatal outcome in patients with placental abruption with and without antepartum hemorrhage. Int J Gynaecol Obstet. 2001;75:193-4.
22. Aliyu MH, Salihu HM, Lynch O, et al. Placental abruption, offspring sex, and birth outcomes in a large cohort of mothers. J Matern Fetal Neonatal Med. 2012;25:248-52.
23. Major CA, de Veciana M, Lewis DF, et al. Preterm premature rupture of membranes and abruptio placentae: is there an association between these pregnancy complications? Am J Obstet Gynecol. 1995;172:672-6.
24. Mackenzie AP, Schatz F, Krikun G, et al. Mechanisms of abruption-induced premature rupture of the fetal membranes: Thrombin enhanced decidual matrix metalloproteinase-3 (stromelysin-1) expression. Am J Obstet Gynecol. 2004;191:1996-2001.
25. Spinillo A, Fazzi E, Stronati M, et al. Severity of abruptio placentae and neurodevelopmental outcome in low birth weight infants. Early Hum Dev. 1993;35:45-54.
26. Li DK, Wi S. Maternal placental abnormality and the risk of sudden infant death syndrome. Am J Epidemiol. 1999;149:608-11.
27. Riihimaki O, Metsaranta M, Ritvanen A, et al. Increased prevalence of major congenital anomalies in births with placental abruption. Obstet Gynecol. 2013;122:268-74.
28. Bajwa SK, Singh A, Bajwa SJ. Contemporary issues in the management of abnormal placentation during pregnancy in developing nations: An Indian perspective. Int J Crit Illn Inj Sci. 2013;3:183-9.
29. RCOG. Placenta praevia, placenta praevia accreta and vasa praevia: diagnosis and management. RCOG Green-top Guideline No. 27. London, United Kingdom: Royal College of Obstetricians and Gynaecologists; 2011.
30. Balayla J, Wo BL, Bédard MJ. A late-preterm, early-term stratified analysis of neonatal outcomes by gestational age in placenta previa: defining the optimal timing for delivery. J Matern Fetal Neonatal Med. 2015;28(15):1756-61.
31. Ananth CV, Smulian JC, Vintzileos AM. The association of placenta previa with history of cesarean delivery and abortion: a meta-analysis. Am J Obstet Gynecol. 1997;177:1071-8.
32. Oyelese Y, Smulian JC. Placenta previa, placenta accreta, and vasa previa. Obstet Gynecol. 2006;107:927-41.
33. Ananth CV, Smulian JC, Vintzileos AM. The effect of placenta previa on neonatal mortality: a population-based study in the United States, 1989 through 1997. Am J Obstet Gynecol. 2003;188:1299-304.
34. Crane JM, Van den Hof MC, Dodds L, et al. Maternal complications with placenta previa. Am J Perinatol. 2000;17:101-5.
35. Tuzović L, Djelmis J, Ilijić M. Obstetric risk factors associated with placenta previa development: case-control study. Croat Med J. 2003;44:728-33.
36. Miller DA, Chollet JA, Goodwin TM. Clinical risk factors for placenta previa-placenta accreta. Am J Obstet Gynecol. 1997;177:210-4.
37. Crane JM, van den Hof MC, Dodds L, et al. Neonatal outcomes with placenta previa. Obstet Gynecol. 1999;93:541-4.
38. Salihu HM, Li Q, Rouse DJ, et al. Placenta previa: neonatal death after live births in the United States. Am J Obstet Gynecol. 2003;188:1305-9.
39. Schneiderman M, Balayla J. A comparative study of neonatal outcomes in placenta previa versus cesarean for other indication at term. J Matern Fetal Neonatal Med. 2013;26:1121-7.
40. Lin C, Wang S, Hsu Y, et al. Risk for respiratory distress syndrome in preterm infants born to mothers complicated by placenta previa. Early Hum Dev. 2001;60:215-24.
41. Harper LM, Odibo AO, Macones GA, et al. Effect of placenta previa on fetal growth. Am J Obstet Gynecol. 2010;203:330.e1-5.
42. Raisanen S, Kancherla V, Kramer MR, et al. Placenta previa and the risk of delivering a small-for-gestational-age newborn. Obstet Gynecol. 2014;124:285-91.
43. Ananth CV, Demissie K, Smulian JC, et al. Relationship among placenta previa, fetal growth restriction, and preterm delivery: a population-based study. Obstet Gynecol. 2001;98:299-306.
44. Heller HT, Mullen KM, Gordon RW, et al. Outcomes of pregnancies with a low-lying placenta diagnosed on second-trimester sonography. J Ultrasound Med. 2014;33:691-6.
45. Pradhan S, Tuladhar A, Shrestha A, et al. Sonographic assessment of placental migration in second trimester low lying placenta. Nepal Med Coll J. 2012;14:331-3.
46. Copland JA, Craw SM, Herbison P. Low-lying placenta: who should be recalled for a follow-up scan? J Med Imaging Radiat Oncol. 2012;56:158-62.
47. Love CD, Wallace EM. Pregnancies complicated by placenta praevia: what is appropriate management? Br J Obstet Gynaecol. 1996;103:864-7.
48. Towers CV, Pircon RA, Heppard M. Is tocolysis safe in the management of third-trimester bleeding? Am J Obstet Gynecol. 1999;180:1572-8.
49. Besinger RE, Moniak CW, Paskiewicz LS, et al. The effect of tocolytic use in the management of symptomatic placenta previa. Am J Obstet Gynecol. 1995;172:1770-5.
50. Sharma D, Spearman P. The impact of cesarean delivery on transmission of infectious agents to the neonate. Clin Perinatol. 2008;35:407-20.

51. Publications Committee, Society for Maternal-Fetal Medicine, Belfort MA. Placenta accreta. Am J Obstet Gynecol. 2010;203:430-9.
52. D'Antonio F, Iacovella C, Bhide A. Prenatal identification of invasive placentation using ultrasound: systematic review and meta-analysis. Ultrasound Obstet Gynecol. 2013;42:509-17.
53. Belfort MA. Indicated preterm birth for placenta accreta. Semin Perinatol. 2011;35:252-6.
54. Wu S, Kocherginsky M, Hibbard JU. Abnormal placentation: twenty-year analysis. Am J Obstet Gynecol. 2005;192:1458-61.
55. Warshak CR, Ramos GA, Eskander R, et al. Effect of predelivery diagnosis in 99 consecutive cases of placenta accreta. Obstet Gynecol. 2010;115:65-9.
56. Eller AG, Porter TF, Soisson P, et al. Optimal management strategies for placenta accreta. BJOG. 2009;116:648-54.
57. Silver RM, Landon MB, Rouse DJ, et al. Maternal morbidity associated with multiple repeat cesarean deliveries. Obstet Gynecol. 2006;107:1226-32.
58. Usta IM, Hobeika EM, Musa AA, et al. Placenta previa-accreta: risk factors and complications. Am J Obstet Gynecol. 2005;193:1045-9.
59. Pri-Paz S, Fuchs KM, Gaddipati S, et al. Comparison between emergent and elective delivery in women with placenta accreta. J Matern Fetal Neonatal Med. 2013;26:1007-11.
60. Robinson BK, Grobman WA. Effectiveness of timing strategies for delivery of individuals with placenta previa and accreta. Obstet Gynecol. 2010;116:835-42.
61. Balayla J, Bondarenko HD. Placenta accreta and the risk of adverse maternal and neonatal outcomes. J Perinat Med. 2013;41:141-9.
62. Räisänen S, Georgiadis L, Harju M, et al. Risk factors and adverse pregnancy outcomes among births affected by velamentous umbilical cord insertion: a retrospective population-based register study. Eur J Obstet Gynecol Reprod Biol. 2012;165:231-4.
63. Ebbing C, Kiserud T, Johnsen SL, et al. Prevalence, risk factors and outcomes of velamentous and marginal cord insertions: a population-based study of 634,741 pregnancies. PLoS One. 2013;8:e70380.
64. Rebarber A, Dolin C, Fox NS, et al. Natural history of vasa previa across gestation using a screening protocol. J Ultrasound Med. 2014;33:141-7.
65. Wiedaseck S, Monchek R. Placental and cord insertion pathologies: screening, diagnosis, and management. J Midwifery Womens Health. 2014;59:328-35.
66. Hasegawa J, Arakaki T, Ichizuka K, et al. Management of vasa previa during pregnancy. J Perinat Med. 2015;43(6):783-4.
67. Robinson BK, Grobman WA. Effectiveness of timing strategies for delivery of individuals with vasa previa. Obstet Gynecol. 2011;117:542-9.

# CHAPTER 13

# Neonatal Encephalopathy: An Obstetric Perspective

*Stacy Yadava, Matthew J Garabedian*

## ABSTRACT

Neonatal encephalopathy is a rare neurodevelopmental condition affecting newborn infants. The etiology is often difficult to identify and the pathogenesis is poorly understood. There are multiple maternal, fetal, and environmental factors that can contribute. The ultimate outcome is variable, but infants are at increased risk for neurologic disability. A better understanding of this condition and appropriate management can help to improve the lives of affected infants.

## INTRODUCTION

Neonatal neurologic injury, particularly hypoxic-ischemic encephalopathy (HIE), is an unfortunate occurrence with potentially devastating long-term neurologic outcomes. Frequently, it is difficult for both the family and medical practitioners to understand the underlying pathology and events leading to neurologic injury. Although neonatal encephalopathy (NE) may be relatively benign, it may also be associated with significant long-term neurologic impairment. In such cases, the family is often left wondering why this occurred. Obstetricians frequently are held responsible for these events; however, the true etiology is multifactorial and may not be related to intrapartum events.

Hypoxic-ischemic encephalopathy and NE both refer broadly to neurologic dysfunction in the days immediately following birth. Manifestations vary widely and include depressed tone, hyporeflexia, difficulty feeding, respiratory compromise, altered level of consciousness and seizures.[1]

It is important to note that these terms are used to describe deficits in term and near-term neonates greater than 34 weeks completed gestation as preterm infants may have disabilities secondary to an underdeveloped nervous system.[2] Development of NE is multifactorial with associated maternal, fetal, and intrapartum factors.

The overall incidence of NE is estimated to be 1-8 per 1,000 births.[2] The range is reflective of varying definitions used by multiple investigators. The overall incidence attributable to acute birth hypoxia alone is roughly 1.6 per 10,000. While NE is rare, the potential long-term outcomes can be devastating. Cerebral palsy (CP) is a long-term neurologic injury that has been associated with HIE and NE.[2,3] However, not all cases of CP are associated with intrapartum events. The spastic quadriplegic and dyskinetic subtypes of CP have been associated with birth hypoxia, where other types of CP more strongly correlate with factors other than intrapartum insult.[2] Therefore, it is important to understand the true etiologies and possible treatment options for these neonates.

Definition of terms:
- Hypoxia—decreased oxygenation at the tissue level
- Hypoxemia—low oxygen content in the blood
- Asphyxia—both hypoxia and metabolic acidosis.

## BIRTH ASPHYXIA

While detrimental events during birth have often been cited as the cause of neurologic deficit, recent evidence has shown that birth hypoxia alone accounts for very few cases of NE. A case-control study from Perth, Australia showed that only 4% of infants with NE experienced intrapartum hypoxia alone.[4] The majority of the study subjects had antepartum risk factors only and another subset had antepartum risk combined with evidence of birth hypoxia. These findings suggest that while adverse birth events may contribute to NE, the overwhelming majority of neonates have other risk factors as well.

Birth asphyxia can lead to neurologic insult in the neonate. Any time the flow of oxygen to the fetus is compromised during delivery there is potential for long-term injury. It is important to be able to identify when significant hypoxia has occurred. Multiple organizations have defined four necessary criteria used to define birth asphyxia sufficient to cause CP:[5,6]

1. Evidence of metabolic acidosis on cord blood gases obtained at delivery (umbilical cord pH < 7.0 and base deficit ≥ 12 mmol/L).
2. Early onset of moderate/severe NE in infants born at 34 or more weeks of gestation.
3. Development of spastic quadriplegic or dyskinetic CP.
4. Exclusion of other identifiable etiologies.

Further findings that are suggestive of an intrapartum event include sudden and prolonged fetal bradycardia, Apgar score <6 after 5 minutes of life, early evidence of multisystem involvement, and early imaging findings consistent with acute cerebral injury. Spastic quadriplegic and dyskinetic CP are more likely to be related to intrapartum hypoxia.[7] It is important to note that most infants with NE do not develop CP, and many children with CP did not have encephalopathy.[2,6] While they are commonly discussed together, the two clinical syndromes may represent different underlying processes rather than a continuum of neurologic deficit.

Cord blood gases should be collected after any delivery where there is concern for hypoxia, such as depressed neonatal tone, low Apgar scores, or need for neonatal resuscitation. The confirmation of metabolic acidosis suggests insufficient oxygen supply to the neonate. While pH of less than 7.2 is used as the cutoff for acidosis, data suggest that pH is suggestive of poor outcome only at levels less than 7.0.[1,3,8] At this level of acidosis, an increase in death, seizure and need for ICU level care was observed. Base deficit of >16 mmol/L has also been correlated with poor outcomes. Forty percent of infants with a cord blood base deficit of >16 will have neonatal health complications including renal, respiratory, and neurologic sequelae. Acidosis that is less severe is not likely to cause disability. Furthermore, documentation of a normal umbilical artery pH excludes birth asphyxia.

## ANTEPARTUM RISK FACTORS

### Maternal Factors

Both maternal and fetal factors can place the newborn at increased risk of encephalopathy. Antepartum factors have been carefully evaluated for linkage to both NE and CP to identify possible causal relationships that occurred prior to birth.

Many maternal demographic factors correlate with NE. The Perth case-control study looked at the relationships between maternal characteristics and fetal outcomes.[4] These include maternal age and socioeconomic status among others. The likelihood of encephalopathy increases with maternal age; the difference is most notable in women ≥35 years of age (adjusted odds ratio (OR) 6.01, 95% confidence interval (CI) 1.28-28.15). Mothers who are unemployed (OR 3.60, 95% CI 1.43-10.28), a housewife (OR 2.48, 95% CI 1.14-5.39), or employed as a manual laborer (OR 3.84, 95% CI 1.43-10.28) are also at increased risk. Interestingly, a small amount of alcohol consumption during pregnancy may have a protective effect. The relationship between these measures and NE has not been well studied, however, they may serve as markers of increased maternal stress. Higher stress levels experienced by these women during pregnancy may be detrimental to the developing neonate.

Maternal medical conditions that notably increase the risk of NE include maternal thyroid disease (OR 9.70, 95% CI 1.97-47.91), severe preeclampsia (OR 6.30, 95% CI 2.25-17.62), and moderate or severe bleeding during pregnancy (OR 3.57, 95% CI 2.25-17.62).[3] Preeclampsia, maternal hypertension, and bleeding during pregnancy can all lead to utero-placental insufficiency of varying degrees, potentially compromising blood flow to the developing fetus. Bleeding associated with placental abruption can be especially devastating given the potential for a large amount of acute blood loss and decreased blood flow the fetus. Maternal thyroid function is necessary for appropriate neurologic development in the newborn, and insufficiently treated thyroid disease during pregnancy can negatively influence neurologic function. Thrombophilia also increases the risk of encephalopathy. This is attributed to the formation of blood clots in the placental circulation, limiting exchange of oxygen and nutrients. As areas of the placenta become ischemic, there is less surface area for exchange with the developing fetus. Intrauterine growth restriction (IUGR) with birth weight <3rd percentile, another sign of compromised placental function, is also strongly correlated with NE. A family history of seizures also increases the risk for NE (OR 2.73, 95% CI 1.16-6.41). This familial distribution implies a possible hereditary component to early neurologic function.[4,9] As seizure is one of the defining features of

NE, any neonate at increased risk of seizure will also be at risk for NE. Outcomes following in vitro fertilization (IVF) are newly identified given recent advances in technology. Following conception with IVF, the pregnancy is at risk for multiple adverse outcomes including perinatal mortality, low birth weight, preterm delivery, and NE.[9,10] The reasons behind these findings are unknown but may be related to the underlying cause of infertility or the IVF procedure itself.

Infection during pregnancy or labor and delivery is another risk factor for NE. Chorioamnionitis has long been known to increase the risk of CP but other more indolent infections also appear to contribute.[4,9,11] In a cohort study of term neonates, 38% of spastic tetraparesis was contributed to by chorioamnionitis in the absence of any other identifiable cause.[11] In addition to the well-known teratogenic viruses such as CMV and rubella, other viruses may compromise fetal status through maternal fever and activation of the inflammatory response.[12] Many neonates who develop neurologic deficits in the setting of intrauterine infection do not show evidence of neonatal sepsis supporting a case for reactivation or less virulent organisms.[12] There is some evidence that intrauterine infection may even bridge pregnancies. Increased levels of inflammatory cytokines are seen in infants who later develop CP.[12,13] While this may be evidence of infection, it is important to note that cytokines are nonspecific and may be elevated in a variety of other conditions. Because of potential adverse outcomes, it is important to promptly identify and treat intrauterine infection with antipyretics and antibiotics. While treatment can reduce the risk of poor outcome, viral and early antepartum infections may go unidentified.

## Fetal Factors

The most common infant characteristic associated with encephalopathy is being born small for gestational age (SGA), defined as <10th percentile of birth weight for estimated gestational age.[14,15] In multiple studies, the rate of SGA amongst infants with NE is 16–17%.[4,14,16] It is perhaps not surprising then that IUGR, a term used to describe fetuses *in utero* with an estimated fetal weight measuring less than the 10th percentile for gestational age, is also associated with NE. Both SGA and IUGR can be signs of placental insufficiency, but can also be due to normal development of a constitutionally small baby.

In cases of multifetal gestation, fetuses are forced to share limited resources. Twins and higher order multiples are at increased risk of low birth weight and preterm delivery, both of which are independent risk factors for neurodevelopmental disability. However, in studies controlling for birth weight and gestational age, there is still evidence that multiples have worse neurodevelopmental outcomes than singleton counterparts. The relative rate of the development of CP for twins ≥2,500 g is reportedly 3.3—5.5 compared to singletons.[9,17] Monochorionic twins seem to account for most of the impairment. This is likely secondary to intrauterine competition for placental blood flow. The development of twin-twin transfusion syndrome and death of a cotwin further increases the risk of adverse outcome for monochorionic twins.

Any congenital structural abnormalities or malformations outside the nervous system will increase the risk for encephalopathy.[2] These may be due to underlying chromosomal aberrations or isolated defects. Many researchers exclude these infants from studies on encephalopathy as they have a baseline increase in risk secondary to abnormal development.

Extremes of gestational age put a neonate at risk, including both preterm and post-term deliveries. The probability increases in births at less than 37 weeks gestational age, and again at 41 weeks or greater.[4,9] At less than 37 weeks, complete development of the nervous system may not be accomplished. Roughly half of all cases of CP are seen in preterm and very preterm infants, lending further support to the importance of term development.[14] Yet more time in utero is not always better; by 42 weeks gestation the likelihood of NE significantly increases. These two outliers illustrate the need for prenatal care to aid in achieving term gestation and appropriate induction of labor for the avoidance of post-term pregnancies.

Nonvertex presentation such as breech and transverse has also been affiliated with NE, likely because of the stress of delivery and need for cesarean delivery.[2] In a cohort study of 245 Norwegian infants born with CP, breech presentation increased the likelihood of CP with an OD of 3.6 (95% CI 2.4-5.3).[18] Vaginal breech extraction has the associated risk of head entrapment. In the instance of head entrapment, an acute decrease in blood flow to the brain occurs. This can lead to hypoxic brain injury if prolonged. Scheduled cesarean delivery for breech presentation eliminates the risk of head entrapment and can improve fetal outcomes.[19] Fetal malpresentation can also be affiliated with abnormalities of the fetal or maternal anatomy. These abnormalities may affect placentation and appropriate blood flow through the umbilical cord. Even in fetuses presenting vertex, suboptimal fetal head position can both prolong the delivery and increase the need for cesarean delivery or instrumentation. Occiput posterior position of the fetal head carries a threefold risk of NE.[2]

## ■ INTRAPARTUM

Intrapartum events which contribute to NE have been closely examined. It is imperative that the obstetric practitioner understands these events, their contribution to HIE and NE, and how to minimize the risk of intrapartum injury. Identification of risk factors for intrapartum injury should prompt appropriate, evidence-based intervention.

The value of electronic fetal heart rate monitoring (EFM) remains a subject of debate. There is ongoing discussion as to how to classify fetal heart rate (FHR) abnormalities and application to clinical decisions. In many developing countries, it is not feasible to use continuous electronic monitoring and intermittent auscultation serves as an alternative means to assess fetal status. When intermittent auscultation is used in lieu of continuous monitoring, there is a twofold increase in neonatal ICU admissions and an increase in neonatal seizure.[20] Yet even with these risks there appears to be no difference in overall mortality or development of CP. Furthermore, there is data to show that continuous monitoring increases the rate of cesarean delivery and operative vaginal delivery without a corresponding reduction in rate of CP.[20] Cesarean delivery and operative deliveries pose other potential complications to both mother and infant.

Evidence relating non-reassuring FHR tracings to CP is disappointing. While reassuring FHR patterns are predictive of good outcome, the reverse is not true for non-reassuring tracings. The positive predictive value for "non-reassuring fetal status" is 0.14%, which means 1–2/1,000 neonates with non-reassuring FHR will later develop CP.[21] Additional information, however, may be obtained from FHR tracings, such as the presence of severe late decelerations, does provide evidence suggestive of acidemia.[22] Given the overall poor correlation to long-term neurologic outcome, American College of Obstetricians and Gynecologists (ACOG) guidelines suggest that low-risk pregnancies be managed with either continuous EFM or intermittent auscultation.[20] If performed correctly, intermittent auscultation provides an accurate assessment of fetal wellbeing. This method is especially useful in many countries that lack the resources to implement universal continuous monitoring. Deliveries complicated by high-risk conditions (diabetes, preeclampsia, etc.) should be monitored continuously.

When continuous EFM is used, the tracing should be observed for evidence of fetal acidosis. Ongoing acidemia in the fetus carries the potential for poor neurologic outcome. The most reliable sign of acidemia is decreased beat-to-beat variability.[23] The presence of moderate variability in the FHR tracing virtually excludes a fetal arterial pH <7.1.[22] If good variability is maintained, umbilical artery pH will be greater than 7.0 in 97% of cases, even in the presence of variable or late decelerations.[20]

In contrast, roughly one-third of infants with intrapartum FHR tracings demonstrating a decrease in variability for more than 1 hour will be acidotic on delivery.[20] These findings suggest that decelerations may be observed for some time as long as the variability is maintained. In an otherwise uncomplicated pregnancy, increased tolerance for FHR aberrations may reduce the rate of cesarean and operative vaginal delivery. When variability is lost, imminent delivery should be considered.

In an effort to standardize intrapartum interpretation of FHR tracings, ACOG and NIH/NICHD have developed a three-tiered system of interpretation.[20] In this system, FHR tracings are analyzed for baseline, variability, presence of accelerations/decelerations, and assigned category I, II, and III. Category III tracings are non-reassuring and indicate the need for swift delivery.[24] A significant limitation of this system is that the designation of a category II FHR pattern poorly identifies an appropriate level of concern for acidemia. The majority of intrapartum FHR tracings are category II.[16] The management of category II FHR tracings is difficult given the uncertain link to academia.[25] Roughly 32% of primary cesarean sections are performed for non-reassuring FHR with the majority of the tracing category II.[26] Alternative systems for interpretation have been proposed to better identify fetuses at risk for intrapartum injury and provide guidance for labor management.[22]

Other intrapartum events that can impact neonatal outcome include cord prolapse, shoulder dystocia, and uterine rupture. Umbilical cord prolapse is a rare but potentially devastating occurrence. Depending on the fetal position and amount of cord compression, the prolapse can lead to a sudden lack of blood flow to the fetus resulting in severe ischemia. Delivery should be accomplished as soon as possible either via impending vaginal delivery or emergency cesarean section. Upward pressure on the presenting fetal part or backfilling the bladder may help to relieve cord compression. Prolapse is associated with an approximately 8% risk of neonatal death, and low Apgar scores (<7 at 5 minutes) are seen in roughly half of cases.[27] However, of surviving neonates, the majority of infants will have normal neurologic outcomes following cord prolapse.

Shoulder dystocia can similarly limit the blood supply to the fetus. When the head is delivered and the body is not, the umbilical cord is compressed and there is potential for hypoxic-ischemic injury. An emphasis on training drills and knowledge of delivery maneuvers may help to reduce the complications following shoulder dystocia for infants and mother alike. Prolonged time to delivery of the body carries a worse prognosis. Improper use of maneuvers by the provider and fetal macrosomia can both contribute to a delay in delivery. Fetal macrosomia >4 kg was seen in 75% of fatal cases in one review.[28] The vast majority of those autopsied showed evidence of acute hypoxic injury.

Uterine rupture is another potentially life-threatening labor event. Given the commonality of cesarean delivery, there is a corresponding population of women attempting vaginal birth after previous cesarean section with subsequent pregnancies. Previous uterine surgery is an inciting factor for possible rupture. With one prior low transverse cesarean section, the risk or rupture has been widely noted as <1%. Time to delivery is again of utmost importance to preserve neonatal outcome. Cases of ongoing neurologic deficit are seen with incident-to-delivery intervals of >30 minutes.[29] Thus, the ability to recognize uterine rupture using intrapartum monitoring is recommended during trial of labor after cesarean section.

Continuous heart rate monitoring can help to identify a distressed fetus and aid providers in making delivery decisions. In cases of non-reassuring FHR patterns, operative vaginal or emergency cesarean delivery is often considered.[20,22] When both of these delivery methods are evaluated, a more than twofold increase in NE is seen. Emergency cesarean section and instrumental vaginal delivery are markers for the development of NE. However, because these procedures are performed when fetal distress is already present, it is impossible to make any causative associations. It was previously thought that infants with tight nuchal cords were at increased risk for adverse outcome and CP. More recent evidence has shown no difference in neonatal outcomes amongst babies born with nuchal cords.[30]

In contrast to the outcomes associated with emergency cesarean delivery, there is some evidence to suggest scheduled elective C-section is protective against NE.[4] This practice minimizes fetal exposure to the stresses of labor. However, neonates born following a prelabor cesarean are at increased risk of more common, but less catastrophic, morbidities, such as respiratory distress syndrome (RDS).[31] There is much debate as to whether or not elective cesarean sections should be performed. An opinion issued by ACOG in 2003 leaves the question open stating that if the surgery is desired and does not impose increased risk to the patient, it may be ethically performed.[32] However, given the rarity of NE, this beneficial effect is likely overshadowed by the surgical risks, more difficult maternal recovery, and potential complications in an otherwise uncomplicated pregnancy. Additionally, currently there is much attention on avoidance of cesarean delivery given not only the short term, but also the long-term associated morbidities, such as placenta accreta.[24,33]

### ■ OUTCOMES

Developmental outcomes vary significantly among infants with NE. Much of this variation is linked to the severity of symptoms with mild NE consistently associated with positive outcomes and severe NE leading to negative outcomes.[34] The scaling of NE is thus of important prognostic value and is accomplished using one of multiple grading scales. Although there is a large amount of heterogeneity within each category, overall outcome trends are evident. Decreased IQ, poor scholastic performance, memory, language, attention, and visuospatial deficits have all been observed as these children age.

Cerebral palsy is perhaps the most feared developmental outcome in affected neonates. Roughly, one-third of CP cases come from neonates affected by encephalopathy.[14] In newborns with evidence of encephalopathy, long-term neurologic status is difficult to predict. In an effort to identify those at greatest risk, associations between CP and multiple parameters have been examined. Apgar scores have been evaluated as possible predictors of neurologic outcome. In a large study of approximately 235,000 Norwegian neonates, those with APGAR scores <3 at 5 minutes of life had a 38% rate of death prior to 8 years of age and a 7% incidence of CP.[35] However, the majority of children later diagnosed with CP had 5 minutes Apgar score of 7-10.

In a population of neonates with encephalopathy, Apgar scores at 10 minutes were related to the severity of long-term neurologic disability with Apgar <3 associated with 76--82% mortality or moderate-severe disability.[36] Therefore while Apgar score seems to have limited prognostic value amongst the general newborn population, it may have increased predictive power in those with NE.

Multiple other techniques have been evaluated for their ability to predict outcomes in neonates with encephalopathy. Bedside neurologic examination, electroencephalogram (EEG), ultrasound, and magnetic resonance imaging (MRI) have all been used to assess the extent of brain damage. Findings from these studies have varying degrees of correlation with long-term neurologic outcome.

Prior to the increased use of EEG and MRI, heavy reliance was placed on the neurologic examination and other clinical findings. Ultrasound has long been used as an available and efficient imaging modality for evaluation of the neonatal brain. Recent evidence suggests bedside neurologic examination and cerebral ultrasound both perform poorly as prognostic tools.[37]

Electroencephalogram can be performed within the first week of life and produces dependable results. MRI has also emerged as a useful tool for evaluation of brain damage. While MRI can also be performed early on, the evidence of brain injury can be more prominently seen toward the end of the first week of life. Both of these studies were found to have sensitivity and specificity of >90% in predicting neurologic deficit after 18 months.[38] As technology continues to advance, both of these studies have shown to be useful in neonates with evidence of encephalopathy.

## NEW TREATMENT ADVANCES

Historically, the focus has been on prevention of NE. As described above, there is limited ability to modify intrapartum events leading to neurologic injury. While continued advances to improve recognition of fetuses at risk and to develop interventions that may improve outcomes, currently there does exist potential treatment modalities for affected infants. Emerging treatments have been shown to diminish the rate of death and neurologic deficit from NE.

One antepartum intervention available for the obstetrician is magnesium sulfate. The use of magnesium sulfate in preterm infants at risk of imminent delivery has been shown to decrease rates of severe CP (relative risk (RR) 0.55, 95% CI 0.32–0.95).[38,39] The evidence suggests use in preterm fetuses up to 32 weeks gestation is beneficial. With few adverse maternal outcomes mostly limited to the side effects of magnesium sulfate, the drug remains a good option for at risk pregnancies.

Antenatal corticosteroids have been administered to women at risk for preterm birth for many years. The major benefits include a reduction in rates of RDS, intraventricular hemorrhage, and necrotizing enterocolitis. There is conflicting evidence for use of corticosteroids to reduce the incidence of CP.[40,41] Large cohort studies have shown improved neonatal survival and a decrease in clinically evident white matter injury. The rates of CP are slightly improved in preterm infants who receive steroids but the difference is not statistically significant (OR 0.82, 95% CI 0.58–1.15).[42]

One promising therapy is the use of hypothermia to limit the severity of neurologic deficit. Cooling methods can be limited to the head with use of a "cool cap" or cooling blankets to induce whole body hypothermia. A Cochrane review of multiple studies using cooling compared to standard of care found a significant reduction in both morbidity and mortality in the treatment group.[42] Neurodevelopment was measured out to 18 months of age. The number needed to treat for additional benefit was only 7–8 neonates. Noted adverse outcomes of cooling are sinus bradycardia and thrombocytopenia.

Both whole body cooling and the use of "cool caps" have shown to provide benefit to affected neonates.[43] Initial research protocols were designed for induction of hypothermia within 6 hours of delivery if HIE was suspected and ongoing cooling for 72 hours. Follow-up at 18 months showed a decrease in death and severe disability. These results have been reproduced in several studies. The exact underlying mechanism is not well understood but cooling is thought to prevent brain damage by reducing the number of free radicals and slowing cellular metabolism. It is important to perform cooling in a well-monitored environment like the neonatal intensive care unit to ensure appropriate temperature control. Side effects include bradycardia, prolonged clotting time, and immune suppression.

Hypothermic treatment requires close monitoring and expensive equipment. Given these limitations, it is limitedly available in large tertiary neonatal care units. With more and more evidence to support the benefits of cooling, it should ideally be made available to newborns worldwide. Currently, groups are attempting to develop a more affordable apparatus which can achieve the same cooling effects. The prevention of ongoing neurologic deficit can save a large amount of future healthcare spending.

Another treatment on the horizon is the use of systemic erythropoietin. There are promising results in animal studies showing a protective effect against neurologic hypoxic-ischemic injury.[44] While the exact mechanism has not been illustrated, erythropoietin acts to dampen the inflammatory cascade and also has vasogenic effects. The first drug safety trials are being conducted in human infants and the drug may have promising benefits for the future.

As research continues to expand our understanding both of the mechanism of injury and potential pathways for treatment and prevention, management of neonates with encephalopathy will continue to advance. For now an ongoing focus on prevention and risk factor modification is important, especially in resource poor regions lacking access to therapeutic modalities. With the constant development of newer technology at lower costs, the outcomes for these infants will improve.

## REFERENCES

1. Nelson KB, Leviton A. How much of neonatal encephalopathy is due to birth asphyxia? Am J Dis Child. 1991;145(11):1325-31.
2. Hankins GD1, Speer M. Defining the Pathogenesis and Pathophysiology Neonatal Encephalopathy and Cerebral Palsy. Obstetric Gynecol. 2003;102(3):628-36..
3. Graham EM, Ruis KA, Hartman AL, et al. A systematic review of the role of intrapartum hypoxia-ischemia in the causation of neonatal encephalopathy. Am J Obstetr Gynecol. 2008;199(6):587-95.
4. Badawi N, Kurinczuk JJ, Keogh JM, et al. Antepartum risk factors for neonatal encephalopathy: the Western Australian case-control study. BMJ. 1998;317:1549-53.
5. MacLennan A. A template for defining a causal relationship between acute intrapartum events and cerebral palsy: international consensus statement. BMJ. 1999;319:1054-9.
6. Committee on Obstetric Practice, American College of Obstetricians and Gynecologists. ACOG Committee Opinion. Number 326, 2005. Inappropriate Use of the Terms Fetal Distress and Birth Aspyxia. Obstet Gynecol. 2005;106(6):1469-70.

7. Nelson KB, Grether JK. Potentially asphyxiating conditions and spastic cerebral palsy in infants of normal birth weight. Am J Obstet Gynecol. 1998;179: 507-13.
8. ACOG Committee Opinion No. 138: Utility of umbilical cord blood acid-base assessment. Int J Gynecol Obstet. 1994;45:303-4.
9. Martinez-Biarge M, Diez Sebastian J, Wusthoff CJ, et al. Antepartum and Intrapartum Factors Preceding Neonatal Hypoxic-Ischemic Encephalopathy. Pediatrics. 2013;132(4):e952-9.
10. Jackson RA, Gibson KA, Wu YW, et al. Perinatal outcomes in singletons following in vitro fertilization: a meta-analysis. Obstetr Gynecol. 2004;103(3):551-63.
11. Wu YW, Escobar GJ, Grether JK, et al. Chorioamnionitis and cerebral palsy in term or near-term infants. JAMA. 2003;290:2677-84.
12. Nelson KB, Willoughby RE. Infection, inflammation and the risk of cerebral palsy. Curr Opin Neurol. 2000;13(2):133-9.
13. Girard S, Kadhim H, Roy M, et al. Role of Perinatal Inflammation in Cerebral Palsy. Pediatr Neurol. 2009;40(3):168-74.
14. Nelson KB, Bingham P, Edwars E, et al. Antecedents of Neonatal Encephalopathy in the Vermont Oxford Network Encephalopathy Registry. Pediatrics. 2012;130(5):878-86.
15. ACOG Practice Bulletin No. 204: Fetal Growth Restriction. Obstetrics & Gynecology: February. 2019;133(2):e97-e109.
16. West CR, Curr L, Battin MR, et al. Antenatal antecedents of moderate or severe neonatal encephalopathy in term infants- a regional review. Australia New Zealand J Obstetr Gynecol. 2005;45:207-10.
17. Lorenz JM. Neurodevelopmental Outcomes of Twins. Semin Perinatol. 2012;36(3):201-12.
18. Andersen G, Irgens L, Skranes J, et al. Is breech presentation a risk factor for cerebral palsy? A Norwegian birth cohort study. Dev Med Child Neurol. 2009;51(11):860-5.
19. Hannah ME, Hannah WJ, Hewson SA, et al. Planned cesarean section versus planned vaginal birth for breech presentation at term: a randomised multicenter trial. Lancet. 2000;356(9239):1375-83.
20. Kumar S, Paterson-Brown S. Obstetric aspects of hypoxic ischemic encephalopathy. Early Hum Dev. 2010;86(6):339-44.
21. American College of Obstetricians and Gynecologists. ACOG Practice Bulletin Number 106. Intrapartum Fetal Heart Rate Monitoring: Nomenclature, Interpretation and General Management Principles Obstet Gynecol. 2009;114(1):192-202.
22. Parer JT, Ikeda T. A framework for standardized management of intrapartum fetal heart rate patterns. American J Obstetr Gynecol. 2007:197(1):26.e1-6.
23. Williams KP, Galerneau F. Intrapartum fetal heart rate patterns in the prediction of neonatal acidemia. Am J Obstetr Gynecol. 2003;188(3):820-3.
24. American College of Obstetricians and Gynecologists; Society for Maternal-Fetal Medicine. Obstetric Care Consensus No. 1. Safe prevention of the primary cesarean delivery. Obstet Gynecol. 2014;123:693-711.
25. Cahill AG, Roehi KA, Obido AO, et al. Association and prediction of neonatal acidemia. AmJ Obstetr Gynecol. 2012;207(3):206.e1-e8.
26. Barber EL, Lundsberg LS, Belanger K, et al. Indications Contributing to the Increasing Cesarean Delivery Rate. Obstet Gynecol. 2011;118(1):29-38.
27. Huang JP, Chen CP, Chen CP, et al. Term pregnancy with umbilical cord prolapse. Taiwan I Obstet Gynecol. 2012;51(3):375-8.
28. Hope P, Breslin S, Lamon L, et al. Fatal shoulder dystocia: a review of 56 cases reported to the Confidential Enquiry into Stillbirths and Deaths in Infancy. Br J Obstetr Gynaecol. 1998;105:1256-61.
29. Holmgren C, Scott J, Porter T, et al. Uterine Rupture with Attempted Vaginal Birth after Cesarean Delivery: Decision-to-Delivery Time and Neonatal Outcome. Obstetr Gynecol. 2012;119(4):725-31.
30. Henry E, Andres RL, Christensen RD. Neonatal outcomes following a tight nuchal cord. J Perinatol. 2013;33:231-4.
31. Gerten KA, Coonrod DV, Bay RC, et al. Cesarean delivery and respiratory distress syndrome: does labor make a difference? Am J Obstet Gynecol. 2005;193(3 Pt 2):1061-4.
32. American College of Obstetricians and Gynecologists. ACOG Committee Opinion Number 559. Cesarean Delivery on Maternal Request. Obstet Gynecol. 2013;121(4):904-7..
33. Silver RM, Landon MB, Rouse DJ, et al. Maternal morbidity associated with multiple repeat cesarean deliveries. Obstetri Gynecol. 2006;107(6):1226-32.
34. Van Handell M, Swaab H, de Vires LS, et al. Long-term cognitive and behavioral consequences of neonatal encephalopathy following perinatal asphyxia: a review. Euro J Pediatr. 2007;166(7):645-54.
35. Most D, Lie RT, Irgens LM, et al. The association of Apgar score with subsequent death and cerebral palsy: A population-based study in term infants. J Pediatr. 2001;138(6):798-803.
36. Laptook AR, Shankaran S, Ambalavanan N, et al. Outcome of term infants using apgar scores at 10 minutes following hypoxic-ischemic encephalopathy. Pediatrics. 2009;124(6):1619-26.
37. Van Laerhoven H, de Haan T, Offringa M, et al. Prognostic Tests in Term Neonates with Hypoxic-Ischemic Encephalopathy: A Systematic Review. Pediatr. 2013;131(88):88-98.
38. Rouse DJ, Hirtz DG, Thom E, et al. A Randomized, Controlled Trial of Magnesium Sulfate for the Prevention of Cerebral Palsy. New Eng J Med. 2008;359(9):895-905.
39. Crowther CA, Hiller JE, Doyle LW, et al. Effect of Magnesium Sulfate Given for Neuroprotection Before Preterm Birth. JAMA. 2003;290(20):2669-76.
40. Foix-L'Helias L, Marret S, Ancel PY, et al. Impact of the use of antenatal corticosteroids on mortality, cerebral lesions and 5-year neurodevelopmental outcomes of very preterm infants: the EPIPAGE cohort study. BJOG. 2008;115(2):275-82.
41. Eriksson L, Haglund B, Ewald U, et al. Short and long-term effects of antenatal corticosteroids assessed in a cohort of 7.,827 children born preterm. ACTA Obstet Gynecol Scand. 2008;88(8):933-8.
42. Jacobs SE, Berg M, Hunt R, et al. Cooling for newborns with hypoxic ischaemic encephalopathy. Cochrane Database Syst Rev. 2013;(1):CD003311.
43. Gluckman PD, Wyatt JS, Azzopardi D, et al. Selective head cooling with mild systemic hypothermia after neonatal encephalopathy: multicentre randomised trial. Lancet. 2005;365(9460):663-70.
44. Xiong T, Qu Y, Mu D, et al. Erythropoietin for neonatal brain injury: opportunity and challenge. Int J Deve Neurosci. 2011;29(6):583-91.

# SECTION 4

# Normal Newborn Care

- Newborn Physical Examination
  *Cherry C Uy*

- Caring for Families through Pregnancy Loss or Death of an Infant
  *Donna F Wallerstein*

- Circumcision
  *Stephen Harris*

- Couplet Care and Common Nursery Issues
  *Priya Jegatheesan, Sudha Rani Narasimhan, Dongli Song*

# CHAPTER 14

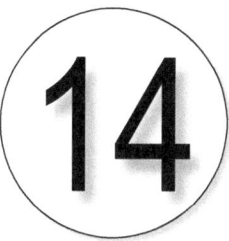

# Newborn Physical Examination

*Cherry C Uy*

## ABSTRACT

The physical examination of the newborn is performed immediately after birth in order to assess the infant's health and comfort. First careful observation is employed, then a gentle hands-on examination to check for physical and neurologic health. Most infants will be healthy, but for those who are not, an astute clinician can spot possible issues and refer the parents to specialists to best care for their baby's individual needs.

## NEWBORN PHYSICAL EXAMINATION

The newborn physical examination should be done in a well-lit environment and in a systematic manner to ensure that nothing obvious is missed. Although most newborn examinations reveal normal findings, these examinations may reveal important facts that need immediate attention. Furthermore, a newborn physical examination can help establish a baseline for comparison, if an issue comes up at a later time.

The sequence of examination and assessment is a matter of personal preference; however, it is best to observe the infant's general appearance in an undisturbed condition. By simple observation and without touching the patient, an examiner is able to get information about size, symmetry, color, breathing, posture, abnormality of movement, and other vital information. It is important to remember that evaluations that require a quiet state, such as listening to the chest and heart sounds, have to be done first. These should then be followed by evaluations that are not dependent on an undisturbed state for an accurate interpretation.

### Gestational Age Assessment

Initial assessment of a newborn infant should include a maturity rating. The gestational age by date provided by the obstetrician has to be validated by a good physical and neurological maturity assessment. This assessment is an important part of the evaluation, especially if the dates of pregnancy are uncertain. The most commonly used technique of gestational assessment is the *Ballard Maturational Assessment* or simply the *Ballard Score*. The assessment is divided into physical and neurological criteria, wherein scores are assigned to specific criteria. The sum of all these scores is given an equivalent gestational age for the infant, ranging from 26 weeks to 44 weeks.[1] The New Ballard Score sheet[2] is an expanded version of the original Ballard Maturation Assessment tool to include extremely premature infants up to 20 weeks.[3]

### Physical Assessment

Examinations performed in a systematic manner will ensure full and complete evaluation. The exact order is not important, but examinations usually proceed from head to toe. Those examinations that disturb the infant, the most should be reserved for last. Basic information about the infant's delivery is an important part of the assessment. Infants born via vaginal delivery may have physical findings that are not normally seen in infants delivered via cesarean section.

Examinations should include evaluating body measurements, i.e. birth weight versus current weight, and length and head circumference. Vital signs are an integral part of the physical examination. Timing of the evaluation has to be documented, since there are clinical and physical findings that may be considered normal or transitional immediately after birth but may be considered abnormal later.

When first approaching a newborn, an examiner should not immediately disturb the infant. A wealth of information is gathered by simply quietly looking at an infant.

- *Overall size of the infant:* Head size relative to body size will give you an idea of cranial and/or intracranial abnormality. Symmetry of the chest and abdominal distention is easily discernible.
- *Posture:* Newborn's posture at rest is reflective of in-utero position. Normal flexion and active movements of the extremities are suggestive of good muscle tone, and lack thereof is indicative of hypotonicity. Abnormal movements may be suggestive of birth injury or congenital abnormality.
- *Congenital abnormalities of the face and extremities.*
- *Skin features*: Acrocyanosis is physiologic and considered benign, whereas generalized/central cyanosis is pathologic and needs immediate attention. Jaundice, pallor, rashes, birthmarks, and other skin discolorations will need further attention.
- *Breathing pattern*: An infant in distress will show some or all of the following: tachypnea, retractions, audible grunting, or stridor.
- *Spontaneous movements:* Well-coordinated and purposeful movement is what a newborn infant should be showing. Facial twitching and repetitive movements are considered abnormal and need further evaluation.

After careful observation and visual inspection have been completed, the examiner may now proceed to a more hands-on part of the physical examination.

## General Examination

After delivery, a careful general examination can easily reveal congenital anomalies, birth injury, and cardiorespiratory disorders that will affect transition to extrauterine life. Presence of one detectable congenital anomaly should prompt further evaluation for other associated malformations.

Examination may begin by evaluating birth weight. An infant's birth size can be categorized as—(1) small for gestational age (SGA) (birth weight below the 10th percentile), (2) appropriate for gestational age (birth weight between 10th percentile and 90th percentile), or (3) large for gestational age (LGA) (birth weight above the 90th percentile). The infant may also be classified as symmetric (head size correlates with body size) or asymmetric (head size is disproportionately larger than body size). Different factors affecting symmetry of growth in SGA infants have to be taken into consideration for further management. Just like in SGA infants, factors causing LGA, such as maternal diabetes, also have to be considered as this may affect further transition to extrauterine life.

### Skin and Integumentary System

The skin has to be examined for any findings that may indicate underlying disorder. Many skin lesions can be seen in newborns. Although these findings are typically benign and self-limiting, differential diagnosis may include conditions that require immediate attention and treatment. Skin pigmentations such as hemangiomas, Mongolian spots, macular stains, and congenital nevi are common. Erythema toxicum, miliaria, benign pustular melanosis, and sucking blister are among the list of common benign lesions that can be confused with pathologic skin lesions. The most commonly confused diagnoses are congenital herpes infection and staphylococcal skin infection in cases of sucking blister and benign pustular melanosis. Sucking blister is present at birth and is a result of sucking of the affected area/s *in utero.*

The skin color must be examined for jaundice, and if an infant is clinically jaundiced, bilirubin level has to be part of the initial evaluation. The level should be correlated with the hours of life of the newborn and plotted against the guideline published by the American Academy of Pediatrics (Bilirubin Nomogram). Jaundice is best assessed in the presence of natural lighting; it is always considered pathologic and warrants further evaluation if noted in the first 24 hours of life.

Newborn nails are normally soft and flexible. Some infants are born with triangular-shaped nails mostly affecting the toenails, the "big toe" in particular. This condition is considered related to a faster growth of the nail matrix in its central portion and then proceeding laterally.[4]

### Head and Neck

Abnormalities involving the head and neck can quickly become evident during the initial examination. A thorough inspection should reveal the size, shape, and presence of any unusual mass or lesion, as well as evidence of trauma. Skull defects or unusual scalp lesions are also typically evident with careful inspection. Although uncommon, findings such as meningocele and encephalocele warrant immediate neurosurgical consultation. Cutis aplasia is a congenital absence of the epidermal layer of the skin, most commonly seen as a solitary defect on the scalp. The lesion may appear as an eroded or ulcerated defect or a healed, membranous, and atrophic scalp lesion associated with alopecia. It is more common for this condition to be a benign isolated finding; however, it can be associated with genetic syndromes and chromosomal anomalies.

Extracranial findings associated with labor and vaginal birth may be seen after delivery. Careful inspection and examination may reveal more obvious evidence of traumatic delivery. Common findings include:
- *Caput succedaneum:* Scalp swelling or edema noted over the presenting part of the head. It is present at birth and crosses the suture lines, and typically resolves within 24–48 hours.
- *Cephalohematoma*: Bleeding between the periosteum and skull. This can be differentiated from caput succedaneum because swelling is localized and limited by the boundaries of individual bones.
- *Subgaleal hemorrhage:* Bleeding between the epicranial aponeurosis and the periosteum **(Fig. 1)**. These areas extend anteriorly from the orbital ridges to the nape of the neck posteriorly and to the level of the ears laterally. When filled just to 1 cm thickness, this space can hold as much as 260 milliliters of blood and cause severe hypovolemia and hemorrhagic shock.[5] Diagnosis is generally clinical, coupled with a high level of suspicion for patients with risk factors such as presence of instrumentation during the delivery. Bleeding into the subgaleal space may be insidious and not readily evident until several hours after delivery. Findings include boggy, fluctuant mass that may be associated with increasing head circumference. Early recognition and immediate intervention are critical as this condition is potentially fatal.

Anterior and posterior fontanels and all suture lines have to be palpated and evaluated for evidence of increased intracranial pressure, such as bulging fontanels or widening of suture separation. There are four suture lines in the skull, namely (1) coronal, (2) sagittal, (3) lambdoid, and (4) metopic. Passage through the birth canal may result in asymmetry of the skull due to overlapping sutures called "molding." This is a temporary condition and should resolve in 2–3 days. Presence of fixed, nonmobile suture lines after birth, continued presence of immobile overlapping sutures, a palpable ridge beyond a few days of life, or an absence of a "soft spot" may be indicative of premature closure of the sutures called craniosynostosis. The most common type of premature suture closure is sagittal synostosis, resulting in a head shape that is long and narrow with a widened forehead. Multiple factors have been implicated in premature suture closure, including several genetic mutations resulting in syndromic craniosynostosis. Craniotabes is a condition where the skull is soft and depressible. It is seen mostly in occipital and parietal bones. Although, it may be normally seen in newborns, it is more common in premature infants and in conditions that affect bone growth such as rickets, malnutrition, hypophosphatasia, and other genetic disorders.

### Face, Eyes, Ears, Nose, and Throat

When evaluating the face, one should pay close attention to facial symmetry. Facial asymmetry may not be apparent when an infant is quiet and sleeping. It is more obvious during facial movements such as crying and yawning. True facial palsy has to be differentiated from asymmetric crying facies (ACF). Facial palsy is a result of injury to the seventh cranial nerve that can happen before or during

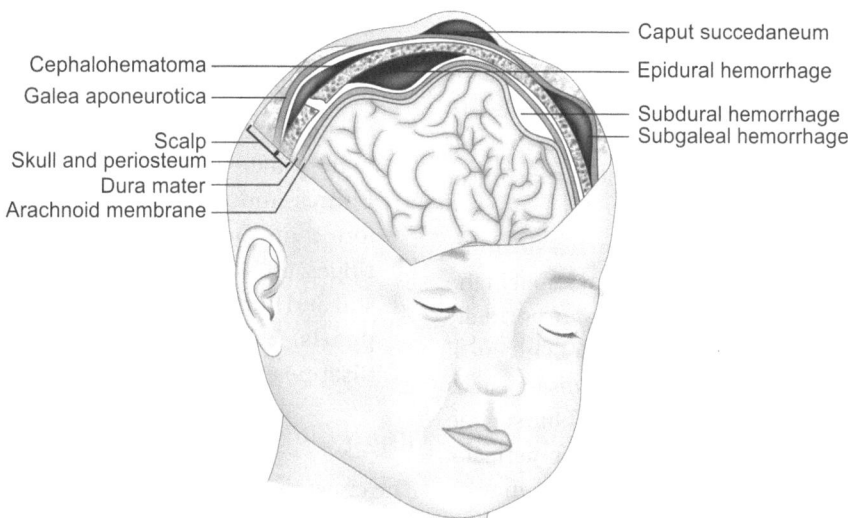

**Fig. 1:** Scalp and soft tissue injury: frequent sites of birth trauma.

delivery, with or without instrumentation. Most of the time, the cause of facial palsy is unknown. It presents with decreased movement of the affected side of the face and is characterized by an inability to close the eyes, loss of the nasolabial folds and an inability to contract the lower facial muscle causing the appearance of "drooping mouth" on the unaffected side. In severe cases, there is no facial movement from the forehead to the chin. In contrast, ACF is due to hypoplasia or congenital absence of the depressor anguli oris muscle. In this condition, since the muscle specifically controlling movement of one side of the mouth is affected, just like in facial palsy, there is asymmetry of the face when crying, more often on the left side. However, the seventh cranial nerve is normal, so the muscles controlling movement of the upper face are intact. Thus, the forehead wrinkles, the eyes close normally, and the nasolabial folds are normal. ACF is typically a benign condition but may be associated with other congenital anomalies.

Eye examination can be challenging in newborns because their eyes are typically closed and they often have eyelid edema. Eversion of the eyelid often happens when force is applied to open the eyes. Most infants, when held vertically in a room with dim lighting, will open their eyes spontaneously and this will allow the examiner to look at the red reflex. Red reflex refers to the reddish-orange reflection of light from the retina and can be seen by focusing on the pupil using an ophthalmoscope held 12-18 inches from the newborn's eyes. Lack of red reflex, presence of dark spots, or presence of white reflex (leukocoria) is an indication to refer to an ophthalmologist.[6] White reflex can be evidence of congenital cataract and retinoblastoma.

The examiner should note symmetry, slant, spacing, and width of the palpebral fissures, appearance of the sclera and conjunctiva, and eye movements. Conjunctival hemorrhages are common after vaginal delivery and if not associated with other findings do not indicate birth trauma. An abnormally wide interpupillary distance (hypertelorism) is associated with genetic and chromosomal syndromes. Pupils are normally round and actively constrict in response to light; however, pupillary reaction to light is generally absent in infants less than 30 weeks gestation.[7] Coloboma is a defect in one of the segments of the eye. Iris coloboma is the most common and usually presents as a black hole or a split in the iris; it gives the pupil an irregular shape. Sclerae are normally white and clear but they sometimes may appear light blue if underdeveloped. This discoloration will usually disappear as the infant gets older. However, presence of deep blue sclerae in an infant warrants evaluation for osteogenesis imperfecta. Corneal opacity or cloudiness, though uncommon, may be the only presentation of congenital glaucoma and warrants an urgent ophthalmology referral.

Ears have to be inspected for position, rotation, size, and appearance. Ears are in a normal location, if the helixes are at the level of the outer canthus of the eye. They are low-set, if they are below this level. Ears are posteriorly rotated, if they deviate more than 10° from the vertical axis of the head. Low-set ears are often posteriorly rotated, reflecting an arrest in normal fetal ear development. Ears should also be inspected for dysplastic features, clefts, pits, or tags. The presence of preauricular skin tags and/or ear pits is associated with significantly higher incidence of hearing impairment.[8]

The nose should be examined for patency. Newborn infants are obligate nose breathers and are not typically able to breathe through their mouth. Patency can be confirmed by gently passing a feeding tube via both nares.

The mouth has to be assessed for its size and shape. The maxilla and mandible have to be proportional and appropriately developed. A small jaw, also called mandibular hypoplasia or micrognathia, although not always pathological, can be a cause of breathing or feeding problems. This condition can also be associated with some genetic abnormalities or syndromes. A genetic workup may be warranted, if associated with other anomalies.

The mouth and pharynx have to be examined using a tongue depressor. Complete visualization of the inside of the mouth and oropharynx is important for identifying oral clefts. Cleft lip may or may not be associated with cleft palate. Cleft palate may involve the hard or soft palate, or both. Soft palate cleft is harder to see without a good depression of the tongue; occasionally, only the uvula is cleft. Cleft lip and palate may be unilateral or bilateral.

There are some findings that are normal and unique to the newborn's mouth:
- Natal teeth often occur in pairs and most commonly appear as lower central incisors. Natal teeth can be covered with membranous tissue and appear as bumps in the gum; they are conical and yellowish with hypoplastic enamel and have little root.[9] They need to be extracted, if they are loose because of the risk of aspiration.
- Epstein's pearls are white, benign, painless nodules seen in the palate of newborns.
- Bohn's nodules are white, firm mucous gland cysts found on the buccal or lingual aspects of the dental ridges; they are occasionally found at the junction of the soft and hard palate and can be confused with Epstein's pearls. Both Epstein's pearls and Bohn's nodules disappear few months after birth.

## Chest

The chest should be evaluated for its shape and symmetry. The ribs of a newborn are flexible and the chest wall is generally more compliant, resulting in slight retractions during respirations. A small thorax or bell-shaped chest can suggest hypoplastic lungs, neurologic abnormalities, or some sort of dwarfism. Pectus excavatum (funnel chest) is characterized by a "sunken" appearance of the anterior chest and is the most common deformity of the chest wall. Pectus carinatum (pigeon chest) is a form of deformation characterized by protrusion of the sternum and ribs. Breast enlargement is common in newborns and is independent of sex; it usually occurs in the first week of life and resolves without treatment in few weeks. Supernumerary nipples are pigmented, non-glandular spots along the nipple line and are more common in African-American infants.

Breathing pattern and rate should be observed for evidence of distress. Normal respiratory rate is between 40 times and 60 times per minute. Respirations should be easy and unlabored; presence of tachypnea, grunting, and retractions is evidence of respiratory distress.

Palpation of the chest reveals an area of pulsation often prominent in premature infants due to the thin chest wall; this point of maximal impulse is normally found at the left lower sternal border in newborns. Hyperdynamic precordium can be observed in patients who are tachycardic or those with heart disease related to volume overload or hypertrophy of the ventricles.

Auscultation of the chest would allow an examiner to evaluate the infant's heart and lungs. This has to be done when the infant is in a relaxed and quiet state. Complete evaluation should include auscultation of the entire chest, the precordium, back, and the axillary area. Normal breath sounds are bronchovesicular and equal on both sides; abnormal lung sounds, such as the presence of crackles, rhonchi, wheezes, and stridor should prompt more evaluation. In newborn infants, upper airway transmitted sounds are common and have to be differentiated from abnormal breath sounds.

Heart sounds are created when the heart valves close, and they are heard best along the left sternal border. Dextrocardia will make the heart sounds shift to the right. Murmurs are created by turbulence of blood flow that occurs inside or outside the heart, as blood flows across valves or blood vessels. These can be classified as benign (physiologic) or abnormal (pathologic) murmurs. They are also characterized by the quality and intensity of the sound created and can be described based on location, transmission, radiation, and when in the cardiac cycle, they occur. Murmurs are typically graded on scale of I-VI. The quality and intensity of the murmur can give clues to whether the murmur is a physiologic or pathologic murmur. Innocent murmurs are typically soft, grade II, or less in intensity, and occur during systole. The most commonly heard murmur during the newborn period is physiologic or transitional.

## Abdomen

The abdomen should be evaluated in a quiet state. Gross inspection should reveal a flat to globular abdomen that is not tense and not discolored in a normal term infant. Distention is abnormal, and if severe, is characterized by tight, shiny looking skin with prominent, and engorged superficial vessels. Furthermore, distention may indicate conditions like intestinal obstruction, organomegaly, or ascites. Scaphoid abdomen may suggest diaphragmatic hernia. Separation of the rectus abdominis muscle, called diastasis recti, is common and typically results in longitudinal midline gap, with protrusion in the abdominal wall. It is a purely cosmetic condition with no known associated morbidity. More serious abdominal wall defects such as omphalocele (abdominal contents remain outside the abdomen inside a protective sac) and gastroschisis (abdominal contents freely protrude outside) will be very evident during an examination.

Palpation of the abdomen should be done in a quiet, noncrying state using warm hands, and with the infant's knee in flexed position. Giving the infant a pacifier may help relax the abdominal musculature. The examination must begin superficially and proceed to deeper palpation without causing any discomfort. The infant must be observed for any signs of discomfort as the palpation progresses to identify tender areas of the abdomen.

Most astute examiners will be able to identify the presence of intra-abdominal mass or organomegaly by careful and gentle palpation. The liver edge is normally palpable 1-3 cm below the right subcostal margin, the kidneys may be palpable by placing the fingertips above and below the lower quadrants and applying moderate but gentle pressure, and the left kidney is more easily palpable. A full urinary bladder is palpable as a firm, globular lower abdominal mass. Any other palpable abdominal mass requires further investigation. More common abdominal masses in the newborn include enlarged kidneys, indicating hydronephrosis or cystic kidney disease, neuroblastoma, and teratomas.

## The Back

The area over the lumbosacral spine should be examined for any pits, dimples, skin tethering, cutaneous hemangiomata, or other unusual findings suggestive of occult spinal dysraphism.

## Genitalia

Genitalia are typically inspected immediately after birth in order to assign the gender of the newborn. Any ambiguity will need to be addressed and explained to the parents immediately so as to allay parental anxiety. The appearance of genitalia varies with gestational age:

- *Female genitalia*: The labia minora and clitoris are both prominent in preterm infants. As the infant approaches term, however, the labia majora become larger and more prominent while the clitoris becomes less prominent. The vaginal opening should be easily visible upon inspection. Many infants will have a hymenal tag, representing a normal and redundant portion of the hymen that protrudes from the vagina at birth and disappears after several weeks. A white-milky vaginal discharge seen in the first 1-2 weeks of life is a physiologic manifestation of withdrawal from maternal hormones and can be blood-tinged sometimes. Careful separation of the labia minora is needed to document a normal vaginal opening. Imperforate hymen can lead to hydrometrocolpos, which typically presents as a bulging hymen due to accumulation of cervical and endometrial gland secretions.[10]
- *Male genitalia* have to be assessed based on penile length, location of urethral meatus, the appearance of the scrotum, and presence of testes.

Normal penile length of the newborn is 3.5 ± 0.4 cm.[11] The examiner should conduct measurement of penile length by measuring a gently stretched penis. Using this proper technique, micropenis in a newborn is defined as penile length of <2 cm. Easy retraction of the foreskin in usually not possible; it is usually adherent and should not be forcefully retracted. The location of the urethral meatus has to be determined and can be defined as: (1) hypospadias, where the urethral opening is displaced into the ventral surface of the penis, and (2) epispadias, where the urethral opening is found on the dorsal surface of the penis. Epispadias is rare and can be associated with bifid penis and bladder extrophy.

Testes should be palpable in the scrotal sac in term infants and late preterm infants. Cryptorchidism, or undescended testes, is the most common congenital malformation in males and occurs in 2-9% of newborn boys.[12] In term infants, the scrotum has prominent rugae; in premature infants the scrotum has less rugae and becomes smoother as it gets closer to the perineal attachment.

## Anus

Anal patency and location have to be inspected during the initial examination. A patent anteriorly displaced anus may go unnoticed. An imperforate anus may occur in several forms. One form is where the rectum may have an opening in other structures, such as the urethra, vagina, base of the penis, or scrotum. Another form can be just a narrowing or stenosis versus total absence of anal opening.

## Extremities

The hands and feet have to be inspected for malformation or deformation. Congenital malformation commonly affects the extremities, and most frequently the fingers. The most common form is polydactyly, which means many fingers. The extra digit is usually a remnant of soft tissue but can occasionally be a fully functioning finger. It is most common in the ulnar (small finger) side, also called postaxial polydactyly, and less common in the radial (thumb) side, called preaxial polydactyly. Syndactyly is a condition wherein two or more digits are fused; it most commonly affects the toes. Both polydactyly and syndactyly can occur in normal newborns, but both are commonly associated with various genetic syndromes. Single palmar crease is common in trisomy 21 but can be seen in the normal population as well.

Long bone fracture is sometimes seen in newborns, particularly in LGA infants with a history of difficult delivery. The most common fractures are those of the clavicle, humerus, and femur. Multiple fractures at birth should raise the suspicion of osteogenesis imperfecta. Palpable crepitus over the clavicle is suggestive of clavicular fracture. Decreased movement of one extremity should raise the possibility of fracture or nerve injury such as brachial plexus injury; in this case, the pattern of injury depends on nerve involvement.

The hips should be evaluated to detect developmental abnormalities such as dislocated or improperly formed hip (dysplasia). Using the Ortolani and Barlow maneuvers, different degrees of developmental hip dysplasia may be detected. The examiner performs these maneuvers by keeping the infant's hip flexed 90°, while the examiner places his or her thumbs on the medial proximal thigh and the long fingers over the greater trochanter. The Barlow maneuver is a test that elicits a "dislocatable" hip by adducting the hip while applying gentle posterior pressure on the thighs and knees. The dislocation is confirmed by "relocating" the hip using the Ortolani maneuver. The examiner should perform the Ortolani test by abducting the infant's thigh and leg while applying gentle pressure on the greater trochanter. A positive test will give an audible or palpable "clunk" resulting from the femoral head moving back into the acetabulum.[13]

## Neurologic Examination

Many of the neurologic responses and behavioral features of the newborn infant depend on the maturational processes. Depending on the level of maturity of the newborn, elicited responses vary in the following ways:

- Preterm infants will have very different responses compared to their term counterparts.

- The quality of response can be highly affected by level of wakefulness.
- Abnormal neurologic signs may be seen, but are often transient.

In a neurologic examination, observation without disturbing the infant is the first approach. Evaluations that require the most disturbances should be saved for last. Just through simple observation, the examiner will be able to see overall quality and symmetry of spontaneous and stimulated movements. Normal movement patterns are typically variable. Therefore, repetitive and stereotypical movements should raise concerns for possible neurologic abnormalities, such as seizures that may present as repetitive motion of lip smacking or bicycling movements of the lower extremities. Asymmetric movements may indicate focal brain injury or specific nerve injury. Jitteriness can be a normal and transient finding, but may indicate neurologic dysfunction if persistent or severe.

Evaluation of an infant's tone is a critical part of newborn examination. Tone is gestational age-dependent, showing increasing response even in the range of term gestation from 37 weeks to 40 weeks. Resting posture between term and preterm infants is very different. Infants born between 38 weeks and 40 weeks have a posture that is characterized by strongly flexed arms and legs. Whereas, an infant born at 28 weeks gestation will have minimal limb flexion as well as minimal resistance to passive manipulation (*see* **Fig. 1**).[14]

Common passive manipulations used to evaluate overall tone of a term newborn are as follows:
- *Eliciting an absence of head lag*: This can be achieved by pulling the infant by the arms from a supine to a sitting position. The head should remain aligned with the body.
- *Horizontal suspension*: The examiner's hand supports the infant in prone position. A normal response from the infant would then be lifting his or her head to maintain neck and trunk alignment for a short period of time.
- *Vertical suspension*: The examiner should hold the infant under both axillae in a vertical position. The infant should then be able to hold his or her head straight and demonstrate active flexion of the hips, knees, and ankles. A hypotonic infant's head will fall forward; his or her lower extremities will dangle without active flexion; and the infant will "slip through" the hands of the examiner.

Hypotonia is the most common neurologic abnormality found in newborn infants. Hypotonia associated with weakness and/or contractures should raise the suspicion of neuromuscular disorders, whereas hypotonia without evidence of weakness and normal or increased reflexes suggests central nervous system (CNS) involvement. Other abnormal signs that suggest CNS involvement in the neonatal period are abnormal posturing of the hands and feet (i.e. fisting), abnormal movements such as seizures, persistent or severe jitteriness, tremors or clonus, and abnormal eye movements. Sucking abnormalities are very nonspecific and may signify either neuromuscular or CNS involvement.[15,16]

### *Primitive Reflexes*

Primitive reflexes are reflexes present in normal newborn infants. They originate in the CNS, specifically the brainstem. They are automatic movements that begin as early as 25 weeks gestation. These movements are normal in the newborn period but disappear as the child achieves normal neurologic development. Some of the most commonly tested primitive reflexes are in **Table 1**. In extremely premature infants, the Moro reflex consists only of opening of the hand; complete Moro reflex is not manifested until late gestation. The sucking reflex is present around 27 weeks but not coordinated with breathing and swallowing until around 33–34 weeks.[14] The examiner can elicit the rooting reflex by gently stroking the angle of the infant's lips and the infant will actively turn his or her head to the stimulated side.

## Infants with Hypoxic-ischemic Encephalopathy

Physical examination, especially the neuromuscular component, varies with sleep-wake cycles and disease state. Hypoxic-ischemic encephalopathy (HIE) due to perinatal asphyxia is an important cause of neurodevelopmental disability. Evidence has shown that brain cooling in patients with moderate-to-severe HIE improves survival and neurodevelopmental outcomes.[17] Newborn infants

**TABLE 1:** Criteria for identifying moderate to severe encephalopathy.

| Category | Moderate encephalopathy | Severe encephalopathy |
| --- | --- | --- |
| Level of consciousness | Lethargic | Stupor or coma |
| Spontaneous activity | Decreased activity | No activity |
| Posture | Distal flexion, complete extension | Decerebrate |
| Tone | Hypotonia (focal or general) | Flaccid |
| Primitive reflexes: | | |
| – Suck | Weak | Absent |
| – Moro | Incomplete | Absent |
| Autonomic system: | | |
| – Pupils | Constricted | Deviated, dilated, or nonreactive to light |
| – Heart rate | Bradycardia | Variable |
| – Respiration | Periodic breathing | Apnea |

who have evidence of an acute perinatal event, such as difficult extraction, abruptio placenta, cord prolapse, or uterine rupture and a 10-minute Apgar score of ≤ 5 should be evaluated for clinical and neurologic criteria for initiation of therapeutic hypothermia. Clinical and biochemical criteria include—(1) cord pH or any postnatal blood gas within the first hour of life with pH ≤7.0 and/or base deficit of ≥16, and (2) continued need for ventilation initiated at birth for at least 10 minutes. Neurologic evaluation must be conducted as soon as the infant is stabilized and adequately resuscitated. Neurologic criteria are based on five major categories of the stage II and III modified Sarnat score—(1) level of consciousness, (2) activity, (3) neuromuscular control, (4) primitive reflexes, and (5) autonomic function **(Table 1)**.[18] Presence of three or more of the aforementioned signs, or presence of seizures, would qualify the infant for brain cooling. Infants with moderate encephalopathy are typically described as lethargic and hypotonic with decreased overall activity. They have weak suck, incomplete Moro reflex, and irregular respiratory effort. In contrast, a severely encephalopathic infant will be apneic, comatose, and flaccid, with absent primitive reflexes (Moro and suck). Their pupils are typically nonreactive to light; fixed and dilated pupils are a very ominous sign. In the context of suspected neurological injury, e.g. hypoxic ischemic encephalopathy, serial neurological examination is important, as a neonate may appear quite different neurologically at different stages of its sleep/wake cycle.

## CONCLUSION

The newborn physical examination should be done in a well-lit environment and includes quiet observation of the infant's appearance and movements and a gentle physical examination. Experienced clinicians often have seen variations of normal and are adept at picking up subtle changes in infant vital signs and behavior. In addition, the standardized neurological examination is recognized as important in an era of total body cooling for infant neuroprotection in infants with HIE (see chapter on Neonatal Encephalopathy). Whether an examination reveals normal findings or brings up issues, the newborn physical examination will help establish a baseline for the infant's health in the future.

## REFERENCES

1. Ballard JL, Novak KK, Driver M. A simplified score for assessment of fetal maturation of newly born infants. J. Pediatr. 1979;95(5 Pt 1):769-74.
2. Khan O, Garcia-Sosa R, Hageman J, et al. Core Concepts: Neonatal Neurological Examination. Neo Reviews. 2014;15(8):e316-24.
3. Ballard JL, Khoury JC, Wedig K, et al. New Ballard Score expanded to include extremely premature infants. J Pediatr. 1991;119(3):417-23.
4. Milano A, Cutrone M, Laforgia N, et al. Incomplete development of the nail of the hallux in the newborn. Dermatology Online J. 2010;16(6):1.
5. Plauché WC. Subgaleal hematoma. A complication of instrumental delivery. JAMA. 1980;244(14):1597-8.
6. Section in Ophthalmology, AAP. Red Reflex Examination in Infants. Pediatrics. 2002;109(5):980-1.
7. Robinson J, Fielder AR. Pupillary diameter and reaction to light in preterm neonates. Arch Dis Child. 1990;65(1 Spec No):35-8.
8. Roth DA, Hildesheimer M, Bardenstein S, et al. Preauricular skin tags and ear pits are associated with permanent hearing impairment in newborns. Pediatrics. 2008;122:e884.
9. Leung KC, Robson WL. Natal teeth: a review. J Natl Med Assoc. 2006;98(2): 226-8.
10. Vitale V, Cigliano B, Vallone G. Imperforate hymen causing congenital hydrometrocolpos. J Ultrasound. 2013;16(1):37-9.
11. Hatipoğlu N, Kurtoğlu S. Micropenis: etiology, diagnosis and treatment approaches. J Clin Res Pediatr Endocrinol. 2013;5(4):217-23.
12. Bay K, Main KM, Toppari J, et al. Testicular descent: INSL3, testosterone, genes and the intrauterine milieu. Nat Rev Urol. 2011;8:187-96.
13. French LM, Dietz FR. Screening for developmental dysplasia of the hip. Am Fam Physician. 1999;60(1):177-84.
14. Dubowitz L, Ricciw D, Mercuri E. The Dubowitz neurological examination of the full-term newborn. Ment Retard Dev Disabil Res Rev. 2005;11(1):52-60.
15. Mercuri E, Ricci D, Pane M, et al. The neurological examination of the newborn baby. Early Hum Dev. 2005;81(12):947-56.
16. Hill A. Neonatal hypotonia. In: Maria BL (Ed). Current management in child neurology, 3rd Edition. Ontario: BC Decker Inc.; 2005. pp. 528-34.
17. Shankaran S. Outcomes of hypoxic-ischemic encephalopathy in neonates treated with therapeutic Hypothermia. Clin Perinatol. 2014;41(1):149-59.
18. Shankaran S, Laptook AR, Ehrenkranz RA, et al. Whole-body hypothermia for neonates with hypoxic-ischemic encephalopathy. N Engl J Med. 2005;353:1574-84.

CHAPTER

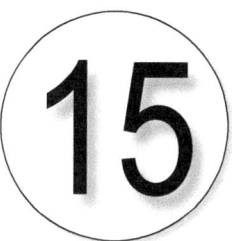

# Caring for Families through Pregnancy Loss or Death of an Infant

*Donna F Wallerstein*

## ABSTRACT

This chapter explores the difficult role of healthcare providers for families in the midst of grief. Identifying various aspects of grief and how to provide compassionate care is highlighted.

## INTRODUCTION TO BEREAVEMENT

*"There is no footprint too small to leave an imprint on this world"*

—Author unknown

Caring for mothers and young children is often thought to be one of the most joyful and satisfying areas of medical practice. As caregivers, we delight in bringing new life to the world and are often witnesses to private moments of joy and love and to the wonder of new eyes. Furthermore, as caregivers, we feel some responsibility and ownership of successfully establishing a family and we are invested in this new life before us. But despite our best care and intentions, sometimes we do not have a new life, sometimes babies are lost early in pregnancy and sometimes lost after a difficult delivery or die due to illness or disease or unknown causes very early in life. What do we say to these parents? For they are still parents, even though there is no baby. This chapter will explore the various types of loss of a child and stages of grief that caregivers may expect to see. We will discuss effects of grief on marriage and family and on decisions about subsequent pregnancies. Cultural variations and societal influences will also be reviewed.

## ROLE OF THE FAMILY AND FAMILY/CHILD DYNAMICS

*"All families have their secrets, most people would never know them, but they know there are spaces, gaps where the answers should be, where someone should have sat, where someone used to be. A name that is never uttered, or uttered just once and never again. We all have our secrets"*

—Cecelia Ahern, The Book of Tomorrow

Alicia and Tom have been married for 1 year and both are in their late twenties. Alicia works part-time at the local school as a teacher's helper and Tom works full-time at a construction company. They are living with Alicia's parents while trying to save money for a home of their own. Alicia's father is retired and her mother is a homemaker. Alicia recently missed her period and went to the doctor for a pregnancy test, which confirmed her pregnancy. The doctor has recommended an ultrasound to see when the baby will be due. When Alicia and Tom talk about the news, they are excited, nervous and wonder what her parents will say about becoming grandparents and whether they should continue living with her parents or begin searching for a place of their own. They wonder if they can afford for Alicia to stay home with the baby or if they will need to hire someone to care for the baby so that Alicia can continue working. They begin to discuss whether a boy or girl would be preferable and start to think about things a baby will need. After 2 days, Alicia returns to the doctor with Tom for the ultrasound. However, the ultrasound shows that there is an empty sac with no heartbeat present. There will be no new baby.

Mary and Ed have three teenage children and have been married for 18 years. When their youngest child entered high school last year, Mary returned to work and this year, the family took a weeklong holiday trip thanks to the increased family income. They are both 39 years old and stopped using birth control 3 years ago because they thought Mary was "too old" to have any more children. They are very surprised when they learn that she is not going through menopause but is now nearly 5 months pregnant. Unfortunately, her ultrasound shows a number of malformations in the fetus and the doctor tells them that the baby is unlikely to survive. They are considering whether to end the pregnancy or wait for a natural miscarriage.

Karla is 16 years old and attends high school. She is involved in her school debate team and thinks she might like to be a lawyer someday. She has been seeing a classmate, Brian, for the last 6 months. Karla and Brian have been sexually active for the past 4 months and uses condoms for contraception "sometimes". Karla has not had a period for more than 6 weeks and has had a positive home pregnancy test. She is afraid to tell her parents, and she and Brian have been arguing about what to do. Karla thinks she wants to keep the baby, but Brian wishes she would just have an abortion. Brian reluctantly accompanies Karla to the prenatal clinic, where they learn that there is no fetal heartbeat and Karla may need to have a procedure to remove the remains of the pregnancy.

These three cases represent a few scenarios of early to mid-pregnancy miscarriage for families and couples at different stages of life. Miscarriage can occur at any age and although older mothers are more likely to miscarry, younger women also have miscarriages.[1]

## MEANING OF PREGNANCY

*"Whether your pregnancy was meticulously planned, medically coaxed, or happened by surprise, one thing is certain—your life will never be the same"*

—**Catherine Jones**

For the couples above, pregnancy can mean very different things. For Alicia and Tom, a baby could represent the natural progression of life for them and for their parents. A baby could be a good excuse to move into a home of their own and could represent the attainment of adulthood and responsibility.[2] Alternatively, a pregnancy could be a disappointment since they are trying to save money. A baby could be a burden to them at this stage in their lives. The grandparents may also have varying reactions. Perhaps they feel they are "too young" to have grandchildren. Or they may wonder how much childcare they will be expected to contribute. Or perhaps they look forward to new life and another chance to interact with children without bearing the full responsibility for their care and upbringing.

Mary and Ed may be relieved, sad, or confused about their unexpected pregnancy and almost immediate loss. They were surprised to be pregnant again after so many years and were enjoying having teenagers and a bit more freedom. A new baby may have meant starting over or may have been a sign that they are "not too old" or still young.

Karla and Brian may feel relieved, sad, or very glad about the news of the miscarriage. Karla may be afraid of a medical procedure and may dread telling her parents. She may wonder how they will pay for the medical procedure or may worry about missing school or having pain. Brian may feel very glad or he may be surprised by sadness. He may wonder if this means something is wrong with him—maybe he isn't able to make a normal baby?

All pregnancies are small buds on a family tree. Whether the tree has many branches or few, each new potential life affects the position of the other branches in some way. With a new life, children become parents, parents become grandparents, and a child becomes brother or sister. Other family members receive new titles as well—aunt, uncle, or cousin, for example. Along with the new title, new expectations arise for interactions and behaviors.

## MEANING OF PREGNANCY TO THE COMMUNITY

*"The experience of birth is vast. It is a diverse tapestry woven by cultural customs, shaped in personal choices, affected by biological factors, and marked by political circumstances. Yet the nature of birth itself prevails in elegant design of simple complexity"*

—**Harriette Hartigan**

Just as various family members assume different roles and expectations upon learning of a pregnancy, so do other community members. A man may suddenly have greater stature in the community because he will now also be a father. Others outside the family may view him differently than before—he may be assumed to be more responsible, manlier, or more capable than before. He may be given more responsibility in the workplace, or he may be expected to need time off from work to help care for his partner and child. Women may experience similar changes and may be viewed as more nurturing or more mature when others learn of the pregnancy. In the same fashion, the community may also make assumptions when a pregnancy is lost, neighbors may wonder if the loss was natural or provoked. Others may wonder what is "wrong" with either the father or mother to cause the baby to be lost. Some may wonder if the parents used drugs or drank alcohol, which caused the baby to be lost. Some cultures may label the couple as "barren" or "unfit" because of the pregnancy loss or may see the loss of the pregnancy as a sign of personal weakness of the parents.[3]

# CHAPTER 15: Caring for Families through Pregnancy Loss or Death of an Infant

## CULTURAL CONSIDERATIONS

*"There were once a man and a woman who had long, in vain, wished for a child..."*

—The Brothers Grimm, Rapunzel

Around the world in various communities, the roles of parents and children play an important part in shaping cultural identity. From ancient times, stories about families have been a tool to shape cultural identity as well as illustrating gender roles and roles of mothers, fathers, children, and siblings. Stories often begin—"once upon a time, there was a man with seven strong sons..." or "Once upon a time, a poor orphan lived in the streets..." Often men with many sons are portrayed as blessed or wealthy, while orphans are often seen as poor or diminished in some way, even if they have riches. These portrayals of families and children are seen in stories from many different lands and shape our ideas of what it means to be fully human.

In the same way, there are many stories of families who could not have children and who sometimes resorted to magical means to have a child. In stories, often mothers, but also fathers, would make bargains with witches or other magical beings to end their infertility. In almost every story of this type, the punishment for dealing in magic is almost always the loss of the child for some period of time. Being unable to have a child is portrayed as unnatural, and, therefore, unnatural means must be employed to attain a child; however, this cannot be accomplished without sacrifice. The sacrifices in these stories are also subtle reminders that bearing a child means a change in lifestyle.[4]

These well-known stories cement cultural fears of infertility and miscarriage, and even in modern times, persist in our cultures, causing parents to feel shame, fear, and anger at the betrayal of their bodies.[5]

One woman cried after her third miscarriage, "What is wrong with me? Why won't my body hold the child?" Women often assume that their bodies are defective in some way, causing them to lose child after child. Others may assume they are being punished for past transgressions—one woman thought that her miscarriages were punishment for an abortion she had had at age 16.

## ROLE OF THE HEALTHCARE PROVIDER

*"Healing is a matter of time, but it is sometimes also a matter of opportunity"*

—Hippocrates

While working with mothers and fathers who have either lost a pregnancy or a newborn, cultural considerations must come into play. The healthcare provider must first recognize the culture of the community as well as the hierarchy of the family. The family leader may be the spokesperson for the family and the family leader can differ from culture to culture.

In some cultures, such as the Roma or Gypsy culture, the maternal grandfather or older relative is the head of the family, and this member heavily influences healthcare decisions for other members of the family.[6] A young Romani couple presented to our clinic after having two pregnancies identified with abnormalities and ultimately miscarried. The father of the wife came to the medical appointment with the young couple and asked many questions about the testing we proposed and the possible information that could be gained. Even though the husband and wife were present at the meeting, the wife's father made the final decision to allow the testing and his daughter complied with his wishes.

Another young couple of East Indian ancestry finally had a son after having several miscarriages. When they came to the clinic with their new baby, he was wearing a bracelet made of red string and his eyes were outlined with kohl. The young couple explained that the husband's mother had given the baby these things for protection from the evil that had caused the other children to be lost. In this family, the husband's mother acted as the decision-maker.

When working to provide compassionate care to a family and to ensure that health information is given full consideration, the healthcare provider must identify the family spokesperson and then include that individual in the meetings. In Western medicine, the focus is often on the individual patient (usually, the mother who has lost a pregnancy); however, this one-on-one care model does not always meet the needs of couples or families, who have a very different model for decision-making.

## MISCARRIAGE

*"Sometimes the smallest things take up the most room in your heart"*

—AA Milne

Miscarriage is broadly defined as the loss of any pregnancy from conception through full term. However, the causes of pregnancy loss at different stages of pregnancy are usually not the same. Therefore, miscarriage is generally divided into stages:

- Early miscarriage is defined as a loss prior to 20 weeks gestation; however, in practice, early miscarriage is more likely to be a loss at less than 15 weeks gestation (first trimester miscarriage).
- Mid-trimester miscarriage or second trimester loss (>14–<28 weeks gestation) is less common, but may be perceived as more traumatic.
- Third trimester miscarriage is any loss greater than 28 weeks gestation and may also be referred to as intrauterine fetal demise (IUFD) or stillbirth.[7] Both patients and caregivers can have very different reactions to these different types of losses.

## Causes of Miscarriage

Early miscarriage occurs in approximately 15% of all recognized pregnancies.[8] Therefore, about one in every seven women can be expected to have at least one miscarriage. Of early miscarriages, chromosome abnormalities account for approximately 50% of these losses. Other common causes of first trimester loss include hormone imbalances (such as luteal phase defects or thyroid dysfunction), anatomic variations (bicornuate or septate uterus), and infectious etiologies (cytomegalovirus). Rarely, teratogens like treatment with chemotherapy or radiation may contribute to early loss.[9] In many cases, the cause of an early miscarriage is never determined.

There is some overlap with causation between first and second trimester loss; chromosome abnormalities still play a significant role in second trimester loss, although not as great as in the first trimester. Congenital anomalies such as heart defects may also cause mid-trimester loss. Cervical insufficiency can cause second trimester loss, as can infectious or immunologic factors (Rh sensitization). Placental abruption can occur as a result of maternal hypertension, teratogen exposure, trauma, or inherited thrombophilia factors. Chronic maternal illness such as uncontrolled diabetes or lupus may also contribute to miscarriage.[10]

Third trimester loss or stillbirth can occur due to all of the factors previously noted as well as cord accidents (nuchal cord). Stillbirth occurs in about one in every 160 pregnancies and 76.2% of all stillbirths occur in South Asia and sub-Saharan Africa.[11]

As noted above, a significant percentage of the world's stillbirths occur in areas with high poverty rates, as compared to areas with more available resources. However, even in countries with low poverty rates and many available resources for diagnosis and treatment, many miscarriages and stillbirths remain unexplained.

## Sudden Infant Death Syndrome and Sudden Unexpected Infant Death Syndrome

Often referred to as "crib death" or "cot death," sudden infant death syndrome (SIDS) occurs primarily in healthy-appearing infants between 1 month and 12 months of age. Most deaths occur between 2 months and 4 months of age. Sudden unexpected infant death syndrome (SUIDS) is the term used at the beginning of an investigation for the sudden death of an infant. SIDS is the term used after a thorough investigation still cannot identify the cause of the infant death.[12] SUIDS can occur for a variety of reasons, including suffocation or previously undetected heart disease. Unexplained infant death is incredibly difficult for both parents and medical professionals. When the cause of a death cannot be determined, parents may begin to question even the smallest of actions and may lose confidence in themselves, their spouse, or their medical caregiver.

## STAGES OF GRIEF

In all of the above cases—early miscarriage, second trimester miscarriage, third trimester miscarriage/stillbirth, and infant death, various stages of grief may occur. The following stages of grief were well defined by Elisabeth Kübler-Ross in her book *On Death and Dying* first published in 1969:[13]

- Stage 1—denial and isolation
- Stage 2—anger
- Stage 3—bargaining
- Stage 4—depression
- Stage 5—acceptance.

While *on Death and Dying* is written about the stages of grief an individual goes through while contemplating one's own death, the same stages of grief can be seen in parents and families who have lost a pregnancy or a child.

When first told "there is no heartbeat" on fetal ultrasound, a young couple may experience disbelief—"Can we come back in a week for another ultrasound? May be it is just too early to see." Once the couple internalizes the loss, they may choose to isolate themselves from family and friends—"How can I tell my mother that she is not going to have a grandchild?" or "How can I face my pregnant best friend?"

This isolation can quickly turn to anger—"Why can my sister have healthy children and I cannot?" Anger may be directed internally—"Why didn't I take my vitamins?" or at family—"I hate my sister!" or at the medical team—"Why didn't my doctor do something to save my baby?" Blame of self or others is often a part of the anger stage and can lead to even more isolation.

The third stage of grief after a loss is often intense bargaining. We recently had a young couple present to the emergency room with a newborn infant who had died at home hours after his birth. In the weeks since his death, the young couple has been seeking answers everywhere—requesting more laboratory tests, taking vitamin supplements, and carefully avoiding another conception for at least 3 months. They are actively bargaining that by doing all of these things, their next baby will live.

Depression can be the longest lasting and most pervasive of all the grief reactions. Depression can manifest as disinterest in normal daily activities, even avoiding bathing or regular meals. Others who are depressed may instantly return to their regular work routine, cheerfully maintaining "I am fine," while avoiding the intense sadness that can overwhelm them in moments alone. Depression may last from weeks to months and can be aggravated by the inability of others to empathize with their pain, particularly over many months.

Finally, acceptance of the loss comes to the parents and family. Acceptance may be apparent when a mother verbalizes her loss to a newly pregnant friend: "Even though I lost my baby, I can feel happy for you now." Acceptance can also be apparent, when a couple says, "we are ready to try for another pregnancy now, even though we are still afraid." Alternatively, acceptance may be the moment when a couple can say, "we are complete together; we have decided not to try to have a baby".

### Gender Differences in Grief

*"It inspires me to be in the space inhabited by our children's spirits and by our shared grief, a sharing which helps us all heal and continue living"*

—**Bill Brown**

Just as in many other areas of life, men and women often react very differently to the loss of a pregnancy or death of a child. However, each individual is unique, regardless of gender, and in some families, traditional gender roles may be reversed. In general, women have both intense physical reactions to the loss of a pregnancy (hormone levels fluctuate, bleeding occurs, and breasts may be engorged), as well as intense emotional reactions (crying, sadness, and rage). While males do not have the physical responses, their emotional responses may be equally strong. However, in many cultures, openly crying is not an acceptable male reaction, and fathers may feel that their emotions are not recognized because they are not allowed to express them.[14] Fathers may also feel pressure to be supportive and "strong" for their partner—fathers are expected to care for the mother, providing both physical support and sustenance as well as emotional support. In one support group, a newly bereaved father says, "I don't know what to say to the people at work—I was supposed to take a leave for 6 weeks after our baby was born, but now that he is gone, I want to go back to work. How can I tell my boss what happened?"

Grief may last for different amounts of time for mothers and fathers. Women may openly express their grief for a longer period of time, while fathers may feel that "life goes on" and that it is time to go back to a prepregnancy routine. Even family members may feel that a mother's grief has lasted "too long" and become bothered by her inability to stop thinking and talking about her loss. This can lead to more emotional distance between family members and can lead to further isolation of the mother. One young mother said: "I know my family is tired of my sadness—they try to change the subject every time, I bring up Kailey. But I just want to talk about her—I know they never saw her, but she is so real to me and I am afraid that if I don't talk about her, I will forget her."

### Sibling Grief

*"The sharp knife of a short life..."*

—**The Band Perry**

Because children have a fluid sense of time and often have little to compare the loss of a sibling or a possible sibling to, their grief reactions may seem unusual to adults. At age 5, Sandra loses her mother in a car accident. After the funeral, family and friends come to the home and find Sandra and her brother still dressed in their funeral clothes, happily laughing and playing together in the yard. This seeming obliviousness to loss is normal for children who have more episodic reactions. For young children particularly, the permanence of death is not realized and so they do not understand the adult reactions of profound sadness. However, children often do feel compassion for the grief of others and will attempt to comfort a sad parent.[15]

Some children will also seek to blame themselves for the loss of a pregnancy or new baby, thinking, "I didn't want a sister and that made the new baby go away". Other children may develop fears when told "the baby died because he was sick"—children may fear even minor illness, thinking, "if I get sick, I will die, too". The loss of a sibling or potential sibling can profoundly affect a child and can color responses to pregnancy, childbirth, and child rearing far into the future. Children whose siblings died at a young age may feel a greater responsibility to succeed or to be good students or to be just "good".

## ROLE OF HEALTHCARE PROVIDERS

*"...above all, do no harm"*

—**Hippocrates**

As professionals, we often see our role as that of "helper" or "problem-solver". We look for answers to the miscarriage or the newborn death, both for the patient, the families, and for ourselves. If we can name the cause of the problem, then surely we can fix it. Like the patients, we are frustrated when all of our tests return normal results and we cannot provide answers. As caregivers, we sometimes forget that even if we solve the problem by identifying the cause of the loss, we cannot solve the real problem: this particular pregnancy, this particular baby, unique, and special, is gone forever. We must learn to feel our own grief so that we can help our patients bear their grief. No matter what we do, we cannot "solve" the real problem. The first step in caring for bereaved patients is to recognize this truth.

When we admit that we cannot make the situation better, we can then clearly say to parents—"I am so sorry for the loss of your child."

The next step in our caregiver journey to facilitate healing is to allow ourselves to stop talking. In our zeal to say something, anything useful, we sometimes say the wrong thing. We find ourselves repeating platitudes such as "you are young and can always have another baby." Our own words mock us—"another baby" is clearly different than this baby—the parents can never have this baby again. And once we acknowledge this truth to ourselves and to the parents, we create an opportunity to bond with our patients and to be allowed the privilege of sharing their grief.

Once we have acknowledged that a unique life is no more, we can help families to create lasting memories for themselves. Sometimes, a pregnancy is lost very early and there are no physical reminders. In these cases, we can encourage parents to take an action to honor the spirit of their child such as plant a tree or light a candle. Cultures and faith traditions around the world have a wide variety of rituals to honor the spirits or memories of those who have died and those same rituals can serve as a source of comfort to those who have lost pregnancies at any stage.[16]

In our clinic, we had a young Jewish couple that suffered an intrauterine demise of their first pregnancy at about 34 weeks of pregnancy. Although they were saddened by the loss, their religious tradition deemed that one who had never breathed never truly existed, and the young parents decided not to look at their child after she was delivered. It helped the young couple that a friend did look at their child and was able to describe her beautiful features to them. Although their faith did not permit them to look upon their child, it allowed others to bring comfort to them. There are many creative ways to provide comfort and support to parents and families while still honoring their wishes and traditions.

For pregnancies that are more advanced, we may have physical mementos to give to parents such as ultrasound images or photos of the baby taken after the loss. Sometimes we have a name card or a lock of hair, a handprint or a footprint to give to parents to keep. Physical objects serve as reminders that the father and mother are also still parents, even if there is no new baby.[17]

As in all areas of healthcare, being truly present for our patients is the greatest healing that we can provide. A telephone call after the family goes home, just to inquire how they are doing, can be a great comfort. We can also facilitate support groups for families, helping families to meet other families who have also lost a child or a pregnancy. For families with internet access, there are many online forums and support groups; this can be very helpful for families who may not have nearby community resources.

## ■ MOVING FORWARD

*"Weeping may endure for a night, but joy comes in the morning"*

—**Psalm 30:5**

As caregivers, our wish for all patients and all families is to move through the experience of grief and emerge with a sense of peace and acceptance, strengthened but not hardened. Healing for different patients may come in different forms, but helping families achieves their goal of a healthy pregnancy and healthy child is a powerful motivator. The majority of couples who lose a pregnancy elect to try again.[18] Women and families recognize that reproductive life is limited and the urge to end reproductive life on a positive note is almost overwhelming.

Healing for some couples is rapid and some are ready to try to conceive very quickly after a loss. For others, the grief process lasts a year or more before they gain the strength and courage to try again. Almost all couples that have lost a pregnancy have an altered perspective on the following pregnancy. Women and men describe feeling fearful and cautious. Many refuse to tell anyone about the pregnancy until they are past the time that the last pregnancy was lost. Some couples have difficulty bonding before the baby is actually born and feel detached from the pregnancy, often using different words to describe the pregnancy—they may refuse to say the word "baby" and call it "the pregnancy" or "the fetus" to distance themselves from the experience. This fear is a result of the loss of innocence—before, they were not really aware that something could go terribly wrong, and now they are all too aware of how tentative a pregnancy or a life may be.

As caregivers, we can express our condolences to grieving parents, we can identify decision-makers in the family, we can direct patients to culturally appropriate ways to hold on to memories of their pregnancy or child, we can listen to them when others will not, and we can direct our patients to others for mutual support and comfort. We must be able to give our patients the tools they need to heal; we cannot heal them, but we can help them.

## ■ COME TO THE EDGE

*Come to the edge, he said.*
*They said: We are afraid.*
*Come to the edge, he said.*
*They came.*
*He pushed them, and they flew.*

— **Guillaume Apollinaire**

## ■ REFERENCES

1. Grande M, Borrell A, Garcia-Posada R, et al. The effect of maternal age on chromosomal anomaly rate and spectrum in recurrent miscarriage. Hum Reprod. 2012;27(10):3109-17.
2. Darvil R, Skirton H, Farrand P. Psychological factors that impact on women's experiences of first-time motherhood: a qualitative study of the transition. Midwifery 2010;26(3):357-66.

3. Hollos M, Whitehouse B. Women in limbo: Life course consequences of infertility in a Nigerian community. Hum Fertil (Camb). 2014;13:1-4.
4. Young J. Once upon a time: How fairy tales shape our lives. Inside Journal magazine; Fall 1997.
5. Tseng YF, Chen CH, Wang HH. Taiwanese women's process of recovery from stillbirth: a qualitative descriptive study. Res Nurs Health. 2014;37(3):219-28.
6. Sutherland A. Gypsies and heath care. Wes J Med. 1992;157(3):276-80.
7. Ammon Avalos L, Galindo C, Li DK. A systematic review to calculate background miscarriage rates using life table analysis. Birth Defects Res A Clin Mol Teratol. 2012;94(6):417-23.
8. Pregnancy Loss. March of Dimes, September 2009/February 2010.
9. Selig BP, Furr JR, Huey RW, et al. Cancer chemotherapeutic agents as human teratogens. Birth Defects Res A Clin Mol Teratol. 2012;94(8):626-50.
10. Michels C, Tiu AY. Second trimester pregnancy loss. Am Fam Physician. 2007;76(9);1241-346.
11. Cousens S, Blencowe H, Stanton C, et al. National, regional, and worldwide estimates of stillbirth rates in 2009 with trends since 1995: a systematic analysis. Lancet. 2011;377(9774);1219-30.
12. Vermont Department of Health. Sudden Unexpected Death of an Infant. [online] Available from http://healthvermont.gov/family/SUDI/index.aspx [Last accessed September, 2019].
13. Kübler-Ross E. On Death and Dying. New York: Macmillan; 1969.
14. The Art of Manliness. Burnham, B. Loss, Grief and manliness: What every man should know about losing a loved one. [online] Available from http://www.artofmanliness.com/2009/08/04/loss-grief-and-manliness-what-every-man-should-know-about-losing-a-loved-one/ [Last accessed September, 2019].
15. Sood AB, Razdan A, Weller EB, et al. Children's reactions to parental and sibling death. Curr Psychiatry Rep. 2006;8(2):115-20.
16. Maoz B, Lauden A, Ben-Zion I. (A psychosocial view of a number of Jewish mourning rituals during normal and pathological grief). Harefuah. 2004;143(4):287-90.
17. Murphy F, Jerrell J. Negotiating the transition: caring for women through the experience of early miscarriage. J Clin Nurs. 2009;18(11):1583-91.
18. Smith LF, Ewings PD, Quinlan C. Incidence of pregnancy after expectant, medical, or surgical management of spontaneous first trimester miscarriage: long term follow-up of miscarriage treatment (MIST) randomised control trial. BMJ. 2009;339:b3827.

## SUGGESTED READING

1. Adolsson A, Larsson PG. Applicability of general grief theory to Swedish women's experience after early miscarriage, with factor analysis of Bonanno's taxonomy, using the Perinatal Grief Scale. Ups J Med Sci. 2010;115(3):201-9.
2. Bayrampour H, Heaman M. Comparison of demographic and obstetric characteristics of Canadian primiparous women of advanced maternal age and younger age. J Obstet Gynaecol Can. 2011;33(8):820-9.
3. Brier N. Grief following miscarriage: a comprehensive review of the literature. J Womens Health (Larchmt). 2008:17(3):451-64.
4. Buglass E. Grief and bereavement theories. Nurs Stand. 2010;24(41):44-7.
5. Day G. Good grief: bereavement literature for young adults and A Monster Calls. Med Humanit. 2012;38(2):115-9.
6. Holyoake DD. Once upon a time there was an angry lion: using stories to aid therapeutic care with children. Nurs Child Young People. 2013;25(7):24-7.
7. Hoppes S. When a child dies the world should stop spinning: an autoethnography exploring the impact of family loss on occupation. Am J Occup Ther. 2005;59(1):78-87.
8. Love AW. Progress in understanding grief, complicated grief, and caring for the bereaved. Contemp Nurse. 2007;27(1):73-83.
9. Seller M, Barnes C, Ross S, et al. Grief and mid-trimester fetal loss. Prenat Diagn. 1993;13(5):341-8.
10. Snowdon C, Brocklehust P, Tasker R, et al. Death, bereavement and randomised controlled trials (BRACELET): a methodological study of policy and practice in neonatal and paediatric intensive care trials. Health Technol Assess. 2014;18(42):1-410.
11. Stirtzinger RM, Robinson GE, Stewart DE, et al. Parameters of grieving in spontaneous bortion. Int J Psychiatry Med. 1999;29(2):235-49.
12. Wheeler Sr, Austin JK. Impact of early pregnancy loss on adolescents. MCN Am J Matern Child Nurs. 2001:26(3)154-9.

# CHAPTER 16

# Circumcision

Stephen Harris

## ■ INTRODUCTION

Circumcision, the surgical removal of the penile prepuce (foreskin), is one of the most common procedures done worldwide. The historical practice of circumcision demonstrates three justifications advanced for the procedure: (1) religious/ritual, (2) secular, and (3) medical. Over the millennia, these justifications have often merged in societies or groups that practice circumcision. After reviewing its history, we will discuss the medical procedure and its medical indications, as a treatment or prophylaxis, in the context of its risks.

## ■ HISTORY

Egyptian tomb and temple paintings and reliefs, and their accompanying hieroglyphic texts, suggest that circumcision was a ritual practice beginning in the Sixth Dynasty (2345–2181 BC).[1-5] The lighter-skinned, priestly class males submit as young adults as part of their symbolic, sacrificial initiation to a group that ensures society's purity and fertility **(Fig. 1)**. By the fifth century BC, when the Greek historian Herodotus visited Egypt, circumcision had become a far more widespread, secular practice, done among all social classes, "for the sake of cleanliness."[1-5]

According to the Old Testament, God commands Abraham at age 99 to circumcise himself and his son, Ishmael, and advises him that Sarah, his wife, will miraculously give birth to another son (Isaac) whom Abraham also must circumcise.[6] To this day, circumcision remains a distinctly religious practice among Jews, the bond between an individual Jewish man and God, and between the entire Jewish people and God: This is my covenant, which you shall keep, between me and you and your seed after you; Every man child among you shall be circumcised ... He that is eight days old shall be circumcised ... And the uncircumcised man child whose flesh of his foreskin is not circumcised, that soul shall be cut off from his people; he has broken my covenant.[7]

While circumcision is not mentioned in the Koran, it is described in the collected oral tradition of Mohammad's teachings (the hadith or sunnah), and has been a ritual

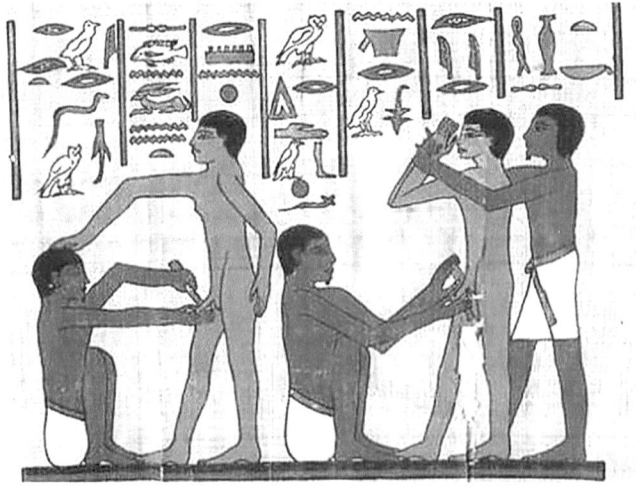

**Fig. 1:** Ancient Egyptian depiction of circumcision *(For color version see Plate 1)*.
*Source:* Anonymous (https://commons.wikimedia.org/wiki/File:Circumcision_Sakkara_3.jpg), Circumcision Sakkara 3 (https://commons.wikimedia.org/wiki/Template:PD-old).

practice since the inception of Islam. The timing of the practice varies among Muslim traditions—from the 8th day, to the time a boy can recite the Koran, to the onset of puberty, to the preparation for the Haj. As the Arab Muslim caliphate and then the Ottoman Empire extended the reach of Islam, circumcision became a common practice in North Africa, Persia, Turkey, and Southeast Asia.[1-5]

There is anthropologic evidence that circumcision developed independently, as ritual practices, among some animist cultures in sub-Saharan Africa, aboriginal people of the Pacific Islands, and some Native American tribes.[1-5]

Circumcision was vehemently deplored in Christendom, so it is ironic that circumcision as a medical practice first gained traction in the sexually repressed Victorian England, as a "cure" for masturbation.[8-10] Innumerable serious medical conditions—epilepsy, developmental delay, "crib death," paralysis, tuberculosis, and sexually transmitted infections (STIs)—were blamed on the foreskin, masturbation, or both. Circumcision became an important preventative measure and cure. In 1860, Dr Athol Johnson wrote in Lancet "In cases of masturbation we must break the habit by inducing such a condition of the parts as will cause too much local suffering to allow of the practice. Circumcision should not be performed under chloroform, so that the pain experienced may be associated with the habit we wish to eradicate."[10] Physicians in the United States accepted these British beliefs and practices. Abraham Wolbarst, writing in JAMA in 1914, said "It is generally accepted that irritation derived from a tight prepuce may be followed by convulsions and epilepsy. It is therefore not at all improbable that in many infants who die in convulsion the real cause of death is a long or tight prepuce. It is the moral duty of every physician to encourage circumcision in the young."[11] Wolbarst was the first to suggest circumcision as a preventive measure for penile cancer, and he strongly advocated universal neonatal circumcision for hygienic purposes.[11] Under these influences, the rates of circumcision in the United States, Britain, and Europe grew from less than 5% in 1860 to over 60% by the end of World War II.[12]

When Britain implemented nationalized health insurance, it began rigorous study the efficacy of many medical procedures, and determined that routine circumcision should not be covered. As the procedure fell out of universal medical favor from the 1950s onward, however, it remained very popular as a secular practice— to promote cleanliness and to ensure that the newborn "looked like dad" or other boys in the community.[13] The incidence peaked at approximately 90% in the United States in the 1970s.[12]

Current worldwide rates range from less than 20% (Central and South America, Europe, India, China) to more than 80% (the Muslim world and much of Africa), with North American and Australia somewhere in between **(Fig. 2)**.[14]

## Male Circumcision Prevalence (December 2006)

The rate in the United States has fallen to approximately 58% in 2010 due to the sexual revolution of the 1970s, the influx of immigrants from regions that do not practice circumcision, and statements from medical societies such as the American Academy of Pediatrics (AAP). The AAP's position has shifted 180 degrees from 1971 to 2012. In 1971, it found "no valid medical indication for circumcision in the neonatal period. In 2006, it reaffirmed a more nuanced position from 1999, recognizing that "newborn circumcision has potential medical benefits and advantages as well as disadvantages and risks." Its most recent, 2010 statement, that "the health

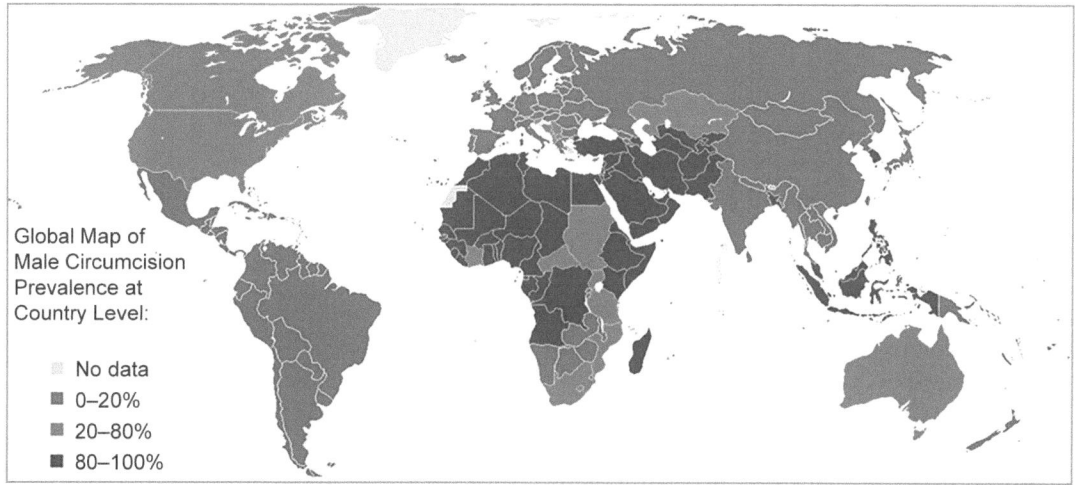

**Fig. 2:** Global map of male circumcision *(For color version see Plate 2)*.
*Source:* WHO. London School of Hygiene and Tropical Medicine, the World Health Organization and the Joint United Nations Programme on HIV/AIDS (UNAIDS). Geneva: WHO; 2007.

benefits of newborn male circumcision outweigh the risks," has been met with considerable controversy.[15-20]

Over the past 30 years, groups opposed to circumcision, such as the National Organization of Circumcision Information Resource Centers (NOCIRC) and Genital Autonomy, have engaged in public protests, political advocacy, and spirited debates in the lay press and medical literature with proponents of the procedure. These anticircumcision groups often make moral analogies between routine male circumcision and generally repugnant practices that may have or have had a religious or cultural basis: female genital cutting, foot binding, widow burning, and slavery.[21,22]

## THE FORESKIN AND THE PROCEDURE

During the first trimester, the foreskin begins to grow over the head of the penis, and should completely and symmetrically cover the glans by the middle of the second trimester. The epithelium of the glans and the foreskin fuse, and begin the slow process of separation after birth. Babies born with any genital anomaly should not be circumcised until there has been a full urologic evaluation (e.g. hypospadias, which in mild to moderate cases presents as a non-circumferential or missing foreskin, giving an appearance that the baby has been "born circumcised.").[16]

Histologically, the foreskin has blood vessels, nerves, mucus-producing cells, smooth muscle, and skin. The foreskin covers the glans and meatus, except when the penis is erect. Debate exists about its function beyond merely "covering" or "protecting" the glans.[16] Opponents to newborn circumcision generally emphasize its potential contribution to sexual pleasure, pointing to its specialized nerve cells and lubricating properties, as well as the fact that the glans epithelium of a circumcised penis becomes cornified (fully keratinized) after the foreskin is removed.[23]

### Technique

Typically, the newborn will not have been fed for an hour or two prior to the procedure, to lessen the chance of vomiting and aspiration. Depending on local medical tradition, circumcision is performed by a specially trained pediatrician, obstetrician-gynecologist, family medicine physician, surgeon, or urologist who has discussed the procedure with the parent(s), ensured there is no family history of bleeding disorders, and obtained informed consent. The penis should have been inspected previously to ensure normal genitalia and to select the proper instrument size. Depending on the training of the practitioner, the infant will be immobilized hand and foot, feet only, or simply held on another person's lap during the procedure. Sterile procedure is used.

While anesthesia is often not provided during a ritual circumcision, it is mandatory for a medical circumcision. Clear evidence shows that newborns experience pain, that proper analgesia is safe, and that it clearly reduces the subjective and objective measures of newborn pain during a circumcision. Nonpharmacologic interventions, such as oral sucrose, are not alone sufficient, because they have been shown to be no different than placebo or environmental modifications to make the infant comfortable. Topical agents, such as 4% lidocaine or 2.5% lidocaine/2.5% prilocaine reduce pain significantly; the 4% lidocaine may be preferable because it works faster (30 minutes as opposed to 60 minutes after application), does not have the theoretical risk of methemoglobinemia, and has less incidence of local skin reactions such as erythema, swelling, and blistering. Doral penile nerve block, typically 1% lidocaine *without epinephrine*, is more effective than topical agents at reducing pain during and after circumcision, but requires more special training than topical analgesia.[16,24-27]

Medical circumcisions generally use one of three instruments: (1) the Gomco clamp, (2) the Mogen clamp, and (3) the Plastibell.[28-32]

All three techniques begin by sterilizing the penis, scrotum and groin with iodine, and then applying hemostats to the foreskin at "10 and 2 o'clock" as one looks down at the dorsal side of the penis (**Fig. 3**). (Before analgesia became commonplace, the infant would begin screaming inconsolably as soon as the first hemostat was applied.) Pulling these hemostats away from the glans allows for insertion of a blunt metal probe to lyse the adhesions between the foreskin and the glans, the fused epithelia that naturally separate in the first few years of life. Once the glans and foreskin are separated, the techniques diverge.

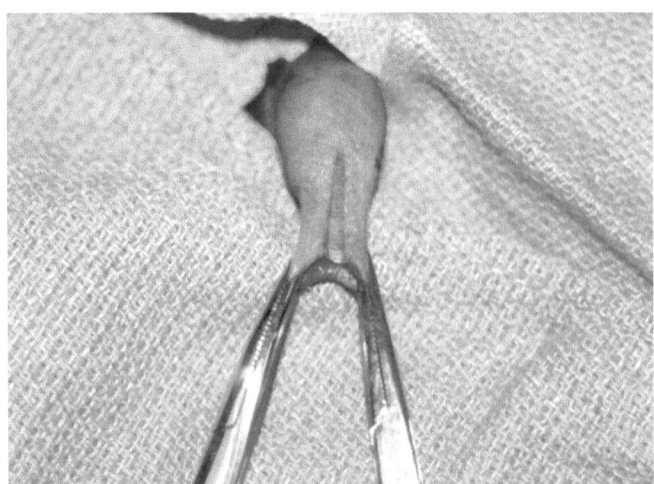

**Fig. 3:** Applying hemostats to the foreskin in preparation for circumcision *(For color version see Plate 2)*.

Those who use the Gomco clamp or Plastibell will affix a hemostat longitudinally at "12 o'clock" about two-thirds of the distance to where the practitioner estimates the corona to be. Upon removal of this hemostat, there is a line of crushed tissue along which the circumciser makes a straight cut, which then allows the entire glans to be exposed by retracting the foreskin down to the corona. (By crushing the tissue, there is very little bleeding.) Then, the metal bell of the Gomco or the plastic bell of the Plastibell is placed over the glans to protect it from being cut and the retracted foreskin is pulled back over the bell **(Fig. 4)**.

Those who use a Gomco should ensure that the size of the bell matches the size of the base of the clamp before placing the base over the bell.[33] Once placed, the skin is adjusted to ensure symmetry and amount of foreskin to remove, the hinge arm of the clamp is fixed, and the nut of the clamp is tightened, crushing the foreskin and its nerves and blood vessels between the metal bell and metal base of the clamp **(Fig. 5)**. After about 5 minutes, the foreskin is cut with a scalpel, the nut, base, and bell are removed, and gauze with petrolatum is applied to the glans **(Figs. 6 and 7)**.

Using a Plastibell, the surgeon ties a string or suture very tightly around the foreskin, crushing it against the groove at the base of the Plastibell. The remaining plastic bell, skin, and tie covering the glans fall off in approximately 3–7 days. Since the plastic bell covers the healing wound, there is no raw tissue exposed to the diaper, urine, and stool, and no petrolatum gauze or specific aftercare is required.

Using a Mogen, the guillotine-like clamp is placed over the foreskin stretched outward from the corona by the hemostats, and the arm is closed, crushing the foreskin. The foreskin distal to the clamp is cut with a scalpel, the clamp arm is lifted, the device removed, and petrolatum gauze applied.

The infant can feed immediately after the circumcision. Most babies do not have issues with urination after the

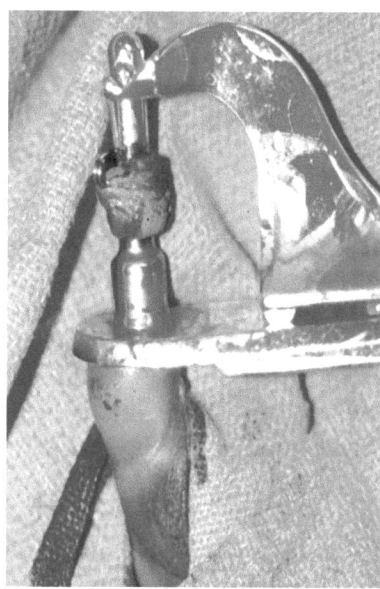

**Fig. 5:** Use of the Gomco clamp *(For color version see Plate 2)*.

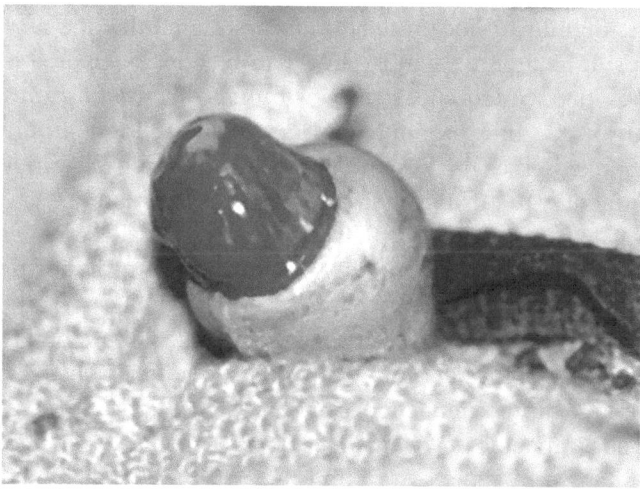

**Fig. 6:** The newly cirumcised penis *(For color version see Plate 2)*.

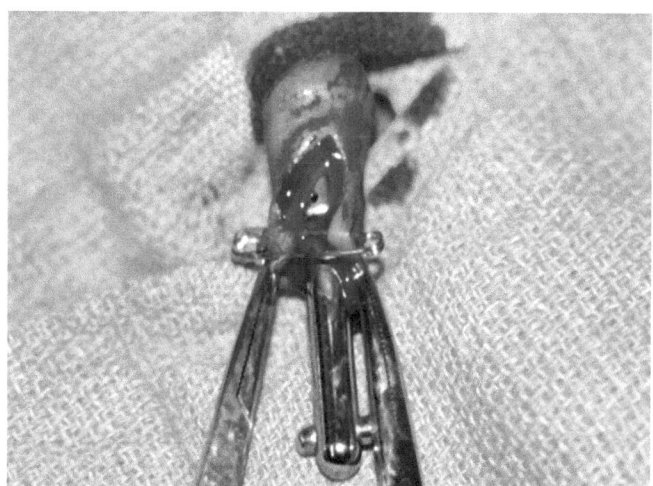

**Fig. 4:** An incision is made where the hemostat has created the linear crushed foreskin tissue *(For color version see Plate 2)*.

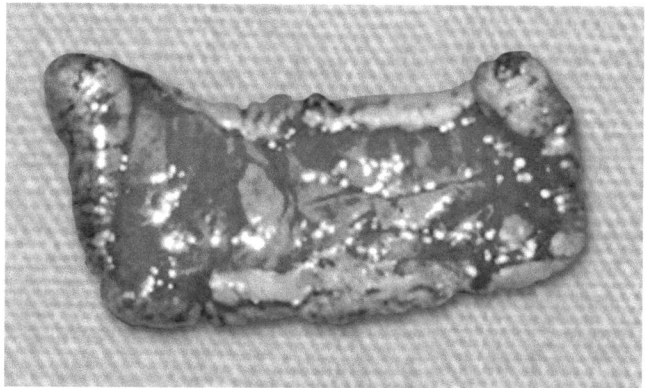

**Fig. 7:** The residual foreskin *(For color version see Plate 3)*.

procedure and do not need acetaminophen or ibuprofen. No matter the method, the glans often looks red, raw, and bruised for several days as healing and granulation occurs. Most recommend frequent and generous application of petrolatum and gauze coverage to the freshly circumcised penis for several days.

## Adverse Effects

Apart from the pain experienced by the newborn, circumcision generally is a safe procedure with few adverse effects. Still, cutting always carries the dual risks of bleeding and infection. All babies bleed during and immediately after a circumcision—most very little, which stops spontaneously or with direct pressure. Bleeding that does not stop with application of hemostatic gauze requires intervention, typically suturing by a consulting urologist or surgeon. The rate of bleeding requiring intervention is approximately 0.1% (1 in 1,000), and will likely occur if one uses a Gomco where there is a mismatch between the size of the bell and the clamp, resulting in incomplete hemostasis. There are case reports of hemorrhage requiring blood transfusions or resulting in death in infants with bleeding diatheses.[33-34]

Significant local infection or systemic infection as a result of circumcision is rarer than bleeding. The area is prepped with iodine, sterile instruments, and procedures are used, and the penis has an excellent blood supply that addresses the local inflammation. The rate of serious infection requiring intervention is approximately 0.01–0.05% (1 in 5,000–10,000). There are reports of necrotizing fasciitis and sepsis requiring intravenous antibiotics or resulting in death.[33]

Meatal stenosis, stricture of the most distal urethra, is far more common among circumcised adult males. The precise causal connection to circumcision is debated. Many believe that the uncovered meatus can become chronically inflamed by repetitive rubbing against the diaper, which over many years can lead to narrowing. Some suggest an immunologic cause triggered by inflammation that leads to lichen sclerosis and narrowing over time. In some, this narrowing remains completely asymptomatic and is only noticed during an examination for other reasons. In others, the narrowing may cause a reduction or diversion of the urinary stream that may or may not be bothersome, but may also be significant enough to require dilations or a meatotomy to relieve obstruction. Those with proven lichen sclerosis may have recurrent obstruction requiring ureteroplasty. Estimates of meatal stenosis caused by circumcision range widely, from 0.01% to 10%, depending on how one defines the condition.[33,35,36]

The urologic literature summarizes a multitude of complications and surgical misadventures that require intervention from minor revision to major reconstruction. These include partial and complete glans amputation, urethrocutaneous fistula and urethral injury, skin bridges and adhesions that cause painful erections, glans buried beneath the circumferential wound as it heals, and redundant foreskin that gives the appearance that the boy was not circumcised.[33,37-40]

All of the adverse events are more frequent when the procedure is done by non-medical personnel.

Finally, while difficult to study, one must regard seriously the claim that circumcision may reduce male sexual pleasure. After all, reducing pleasure or desire was the very reason given by Victorian physicians for medical circumcision in the first place, and the foreskin definitely contains nervous tissue and cells that lubricate. There are subjective testimonies of men who have undergone plastic surgery, which claim enhanced sexual pleasure after the "foreskin restoration" procedure.[41] Still, studies using objective surrogate measures of pleasure, such as the International Index of Erectile Function, pudendal nerve evoked potential, and intravaginal ejaculatory latency times suggest that men circumcised as babies do not differ from uncircumcised men in these sensation end points.[42]

## MEDICAL INDICATIONS

Medical providers are certainly entitled to their own personal opinion regarding circumcision performed for religious/ritual or secular practices. As a medical professional, however, providers should focus on discussing the strictly medical indications as they compare to the risk/benefit profile of the procedure.

### Circumcision as Treatment of Acquired Conditions

Phimosis is the inability to retract the foreskin to the corona of the glans. About 95% of male newborns are born with a physiologic phimosis, since the epithelial layers of the foreskin and glans are fused in utero. At age one, about 50% of boys can have their foreskins easily retracted; by age three, about 95% can retract the foreskin; and more than 99% of young men can retract their foreskins by age 17. The general guidance to parents of uncircumcised boys is to leave the foreskin alone until the boy is able to retract it himself; only simple, daily external cleaning is required.[16,43]

Most consider the inability to retract the foreskin as normal until after age 5 and unless there is "pathological phimosis," there is no reason to intervene medically even after that age. Pathological phimosis may become present if a boy has recurrent infections of the glans and foreskin (balanoposthitis) or other chronic dermatologic conditions (e.g. lichen sclerosis et atrophicus), which can cause scarring over time, leading to inability to normally retract the foreskin and painful erections.[44-47] Even without infections and/or scarring, a tight phimosis may become symptomatic for a boy whose foreskin balloons painfully during urination.

Prior to circumcising a boy with pathological or painful phimosis, most recommend a 1-2 month course of moderate to high potency topical steroids (e.g. clobetasol propionate 0.05% or betamethasone valerate 0.05% cream), applied once daily along with "stretching exercises" (gentle retraction of the foreskin to the point where it begins to become uncomfortable). Studies show success rates of 70-95% with steroid cream and stretching, although these studies have been criticized for selection bias. Since phimosis rarely an urgent condition, it is reasonable to attempt steroids and stretching prior to surgical referral.[44-47]

As will be discussed later, uncircumcised boys have a greater risk of urinary tract infection (UTI). It is unclear at what point a boy with recurrent UTI should be referred for circumcision, but it seems prudent to do so after the first or second UTI if he has a significant chronic bladder or kidney condition (e.g. high grade reflux, renal scars, and congenital malformations).

## Circumcision as Prophylaxis

Proponents of neonatal circumcision advocate for the procedure on public health grounds to reduce the risk of urinary tract and viral STIs (e.g. HIV, HSV, and HPV) and their complications (AIDS, penile and cervical cancer).

The most recent, 2010, policy statement from the American Academy of Pediatrics states that these benefits outweigh the risks to the individual neonate.[15,16] While it is difficult to quantify some of the risks, such as pain, meatal stenosis, surgical misadventure, and possibly reduced sexual pleasure, one can counsel parents that the easily quantifiable risks of bleeding and infection are indeed very, very low.[15,16]

From a public health standpoint, one must look carefully at the epidemiology. Like other medications and procedures advocated as "good for all" (e.g. Vitamin K injection at birth to prevent hemorrhagic disease of the newborn, erythromycin eye ointment to prevent gonococcal neonatorum, and vaccines to prevent serious childhood and adult infections), one must balance the number needed to circumcise to prevent a particular disease against the number of adverse events likely to occur for every person spared a particular disease.[15,16,44-47]

## UTI and its Complications

While no large randomized controlled study demonstrates reduced UTI prospectively through circumcision, excellent meta-analyses of numerous case control and cohort studies show that circumcision reduces the rate of urinary tract infection in the first year of life from 1 per 100 to 1 per 1,000 male infants. This ten-fold risk reduction falls to a risk reduction of six-fold from age 1-16, where the incidence is much less common.[48-50]

The value of circumcision for UTI depends on the disease you are trying to prevent. Estimates are that one must circumcise 150 newborns to prevent one UTI in the first year of life. This is an easily treated, typically self-limited disease without sequelae. Using a 0.08% risk of serious bleeding and 0.06% risk of infection per circumcision, one would expect one patient to bleed for every 8 UTIs prevented and one to become infected for every 11 UTIs prevented.

Those who advance circumcision on public health grounds to prevent UTI do so to reduce the risk of recurrent UTI, especially in patients with high grade vesicoureteral reflux, which can cause renal scars and, rarely, chronic renal failure and its complications. Estimates are that one must circumcise about 50,000 newborns to prevent one case of chronic renal failure from recurrent UTI— 40 patients would bleed and 30 become infected to prevent one case of chronic renal disease, and an unknown number of newborns would also experience the adverse effects listed above that are difficult to quantify.

Whether these risk/benefit calculations support universal as opposed to targeted circumcision (e.g. in a patient with recurrent UTI or known reflux or renal scar) continues to be subject of debate.

## STIs and their Complications

The preputial space between the foreskin and glans is a warm, moist, and seemingly fertile area for the growth of microorganisms, and it was long-standing belief in the early and mid-20th century that circumcision reduced the chances of acquiring common sexually transmitted diseases such as gonorrhea and syphilis. The balance of over 50 years of research, however, shows no impact from circumcision on the incidence of these diseases, or on the rate of chlamydia, the most common STI.[51-55]

Viral STIs—herpes simplex virus (HSV), human papillomavirus (HPV), and human immunodeficiency virus (HIV)—are a different story. The balance of 20 years of research shows that circumcised men acquire these viral STIs at a lower rate that those who are uncircumcised. HSV alone is a lifelong, burdensome infection, but it also independently raises one's risk of acquiring HIV, which is life altering to life threatening, depending on one's access to anti-retroviral therapy. Multiple sexually transmitted HPV serotypes infect the anogenital and pharyngeal regions— infection may be subclinical, cause papillomas, or progress to invasive cancers of the cervix, penis, and throat.[56-62]

Despite these findings, one cannot immediate conclude that universal neonatal circumcision—on individual or public health grounds—is a wise recommendation without looking carefully at the data. Clearly, no one recommends circumcision as an exclusive measure to prevent any of these STIs: circumcised men must still wear condoms, practice safe sex, and, ideally, be vaccinated against HPV.

Three excellent randomized studies on HIV negative adult African men showed that HIV acquisition 2 years after circumcision was 1-2% compared to 2-4% in the control group that remained uncircumcised (risk reduction about 50% in each study). There was a 2-4% rate of adverse events following the circumcision.[63-65] Based on this data, the World Health Organization began campaigns to increase the availability of circumcision in Africa.

Many have cautioned that the promising results from Africa cannot necessarily be applied elsewhere. First, outside of the Africa, the prevalence of HIV is substantially lower (e.g. 15-25% in many areas of Africa versus under 5% in most of the rest of the world): the number needed to circumcise to prevent one case of HIV would be much higher.[66-71]

Second, the baseline rate of circumcision in Africa is very low, so the impact of a circumcision program would be expected to be higher than in a country where the rate of circumcision is already high.[66-71]

Third, the mode of transmission of HIV in Africa is mostly heterosexual (80% of cases in Africa compared to 25% in the United States), as to in Europe and the United States where 60% of the cases are transmitted by men having sex with men. While the African studies show a 50-60% risk reduction post-circumcision for men who have sex with an HIV positive woman, similarly well done studies on HIV negative adult African women showed that circumcising their HIV positive partner actually increased the woman's risk of acquiring HIV (18% compared to 12% if the male partner remained uncircumcised). Circumcision protects the male having insertive sex with an HIV positive woman, not a woman having receptive sex with an HIV positive man.[72] Finally, several studies show that circumcision status does not affect the acquisition of HIV by men who have sex with HIV positive men. Some have suggested that this difference is due to the fact that the HIV load in the anus of one who is HIV positive is 100-times the vaginal viral load in an HIV positive woman.[73-75]

A program of circumcision in a region where the transmission in mostly non-heterosexual would likely have a much lower impact on the rates of HIV acquisition. One study modeling the impact of a universal circumcision program in the United States—taking into account lifetime risk of HIV acquisition and pre-existing circumcision prevalence—estimated that 300 males needed to be circumcised to prevent one male from acquiring HIV, and for every 4-5 HIV cases prevented, one male would suffer clinically significant bleeding or infection from the circumcision. This model also showed substantial ethnic variation, unlikely to be useful in designing a widespread public health proposal.[76]

In counseling a parent, then, one can say that circumcision probably does reduce the risk of their son acquiring HIV from an HIV positive woman, and that the magnitude of the risk reduction depends on the baseline rate of HIV where the son will live.[77,78] It is unlikely to be higher than a risk reduction from ~3-4% to 1-2%, as the studies found in Africa, where HIV is rife. And it certainly would not be high enough that their son could forego using condoms to prevent HIV and other sexually transmitted infections. Public health planners, in considering a recommend for universal circumcision, must acknowledge a complex set of considerations related to ethnic variations in HIV prevalence, HIV acquisition risk, sexual practice, baseline circumcision rates, as well as the fact that it is unlikely to protect women or men who have sex with men.

## REFERENCES

1. Angulo JC, García-Díez M. Male genital representation in paleolithic art: erection and circumcision before history. Urology. 2009;74(1):10-4.
2. Massry SG. History of circumcision: a religious obligation or a medical necessity. J Nephrol. 2011;17:S100-2.
3. Gollaher DL. Circumcision: a history of the world's most controversial surgery. New York: Basic Books; 2000.
4. Paige KE. The Ritual of Circumcision. Hum Nat. 1978;1:40-8.
5. Dunsmuir WD, Gordon EM. The history of circumcision. Br J Urol. 1999; 83:1-12.
6. Genesis, Chapter 17, Old Testament Bible, American King James Version, American Bible Society, 2000.
7. Genesis, Chapter 17, Verses 10-14, American King James Version, American Bible Society, 2000.
8. Moscucci O. Clitoridectomy, Circumcision and the Politics of Sexual Pleasure in Mid-Victorian Britain. In: Miller AH, Adams JE (Eds). Sexualities in Victorian Britain. Indiana: Indiana University Press; 1996.
9. Hutchinson J. On circumcision as a Preventive of Masturbation. Arch Surg. 1890;2:267-9.
10. Johnson A. An injurious habit occasionally met with in infancy and early childhood. Lancet. 1860;1:344-5.
11. Wolbarst AL. Universal Circumcision as Sanitary Measure. JAMA. 1914;62:92-7.
12. Morris BJ, Bailis SA, Wiswell TE. Circumcision Rates in the United States: Rising or Falling? What Effect Might the New Affirmative Pediatric Policy Statement Have? Mayo Clin Proc. 2014;89:677-86.
13. Gairdner D. The Fate of the Foreskin. Br Med J. 1949;2:1433-7.
14. WHO. Joint United Nations Programme on HIV/AIDS, WHO, London School of Hygiene and Tropical Medicine. Male Circumcision: Global Trends and Determinants of Prevalence, Safety, and Acceptability. Geneva: World Health Organization Press; 2007.

15. American Academy of Pediatrics Task Force on Circumcision. Circumcision Policy Statement. Pediatrics. 2012;130:585-6.
16. American Academy of Pediatrics Task Force on Circumcision. Technical Report: Male Circumcision. Pediatrics. 2012;130:e756-85.
17. American Academy of Pediatrics Committee on Fetus and newborn. Report of the Ad Hoc Task Force on Circumcision. Pediatrics. 1989;84:388-91.
18. American Academy of Pediatrics Task Force on Circumcision. Circumcision Policy Statement. Pediatrics. 1999;103:686-93.
19. American Academy of Pediatrics Committee on Fetus and newborn. Report of the Ad Hoc Task Force on Circumcision. Pediatrics. 1975;56:610-1.
20. American Academy of Pediatrics Committee on Fetus and newborn. Standards and Recommendations for Hospital Care of Newborn Infants, 5th edition. Evanston: American Academy of Pediatrics; 1971.
21. National Organization of Circumcision Information Resource Centers. Answers to Your Questions about NOCIRC. San Anselmo, California: NOCIRC;2014.
22. Helsinki Declaration. 2012 Helsinki Declaration of the Right to Genital Autonomy. [online] Available from www.genitalautonomy.org. [Last Accessed November, 2019].
23. Taylor JR, Lockwood AP, Taylor AJ. The prepuce: specialized mucosa of the penis and its loss to circumcision. Br Urol. 1996;77:291-5.
24. Bellieni CV, Alagna MG, Buonocore. Analgesia for infants' circumcision. Ital J Pediatr. 2013;39:38.
25. Butler-O'Hara M, LeMoine C, Guillet R. Analgesia for neonatal circumcision: a randomized controlled trial of EMLA cream versus dorsal penile nerve block. Pediatrics. 1998;101:E5.
26. Stevens B, Yamada J, Ohlsson A. Sucrose for analgesia in newborn infants undergoing painful procedures. Cochr Data Syst Rev. 2010:CD001069.
27. Lehr VT, Cepeda E, Frattarelli DA, et al. Lidocaine 4% cream compared with lidocaine 2.5% and prilocaine 2.5% or dorsal penile block for circumcision. Am J Perinatol. 2005;22:231-7.
28. Gee WF, Ansell JS. Neonatal circumcision: a ten year overview: with comparison of the Gomco clamp and the Plastibell device. Pediatrics. 1976;58:824-7.
29. Mahomed A, Ogston K. Gomco circumcision. J Pediatr Surg. 2002;37:683.
30. Kurtis PS, DeSilva HN, Bernstein BA, et al. A comparison of the Mogen and Gomco clamps in combination with dorsal penile nerve block in minimizing the pain of neonatal circumcision. Pediatrics. 1999;103:E23.
31. Thornton J. A randomized trial of Mogen clamp versus Plastibell for neonatal male circumcision in Botswana. J Acquir Immune Defic Syndr. 2013;64:e12-3.
32. Freeman JJ, Spencer AU, Drongowski RA, et al. Newborn circumcision outcomes: are parents satisfied with the results? Pediatr Surg Int. 2014;30:333-8.
33. Weiss HA, Larke N, Halperin D, et al. Complications of circumcision in male neonates, infants and children: a systematic review. BMC Urology. 2010;10:2.
34. Feinberg AN, Brust RA, Walker TA. Bleeding at circumcision: patient or operator issue? Clin Pediatr. 2010;49:760-3.
35. Stewart L, McCammon K, Metro M, et al. SIU/ICUD Consultation on Urethral Strictures: Anterior urethra-lichen sclerosus. Urology. 2014;83:S27-30.
36. Pieretti RV, Goldstein AM, Pieretti-Vanmarcke R. Late complications of newborn circumcision: a common and avoidable problem. Pediatr Surg Intern. 2010;26:515-8.
37. Bode CO, Ikhisemojie S, Ademuyiwa AO. Penile injuries from proximal migration of the Plastibell circumcision ring. J Pediatr Urol. 2010;6:23-7.
38. Sherman J, Borer JG, Horowitz M, et al. Circumcision: successful glanular reconstruction and survival following traumatic amputation, J Urol. 1996;156: 842-4.
39. Strimling BS. Partial amputation of glans penis during Mogen clamp circumcision. Pediatrics. 1996;97:906-7.
40. Gesundheit B, Grisaru-Soen G, Greenberg D, et al. Neonatal genital herpes simplex virus type 1 infection after Jewish ritual circumcision: modern medicine and religious tradition. Pediatrics. 2004;114:e259-63.
41. NOCIRC of Michigan. Restore Yourself-A Handy Kit for Circumcised Men. [online] Available from http://www.nocircofmi.org/Portals/0/Documents/Pamphlets/RestoreYourselfPamphlet.pdf. [Last Accessed November, 2019].
42. Morris BJ, Krieger JN. Does male circumcision affect sexual function, sensitivity, or satisfaction?—a systematic review. J Sex Med. 2013;10:2644-57.
43. American Academy of Pediatrics. Care for an Uncircumcised Penis. [online] Available from www.healthchildren.org. [Last Accessed November, 2019].
44. Elmore JM, Baker LA, Snodgrass WT. Topical steroid therapy as an alternative to circumcision for phimosis in boys younger than 3 years. J Urol. 2002;168:1746-7.
45. Ashfield JE, Nickel KR, Siemens DR, et al. Treatment of phimosis with topical steroids in 194 children. J Urol. 2003;169:1106-8.
46. Yang SS, Tsai YC, Wu CC, et al. Highly potent and moderately potent topical steroids are effective in treating phimosis: a prospective randomized study. J Urol. 2005;173(4):1361-3.
47. Zampieri N, Corroppolo M, Camoglio FS, et al. Phimosis: stretching methods with or without application of topical steroids? J Pediatr. 2005;147:705-6.
48. Jagannath VA, Fedorowicz Z, Sud V, et al. Routine neonatal circumcision for the prevention of urinary tract infections in infancy. Coch Data Syst Rev. 2012:CD009129.
49. Morris BJ, Wiswell TE. Circumcision and lifetime risk of urinary tract infection: a systematic review and meta-analysis. J Urol. 2013;189:2118-24.
50. Singh-Grewal D, Macdessi J, Craig J. Circumcision for the prevention of urinary tract infection in boys: a systematic review of randomised trials and observational studies. Arch Dis Child. 2005;90:853-8.
51. Dickson NP, van Roode T, Herbison P, et al. Circumcision and risk of sexually transmitted infections in a birth cohort. J Pediatr. 2008;152:383-7.
52. Tobian AA, Serwadda D, Quinn TC, et al. Male Circumcision for the Prevention of HSV-2 and HPV Infections and Syphilis. N Engl J Med. 2009;360:1298-309.
53. Mehta SD, Moses S, Agot K, et al. Adult male circumcision does not reduce the risk of incident Neisseria gonorrhoeae, Chlamydia trachomatis, or Trichomonas vaginalis infection: results from a randomized, controlled trial in Kenya. J Infect Dis. 2009;200:370-8.
54. Fergusson DM, Boden JM, Horwood LJ. Circumcision status and risk of sexually transmitted infection in young adult

males: an analysis of a longitudinal birth cohort. Pediatrics. 2006;118:1971-7.
55. Long SS. Population-based study of effect of circumcision on rates of common sexually transmitted infections (STIs). J Pediatr. 2008;152:A3.
56. Albero G, Castellsagué X, Giuliano AR, et al. Male circumcision and genital human papillomavirus: a systematic review and meta-analysis. Sex Transm Dis. 2012;39:104-13.
57. Castellsagué X, Bosch FX, Muñoz N, et al. Male circumcision, penile human papillomavirus infection, and cervical cancer in female partners. N Engl J Med. 2002;346:1105-12.
58. Chelimo C, Wouldes TA, Cameron LD, et al. Risk factors for and prevention of human papillomaviruses (HPV), genital warts and cervical cancer. J Infect. 2013;66:207-17.
59. Lu B, Wu Y, Nielson CM, et al. Factors associated with acquisition and clearance of human papillomavirus infection in a cohort of US men: a prospective study. J Infect Dis. 2009;199:362-71.
60. Auvert B, Sobngwi-Tambekou J, Cutler E, et al. Effect of male circumcision on the prevalence of high-risk human papillomavirus in young men: results of a randomized controlled trial conducted in Orange Farm, South Africa. J Infect Dis. 2009;199:14-9.
61. Mehta SD, Moses S, Agot K, et al. Medical male circumcision and herpes simplex virus 2 acquisition: posttrial surveillance in Kisumu, Kenya. J Infect Dis. 2013;208:1869-76.
62. Larke NL, Thomas SL, dos Santos Silva I, et al. Male circumcision and penile cancer: a systematic review and meta-analysis. Can Causes Contr. 2011;22:1097-110.
63. Auvert B, Taljaard D, Lagarde E, et al. Randomized, controlled intervention trial of male circumcision for reduction of HIV infection risk: the ANRS 1265 Trial. PLoS Med. 2005;2:e298.
64. Bailey RC, Moses S, Parker CB, et al. Male circumcision for HIV prevention in young men in Kisumu, Kenya: a randomised controlled trial. Lancet. 2007;369:643-56.
65. Gray RH, Kigozi G, Serwadda D, et al. Male circumcision for HIV prevention in men in Rakai, Uganda: a randomised trial. Lancet. 2007;369:657-66.
66. Mehta SD, Moses S, Agot K, et al. The long term efficacy of medical male circumcision against HIV acquisition. AIDS. 2013;27(18):2899-907.
67. Denniston GC, Hill G. Male circumcision in HIV prevention. Lancet. 2007;369:1598.
68. Brewer DD, Potterat JJ, Brody S. Male circumcision in HIV prevention. Lancet. 2007;369:1597.
69. Leibowitz AA, Desmond K, Belin T. Determinants and policy implications of male circumcision in the United States. Am J Public Health. 2009;99:138-45.
70. Arora P, Nagelkerke NJ, Jha P. A systematic review and meta-analysis of risk factors for sexual transmission of HIV in India. PLoS One. 2012;7:e44094.
71. Newell ML, Bärnighausen T. Male circumcision to cut HIV risk in the general population. Lancet. 2007;369(9562):617-9.
72. Wawer MJ, Makumbi F, Kigozi G, et al. Circumcision in HIV-infected men and its effect on HIV transmission to female partners in Rakai, Uganda: a randomised controlled trial. Lancet. 2009;374:229-37.
73. Wiysonge CS, Kongnyuy EJ, Shey M, et al. Male circumcision for prevention of homosexual acquisition of HIV in men. Coch Data Syst Rev. 2011:CD007496.
74. Millett GA, Flores SA, Marks G, et al. Circumcision status and risk of HIV and sexually transmitted infections among men who have sex with men: a meta-analysis. JAMA. 2008;300:1674-84.
75. Templeton DJ, Millett GA, Grulich AE. Male circumcision to reduce the risk of HIV and sexually transmitted infections among men who have sex with men. Curr Opin Infect Dis. 2010;23:45-52.
76. Sansom SL, Prabhu VS, Hutchinson AB, et al. Cost-effectiveness of newborn circumcision in reducing lifetime HIV risk among U.S. males. PLoS One. 2010;5:e8723.
77. Siegfried N, Muller M, Deeks JJ, et al. Male circumcision for prevention of heterosexual acquisition of HIV in men. Coch Data Syst Rev. 2009:CD003362.
78. Perera CL, Bridgewater FH, Thavaneswaran P, et al. Safety and efficacy of nontherapeutic male circumcision: a systematic review. Ann Fam Med. 2010;8:64-72.

# CHAPTER 17

# Couplet Care and Common Nursery Issues

Priya Jegatheesan, Sudha Rani Narasimhan, Dongli Song

## ABSTRACT

Keeping the mother-infant dyad together and optimizing care in the postpartum unit is essential to improve short and long-term outcomes in mothers and children. This can be accomplished through maternal and newborn-care practices that promote bonding and successful breastfeeding. Optimal neonatal screening methods and management strategies should be employed in order to prevent and/or treat hypoglycemia, sepsis, and hyperbilirubinemia in asymptomatic infants while keeping them with the mother and minimizing mother-infant separation.

## INTRODUCTION

Early mother-infant separation for more than a week may have negative impact on the quality of the dyad's relationship.[1] Mother-infant separation during the postpartum period has been shown to interfere with establishing successful breastfeeding.[2] Lack of precise methods to identify infants at risk of adverse effects due to hypoglycemia, sepsis or hyperbilirubinemia leads to a lower threshold for evaluation and treatment of these conditions. Policies, protocols, and practices related to screening and management of hypoglycemia, sepsis, and bilirubin in healthy asymptomatic newborns may inadvertently lead to mother-infant separation and adversely affect maternal and infant bonding.

Couplet care to promote mother-infant bonding may be even more critical in special populations who are exposed to substances in utero and are at risk for neonatal withdrawal syndrome after birth. This is particularly true in mothers with opiate use disorder in treatment programs who are committed to sobriety.

## SKIN-TO-SKIN

The minutes and hours after birth are critical to mother-infant bonding, but separation of mother and infant after birth is common, even though the World Health Organization recommends immediate skin-to-skin (STS) contact after birth.[3] Decreasing mother-infant separation should be a goal to promote maternal bonding and establish successful breastfeeding, thus optimizing newborn care.

Newborns should be placed STS immediately after birth to help with the natural transition; the infant should be placed on mother's abdomen while remaining connected to the mother by the umbilical cord. After cutting the cord, the stable newborn should be placed directly on the chest of the mother (STS). A blanket may be placed over the infant and mother to maintain euthermia.

Immediate STS is defined as placement of the infant on the mother within 10 minutes of birth, while early STS contact begins 10 minutes to 24 hours after birth. STS contact with mothers allows newborns to experience nine instinctive stages, an intricate weave of maternal hormones and newborns' reactions to their mother.[4] In a 2016 Cochrane review, women who had STS contact with their infant were more likely to be breastfeeding at 1-4 months after delivery, and also breastfed their infants longer.[5]

In addition, infants who experienced STS contact with their mothers had better physiological stabilization and higher blood glucose levels, with no adverse effects reported.[5]

Maternal practices can have a profound effect in promoting successful breastfeeding and optimal care for the newborn. Cesarean section (C-section) deliveries pose challenges to accomplishing immediate or early STS. The sterile environment, limitations of space, and ongoing surgery can be barriers to achieving STS in the operating room. However, these newborn infants need particular attention for successful breastfeeding since C-section is associated with breastfeeding difficulties.[6] Immediate or early STS contact in C-section deliveries (while still in the operating room) may increase breastfeeding success, defined by reduced formula supplementation in the hospital, increased bonding, decreased time to first breastfeeding, and improved maternal satisfaction.[7] There have been no adverse effects of positioning of infant during STS contact in C-section births.[8] Early/immediate STS can be performed safely in C-section deliveries with the collaboration of all parties involved.[9] Education of staff, mothers and family members is key to achieving early or immediate STS contact for all mother-infant couplets, including C-section births.[10]

Mothers should be encouraged to continue STS throughout the birth hospitalization as well as early postdischarge days, helping to ensure baby's access to breastfeed by an "on demand" schedule rather than by feeding on a strict schedule. On-demand feedings will help maintain mother's milk supply and will allow mothers to learn their babies' cues. Interestingly, schedule fed babies may have a poorer cognitive and academic outcome in childhood years when compared to demand fed babies.[11] Continued and prolonged STS will also increase maternal/infant bonding; increased levels of oxytocin are found in infants, mothers, and fathers during STS contact. Parents with higher levels of oxytocin have increased synchrony, bonding, and responsiveness to their newborns.[12]

## HYPOGLYCEMIA SCREENING

Hypoglycemia screening is recommended for all symptomatic newborns and asymptomatic newborns who are at risk for hypoglycemia (i.e. preterm, small for gestational age, large for gestational age, and infants of diabetic mothers). Because of concern for potential adverse long-term neurological sequelae as a result of persistent hypoglycemia, screening and treating appropriate infants is essential.[13]

There is no consensus regarding the minimum glucose values to define and treat asymptomatic hypoglycemia.[14]

The Pediatric Endocrine Society (PES) suggests that neonatal hypoglycemia in high-risk newborns is a hypoketotic state and therefore recommends a target threshold of more than 50 mg/dL for less than 48 hours.[15] However, many studies use a single value of 47 mg/dL as the threshold based on a study in preterm infants (<1,850 g) proposing a blood glucose level of less than 47 mg/dL as a critical value associated with adverse neurodevelopmental sequelae.[16] A recent noninferiority trial comparing hypoglycemia threshold of less than 37 mg/dL and less than 47 mg/dL showed that in infants who have moderate hypoglycemia (<37 mg/dL) after 3 hours of life, there was no difference in the 18 month neurodevelopmental outcome.[17] The American Academy of Pediatrics (AAP) clinical report suggests lower glucose values are acceptable because they are transient during the first few hours of life. In fact, the AAP proposes time-sensitive thresholds (<40 mg/dL at 0-4 h and <45 mg/dL at 4-24 h) for the definition of hypoglycemia.[18] While differing recommendations from the AAP and PES leads to variations in practice, the fundamental aim is to reduce the risk for potential brain injury and adverse long-term neurological sequelae.

The majority of centers use intermittent blood glucose checks to detect hypoglycemia. Based on expert opinions,[18] blood glucose monitoring should continue until it is established that the infant is no longer at risk for developing hypoglycemia.[18] Unfortunately, this could lead to overscreening, resulting in unnecessary painful procedures. More importantly, intermittent glucose monitoring may underestimate the true number of hypoglycemic episodes when compared to continuous interstitial glucose monitoring used in a research setting.[19] However, continuous glucose monitoring is invasive, has not been associated with improved outcomes, and is not yet approved for routine clinical use in newborns.[20]

One way to avoid unnecessary testing and promote optimal glycemic control is to encourage and support frequent, effective breastfeeding, thereby preventing transient hypoglycemia. While controversies about the definition and treatment of neonatal hypoglycemia continue, the focus should be on delivery room practices to promote successful transition of the newborn to extrauterine life. This includes implementing delayed (physiologic) cord clamping to optimize neonatal cardiopulmonary transition,[21] optimal thermoregulation, early STS, and early breastfeeding. Early and prolonged STS not only increases in-hospital breastfeeding rates, it also decreases hypoglycemia.[22,23] The AAP also recommends initiating early breastfeeding, checking the blood glucose level after the first successful breastfeeding,[18] and continuing frequent feeds to prevent hypoglycemia.

## SCREENING FOR SEPSIS IN AT RISK NEWBORNS

Early-onset sepsis (EOS) is defined as culture-proven infection occurring within a week after birth; 95% of cases are diagnosed in the first 48 hours of life.[24] EOS is a major newborn morbidity, and is associated with high mortality. The current incidence of EOS in the United States is ~0.77 per 1,000 live births, with 0.22 per 1,000, and 0.16 per 1,000 live births due to group B *Streptococcus* (GBS) and *Escherichia coli* EOS respectively.[25] The incidence varies based on gestational age, with premature infants (<34 weeks) having a much higher risk of EOS. The case mortality rates range from 7 to 11%; higher mortality is seen in preterm infants, (2% in term infants vs 19% in preterm infants), black infants (1.6% in nonblack infant vs 24.4% in black infants), and infants with *E. coli* EOS.[24-26]

The primary source of the bacterial isolate is in the blood, with a small (5-10%) percentage isolated in cerebrospinal fluid. Group B streptococcus is the most common organism causing EOS, accounting for ~40% of EOS. With the implementation of screening-based GBS prophylaxis guidelines in 1997, the incidence of EOS due to GBS has decreased from about 1.5 per 1,000 live births in 1997 to ~0.2 per 1,000 live births in 2015.[25,27] In the same period, *E. coli* has become an increasingly important cause of mortality due to EOS, especially among the preterm population. A 2008 study reported an increase in ampicillin-resistant *E. coli* sepsis with use of ampicillin for GBS prophylaxis, especially in preterm infants.[28] Another study evaluating EOS from 1990 to 2007 has shown a decrease in the overall causes of EOS, GBS EOS, and no change in ampicillin-resistant *E. coli* EOS rates.[27] The proportion of ampicillin-resistant *E.coli* EOS of all EOS increased and was associated with peripartum ampicillin exposure.

Perinatal risk factors for sepsis include GBS colonization with inadequate maternal prophylaxis, maternal fever, chorioamnionitis, and prolonged (>18 h) rupture of membranes. Centers for Disease Control and Prevention (CDC) recommendations for prevention of perinatal GBS disease have been revised several times over the past decades.[29-31] The 2010 CDC guideline recommends evaluation and antibiotic therapy for infants whose mothers had chorioamnionitis; limited evaluation with complete blood count (CBC) and blood culture for those born at less than 37 weeks gestation or prolonged rupture of membranes; and observation alone for infants with inadequate GBS prophylaxis.[32] The policy of treatment of all newborns born to mothers with chorioamnionitis has resulted in neonatal intensive care unit (NICU) admission and antibiotic therapy of 60–1,400 asymptomatic newborns for each infected asymptomatic newborn.[33] The most recent AAP clinical report replacing the 2010 CDC guidelines[34] provides three different approaches to the care of newborns at risk for sepsis: (1) Categorical risk assessment as described in the previous versions of CDC guidelines, (2) Multivariate risk assessment using the neonatal sepsis calculator, and (3) Enhanced clinical observation. The categorical risk assessment approach has led to overtreatment with antibiotics in very low risk infants.

The neonatal sepsis calculator is an online tool that was developed (based on a multivariate regression model of all perinatal risk factors) to guide management of newborns at risk for sepsis.[35] Subsequently, the calculator has been revised to include clinical signs and symptoms in the first few hours of life.[36,37] Implementing the sepsis calculator has been shown to reduce laboratory testing by 70% and antibiotics use by 50%.[38] One study showed that using the sepsis calculator reduced laboratory evaluation (i.e. CBC, blood culture, C-reactive protein) and antibiotic exposure by 80% in the maternal chorioamnionitis population, without increasing readmissions for EOS.[39] CBC is commonly used to screen newborns for sepsis. After the first 4 hours of life, a low white blood cell count, low absolute neutrophil count, and elevated immature to total neutrophil ratio are associated with increased likelihood of infection.[40] However, the likelihood ratios or specificity of these abnormal values to rule out EOS may be low.[41,42] The low specificity of laboratory-based EOS screening has contributed to unnecessary EOS treatment and early mother-infant separation, which has been shown to delay initiation of breastfeeding and increase formula supplementation.[43]

Recent active bacterial core surveillance data have shown that 48% of the cases with EOS did not have any risk factor that required intrapartum antibiotic prophylaxis.[24] Hence, the categorical or the multivariate risk-based assessments would not capture these infants. Using physical examination alone instead of risk factor and laboratory evaluation for sepsis screening has been shown to be effective in identifying infants with EOS.[44] Standardized physical examination and close observation in the first 48 hours for all newborns to identify any signs of infection is the optimal approach to identify all infants with EOS while minimizing unnecessary laboratory evaluations, mother-infant separation, and antibiotic exposure. This approach identifies infants who do not have perinatal risk factors for sepsis but who go on to develop EOS. A coordinated effort between nursing staff and physicians is necessary to act upon the signs of infection identified in a timely manner. For at-risk populations, serial newborn evaluation in highly-resourced perinatal centers shows promise for reducing mother-infant separation.[45,46] Novel approaches with noninvasive monitoring[47] may further aid in reducing the duration of mother-infant separation.

## HYPERBILIRUBINEMIA SCREENING

Neonatal jaundice, due to transient buildup of bilirubin in the blood, is the most common diagnosis in newborns, affecting over 60% of term infants and 80% of preterm infants.

Bilirubin, a byproduct of hemoglobin breakdown in the blood, is a beneficial antioxidant at low levels, but a neurotoxin at higher levels that can cause brain damage and even death. Survivors suffer a spectrum of bilirubin-induced neurological dysfunction (BIND), from classic kernicterus to neurodevelopmental impairments in preterm infants.[48-50]

Despite the availability of prevention strategies and treatments, BIND, and related deaths still occur in high-income countries with well-established medical systems, with a disproportionately high burden persisting in low- and middle-income countries. According to the 2016 Global Burden of Disease report, hyperbilirubinemia-caused early neonatal death (within 0–6 days) ranked as the 7th most common cause of death globally, 7th in sub-Saharan Africa, 8th in South Asia, 9th in West Europe, and 13th in North America.[51] Key reasons exist to explain why bilirubin-induced brain injury and death continue to occur: the current diagnostic method does not accurately determine which newborns require treatment, and necessary treatment fails to be provided in a timely manner.

The main preventive strategy is to closely monitor newborns' bilirubin levels and assess their risk for BIND.[52-55] Traditionally, clinicians estimated the severity of jaundice based on degree of yellowing in the skin, which is now known to be inaccurate. More recently, International Pediatric Organizations have recommended universal screening for neonatal hyperbilirubinemia within the first days of life by either measuring transcutaneous bilirubin (TcB) level or total serum bilirubin (TSB) level.[52] Infants whose TcB level reaches the recommended threshold for phototherapy[56,57] require a confirmatory TSB test to determine if treatment is indicated.[58,59]

Neonatal jaundice peaks at 3–5 days of life, which presents a challenge to identifying newborns at risk for BIND, particularly in areas where infants are not routinely medically evaluated within 1–3 days after discharge. To overcome this difficulty, a recently developed smartphone app, BiliCam, obtains images of a newborn's skin and transmits them to a computer center for analysis by machine learning algorithm.[60] This innovative internet-based technology has been shown to give accurate estimates of TSB levels, facilitating remote screening of newborns for hyperbilirubinemia.

Currently, the only diagnostic blood test to determine infants' susceptibility for BIND is TSB. Unfortunately, TSB lacks both sensitivity and specificity to discriminate the precise thresholds between safe and worrisome TSB levels in jaundiced infants.[61-66] The false negative rate of TSB tests for BIND is ~8–10%, leading to treatment being delayed or withheld. The false positive rate of TSB is ~50–80%, leading to overdiagnosis of hyperbilirubinemia, unnecessary treatment, delayed hospital discharge after birth, and unnecessary rehospitalization in the first week of life. In the US, each year approximately 2% of all newborns (80,000) are readmitted to the hospital for treatment of hyperbilirubinemia. It causes significant maternal anxiety, interference with breastfeeding, and disruption to mother-infant bonding. Early mother-infant attachment is increasingly recognized as critical to enhancing both mother and child's long-term psychological health and reducing maternal postpartum depression. Accurate diagnosis and treatment of jaundiced newborns results in better outcomes and cost savings, thus improving value.

Phototherapy treatment of jaundice is no longer considered benign. Aggressive phototherapy is associated with higher rates of death in extremely premature infants.[67] Recent studies also show an association between phototherapy and increased risk of both cancer and seizures.[68,69] Exchange transfusion, a procedure reserved for treatment of severe hyperbilirubinemia, requires blood products and highly invasive procedures with potentially serious complications, including death.

The severe limitations of using TSB to guide therapy for diagnosis and treatment of hyperbilirubinemia are widely recognized. Many studies have shown that only a small fraction (<1%) of the total bilirubin—unbound bilirubin or free bilirubin ($B_f$)—in the blood can enter the brain and lead to neurological damage. As a result, measurement of $B_f$ is considered critical in determining the risk for BIND in jaundiced infants.[70-77] Measurement of $B_f$ as well as bilirubin binding parameters will allow clinicians to practice precision and personalized management to minimize both brain injury and unnecessary treatment.[78-81]

## PERINATAL SUBSTANCE EXPOSURE AND NEONATAL OPIATE WITHDRAWAL SYNDROME

According to a Substance Abuse and Mental Health Services Administration (SAMHSA) survey of pregnant women, 5.9% reported the use of an illicit substance, 8.5% reported the use of alcohol, and 16% reported smoking cigarettes.[82] These rates are about half that of age-matched nonpregnant women, suggesting that pregnancy is a motivating factor for many of these women to stop using substances. When infants are born dependent upon substances their mother used during pregnancy, they may show symptoms of neonatal abstinence syndrome (NAS) as they withdraw. The term neonatal opioid withdrawal syndrome (NOWS) refers specifically to infant withdrawal from opioids. The national rise in opiate use disorder has led to an increase in NAS/NOWS.[83-85]

Newborns exposed to substances in utero are at risk for symptoms of NAS/NOWS:[86] increased fussiness, irritability, tone abnormalities, difficulty feeding, lack of sleep, sweating, sneezing, etc. These symptoms significantly overlap between signs/symptoms of toxidromal versus withdrawal effect of substances, especially in polysubstance use. Infants affected by stimulants such as methamphetamine usually present with toxidromal effect manifesting with signs of central nervous system irritation immediately after birth, symptoms that gradually improve over the next few days. Newborns exposed to short-acting opiates (e.g. heroin, oxycontin) may start showing signs of withdrawal effect as early as 4–6 hours after birth, whereas infants exposed to a long-acting opiate such as methadone may not develop signs of withdrawal until 72 hours or longer. Understanding the prenatal history and progression of symptoms is necessary to delineate opiate withdrawal symptoms that require additional treatment. Regardless of the situation, the most critical intervention is for the mother to be able to respond to the infant's cues, provide supportive care, and to promote mother-infant attachment/bonding.[87,88] Nonpharmacological interventions such as holding, cuddling, sucking, STS, breastfeeding,[89] and decreasing environmental stimulation are the first line of treatment and have been shown to reduce the need for pharmacological treatment.[90,91] Recently, California perinatal and maternal quality care collaboratives jointly released a toolkit addressing best practices to support and improve care of substance exposed mothers and newborns.[92]

Multiple quality improvement efforts have been initiated in national and statewide collaboratives to decrease the burden of prolonged NICU stay for NAS/NOWS.[91,93,94] Rooming-in with mother is an essential measure to reduce the need for pharmacological treatment[95-99] and alleviate maternal anxiety and fear.

A new NAS/NOWS scoring tool, Eat, Sleep, Console (ESC), is a functional assessment tool that evaluates the newborn's ability to eat, sleep between feedings, and be comforted.[100-102] The ESC tool involves implementing nonpharmacological interventions to optimize the newborn's ability to function, emphasizing maternal/caregiver involvement and promoting caregiver rest and self-care. ESC has been shown to significantly reduce the need for pharmacological treatment and duration of hospital stay for NAS/NOWS. Caregiver education on consoling support interventions adapted from the newborn behavior observation scale is integral to empowering the mother to care for her infant. This education is essential and helpful for all mother-infant dyads exposed to substances, not just those at risk for NAS/NOWS.

Promoting family-centered care for these newborns requires understanding of all the maternal challenges associated with substance use disorder, which is often associated with comorbidities such as mental illness, trauma, and history of violence. More than 50–90% of pregnant women with substance use disorder have a history of physical or sexual abuse. Providing trauma-informed care and universal precautions to prevent retraumatization is essential for maternal well-being and builds trust between the mother and healthcare providers. Compassionate care for the mother is necessary to empower her to optimize care of the newborn: "nurture the mother and nurture the baby." A multidisciplinary team including psychologists, addiction specialists, clinical and medical social workers, and peer support is necessary to assist mothers during their birth hospitalization and after discharge. It is essential to connect them to resources in the community. In Canada, multiservice holistic programs for pregnant and parenting women with substance use have shown that obtaining help with substance use was the central theme of the women participating in the program.[103] Participation in these programs led to a reduction in substance use, improved housing, strengthened mother-infant bonding, and promoted wellness.

## CONCLUSION

Mother-infant couplet care minimizing mother-infant separation is essential to optimal newborn outcomes. Practices essential to mother-infant bonding include early, frequent breastfeeding and STS practices, which promote both maternal and infant mental and physical health. In addition, carefully considered screening and management protocols should be employed for hypoglycemia, sepsis, and hyperbilirubinemia. Finally, for infants with risk of NAS/NOWS, use of nonpharmacological interventions by the mother to minimize risk of opiate withdrawal are recommended whenever possible. These policies and practices will minimize mother-infant separation, reduce unnecessary interventions, and optimize mother-infant well-being.

## REFERENCES

1. Howard K, Martin A, Berlin LJ, et al. Early mother-child separation, parenting, and child well-being in early head start families. Attach Hum Dev. 2011;13(1):5-26.

2. Gomez-Pomar E, Blubaugh R. The Baby Friendly Hospital Initiative and the ten steps for successful breastfeeding. a critical review of the literature. J Perinatol. 2018;38(6):623-32.
3. Abdulghani N, Edvardsson K, Amir LH. Worldwide prevalence of mother-infant skin-to-skin contact after vaginal birth: a systematic review. PLoS One. 2018;13(10):e0205696.
4. Widström AM, Brimdyr K, Svensson K, et al. Skin-to-skin contact the first hour after birth, underlying implications and clinical practice. Acta Paediatr. 2019;108(7):1192-204.
5. Moore ER, Bergman N, Anderson GC, et al. Early skin-to-skin contact for mothers and their healthy newborn infants. Cochrane Database Syst Rev. 2016;11:CD003519.
6. Hobbs AJ, Mannion CA, McDonald SE, et al. The impact of caesarean section on breastfeeding initiation, duration and difficulties in the first four months postpartum. BMC Pregnancy Childbirth. 2016;16:90.
7. Stevens J, Schmied V, Burns E, et al. Immediate or early skin-to-skin contact after a caesarean section: a review of the literature. Matern Child Nutr. 2014;10(4):456-73.
8. Havranek T, Shtzkin E, Chuang M, et al. Respiratory outcomes after neonatal prone versus supine positioning following scheduled cesarean delivery: a randomized trial. J Matern Fetal Neonatal Med. 2019:1-7.
9. Crenshaw JT, Adams ED, Gilder RE, et al. Effects of skin-to-skin care during cesareans: a quasiexperimental feasibility/pilot study. Breastfeed Med. 2019;14(10):731-43.
10. Allen J, Parratt JA, Rolfe MI, et al. Immediate, uninterrupted skin-to-skin contact and breastfeeding after birth: a cross-sectional electronic survey. Midwifery. 2019;79:102535.
11. Iacovou M, Sevillla A. Infant feeding: the effects of scheduled vs on-demand feeding on mothers well-being and children's cognitive development. Eur J Public Health. 2013;23(1):13-9.
12. Scatliffe N, Casavant S, Vittner D, et al. Oxytocin and early parent-infant interactions: a systematic review. Int J Nurs Sci. 2019;6(4):445-53.
13. Wickstrom R, Skiold B, Petersson G, et al. Moderate neonatal hypoglycemia and adverse neurological development at 2-6 years of age. Eur J Epidemiol. 2018;33(10):1011-20.
14. Tin W. Defining neonatal hypoglycaemia: a continuing debate. Semin Fetal Neonatal Med. 2014;19(1):27-32.
15. Thornton PS, Stanley CA, De Leon DD, et al. Recommendations from the Pediatric Endocrine Society for Evaluation and Management of Persistent Hypoglycemia in Neonates, Infants, and Children. J Pediatr. 2015;167(2):238-45.
16. Lucas A, Morley R, Cole TJ. Adverse neurodevelopmental outcome of moderate neonatal hypoglycaemia. BMJ. 1988;297(6659):1304-8.
17. van Kempen A, Eskes PF, Nuyetemans D, et al. Lower versus traditional treatment threshold for neonatal hypoglycemia. N Engl J Med. 2020;382:534-44.
18. Committee on Fetus and Newborn; Adamkin DH. Postnatal glucose homeostasis in late-preterm and term infants. Pediatrics. 2011;127(3):575-9.
19. Harris DL, Battin MR, Weston PJ, et al. Continuous glucose monitoring in newborn babies at risk of hypoglycemia. J Pediatr. 2010;157(2):198-202.e1.
20. Shah R, McKinlay C, Harding JE. Neonatal hypoglycemia: continuous glucose monitoring. Curr Opin Pediatr. 2018;30(2):204-8.
21. Vali P, Mathew B, Lakshminrusimha S. Neonatal resuscitation: evolving strategies. Version 2. Matern Health Neonatol Perinatol. 2015;1:4.
22. Chiruvolu A, Miklis KK, Stanzo KC, et al. Effects of skin-to-skin care on late preterm and term infants at-risk for neonatal hypoglycemia. Pediatr Qual Saf. 2017;2(4):e030.
23. Dalsgaard BT, Rodrigo-Domingo M, Kronborg H, et al. Breastfeeding and skin-to-skin contact as non-pharmacological prevention of neonatal hypoglycemia in infants born to women with gestational diabetes; a Danish quasi-experimental study. Sex Reprod Healthc. 2019;19:1-8.
24. Nanduri SA, Petit S, Smelser C, et al. Epidemiology of invasive early-onset and late-onset group B streptococcal disease in the United States, 2006 to 2015: multistate laboratory and population-based surveillance. JAMA Pediatr. 2019;173(3):224-33.
25. Schrag SJ, Farley MM, Petit S, et al. Epidemiology of invasive early-onset neonatal sepsis, 2005 to 2014. Pediatrics. 2016;138(6):e20162013.
26. Weston EJ, Pondo T, Lewis MM, et al. The burden of invasive early-onset neonatal sepsis in the United States, 2005-2008. Pediatr Infect Dis J. 2011;30(11):937-41.
27. Puopolo KM, Eichenwald EC. No change in the incidence of ampicillin-resistant, neonatal, early-onset sepsis over 18 years. Pediatrics. 2010;125(5):e1031-8.
28. Bizzarro MJ, Dembry L, Baltimore RS, et al. Changing patterns in neonatal Escherichia coli sepsis and ampicillin resistance in the era of intrapartum antibiotic prophylaxis. Pediatrics. 2008;121(4):689-96.
29. Prevention of perinatal group B streptococcal disease: a public health perspective. Centers for Disease Control and Prevention. MMWR Recomm Rep. 1996;45(RR-7):1-24.
30. Schrag S, Gorwitz R, Fultz-Butts K, et al. Prevention of perinatal group B streptococcal disease. Revised guidelines from CDC. MMWR Recomm Rep. 2002;51(RR-11):1-22.
31. Verani JR, McGee L, Schrag SJ, et al. Prevention of perinatal group B streptococcal disease—revised guidelines from CDC, 2010. MMWR Recomm Rep. 2010;59(RR-10):1-36.
32. Committee on Infectious Diseases; Committee on Fetus and Newborn; Baker CJ, et al. Policy statement—Recommendations for the prevention of perinatal group B streptococcal (GBS) disease. Pediatrics. 2011;128(3):611-6.
33. Wortham JM, Hansen NI, Schrag SJ, et al. Chorioamnionitis and culture-confirmed, early-onset neonatal infections. Pediatrics. 2016;137(1):e20152323.
34. Puopolo KM, Lynfield R, Cummings JJ, et al. Management of infants at risk for group B Streptococcal disease. Pediatrics. 2019;144(2): e20191881.
35. Puopolo KM, Draper D, Wi S, et al. Estimating the probability of neonatal early-onset infection on the basis of maternal risk factors. Pediatrics. 2011;128(5):e1155-63.
36. Escobar GJ, Puopolo KM, Wi S, et al. Stratification of risk of early-onset sepsis in newborns ≥ 34 weeks' gestation. Pediatrics. 2014;133(1):30-6.
37. Kuzniewicz MW, Walsh EM, Li S, et al. Development and implementation of an early-onset sepsis calculator to guide antibiotic management in late preterm and term neonates. Jt Comm J Qual Patient Saf. 2016;42(5):232-9.
38. Kuzniewicz MW, Puopolo KM, Fischer A, et al. A quantitative, risk-based approach to the management of neonatal early-onset sepsis. JAMA Pediatr. 2017;171(4):365-71.

39. Sharma V, Adkisson C, Gupta K. Managing infants exposed to maternal chorioamnionitis by the use of early-onset sepsis calculator. Glob Pediatr Health. 2019;6:2333794X19833711.
40. Newman TB, Puopolo KM, Wi S, et al. Interpreting complete blood counts soon after birth in newborns at risk for sepsis. Pediatrics. 2010;126(5):903-9.
41. Newman TB, Draper D, Puopolo KM, et al. Combining immature and total neutrophil counts to predict early onset sepsis in term and late preterm newborns: use of the I/T2. Pediatr Infect Dis J. 2014;33(8):798-802.
42. Hornik CP, Benjamin DK, Becker KC, et al. Use of the complete blood cell count in early-onset neonatal sepsis. Pediatr Infect Dis J. 2012;31(8):799-802.
43. Mukhopadhyay S, Liberman ES, Puopolo KM, et al. Effect of early-onset sepsis evaluations on in-hospital breastfeeding practices among asymptomatic term neonates. Hosp Pediatr. 2015;5(4):203-10.
44. Cantoni L, Ronfani L, Da Riol R, et al. Physical examination instead of laboratory tests for most infants born to mothers colonized with group B Streptococcus: support for the Centers for Disease Control and Prevention's 2010 Recommendations. J Pediatr. 2013;163(2):568-73.
45. Joshi NS, Gupta A, Allan JM, et al. Clinical monitoring of well-appearing infants born to mothers with chorioamnionitis. Pediatrics. 2018;141(4):e20172056.
46. Joshi NS, Gupta A, Allan JM, et al. Management of chorioamnionitis-exposed infants in the newborn nursery using a clinical examination-based approach. Hosp Pediatr. 2019;9(4):227-33.
47. Fairchild KD. Predictive monitoring for early detection of sepsis in neonatal ICU patients. Curr Opin Pediatr. 2013;25(2):172-9.
48. Le Pichon JB, Riordan SM, Watchko J, et al. The neurological sequelae of neonatal hyperbilirubinemia: definitions, diagnosis and treatment of the kernicterus spectrum disorders (BINDs). Curr Pediatr Rev. 2017;13(3):199-209.
49. Bhutani VK, Wong RJ, Stevenson DK. Hyperbilirubinemia in preterm neonates. Clin Perinatol. 2016;43(2):215-32.
50. Watchko JF, Tiribelli C. Bilirubin-induced neurologic damage—mechanisms and management approaches. N Engl J Med. 2013;369(21):2021-30.
51. Olusanya BO, Teeple S, Kassebaum NJ. The Contribution of Neonatal Jaundice to Global Child Mortality: Findings from the GBD 2016 Study. Pediatrics. 2018;141(2):e20171471.
52. American Academy of Pediatrics Subcommittee on Hyperbilirubinemia. Management of hyperbilirubinemia in the newborn infant 35 or more weeks of gestation. Pediatrics. 2004;114(1):297-316.
53. Maisels MJ, Watchko JF, Bhutani VK, et al. An approach to the management of hyperbilirubinemia in the preterm infant less than 35 weeks of gestation. J Perinatol. 2012;32(9):660-4.
54. Kuzniewicz MW, Escobar GJ, Newman TB. Impact of universal bilirubin screening on severe hyperbilirubinemia and phototherapy use. Pediatrics. 2009;124(4):1031-9.
55. Bhutani VK, Meng VK, Knauer Y, et al. Extreme hyperbilirubinemia and rescue exchange transfusion in California from 2007 to 2012. J Perinatol. 2016;36(10):853-7.
56. Stanford Children's Health, Lucile Packard Children's Hospital Stanford (2020). Premie BiliRecs: A tool for treatment of indirect hyperbilirubinemia in pre-term infants. [online] Available from: https://pbr.stanfordchildrens.org/ [Last accessed July, 2020].
57. BiliToolTM. (2019). BiliTool is designed to help clinicians assess the risks toward the development of hyperbilirubinemia or "jaundice" in newborns over 35 weeks gestational age. [online] Available from: http://bilitool.org/ [Last accessed July 2020].
58. Bhutani VK, Gourley GR, Adler S, et al. Noninvasive measurement of total serum bilirubin in a multiracial predischarge newborn population to assess the risk of severe hyperbilirubinemia. Pediatrics. 2000;106(2):E17.
59. Taylor JA, Burgos AE, Flaherman V, et al. BORN Investigators. Utility of decision rules for transcutaneous bilirubin measurements. Pediatrics. 2016;137(5):e20153032.
60. Taylor JA, Stout JW, de Greef L, et al. Use of a Smartphone App to Assess Neonatal Jaundice. Pediatrics. 2017;140(3):e20170312.
61. Holtzman NA. Management of hyperbilirubinemia: quality of evidence and cost. Pediatrics. 2004;114(4):1086-8.
62. Wennberg RP, Ahlfors CE, Bhutani VK, et al. Toward understanding kernicterus: a challenge to improve the management of jaundiced newborns. Pediatrics. 2006;117(2):474-85.
63. Ahlfors CE. Predicting bilirubin neurotoxicity in jaundiced newborns. Curr Opin Pediatr. 2010;22(2):129-33.
64. Watchko JF, Maisels MJ. The enigma of low bilirubin kernicterus in premature infants: why does it still occur, and is it preventable? Semin Perinatol. 2014;38(7):397-406.
65. Chang PW, Newman TB, Maisels MJ. Update on predicting severe hyperbilirubinemia and bilirubin neurotoxicity risks in neonates. Curr Pediatr Rev. 2017;13(3):181-7.
66. Das S, van Landeghem FKH. Clinicopathological Spectrum of Bilirubin Encephalopathy/Kernicterus. Diagnostics (Basel). 2019;9(1):24.
67. Morris BH, Oh W, Tyson JE, et al. Aggressive vs. conservative phototherapy for infants with extremely low birth weight. N Engl J Med. 2008;30;359(18):1885-96.
68. Newman TB, Wu YW, Kuzniewicz MW, et al. Childhood seizures after phototherapy. Pediatrics. 2018;142(4):e20180648.
69. Wickremasinghe AC, Kuzniewicz MW, Grimes BA, et al. Neonatal phototherapy and infantile cancer. Pediatrics. 2016;137(6):e20151353.
70. Funato M, Tamai H, Shimada S, et al. Vigintiphobia, unbound bilirubin, and auditory brainstem responses. Pediatrics. 1994;93(1):50-3.
71. Amin SB, Ahlfors C, Orlando MS, et al. Bilirubin and serial auditory brainstem responses in premature infants. Pediatrics. 2001;107(4):664-70.
72. Ahlfors CE, Parker AE. Unbound bilirubin concentration is associated with abnormal automated auditory brainstem response for jaundiced newborns. Pediatrics. 2008;121(5):976-8.
73. Ahlfors CE, Amin SB, Parker AE. Unbound bilirubin predicts abnormal automated auditory brainstem response in a diverse newborn population. J Perinatol. 2009;29(4):305-9.
74. Morioka I, Nakamura H, Koda T, et al. Serum unbound bilirubin as a predictor for clinical kernicterus in extremely low birth weight infants at a late age in the neonatal intensive care unit. Brain Dev. 2015;37(8):753-7.
75. Amin SB, Saluja S, Saili A, et al. Chronic auditory toxicity in late preterm and term infants with significant hyperbilirubinemia. Pediatrics. 2017;140(4):e20164009.

76. Amin SB, Wang H. Bilirubin albumin binding and unbound unconjugated hyperbilirubinemia in premature infants. J Pediatr. 2018;192:47-52.
77. van der Schoor LW, Dijk PH, Verkade HJ, et al. Unconjugated free bilirubin in preterm infants. Early Hum Dev. 2017;106-107:25-32.
78. Ahlfors CE. The bilirubin binding panel: a Henderson-Hasselbalch approach to neonatal hyperbilirubinemia. Pediatrics. 2016;138(4):e20154378.
79. Ahlfors CE, Bhutani VK, Wong RJ, et al. Bilirubin binding in jaundiced newborns: from bench to bedside? Pediatr Res. 2018;84:494-8.
80. Wennberg RP. Commentary: Bench to bedside—one step closer? Pediatr Res. 2018;84(4):483-4.
81. Morioka I. Hyperbilirubinemia in preterm infants in Japan: new treatment criteria. Pediatr Int. 2018;60(8):684-90.
82. SAMHSA (2013). Results from the 2012 National Survey on Drug Use and Health: Summary of National Findings. [online] Available from: https://store.samhsa.gov/product/Results-from-the-2012-National-Survey-on-Drug-Use-and-Health-NSDUH-/SMA13-4795 [Last accessed July, 2020].
83. Patrick SW, Schumacher RE, Benneyworth BD, et al. Neonatal Abstinence Syndrome and Associated Health Care Expenditures: United States, 2000-2009. JAMA. 2012;307(18):1934-40.
84. Patrick SW, Davis MM, Lehmann CU, et al. Increasing incidence and geographic distribution of neonatal abstinence syndrome: United States 2009 to 2012. J Perinatol. 2015;35(8):667.
85. Pryor JR, Maalouf FI, Krans EE, et al. The opioid epidemic and neonatal abstinence syndrome in the USA: a review of the continuum of care. Arch Dis Child Fetal Neonatal Ed. 2017;102(2):F183-7.
86. Hudak ML, Tan RC, Committee on Drugs, et al. Neonatal drug withdrawal. Pediatrics. 2012;129(2):e540-60.
87. Kondili E, Duryea DG. The role of mother-infant bond in neonatal abstinence syndrome (NAS) management. Arch Psychiatr Nurs. 2019;33(3):267-74.
88. Velez M, Jansson LM. The Opioid dependent mother and newborn dyad: non-pharmacologic care. J Addict Med. 2008;2(3):113-20.
89. Wu D, Carre C. The Impact of Breastfeeding on Health Outcomes for Infants Diagnosed with Neonatal Abstinence Syndrome: A Review. Cureus. 2018;10(7):e3061.
90. Mangat AK, Schmölzer GM, Kraft WK. Pharmacological and non-pharmacological treatments for the Neonatal Abstinence Syndrome (NAS). Semin Fetal Neonatal Med. 2019;24(2):133-41.
91. Whalen BL, Holmes AV, Blythe S. Models of care for neonatal abstinence syndrome: What works? Semin Fetal Neonatal Med. 2019;24(2):121-32.
92. MBSEI Toolkit. (2020). Mother & Baby Substance Exposure Toolkit. [online] Available from: https://nastoolkit.org/ [Last accessed July, 2020].
93. Wachman EM, Grossman M, Schiff DM, et al. Quality improvement initiative to improve inpatient outcomes for Neonatal Abstinence Syndrome. J Perinatol. 2018;38:1114-22.
94. Patrick SW, Schumacher RE, Horbar JD, et al. Improving care for neonatal abstinence syndrome. Pediatrics. 2016;137(5):e20153835.
95. MacVicar S, Kelly LE. Systematic mixed-study review of nonpharmacological management of neonatal abstinence syndrome. Birth. 2019;46(3):428-38.
96. MacMillan KDL, Rendon CP, Verma K, et al. Association of Rooming-in with Outcomes for Neonatal Abstinence Syndrome: A Systematic Review and Meta-analysis. JAMA Pediatr. 2018;172(4):345-51.
97. Holmes AV, Atwood EC, Whalen B, et al. Rooming-in to treat neonatal abstinence syndrome: improved family-centered care at lower cost. Pediatrics. 2016;137(6):e20152929.
98. Newman A, Davies GA, Dow K, et al. Rooming-in care for infants of opioid-dependent mothers: implementation and evaluation at a tertiary care hospital. Can Fam Physician. 2015;61(12):e555-e561.
99. McKnight S, Coo H, Davies G, et al. Rooming-in for infants at risk of neonatal abstinence syndrome. Am J Perinatol. 2016;33(5):495-501.
100. Grossman MR, Lipshaw MJ, Osborn RR, et al. A novel approach to assessing infants with neonatal abstinence syndrome. Hosp Pediatr. 2018;8(1):1-6.
101. Grossman M, Seashore C, Holmes AV. Neonatal abstinence syndrome management: a review of recent evidence. Rev Recent Clin Trials. 2017;12(4):226-32.
102. Grisham LM, Stephen MM, Coykendall MR, et al. Eat, sleep, console approach: a family-centered model for the treatment of neonatal abstinence syndrome. Adv Neonatal Care. 2019;19(2):138-44.
103. Hubberstey C, Rutman D, Schmidt RA, et al. Multi-service programs for pregnant and parenting women with substance use concerns: women's perspectives on why they seek help and their significant changes. Int J Environ Res Public Health. 2019;16(18):3299.

# SECTION 5

# Disorders of Structure and Function in the Fetus and Neonate

- Prenatal Diagnosis
  *Robert L Wallerstein*
- Birth Defects
  *Robert L Wallerstein*
- Inborn Errors of Metabolism and Newborn Screening
  *Gregory M Enns*
- Common Surgical Conditions of the Neonate
  *Stephanie D Chao, Julie R Fuchs*
- Point-of-Care Testing in Newborn Screening: Hearing Loss and Critical Congenital Heart Disease
  *Rebecca Barnett*

# CHAPTER 18

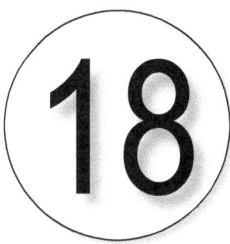

# Prenatal Diagnosis

Robert L Wallerstein

## ABSTRACT

Prenatal diagnosis is the area of medicine concerned with the identification of birth defects and genetic disorders during pregnancy. This specialty utilizes multiple modalities including imaging, specialized procedures, and laboratory analysis. Genetic counseling is an essential component of prenatal diagnosis so that patients and their families will have a clear understanding of testing options and their implications. The goal of prenatal diagnosis is to provide an accurate diagnosis so that individualized pregnancy management can be provided. Pregnancy termination, while an option for many families, is not an obligatory recommendation for an affected pregnancy. Prenatal diagnosis of a birth defect can allow for preparation for an affected child and establishment of management planning for pregnancy and delivery.

## PRENATAL DIAGNOSIS (TABLE 1)

Prenatal diagnosis refers to a variety of testing modalities used to evaluate the fetus for diseases and conditions prior to delivery. The aim is to detect birth defects prior to delivery to assist with management. Prenatal diagnosis is organized in many different ways in different settings. For much of prenatal diagnosis, the goal is to confirm a diagnosis during a time period when pregnancy termination of serious anomalies is still available. Irrespective of the availability of pregnancy termination, prenatal diagnosis is helpful because prenatal detection of a variety of conditions can help with individualization of pregnancy and delivery planning and management. As an example, identification of a lethal chromosome defect such as trisomy 18 could lead to plans of care including limited fetal monitoring during labor, reservation of cesarean section for maternal indications only, and offering comfort care for the infant instead of full resuscitation.[1-3]

Prenatal diagnosis may include a variety of technologies. Ultrasound imaging, chorionic villus sampling (CVS), amniocentesis, and nuchal translucency (NT) measurement may be used in combination with a variety of biochemical,

**TABLE 1:** Common prenatal tests.

| Common prenatal tests | |
|---|---|
| First-trimester | • Beta-hCG (beta-human chorionic gonadotropin)<br>• PAPP-A (pregnancy-associated plasma protein A)<br>• NT (nuchal translucency)<br>• CVS (chorionic villus sampling)<br>• Chromosome analysis/chromosome microarray<br>• Cell-free DNA (can be performed any time after 10 weeks gestation) |
| Second-trimester | • AFP (alpha-fetoprotein)<br>• uE3 (unconjugated estriol)<br>• Inhibin A<br>• hCG<br>• Amniocentesis<br>• Amniotic fluid AFP/acetylcholinesterase<br>• Acetylcholinesterase assays<br>• Chromosome analysis/chromosome microarray |

cytogenetic, and molecular tests.[4,5] Using all of these modalities together makes it possible to prenatally diagnose a wide variety of conditions.[6] Many prenatal diagnosis screening programs focus on more common genetic conditions such as Down syndrome and neural tube defects.[7-9] The incidence of Down syndrome worldwide is approximately 1:600, and the incidence of neural tube defects varies in different locations but is approximately 1:1,000. Historically, the first prenatal screening tests consisted of second trimester AFP (alpha-fetoprotein), low levels of which are associated with Down syndrome and elevated levels of which are associated with neural tube defects and other structural malformations. Biochemical maternal serum screening tests, encompassing AFP, hCG (human chorionic gonadotropin), PAPP-A (pregnancy-associated plasma protein A), uE3 (unconjugated estriol), and inhibin A, identified increased risk for birth defects and were followed up with ultrasound and definitive testing such as CVS and amniocentesis, where chromosome analysis was performed. Amniotic fluid AFP and acetylcholinesterase assays assisted in follow-up diagnosis.[10]

This initial scheme for prenatal diagnosis has expanded and currently encompasses maternal serum screening with markers in both first trimester (maternal serum PAPP-A and beta-hCG) and second trimester (AFP, hCG, uE3, and inhibin A) as well as ultrasound in the first trimester to include a NT measurement and second trimester ultrasound. Amniocentesis is still used as well as cell-free DNA, in which maternal blood is tested for cell-free fetal DNA to help diagnose chromosome abnormalities. Prenatal diagnosis initially most often was performed for pregnancies at higher risk due to advanced maternal age or family history, but recently has become more routinely available for additional indications. At the present time, pregnant women of all ages and family histories should be offered screening for birth defects. Screening typically begins with biochemical marker screening, with additional testing available for higher risk patients. The American College of Obstetrics and Gynecology has issued a statement that invasive testing such as amniocentesis should be made available to all pregnant women. Depending on the center and the location, however, screening options have different availabilities.[11,12]

## INVASIVE DIAGNOSTIC TESTING

### Chorionic Villus Sampling

Chorionic villus sampling typically is performed between 10 weeks and 14 weeks gestation, and allows sampling of placental tissue by direct biopsy. CVS can be performed either transabdominally or transcervically; the best approach is determined by the practitioner through ultrasound. The risk of pregnancy loss with the CVS procedure is operator-dependent, but is typically less than 1%. There was initially concern that CVS led to limb reduction, but this has been determined to be the case only when the procedure is performed prior to 10 weeks gestation, at which time the risk of limb reduction defects is 1-2%. A variety of genetic testing can be performed through CVS. Predominantly, CVS is done for diagnosis of chromosomal disorders. Other molecular genetic and biochemical testing can be performed as appropriate based on the family history.[13]

### Amniocentesis

Amniocentesis for genetic diagnosis is usually performed between 16 weeks and 18 weeks gestation, and typically can be performed safely up to 24 weeks gestation. This procedure is performed by inserting a needle into the amniotic sac using ultrasound guidance and aspirating amniotic fluid. The risk of miscarriage from amniocentesis is less than 1:300, and a recent study quotes a risk of 1:1,200. Complications are very uncommon. The cells obtained in the amniotic fluid, which are a mixed collection of cells (maternal and fetal), can be used for cytogenetic analysis and the fluid can be used for measurement of AFP. Again, there is a wide variety of testing that can be performed, if there is a specific indication.[14,15]

## GENETIC COUNSELING

An important point to emphasize is that genetic counseling should accompany prenatal diagnosis, as prenatal diagnosis provides information for couples and decision-making based on that information is very individualized. It is strongly recommended that couples be allowed to make their own decisions about pregnancy continuation or termination, if a fetal abnormality is detected. It is only through genetic counseling that this can be accomplished. In many settings, counseling is performed by a Masters level genetic counselor, who is specially trained and, in many instances, certified and licensed in genetic counseling. The process of genetic counseling consists of obtaining a detailed family history and providing a careful explanation of the risks, benefits, alternatives, and limitations of the information that prenatal diagnosis can provide. There are both medical as well as psychosocial aspects to decision-making following prenatal diagnosis, and only with the provision of genetic counseling is this process done in a compassionate and ethical manner.[16,17] Genetic counseling is a dynamic communication process between patients and their providers to help families understand the genetic implications of their situation. Sensitivity to cultural issues is of paramount importance in helping families both accept and process complex information in ways that they can use the information most appropriately.

## First-trimester Diagnosis

Typically, the second trimester is when most birth defects and conditions are diagnosed. However, due to families wishing to have earlier diagnosis, modalities have been developed for first trimester diagnosis. A newer modality is that of biochemical screening in combination with NT measurement. NT refers to an ultrasonographic lucency in the posterior fetal neck. This typically is measured as a part of the combined screening program when the fetal crown-rump length is between 45 mm and 84 mm. NT is not measured beyond a gestational age of 14 weeks (or a maximum crown-rump length of 84 mm) because NT begins to regress after this stage, as there is reduction of placental resistance in the beginning fetal renal function. This measurement can help indicate a risk for Down syndrome as well as create a patient-specific risk profile when combined with biochemical markers. An increased NT measurement is associated with an increased risk of fetal cardiac defects, syndromic problems, and chromosomal conditions. The 99th percentile is approximately 3.5 mm and does not change significantly with crown-rump length. This measurement is used as a cutoff often in considering normality. Approximately, 1% of pregnancies will have a fetal NT above 3.5 mm. The significance of this is an increased risk for chromosomal abnormalities, and it is strongly associated with trisomy 21, trisomy 18, trisomy 13, Turner syndrome, and triploidy, in descending order. In the presence of a normal karyotype, an NT measurement of ≥3.5 mm is also associated with a range of structural malformations, which shows a high risk of cardiac defects, rare genetic syndromes, and poor pregnancy outcome with miscarriage. The pathophysiology of enlarged NT is complex and unlikely to be related to a single underlying mechanism. Potential mechanisms include cardiac dysfunction, venous congestion in the head and neck, failure of lymphatic drainage, an alteration of the composition of extracellular matrix, congenital infection, and fetal anemia. In terms of cardiac defects, the risk of heart defect increases with NT thickness **(Table 2)**.

The risk of fetal chromosome abnormalities increases with increasing NT thickness as well **(Table 3)**. Using NT alone, 70% of Down syndrome fetuses can be detected. In combination with biochemical markers, this detection rate increases significantly.[18-22]

**TABLE 2:** Nuchal translucency measurement and risk of heart defect.[18]

| Nuchal translucency thickness | Risk of heart defect in fetus |
|---|---|
| ≤3.4 mm | 4 in 1,000 |
| 3.5–4.4 mm | 27 in 1,000 |
| 4.5–5.4 mm | 43 in 1,000 |
| 5.5–6.4 mm | 63 in 1,000 |
| ≥6.5 mm | 169 in 1,000 |

**TABLE 3:** Nuchal translucency measurement and risk of chromosome abnormalities.[23]

| Nuchal translucency thickness | Risk of chromosome abnormalities |
|---|---|
| 3 mm | 3 × background risk for maternal age |
| 4 mm | 18 × background risk |
| 5 mm | 28 × background risk |
| ≥6 mm | 36 × background risk |

## Second-trimester Serum Screening

Second trimester serum screening is a modality that includes both triple and quadruple screens. Additionally, maternal serum AFP in the mid-1980s was used to screen for Down syndrome and neural tube defects. hCG and uE3 testing were added, resulting in a triple screen, and subsequent to that Inhibin A testing was added, yielding the quadruple screen. These results are calculated using an algorithm that corrects for age, race, weight, and diabetic status. The Agency for Healthcare Research and Quality recommended that all pregnant women be offered maternal serum screening in 1996. The cutoffs are typically set such that the screen positive rate is approximately 5%, and as such the detection rate for Down syndrome using this modality alone is 81%. In women older than 35 years of age, combined screening detects approximately 90% of Down syndrome pregnancies. For all women, the detection rate of combined screening for trisomy 18 is 90%. Further efforts to improve detection rates of chromosome abnormalities led to the combining of first and second trimester modalities, resulting in detection rates for Down syndrome improving to 92–96% with a false positive rate of approximately 5%. Integrated screening involves using the PAPP-A analyte in the first trimester with NT, and then the quadruple screen in the second trimester. A single risk determinant is made using all the data. Stepwise sequential screening combines first trimester as well as NT testing with an age-associated risk, and subsequently the second trimester determination is made, but it is reported after the first trimester studies. This process is in contrast to the integrated screen, which does not give a risk estimate until all data are obtained.

Second trimester ultrasound is useful for detecting many structural fetal abnormalities of almost any part of the anatomy ranging from brain anomalies, facial clefting, neural tube defects, abdominal wall defects, limb deformities, renal anomalies, and congenital heart defects. Fetal echocardiography, which is a focused study of the fetal heart that is useful in detecting congenital heart defects, may also be employed.

The amount of testing that can be performed on fetal tissue from CVS or amniocentesis is growing exponentially and depends on the family history and scenario. The typical studies are cytogenetics for chromosome abnormalities. The availability of chromosome microarray is increasing. This test can detect smaller chromosome duplications and deletions. Chromosome microarray does not detect translocations or other balanced rearrangements. Depending on its availability, some centers are offering chromosome microarray routinely, while others are using this technology only when there is an identified fetal anomaly.[24-27]

## Following Prenatal Diagnosis

In the advent of an abnormal result, whether it is via ultrasound or genetic testing, genetic counseling should be provided to help the family understand the result and to make appropriate decisions. There is benefit for families who chose to continue to the pregnancy in terms of preparation for birth of an affected child, and there is also benefit to the medical team to be ready for a child with special health needs in the newborn period. For those families who elect to terminate, the availability of termination is variable depending on the location. In the United States, termination is legal up to 24 weeks of gestation and in selected circumstances may be available after that time for lethal anomalies, but availability varies in different geographic settings both in the United States and around the world.[28,29]

Increased availability of the above-mentioned prenatal diagnosis modalities has created an opportunity for better fetal evaluation as time goes on and more pregnancies have increased surveillance. In many settings, it is routine to offer screening as well as detailed ultrasound for every pregnancy. With current pregnancy monitoring, the increased detection of birth defects will lead to individualized care plans and improved outcomes.[30]

## REFERENCES

1. Kapoor S, Gupta S, Kabra M. Prenatal screening: perspective for the pediatrician. Indian Pediatr. 2014;51(12):959-62.
2. Cleary-Goldman J, Morgan MA, Malone FD, et al. Screening for Down syndrome: practice patterns and knowledge of obstetricians and gynecologists. Obstet Gynecol. 2006;107(1):11-7.
3. Gagnon A, Wilson RD, Allen VM, et al. Society of Obstetricians and Gynaecologists of Canada. Evaluation of prenatally diagnosed structural congenital anomalies. J Obstet Gynaecol Can. 2009;31(9):875-81.
4. Benson CB, Doubilet PM. The history of imaging in obstetrics. Radiology. 2014;273(2 Suppl):S92-110.
5. Brezina PR, Kearns WG. The evolving role of genetics in reproductive medicine. Obstet Gynecol Clin North Am. 2014;41(1):41-55.
6. Hardisty EE, Vora NL. Advances in genetic prenatal diagnosis and screening. Curr Opin Pediatr. 2014;26(6):634-8.
7. Skjøth MM, Draborg E, Pedersen CD, et al. Providing information about prenatal screening for Down syndrome: a systematic review. Acta Obstet Gynecol Scand. 2015;94(2):125-32.
8. Salih MA, Murshid WR, Seidahmed MZ. Epidemiology, prenatal management, and prevention of neural tube defects. Saudi Med J. 2014;35 (Suppl 1):S15-28.
9. Wilson RD; SOGC Genetics Committee; special contributor. Prenatal screening, diagnosis, and pregnancy management of fetal neural tube defects. J Obstet Gynaecol Can. 2014;36(10):927-42.
10. Russo ML, Blakemore KJ. A historical and practical review of first trimester aneuploidy screening. Semin Fetal Neonatal Med. 2014;19(3):183-7.
11. Chitayat D, Langlois S, Wilson RD, et al. Prenatal screening for fetal aneuploidy in singleton pregnancies. J Obstet Gynaecol Can. 2011;33(7):736-50.
12. Audibert F, Gagnon A, Genetics Committee of the Society of Obstetricians and Gynaecologists of Canada, et al. Prenatal screening for and diagnosis of aneuploidy in twin pregnancies. J Obstet Gynaecol Can. 2011;33(7):754-67.
13. Maruotti GM, Frisso G, Calcagno G, et al. Prenatal diagnosis of inherited diseases: 20 years' experience of an Italian Regional Reference Centre. Clin Chem Lab Med. 2013;51(12):2211-7.
14. Willner JP. Reproductive genetics and today's patient options: prenatal diagnosis. Mt Sinai J Med. 1998;65(3):173-7.
15. Ball RH. Invasive fetal testing. Curr Opin Obstet Gynecol. 2004;16(2):159-62.
16. Stembalska A, Slezak R, Pesz K, et al. Prenatal diagnosis-principles of diagnostic procedures and genetic counseling. Folia Histochem Cytobiol. 2007;45(Suppl 1):S11-6.
17. Van McCrary S, Green HC, Combs A, et al. A delicate subject: The impact of cultural factors on neonatal and perinatal decision making. J Neonatal Perinatal Med. 2014;7(1):1-12.
18. Jelliffe-Pawlowski LL, Norton ME, Shaw GM, et al. Risk of congenital heart defects by nuchal translucency norms. Am J Obstet Gynecol. 2015;212(4):518.e1-10.
19. Huang T, Dennis A, Meschino WS, et al. First trimester screening for Down syndrome using nuchal translucency, maternal serum pregnancy-associated plasma protein A, free-β human chorionic gonadotrophin, placental growth factor and α-fetoprotein. Prenat Diagn. 2015;35(7):709-16.
20. Latendresse G, Deneris A. An update on current prenatal testing options: first trimester and noninvasive prenatal testing. J Midwifery Womens Health. 2015;60(1):24-36.

21. Lund IC, Christensen R, Petersen OB, et al. Chromosomal microarray in fetuses with increased nuchal translucency. Ultrasound Obstet Gynecol. 2015;45(1):95-100.
22. Wallerstein R, Jelks A, Garabedian MJ. A new model for providing cell-free DNA and risk assessment for chromosome abnormalities in a public hospital setting. J Pregnancy. 2014;2014:962720.
23. Wright D, Syngelaki A, Bradbury I, et al. First-trimester screening for trisomies 21, 18, and 13 by ultrasound and biochemical testing. Fetal Diagn Ther. 2014;35(2):118-26.
24. Alldred SK, Deeks JJ, Guo B, et al. Second trimester serum tests for Down's Syndrome screening. Cochrane Database Syst Rev. 2012;6:CD009925.
25. Malone FD, Canick JA, Ball RH, et al. First-trimester or second-trimester screening, or both, for Down's syndrome. N Engl J Med. 2005;353(19):2001-11.
26. Rumi Kataguiri M, Araujo Júnior E, Silva Bussamra LC, et al. Influence of second-trimester ultrasound markers for Down syndrome in pregnant women of advanced maternal age. J Pregnancy. 2014;2014:785730.
27. Chasen ST. Maternal serum analyte screening for fetal aneuploidy. Clin Obstet Gynecol. 2014;57(1):182-8.
28. Lafarge C, Mitchell K, Fox P. Termination of pregnancy for fetal abnormality: a meta-ethnography of women's experiences. Reprod Health Matters. 2014;22(44):191-201.
29. Hern WM. Fetal diagnostic indications for second and third trimester outpatient pregnancy termination. Prenat Diagn. 2014;34(5):438-44.
30. Arbour L, Melnikov V, McIntosh S, et al. The current state of birth outcome and birth defect surveillance in northern regions of the world. Int J Circumpolar Health. 2009;68(5):443-58.

# CHAPTER 19

# Birth Defects

*Robert L Wallerstein*

## ABSTRACT

Birth defects encompass a wide and diverse group of structural congenital disorders. The World Health Organization estimates that 1 in 33 infants is born with a birth defect, and this results in approximately 3.2 million birth defect-related disabilities every year. An estimated 270,000 newborns die every year during the first 28 days of life from birth defects. Birth defects can result in long-term disability, which can have significant impact on individuals, families, and society.[1-3] There are many different causes of birth defects; those caused by exposures (such as infections) or inadequate intake of dietary factors (for instance, folic acid or iodine) can be prevented.[4] However, many other birth defects occur spontaneously and therefore are more challenging to detect.

Prenatal diagnosis strategies are devised to look for common birth defects. The prenatal identification of birth defects is becoming easier as more healthcare facilities worldwide have increasing access to technology such as ultrasound.[5,6]

## INTRODUCTION

Birth defects are important causes of childhood death, chronic illness, and disability in many countries. In 2010, the World Health Assembly adopted a resolution to promote primary prevention of birth defects and the health of children with congenital anomalies by four different actions: (1) developing and strengthening registration and surveillance systems; (2) developing expertise and building capacity; (3) strengthening research and studies on etiology, diagnosis, and prevention; and (4) promoting international cooperation. At the time of this assembly in 2010, 2.7 million neonatal deaths due to birth defects had occurred in 193 countries.[1]

## CAUSES AND RISK FACTORS

Approximately half of all congenital anomalies occur spontaneously and cannot be linked to a specific factor. Maternal age is related to chromosome abnormalities, as women who are over the age of 35 years have an increased chance for trisomies such as trisomy 13, 18, and 21. Women of this age also have an increased risk for miscarriage and stillbirth.[7] Consanguinity can increase the incidence of rare autosomal recessive birth defects.[8] Certain populations are genetic isolates with increased risk for certain birth defects, examples of which include Tay–Sachs disease in the Ashkenazi Jewish community, hemoglobinopathies in the Arab community, and congenital nephrosis in the Finnish community.[9] Another cause of birth defects is maternal exposure to environmental agents such as pesticides, medications, alcohol, tobacco, and other drugs.[10] Women with decreased dietary folate intake have an increased risk of neural tube defects such as spina bifida and anencephaly, as well as other birth defects.[11] Maternal infections such as syphilis and rubella can also cause birth defects and intellectual disability.[12] Lastly, socioeconomic factors can play a role in the appearance of birth defects as women of lower socioeconomic status are at increased risk for issues relating to nutrition and exposure.[13]

The most common birth defects are congenital heart defects, neural tube defects, and Down syndrome. Congenital heart defects are thought to be multifactorial conditions; they can be related to genetic syndromes and chromosome abnormalities, but in the majority of cases, they are isolated birth defects.[14] The congenital heart defect rate in the general population is close to 1%, and there is a wide degree of severity depending on the specific defect that is present.[15] Prenatal diagnosis of congenital heart defects is available by careful ultrasonography of the fetal heart, which is predominantly done in the second and third trimesters.[16] In most cases there is not a specific genetic factor identifiable. However, if a congenital heart defect is identified on ultrasound, the risk of a chromosome abnormality is approximately 20% as other defects cannot always be detected and it may represent the syndromic presentation.[17]

Neural tube defects are also multifactorial in nature. They are related to maternal folic acid metabolism.[18] Prenatal diagnosis by maternal serum alpha fetoprotein and prenatal ultrasound has increased detection of these anomalies. Neural tube defects can be related to genetic syndromes in some cases, such as chromosome abnormalities, but in these cases the neural tube defects are also associated with other abnormalities such as Meckel–Gruber syndrome, which is a triad of neural tube defects, renal anomalies, and polydactyly. This would be an example of a multisystem genetic syndrome presenting with a common birth defect.[19,20]

The third most common birth defect is that of Down syndrome, a chromosome abnormality that is related to trisomy 21. About 95% of individuals with Down syndrome have a straightforward trisomic karyotype. Approximately 3% have a familial translocation often involving chromosomes 21 and 14, but in these cases, the birth defect can involve chromosome 21 and other chromosomes. The remaining 2% are de novo translocations.[21] Individuals with Down syndrome have intellectual disabilities and are at high risk for congenital heart defects, which is seen in approximately 50% of individuals. Half of the congenital heart defects in individuals with trisomy 21 are endocardial cushion defects or atrioventricular canal defects. Individuals with Down syndrome can also have hypothyroidism, bowel obstruction, and significant hypotonia.[22]

As can be seen from a review of these common birth defects, typically any birth defects affect a number of body systems, and therefore, require complex medical care by different medical specialties. The cost and utilization of resources is great for these individuals.[23]

Birth defects can be divided by etiology. They can have single gene abnormalities that are autosomal recessive, autosomal dominant or X-linked etiologies. There also can be chromosomal disorders as well as multifactorial disorders.[24]

Many individuals who have birth defects also suffer from functional issues with intellectual disability and functional impairments such as inborn errors of metabolism or other medical concerns such as hematologic issues. Therefore, the identification and treatment of these conditions, in addition to maintenance of registries and support groups, are of worldwide interest.[25]

## EVALUATION OF A CHILD WITH BIRTH DEFECTS

In order to approach treatment of a child with birth defects,[26,27] healthcare providers should consider the following.

### Prenatal History

In order to understand the full history of a child with birth defects, healthcare providers should first interview the parents and review medical records to identify any issues found during the pregnancy, with attention to pregnancy testing, imaging and maternal health and exposure history. The prenatal history can alert the practitioner to growth issues, suspicion of anomalies during pregnancy, and test results that may rule in or rule out certain diagnoses.

### Family History

The family history is another important tool. Constructing a three-generation pedigree with special attention to infants born with birth defects, early deaths, or recurrent pregnancy losses is the standard practice. Reviewing the presence or absence of congenital anomalies and disabilities is also helpful. Healthcare practitioners should ask about consanguinity and degree of relationship between parents to identify if recessive disorders are likely. This information is often taken down by a genetic counselor, but can also be obtained by any medical personnel. The analysis of a three-generation family history with particular attention to neonatal issues can be quite illustrative in terms of narrowing a diagnostic opinion about an affected individual. Issues that providers need to note are family members with a similar presentation, other birth defects in the family, history of intellectual disability, and family history of consanguinity. These factors are typically recorded in a graphic form as a pedigree **(Fig. 1)** and are an important part of the overall evaluation.

### Review Medical Course

Review of the child's medical course with results of all imaging and testing to date is important to help in establishing the child's status and what is currently known.

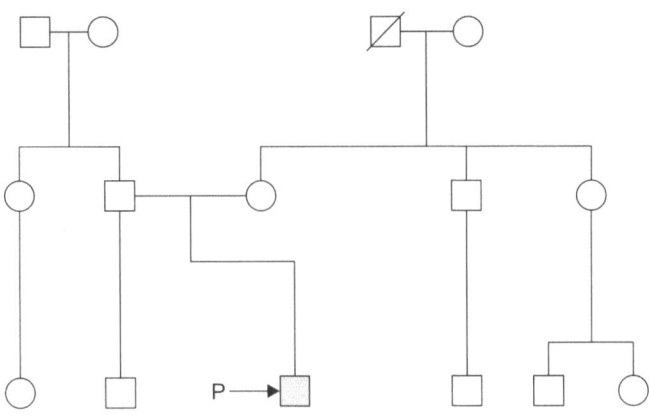

**Fig. 1:** Three-generation pedigree.

## Careful Physical Examination

The physical examination of the child with birth defects should include growth (head circumference, length, and weight) and anthropomorphic traits. A dysmorphology examination looks at the facial and physical features of a child and evaluates for differences beyond normal variation. These traits should be documented as findings for diagnostic evaluation.

## Formulation of Possible Diagnoses

When the preceding steps are completed, the information needs to be integrated to see if it suggests a known constellation of findings or syndrome. This can be done by literature review and also by looking at databases to search for the findings. The main database for such research is the Online Mendelian Inheritance in Man (OMIM) website (http://www.ncbi.nlm.nih.gov/omim) where various features in combination can be assessed for single gene disorders.[28]

## Consideration of Genetic Tests

Diagnoses can also be aided by laboratory studies. The classic way to identify a child with birth defects is through a chromosome study with a routine karyotype to rule out trisomies or other structural chromosome abnormalities. However, recent practice has yielded additional, more effective tests. For example, chromosome microarray, also referred to as comparative genomic hybridization, has shown significant utility for evaluating children with birth defects. Chromosome microarray can identify structural chromosome changes related to birth defects and developmental disabilities and is now often used as a first-line test. One of the differences between a routine karyotype chromosome study and a comparative genomic hybridization is that the comparative genomic hybridization cannot identify balanced rearrangements where there is no missing or extra material. The chromosome microarray, by comparison, is predominantly designed to identify missing or extra material. If comparative genomic hybridization is done alone; however, it can miss those balanced rearrangements. For example, the test could miss a balanced translocation, not revealing that the family has risk for other chromosomal disorders. The limitation of the routine karyotype is that extra or missing pieces of chromosomal material detected are shown with much lower resolution than the comparative genomic hybridization.[29-31]

In addition to the above-mentioned chromosome studies, there are multitudes of genetic tests looking at hundreds, if not thousands, of genetic disorders. These are targeted assays that can look at a specific gene to find point mutations or other rearrangements that would not be identified on a chromosome or comparative genomic hybridization analysis. Administering tests require skilled personnel to guide testing in an efficient and cost-effective manner.

A new technology that will get more and more use in the years ahead is that of whole exome screening (WES). This is a test in which all of the known genes are sequenced by massively parallel sequencing to look for occult genes. In recent years, this test has become more clinically available, but still is predominantly available only in specialized centers. Its limited availability is partly related to technology availability and partly related to cost. The benefits of this approach is that WES can find abnormalities in genes that are not specifically being requested and it can uncover occult genetic issues. Concerns about WES are that genes that may not be related to the current clinical indication are sequenced, identifying other factors that may cause additional concern and distress. For example, the test could reveal that a child who has birth defects also has a gene that is associated with an increased chance of breast cancer. This finding, while perhaps not having implications for the child until adulthood, may have immediate further implications for other family members. Regardless, the results would be reported to the family, possibly causing much concern unrelated to the original purpose for the genetic test. Many professional societies that regulate genetics are currently working on guidelines to help with reporting. Genetic counseling is important for families undergoing genetic testing, particularly this type of analysis, to help them understand the limitations, risks, and benefits of the information that will be gleaned from the results.[32]

## Planning for Medical Management

The need for a specific diagnosis is important for the prognosis of the patient, counseling for the family, and for ongoing medical management. If a chromosome abnormality is identified, specific data can be accessed about prognosis and plans made for surveillance. Plans for care can then be established that meet the specific needs of the individual to help maximize developmental and medical outcomes in the future. This has implications for healthcare resource allocation. The child with birth defects is typically a consumer of complex medical services that include genetics and genetic counseling, pediatrics, pediatric neurology, pediatric surgery, pediatric cardiology, pediatric gastroenterology, and pediatric endocrinology, among many others. Geneticists and genetic counselors are uniquely trained to help manage these individuals and can help prepare ongoing care plans. An issue that is becoming more prevalent, as medical technology improves, is that there is increased survival of individuals with birth defects, and so medical resource planning needs to take into consideration providing appropriate resources for these individuals as they enter adulthood in terms of resources and transitioning to adult services.[33-35]

## CASE STUDIES

The following vignettes illustrate the diverse nature of birth defects and their presentation.

### Case 1

Prenatal ultrasound in the third trimester showed limb length of the fetus to be less than the fifth percentile. The parents were in good health and of Central American ancestry. The father was 5 feet 4 inches (1.63 m) in height, and the mother was 4 feet 10 inches (1.47 m) in height. There was no family history of birth defects, intellectual disabilities, or infant deaths. The infant, born term, went to the regular nursery where an initial examination showed no dysmorphic features, but did show rhizomelic shortening of all four extremities. During the first day of life, the baby developed respiratory distress requiring positive pressure support. A skeletal survey was performed showing and suggesting a diagnosis of Jeune asphyxiating thoracic dystrophy. Genetic testing was performed and two mutations were identified in the *DYNC2H1* gene, which confirmed the clinical diagnosis. Jeune asphyxiating thoracic dystrophy is an autosomal recessive condition and as such confers 25% recurrence for future pregnancies. Because mutations were identified in this infant, prenatal diagnosis for future pregnancies would be available by either chorionic villus sampling at 10–14 weeks or amniocentesis at 16–20 weeks. The overall prognosis for this syndrome is poor; although there are long-term survivors and the course is variable.[36]

### Case 2

A routine prenatal ultrasound showed enlarged cerebral ventricles at 18 weeks gestation. Amniocentesis was elected. Chromosome studies showed that there was a deletion on chromosome 17. Parental studies were normal, indicating that this was a de novo chromosome deletion. The family elected to continue the pregnancy. Ventricles continued to enlarge. At 34 weeks gestation, the head circumference was 38 weeks size. The infant, delivered by cesarean section, had no respiratory distress and went to the regular nursery. Initially the head circumference decreased in size, but subsequently continued to enlarge, necessitating ventriculoperitoneal shunting. The family was advised about the high risk for developmental disabilities and the need for future close follow-up.

### Case 3

An infant delivered at 37 weeks gestation had a small mandible, a U-shaped cleft, and distinctive dysmorphic features. The baby went to the regular nursery and had a trial on room air but developed respiratory distress, requiring positive pressure support. Further examination showed small palpebral fissures, dysplastic ears, a small mandible, and a tongue that slid back occluding the airway. A clinical diagnosis of Pierre Robin was made. Chromosome studies showed duplication on chromosome 6. Craniofacial intervention was planned with mandibular distraction. The infant did well, with a more stable airway resulting. As a diagnosis of Pierre Robin carries a high risk for developmental disabilities, a protocolized schedule of regular and careful follow-up was established.[37]

## CONCLUSION

The field of genetics continues to grow and, as such, the knowledge and experience with individuals born with birth defects continues to expand as well to provide improved care and outcomes.

An important part of care for individuals with birth defects is that of genetic counseling. Genetic counseling is a process in which individuals are given information to help them adjust to their individual situations regarding a genetic issue or birth defect. Genetic counselors deal with medical information as well as emotional considerations in a context of cultural sensitivity to each family's needs. Genetic counseling is very important for these families because this process helps to deal with reproductive concerns and recurrence risks. Prenatal diagnosis is also addressed by genetic counseling to help families understand what the chances are of a specific birth defect recurring and their options for diagnosis in a future pregnancy. Multiple options are reviewed during genetic counseling to include prenatal diagnosis, contraception, pregnancy management, adoption, and medical management.[38]

Children with birth defects often require a multidisciplinary team for their diagnosis and management. This continues throughout the child's lifetime. Many organ systems can be affected and an approach caring for the child and family can be generated through coordination of care.[39-42]

## REFERENCES

1. World Health Organization. (2016). Birth Defects: Report by the Secretariat. [online] Available from http://apps.who.int/gb/ebwha/pdf_files/WHA63/A63_10-en.pdf [Last accessed September, 2019].
2. Castillo Taucher S. [Services for the care and prevention of birth defects. Reduced report of a World Health Organization and March of Dimes Foundation meeting]. Rev Med Chil. 2007;135(6):806-13.
3. Verma IC, Puri RD. Global burden of genetic disease and the role of genetic screening. Semin Fetal Neonatal Med. 2015;20(5):354-63.
4. Thong MK. Birth defects registries in the genomics era: challenges and opportunities for developing countries. Front Pediatr. 2014;2:60.
5. Marteau T. Towards informed decisions about prenatal testing: a review. Prenat Diagn. 1995;15(13):1215-26.
6. Leung KY, Poon CF, Teotico AR, et al. Recommendations on routine mid-trimester anomaly scan. J Obstet Gynaecol Res. 2015;41(5):653-61.
7. Gill SK, Broussard C, Devine O, et al. Association between maternal age and birth defects of unknown etiology: United States, 1997-2007. Birth Defects Res A Clin Mol Teratol. 2012;94(12):1010-8.
8. Majeed-Saidan MA, Ammari AN, AlHashem AM, et al. Effect of consanguinity on birth defects in Saudi women: results from a nested case-control study. Birth Defects Res A Clin Mol Teratol. 2015;103(2):100-4.
9. Khlat M, Khoury M. Inbreeding and diseases: demographic, genetic, and epidemiologic perspectives. Epidemiol Rev. 1991;13:28-41.
10. Al-Hadithi TS, Al-Diwan JK, Saleh AM, et al. Birth defects in Iraq and the plausibility of environmental exposure: A review. Confl Health. 2012;6(1):3.
11. Czeizel AE, Vereczkey A, Szabó I. Folic acid in pregnant women associated with reduced prevalence of severe congenital heart defects in their children: a national population-based case-control study. Eur J Obstet Gynecol Reprod Biol. 2015;193:34-9.
12. Toda K, Reef S, Tsuruoka M, et al. Vaccine. Congenital rubella syndrome (CRS) in Vietnam 2011-2012-CRS epidemic after rubella epidemic in 2010-2011. Vaccine. 2015;33(31):3673-7.
13. Wham CA, Teh R, Moyes S, et al. Health and Social Factors Associated with Nutrition Risk: Results from Life and Living in Advanced Age: A Cohort Study in New Zealand (LiLACS NZ). J Nutr Health Aging. 2015;19(6):637-45.
14. Cowan JR, Ware SM. Genetics and genetic testing in congenital heart disease. Clin Perinatol. 2015;42(2):373-93.
15. Hoffman J, Kaplan S. The incidence of congenital heart disease. J Am Coll Cardiol. 2002;39(12):1890-900.
16. Holland BJ, Myers JA, Woods CR Jr. Prenatal diagnosis of critical congenital heart disease reduces risk of death from cardiovascular compromise prior to planned neonatal cardiac surgery: a meta-analysis. Ultrasound Obstet Gynecol. 2015;45(6):631-8.
17. Tang S, Lv J, Chen X, et al. Prenatal Diagnosis of DNA Copy Number Variations by Genomic Single-Nucleotide Polymorphism Array in Fetuses with Congenital Heart Defects. Fetal Diagn Ther. 2016;39(1):64-73.
18. Salih MA, Murshid WR, Seidahmed MZ. Classification, clinical features, and genetics of neural tube defects. Saudi Med J. 2014;35 (Suppl 1):S5-S14.
19. Wilson RD; SOGC Genetics Committee; Special Contributor. Prenatal screening, diagnosis, and pregnancy management of fetal neural tube defects. J Obstet Gynaecol Can. 2014;36(10):927-39.
20. Barisic I, Boban L, Loane M, et al. Meckel-Gruber Syndrome: a population-based study on prevalence, prenatal diagnosis, clinical features, and survival in Europe. J Hum Genet. 2015;23(6):746-52.
21. Skotko BG, Capone GT, Kishnani PS. Postnatal diagnosis of Down syndrome: synthesis of the evidence on how best to deliver the news. Pediatrics. 2009;124(4):e751-8.
22. Weijerman ME, van Furth AM, Vonk Noordegraaf A, et al. Prevalence, neonatal characteristics, and first-year mortality of Down syndrome: a national study. J Pediatr. 2008;152(1):15-9.
23. Tilford JM, Robbins JM, Hobbs CA. Improving estimates of caregiver time cost and family impact associated with birth defects. 2001;64(Suppl 1):S37-41.
24. Hobbs CA, Chowdhury S, Cleves MA, et al. Genetic epidemiology and nonsyndromic structural birth defects: from candidate genes to epigenetics. JAMA Pediatr. 2014;168(4):371-7.
25. Petterson B, Bourke J, Leonard H, et al. Co-occurrence of birth defects and intellectual disability. Paediatr Perinat Epidemiol. 2007;21(1):65-75.
26. Jones KL, Adam MP. Evaluation and diagnosis of the dysmorphic infant. Clin Perinatol. 2015;42(2):243-61.
27. Lidral AC, Murray JC. Genetic approaches to identify disease genes for birth defects with cleft lip/palate as a model. Birth Defects Res A Clin Mol Teratol. 2004;70(12):893-901.
28. Hamosh A, Scott AF, Amberger J, et al. Online Mendelian Inheritance in Man (OMIM), a knowledgebase of human genes and genetic disorders. Nucleic Acids Res. 2002;30(1):52-5.
29. Sullivan PK, Tattini CD. Early evaluation and management of craniofacial dysmorphology. Med Health R I. 2001;84(12):392-4.
30. Godfrey E, Clark P. Developing standards for chromosomal microarray testing counselling in paediatrics. Acta Paediatr. 2014;103(6):574-7.
31. Faucett WA, Savage M. Chromosomal microarray testing. JAAPA. 2012;25(1):65-6.
32. Resta N, Memo L. Chromosomal microarray (CMA) analysis in infants with congenital anomalies: when is it really helpful? J Matern Fetal Neonatal Med. 2012;25(Suppl 4):124-6.
33. Nagy PL, Mansukhani M. The role of clinical genomic testing in diagnosis and discovery of pathogenic mutations. Expert Rev Mol Diagn. 2015;15(9):1101-5.

34. Iglesias A, Anyane-Yeboa K, Wynn J, et al. The usefulness of whole-exome sequencing in routine clinical practice. Genet Med. 2014;16(12):922-31.
35. Sharma R. Birth defects in India: Hidden truth, need for urgent attention. Indian J Hum Genet. 2013;19(2):125-9.
36. Keppler-Noreuil KM, Adam MP, Welch J, et al. Clinical insights gained from eight new cases and review of reported cases with Jeune syndrome (asphyxiating thoracic dystrophy). Am J Med Genet A. 2011;155A(5):1021-32.
37. Monlleó IL, Barros AG, Fontes MI, et al. Diagnostic implications of associated defects in patients with typical orofacial clefts. J Pediatr (Rio J). 2015;91(5):485-92.
38. Hodgson JM, Metcalfe SA, Aitken M, et al. Improving family communication after a new genetic diagnosis: a randomised controlled trial of a genetic counselling intervention. BMC Med Genet. 2014;15:33.
39. Ling EW, Sosuan LC, Hall JC. Congenital anomalies: an increasingly important cause of mortality and workload in a neonatal intensive care unit. Am J Perinatol. 1991;8(3):164-9.
40. Smith AJ, Oswald D, Bodurtha J. Trends in Unmet Need for Genetic Counseling Among Children With Special Health Care Needs, 2001-2010. Acad Pediatr. 2015;15(5):544-50.
41. Adams-Chapman I, Hansen NI, Shankaran S, et al. Ten-year review of major birth defects in VLBW infants. Pediatrics. 2013;132(1):49-61.
42. Calzolari E, Barisic I, Loane M, et al. Epidemiology of multiple congenital anomalies in Europe: a EUROCAT population-based registry study. Birth Defects Res A Clin Mol Teratol. 2014;100(4):270-6.

CHAPTER

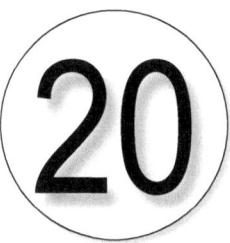

# Inborn Errors of Metabolism and Newborn Screening

*Gregory M Enns*

## ABSTRACT

The clinician must have a high index of suspicion and consider inborn errors of metabolism (IEMs) in all neonates with nonspecific features of distress *upon initial presentation*. Rapid diagnosis and treatment can prevent death or significant morbidity in many instances. Common neonatal findings in children with IEMs include irritability, poor feeding, hypotonia, apnea, and seizures. Other nonspecific clinical features include hypothermia, tachypnea, and lethargy. In more severely affected neonates, there may be an inexorable progression from lethargy to coma and death. Standard laboratory tests often provide the first clues to the possibility of an underlying metabolic disease in a symptomatic neonate. Neonates presenting in a metabolic crisis secondary to an underlying IEM require management in an intensive care setting. Although tandem mass spectrometry (MS/MS) newborn screening has the potential to provide physicians caring for acutely ill infants with critical diagnostic information, neonates may present with clinical symptoms before results of the screen are reported.

## INTRODUCTION

Inborn errors of metabolism, although rare individually, have an aggregate incidence of approximately 1 in 1,000.[1,2] Nevertheless, these conditions tend to be considered only after more common causes of neonatal distress have been excluded. Because affected neonates are at high risk of morbidity or mortality, appropriate treatment should be started as soon as possible.[3-6] Although newborn screening by MS/MS is becoming the international standard, such testing takes time and, furthermore, only screens for a limited number of disorders.[7,8] Therefore, the clinician must have a high index of suspicion and consider IEMs in all neonates with nonspecific features of distress *upon initial presentation*. Rapid diagnosis and treatment can prevent death or significant morbidity in many instances.

Neonates exhibit signs and symptoms of distress in a nonspecific manner without regard to the origin of illness. Clinical features of neonatal distress such as apnea or tachypnea, feeding difficulties, vomiting, jaundice, failure to thrive, seizures, hypotonia or hypertonia, lethargy, or coma represent responses to diseases in one of two broad categories—(1) disorders resulting from causes such as sepsis, hypoxemia, toxins, trauma, or congenital structural brain abnormalities; or (2) disorders caused by an IEM. In practice, neonates who have an underlying IEM may be initially misdiagnosed as having sepsis. However, by obtaining appropriate simple laboratory investigations immediately, such as blood gases, glucose, electrolytes, lactate, and ammonia, and urinalysis for ketones and glucose, the astute clinician may not only determine the likelihood of a metabolic disorder being present, but also narrow the differential diagnosis with respect to the type of IEM.[3,9]

## INHERITANCE

The family history is an important part of the assessment of any neonate suspected of having an IEM. Autosomal recessive inheritance is most commonly encountered in these conditions, although X-linked (e.g. ornithine transcarbamylase deficiency) or maternal (mitochondrial) inheritance may also occur. An affected relative with a similar presentation may provide a significant diagnostic clue. Special attention should be given to stillbirths, unexplained deaths, and neurologic diseases or delayed development of any degree or severity. Consanguinity increases the likelihood of an autosomal recessive condition. Mitochondrial inheritance is suggested by affected females transmitting the disease to all children, while no transmission occurs from affected males. Additionally, in suspected mitochondrial disease with maternal inheritance, a matrilineal history of diabetes or hearing loss may be present in oligosymptomatic individuals. It should be noted, however, that the majority of mitochondrial disorders in children demonstrate autosomal recessive inheritance.[10] Maternal illness in pregnancy has also been associated with specific metabolic disorders and may yield a clue to the presence of an inborn error of metabolism in a neonate. For example, acute fatty liver of pregnancy and hemolysis, elevated liver enzymes, and low platelets (HELLP) syndrome may occur in a heterozygous mother carrying a fetus with a fatty acid oxidation defect.[11]

## SIGNS AND SYMPTOMS

The onset of symptoms of biochemical genetic disorders may be prenatal, perinatal, or postnatal, appearing after an interval period of apparent good health.[3,4] In most cases, pregnancy is unremarkable, although maternal liver disease may be seen in some cases in which the fetus is affected by a fatty acid oxidation disorder (FAOD), and complications such as fetal ascites or nonimmune hydrops may occur in other IEMs.[3,11] The neonate may appear well until subjected to a catabolic insult, such as infection or fasting, or an excessive protein or carbohydrate load. Following exposure to a stressor, the child may become strikingly ill suddenly, and can present with sudden infant death of unexplained etiology. The absence of a normal period, however, does not exclude an IEM or other genetic disorder, such as a congenital myopathy, from diagnostic consideration. Neonatal distress from asphyxia or complications of prematurity may constitute environmental stress that unmasks an underlying metabolic disease. On the other hand, various IEMs may mimic hypoxic-ischemic encephalopathy even in the absence of exogenous stress.[12,13] Presentations of selected IEMs presenting in the perinatal or neonatal period are summarized in **Box 1**.

Common neonatal findings in children with IEMs include irritability, poor feeding, hypotonia, apnea, and seizures. Other nonspecific clinical features include hypothermia, tachypnea, and lethargy. In more severely affected neonates, there may be an inexorable progression from lethargy to coma and death. In some cases, dysmorphic

> **BOX 1:** Inborn errors of metabolism with presentation in the perinatal or neonatal period.
>
> *Encephalopathy without metabolic acidosis:*
> - Urea cycle disorders*
> - Maple syrup urine disease
> - Mevalonic acidemia
>
> *Seizures:*
> - Glycine encephalopathy
> - Molybdenum cofactor/sulfite oxidase deficiency
> - Pyridoxine-dependent seizures (*ALDH7A1* deficiency)
> - Pyridoxamine 5'-phosphate oxidase deficiency (*PNPO* deficiency)
> - Glucose transporter (GLUT-1) deficiency
> - Guanidinoacetate methyltransferase (GAMT) deficiency
> - Cathepsin D deficiency (congenital neuronal ceroid lipofuscinosis)
> - Early infantile epileptic encephalopathies (EIEE)**
> - 3-Phosphoglycerate dehydrogenase deficiency
> - 4-Aminobutyrate aminotransferase (GABA transaminase) deficiency
> - Mitochondrial glutamate transporter deficiency (*SLC25A22* deficiency)
> - Biotinidase deficiency
>
> *Encephalopathy with metabolic acidosis:*
> - Organic acidemias†
> - Fatty acid oxidation disorders‡
> - Congenital lactic acidoses§
>
> *Hypotonia:*
> - Congenital disorders of glycosylation
> - Congenital lactic acidoses§
> - Congenital muscular dystrophies
> - Glycine encephalopathy
> - Organic acidemias†
> - Peroxisomal disorders
> - Sulfite oxidase/molybdenum cofactor deficiency
> - Urea cycle disorders.*
>
> *Cardiomyopathy:*
> - Fatty acid oxidation disorders‡
> - Mitochondrial disorders
> - Pompe disease
> - I-cell disease
>
> *Liver disease:*
> - α-1-antitrypsin deficiency
> - Bile acid synthesis defects
> - Fatty acid oxidation disorders‡
> - Galactosemia
> - Glycogen storage disease type IV
> - Mitochondrial disorders
> - Neonatal hemochromatosis
> - Niemann-Pick disease type C
> - Tyrosinemia
>
> *Dysmorphic features:*
> - Congenital disorders of glycosylation
> - Cholesterol biosynthetic defects§§
> - Congenital lactic acidoses§
> - Congenital muscular dystrophies
> - Lysosomal storage disorders
> - Multiple acyl-CoA dehydrogenase deficiency
> - Peroxisomal disorders
>
> *Contd...*

*Contd...*

*Hypoglycemia:*
- Congenital disorders of glycosylation
- Congenital lactic acidosis§
- Fatty acid oxidation disorders‡
- Glycogen storage disease
- Gluconeogenesis disorders#
- Hyperinsulinism
- Organic acidemias.†

*Notes:*
*Argininosuccinic acid lyase deficiency, carbamoyl phosphate synthetase deficiency, citrullinemia, and ornithine transcarbamylase deficiency.
**Defects in a number of genes have been associated with an EIEE, or Ohtahara syndrome, phenotype, including *ARX*, *CDKL5*, *KCNQ2*, *MAGI2*, *PLCβ1*, *PNPO*, *SLC25A22*, *SCNA1*, *SPTAN1*, and *STXBP1*.
†Methylmalonic acidemia, propionic acidemia, isovaleric acidemia, and holocarboxylase synthetase deficiency.
‡Carnitine translocase deficiency, carnitine-acylcarnitine translocase deficiency, carnitine palmitoyltransferase deficiency, long-chain 3-hydroxy-acyl-CoA dehydrogenase deficiency, trifunctional protein deficiency, and very long-chain acyl-CoA dehydrogenase deficiency.
§Mitochondrial disorders, pyruvate dehydrogenase deficiency, and pyruvate carboxylase deficiency.
§§Conradi-Hunermann syndrome, desmosterolosis, mevalonic acidemia, and Smith-Lemli-Opitz syndrome.
#Fructose 1,6- bisphosphatase deficiency and phosphoenolpyruvate carboxykinase deficiency.

features may be present, but in most IEMs specific physical abnormalities are not apparent. More limited symptoms, often in the form of generalized or partial seizures, may also occur. These can include staring spells, unusual eye movements, tremulousness, or myoclonus, and various combinations of tone abnormalities, lethargy, and a weak cry. Electroencephalography may show a nonspecific diffuse encephalopathy or a variety of other findings, such as a burst-suppression pattern or hypsarrhythmia.[14] Unless an IEM is suspected, the neonate may be initially misdiagnosed as having perinatal asphyxia.

A concomitant acquired disorder may confound the diagnosis of an inherited metabolic disease. For example, neutropenia or pancytopenia secondary to bone marrow suppression is a relatively common feature of organic acidemias, and this can lead to an increased susceptibility to infection. *Escherichia coli* sepsis is frequent in infants with galactosemia, and the inanition and jaundice of that disorder when untreated might wrongly be ascribed solely to sepsis.[15] Other examples of acquired conditions that may complicate the presentation of a metabolic disorder include pulmonary hemorrhage or primary respiratory alkalosis in urea cycle defects, or intracranial hemorrhage in congenital disorders of glycosylation.[16,17]

## PHYSICAL FINDINGS

Although some IEMs have associated dysmorphic features, a lack of abnormal physical findings is generally encountered in neonates who have an underlying IEM. Nevertheless, certain clinical features may yield important clues to support a diagnosis of an inherited biochemical disorder. Nonimmune hydrops or ascites may be seen in erythrocyte enzymopathies that cause hemolysis, some lysosomal storage disorders, congenital disorders of glycosylation, glycogen storage disorder type IV, and mitochondrial disorders.[3] Abnormal, brittle hair may occur in some urea cycle defects (argininosuccinic aciduria and citrullinemia), holocarboxylase synthetase deficiency, and Menkes syndrome. An ocular examination may reveal neonatal cataracts (galactosemia, glucose-6-phosphate dehydrogenase deficiency, and some mitochondrial or peroxisomal disorders), lens dislocation (sulfite oxidase or molybdenum cofactor deficiency), optic atrophy (mitochondrial disease), or retinitis pigmentosa (peroxisomal or mitochondrial disorders, and congenital disorders of glycosylation). Hepatomegaly may be present in hepatorenal tyrosinemia, carbohydrate disorders [galactosemia and glycogen storage disease (GSD)], peroxisomal disorders, some lysosomal storage disorders, inborn errors of bile acid metabolism, neonatal hemochromatosis, or mitochondrial disease. A distinctive odor has been associated with several organic acidemias, including branched-chain α-ketoacid dehydrogenase deficiency (maple syrup), and isovaleric acidemia or multiple acyl-CoA dehydrogenase deficiency (sweaty).

## CLINICAL PRESENTATIONS

Although a paucity of physical findings is generally encountered in neonates who have an underlying IEM, certain clinical presentations deserve specific mention, including—(1) encephalopathy without metabolic acidosis; (2) encephalopathy with metabolic acidosis; (3) cardiomyopathy; (4) hepatic disease; (5) dysmorphic features; and (6) hypoglycemia.

## ENCEPHALOPATHY WITHOUT METABOLIC ACIDOSIS

Neurological deterioration is a relatively common presentation of IEMs with a neonatal onset. Because the clinical presentation is nonspecific, the neonate may be misdiagnosed initially as having sepsis.[18] Therefore, for any neonate suspected of having sepsis, simple laboratory studies as listed in **Box 2** are recommended. Maple syrup urine disease (MSUD) typically presents in the first few days to weeks of life with nonspecific clinical features, such as poor feeding, emesis, lethargy, hypotonia, and opisthotonus. Bicycling movements or seizures may supervene as the disease course progresses. Although ketosis occurs, significant metabolic acidosis is typically absent at the time of presentation. The early clinical course of patients with urea cycle disorders is similar to that in MSUD, although respiratory alkalosis and significant hyperammonemia are hallmarks of this category of disease and are absent in MSUD. Transient hyperammonemia of the newborn (THAN) may also cause neonatal hyperammonemia. THAN tends to occur in the first day of life, while urea cycle disorders typically present after day of life one.

A growing number of IEMs are characterized by neurological deterioration and seizures, in the absence of abnormal findings upon routine biochemical analysis of blood and urine (**Table 1**).[3,4,12,19] The nonspecific clinical features of these conditions may resemble those encountered in perinatal asphyxia. However, unlike acute asphyxia, there is often absent or limited history of birth trauma and patients appear normal for at least a short time. If the degree of neonatal encephalopathy appears to be greater than expected from careful review of the perinatal history, an inborn error or other genetic condition, such as a congenital myopathy or an early infantile epileptic encephalopathy (EIEE), should be a strong consideration.[12] Because these conditions require specialized testing, often in cerebrospinal fluid (CSF), it is important to save a sample if a more common cause for neonatal seizures is not identified. Because many of these conditions are treatable, at least to some extent, establishing a diagnosis is clearly important.

Peroxisomal disorders, such as Zellweger syndrome or neonatal adrenoleukodystrophy, may be associated with profound hypotonia and seizures, in the absence of significant routine laboratory findings. Other clinical features include neuronal migration defects, craniofacial

**BOX 2:** Initial clinical laboratory studies.

- Blood gas
- Ammonia
- Lactate
- Electrolytes (anion gap)
- Glucose
- Blood urea nitrogen
- Liver function tests
- Urinalysis (ketones, reducing substances)

**TABLE 1:** Evaluation and treatment of select disorders associated with seizures.

| Disorder | Diagnosis* | Therapy |
| --- | --- | --- |
| Aromatic amino acid decarboxylase deficiency | CSF neurotransmitters | Dopaminergic agonists<br>Monoamine oxidase inhibitors<br>Vitamin $B_6$ |
| Glycine encephalopathy† | ↑ CSF to plasma glycine ratio<br>*GLDC*, *AMT*, and *GCSH* sequencing | Sodium benzoate<br>Dextromethorphan |
| Pyridoxine-dependent seizures | *ALDH7A1* sequencing<br>↑ pipecolic acid, α-aminoadipic semialdehyde, piperideine-6-carboxylate in urine, plasma, and CSF | Vitamin $B_6$ |
| Pyridoxamine 5'-phosphate oxidase | *PNPO* sequencing | Pyridoxal-5'-phosphate |
| Glucose transporter deficiency | ↓ CSF glucose, *SLC2A1* sequencing | Ketogenic diet |
| Guanidinoacetate methyltransferase deficiency | ↓ brain creatine on MRS<br>↑ plasma and urine Guanidinoacetate | Creatine<br>Ornithine<br>Low arginine diet |
| 3-Phosphoglycerate dehydrogenase deficiency | ↓ CSF serine | Serine + glycine |
| Mitochondrial glutamate transporter deficiency | ↓ CSF and serum glutamine<br>*SLC25A22* sequencing | Anticonvulsants |
| Biotinidase deficiency | Serum enzyme testing<br>*BTD* sequencing | Biotin |
| Early infantile epileptic encephalopathies (EIEE)‡ | Gene sequencing | Vigabatrin (*STXBP1*)<br>Phenobarbital (*KCNQ2*, *KCNQ3*) |

(CSF: cerebrospinal fluid; MRS: magnetic resonance spectroscopy; IEM: inborn errors of metabolism).
Notes:
*Diagnosis of these conditions requires specialized biochemical or genetic testing. Routine biochemical analysis of plasma or urine is often normal.
†Although benzoate and dextromethorphan may have some positive effects on seizure control, the prognosis for glycine encephalopathy is poor with affected children typically not walking or talking.
‡EIEEs are caused by defects in genes coding for proteins with diverse neurological roles, such as cell signaling or ion channel function. Although the great majority of these conditions are not strictly classified as IEMs, they are included because they may have a similar presentation to IEMs that are associated with seizures as a prominent clinical feature. Treatment is mostly supportive, although specific anticonvulsants have been found to be effective in some of these conditions.

dysmorphism, pigmentary retinopathy, hepatomegaly, jaundice, and renal cysts. Care is supportive.

## ENCEPHALOPATHY WITH METABOLIC ACIDOSIS

A significant metabolic acidosis is a prominent feature of organic acidemias, and may be seen in fatty acid oxidation defects and primary lactic acidemias, such as pyruvate dehydrogenase deficiency or mitochondrial disorders. Organic acidemias with a neonatal presentation characterized by neurological deterioration and significant metabolic acidosis are virtually indistinguishable from each other on clinical grounds. Blood ammonia levels may reach or surpass those encountered in urea cycle disorders. Neutropenia, thrombocytopenia, or pancytopenia is common, and, consequently, sepsis or a bleeding diathesis may supervene. The nonspecific sweet smell of ketone bodies may be detected, although some organic acidemias have more distinctive odors.

Approximately 5% of unexplained sudden deaths in the first year of life may be attributed to FAODs.[20] Although encephalopathy may dominate the clinical picture, multi-organ system involvement is common, with infants showing various degrees of cardiac, skeletal muscle, and hepatic involvement. Hyperammonemia and lactic acidosis may occur, and are often associated with significant hypoglycemia. Whereas ketosis is relatively common in organic acidemias, FAODs are characterized by hypo- or nonketotic hypoglycemia. Cardiomyopathy, arrhythmias, or both are particularly common in long-chain defects such as carnitine-acylcarnitine translocase deficiency, very-long-chain acyl-CoA dehydrogenase deficiency or long-chain 3-hydroxyacyl-CoA dehydrogenase deficiency. Hepatomegaly and hepatocellular dysfunction are often encountered in FAODs with neonatal presentation.

Neonatal lactic acidosis is commonly encountered in disorders of pyruvate metabolism and mitochondrial disorders, and also may be seen in some FAODs, organic acidemias, glycogen storage disorders, and disorders of gluconeogenesis. Severe hypotonia, seizures, and brain abnormalities, including cerebral and cerebellar atrophy, agenesis of the corpus callosum, or Leigh syndrome may occur in pyruvate dehydrogenase complex deficiency.[21] Virtually any organ system may be affected, either in isolation or in any combination, in neonates with mitochondrial disease. However, involvement of the neuromuscular system, including basal ganglia involvement, hypotonia, and seizures, is especially common. Mitochondrial disease is also characterized by relatively frequent occurrence of prematurity, intrauterine growth retardation, polyhydramnios or oligohydramnios, hypotonia requiring ventilatory support, poor feeding, and emesis.[18,22,23]

## CARDIOMYOPATHY

Long-chain fatty acid oxidation defects and mitochondrial disorders are significant causes of neonatal cardiomyopathy and arrhythmias.[24] Cardiomyopathy may also be seen in congenital disorders of glycosylation, although pericardial effusion appears to be more common.[25] The infantile form of Pompe disease typically presents after 1 month of age with muscle weakness and a rapidly progressive cardiomyopathy, but may occasionally present in the neonatal period.[26] Electrocardiography may show large QRS complexes and a short PR interval, secondary to the electrical conductive properties of glycogen. Several other lysosomal storage disorders may lead to cardiomyopathy, but thickened cardiac valves secondary to accumulation of complex macromolecules are more common and tend to develop in later childhood.[27]

## LIVER DISEASE

Parenchymal liver disease and associated liver dysfunction may be a prominent feature of a variety of IEMs. Clinical findings will include various degrees of hepatomegaly, jaundice, and coagulopathy.[28] Neonatal hemochromatosis and mitochondrial disorders, including a number of conditions that cause mitochondrial DNA depletion syndrome, can present with significant hepatocellular disease in the first week of life, although mitochondrial disorders can have an initial presentation at any age. Neonates with classic galactosemia often have a history of persistent hyperbilirubinemia, hepatomegaly, hepatocellular dysfunction, and renal disease. Neonates with α-1-antitrypsin deficiency may also have persistent jaundice that may progress to cirrhosis over a period of months. Cholestasis, with a presentation after week 3 of life, may be the presenting feature of α-1-antitrypsin deficiency, disorders of bile acid synthesis, and Niemann-Pick disease type C.[3] Cholestatic jaundice and multiple organ system involvement, including pericardial effusion, cardiomyopathy, protein-losing enteropathy, and abnormal fat distribution are characteristics of congenital disorder of glycosylation type I.

Severe hepatocellular dysfunction is characteristic of hereditary tyrosinemia type I, and may be seen in fatty acid oxidation defects during metabolic decompensation triggered by catabolic illness, such as a viral infection.[24] Hereditary fructose intolerance presents in the newborn period with acute liver dysfunction only if an affected infant is exposed to fructose. Hepatomegaly associated with hypoglycemia and lactic acidemia is seen of some disorders of gluconeogenesis.[28]

## DYSMORPHIC FEATURES

Infants with peroxisomal biogenesis disorders may have facial dysmorphism, including large anterior fontanelle, broad nasal bridge, flattened facies, epicanthic folds and flattened facial profile, and other findings, such as hypotonia, seizures, and liver dysfunction, at birth. Short limbs, joint contractures, and epiphyseal stippling are characteristics of rhizomelic chondrodysplasia punctata.[29] Pyruvate dehydrogenase deficiency, cholesterol biosynthetic disorders (mevalonic aciduria, Smith-Lemli-Opitz syndrome), 3-hydroxyisobutyric aciduria, multiple acyl-CoA dehydrogenase deficiency (glutaric aciduria type II), D-2-hydroxyglutaric aciduria, and mitochondrial disorders may also be associated with dysmorphic features.[29,30] Children with some forms of congenital disorders of glycosylation have strabismus, inverted nipples, and unusual subcutaneous fat pads, often with supra-iliac fat pads and buttock lipodystrophy.[31] The coarse features typical of lysosomal storage disorders evolve in infancy and early childhood, but some these conditions may present in the neonatal period with nonimmune hydrops.[32] Nonimmune hydrops may be encountered in a number of other conditions, including a variety of IEMs (**Box 3**).[33]

## HYPOGLYCEMIA

Neonatal hypoglycemia may be caused by a variety of endocrine and biochemical disorders and may be life-threatening.[34] Prominent hepatomegaly suggests a GSD. The liver is typically normal in size in glycogen synthase deficiency, which is sometimes referred to as GSD type 0. Multiorgan failure and hypo- or nonketotic hypoglycemia are seen in FAODs. Disorders of ketone body synthesis are also associated with hypo- or nonketotic hypoglycemia. Increased lactate, in addition to hypoglycemia, is present in GSDs, disorders of gluconeogenesis, such as fructose 1,6-bisphosphatase deficiency, some FAODs or organic acidemias, and mitochondrial disorders. Hyperinsulinism has been found in congenital disorders of glycosylation, as well as in the hyperinsulinism-hyperammonemia syndrome (HIHA). HIHA is an autosomal dominant condition caused by glutamate dehydrogenase hyperactivity. Congenital hyperinsulinism is etiologically heterogeneous and may be found, e.g. in cases of inappropriate insulin secretion by the Langerhans islet β cells or dysfunction of the pancreatic ATP-sensitive potassium channel.[34] Hypoglycemia in association with cholestasis may be seen in FAODs or adrenal or pituitary insufficiency.[3]

## BASIC LABORATORY INVESTIGATIONS

Standard laboratory tests, including blood gases, electrolytes, glucose, lactate, ammonia levels, and urinalysis, often provide the first clues to the possibility of an underlying metabolic disease in a symptomatic neonate. Although the presence of a specific inborn error of metabolism cannot be confirmed until specialized biochemical genetic laboratory results are available, a diagnosis may at least be suspected, and an inborn error disease category reasonably hypothesized, on the basis of simple studies and the clinical presentation. Because the physician must initiate appropriate therapy without delay, and without an established final diagnosis, obtaining appropriate laboratory tests is a critical part of the evaluation of a neonate suspected of having an IEM (*see* **Box 2**).

Evaluating blood electrolytes allows for the calculation of the anion gap. The term "anion gap" is a misnomer because of the implication that there is a disequilibrium between cation and anion concentrations. However, the body is in electrochemical neutrality. In other words, if the concentrations of all the serum cations are added together, the sum would equal the concentration of total serum anions.[35] The anion gap is most often estimated according to the formula $[Na^+] - ([Cl^-] + [HCO_3^{2-}])$. A normal anion gap is approximately 8–16 mEq/L. However, the *actual* concentration of unmeasured anions (UA), including proteins, lactate, ketone bodies, inorganic phosphate and sulfate, and organic acids, and excluding chloride and bicarbonate, is about 23 mEq/L.[35] Because the body is in electroneutrality, the total cation concentration ($[Na^+]$ + the

---

**BOX 3:** Conditions associated with nonimmune hydrops.

- Lysosomal storage disorders*
- Cholesterol biosynthesis defects†
- Congenital disorders of glycosylation
- Fatty acid oxidation disorders‡
- Glycogen storage disease type IV
- Mitochondrial disorders§
- Neonatal hemochromatosis
- Peroxisomal disorders
- RBC enzyme defects#
- Transaldolase deficiency

Notes:
*Farber disease, galactosialidosis, Gaucher disease type 2, $G_{M1}$-gangliosidosis, I-cell disease, infantile sialic acid storage disease, sialidosis, mucopolysaccharidosis types IVa and VII, multiple sulfatase deficiency, Niemann-Pick disease types A and C, and Wolman disease.
†Conradi-Hunermann syndrome, Greenberg syndrome, and Smith-Lemli-Opitz syndrome.
‡Carnitine translocase deficiency, long-chain-3-hydroxy-acylCoA dehydrogenase deficiency.
§Various respiratory chain subunit deficiencies, Pearson marrow-pancreas syndrome.
#Glucose-6-phosphate dehydrogenase deficiency, glucose-6-phosphate isomerase deficiency, and pyruvate kinase deficiency.

concentration of unmeasured cations [UC]) and the total anion concentration ([Cl$^-$] + [HCO$_3^{2-}$] + the concentration of UA) must equal one another. This produces the following equation: [Na$^+$] + [UC] = [Cl$^-$] + [HCO$_3^{2-}$] + [UA]. Further rearrangement yields the following: [Na$^+$] − ([Cl$^-$] + [HCO$_3^{2-}$]) = [UA] − [UC]. In summary, the clinically used "anion gap" actually represents the difference in concentration between UA and UC.[35]

It follows that an increased anion gap is caused by either an increase in the concentration of UA, or a decrease in the concentration of UC. An increased anion gap is typical of an underlying metabolic acidosis caused by IEMs. Organic acids that titrate bicarbonate, such as ketone bodies (acetoacetate and β-hydroxybutyrate), lactate, and acids produced secondary to specific inherited enzymopathies, e.g. derivatives of methylmalonic, and propionic or isovaleric acid, are the usual cause of such an increase in anion gap.

On the other hand, the anion gap is normal when metabolic acidosis occurs as a result of bicarbonate loss. This is because of a concomitant increase in plasma chloride concentration. Such a hyperchloremic metabolic acidosis may be caused by kidney disease that leads to renal tubular acidosis or diarrhea leading to increased intestinal bicarbonate loss. A decreased anion gap is relatively rarely seen in clinical practice, but may be caused by hypoalbuminemia.[35]

A neonatal metabolic acidosis with increased anion gap may be caused by an abnormal accumulation of lactic acid. Any condition that causes tissue hypoxia or ischemia, including sepsis, decreased cardiac output, pulmonary hypertension, or severe anemia may cause lactic acidemia. In such instances, the lactic acidemia tends to resolve relatively quickly once the etiology of the disturbance is treated. More persistent neonatal lactic acidemia may be encountered in mitochondrial disorders, some organic acidemias, and disorders of pyruvate metabolism, fatty acid oxidation, or gluconeogenesis.

Regardless of the underlying cause of illness, hypoglycemia is common in the sick neonate. If hypoglycemia is associated with illness unrelated to an IEM or endocrine disorder, administration of glucose at, or slightly above, the basal neonatal glucose oxidation rate is typically adequate to resolve the issue. On the other hand, IEMs may cause hypoglycemia that is more difficult to treat, requiring high levels of IV glucose. The presence of urine ketones in the neonate is unusual. If hypoglycemia is present in conjunction with ketosis and an increased anion gap metabolic acidosis, an organic acidemia is a diagnostic consideration. MSUD may also be associated with ketosis and hypoglycemia, but significant metabolic acidosis is not typical. Hypoketotic hypoglycemia is seen in hyperinsulinism and FAODs.

Hyperammonemia is a life-threatening condition that may occur in the absence of other obvious biochemical laboratory derangements. A respiratory alkalosis secondary to central stimulation of ventilation by ammonium is often present. All infants with altered consciousness or suspected sepsis should have an ammonia level checked without delay. Urea cycle disorders are a relatively common etiology for significant neonatal hyperammonemia (>200 μmol/L and often ≥2,000 μmol/L). However, infants with THAN, organic acidemias (e.g. methylmalonic or propionic acidemias), and some fatty acid oxidation defects (especially long-chain disorders) may have plasma ammonia levels as high as those encountered in urea cycle disorders because of a secondary inhibition of the urea cycle by toxic metabolites. In contrast to organic acidemias, urea cycle disorders are not usually associated with significant metabolic acidosis or ketosis; respiratory alkalosis is typical. Furthermore, blood urea nitrogen (BUN) levels tend to be low in urea cycle disorders, while hyperammonemia with an elevation of BUN is more commonly seen in organic acidemias. In addition, FAODs are more likely to be associated with hypoketotic hypoglycemia, which may be helpful in discriminating these conditions from others that cause hyperammonemia while specific biochemical genetic laboratory results are pending.

## SPECIALIZED LABORATORY INVESTIGATIONS

In order to arrive at a final diagnosis of an IEM, specialized laboratory tests, typically only performed at certain centers with specific expertise in IEM management, are required (**Box 4**). In some instances, more detailed evaluations are needed in order to arrive at the underlying diagnosis, especially if the neonate has an encephalopathic presentation without metabolic acidosis or hyperammonemia. Such neonates may have signs and symptoms more commonly associated with perinatal asphyxia, but the specialized tests shown in **Box 4** typically yield normal results.[12] Therefore, other studies may be needed, including analysis of neurotransmitter, amino acid, and lactate levels in CSF, or genetic testing, including sequencing of genes associated with EIEE or congenital myopathies (*see* **Table 1**). Collecting blood, urine, and CSF samples at the same time is ideal.

**BOX 4:** Initial specialized biochemical laboratory studies.

- Quantitative plasma amino acids
- Plasma total, free and esterified carnitine
- Plasma acylcarnitine profile
- Urine organic acids

## NEUROIMAGING FINDINGS

Although in many cases brain findings may be nonspecific, in some instances neuroimaging may provide important clues to the presence of an IEM. Magnetic resonance imaging (MRI) may show abnormal hyperintense signal in the basal ganglia in mitochondrial disease, pyruvate dehydrogenase deficiency, urea cycle disorders, and organic acidemias.[36,37] Caudate nucleus and putamen involvement, as well as enlarged frontotemporal CSF spaces and wide Sylvian fissures, may occur in glutaric acidemia type I.[37,38] White matter abnormalities are seen in MSUD, peroxisomal disorders, serine deficiency disorders, and glycine encephalopathy. Diffuse edema is present in urea cycle disorders and sulfite oxidase deficiency. Subependymal cysts may be seen in pyruvate dehydrogenase deficiency, mitochondrial disorders, and peroxisomal disorders. Early MRI in congenital disorders of glycosylation may appear normal, but this condition is often associated with pontocerebellar hypoplasia. Other causes of cerebellar hypoplasia include sulfite oxidase deficiency, pyruvate dehydrogenase deficiency, glycine encephalopathy, multiple acyl-CoA dehydrogenase deficiency, and peroxisomal disorders. More classic findings associated with perinatal asphyxia, such as encephalomalacia with cystic changes, have been described in a number of IEMs, including mitochondrial disorders, sulfite oxidase/molybdenum cofactor deficiency, urea cycle disorders, glycine encephalopathy, and pyridoxine-responsive seizures.[37] Magnetic resonance spectroscopy may show a lactate doublet in mitochondrial disorders or pyruvate dehydrogenase deficiency, or an absent or abnormally low creatine peak in disorders of creatine synthesis or transport.[37]

## MANAGEMENT

Neonates presenting in a metabolic crisis secondary to an underlying IEM require management in an intensive care setting. Supportive measures, such as intubation and ventilation, circulatory support, rehydration and correction of hypoglycemia and electrolyte, and calcium and phosphate imbalances must be initiated without delay. In addition, prompt attention to concomitant sepsis and administration of IV fluids in order to provide adequate caloric support and prevent catabolism are critical initial therapeutic measures.[39] Insertion of a central venous catheter in order to provide high-concentration dextrose fluids or total parenteral nutrition is often needed. Such a line may also serve as a means to provide extracorporeal dialysis if needed.[39] Specific therapies for select IEMs are shown in **Table 2**.

**TABLE 2:** Specific therapies for select inborn errors of metabolism.

| Disorder | Therapy |
|---|---|
| Galactosemia | Galactose restriction |
| Hereditary tyrosinemia | Nitisinone |
| Holocarboxylase synthetase deficiency | Biotin |
| Isovaleric acidemia | Limit protein*<br>Carnitine<br>Glycine |
| Methylmalonic acidemia | Limit protein*<br>Carnitine<br>Vitamin $B_{12}$ |
| Neonatal seizures | See **Table 1** |
| Urea cycle disorders | Limit protein*<br>Alternative pathway therapy |

*Note:*
*NB: Although a low-protein diet is a common part of the management of these conditions, over restriction of protein intake is associated with catabolism and worsening of disease; a careful nutritional balance must be maintained under the guidance of an experienced biochemical genetics team. Medical foods that restrict protein or specific amino acids associated with a given disorder are typically used in chronic management.

As a general principle, any component of food that may have precipitated or contributed to the metabolic decompensation is stopped, and high-caloric oral, enteral, or IV supplementation is provided. Initially, IV fluids with age-appropriate electrolytes and dextrose are most commonly given, although IV fat emulsions may be used in some instances to increase caloric intake.[3] Fat emulsions, however, should be avoided if an underlying FAOD is suspected. If hyperglycemia occurs as a result of the high-concentration dextrose infusion, an insulin drip may be started along with close monitoring of glucose levels. It must be emphasized that although initially protein is stopped in many IEMs presenting in the newborn period, e.g. urea cycle disorders, organic acidemias, and MSUD, reintroduction of protein nutrition within approximately 24 hours is essential in order to prevent catabolism and promote normal growth.

Intravenous infusion of sodium benzoate plus sodium phenylacetate, along with infusion of arginine HCl, may successfully treat some cases of hyperammonemia secondary to urea cycle disorders.[40] This has been termed alternative pathway therapy because benzoate conjugates with glycine and phenylacetate conjugates with glutamine, yielding compounds that bypass the urea cycle and are directly excreted in the urine, hence, providing an alternative pathway for nitrogen elimination. However, in cases of significant hyperammonemia, metabolic acidosis, or both, hemodialysis or various forms of hemofiltration may be needed. In general, toxic metabolites (ammonia, leucine, and organic acids) should be removed as quickly as possible. Therefore, if significant hyperammonemia is present, it is typical for preparations for dialysis to occur alongside starting alternative pathway therapy. Although peritoneal dialysis has been used to treat IEMs in the past, better clearance of toxins is achieved by hemodialysis or other extracorporeal blood purification techniques.[41]

If an organic acidemia is suspected, IV supplementation with carnitine is often performed, because in these conditions abnormal acylcarnitine species accumulate and are excreted in the urine, lowering body levels of carnitine. Carnitine supplementation has also been used for the treatment of FAODs, although there appears to be a theoretical risk in some long-chain disorders.[42] Glycine supplementation, in addition to carnitine, is used to treat isovaleric acidemia.

Because some IEMs are vitamin-responsive, high-dose vitamin or cofactor supplementation is another common therapeutic modality. Intramuscular vitamin $B_{12}$ is commonly used if an underlying organic acidemia is a diagnostic consideration, because $B_{12}$-responsive methylmalonic acidemia may present in the newborn period. Similarly, holocarboxylase synthetase deficiency may present in neonates with metabolic acidosis and elevated lactate and is responsive to biotin supplementation. Thiamine (pyruvate dehydrogenase deficiency and MSUD) and riboflavin (multiple acyl-CoA dehydrogenase deficiency) have also been used as therapies for neonates with metabolic decompensation, although vitamin-responsive forms of these IEMs tend to present later in childhood.

Isolated seizures that are amenable to treatment represent an important category of neonatal metabolic disease (*see* **Table 1**). Pyridoxine-dependent epilepsy secondary to antiquitin deficiency (α-amino adipic semialdehyde dehydrogenase deficiency) is caused by defective lysine catabolism that causes a secondary deficiency of vitamin $B_6$. Severe epilepsy unresponsive to conventional anticonvulsants is typical, although seizures will usually stop after pyridoxine supplementation. Pyridox(am)ine 5′-phosphate oxidase deficiency presents similarly, but is resistant to pyridoxine supplementation; treatment with pyridoxal 5′-phosphate controls seizures and early institution of therapy improves prognosis. Disorders of serine biosynthesis may present with intrauterine growth retardation and microcephaly, but seizures are common. Supplementation with serine and glycine must be started soon after birth in order to control seizures and maximize developmental outcome.[14]

## NEWBORN SCREENING

In the early 1960s, newborn screening for phenylketonuria was made possible by the development of the bacterial inhibition assay by Dr Robert Guthrie. Other disorders, including congenital hypothyroidism, galactosemia, and hemoglobinopathies, were slowly added to the newborn screening menu as assays for each condition became available. However, in the 1990s with the development of tandem mass spectrometry (MS/MS), the paradigm of laborious addition of new diagnostic tests "one at a time" was replaced by a method that allowed detection of >40 analytes virtually simultaneously in a matter of minutes.[43] Newborn screening using MS/MS has become the standard in developed nations, and some developing countries.[44] MS/MS has the ability to detect a number of IEMs by analyzing a filter paper newborn blood spot, including organic acidemias, FAODs and some amino acid, and urea cycle disorders.

Although MS/MS newborn screening has the potential to provide physicians caring for acutely ill infants with critical diagnostic information, neonates may present with clinical symptoms before results of the screen are reported. Therefore, physicians must have a high index of suspicion for an underlying IEM in neonates presenting with characteristic signs and symptoms and start therapy before initial screening results are known. This is especially true for neonates who have organic acidemias or urea cycle defects, because presentation in the first week of life is relatively common in these conditions.

Despite the widespread use of MS/MS newborn screening, public health programs in countries employing this technology have not reached consensus on the implementation of bloodspot screening. For example, the number of conditions for which screening is recommended ranges from 5 to over 50 depending on regional philosophy related to newborn screening. False positive results are more likely to occur in systems using a high number of tests, whereas devastating consequences of not screening for a potentially treatable condition may occur in countries screening for a limited number of conditions.[44] Some conditions may exhibit only mild or intermittent excretion of metabolites, so false negative results are an unavoidable part of any newborn screening program. On the other hand, it is important to realize that positive screening results require confirmation by definitive testing by a specialized diagnostic laboratory.[45]

Because of the success of MS/MS screening in reducing neonatal morbidity and mortality, there is increasing interest in starting newborn screening programs in developing countries. Most programs have focused on congenital hypothyroidism as an initial screening condition, although MS/MS for IEMs has also been implemented by some developing programs.[44,46] However, additional challenges related to health and political priorities, geography, cultural and religious attitudes, economic issues, and government stability have resulted in relatively slow uptake of MS/MS screening in developing health systems.[46] Nevertheless, with the continued success of newborn screening programs in improving the health of children, MS/MS dried bloodspot technology will likely continue to spread.

## REFERENCES

1. Applegarth DA, Toone JR, Lowry RB. Incidence of inborn errors of metabolism in British Columbia, 1969-1996. Pediatrics. 2000;105(1):e10.
2. Sanderson S, Green A, Preece MA, et al. The incidence of inherited metabolic disorders in the West Midlands, UK. Arch Dis Childhood. 2006;91(11):896-9.
3. Leonard JV, Morris AA. Diagnosis and early management of inborn errors of metabolism presenting around the time of birth. Acta Paediatrica. 2006;95(1):6-14.
4. Saudubray JM, Sedel F, Walter JH. Clinical approach to treatable inborn metabolic diseases: an introduction. J Inherited Metabol Dis. 2006;29(2-3):261-74.
5. Pearl PL. New treatment paradigms in neonatal metabolic epilepsies. Journal of inherited metabolic disease. 2009;32(2):204-13.
6. van Karnebeek CD, Stockler S. Treatable inborn errors of metabolism causing intellectual disability: a systematic literature review. Molr Genet Metab. 2012;105(3):368-81.
7. McCabe LL, Therrell BL Jr, McCabe ER. Newborn screening: rationale for a comprehensive, fully integrated public health system. Mol Genet Metab. 2002;77(4):267-73.
8. Scala I, Parenti G, Andria G. Universal screening for inherited metabolic diseases in the neonate (and the fetus). J Matern Fetal Neonatal Med. 2012;25(Suppl 5):4-6.
9. Burton BK. Inborn errors of metabolism in infancy: a guide to diagnosis. Pediatrics. 1998;102(6):E69.
10. Schaefer AM, Taylor RW, Turnbull DM, et al. The epidemiology of mitochondrial disorders--past, present and future. Biochim Biophys Acta. 2004;1659(2-3):115-20.
11. Browning MF, Levy HL, Wilkins-Haug LE, et al. Fetal fatty acid oxidation defects and maternal liver disease in pregnancy. Obstetr Gynecol. 2006;107(1):115-20.
12. Enns GM. Inborn errors of metabolism masquerading as hypoxic-ischemic encephalopathy. Neo Reviews. 2005;6(12):e549-e58.
13. Greene CL, Goodman SI. Catastrophic metabolic encephalopathies in the newborn period. Evaluation and management. Clin Perinatol. 1997;24(4):773-86.
14. Rahman S, Footitt EJ, Varadkar S, et al. Inborn errors of metabolism causing epilepsy. Dev Med Child Neurol. 2013;55(1):23-36.
15. Levy HL, Sepe SJ, Shih VE, et al. Sepsis due to Escherichia coli in neonates with galactosemia. New Eng J Med. 1977;297(15):823-5.
16. Sheffield LJ, Danks DM, Hammond JW, et al. Massive pulmonary hemorrhage as a presenting feature in congenital hyperammonemia. J Pediatr. 1976;88(3):450-2.
17. Cohn RD, Eklund E, Bergner AL, et al. Intracranial hemorrhage as the initial manifestation of a congenital disorder of glycosylation. Pediatrics. 2006;118(2):e514-21.
18. Honzik T, Tesarova M, Magner M, et al. Neonatal onset of mitochondrial disorders in 129 patients: clinical and laboratory characteristics and a new approach to diagnosis. J Inherit Metab Dis. 2012;35(5):749-59.
19. Van Hove JL, Lohr NJ. Metabolic and monogenic causes of seizures in neonates and young infants. Mol Genet Metab. 2011;104(3):214-30.
20. Boles RG, Buck EA, Blitzer MG, et al. Retrospective biochemical screening of fatty acid oxidation disorders in postmortem livers of 418 cases of sudden death in the first year of life. J Pediatr. 1998;132(6):924-33.
21. DeBrosse SD, Okajima K, Zhang S, et al. Spectrum of neurological and survival outcomes in pyruvate dehydrogenase complex (PDC) deficiency: lack of correlation with genotype. Mol Genet Metab. 2012;107(3):394-402.
22. von Kleist-Retzow JC, Cormier-Daire V, Viot G, et al. Antenatal manifestations of mitochondrial respiratory chain deficiency. J Pediatr. 2003;143(2):208-12.
23. Gibson K, Halliday JL, Kirby DM, et al. Mitochondrial oxidative phosphorylation disorders presenting in neonates: clinical manifestations and enzymatic and molecular diagnoses. Pediatrics. 2008;122(5):1003-8.
24. Houten SM, Wanders RJ. A general introduction to the biochemistry of mitochondrial fatty acid beta-oxidation. J Inherit Metab Dis. 2010;33(5):469-77.
25. Truin G, Guillard M, Lefeber DJ, et al. Pericardial and abdominal fluid accumulation in congenital disorder of glycosylation type Ia. Mol Genet Metab. 2008;94(4):481-4.
26. van den Hout HM, Hop W, van Diggelen OP, et al. The natural course of infantile Pompe's disease: 20 original cases compared with 133 cases from the literature. Pediatrics. 2003;112(2):332-40.
27. Gilbert-Barness E. Review: Metabolic cardiomyopathy and conduction system defects in children. Ann Clin Lab Sci. 2004;34(1):15-34.
28. Clayton PT. Inborn errors presenting with liver dysfunction. Semin Neonatol. 2002;7(1):49-63.
29. Clayton PT, Thompson E. Dysmorphic syndromes with demonstrable biochemical abnormalities. J Med Genet. 1988;25(7):463-72.
30. Cormier-Daire V, Rustin P, Rötig A, et al. Craniofacial anomalies and malformations in respiratory chain deficiency. Am J Med Genet. 1996;66(4):457-63.
31. Freeze HH. Genetic defects in the human glycome. Nat Rev Genet. 2006;7(7):537-51.
32. Moreno CA, Kanazawa T, Barini R, et al. Non-immune hydrops fetalis: A prospective study of 53 cases. Am J Med Genet A. 2013;161A(12):3078-86.
33. Whybra C, Mengel E, Russo A, et al. Lysosomal storage disorder in non-immunological hydrops fetalis (NIHF): more common than assumed? Report of four cases with transient NIHF and a review of the literature. Orphanet J Rare Dis. 2012;7:86.
34. Valayannopoulos V, Romano S, Mention K, et al. What's new in metabolic and genetic hypoglycaemias: diagnosis and management. Euro J Pediatr. 2008;167(3):257-65.
35. Oh MS, Carroll HJ. The anion gap. New Eng J Med. 1977;297(15):814-7.
36. Hoon AH Jr, Reinhardt EM, Kelley RI, et al. Brain magnetic resonance imaging in suspected extrapyramidal cerebral

palsy: observations in distinguishing genetic-metabolic from acquired causes. J Pediatr. 1997;131(2):240-5.
37. Poretti A, Blaser SI, Lequin MH, et al. Neonatal neuroimaging findings in inborn errors of metabolism. J Magn Reson Imaging. 2013;37(2):294-312.
38. Hendriksz CJ. Inborn errors of metabolism for the diagnostic radiologist. Pediatr Radiol. 2009;39(3):211-20.
39. Ogier de Baulny H. Management and emergency treatments of neonates with a suspicion of inborn errors of metabolism. Semi Neonatol. 2002;7(1):17-26.
40. Enns GM, Berry SA, Berry GT, et al. Survival after treatment with phenylacetate and benzoate for urea-cycle disorders. New Eng J Med. 2007;356(22):2282-92.
41. Schaefer F, Straube E, Oh J, et al. Dialysis in neonates with inborn errors of metabolism. Nephrol Dial Transplant. 1999;14(4):910-8.
42. Spiekerkoetter U, Lindner M, Santer R, et al. Treatment recommendations in long-chain fatty acid oxidation defects: consensus from a workshop. J Inherit Metab Dis. 2009;32(4):498-505.
43. Garg U, Dasouki M. Expanded newborn screening of inherited metabolic disorders by tandem mass spectrometry: clinical and laboratory aspects. Clin Biochem. 2006;39(4):315-32.
44. Wilcken B. Newborn screening: how are we travelling, and where should we be going? J Inherit Metab Dis. 2011;34(3):569-74.
45. Coman D, Bhattacharya K. Extended newborn screening: an update for the general paediatrician. J Paediatr Child Health. 2012;48(2):E68-72.
46. Therrell B, Padilla CD. Barriers to implementing sustainable national newborn screening in developing health systems. Int J Pediatr Adolesc Med. 2014;1:49-60.

# CHAPTER 21

# Common Surgical Conditions of the Neonate

*Stephanie D Chao, Julie R Fuchs*

## ABSTRACT

Neonates sometimes require surgical intervention. Accurate diagnosis and medical stabilization are crucial to a successful outcome. Surgical patients require collaboration of neonatologists, pediatric surgeons, pediatric radiologists, and pediatric anesthesiologists, among others, and often a multidisciplinary approach. In this chapter, we review neonatal surgical diseases.

## ESOPHAGEAL ATRESIA AND TRACHEOESOPHAGEAL FISTULA

### Clinical Presentation

Esophageal atresia (EA), with or without tracheoesophageal fistula (TEF), affects ~1 in 2,500–4,000 live births.[1] EA is inconsistently diagnosed prenatally. Findings on prenatal ultrasonography include an absent or small stomach bubble and maternal polyhydramnios.[2] Infants without antenatal identification typically become symptomatic within hours of birth. Early symptoms reflect the infant's inability to handle oral secretions. Respiratory symptoms and excessive salivation develop with drooling, coughing, choking, or cyanosis. If feeding is attempted, patients may gag and regurgitate with possible aspiration. Inability to pass an orogastric or nasogastric (NG) tube into the stomach is virtually pathognomonic.

In EA with TEF, the presence of significant communication with the tracheobronchial tree may lead to rapid respiratory decline. Each breath leads to increased gastric distention with reflux into the respiratory tree. Aspiration of secretions from the upper pouch can exacerbate respiratory symptoms.[3]

In the rarer TEF without atresia (H-type fistula), diagnosis is delayed for days to months until the infant presents with recurrent pneumonias or with choking or cyanosis during feeding.

### Pathophysiology

The exact mechanism of the pathogenesis of EA/TEF malformations remains poorly understood. The trachea and esophagus originate from the primitive foregut. Many theories that attempt to explain EA/TEF malformations describe the early formation of a tracheoesophageal septum, and the failure of normal migration and separation into separate respiratory and digestive tubes. Interruption of normal development may stem from extrinsic intrathoracic compression, epithelial compression, differential growth, or vascular occlusion. An animal model utilizing Adriamycin teratogenicity on the developing rat embryo has helped researchers gain better insight into the pathogenesis of EA/TEF.[4]

Anatomic patterns of EA/TEF malformations (**Figs. 1A to E**)[5] were first described in 1953. Type C represents ~85% of cases[3] and features a blind proximal esophageal pouch with distal TEF. The distal esophagus usually arises posteriorly from the trachea, at the level of the carina. Type A is next most common defect (~8.5%) with a pure EA with no fistula to the trachea.

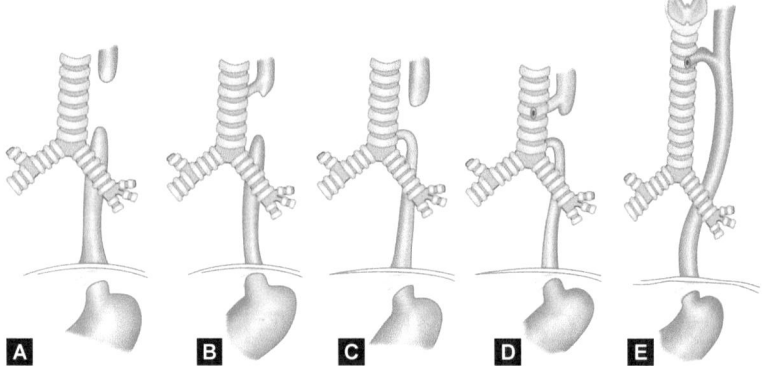

Figs. 1A to E: Gross classification of tracheoesophageal fistulas.[5]

## Diagnosis

The diagnosis of EA is made by passing an orogastric or NG catheter that meets resistance at 8–11 cm from the mouth or nose. Chest radiograph reveals the NG at the thoracic inlet (near the 2–4th vertebral body). If the diagnosis remains unclear, a small amount (0.5–1 mL) of contrast via catheter and the resultant meniscus on radiograph is confirmatory (although rarely done as contrast carries the risk of aspiration). Plain radiograph of the abdomen demonstrating a gastric air bubble/distal bowel gas suggests distal fistula. Conversely, a gasless abdomen raises suspicion of pure EA or proximal fistula only. Bronchoscopy at time of operative repair is often the definitive means of confirming the diagnosis.[6]

H-type TEF is difficult to diagnose. Routine fluoroscopic upper gastrointestinal (UGI) may miss the subtlety of a small H-type fistula. When this malformation is suspected, a "pull-back" tube esophagram with barium is necessary to demonstrate the small communication, frequently performed in the prone position.[3]

Associated anomaly frequency with EA/TEF ranges from 30% to >50%. Approximately 20% of infants with EA/TEF also demonstrate VACTERL anomalies (vertebral, anal, cardiac, tracheoesophageal, renal, and limb deformities).[7] Noninvasive studies include radiographs to assess the vertebral bodies and limbs, echocardiogram (to exclude congenital heart disease and exclude right-sided aortic arch), and abdominal ultrasound/renal investigation to rule out genitourinary anomalies.

## Treatment

Stabilization of respiratory status with a suction catheter in the proximal pouch, upright patient positioning, and proper airway management must be immediately implemented. Spontaneously breathing is preferred as mechanical ventilation increases airflow through a distal fistula, worsening gastric distention, and causing rupture in a few patients. Close monitoring in a neonatal intensive care unit (NICU) is ideal.

If an infant does not require mechanical ventilation, minimizing gastric distention via the fistula, emergent operation is rare, allowing time for additional studies, particularly echocardiogram. The primary goals at the time of operation are expeditious identification, division of the fistula, and primary repair. Initial approach includes rigid bronchoscopy to identify the fistula and rule out less common proximal fistulas. The standard open approach is via a right thoracotomy unless right-sided aortic arch is identified on preoperative imaging (in which case a left thoracotomy is used). Dissection occurs in a retropleural or transpleural manner. Once adequate exposure is achieved, the proximal pouch, distal esophagus, trachea, and vagus nerve are identified. The fistula is isolated and ligated, carefully avoiding narrowing the trachea. Meticulous dissection of proximal and distal esophagus is undertaken to mobilize both ends to attempt primary anastomosis. An H-type fistula can be divided and ligated via a right cervical approach and an autologous tissue interposition placed between both ends to prevent recurrence.

In "long-gap" atresia (a gap >~6 vertebral bodies), the distance between esophageal segments is too long for primary anastomosis. Commonly seen in pure EA without fistula (type A), a gastrostomy tube may be placed as a temporizing measure to allow infant growth while waiting for the gap to lessen, often resulting in successful primary anastomosis with delayed repair. Other options to lengthen the esophagus include routine dilatation, the application of extrathoracic or intrathoracic gradual traction (Foker technique), and circular myotomy. Ultimately, if the gap is not overcome, esophageal conduit is necessary, including gastric tube, gastric pull-up, and colonic/jejunal interposition grafts.

Increasingly, minimally invasive approaches to thoracoscopic EA/TEF repair are gaining popularity. Early studies were limited to retrospective series which demonstrated noninferiority to traditional open surgery when performed by experienced minimally invasive surgeons.[8] Complication and recurrence rates were similar, with longer operative times and higher peak intraoperative partial pressure of carbon dioxide (pCO$_2$) values observed in thoracoscopy. Further benefits may include shorter hospital stay and decreased risk of musculoskeletal deformities (such as scoliosis) consequent to newborn thoracotomy.[9,10]

## Complications

Anastomotic leak is a relatively common complication in the early postoperative period. Most will close spontaneously with adequate nutrition and drainage. However, leaks predispose patients to esophageal strictures after healing which may require repeated esophageal balloon dilation and less commonly, reoperation. Gastroesophageal reflux, tracheomalacia, and abnormal esophageal peristalsis resulting in dysphagia are late consequences seen commonly post-EA/TEF repair. Despite short- and long-term consequences, survival is high and most adults with childhood EA/TEF repair perceive their quality of life as favorable.[11,12]

## ■ CONGENITAL DIAPHRAGMATIC HERNIA

### Clinical Presentation

Congenital diaphragmatic hernia (CDH) affects 1 in 2,000–5,000 live births per year. CDH had been associated with high mortality rates, but with better understanding of physiology and NICU practice improvement, survival is now ~70–95%.[13]

Multidisciplinary care teams including obstetricians, neonatologists, and pediatric surgeons are required for optimal plan and delivery of CDH infants, who present with respiratory distress. The degree of respiratory distress correlates with size of defect and amount of visceral herniation, but most importantly lung hypoplasia. Breath sounds may be absent or asymmetric. Neonates often require intubation and cardiopulmonary support.

### Pathophysiology

The diaphragmatic defect is usually posterolateral (Bochdalek type) due to failure of proper closure of the pleuroperitoneal canals at approximately 8 weeks' gestation. This failure of membrane closure results in a prominent anterior rim of diaphragm, with diminutive posterior and lateral rims. Approximately 90% of CDHs occur in the left hemidiaphragm.[3] Abdominal contents herniate through the defect during embryonic development, impairing normal lung development. The resultant pulmonary hypoplasia (primarily ipsilateral lung, but to a lesser extent contralateral) is characterized by abnormal bronchiolar branching, diminished alveolar surface area, and altered pulmonary vasculature. After birth, the infant's physiology is complicated by pulmonary hypertension.[14] Intestinal nonrotation is common as the bowel protrudes into the thoracic cavity rather than undergoing its normal rotation and abdominal fixation.

The less common Morgagni-type CDH (failure of closure of septum transversum) often presents in later childhood with fewer respiratory symptoms. Few CDH cases are associated with genetic defects, such as *WT1* gene mutation. Patients with Fryns syndrome or chromosomal abnormalities have poorer outcomes.[15]

### Diagnosis

Two-thirds of CDH diagnoses occur prenatally. Fetal ultrasound or magnetic resonance imaging (MRI) demonstrates abdominal contents within the thorax. Fetal echocardiography and genetic testing is recommended when CDH diagnosis may assist in family counseling. Herniation of liver into the chest in a left-sided CDH portends a poorer prognosis. Calculating a lung-to-head ratio may predict survival.[16]

At birth, a chest radiograph is usually diagnostic. Herniated intestine is seen in the chest with paucity of bowel gas in the abdomen. Other confirmatory studies are unnecessary. Echocardiography helps quantify the degree of pulmonary hypertension and exclude intrinsic cardiac defects.

### Treatment

#### Initial Management

Prenatally diagnosed CDH infants should deliver at tertiary care centers with access to multidisciplinary teams including neonatologists and pediatric surgeons, and in proximity to extracorporeal membrane oxygenation (ECMO). Neonates with CDH require medical stabilization at birth with a nasogastric tube or orogastric tube (OGT) inserted to decompress herniated stomach and bowel. Most infants require mechanical ventilation. Permissive hypercapnia decreases barotrauma. Although surfactant and inhaled nitric oxide are employed to improve oxygenation, neither has been demonstrated in large trials to improve survival in infants with CDH.[17] ECMO may be required when standard ventilation fails, and limited to neonates weighing >2 kg and gestational age >34 weeks without moderate to severe intracranial hemorrhage or other lethal anomalies.

## Surgical Intervention

Infants benefit from delaying repair following stabilization of cardiopulmonary status. It is prudent to observe beyond 48 hours [allowing pulmonary artery (PA) pressures to deescalate] to optimize timing of surgical repair, which may be days from delivery.

Transabdominal surgical repair is typical. The diaphragmatic remnant edge may be rolled with careful dissection to unfurl. Small defects are repaired primarily by suture repair. Larger defects require patch repair, most commonly using a Gore-Tex synthetic patch.

Many centers now use thoracoscopic CDH repair to lower morbidity and postoperative pain. Studies show equivalence to traditional open repairs in terms of time to enteral feeds and length of hospital stay, with cosmetic benefit.[18] However, long-term data are limited. Thoracoscopy worsens pulmonary hypertension and pCO2 intraoperatively, and is poorly tolerated by some. Higher recurrence rates may occur in thoracoscopic repair. Randomized controlled trials (RCTs) are required to optimize surgical approach.[9]

## DUODENAL OBSTRUCTION

### Clinical Presentation

Duodenal obstruction has many causes, duodenal atresia being the most common. It affects ~1 in 6,000–10,000 live births.[19,20] Antenatal diagnosis is suggested by the presence of a "double bubble" (dilated stomach and proximal duodenum) on prenatal ultrasound and maternal polyhydramnios.

Prenatally undiagnosed infants present early with feeding intolerance and emesis, which is bilious as the obstruction is usually distal to the ampulla of Vater. Occasionally, it is nonbilious. OGT placement results in high volume output. Approximately half will pass meconium normally.[20] Abdominal distention is rare or subtle because of proximal obstruction.

### Pathophysiology

Duodenal atresia has three variants. Type I atresia is a duodenal wall in continuity with a web obstructing luminal flow. In Type II atresia, proximal and distal duodenum are connected by a thin fibrous cord. In Type III atresia, proximal and distal duodenum are separated, associated with a V-shaped gap in the intervening mesentery. Although distal intestinal atresias are believed vascular accidents in utero, duodenal atresia is widely believed a failure of intestinal recanalization. Between 5 weeks and 8 weeks gestation, epithelial proliferation occludes the developing foregut. The foregut recanalizes at 10 weeks. Less common causes of duodenal obstruction include annular pancreas, preduodenal portal vein, and peritoneal bands (Ladd's bands) associated with intestinal malrotation.

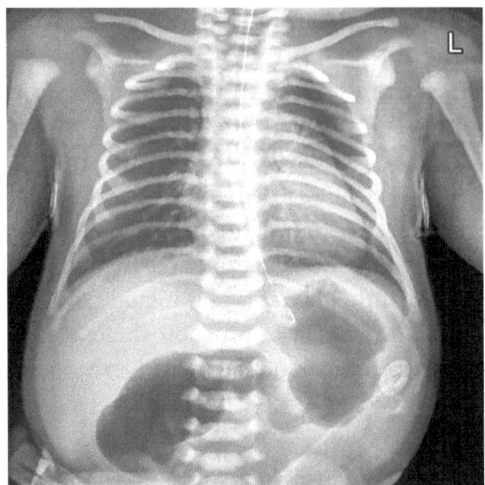

**Fig. 2:** Radiograph depicting the "double bubble" of duodenal atresia.

### Diagnosis

The presence of a "double bubble" sign on plain abdominal radiograph is pathognomonic for duodenal obstruction (**Fig. 2**). More distal intestinal gas represents incomplete obstruction, such as duodenal web. When diagnosis is unclear from plain radiograph, an UGI oral contrast fluoroscopy is performed and contrast stops abruptly at the smooth atretic proximal duodenal pouch. In incomplete obstruction, a thin streak of contrast flows into and opacifies the jejunum. UGI distinguishes duodenal atresia from intestinal malrotation, which requires immediate operation.

Duodenal atresia is associated with other congenital anomalies in ~60% of cases. Approximately 25% of cases are associated with congenital cardiac anomalies.[21] Echocardiogram excludes anomalies that pose significant morbidity and mortality risk. Abdominal ultrasonography excludes other associated anomalies (i.e. genitourinary). Chromosomal studies are useful, albeit not urgent. Trisomy 21 (Down syndrome) is most commonly associated with duodenal atresia (28%). Other associated anomalies include malrotation, TEF, and anorectal malformations (ARMs).[21]

### Treatment

Infants suspected of having duodenal obstruction should have an OGT placed at birth for gastric decompression until surgery.

A transverse right upper quadrant incision was traditional, while laparoscopic approaches have become increasingly popular. A Kocher maneuver is performed to completely mobilize the duodenum. Once free, a diamond duodeno-duodenostomy may be performed (proximal transverse and distal longitudinal incisions).[22] This approach is used for duodenal atresia, preduodenal portal vein, and annular pancreas. If there is large size discrepancy between the two ends, a tapering duodenoplasty is performed, resecting the antimesenteric side of the dilated bowel to hasten postoperative bowel function and prevent stasis. In certain Type I atresias, excision of the mucosal web is possible if the ampulla can be safely avoided. Regardless of procedure, careful identification of the bile duct insertion is important to prevent injury or ampullary occlusion.[20,23]

## JEJUNOILEAL AND COLONIC ATRESIAS

### Clinical Presentation

Jejunoileal atresias are now associated with a survival rate of ~90%.[24] Neonates present shortly after birth with abdominal distention. Most patients present with bilious emesis or failure to pass meconium.

Small intestinal atresias are classified into four types:
- *Type I*: Short-segment stenosis or membranous web occluding the lumen.
- *Type II*: Serosal surface gap, sometimes separated by fibrous cord **(Fig. 3)**.
- *Type IIIa*: Serosal gap with associated V-shaped mesenteric defect.
- *Type IIIb*: "Apple-peel" or "Christmas tree" atresia. Usually in proximal jejunum followed by narrow-caliber blind distal intestine without mesenteric fixation. Ileocolic arterial blood supply usually tenuous.
- *Type IV*: Multiple atresias.[25]

Colonic atresias are incredibly rare, comprising <1% of all intestinal atresias.

### Pathophysiology

Atresia and small intestine stenosis (except duodenum) and colon are believed caused by vascular accidents in utero. Vascular accidents may be due to hernia, volvulus, gastroschisis, or intussusception. The causative events are believed to occur relatively late in utero. Associated anomalies are rare.

### Diagnosis

Prenatal echogenic or distended loops of bowel may suggest diagnosis. After birth, plain abdominal radiographs typically demonstrate distended loops of small bowel with a lack of gas in the colon or rectum. Intra-abdominal calcifications suggest fetal bowel perforation with meconium peritonitis. A contrast enema usually demonstrates small caliber colon (microcolon), a result of disuse, and may demonstrate failure to reflux beyond an obstructed segment. Obtaining UGI with small bowel follow-through is of little value unless atresia is very proximal. Persistently fixed and dilated small intestinal loop mandates operative exploration.[26]

### Treatment

After initial stabilization with NG decompression and intravenous fluids, and a brief period of observation, operation proceeds to prevent intestinal perforation or volvulus of the massively dilated proximal segment of bowel.

The greatest potential morbidity for infants with intestinal atresia is risk of developing short bowel syndrome (SBS). Operative repair goals include vigilance for multiple atresias, re-establishing bowel continuity, and preserving bowel length and ileocecal valve. In the rare case of acute perforation or an unstable patient, a staged repair is indicated. Enterostomy, sometimes multiple, is created during initial exploration with intestinal continuity established weeks later.

In standard atresia, the largest, most bulbous segment of proximal bowel is removed, allowing end-to-end or end-to-back anastomosis. If there is a massive caliber discrepancy between proximal (dilated) bowel and distal segment, a tapering enteroplasty may be required to complete primary anastomosis and may help restore function to the proximal dilated bowel. A number of methods are used to preserve and maximize the functionality of bulbous dilated bowel to prevent SBS. The Bianchi procedure is longitudinal division of dilated bowel with the splitting of its mesentery and subsequent end-to-end anastomosis of the resultant two segments. An alternative bowel lengthening procedure gaining popularity is the serial transverse enteroplasty procedure (STEP),[27] which entails alternating serial firing of a gastrointestinal anastomosis (GIA) stapler perpendicular to the long axis of the bowel. Alternating the direction of the stapler from side to side creates a channel of bowel both smaller in diameter and longer in length than the original

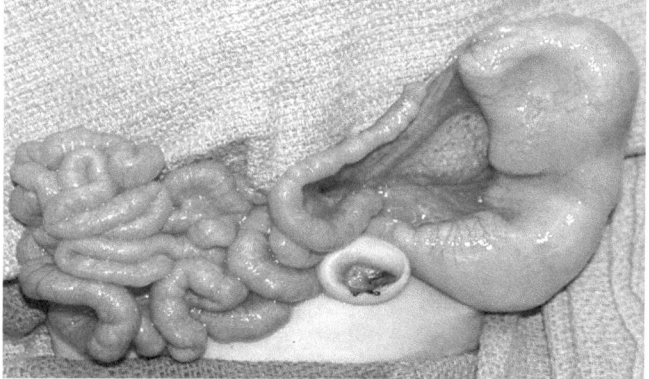

**Fig. 3:** Type II intestinal atresia *(For color version see Plate 3)*.

bowel.[27] Although most commonly applied to patients with SBS (from other causes) with resultant dilatation in order to lengthen the bowel, they have been used in select cases of severe atresia.

Ileal atresia with standard end-to-end repair generally fares well, without long-term intestinal function issues. More proximal atresia (jejunal) babies require additional time to achieve full feeds and prolonged parenteral nutrition.

## ABDOMINAL WALL DEFECTS

### Clinical Presentation

Abdominal wall defects include umbilical hernia, omphalocele, and gastroschisis. Of the three, umbilical hernias are the most common. A fascial defect at the umbilicus results in abdominal content protrusion covered by skin or a palpable umbilical ring. Most children are asymptomatic and incarceration is rare.

Omphalocele is a midline defect at the umbilical ring through which evisceration of bowel and often liver occurs. Abdominal viscera are covered by a translucent membrane or sac composed of fused peritoneum and amnion. The umbilical cord inserts centrally into this sac. Omphaloceles typically measure 2–10 cm in diameter. Giant omphaloceles are larger than 10 cm. Up to 70% of omphaloceles are associated with other congenital anomalies, genetic syndromes, or chromosomal defects.[28]

Gastroschisis is an abdominal wall defect just lateral to the insertion of the umbilical cord, usually on the right. Abdominal viscera including bowel, stomach, and gonads are commonly exposed. Without covering for the eviscerated bowel, exposure to the surrounding amniotic fluid results in inflamed, thickened, and often matted bowel.

### Pathophysiology

Omphalocele results from failure of normal physiologic herniation and reduction of the intestines at 6–10 weeks' gestation. Failure of proper midline fusion is also associated with more extensive midline defects such as cephalic fold defects found in pentalogy of Cantrell—sternal cleft, omphalocele, intracardiac defects, ectopia cordis, and anterior diaphragmatic hernia.[29]

Gastroschisis is believed secondary to ischemic insult to the right umbilical vein or early in utero rupture of cord hernia. Because gastroschisis likely arises from disruption, rather than a developmental defect, it is typically not associated with a genetic syndrome.[28]

### Diagnosis

Both omphalocele and gastroschisis are detectable by second trimester ultrasound. Maternal serum alpha-fetoprotein (AFP) can be elevated, with higher elevations observed in gastroschisis. Early diagnosis optimizes postnatal care.[28,29]

### Treatment

At birth, immediate care of both omphalocele and gastroschisis minimizes fluid and heat loss, with careful handling of the exposed bowel. The bowel is moistened with warm sterile saline and covered. Care is maintained to avoid rupture of the omphalocele sac. A plastic bowel bag or wrap is required transiently. The neonate may require transport to a pediatric surgery specialty care center. Immediately after birth, appropriate fluid resuscitation, antibiotics, and OGT decompression are indicated before reduction of intestinal contents.[30]

Primary closure feasibility depends on the available abdominal wall, often significantly diminished without having needed to accommodate the fetal bowel.[30] With small defects, primary closure is achievable. Biologic and synthetic prostheses are used as temporary or permanent patches for closure for abdominal defects too large for primary closure.

For gastroschisis, a silo may be placed when the herniated viscera are not immediately abdominally reducible at birth. It may be constructed from Dacron-reinforced Silastic sheets sewn to the fascial edge. Alternatively, a preformed, single piece spring-loaded silo may be placed over the bowel, with the base serving as anchor under the fascial edge **(Fig. 4)**. Over several days, bowel edema improves and abdominal contents are gradually reduced into the abdomen. The abdomen stretches to accommodate the new contents.[31] Caution is taken to avoid rapid reduction, which may compromise pulmonary function and/or diminish abdominal venous return. It is important to maintain a gentle silo angle to prevent mesenteric vessel

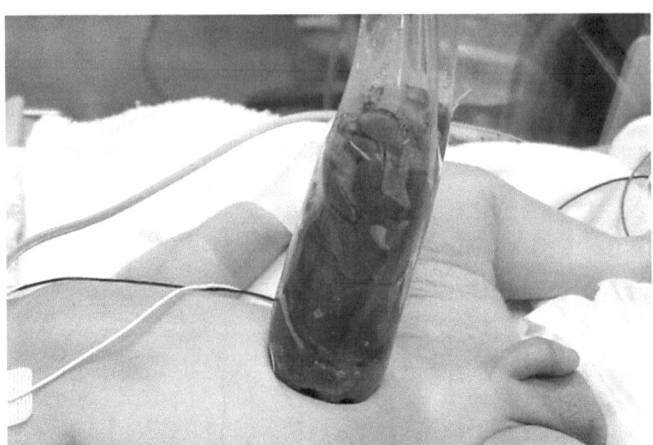

**Fig. 4:** Preformed spring-loaded silo used in gastroschisis reduction at bedside *(For color version see Plate 3)*.

kinking. Preformed silo use permits definitive abdominal wall closure electively. In a prospective RCT, preformed silo use compared to primary closure demonstrated no difference between groups with respect to length of time on total parenteral nutrition, length of stay, or sepsis or necrotizing enterocolitis (NEC) frequency. There was; however, a trend toward fewer ventilator days.[32] Newer techniques include sutureless patch closure using the umbilical cord or a temporary dressing over the defect and reduced bowel. With this method, the skin eventually closes over the defect, leaving an umbilical hernia which often closes spontaneously over the next few years.[33]

For a giant omphalocele or an unstable neonate, topical agents may be applied to the sac to promote desiccation and eventual epithelialization.[29] Common agents include silver sulfadiazine cream (Silvadene) and bismuth tribromophenate (Xeroform) dressing. A gauze wrap applied with a supportive orthotic device and gentle pressure over time gradually reduces the omphalocele.

The initial short-term goal is to obtain epithelial coverage over the defect. When primary fascial closure is not achieved in the immediate postnatal period or has failed, definitive repair of the ventral hernia is performed. Repair may be delayed for months, even years, to allow correction of other anomalies (e.g. cardiac) and prevent dense adhesions between abdominal viscera and overlying skin.

## Complications

Herniated viscera reduction is carefully balanced with lack of abdominal domain. Abdominal compartment syndrome may result from rapid reduction, leading to reduced lung compliance, impaired venous return, and decreased organ perfusion. If end-organ failure develops, immediate abdominal decompression is undertaken, removing external pressure or reopening of the hernial repair with silo placement.

Necrotizing enterocolitis occurs in ~20% of gastroschisis patients. NEC development is independent of silo placement.[34]

Bowel dysmotility is associated with gastroschisis. Prolonged ileus is due to inflamed bowel resulting from chronic amniotic fluid exposure. When feeding advancement fails over 4-6 weeks, a contrast study may be considered to exclude atresia (~10% of gastroschisis) and other causes of obstruction. Intestinal failure in gastroschisis infants may result from multiple bowel resections for atresia, NEC, or chronic malabsorption and dysmotility. These infants require chronic, partial, or total parenteral nutrition.[35] Adhesive bowel obstruction is a late complication of gastroschisis or omphalocele. Most patients with abdominal wall defects report a good quality of life, but ~50% reported some gastrointestinal symptoms (e.g. regurgitation, constipation, and intermittent abdominal pain).[36,37]

# INTESTINAL MALROTATION

## Clinical Presentation

Intestinal malrotation may be incidental and asymptomatic or present emergently in critically ill children. Up to 80% of patients present in the first few weeks of life, but some present in adulthood. Autopsy studies estimate prevalence of rotational disorders as high as 1% of the population.[38] The classic presentation of malrotation is a previously healthy infant with bilious emesis, which is surgical until proven otherwise. Associated symptoms vary from frequent spit up with feeds to ischemic complications of midgut volvulus, including bloody stools, a firm or distended abdomen, hypovolemia, acidosis, and shock. Bilious emesis is evaluated expeditiously because delay may result in intestinal necrosis, SBS, or death.[39]

## Pathophysiology

Intestinal malrotation occurs due to failure of prenatal progression of intestinal rotation and fixation. The digestive system has infolded endoderm, which forms a single tubular structure at 4 weeks. The vascular supply forms a week later. At 6 weeks, the midgut lengthens and herniates into the umbilical cord. Normal rotation begins within the umbilical cord and completed by 12 weeks when the intestine returns to the abdominal cavity. Ultimately, the intestines complete a 270° counterclockwise rotation. Normal fixation and rotation results in the ligament of Treitz fixed and retroperitonealized in the left upper quadrant, behind and to the left of the superior mesenteric artery (SMA). The mesentery is broadly fixed from the left upper quadrant to right lower quadrant where the cecocolic loop begins.[40]

Abnormal rotation and fixation result in nonrotation, cecocolic malrotation, classic malrotation, and other less severe anomalies. Nonrotation results in small bowel being situated in the right abdomen, with colon on the left. This is the position of the intestine following a Ladd's procedure. In cecocolic malrotation or reverse rotation, cecum and colon are rotated in the reverse direction, with the SMA and duodenum lying anterior to cecum and colon. With this defect, patients are at risk for cecal volvulus and colonic obstruction (acute or chronic), usually occurring after the neonatal period. Classic malrotation is the most common newborn rotational anomaly. The ligament of Treitz is right of midline and the cecum lies in the right upper quadrant. Malrotation is associated with a narrowed mesentery and fibrous peritoneal bands (Ladd's bands) which extend from the colon, across the duodenum, and attach retroperitoneally.[40] Duodenal obstruction may be caused by Ladd's bands, or clockwise midgut twisting may occur due to the narrow pedicle formed by the mesenteric base. Notably, rotation and fixation abnormalities often coexist with heterotaxia, CDH, gastroschisis, and omphalocele.

## Diagnosis

Distressed infants with bilious emesis need no further imaging; immediate operative exploration is performed. In a stable patient, physical examination may be of limited value. Abdominal tenderness may be mild and nonfocal. Abdominal distention may be absent in the case of proximal obstruction.

Radiographic workup should be expeditious. Abdominal radiographs do not confirm the diagnosis; however, there are nonspecific suggestive signs. A "double bubble" indicates duodenal obstruction. Commonly this is attributed to duodenal atresia, but may also represent duodenal compression from Ladd's bands or midgut volvulus (especially when there is a small amount of distal gas). Paucity of gas on a plain radiograph should raise concern for midgut volvulus. UGI with water-soluble contrast optimizes evaluation of bilious emesis. A duodenojejunal junction which fails to cross midline and sits to right of midline indicates malrotation. A sharp tapering or "bird's beak" appearance suggests midgut volvulus.[41,42]

## Treatment

Malrotation management includes initial placement of NG tube for proximal decompression and adequate hydration/fluid resuscitation. Prompt surgical management prevents ischemia from uncorrected midgut volvulus.

Laparoscopic Ladd's procedure is the gold standard for correcting classic malrotation.[43] The key steps include:[39]
- Counter-clockwise derotation of volvulus, if present
- Division of abnormal peritoneal attachments (Ladd's bands)
- Broadening/widening of mesentery
- Positioning of the small bowel to the right and colon to the left of midline
- Appendectomy.

Increasing skill with minimal access techniques means that Ladd's procedure is increasingly laparoscopic. Feasibility and equivalence of the laparoscopic approach for malrotation without torsion has been noted.[44] Laparoscopy has demonstrably decreased time to starting feeds, reaching full feeds, and time to discharge. Operative times with laparoscopy are comparable to traditional open surgery and outcomes are as safe.[45]

# NECROTIZING ENTEROCOLITIS

## Clinical Presentation

Necrotizing enterocolitis occurs mostly in premature infants. Full-term infants who develop NEC often have associated predisposing conditions, such as congenital heart disease, infection, or asphyxia. The overall incidence is ~1:1,000 live births, but higher among infants weighing <1,500 grams (3–10%).[46]

## Pathophysiology

Necrotizing enterocolitis presentation varies, from acute onset with rapid progression to slow indolent. Initial subtle findings include increased apnea, bradycardia, desaturations, temperature instability, or lethargy. The infant exhibits feeding intolerance, abdominal distention, bloody stools, or discoloration of the abdominal wall. Perforated viscus or necrotic bowel is indications for surgery. Pathophysiology is multifactorial, broadly caused by compromised mucosal integrity, intestinal ischemia, pathogenic bacterial colonization, and excess intestinal luminal protein substrate.[3] The initial insult results in disruption of intestinal barrier, bacterial translocation, and hyperimmune response leading to coagulation necrosis and eventually perforation.[46]

Feeding variation is associated with risk of NEC. Delayed introduction of feeds and slow advancement fail to demonstrate decreased risk of NEC.[47] However, standardized feeding protocols for initiation of feeds based on gestation age with standard volumes and concentrations reduce NEC incidence. Human breast milk is known for its universal benefits to the infant, including antimicrobial and anti-inflammatory properties. RCTs demonstrate decreased NEC in infants fed human breast milk compared to formula.[48]

## Diagnosis

Diagnosis of NEC is by plain abdominal radiograph. Findings include pneumatosis intestinalis **(Fig. 5)**, portal venous gas, thickened or fixed bowel loops, and free air. Such changes may also be seen on abdominal ultrasound.

There is no single diagnostic study for NEC. Rather, findings are consistent with sepsis or inflammation. Nonspecific findings include leukocytosis, thrombocytopenia, metabolic acidosis, and elevated C-reactive protein.

## Treatment

The majority of NEC is nonsurgical. Close monitoring with serial abdominal examinations and plain films is mandatory. Initial management starts with bowel decompression and bowel rest. Feeds are immediately stopped and nutrition is provided parenterally. Broad-spectrum antibiotics treatment ranges from 7 days to 14 days.

Perforation is the only absolute indication for surgery. Relative indications include refractory sepsis despite maximal medical support, fixed intestinal loop on abdominal radiograph, and abdominal wall discoloration. Traditionally, surgical management included primary laparotomy with bowel resection and enterostomy formation. However, increasingly NEC is managed with primary peritoneal drainage (PPD), mainly in very low birth weight infants. Originally this strategy was introduced as a temporizing measure until laparotomy, but it is increasingly used as a definitive intervention without subsequent laparotomy. Multiple RCTs comparing PPD with laparotomy fail to demonstrate superiority of either strategy.[49]

## Outcomes and Prognosis

Mortality from NEC is as high as 40%. Survivors face increased risk of poor gastrointestinal and neurodevelopmental outcomes. Stricture formation and recurrence are immediate concerns; ~5% of cases recur and most can be managed nonoperatively. Stricture formation complicates 10–40% managed medically and surgically. Colonic strictures are most common and usually require delayed surgical intervention.[46,48]

Intestinal insufficiency leading to SBS is the most devastating complication of surgically-treated NEC. Intestinal length and absorptive capacity are important factors in determining long-term parenteral nutrition dependence. These infants require a program of intestinal rehabilitation to prevent long-term complications associated with parenteral nutrition, including cholestatic liver disease, recurrent line infections, and poor bone formation, among others. Ultimately, some will require intestinal transplantation.[46,48]

## SACROCOCCYGEAL TERATOMA

### Clinical Presentation

Sacrococcygeal teratoma (SCT) is the most common solid organ newborn tumor, occurring in ~1 in 20,000–40,000 births, with female predominance.[50,51] SCTs are usually diagnosed antenatally. Clinical presentation includes an exophytic, epithelialized lesion arising from the sacral region, sometimes displacing other perineal structures, such as the anus and vagina. SCTs may be entirely internal and present later in life, usually before the age of 3–4 years. Internal SCTs may present later as palpable abdominal masses or due to compression symptoms, including lower extremity pain or weakness (nerve compression), constipation or abdominal distention (rectal displacement), or disorders of bladder emptying (compression of the bladder neck).[52,53]

Currently SCT is classified[54] into four types: Type I (predominantly external), Type II (presenting externally but with significant intrapelvic extension), Type III (predominantly intrapelvic and intra-abdominal mass with external component), and Type IV (presacral mass with no external component)(**Fig. 6**).

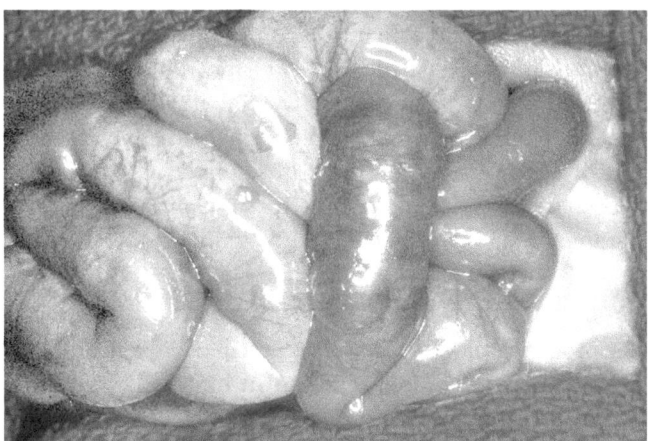

**Fig. 5:** Pneumatosis intestinalis *(For color version see Plate 3).*

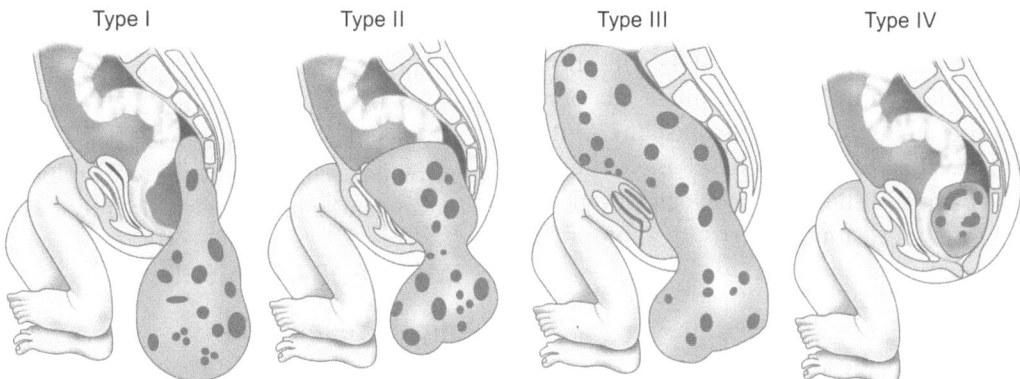

**Fig. 6:** Altman's classification of the four types of sacrococcygeal teratoma.[54]

## Pathophysiology

Teratomas arise from totipotent cells, either primordial germ cells or cells in Henson's node of the primitive streak. At 4-5 weeks' gestation, these cells originate in the allantois of the embryonic yolk sac endoderm and migrate to the genital ridge of the posterior abdominal wall. Extragonadal germ cell tumors result from aberrant migration of these totipotent cells, with the sacrococcygeal region being the most common extragonadal site.[3] SCTs are uniformly attached to the coccyx.

Sacrococcygeal teratomas are histologically classified into three types: benign, mature teratomas; immature (embryonic tissues) without malignant transformation; and malignant (contains mixture of malignant, mature, and immature tissue). Overall, malignancy is found in ~20% of SCTs; the malignancy rate is significantly higher in children resected age >2 months.[55]

## Diagnosis

The majority of SCTs are diagnosed prenatally as early as 16-20 weeks gestation. Characterized by chaotic organization of solid and cystic components, these are highly vascular lesions. Large SCTs can cause arteriovenous shunting and high output cardiac failure. Echocardiography is recommended to exclude high output heart failure, resulting in hydrops. Placentomegaly and fetal hydrops can be detected as early as 28-30 weeks gestation on prenatal ultrasound and may portend poorer prognosis. Large tumors can also result in intratumoral hemorrhage, leading to anemia. Polyhydramnios may also be seen prenatally and elevate risk of premature birth.[50,51]

Prenatal ultrasound may be limited in its evaluation of SCTs due to acoustic shadowing of pelvic bones, and fetal MRI offers important information regarding intrapelvic and cephalad tumor extent. This information is useful in prenatal counseling on its potential functional impact.[51]

After birth, diagnosis is made by physical examination, including rectal examination to exclude presacral mass. Perineal examination evaluates displacement of perineal structures. Abdominopelvic ultrasound is the first mode of imaging used to diagnose suspected SCTs with intrapelvic extension, followed by MRI to evaluate anatomic relationships and exclude meningocele. Baseline AFP is obtained at initial evaluation. Although AFP is elevated in the neonate, normograms distinguish pathologic elevations. AFP is followed through treatment to ensure appropriate postoperative decline.

## Treatment

Fetal SCTs are followed closely with serial imaging; the majority of fetuses have an uneventful prenatal course. Vaginal delivery is possible, but may be complicated by tumor hemorrhage or dystocia due to tumor size. Lethal tumor hemorrhage can occur if not recognized and managed expeditiously. A tumor size of >5 cm (or volume 750 cm$^3$) is an indication for elective cesarean section. The development of hydrops, placentomegaly, or high output cardiac failure prompts emergent cesarean section.[3]

Elective surgery is performed shortly after birth. Depending on SCT type, surgery may start either in the supine or prone approach. Predominantly external SCTs are approached posteriorly with complete resection of the tumor and coccyx, en bloc. The pelvic muscles are preserved and carefully reapproximated at the conclusion of the case. Skin is preserved to ensure closure. In SCTs with a large internal component, tumor resection begins with laparotomy to approach the intra-abdominal component first, with the goal of early control of the middle sacral artery.

Complete resection is the key to SCT management. Chemotherapy with a standardized carboplatin-etoposide-bleomycin or cisplatinum-based regimen has improved mortality of malignant SCTs.[56]

Sacrococcygeal teratoma management has been an early success of fetal surgery. Although limited to a few centers, fetal surgery occurs in cases that meet criteria including absence of maternal contraindication, previable fetus (gestational age 20-30 weeks), favorable tumor stage, fetal hydrops or placentomegaly, fetal high output cardiac failure, normal fetal karyotype, and absence of maternal mirror syndrome (phenomenon of maternal proteinuria, preeclampsia, and edema in which maternal physiologic derangement mirrors that of the fetus).[57]

## Complications and Prognosis

The prognosis of resected SCTs is excellent. Recent advances in chemotherapy have resulted in high malignant SCT survival. Poor outcome prognosticators include older age and larger tumors. Factors associated with high recurrence include incomplete resection, failure to resect the coccyx, and immature/malignant histology. Close follow-up of SCT patients is essential, with routine postoperative rectal examination, AFP monitoring, and imaging.

Long-term morbidity is largely associated with anorectal and urinary complications caused by tumor displacement or associated with surgical resection. This underscores the importance of close follow-up by a multidisciplinary team to prevent and manage pelvic floor dysfunction.[51]

## ■ IMPERFORATE ANUS

### Clinical Presentation

The diagnosis of imperforate anus, often made at birth, is also referred to as "ARM", including all defects associated

> **BOX 1:** Classification of anorectal malformations.
>
> *Male defects:*
> - Perineal fistula
> - Rectourethral bulbar fistula
> - Rectourethral prostatic fistula
> - Rectovesical (bladder neck) fistula
> - Imperforate anus without fistula
> - Rectal atresia and stenosis
>
> *Female defects:*
> - Perineal defects
> - Vestibular fistula
> - Imperforate anus with no fistula
> - Rectal atresia and stenosis
> - Cloaca

with an abnormal anal orifice. Referred to as "low," "intermediate," or "high" malformations, these obsolete terms lack prognostic or therapeutic significance. ARMs range from mildly displaced perineal fistulas to absence of any orifice. **Box 1** represents the common contemporary stratification of ARMs.[58]

Defects common to both males and females include cutaneous perineal fistula, imperforate anus without fistula, and rectal atresia. Perineal fistulas represent the lowest defect with best outcome for continence after repair. The rectum opens anterior to the center of the anal sphincter and is associated with a small bridge of skin known as a "bucket handle" deformity or mucus trapped along the median raphe known as a "string of pearls" defect.[3,59] Imperforate anus without fistula typically occurs with trisomy 21. Although there is absence of fistula, often there is a common wall between rectum and urethra in the male, and rectum and vagina in the female. Rectal atresia is rare, occurring in <1% of ARMs. The perineum looks normal since the anal canal is normally formed. The defect is diagnosed by failure to pass a thermometer beyond the perineum. There is severe stenosis or total atresia. Functional outcomes are good because the sphincter complex is normal.[57,58]

Males may present with fistulas to bulbar urethra, prostatic urethra, or bladder neck. The higher the genitourinary fistula, the poorer the functional outcome after surgery.[3,58]

In females, the most common presentation is a rectovestibular fistula. The rectum inserts in the vestibule, outside the hymen and posterior to the vagina. Rectovaginal fistulas are exceedingly rare, and it has been debated whether or not they truly exist or simply represent a misidentified ARM. Females may also present with a cloaca in which the rectum, urethra, and vagina share a single orifice. When the common channel is less than 3 cm in length, there is greater likelihood of repair without need for laparotomy with improved long-term function.[58]

# PATHOPHYSIOLOGY

Anorectal malformations are developmental anomalies of the hindgut, allantois, and müllerian duct occurring before 7 weeks' of gestation, but a complex understanding of the pathophysiology or embryologic development is lacking. In animal studies, *Sonic Hedgehog* and *Wingless (wnt)* signaling pathways are implicated in ARM development. Other signaling pathways and environmental exposures are implicated in some studies.[60]

Detectable chromosomal anomalies are associated with 4.5–11% of ARMs.[61] Up to 75% of ARM children have other congenital anomalies. These include the VACTERL association (*see* section on TEFs) and the Currarino triad (a caudal regression syndrome characterized by hemisacrum, ARM, and presacral mass).[62]

## Diagnosis

Anorectal malformation diagnosis is made clinically on physical examination. A 24-48 hours observation period is required to identify or exclude a fistula with the passage of meconium in a displaced fecal stream or meconium-tinged urinary stream. A prone cross table lateral radiograph aids in determining the distance of the rectal pouch from the anus based on the location of the rectal air bubble, although predictive value is limited.

During the initial observation period, associated anomalies bear exclusion. This includes renal ultrasound, echocardiogram, and spinal ultrasound to exclude tethered cord. Skeletal survey is performed to exclude limb or vertebral anomalies, and to assess sacral and pelvic development.[58,63]

## Treatment

The immediate consideration after birth is whether to temporize with a colostomy or perform a primary pull-through procedure. Instability of the neonate, a flat perineum, cloaca, absence of fistula, the presence of meconium in the urine, and a high rectal air bubble above the coccyx on cross table radiograph are indications for initial colostomy. When necessary, a divided colostomy is performed. The proximal limb and the distal mucus fistula are separated by a bridge of skin and fascia (contrary to a loop colostomy). This prevents contamination of the urinary tract by the fecal stream in the presence of a rectourinary fistula. A divided colostomy also prevents abnormal dilatation of the rectum, which can complicate a later pull-through procedure. Colonic lavage of the mucus fistula is performed at the time of colostomy creation to prevent future urosepsis and allow for future distal colostogram.[58,62] When the infant is ready for a pull-through procedure,

~4–12 weeks after colostomy, a distal colostogram is useful preoperatively. The colostogram allows better understanding of ARM present, length of bowel available for pull-through, and relationship between the sacrum, coccyx, and rectum. This helps in planning the operative approach. The exact surgery for each ARM is beyond the scope of this chapter. Posterior sagittal anorectoplasty[64] enables best visualization of the entire malformation and muscle sphincter complex. A muscle stimulator identifies the location of maximal muscle contraction. A posterior midline incision is centered over this site and extended through the skin crease and sphincter mechanism. The length of incision varies with the complexity of the ARM, but may start near the coccyx. The rectum is identified and dissected from the genitourinary tract, avoiding injury during dissection of the common wall. The rectum is anchored within the sphincter complex without tension and the anorectoplasty completed, classically with 16 absorbable circumferential interrupted sutures. The perineal body is reconstructed and the remaining skin is closed.[62,63]

A laparoscopic-assisted approach has gained popularity for high malformations.[65] Minimal perineal dissection exposes the rectal pouch, followed by dissecting the common wall and/or dividing the fistula to the urethra. The pelvic floor muscles are identified via laparoscopy and by perineal electrostimulation. A limited incision is made from the perineum (<1 cm) and a trocar is introduced after minimal dissection from the perineum. This perineal trocar forms a passage through the center of the muscle complex through which the previously dissected rectum is grasped and exteriorized to complete the anorectoplasty.

Postoperative care and caretaker involvement are critical to optimize outcomes. Starting 2–3 weeks after anorectoplasty, dilations of the neoanus are started to prevent stricture. Eventually, some children require a bowel management program either for constipation (most commonly) or fecal incontinence. This begins even before the period of toilet training to achieve regularity of bowel movements early in life.[62] Long-term urologic and gynecologic follow-ups are necessary.

## SUMMARY

Advances in pediatric surgery such as laparoscopy, improvements in anesthesia, and newborn care have greatly enhanced quality-of-care and quality-of-life for newborns requiring pediatric surgical intervention. The majority of these conditions are congenital and often diagnosed prenatally. Improvements in perinatal care, development of fetal diagnosis, and specialized treatment centers have all played a role in improving family participation in newborn surgical care. Currently several registries, e.g. CDH Registry, University of California Fetal Consortium, and other pediatric surgical networks are exploring ways to examine variations in practice and care. These approaches are likely to optimize future family-integrated care for newborn surgical patients.

## REFERENCES

1. Sfeir R, Michaud L, Salleron K, et al. Epidemiology of esophageal atresia. Dis Esophagus. 2013;4:354-55.
2. Burge DM, Shah L, Spark P, et al. Contemporary management and outcomes for infants born with oesophageal atresia. Br J Surg. 2013;4:515-21.
3. Dolgin SE, Hamner CE. Surgical Care of Major Newborn Malformations. Singapore: World Scientific Publishing Co.; 2012.
4. Merei JM, Hutson JM. Embryogenesis of tracheoesophageal anomalies: a review. Pediatr Surg Int. 2002;18:319-26.
5. Gross RE. The surgery of infancy and childhood. Philadelphia: WB Saunders; 1953.
6. Coran AG, Adzick NS, Krummel TM, et al. Pediatric Surgery. 7th edition. Philadelphia: Elsevier, Saunders; 2012.
7. Driver CP, Shankar KR, Jones MO, et al. Phenotypic presentation and outcome of esophageal atresia in the era of the spitz classification. J Pediatr Surg. 2001;36(9):1419-21.
8. Szavay PO, Zundel S, Glumenstock G, et al. Perioperative outcome of patients with esophageal atresia and tracheo-esophageal fistula undergoing open versus thoracoscopic surgery. J Laparoendosc Adv Surg Tech A. 2011;21(5):439-43.
9. Dingemann C, Ure B, Dingemann J. Thoracoscopic procedure in pediatric surgery: what is the evidence? Eur J Pediatr Surg. 2014;24(1):14-9.
10. Holcomb GW, Rothenberg SS, Bax KMA, et al. Thoracoscopic repair of esophageal atresia and tracheoesophageal fistula: a multi-institutional analysis. Ann Surg. 2005;242(3):422-30.
11. Deurloo JA, Ekkelkamp S, Hartman EE, et al. Quality of life in adult survivors of correction of esophageal atresia. Arch Surg. 2005;140(10):976-80.
12. Koivusalo A, Pakarinen MP, Turunen P, et al. Health-related quality of life in adult patients with esophageal atresia: a questionnaire study. J Pediatr Surg. 2005;40(2):307-12.
13. Downard CD, Jaksic T, Garza JJ, et al. Analysis of an improved survival rate for congenital diaphragmatic hernia. J Ped Surg. 2003;38:729-32.
14. Badillo A, Gingalewski C. Congenital diaphragmatic hernia: treatment and outcomes. Semin Perinatol. 2014;38:92-6.
15. Bollmann R, Kalache K, Mau H, et al. Associated malformations and chromosomal defects in congenital diaphragmatic hernia. Fetal Diagn Ther. 1995;10(1):53-9.
16. Aspelund G, Fisher JC, Simpson LL, et al. Prenatal lung-head ratio: threshold to predict outcome for congenital diaphragmatic hernia. J Matern Fetal Neonatal Med. 2012;25(7):1011-6.
17. Moya FR, Lally KP. Evidence-based management of infants with congenital diaphragmatic hernia. Semin Perinatol. 2005;29(2):112-7.

18. Tanaka T, Okazaki T, Fukatsu Y, et al. Surgical intervention for congenital diaphragmatic hernia: open versus thoracoscopic surgery. Pediatr Surg Int. 2013;29(11):1183-6.
19. Hemming V, Rankin J. Small intestinal atresia in a defined population: occurrence, prenatal diagnosis and survival. Prenat Diagn. 2007;27(13):1205-11.
20. Fonkalsrud EW, DeLorimier AA, Hays DM. Congenital atresia and stenosis of the duodenum. A review compiled from the members of the Surgical Section of the American Academy of Pediatrics. Pediatrics. 1969;43(1):79-83.
21. Dalla Vecchia LK, Grosfeld JL, West KW, et al. Intestinal atresia and stenosis: a 25-year experience with 277 cases. Arch Surg. 1998;133(5):490-6.
22. Kimura K, Mukohara N, Nishijima E, et al. Diamond-shaped anastomosis for duodenal atresia: an experience with 44 patients over 15 years. J Pediatr Surg. 1990;25(9):977-9.
23. Spigland N, Yazbeck S. Complications associated with surgical treatment of congenital intrinsic duodenal obstruction. J Pediatr Surg. 1990;25(11):1127-30.
24. Stollman TH, de Blaauw I, Wijnen MH, et al. Decreased mortality but increased morbidity in neonates with jejunoileal atresia; a study of 114 cases over a 34-year period. J Pediatr Surg. 2009;44(1):217-21.
25. Grosfeld JL, Ballantine VN, Shoemaker R. Operative management of intestinal atresia and stenosis based on pathologic findings. J Pediatr Surg. 1979;14:368-75.
26. Sato S, Nishijima E, Muraji T, et al. Jejunoileal atresia: a 27-year experience. J Pediatr Surg. 1998;33(11):1633-5.
27. Kim HB, Fauza D, Garza J, et al. Serial transverse enteroplasty (STEP): a novel bowel lengthening procedure. J Pediatr Surg. 2003;38(3)425-9.
28. Christison-Lagay ER, Kelleher CM, Langer JC. Neonatal abdominal wall defects. Semin Fetal Neonatal Med. 2011;16(3):164-72.
29. Islam S. Advances in surgery for abdominal wall defects: gastroschisis and omphalocele. Clin Perinatol. 2012;39(2):375-86.
30. Mann S, Blinman TA, Douglas Wilson R. Prenatal and postnatal management of omphalocele. Prenat Diagn. 2008;28(7):626-32.
31. Stanger J, Mohajerani N, Skarsgard ED. Practice variation in gastroschisis: factors influencing closure technique. J Pediatr Surg. 2014;49(5):720-3.
32. Pastor AC, Phillips JD, Fenton SJ, et al. Routine use of a SILASTIC spring-loaded silo for infants with gastroschisis: a multicenter randomized controlled trial. J Pediatr Surg. 2008;43(10):1807-12.
33. Choi WW, McBride CA, Bourke C, et al. Long-term review of sutureless ward reduction in neonates with gastroschisis in the neonatal unit. J Pediatr Surg. 2012;47(8):1516-20.
34. Schlatter M, Norris K, Uitvlugt N, et al. Improved outcomes in the treatment of gastroschisis using a preformed silo and delayed repair approach. J Pediatr Surg. 2003;38(3):459-64.
35. Friedmacher F, Hock A, Castellani C, et al. Gastroschisis-related complications requiring further surgical interventions. Pediatr Surg Int. 2014;30(6):615-20.
36. van Eijck FC, Wijnen RM, van Goor H. The incidence and morbidity of adhesions after treatment of neonates with gastroschisis and omphalocele: a 30-year review. J Pediatr Surg. 2008;43(3):479-83.
37. van Eijck FC, Hoogeveen YL, van Weel C, et al. Minor and giant omphalocele: long-term outcomes and quality of life. J Pediatr Surg. 2009;44(7):1355-9.
38. Durkin ET, Lund DP, Shaaban AF, et al. Age-related differences in diagnosis and morbidity of intestinal malrotation. J Am Coll Surg. 2008;206:658-63.
39. Shalaby MS, Kuti K, Walker G. Intestinal malrotation and volvulus in infants and children. BMJ. 2013;347-50.
40. Millar AJW, Rode H, Cywes S. Malrotation and volvulus in infancy and childhood. Semin Pediatr Surg. 2003;12(4):229-36.
41. Nehra D, Goldstein AM. Intestinal malrotation: varied clinical presentation from infancy through adulthood. Surgery. 2011;149(3):386-93.
42. Doherty GM, Way LW. Current Surgical Diagnosis and Treatment, 12th edition. New York: Lange Medical Books/McGraw-Hill; 2006.
43. Ladd WE, Gross RE. Abdominal Surgery of Infancy and Childhood. Philadelphia, PA: WB Saunders; 1941.
44. Bass KD, Rothenberg SS, Chang JHT. Laparoscopic Ladd's procedure in infants with malrotation. J Pediatr Surg. 1998;33(2):279-81.
45. Stanfill AB, Pearl RH, Kalvakuri K, et al. Laparoscopic Ladd's procedure: treatment of choice for midgut malrotation in infants and children. J Laparoendosc Adv Surg Tech A. 2010;20(4):369-72.
46. Dominguez DM, Moss RL. Necrotizing enterocolitis. Clin Perinatol. 2012;39(2):387-401.
47. Kennedy KA, Tyson JE, Chamnanvanakij S. Rapid versus slow rate of advancement of feedings for promoting growht and preventing necrotizing enterocolitis in parenterally fed low-birth-weight infants. Cochrance Database Syst Rev. 2000;2:CD001241.
48. Sullivan S, Schanler RJ, Kim JH, et al. An exclusively human milk-based diet is associated with a lower rate of necrotizing enterocolitis than a diet of human milk and bovine milk-based products. J Pediatr. 2010;156(4):562-7.
49. Downard CD, Renaud E, St. Peter SD, et al Treatment of necrotizing enterocolitis: an American Pediatric Surgical Association Outcome and Clinical Trials Committee Systematic Review. J Pediatr Surg. 2012;47:2111-22.
50. Perrelli L, D'Urzo C, Manzoni C, et al. Sacrococcygeal teratoma. Outcome and management. An analysis of 17 cases. J Perinat Med. 2002;30:179-84.
51. Gucciardo L, Uyttebroek A, De Wever I, et al. Prenatal assessment and management of sacrococcygeal teratoma. Prenat Diagn. 2011;31:678-88.
52. Whalen TV, Mahour GH, Landing BH, et al. Sacrococcygeal teratomas in infants and children. Am J Surg. 1985;150:373-75.
53. Koop CE. Abdominal mass in the newborn infant. NEJM. 1973;289(11):569-71.
54. Altman RP, Randolph TG, Lilly JR. Sacrococcygeal teratoma: American Academy of Pediatrics Surgical Section Survey—1973. J Pediatr Surg. 1974;9(3):389-98.

55. Grosfeld JL, Ballantine TV, Lowe D, et al. Benign and malignant teratomas in children: analysis of 85 patients. Surgery. 1976;80(3):297-305.
56. Billmire DF. Malignant germ cell tumors in childhood. Semin Pediatr Surg. 2006;15:30-6.
57. Wilson RD, Hedrick H, Flake AW, et al. Sacrococcygeal teratomas: prenatal surveillance, growth and pregnancy outcome. Fetal Diagn Ther. 2009;25:15-20.
58. Peña A, Hong A. Advances in the management of anorectal malformations. Am J Surg. 2000;180(5):370-6.
59. Ziegler MM, Azizkhan RG, Weber TR. Operative Pediatric Surgery. New York: McGraw-Hill; 2003.
60. Moore SW. Associations of anorectal malformations and related syndromes. Pediatr Surg Int. 2013;29(7):665-76.
61. Marcelis C, de Blaauw I, Brunner H. Chromosomal anomalies in the etiology of anorectal malformations: a review. Am J Med Genet A. 2011;155A(11):2692-704.
62. Martucciello G, Torre M, Belloni E, et al. Currarino syndrome: proposal of a diagnostic and therapeutic protocol. J Pediatr Surg. 2004;39(9):1305-11.
63. Bischoff A, Levitt MA, Peña A. Update on the management of anorectal malformations. Pediatr Surg Int. 2013;29:899-904.
64. deVries PA, Peña A. Posterior sagittal anorectoplasty. J Pediatr Surg. 1982;17(5):638-43.
65. Georgeson KE, Inge TH, Albanese CT. Laparoscopically assisted anorectal pull-through for high imperforate anus: a new technique. J Pediatr Surg. 2000;35(6):927-31.

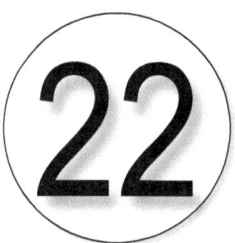

CHAPTER 22

# Point-of-Care Testing in Newborn Screening: Hearing Loss and Critical Congenital Heart Disease

*Rebecca Barnett*

*"The truth is rarely pure and never simple. Modern life would be very tedious if it were either, and modern literature a complete impossibility."*
—**Oscar Wilde; The Importance of Being Earnest**

## ABSTRACT

Newborn point-of-care testing includes novel approaches to screen for congenital disorders of structure and function not detectable by traditional blood spot testing. Two valuable examples include screening for congenital hearing loss and critical congenital heart disease (CCHD). The results of these tests allow the healthcare team and family to build an optimal discharge plan for the patient after birth. This chapter will briefly explore testing, causes of, and treatments for hearing loss and CCHD.

## INTRODUCTION

Much is known about blood spot screening for inborn errors of metabolism, hemoglobinopathies, and rare diseases related to newborn function. These diseases have a cumulative incidence of approximately 1 per 1,000 at birth. Newborn hearing loss and critical congenital heart disease (CCHD) also each have frequencies of ~1 per 1,000 live births. Increased understanding of the genetic basis of these conditions has made detection and counseling critical to early intervention and prevention of disability for affected infants, their families, and society at large.

Advances in noninvasive technology have made screening at the bedside (point-of-care) testing possible. Integration of such processes into the workflow of healthcare delivery systems presents unique challenges in screening not initially recognized when screening was first implemented. Concurrently, advances in infant anesthesia, critical and perioperative care, acoustic amplification, cochlear implants, interventional cardiology, and cardiothoracic surgery have allowed global transfer of these technologies. These advantages make point-of-care screening a topic for inclusion in this book at this time.

Healthcare informatics present an emerging unique and important opportunity for fine-tuning the public health relevance and opportunity for global incorporation into healthcare delivery for newborns. It is very likely that other noninvasive tests shall someday emerge as relevant strategies for preventive and optimization of healthcare, not just in newborns but in other at-risk populations.

## NEWBORN HEARING LOSS

### Historical Perspective

Children with hearing abnormalities may have significant delays in their speech and development compared to children with normal hearing. In 1988, the average age of identification of profoundly deaf children was 2.5 years as reported by the Commission on Education. At that time, there was no technology or infrastructure available to test hearing in newborns. In 1989, the Rhode Island Study Demonstration Project was one of the first large scale studies to evaluate the feasibility of universal newborn hearing screening. Using transient-evoked otoacoustic emissions (TEOAEs), researchers tested a total of 1,850 newborns in both the well-baby nursery and the neonatal intensive care unit (NICU). Their results showed that 497 (27%) infants were referred for rescreening; 81% were rescreened, and 115 infants (6.2% of the total group) received diagnostic audiologic evaluations. Of this group, 11 babies were found to have sensorineural hearing loss (SNHL), 6 with bilateral severe-to-profound loss and 1 with unilateral moderate loss.[1] The work-group expanded to include other states performing universal newborn screening and, by 1993, the National Institutes of Health (NIH) Consensus Conference recommended universal newborn hearing screening. The Joint Commission on Infant Hearing (JCIH), established in late 1969, released a statement in 1994 that endorsed universal hearing screening in the hospital before discharge to improve detection of hearing loss in newborns and infants, stating that all infants with hearing loss must be identified before the age of 3 months and receive intervention by 6 months.[2] The Centers for Disease Control and Prevention (CDC) and state health departments began requesting national data from states on newborn screening in 1999. Currently, it is estimated that over 98% of all newborns in the United States are screened for hearing loss at birth.[3] Universal hearing screening is the standard-of-care not only for the US hospitals and birthing centers but for many countries around the world.[4]

## Prevalence of Hearing Loss

Neonatal hearing loss averages 1.1 per 1,000 US infants with child and adolescent rates demonstrating much variability. Hearing loss is over-represented in low-income households, the Hispanic-American population, and certain familial causes. Genetic causes contribute to a quarter of neonatal hearing loss across studies.[5] A nationwide cohort of 2,186 Dutch NICU newborns 1998–2002 with risk factors (familial hearing loss, fetal infection, craniofacial anomalies, birthweight < 1,500 g, hyperbilirubinemia, ototoxic medications, cerebral complications, severe birth asphyxia, assisted ventilation > 4 days, and syndromes) showed a 3.2% uni- or bilateral hearing loss with multivariate analysis showing only severe birth asphyxia and ventilation > 4 days being independent risk factors for hearing loss.[6] The CDC estimates of the US hearing loss include 1.7 per 1,000 babies screened in 2016 (range 0–11.1 per 1,000 screened). Earlier studies in older children aged 3–17 years based on parental report (1997–2005) had 5 per 1,000 prevalence; 14.9% of aged 6–19 years screened in 1988–2004 for low- or high-frequency loss, in one or both ears, at the minimal 16 decibel hearing level.[3] These studies examining the prevalence of hearing loss highlight the importance of a good understanding of the risk factors associated with hearing loss and the need for an organized newborn hearing program.

## Defining Newborn Hearing Loss Risk Factors and Etiology

Congenital hearing loss is the inability of the ear to convert the vibratory energy of sound into the electrical energy of nerve impulse (**Fig. 1**).[7]

Sound is transmitted via the external auditory canal to the tympanic membrane and ossicles. Then air vibration is translated and amplified to mechanical vibration, which is transmitted to the cochlea, resulting in movement of the cochlear fluids. The cochlear fluid movement alters the shape of the outer hair cells which mediates sound amplification and increases frequency. The movement of the inner hair cells of the cochlea stimulates the adjacent nerve fibers and transmits the electrical signal to the brain (**Fig. 2**). It is important to understand where the problem lies when it comes to congenital hearing loss, as it is characterized as conductive, sensorineural, mixed, or auditory neuropathy. Conductive hearing loss is caused by a problem with the outer or middle ear structures. It can be permanent, such as aural atresia, but is often temporary and is amenable to medical or surgical interventions, such as removing a cerumen impaction or treating a middle ear infection. SNHL is often permanent and represents a problem with the inner ear, cochlea, auditory nerve, or along the central auditory pathway. Auditory neuropathy, or auditory neuropathy spectrum disorder, is a dysfunction of the inner hair cells, auditory nerve or the synapse between the two. Auditory neuropathy is estimated to be 40% from genetic causes with the remainder acquired from risk factors often associated with the NICU population.[8]

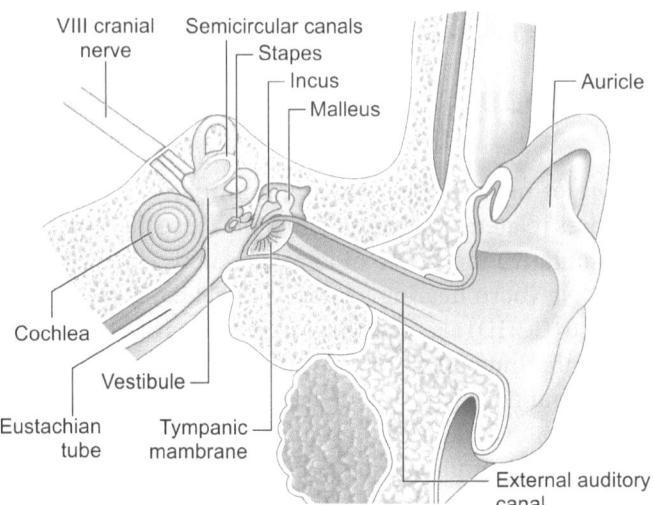

**Fig. 1:** Cross-section of the ear anatomy.

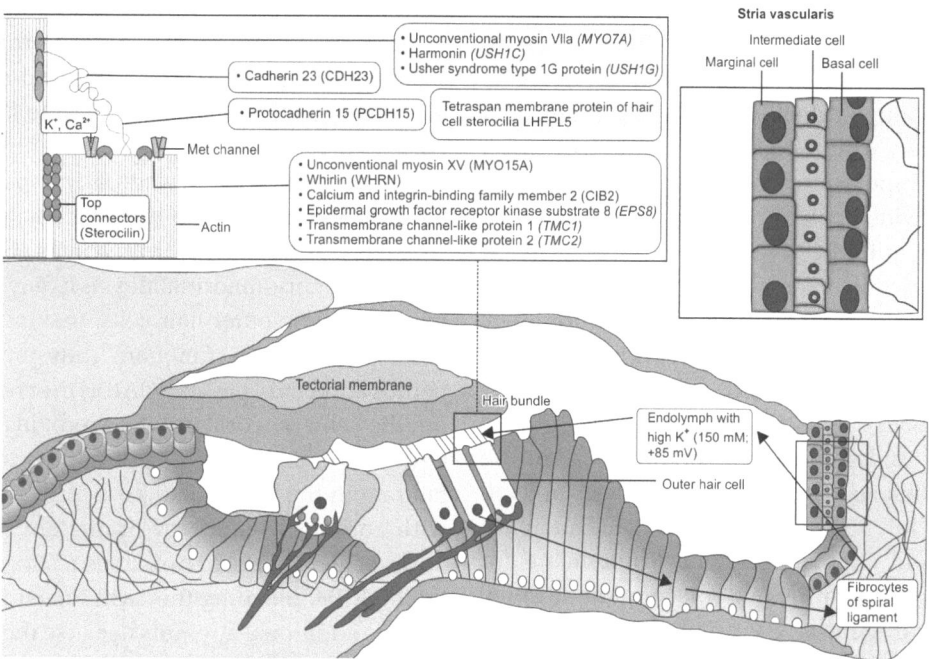

Fig. 2: The stria vascularis and sensory hair cells.

The JCIH periodically reviews current literature and publishes consensus statements regarding infant risk factors and screening practices; the latest statement was published in 2019. In conjunction with the American Academy of Pediatrics (AAP), the JCIH lists the following risk factors for early childhood hearing loss and gives guidance regarding frequency of rescreening beyond the initial newborn screen. Infants with certain or multiple risk factors warrant frequent repeat hearing screens as they may pass the initial hospital hearing screen but present with delayed hearing loss. Having a family history of hearing loss remains a risk factor as genetic causes are so frequent; however, only 1.43% of children with a positive family history have hearing loss.[9] Perinatal risk factors include NICU hospitalization > 5 days, hyperbilirubinemia requiring exchange transfusion, aminoglycoside administration > 5 days, asphyxia or hypoxic-ischemic encephalopathy (HIE), extracorporeal membrane oxygenation (ECMO), *in utero* infections (herpes, rubella, syphilis, toxoplasmosis, cytomegalovirus or CMV, and Zika), and certain congenital anomalies such as craniofacial malformations, microcephaly, acquired hydrocephalus, and temporal bone abnormalities. There are over 400 known syndromes associated with abnormal hearing.[10] Syndromes associated with hearing loss include Jervell and Lange-Nielsen, Usher, Alport, branchio-oto-renal syndrome, Waardenburg, Pendred, CHARGE, VACTERL, Trisomy 21, Treacher Collins, Crouzon, Klippel-Feil, and Goldenhar. Significant risk factors include postnatal events such as culture positive infections leading to SNHL (such as confirmed bacterial/viral meningitis or encephalitis), significant head trauma or skull fractures, chemotherapy, and any caregiver or parental concern regarding the infant's hearing.[11,12] Our goal as neonatal providers should be to prevent hearing loss by judicious use of ototoxic medications, identify risk factors, and ensure appropriate referrals and follow up.

## Mechanisms of Genetic and Acquired Hearing Loss

A diagnosis of hearing loss is followed by determining the possible cause, then treatment is tailored to the individual. While neonatal hearing loss can be acquired, genetic causes are most common. Approximately 120 nonsyndromic genes involved in hearing loss have been identified; ~40% of these genes are autosomal dominant and 60% autosomal recessive. A very small percentage of hearing loss results from X-linked or maternal mitochondrial deoxyribonucleic acid (DNA) inheritance leading to later onset hearing loss.[10] Genetic hearing loss often is due to abnormalities in genes that encode proteins important to inner ear homeostasis and inner hair cell structure and function. Ion transport and electrical signal conduction can be impacted when abnormal proteins are expressed. Half of all severe-to-profound hearing loss is due to a mutation in the *GJB2* gene which encodes for a protein called connexin 26. Mutation in *GJB6* which encodes for connexin 30 is another very common genetic cause of hearing loss. Mutations in the *STRC, CLDN14, MARVELD2, KCNQ4, TECTA, ESPN,* and *OTOF* are other known genetic causes of hearing loss.[7]

Acquired hearing loss in the newborn period is most commonly associated with fetal CMV or rubella infection, although other bacterial and viral infections can be implicated. Even though rubella is considered eradicated from Western society with modern vaccination practices, it still remains an important cause of acquired congenital hearing loss worldwide.

Congenitally acquired CMV is associated with intrauterine growth restriction, microcephaly, cerebral calcifications, chorioretinitis, extramedullary hematopoiesis, jaundice, and thrombocytopenia. While 90% of congenital CMV is asymptomatic,[13] 14% of infants exposed to CMV *in utero* develop SNHL of some type and 3-5% of those develop bilateral moderate-to-profound SNHL.[14] In the US, Utah was the first state to implement hearing targeted CMV screening in July 2013. Currently, Connecticut, Iowa, New York, Utah, and Virginia have state requirements for all newborns who fail their hearing screen in the hospital to be tested for congenital CMV. While this remains controversial, many hospitals across the nation have begun hearing-targeted CMV screening by urine or saliva/cheek swab polymerase chain reaction (PCR) and are proposing legislative mandates.[15] Hearing-targeted CMV screening adds yet another layer of complexity to the newborn screening process when taking into account the costs of testing as well as the follow-up required. Gantt evaluated the cost-effectiveness of targeted screening of congenital CMV in 2016 and estimated a reduction in severe-to-profound hearing loss by 4.2-13% given a modest response to antiviral treatment with a cost of approximately $11 per infant.[16] Emerging evidence continues to build with many sites claiming approximately 6% positive CMV with targeted screening,[17] while other researchers have seen lower yield from newly implemented programs.[18]

## Newborn Hearing Screening Tests and Protocol

### Otoacoustic-evoked Emissions

Otoacoustic emissions (OAE) are expressed when the outer hair cells respond to auditory stimuli. Evoked OAEs occur after the application of a click or low tone stimulus, almost like an echocardiography returning to the middle ear as a vibration. The evoked emission response represents the motion of the tympanic membrane vibrating due to fluid pressure fluctuation generated in the cochlea. These emissions can give a frequency-specific indication of cochlear status and are measured by a small probe in the external auditory canal. The OAE uses hearing thresholds of mild hearing loss (30-35 dB HL), so if the infant has slight to mild (16-25 dB HL) hearing loss they may still pass the OAE. The presence of OAE is highly correlated with normal hearing and normal cochlear function. The absence of OAE indicates cochlear dysfunction, but the test can be affected by abnormal outer or middle ear problems and is very sensitive to middle ear effusions and cerumen or vernix in the ear canal leading to a possible fail in the setting of normal cochlear function. OAE is the most common hearing screen performed in the well-baby population. Testing can be done within 10 minutes and the baby does not have to be asleep. OAE testing is limited in its ability to assess more central auditory abnormalities, as it only measures cochlear function of the outer hair cells, making it less effective in detecting neural dysfunction. Thus, a baby with auditory neuropathy could pass the OAE as the cochlea is functioning but the central neural problem remains undetected by the OAE. Screening with the OAE is likely to result in a higher fail rate in the immediate post-birth period as compared with automated auditory brainstem response (AABR).[4] Many centers perform two-stage testing, as recommended by the JCIH, meaning they will repeat the OAE only once with no additional attempts because the statistical chances of falsely passing increase, and if the infant does not pass, then referral to audiology is recommended.

### Automated Auditory Brainstem Response

Automated auditory brainstem response is a measurement of the electrical potentials formed in response to stimuli that reflect neural activity of the auditory nerve and auditory portions of the brainstem. The AABR is the recommended technology to perform hearing screening in the NICU population, as it tests not only cochlear function but also central nervous system response. The screen is performed by placing electrodes on or near the infant's ears, then presenting test stimuli through an ear probe or earphone. The resulting electrical activity is measured and the screening machine determines if the response is normal. The AABR uses mild-to-moderate hearing thresholds of 40-45 dB HL. The limitation of AABR thresholds is that there is a greater chance of missing babies with hearing thresholds of 25-40 dB HL, it takes longer than OAE, and it is better performed with a calm and quiet infant. Failing an AABR requires further testing and audiologic evaluation. Upon audiologic evaluation, infants undergo a battery of more detailed physiologic audiometry, usually including otoscopy, tympanometry, stapedial acoustic reflex test, OAE, and AABR.[19]

## Treatment Approaches

When considering treatment, the first priority is to protect the rights of the infant by explaining all options to the family, enabling them to make informed decisions regarding their child's ongoing care. It is worthwhile remembering that some people do not consider deafness a disability, and some may not want hearing aids or a surgical solution for their child with hearing loss. Regardless of whether the infant goes on to use hearing aids, a cochlear implant, or neither, families are encouraged to begin communicating with the child through sign language as soon as possible. Early intervention is critical for language development, which, in turn, is critical to the cognitive development of the child. This means that the family will need to learn sign language, as a visual language is the only option for a very young child who is deaf. Healthcare professionals can frame this positively as a family bonding activity. Even families with limited sign language fluency can benefit their children's cognitive and psychosocial growth.[20] Risk of developmental delay is caused not only by the hearing loss itself, but also by delayed language acquisition. Making both visual and oral languages available to a child through family support and exposure to good models of both language modalities primes that child for language acquisition and appropriate cognitive development.[20] Considerations advanced by advocacy groups are vital to optimizing family-integrated care.

Treatment will depend greatly on what type of hearing loss is determined and if it is thought to be syndromic, nonsyndromic, or acquired. Prenatal, birth, and neonatal history as well as the physical examination can lead initial workup of the infant, especially in the syndromic and presumed acquired causes. Initial workup generally includes screening for congenital infections, imaging, and genetic testing with audiology and ear, nose, and throat (ENT) referral. In the past, genetic testing was limited to screening for *GJB2* and *GJB6* mutations; however, there are now next-generation DNA sequencing genetic testing panels available for both syndromic and nonsyndromic associated hearing loss. A 2016 study evaluated 1,119 patients with SNHL who underwent comprehensive genetic testing and found the testing to be diagnostic in 39% of the study subjects, making comprehensive genetic testing the highest yield test in the evaluation of confirmed hearing loss.[21] Genetic counseling and testing also improve the ability to make treatment decisions, as cochlear implantation has limited success in improving hearing loss arising from certain genetic causes, for example.

In the case of acquired hearing loss, treatment will depend on the underlying etiology. For example, randomized controlled trials show that infants with congenital CMV show improved neurodevelopmental outcomes with ganciclovir treatment for 6 months starting in the first month of life and decreased hearing loss in the first 5 years of life.[22] Retrospective observational studies have shown ganciclovir to improve and preserve hearing at the age of 1 year.[23] Toxoplasmosis is treated with spiramycin, pyrimethamine, and sulfadiazine, but the degree of hearing loss from toxoplasmosis and how treatment may impact hearing is less well known. In the cases of rubella, syphilis, and Zika, the mainstay treatment is prevention, early detection, and continued hearing surveillance.

Conventional hearing aids are most often used in confirmed SNHL, but sometimes may be used in conductive hearing loss too when other options are not available or will be performed later in the infant's life. The goal is to fit amplification devices by 4 months of age, according to the JICH. It is important that infants have expedited fitting and frequent follow-up to assure appropriate fit and function of the hearing aid. Present-day hearing aids are digital and customizable to the infant's needs; most infants use the behind the ear style. Hearing gains for these aids range from 35 to 65 dB depending on type of aid used and are programed to the individual's needs. While there are immense advantages to hearing aids and early use, there are also drawbacks including cost, complications with fitting, and cosmetic concerns.

With the disadvantages of typical hearing aids, there has been a lot of excitement about the use of cochlear implants and studies have shown the earlier this is done, the better the outcome. Cochlear implants are not recommended, however, until around 1 year of age, and the need for surgery, high cost, and lack of insurance reimbursement have limited their use somewhat. Currently, the US Food and Drug Administration (FDA) has approved use of cochlear implants in children aged 9 months or older, but many have been implanted younger, off protocol, than the previously approved minimum age of 12 months.[24,25] Cochlear implants are considered the standard-of-care in children with profound congenital hearing loss in families whose goal is development of spoken language. Bilateral cochlear implantation shows improved outcomes over unilateral implantation and when done early, children can achieve nearly equal receptive and expressive language growth when compared to their normal hearing peers.[24,25] Side effects from cochlear implantation may include bleeding, increased risk of meningitis, device malfunction, facial nerve weakness, ringing in the ear, dizziness, and poor hearing result. Although often advertised as a cure, it is more similar to a treatment that requires intense support from otorhinolaryngologists, audiologists specializing in cochlear implantation, years of support from speech therapists, and the family **(Fig. 3)**.

In the case of permanent conductive hearing loss, a bone-anchored hearing aid may be an option, but can be challenging to treat with varying benefits dependent on hearing thresholds. These bone-anchored aids work by using vibratory stimuli to the mastoid bone, thus stimulating the

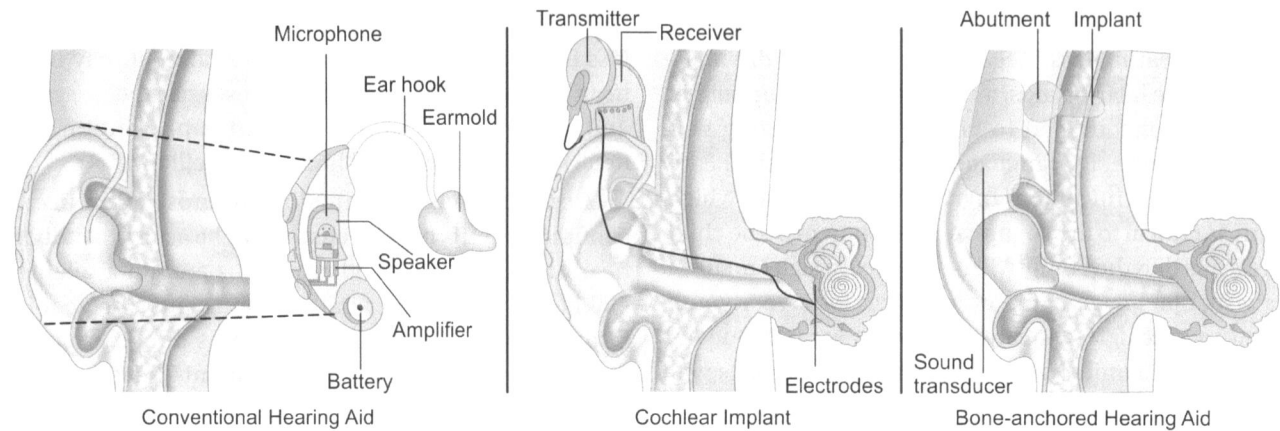

**Fig. 3:** Nonmedical treatments for hearing loss.

cochlea directly. They can also be used in unilateral SNHL. Other surgical options may be successful in improving conductive hearing loss, for example, repair of congenital aural atresia, the tympanic membrane, or ossicles.[7,19]

## Healthcare Delivery and Hearing Programs

It is important to have an institutional program led by audiology, trained screening staff, state mandated reporting of data, and at least annual calibration of the testing equipment. An organized system for referral to audiology and early intervention is essential. Infants with congenital hearing loss without other disabilities can have language development similar to their hearing peers if early intervention is started before 6 months of age.[26] Continued hearing surveillance is paramount, especially in high-risk infants, as only 50% of permanent hearing loss is identified by the newborn screen.[12] This responsibility falls to the medical home to follow high-risk infants and rescreen as necessary according to their risks and to address any parental or caregiver concerns.

Guidelines for pediatric medical home providers are shown in **Flowchart 1** and are adapted from the AAP 2007 statement.[12]

## Newborn Hearing Loss: A Summary

Newborn hearing loss is prevalent and requires early diagnosis as well as prompt referral to audiology for evaluation and treatment. Early intervention is of paramount importance as decades of research support better neurodevelopmental outcomes with early therapy and treatment. There are many potential causes and risk factors that affect the hearing-impaired; thus, the medical team must have a basic understanding of the challenges these infants and their families face.

Despite well-developed universal hearing screening programs in the US, follow-up still remains a challenge. Fortunately, many supporting organizations such as the JCIH, AAP, and the American Speech Language Hearing Association help direct programs and support families of infants with hearing loss. Advances in technology in audiology and otolaryngology as well as genetics continue to further diagnostic and treatment capabilities. In the near future, universal screening protocols may include universal genetic testing and CMV screening as technology continues to develop. Healthcare providers are encouraged to help parents filter through the advice, hearing technologies, therapies, and resources to help their child navigate the world successfully.

## CRITICAL CONGENITAL HEART DISEASE

The second point-of-care screening commonly used at birth is testing for congenital heart disease (CHD). While CHD occurs in 8 per 1,000 live births, about 12.5% of these are critical occurring with a prevalence of 1 in 1,000 live births.[27] CCHD is defined as a structural defect of the heart or great vessels requiring interventional catheterization or heart surgery in the first few days or weeks of life, without which severe morbidity or mortality would ensue. These defects typically include severe hypoxemic conditions (classically detected by obtaining blood arterial oxygen in the 100% oxygen challenge test) readily detected with transcutaneous pulse oximetry. Left ventricular outflow tract obstructive lesions and aortic arch anomalies are more challenging to detect and may be missed with oxygen saturation screening. Additional approaches such as screening with perfusion index show promise during ductal closure only and are not optimal screening methodology.[28,29]

## Historical Perspective and Cost-effectiveness of Universal Critical Congenital Heart Disease Screening

Early research using pulse oximetry to screen for CCHD was first reported in 1995.[30,31] Since that time, much research

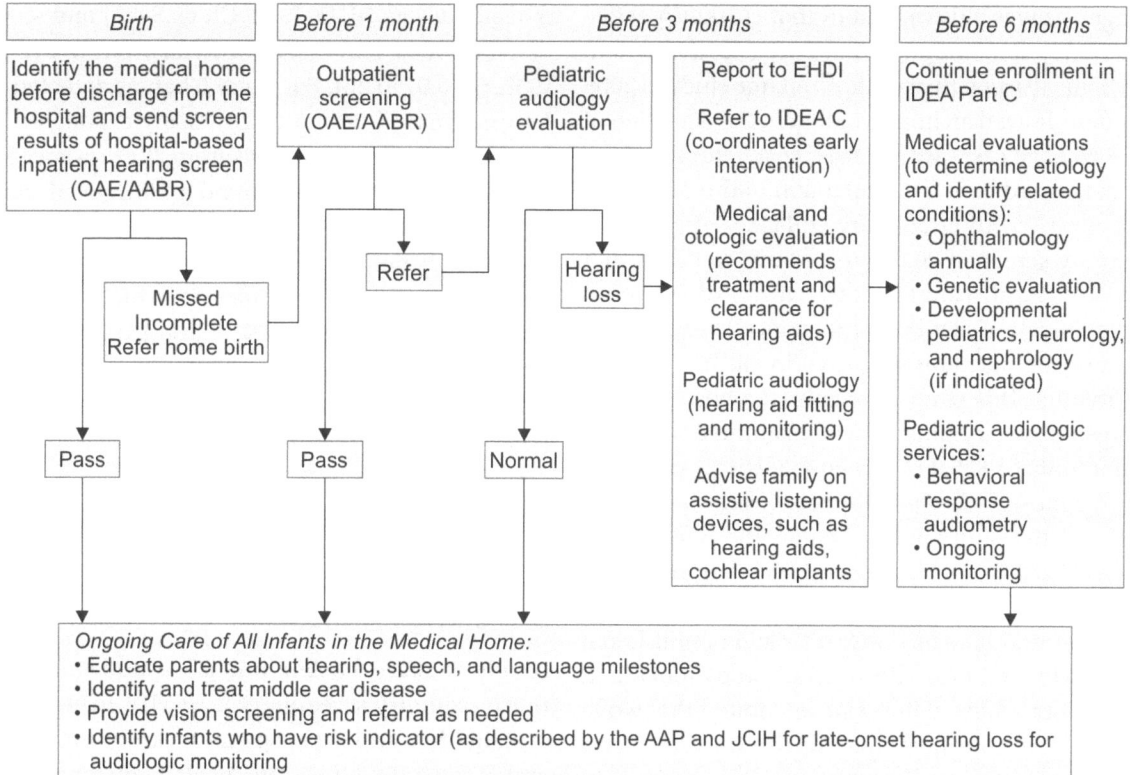

**Flowchart 1:** Guidelines for Newborn Hearing Screening, Diagnosis of Hearing Loss, and Intervention.

(AABR: automated auditory brainstem response; AAP: the American Academy of Pediatrics; EHDI: early hearing and detection and intervention; JCIH: Joint Commission on Infant Hearing; IDEA C: Part C of the Individuals with Disabilities Education Act; OAE: otoacoustic emissions)
*Source:* Adapted from the AAP Universal Newborn Hearing Screening, Diagnosis, and Intervention Guidelines for pediatric medical home providers.[12]

has emerged evaluating the accuracy, cost-effectiveness, and implementation strategies of universal pulse oximetry screening for CCHD and will be discussed throughout this chapter. In 2009, AAP and the American Heart Association (AHA) reviewed growing evidence and concluded that pulse oximetry may improve the detection of CCHD, but they could not recommend universal implementation at that time due to the lack of large population studies.[32] One year later, the US Secretary of Health and Human Services recommended that pulse oximetry for CCHD should be added to the Recommended Uniform Screening Panel (RUSP) in addition to current testing such as metabolic and hearing screening. In 2011, the AAP developed a workgroup and published "Strategies for Implementing Pulse Oximetry Screening for CCHD," recommending universal pulse oximetry screening.[33] Many states began the practice of universal CCHD screening prior to legislative requirements; it was not until 2018 that CCHD screening became a required addition to the RUSP in the United States.[33,34]

Prenatal detection of complex congenital heart defects in the US in 2011 was, at best, 50%.[35] An international birth defect clearinghouse published their retrospective data from 15 different programs during 2000–2014, evaluating 18,243 cases of complex CHD per 8,847,801 births, with a prevalence of 19.1/10,000 (range 10–31/10,000 births). Approximately one-third of the 15 programs had a 50% detection rate with trends of increasing detection.[36] A retrospective study from China reviewed 1,492 cases of CHD, where 583 cases were described as complex CHD and prenatal ultrasound accuracy was 91%.[37] As technology has improved, imaging quality and diagnostic ability have advanced as well. However, there are still modern-day challenges that make prenatal diagnosis difficult and deter women from receiving appropriate prenatal care, such as the increasing rate of maternal obesity, opioid addiction, racial and ethnic disparities in prenatal care, and increasing healthcare costs. Universal pulse oximetry screening for CCHD can be especially helpful in those cases of no prenatal care or limited imaging capacity due to body habitus.

Many industrialized nations, including countries in Europe and the Americas, have begun routine CCHD screening in the last decade. The People's Republic of China hopes to implement universal screening in 2020. There is data to suggest that earlier diagnosis of CCHD is both cost-effective and leads to improved infant outcomes.

A 2005 study used a decision analytical model to evaluate the detection rate in the United Kingdom by pulse oximetry and by screening echocardiogram as key drivers for cost compared to clinical examination alone. They found that timely diagnosis was elusive, and in that current practice model, oximetry screening was not cost-effective due to projected high false positive results.[38] A large study in 2009 out of Sweden showed an improvement in the detection of CCHD to 92% of all cases with at least cost neutral savings for every diagnosed case in comparison to the cost of an infant presenting with circulatory collapse.[28] By 2012, a large UK study screened 20,000 newborns, resulting in a sensitivity of 75% with a low false positive rate of 0.84% and a high detection rate of significant (not critical) heart defects and respiratory or infectious diagnoses in the false positive screened infants. This study determined a cost-effective ratio of pulse oximetry plus clinical examination versus examination only of £25,000 (US equivalent to ~$37,000) per timely diagnosis.[39] The first US cost-effectiveness study in 2013 used a decision analytic model and determined screening would cost approximately $6 per infant and could save 20 infant lives annually with a cost of approximately $40,000 per life year gained.[40] In 2017, China published a decision analytic and cost-effectiveness study looking at averted disability-adjusted life years and found that while examination alone is the most cost-effective, pulse oximetry screening combined with clinical examination resulted in the best health outcomes.[41]

## Supporting Evidence and Screening Approach

When considering universal CCHD screening, the benefits seem to overwhelmingly outweigh the potential risks that were initially speculated, such as increased healthcare use and costs (need for transport to larger center, echocardiograms, and consultations) as well as parental and staff anxiety. In 2011, the AAP published recommendations for a standardized approach to screening and diagnostic follow-up for CCHD in the normal newborn population. The AAP focused on identifying certain ductal dependent, hypoxemic defects: hypoplastic left heart syndrome (HLHS), pulmonary atresia (PA), tetralogy of Fallot (TOF), total anomalous pulmonary venous return (TAPVR), transposition of the great arteries (TGA), tricuspid atresia (TA), and truncus arteriosus. Not listed are coarctation of the aorta (COA) and aortic stenosis (AS), as they are frequently missed due to timing of ductal closure, milder obstruction at time of screening, and earlier newborn discharge. One study found that 7 in 100,000 live births had missed or delayed critical CHD diagnoses, with COA the most commonly missed defect.[42]

Many large meta-analyses have been done evaluating the effectiveness of pulse oximetry screening for CCHD. A Cochrane Review in 2018 published a review of 19 studies using >95% or 95% or greater as the oxygen saturation cutoff in 436,758 infants with a prevalence of CCHD in 6/10,000. Sensitivity was 76.3% (95% CI, 69.5-82) and specificity of 99.9% (95% CI, 99.7-99.9) with a false positive rate of 0.14% (95% CI, 0.07-0.22). For every 5 babies detected there will be one missed case and 14 falsely suspected infants.[43] Another large meta-analysis from 2019 reviewed 5 studies with 404,735 infants and found an improved sensitivity of 92% with pulse oximetry and examination, compared to 53% with examination alone. The specificity was 98% with pulse oximetry and examination, which was equal to the examination alone at 99%.[44] Thangaratinam performed one of the earlier meta-analyses showing similar findings as above and recommended the optimal time for the screening, as there were increased false positives when it was performed before 24 hours of age.[45]

Defects noted upon pulse oximetry screening as listed in the meta-analysis are shown in **Figures 4A and B**.

## Screening Protocol

In July of 2020, the AAP published updated strategies for pulse oximetry screening for CCHD. In this update, the stakeholders and expert panel reviewed current literature and re-examined the protocol allowing for minor changes to improve the ease and accuracy of the screening process while also improving the time to diagnosis. The updated protocol recommends performing the pulse oximetry screen around 24 hours of age or before discharge home from the nursery. Motion-tolerant oximeters that report functional oxygen saturations and are FDA approved for use in newborns with a 2% root mean square accuracy should be used. Healthcare workers who are trained to work with newborns and familiar with the equipment should perform the screen. The pulse oximeter is placed on the right hand for the preductal measurement and on either foot for the postductal measurement. The infant is considered to have passed the screen if pulse oximetry is 95% or more in the right hand and foot with a difference of 3% or less between the two measurements. The infant is considered to have failed the screen if pulse oximetry is 89% or less in either the right hand or foot; that infant requires immediate medical assessment without repeat screening. If an infant has oximetry of 90-94% in either the right hand or foot, or has a difference of 4% or more between the two measurements, the baby needs to be rescreened in 1 hour. Upon the second screening measurement, if the baby has oximetry of 95% or more in the right hand and foot and a difference of 3% or less between the measurements, this is a pass and no further screening is required. If the second measurement shows oximetry of 94% or less in either the right hand or foot, or a difference between the two measurements of 4% or more,

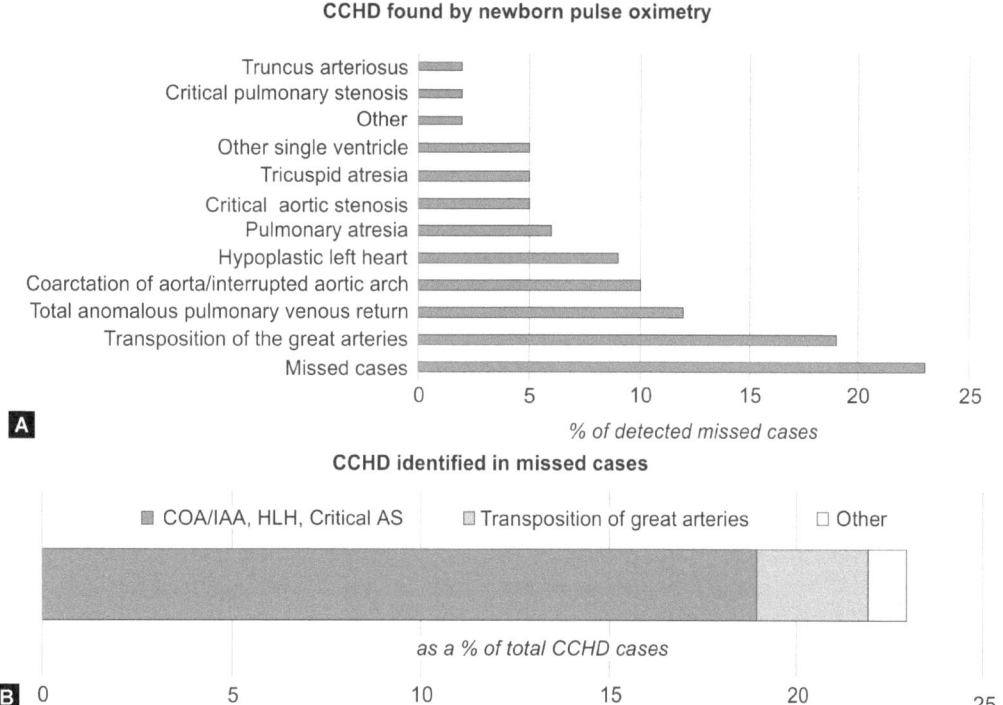

**Figs. 4A and B:** Simplified illustrative distribution of the 114 critical congenital heart disease (CCHD) lesions from 10 studies (excluding three studies that had prenatally diagnosed CCHD) included in the meta-analysis by Thangaratinam et al.[45] Saturation screened, N (190,867); true-positives, n (88); false-negatives, n (26).
(AS: aortic stenosis; CoA/IAA: coarctation of the aorta/interrupted aortic arch; HLH: hypoplastic left heart)
*Source:* Adapted from Govindaswami.[27]

this is a failed screen and the baby requires immediate medical assessment. See **Flowchart 2** for the screening algorithm, adapted from the AAP 2020 statement.[46]

The AAP update continues to recommend a lower limit of oximetry of 95% for both pre- and postductal measurements. Having both measurements is useful in detecting defects with reversed differential cyanosis, for example, TGA with pulmonary hypertension, interrupted aortic arch, or supracardiac TAPVR. In the case of COA, the narrowed area may not be obstructed at time of screening, leading to less hypoxemia, so the postductal saturations could still be normal. The AAP update recommended only rescreening a baby one time, as compared to the previously recommended two repeat screens before assessment.[46] Removing the second repeat screen prioritizes prompt evaluation of the infant who fails the screening; it does not change the sensitivity of the screen and only increases the false positive rate a small amount.[47]

It is helpful to review the function of the patent ductus arteriosus (PDA) in certain types of CCHD and how that would affect pre- and postductal oximetry. The PDA maintains pulmonary blood flow in PA, truncus arteriosus, and TOF. The PDA maintains systemic blood flow in HLHS, persistent pulmonary hypertension of the newborn (PPHN), critical aortic stenosis/coarctation/interrupted aortic arch, and it promotes mixing in TGA. Patterns of findings upon pulse oximetry screening can include having the preductal oximetry higher than the postductal and may be seen in HLHS, pulmonary hypertension, critical aortic stenosis, and COA or interrupted aortic arch. If the postductal saturations are higher than the preductal saturations, typical findings would be TGA or TAPVR. Often the pre- and postductal saturations can be similar and this is often associated with pulmonary atresia, truncus arteriosus, or tetralogy of Fallot. Though screening has been beneficial in detecting CCHD, it is still expected that there will be missed cases and a negative screen does not rule out the possibility of CCHD. Outflow tract obstructions may not be severe enough to have hypoxemia at the time of screening or in cases of CCHD where there may be pulmonary overcirculation the saturations may be normal, producing false negative results. Special considerations have been discussed in the NICU population, as implementing CCHD screening there is fraught with issues, for example, oxygen needs for other medical problems, optimal oxygen saturation limits for premature infants, and timing of screening. Despite the varied population in the NICU, there have been many studies showing pulse oximetry may still be a valuable tool in detecting CCHD with possibly a higher false positive rate and later date that screening occurs.[48-51]

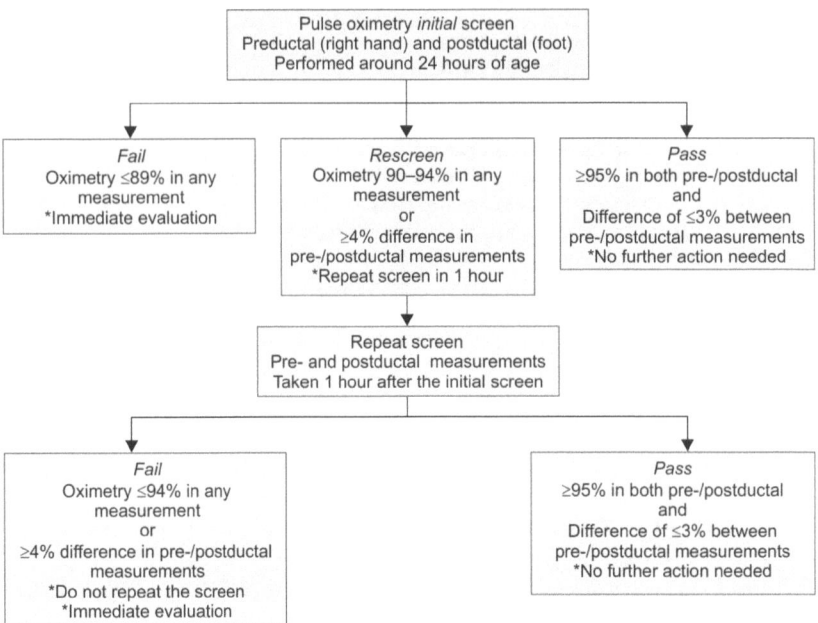

**Flowchart 2:** Newborn CCHD Screening with Pulse Oximetry.

(AAP: the American Academy of Pediatrics; CCHD: critical congenital heart disease)
*Source:* Adapted from the AAP revised algorithm for CCHD screening with pulse oximetry.[46]

It is important that hospitals performing this point-of-care test have a plan that can be quickly launched to evaluate infants who fail the screen. The plan may include transferring the infant to a hospital with an available pediatric cardiologist. Documenting in each patient's chart that screening occurred (and if not, why not), the age at screening, actual pulse oximetry results, and interpretation of pass/fail (if the infant failed, what intervention occurred) are all beneficial to audit protocol adherence as well as individual hospital or state reporting requirements, and possibly national tracking.

## Treatment Approach

Any infant who screens positive, or fails the screen, needs a physical examination by an experienced medical provider to see if there are other risk factors or abnormalities, such as a respiratory problem or sepsis. If the infant fails the screen with saturations of 89% or less, immediate evaluation is needed. If a healthy-appearing infant requires retesting based on saturation levels (90-94%) then fails the rescreen (94% or less), an echocardiogram must be obtained to evaluate for CCHD. Performing a hyperoxia test, electrocardiogram (EKG), four limb blood pressure measurements, and chest X-rays may help augment the workup, but these tests are not to replace or delay obtaining an urgent echocardiogram. Please see Chapter 24, Assessment and Treatment Options for Neonates with Congenital Heart Disease, to review medical and surgical treatment options. Many of the CCHD are isolated defects but special consideration should be taken to evaluate the infant for genetic abnormalities, environmental, and family risk factors. In diagnosing CCHD, upon discussion with the pediatric cardiologist, further studies such as comparative genomic hybridization, karyotype, fluorescent in-situ hybridization studies, and ultrasound may be warranted.

## Critical Congenital Heart Disease: A Summary

While the implementation of universal pulse oximetry screening for CCHD has been shown to be successful in detecting CCHD and reducing early infant cardiac deaths,[46,52] challenges remain in documenting, tracking and confirming that the screening program is successful. Furthermore, implementation of screening in special populations (such as infants born outside the hospital/home births, or NICU populations) poses unique challenges.

## CONCLUSION

Newborn point-of-care testing for critical congenital heart disease and hearing loss screens a majority of infants for congenital disorders of structure and function. Technological advances have made noninvasive screening at bedside (point-of-care) possible. Point-of-care screening occurs in time-sensitive "developmental windows" with high impact for preventing morbidity and mortality, allowing healthcare teams and families to design an appropriate discharge plan for each infant.

Optimal handling of these two newborn conditions, hearing loss and CCHD, will inform future opportunities for

| TABLE 1: Resources on hearing loss. | |
|---|---|
| The American Speech-Language Association (ASHA) | https://www.asha.org/public/hearing/Hearing-Screening/ |
| March of Dimes | https://www.marchofdimes.org/complications/hearing-loss-and-your-baby.asp |
| National Deaf Children's Society | https://www.ndcs.org.uk/information-and-support/childhood-deafness/causes-of-deafness/ |
| National Center for Hearing Assessment and Management, Utah State University | https://www.infanthearing.org |
| Joint Committee on Infant Hearing | https://www.jcih.org |
| National CMV Foundation | https://www.nationalcmv.org |

prevention and management in hospital-based healthcare delivery systems. There may be parallels for relevance for the current coronavirus disease 2019 (COVID-19)/severe acute respiratory syndrome coronavirus 2 (SARS-CoV-2) pandemic and the need for timely screening, optimal healthcare delivery systems, and infrastructure support (e.g., personal protective equipment, ventilators, and ICU beds).

Data from point-of-care testing presents an important opportunity for global incorporation of screening into healthcare delivery. In the future, additional noninvasive bedside tests will no doubt emerge to improve preventative healthcare for newborns.

Organizations which provide resources to the public on children's hearing loss, including knowledge of underlying cause and current testing, can be found in **Table 1**.

## REFERENCES

1. White KR, Vohr BR, Behrens TR. Universal newborn hearing screening using transient evoked otoacoustic emissions: results of the Rhode Island hearing assessment project. Semin Hearing. 1993;14:18-29.
2. Joint Commission on Infant Hearing. 1994 Position Statement. [online] Available from: http://www.jcih.org/JCIH1994.pdf. [Last accessed September, 2020].
3. Centers for Disease Control and Prevention, National Center on Birth Defects and Developmental Disabilities. Hearing Loss in Children: Data and Statistics about Hearing Loss in Children. [online] Available from: https://www.cdc.gov/ncbddd/hearingloss/data.html. [Last accessed September, 2020].
4. van Dyk M, Swanepoel de W, Hall JW 3rd. Outcomes with OAE and AABR screening in the first 48 h: implications for newborn hearing screening in developing countries. Int J Pediatr Otorhinolaryngol. 2015;79(7):1034-40.
5. Mehra S, Eavey RD, Keamy DG Jr. The epidemiology of hearing impairment in the United States: newborns, children, and adolescents. Otolaryngol Head Neck Surg. 2009;140(4):461-72.
6. Hille ET, Van Straaten H, Verkerk PH. Prevalence and independent risk factors for hearing loss in NICU infants. Acta Pædiatrica. 2007;96:1155-8.
7. Korver AM, Smith RJ, Van Camp G, et al. Congenital hearing loss. Nat Rev Dis Primers. 2017;3:16094.
8. Shearer AE, Shen J, Amr S, et al. A proposal for comprehensive newborn hearing screening to improve identification of deaf and hard-of-hearing children. Genet Med. 2019;21:2614-30.
9. Driscoll C, Beswick R, Doherty E, et al. The validity of family history as a risk factor in pediatric hearing loss. Int J Pediatr Otorhinolaryngol. 2015;79(5):654-9.
10. Van Camp G, Smith RJH. Hereditary Hearing Loss Homepage. [online] Available from: https://hereditaryhearingloss.org. [Last accessed September, 2020].
11. Joint Committee on Infant Hearing. Year 2019 Position Statement: Principles and Guidelines for Early Hearing Detection and Intervention Programs. J Early Hearing Detect Interven (JEHDI). 2019;4(2):1-44.
12. American Academy of Pediatrics, Joint Committee on Infant Hearing. Year 2007 Position Statement: Principles and Guidelines for Early Hearing Detection and Intervention Programs. Pediatrics. 2007;120(4):898-921.
13. Goderis J, De Leenheer E, Smets K, et al. Hearing loss and congenital CMV infection: a systematic review. Pediatrics. 2014;134(5):972-82.
14. Grosse SD, Ross DS, Dollard SC. Congenital cytomegalovirus (CMV) infection as a cause of permanent bilateral hearing loss: a quantitative assessment. J Clin Virol. 2008;41(2):57-62.
15. National CMV Foundation (2020). Cytomegalovirus. [online] Available from: https://www.nationalcmv.org. [Last accessed September, 2020].
16. Gantt S, Dionne F, Kozak FK, et al. Cost-effectiveness of Universal and Targeted Newborn Screening for Congenital Cytomegalovirus Infection. JAMA Pediatr. 2016;170(12):1173-80.
17. Diener ML, Zick CD, Browning McVicar S, et al. Outcomes from a Hearing-Targeted Cytomegalovirus Screening Program. Pediatrics. 2017;e20160789.
18. Vancor E, Shapiro ED, Loyal J. Results of a Targeted Screening Program for Congenital Cytomegalovirus Infection in Infants Who Fail Newborn Hearing Screening. J Pediatr Infect Dis Soc. 2019;8(1):55-9.
19. McGrath A, Vohr R. Hearing Loss in the Newborn Infant: Early Hearing Detection and Intervention. NeoReviews. 2017;18(10):e587-97.
20. Humphries T, Kushalnagar P, Mathur G, et al. Support for parents of deaf children: common questions and informed, evidence-based answers. Int J Pediatr Otorhinolaryngol. 2019;118:134-42.
21. Sloan-Heggen CM, Bierer AO, Shearer AE, et al. Comprehensive genetic testing in the clinical evaluation of 1119 patients with hearing loss. Hum Genet. 2016;135(4):441-50.
22. Kimberlin DW, Lin CY, Sanchez PJ, et al. Effect of ganciclovir therapy on hearing in symptomatic congenital cytomegalovirus disease involving the central nervous system: a randomized, controlled trial. J Peds. 2003;143(1):16-25.

23. Pasternak Y, Ziv L, Attias J, et al. Valganciclovir is beneficial in children with congenital cytomegalovirus and isolated hearing loss. J Pediatr. 2018;199:166-70.
24. Miyamoto RT, Colson B, Henning S, Pisoni D. Cochlear implantation in infants below 12 months of age. World J Otorhinolaryngol Head Neck Surg. 2018;3(4):214-8.
25. Dettman SJ, Pinder D, Briggs RJ, et al. Communication development in children who receive the cochlear implant younger than 12 months: risks versus benefits. Ear Hear. 2007;28(2 Suppl):11S-8S.
26. Yoshinaga-Itano C, Coulter D, Thomson V. Developmental outcomes of children with hearing loss born in Colorado hospitals with and without universal newborn hearing screening programs. Semin Neonatol. 2001;6(6):521-9.
27. Govindaswami B, Jegatheesan P, Song D. Oxygen Saturation Screening for Critical Congenital Heart Disease. NeoReviews. 2012;13(12):e724-31.
28. de-Wahl Granelli A, Wennergren M, Sandberg K, et al. Impact of pulse oximetry screening on the detection of duct dependent congenital heart disease: a Swedish prospective screening study in 39,821 newborns. BMJ. 2009;338:a3037.
29. Jegatheesan P, Nudelman M, Goel K, et al. Perfusion index in healthy newborns during critical congenital heart disease screening at 24 hours: retrospective observational study from the USA. BMJ Open. 2017;7(12):e017580.
30. Byrne B, Donohue P, Bawa R, et al. Oxygen saturation as a screening test for critical congenital heart disease [abstract]. Pediatr Res. 1995;379(suppl):198A.
31. Kao BA, Feit LR, Werner JC. Pulse oximetry as a screen for congenital heart disease in newborns [abstract]. Pediatr Res. 1995;37(suppl):216A.
32. Mahle WT, Newburger JW, Matherne GP, et al. Role of pulse oximetry in examining newborns for congenital heart disease: a scientific statement from the AHA and AAP. Pediatrics. 2009;124(2):823-36.
33. Kemper AR, Mahle WT, Martin GR, et al. Strategies for implementing screening for critical congenital heart disease. Pediatrics. 2011;128(5):e1259-67.
34. Glidewell J, Grosse SD, Riehle-Colarusso T, et al. Actions in support of newborn screening for critical congenital heart disease—United States, 2011-2018. MMWR Morb Mortal Wkly Rep. 2019;68(5):107-11.
35. Israel SW, Roofe LR, Saville BR, et al. Improvement in antenatal diagnosis of critical congenital heart disease implications for postnatal care and screening. Fetal Diagn Therapy. 2011;30(3):180-3.
36. Bakker MK, Bergman JEH, Krikov S, et al. Prenatal diagnosis and prevalence of critical congenital heart defects: an international retrospective cohort study. BMJ Open. 2019;9(7):e028139.
37. Qiu X, Weng Z, Liu M, et al. Prenatal diagnosis and pregnancy outcomes of 1492 fetuses with congenital heart disease: role of multidisciplinary-joint consultation in prenatal diagnosis. Sci Rep. 2020;10:7564.
38. Knowles R, Griebsch I, Dezateux C, et al. Newborn screening for congenital heart defects: a systematic review and cost-effectiveness analysis. Health Technol Assess. 2005;9(44):1-152, iii-iv.
39. Ewer AK, Furmston AT, Middleton LJ, et al. Pulse oximetry as a screening test for congenital heart defects in newborn infants: a test accuracy study with evaluation of acceptability and cost-effectiveness. Health Technol Assess. 2012;16(2):v-xiii, 1-184.
40. Peterson C, Grosse SD, Oster ME, et al. Cost-effectiveness of routine screening for critical congenital heart disease in US newborns. Pediatrics. 2013;132(3):e595-603.
41. Tobe RG, Martin GR, Li F, et al. Cost-effectiveness analysis of neonatal screening of critical congenital heart defects in China. Medicine (Baltimore). 2017;96(46):e8683.
42. Aamir T, Kruse L, Ezeakudo O. Delayed diagnosis of critical congenital cardiovascular malformations (CCVM) and pulse oximetry screening of newborns. Acta Pædiatrica. 2007;96:1146-9.
43. Plana MN, Zamora J, Suresh G, et al. Pulse oximetry screening for critical congenital heart defects. Cochrane Database Syst Rev. 2018;(3):CD011912.
44. Aranguren Bello HC, Londoño Trujillo D, Troncoso Moreno GA, et al. Oximetry and neonatal examination for the detection of critical congenital heart disease: a systematic review and meta-analysis. F1000Res. 2019;8:242.
45. Thangaratinam S, Brown K, Zamora J, et al. Pulse oximetry screening for critical congenital heart defects in asymptomatic newborn babies: a systematic review and meta-analysis. Lancet. 2012;379(9835):2459-64.
46. Martin GR, Ewer AK, Gaviglio A, et al. Updated strategies for pulse oximetry screening for critical congenital heart disease. Pediatrics. 2020;146 (1):e20191650.
47. Diller CL, Kelleman MS, Kupke KG, et al. A modified algorithm for critical congenital heart disease screening using pulse oximetry. Pediatrics. 2018;141(5):e20174065.
48. Van Naarden Braun K, Grazel R, Koppel R, et al. Evaluation of critical congenital heart defects screening using pulse oximetry in the neonatal intensive care unit. J Perinatol. 2017;37(10):1117-23.
49. Iyengar H, Kumar P, Kumar P. Pulse-oximetry screening to detect critical congenital heart disease in the neonatal intensive care unit. Pediatr Cardiol. 2014;35:406-10.
50. Goetz EM, Magnuson KM, Eickhoff JC, et al. Pulse oximetry screening for critical congenital heart disease in the neonatal intensive care unit. J Perinatol. 2016;36(1):52-6.
51. Manja V, Mathew B, Carrion V, et al. Critical congenital heart disease screening by pulse oximetry in a neonatal intensive care unit. J Perinatol. 2015;35(1):67-71.
52. Abouk R, Grosse SD, Ailes EC, et al. Association of US State Implementation of Newborn Screening Policies for Critical Congenital Heart Disease with Early Infant Cardiac Deaths. JAMA. 2017;318(21):2111-8.

# SECTION 6

# Cardiorespiratory Disorders

- Extracorporeal Membrane Oxygenation in the Neonate
  *John Patrick Cleary*

- Assessment and Treatment Options for Neonates with Congenital Heart Disease
  *Christina T Sheridan*

- Pulmonary Hypertension in the Neonatal Intensive Care Unit Setting
  *Yueh-Tze Lan*

- Patent Ductus Arteriosus
  *Priya Jegatheesan, Balaji Govindaswami*

- Common Cardiorespiratory Disorders at Birth
  *Kamakshi Devarajan, Balaji Govindaswami*

# CHAPTER 23

# Extracorporeal Membrane Oxygenation in the Neonate

*John Patrick Cleary*

## ABSTRACT

Extracorporeal life support (ECLS) is an adaptation of operative cardiopulmonary bypass (CPB) to allow prolonged support of heart and/or lung function in critically ill patients. The history and present status of ECMO indications and management are described.

## INTRODUCTION

Commonly referred to as extracorporeal membrane oxygenation (ECMO), it has been proven to benefit newborns with hypoxic respiratory failure and shock. In the last 40 years, ECMO has moved from a rare heroic intervention in dying patients to an accepted therapy around the world.

## HISTORY

Early attempts at CPB were led by Dr John Gibbon at Thomas Jefferson University. His work to develop a heart-lung machine began in the 1930s. He first used a roller pump-based circuit in the repair of an atrial septal defect in 1953.[1]

In the same time period, C Walton Lillehei MD was also advancing cardiac surgery in children using controlled cross-circulation, where commonly the parent served as extracorporeal circuit. Despite a possible 200% mortality, his team at the University of Minnesota performed 44 open heart surgeries in 1955, including the first repairs of atrioventricular (AV) canal and tetralogy of Fallot.[2] Operative CPB was limited due to hemolysis and bleeding complications associated with early oxygenators and anticoagulation. It was not well-suited for prolonged support. Dr Theodor Kolobow and colleagues developed a silicone membrane lung that improved the ability to provide prolonged support without excessive hemolysis.[3]

The work of Robert Bartlett MD and his group first in Orange County, California and later at the University of Michigan was pivotal in making ECMO part of newborn care.[4] In 1975, his team brought ECMO from the animal laboratory to the bedside when a newborn with severe hypoxic respiratory failure due to meconium aspiration syndrome (MAS) and pulmonary hypertension was successfully treated over a 3-day period. The story and ongoing life events of Esperanza (Hope), named by her nurses after her immigrant mother quickly left the hospital, have educated and inspired many ECMO team members.[5]

Empiric use of ECMO continued with survival superior to expectations of standard care. This led Dr Bartlett and colleagues to undertake a study with the statistically sound but later controversial design described as "randomized play the winner". With the goal of minimizing morbidity from an intervention, such trials begin with a balanced assignment but increase the likelihood of enrollment to a given arm based upon the ongoing results. Application of this design led to only one patient (who died) being assigned to control therapy, while all 11 patients assigned to ECMO survived.[6] This and related work by Dr Pearl O'Rourke[7] was validated in 1996 when the UK Collaborative ECMO Trial Group demonstrated the effectiveness of neonatal ECMO. This randomized trial enrolled 185 infants with severe respiratory failure before stopping early when a benefit of ECMO was demonstrated. Referral for ECMO was associated with one additional survivor for every three allocated to ECLS.[8]

## THE ESTABLISHMENT OF EXTRACORPOREAL LIFE SUPPORT ORGANIZATION

Following the lead of Dr Bartlett and others, the small number of centers performing ECMO for neonates gradually grew through communication and collaboration. In 1989, this community organized under the structure of the Extracorporeal Life Support Organization (ELSO). ELSO encouraged and facilitated the sharing of data, outcomes, and lessons learned in the use of ECMO. International experience with ECMO led to the establishment of the European Extracorporeal Life Support Organization (EuroELSO) and later an Asia-Pacific chapter of ELSO. Critical to the dissemination of information and standardization of ECMO was the creation of the ELSO registry, which has tracked data on tens of thousands of neonates. The registry allows the comparison of outcomes, complications, and approaches to care.[9] Participating centers can review the database in real time to guide clinical decision-making. Many important publications and clinical decisions have relied on the quality of the ELSO database and the collaborative spirit of ELSO.

## EXTRACORPOREAL MEMBRANE OXYGENATION IN THE NEONATE

While ECLS has expanded to support older children and adults, its original success and most common indication has been in the neonate. The use of neonatal ECMO peaked in 1992 with over 1,500 cases reported to ELSO. Use has fallen to approximately 800 neonatal respiratory cases per year with the introduction of new therapies such as nitric oxide therapy, surfactant, high-frequency oscillatory ventilation (HFOV), and more permissive approaches to ventilation.[10] The ECMO team should play a key role in the safe and thoughtful application of these pre-ECMO therapies. We must be careful that avoiding ECLS not become a goal in itself as the benefit of evolving therapies should be balanced with the proven effects of ECMO. Centers should have a transfer relationship with an ECMO center that allows safe application of evolving therapies without morbidity or mortality associated with the late initiation of ECMO. If an infant is failing conventional therapy (the terms "failure" and "conventional" are challenging to define) and has reversible disease (again, a challenge to define), then ECLS is indicated.

## EXTRACORPOREAL MEMBRANE OXYGENATION FOR RESPIRATORY FAILURE

The most common indication for ECMO in the neonate is respiratory failure complicated by pulmonary hypertension. Since the inception of the ECMO registry, MAS is the most common diagnosis to require ECMO support, with congenital diaphragmatic hernia (CDH), sepsis, respiratory distress syndrome (RDS), and idiopathic persistent pulmonary hypertension of the newborn (PPHN) frequently reported. In recent years; however, CDH and a category labeled "other" are coded as the indication for ECMO more often than MAS.[11]

## WHEN TO USE EXTRACORPOREAL MEMBRANE OXYGENATION

The historical indications for ECMO inform our present therapy but cannot be used as concrete indications, as they were based on the projected likelihood of death with standard therapies which have changed significantly. In the early years of ECMO, an oxygenation index (OI) over 40 predicted death with nearly 90% certainty, while by the time of the UK ECMO trial this same indication for entry in the trial had only 40% mortality in the control group.

$$\text{Oxygenation index} = \text{Mean airway pressure} \times FiO_2 \times 100/PaO_2$$

where,

$FiO_2$: Fraction of inspired oxygen
$PaO_2$: Partial pressure of oxygen.

The OI remains the most common way to communicate the severity of respiratory failure. It is simple to calculate yet incorporates the level of ventilator support along with the degree of intra- or extrapulmonary shunt. An OI over 40 on multiple blood gases for hours is an indication for ECLS at most centers. Schumacher, among others, has suggested that earlier initiation of ECLS when OI is between 25 and 40 may reduce morbidity.[12]

Other potential criteria to initiate ECMO include an alveolar-arterial oxygen gradient ($AaDO_2$) >620 for 4 hours or refractory metabolic acidosis. That acute deterioration is among the most common indications for ECMO reflects the challenge of optimally timing therapy. The decision to initiate ECMO is typically a collaborative decision of the primary neonatal intensive care unit (NICU) treating team and ECLS medical and surgical consultants.

## PRE-EXTRACORPOREAL MEMBRANE OXYGENATION EVALUATION

Before initiating ECLS, an echocardiogram is routinely obtained to rule out congenital heart disease as the cause of hypoxemia. Extra attention must be given to the pulmonary veins as total anomalous pulmonary venous return (TAPVR) with obstruction can mimic lung disease and there are many reports of making this diagnosis after initiating ECLS. In addition, a head ultrasound (US) is routinely performed before ECLS.

## CONTRAINDICATIONS TO EXTRACORPOREAL LIFE SUPPORT

Extracorporeal membrane oxygenation should not be initiated in the setting of lethal malformations or congenital anomalies, severe brain damage or intracranial hemorrhage. ECMO is not offered in the setting of significant prematurity (typically <34 weeks gestational age) due to the likely complication of intracerebral hemorrhage (ICH). Late preterm (34–36$^{6/7}$ weeks' gestational age) infants are more likely to die or have serious neurological complications when placed on ECMO, and therefore the threshold to place an infant on ECLS is typically higher. CPB in the preterm neonate is an area of ongoing research and progress.[13] A weight of less than 2 kilograms is a relative contraindication to ECLS because of anticipated challenges with cannulation. Intraventricular hemorrhage grade 1–2 is another relative contraindication to ECMO.

## MODE OF EXTRACORPOREAL LIFE SUPPORT

When beginning ECLS in the newborn, a decision to support with veno-venous (V-V) versus veno-arterial (V-A) is made. In V-A ECMO, a catheter is placed in the right atrium via the jugular vein to allow drainage of venous blood and a return catheter is placed in the carotid artery optimally positioned with the tip at the aortic arch. For V-V ECMO, a double lumen cannula is placed via the internal jugular vein with the larger venous return ports positioned low in the right atrium and returning arterialized blood directed towards the tricuspid valve.

Veno-venous ECMO has several potential advantages in treating neonatal respiratory failure, perhaps the greatest of which is avoiding ligation of the carotid artery. Returning oxygenated blood to the right side of the heart could directly benefit pulmonary vascular resistance, in contrast to the bypass of V-A ECLS. V-V ECMO avoids the acute reduction in preload and increase in afterload associated with V-A ECMO, which avoids possible cardiac stun on the initiation of ECLS. The maintenance of pulsatile flow to the systemic circulation is another potential benefit.[14]

While V-A ECMO is indicated for cardiac failure, there is a perception that V-A ECLS should be used in the setting of a high pressor requirement in the setting of respiratory failure.

With the initiation of V-V ECMO, the reversal of hypoxia typically lead to improved myocardial performance and inotropes are commonly weaned rapidly. A common bias towards V-A ECLS for CDH is not supported by a number of reports.[15]

Despite the potential benefits of V-V ECMO, the ELSO registry does not demonstrate a difference in outcome between patients treated with V-V or V-A and about two-thirds of the ECMO support reported to the registry remains V-A.

## THE EXTRACORPOREAL MEMBRANE OXYGENATION CIRCUIT

The ECMO circuit **(Fig. 1)** provides temporary support of pulmonary function via an artificial lung and can support heart function in V-A ECLS via a pump which returns blood to the patient. Historically, the majority of ECMO was performed using silicone oxygenators in which blood passes on one side of the silicone and blended sweep gas flows through the silicone to allow gas transfer. Recently, more efficient and lower resistance hollow fiber oxygenators, commonly used in operative CPB, have replaced the silicone lung for most ECLS. Sweep gas flow and composition are adjusted to a target pump arterial blood gas which is returned to the patient. The typical pump used for ECLS has gradually moved from a roller occlusion pump, which pushes fluid forward while compressing a length of tubing, to centrifugal pumps where a spinning element propels blood forward. With both pump types, support is adjusted by manipulating flow.

Additional components of the ECMO circuit include a heat exchanger and devices to monitor flow, pressure, and

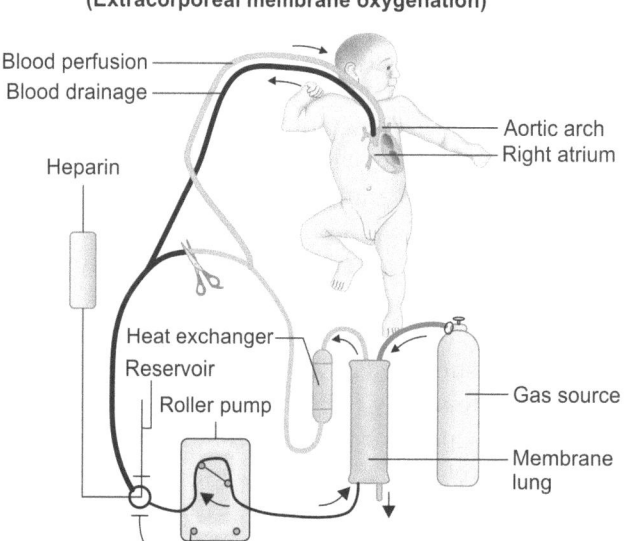

**Fig. 1:** Circuit diagram of infant on ECMO.

saturation. Heparin is used to minimize clotting, but must be monitored closely to avoid bleeding complications. An ECMO specialist or perfusionist typically monitors the circuit as their primary responsibility.

## EXTRACORPOREAL MEMBRANE OXYGENATION MANAGEMENT

When ECMO is initiated, the goal is to normalize oxygen delivery to the tissues by targeting a venous saturation of 70-80 on V-A and a oxygen saturation of arterial blood ($SaO_2$) over 85 on V-V ECMO. Typical pump flows are 80-120 mL/kg/min on V-A ECMO and approximately 20% higher on V-V due to recirculation.[10]

### Lung Rest

Once reproducible oxygenation has been established on ECMO, the ventilator settings should be reduced to minimize ongoing volutrauma and oxygen toxicity. $FiO_2$ is quickly reduced below 0.40 and commonly to 0.21. On synchronized intermittent mandatory ventilation (SIMV) the rate is typically reduced to <15 with peak inspiratory pressure (PIP) decreased to target a tidal volume of 3-5 mL per kilogram. A moderate positive end-expiratory pressure (PEEP) of 8-10 cm/$H_2O$ is recommended to limit volume loss and has been correlated with shorter duration of ECMO.[16] At our center; HFOV at reduced settings is commonly used for rest ventilation in the setting of severe lung disease or air leak syndrome.

### Anticoagulation

A critically ill patient supported with ECMO creates the interaction between a patient at risk for bleeding and a circuit that promotes thrombosis. Heparin is infused continuously (10-40 units/kg/hr) to target an activated clotting time (ACT) of approximately 180-200 seconds. This goal is adjusted based on the presence of bleeding or the recognition of clot in the circuit. Since heparin acts through antithrombin (AT), many centers will monitor antithrombin III (ATIII) levels and administer pooled or recombinant ATIII to target a level >70% of adult norms.[17]

It has long been accepted that ACT is an imperfect measure of adequate heparinization as it is also affected by platelet activity and coagulation factors. Most centers now supplement ACT measurement with the thromboelastography (TEG) and/or anti-Xa assay in addition to frequent measurement of coagulation panels and platelet levels.[18] Attempts to create a less thrombogenic circuit through heparin coating of circuit materials have shown some reduction in fibrinolysis but have not eliminated clotting complications or the need for heparin.[19]

While ECMO has proven to be lifesaving, it can be associated with meaningful complications, the most important of which is central nervous system (CNS) injury. About 5-10% of neonates placed on ECMO will have evidence of CNS hemorrhage or infarction; survival is reduced in this group of infants. Frequent head US is performed while an infant is on ECMO, and a post-ECMO CT scan or MRI is ordered. Cooling was considered a protective measure on ECMO, but based on present data is not recommended.[20]

### Weaning

Extracorporeal membrane oxygenation support is adjusted to target adequate venous saturation for V-A supported patients or arterial saturation for V-V. Duration of ECMO varies with the degree of lung disease and reversibility of pulmonary hypertension, ranging from as little as 3-5 days in patients with PPHN to more than 2 weeks in some patients with CDH. In the modern era, as ECLS has become less common for respiratory failure, evaluation for rare diagnoses such as alveolar capillary dysplasia or surfactant protein B deficiency should be pursued in infants failing to wean from ECLS.[21]

Gradually ventilator support and gas exchange move back to the patient's lungs, hopefully at relatively low levels of support. When flow is minimized, patients on V-A ECLS are commonly trialed off by allowing the circuit flow to continue via a bridge while the arterial and venous catheters are clamped and if successful, the catheters are removed. With V-V ECMO, the sweep gas flow to the artificial lung is reduced and then capped prior to removal of the catheter.[10]

## SPECIAL CONSIDERATION: CONGENITAL DIAPHRAGMATIC HERNIA

As ECMO has become less common for traditional indications such as MAS, ECMO use in patients with CDH has remained relatively stable. Overall survival with and without ECLS is improving after decades of high mortality. ECMO is appealing for patients with lung hypoplasia and potentially reversible pulmonary hypertension who are failing standard therapy. ECLS use varies across centers, but 15-30% of CDH patients receive ECMO, with survival of ECMO treated infants reported between 50% and 70%. Cooperation between ECMO centers via the CDH study group has led to several changes in perioperative CDH management.[22] Delivery room and preoperative management targets minimizing volutrauma either with pressure limited SIMV or HFOV. Permissive hypercapnia and acceptance of preductal saturations in the 70s to 80s in the first hours of life are common practices.

Spontaneous breathing is maintained and practices such as hyperventilation, induced alkalosis, and paralysis have been abandoned. Unlike other neonatal lung diseases associated with PPHN, nitric oxide has not been shown to reduce the need for ECLS in CDH, but is not uncommonly used.[23] Surfactant therapy also has conflicting data in CDH; despite evidence of reduced surfactant pools, a large prospective (though nonrandomized) study showed decreased survival in surfactant-treated infants.[24] Surfactant therapy is typically reserved for infants with radiographic evidence of hyaline membrane disease (HMD).

## Timing of Surgery

If adequate decompression of bowel is maintained, surgery does not improve ventilation and commonly exacerbates pulmonary hypertension. Because of this, surgery is often delayed for several days to allow improvement in pulmonary hypertension. CDH patients who are placed on ECLS typically are repaired on ECMO when support has weaned, or if possible after removal from ECMO.

The net effect of this multifactorial evolution in CDH care has been improved overall survival, with several large centers reporting survival over 80% after decades of >40% mortality.[25]

## SPECIAL CONSIDERATION: CONGENITAL HEART DISEASE

An area of significant increase in ECLS in the neonate has been in patients with congenital heart disease. While it was once considered futile to place an infant on ECMO following CHD surgery, it is now an accepted option in perioperative support. Common indications for ECLS in this population include refractory acidosis and a high pressor requirement. The low cardiac output state commonly improves with 48–72 hours of ECLS. Whenever ECLS is required, reversible surgical problems immediately should be considered and transport on ECMO for imaging or catheterization is common. Technical issues with cannulation and management of CHD on ECLS are important but beyond the focus of this chapter.[26] In rare instances, ECMO is used as a bridge to transplant or to other support devices.

## ANTICIPATED SURVIVAL WITH EXTRACORPOREAL LIFE SUPPORT

Anticipated survival with ECMO varies by diagnosis. As per the ELSO registry https://www.elso.org/Registry/Statistics/InternationalSummary.aspx,[27] patients with respiratory failure commonly wean from support in 5 days. MAS patients have reported survival of 94%, patients with PPHN or RDS have approximately 80% survival, patients with sepsis have a reported 75% survival, and CDH patients have longer ECMO runs (>10 days) and approximately 50% survival.

## COMPLICATIONS AND FOLLOW-UP

While ECMO has proven to be lifesaving, it can be associated with meaningful complications, the most important of which is CNS injury. Neonates placed on ECMO that show evidence of CNS hemorrhage or infarction (5–10%) have reduced survival rates. As with other critically ill newborns, close developmental follow-up is required for this population of infants. Major disability at school age is reported in 15% of ECMO-treated newborns and mild to moderate problems are reported in approximately 35%. These outcomes are similar to matched patients who did not receive ECMO.[27] The developmental prognosis for infants with CDH treated with ECLS is more guarded.[28]

## SUMMARY

Extracorporeal membrane oxygenation is a proven lifesaving therapy for infants with hypoxemic respiratory failure. While progress with other therapies has reduced the frequency of a neonate needing support, ECMO remains an important option in NICU care.

## REFERENCES

1. Fortenberry J. The history and development of extracorporeal support. In: Annich GM, Lynch WR, MacLaren G, Wilson JM, Bartlett RH (Eds). Extracorporeal Cardiopulmonary Support in Critical Care, 4th Edition. Ann Arbor, Michigan: ELSO; 2012.
2. Lillehei CW. History of the development of extracorporeal circulation. In: Arensman RM, Cornish JD (Eds). Extracorporeal Life Support in Critical Care. Boston: Blackwell Publications; 1993.
3. Kolobow T, Zapol W, Pierce JE, et al. Partial extracorporeal gas exchange in alert newborn lambs with a membrane artificial lung perfused via an A-V shunt for periods up to 96 hours. Trans AM Soc Intern Organs. 1968:14:328-34.
4. Bartlett RH, Gazzaniga AB, Toomasian J, et al. Extracorporeal membrane oxygenation (ECMO) in neonatal respiratory failure. 100 cases. Ann Surg. 1986;204(3):236-45.
5. Bartlett RH. Esperanza. Presidential address. Trans Am Soc Artif Intern organs. 1985;31:723-6.
6. Bartlett RH, Roloff DW, Cornell RG, et al. Extracorporeal circulation in neonatal respiratory failure: a prospective randomized study. Pediatrics. 1985;76(4):479-87.
7. O'Rourke PP, Crone RK, Vacanti JP, et al. Extracorporeal membrane oxygenation and conventional medical therapy in neonates with persistent pulmonary hypertension of the newborn: a prospective randomized study. Pediatrics. 1989;84(6):957-63.
8. UK Collaborative ECMO Trial Group. UK collaborative randomized trial of neonatal extracorporeal membrane oxygenation. Lancet. 1996;348(9020):75-82.

9. Domico MB, Ridout DA, Bronicki R, et al. The impact of mechanical ventilation time before initiation of extracorporeal life support on survival in pediatric respiratory failure: a review of the Extracorporeal Life Support Registry. Pediatr Crit Care Med. 2012;13(1):16-21.
10. Suttner DM, Short BL. Neonatal Respiratory ECLS. In: Annich GM, Lynch WR, MacLaren G, Wilson JM, Bartlett RH (Eds). Extracorporeal Cardiopulmonary Support in Critical Care, 4th edition. Ann Arbor, Michigan: ELSO; 2012.
11. Registry of the Extracorporeal Support Organization, Ann Arbor Michigan.
12. Schumacher RE. Extracorporeal membrane oxygenation. Will this therapy continue to be as efficacious in the future? Pediatr Clin North Am. 1993;40(5):1005-22.
13. Reddy VM. Low birth weight and very low birth weight neonates with congenital heart disease: timing of surgery, reasons for delaying or not delaying surgery. Semin Thorac Cardiovasc Surg Pediatr Card Surg Annu. 2013;16(1):13-20.
14. Cornish JD, Heiss KF, Clark RH, et al. Efficacy of venovenous extracorporeal membrane oxygenation for neonates with respiratory and circulatory compromise. J Pediatrics. 1993;122(1):105-9.
15. Guner YS, Khemani RG, Qureshi FG, et al. Outcome analysis of neonates with congenital diaphragmatic hernia treated with venovenous vs venoarterial extracorporeal oxygenation. J Pediatric Surg. 2009;44(9):1691-701.
16. Keszler M, Ryckman FC, McDonald JV Jr, et al. A prospective, multicenter, randomized study of high versus low positive end-expiratory pressure during extracorporeal membrane oxygenation. J Pediatr. 1992;120(1):107-13.
17. Byrnes JW, Swearingen CJ, Prodhan P, et al. Antithrombin III supplementation on extracorporeal membrane oxygenation: impact on heparin dose and circuit life. ASAIO J. 2014;60(1):57-62.
18. Bembea MM, Annich G, Rycus P, et al. Variability in anticoagulation management of patients on extracorporeal membrane oxygenation: an international survey. Pediatr Crit Care Med. 2013;14(2):e77.
19. Urlesberger B, Zobel G, Rödl S, et al. Activation of the clotting system: heparin-coated versus non coated systems for extracorporeal circulation. Int J Artif Organs. 1997;20(12):708-12.
20. Field D, Juszczak E, Linsell L, et al. Neonatal ECMO study of temperature (NEST): a randomized controlled trial. Pediatrics. 2013;132(5):e1247-56.
21. Deshmukh H, Lioy J. The use of early lung biopsy in detection of fatal pulmonary disease in the neonate. J Pediatr. 2014;164(4):934-6.
22. Harting MT, Lally KP. The Congenital Diaphragmatic Hernia Study Group registry update. Semin Fetal Neonatal Med. 2014;19:370-5.
23. Campbell BT, Herbst KW, Briden KE, et al. Inhaled nitric oxide use in neonates with congenital diaphragmatic hernia. Pediatrics. 2014;134(2):e420-6.
24. Cogo PE, Simonato M, Danhaive O, et al. Impaired surfactant protein B synthesis in infants with congenital diaphragmatic hernia. Eur Respir J. 2013;41(3):677-82.
25. Ruano R, Javadian P, Kailin JA, et al. Congenital heart anomaly in newborns with congenital diaphragmatic hernia: a single-center experience. Ultrasound Obstet Gynecol. 2014;45:683-8.
26. Cooper DS, Hirsch JC, Jacobs JP. Pediatric cardiac extracorporeal life support. In: Annich GM, Lynch WR, MacLaren G, Wilson JM, Bartlett RH (Eds). Extracorporeal Cardiopulmonary Support in Critical Care, 4th rdition. Ann Arbor, Michigan: ELSO; 2012.
27. Extracorporeal Life Support Organization. (2019). International Summary. [online] Available from https://www.elso.org/Registry/Statistics/InternationalSummary.aspx [Last accessed September, 2019].
28. McGahren ED, Mallik K, Rodgers BM. Neurologic outcome is diminished in survivors of congenital diaphragmatic hernia requiring extracorporeal membrane oxygenation. J Pediatr Surg. 1997;32(8):1216-20.

CHAPTER 24

# Assessment and Treatment Options for Neonates with Congenital Heart Disease

*Christina T Sheridan*

## INTRODUCTION

Congenital heart defects (CHDs) occur in 0.8% of live births. Advances in technology offer pediatric cardiothoracic surgeons, cardiologists, neonatologists, and maternal-fetal medicine physicians a range of diagnostic and therapeutic options. This chapter educates caregivers to assess, stabilize, and understand the treatment options available to CHD children and families.

## THE ROLE OF FETAL ECHOCARDIOGRAPHY: BEYOND THE FOUR-CHAMBER VIEW

Ultrasound has become invaluable in screening and diagnosis. Portable laptop-sized ultrasound allows practitioners to travel easily to patients. In 2003, nuchal translucency was introduced for screening fetuses 11–13[6/7] weeks' gestation. In conjunction with maternal age and same-day blood tests, the detection rate is 90–95% for trisomy 13, 18, and 21.[1] Cell-free fetal deoxyribonucleic acid (DNA) testing from maternal blood is offered for older mothers, prior child with a trisomy, parental chromosomal abnormality, or other positive screening tests for aneuploidy.[2]

The fetal heart is formed in the first 8 weeks and best imaged for CHD after 17–18 weeks' gestation. In healthy pregnancies, fetal anatomy scans are routinely done at 18–21 weeks. The fetal heart four-chamber view **(Fig. 1)** is inadequate to exclude CHD, as sensitivity for outflow tract **(Fig. 2)** abnormalities is poor. These lesions include dextro-transposition of the great arteries (D-TGA), truncus arteriosus (TA), partial atrioventricular (AV) canal defect, or AV discordance. Demonstrating left ventricular outflow tract (LVOT) with a slight anterior tilt of the transducer from the four-chamber view maximizes detection of significant cardiac defects, since fewer than 25% of CHD occurs in high-risk pregnancies.[3]

A level 2 fetal echocardiogram (echo) **(Table 1)** gives a more detailed structural and functional assessment of the fetal heart and helps in guiding the prenatal care and delivery plan.

First, cardiac situs and axis are determined **(Fig. 3)**. Intracardiac structures are shown by two-dimensional echo, followed by color Doppler, and then pulse/continuous wave Doppler. Since the fetus moves, the provider must

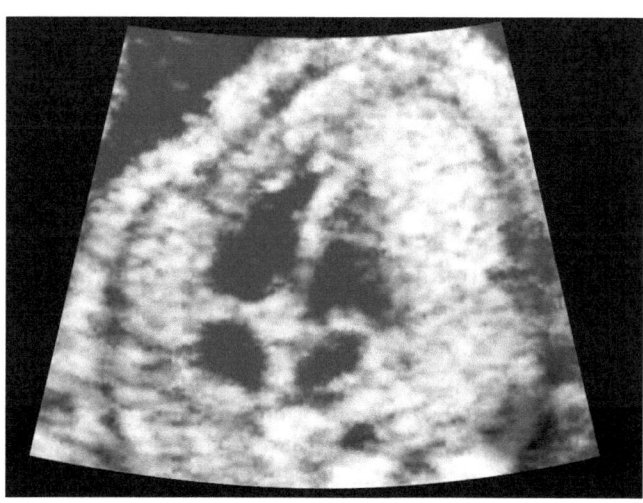

**Fig. 1:** Fetal four-chamber view.

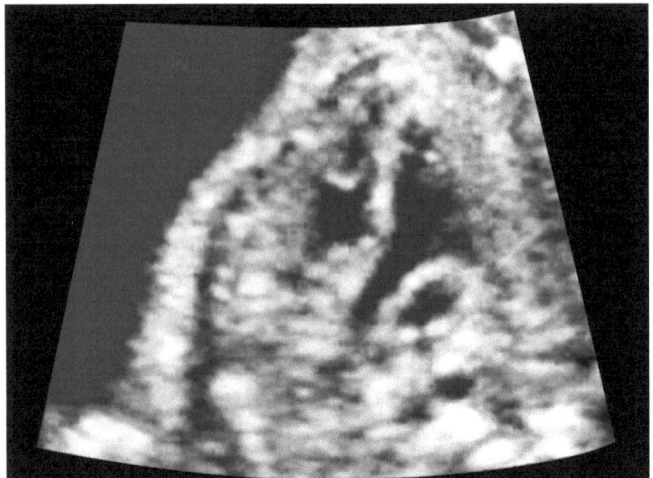

**Fig. 2:** Left ventricular outflow tract is shown in this five-chamber view. Apex of the heart is at 12 o'clock.

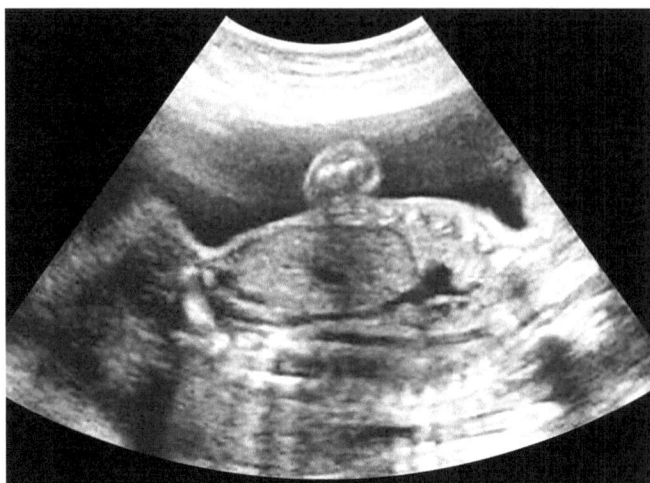

**Fig. 4:** Sagittal view of a fetus in spine-down, supine position, showing clear bicaval and arch views. Head is to the right.

| TABLE 1: Indications for level 2 fetal echocardiogram. ||
| --- | --- |
| *Maternal age >35 years* | *Gestational diabetes* |
| Family history of congenital heart defect | Maternal obesity |
| Abnormal four-chamber view | Twin gestation |
| Fetal arrhythmias | In vitro fertilization |
| Hydrops | Other fetal abnormalities |

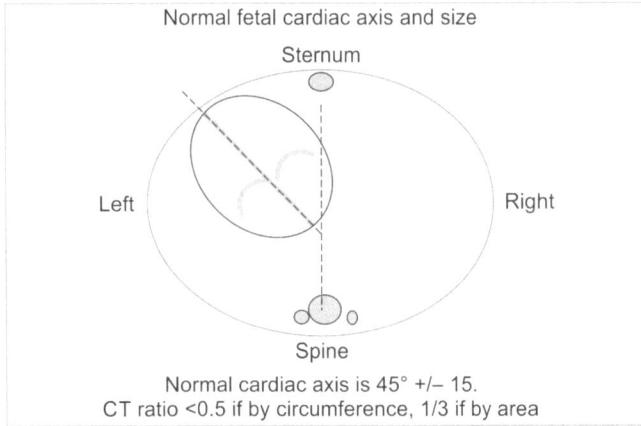

**Fig. 3:** Normal fetal cardiac axis and size (CT: cardiocthoracic).

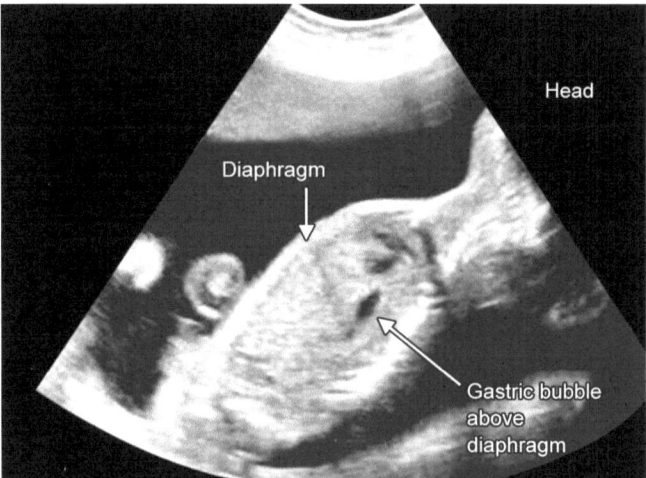

**Fig. 5:** Fetus with varying cardiac axis on serial fetal echoes. Image shows gastric bubble above diaphragm, consistent with congenital diaphragmatic hernia (CDH). When stomach was below diaphragm, cardiac axis was normal; when stomach slid through hernia, cardiac axis was abnormal and rightward (mesocardia).

have sound understanding of the spatial relationship of the anatomy.

Similar to transthoracic echo, fetal echo requires systematic evaluation of the situs, AV and ventriculo-arterial concordance, visualizing all four chambers, outflow tracts, and interrogation of inflow and outflows by color and pulse wave Doppler. In the ideal fetal position, spine-down relative to the transducer, images of the aorta, ductal arch, and descending aorta can be easily obtained. The normal fetal foramen ovale bows and shunts right-to-left, and the ductus arteriosus (DA) is as large as the aorta and shunts right-to-left.

The bicaval view from the subcostal sagittal view shows the superior vena cava (SVC), inferior vena cava (IVC), and descending aortic arch (AA), and is important when evaluating a fetus with suspected congenital diaphragmatic hernia (CDH) **(Figs. 4 and 5)**. Pulmonary veins (PVs) are quite small and receive only about 7% of the combined cardiac outflow in fetal physiology;[4] therefore verifying all four is not realistic. The important and high-yield "three-vessel view" is obtained from the high parasternal short axis and confirms great artery relationship. The three vessels seen are the SVC, aorta, and main pulmonary artery (MPA) with branching pulmonary arteries (PAs). A left SVC, if present, would be seen as a tiny circle to the right of the MPA **(Figs. 6 and 7)**.

Color Doppler enables interrogation of the atrial and ventricular septa, and quantification of valve regurgitation. It also shows the "hockey stick" angulation of the DA and "candy cane" appearance of the true AA. Both the foramen ovale and ductus shunt right-to-left in fetal circulation.

Fetal M-mode, which is a time motion display of the ultrasound wave against a time axis, demonstrates the 1:1 relationship of an atrial-to-ventricular contraction in sinus rhythm, or when atrial ectopy occurs. Pulse wave Doppler assesses inflow and outflow tracts for gradients and evaluates obstruction. A cursor placed at the junction between the mitral and aortic valve in the five-chamber view can calculate the mechanical PR interval. In mothers with known anti-Ro and anti-La antibodies, serial PR intervals assess the fetus at risk for developing heart block **(Fig. 8)**.

## LIMITATIONS OF FETAL ECHOCARDIOGRAM

Fetal echo image quality is limited by maternal obesity, anterior placenta, fetal position, late gestational age, and multiple fetuses. Maternal position change (side-to-side or a short walk) may encourage fetal position change. Small atrial and ventricular septal defects (VSDs), minor valve abnormalities, and ductal or arch anomalies may be missed in the fetus due to differences in fetal circulation and right-to-left shunting at the atrial and ductal level. If interrogation of the fetal heart is incomplete or suboptimal, newborn postnatal echo is recommended.

## USEFUL TOOLS

Nomograms and z-score calculators are available online and helpful when reporting on valve and vessel diameters. A friendly web calculator is Parameter-Z,[5] where z-scores are computed from prior published fetal/pediatric heart series. By entering the gestational age (GA), femur length, and valve diameters, the z-scores are then obtainable.

## WHEN STRUCTURAL CARDIAC DEFECTS ARE FOUND

Counseling CHD expectant parents takes time and practice. A genetic counselor is integral, especially if other abnormalities are found. Some parents decide to terminate the pregnancy once they have been informed about the genetic and anatomic workup. Serial echo assessments allow for additional opportunities to get more anatomical detail, while monitoring of interval chamber or valve growth, especially if there are concerns for valve stenosis, valve regurgitation or an arrhythmia. If anatomical details remain stable, and the CHD type does not require prostaglandins (PGE) at birth, the pediatric cardiologist can safely advise the parents to a vaginal delivery at term at a nearby hospital. However, if the type of heart defect in the fetus is complex

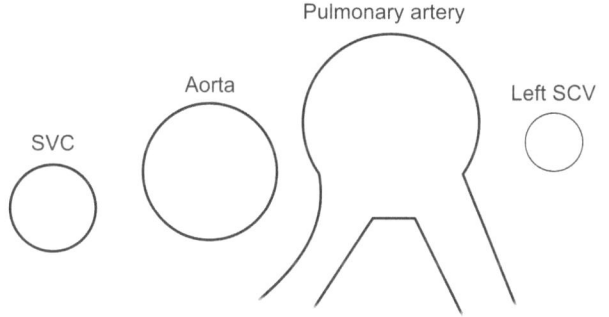

**Fig. 6:** Relative size and relationship of great vessels (schematic view of fetal chest) (SVC: superior vena cava).

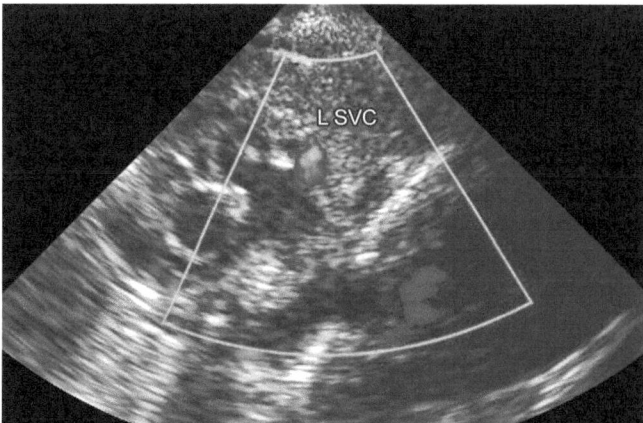

**Fig. 7:** High parasternal transverse three-vessel view of fetal chest in two-dimensional (2D), confirming relationship of the great vessels and their relative size to one another. A persistent left superior vena cava (SVC) would be seen as a small circle on the other side of the pulmonary artery (PA) *(For color version see Plate 3)*.

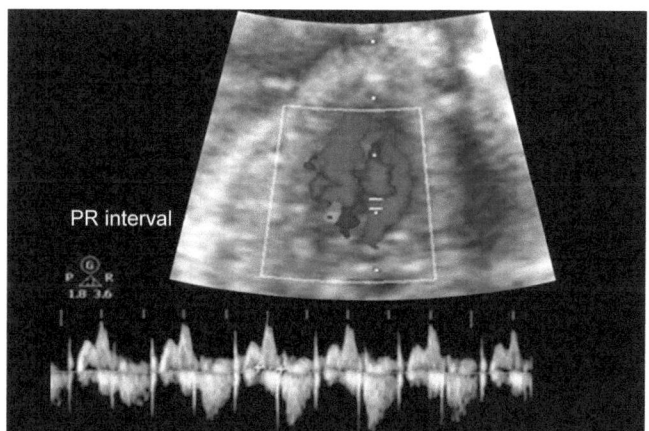

**Fig. 8:** Mechanical PR interval in a fetus. Doppler gate is placed at the junction of mitral and aortic valves. The mechanical PR interval (in milliseconds) is measured from beginning of the A wave of mitral valve to the beginning of the left ventricular outflow tract (LVOT) signal *(For color version see Plate 3)*.

and may require PGE or another early intervention, it would be appropriate to refer the mother to a specialized fetal center around 30–32 weeks of gestation to plan for her newborn's delivery with an informed obstetric, neonatal intensive care unit (NICU), and pediatric cardiology team ready. For instance, fetuses with isolated aortic stenosis can progress to a hypoplastic left heart syndrome (HLHS). Few centers have the capability and experience to perform fetal intervention to balloon-dilate the aortic valve to prevent HLHS.[6] Refractory hydrops or premature ductal closures are other indications for emergent delivery. The majority of fetuses with single ventricle complexes and D-TGA variants are born at term and delivered vaginally.

Types of CHD that are best managed prenatally or from birth at a tertiary care center include those with single ventricle physiology [i.e. HLHS, double outlet right ventricle (DORV), heterotaxy syndrome with unbalanced AV canal, or severe Ebstein's], transposition complexes, severe aortic or pulmonic stenosis, or tetralogy of Fallot (TOF) variants, particularly with absent pulmonary valves. With complex CHD, there may be increased risk of prematurity and fetal demise. Planning for delivery at a tertiary care center allows for prompt administration of prostaglandin E1 (PGE1) and surgical intervention if needed. Meeting members of the care team, including neonatologists, pediatric cardiologists, cardiothoracic surgeon, and social workers can help parents prepare for delivery and subsequent NICU course. In some centers, newborns with known critical pulmonary stenosis or pulmonary atresia with an intact ventricular septum are evaluated in the catheterization laboratory immediately after birth for radiofrequency perforation or balloon valve dilation,[7,8] or to perform a hybrid procedure in stage 1 palliation of the single ventricle repair.[9]

## ■ MANAGING FETAL ARRHYTHMIAS

With an incidence of ~0.3%, fetal arrhythmias detected during routine obstetrics (OB) visits, should prompt evaluation of fetal cardiac anatomy.[10,11] Associated cardiac defects include left atrial isomerism, Ebstein's anomaly, AV discordance, and cardiac tumors. Fetal tachycardia, defined as ventricular fetal heart rate (FHR) >180, is most pathologic when rates are higher (>200) and without variability. The most common causes are supraventricular tachycardia (SVT) or atrial flutter with varying degrees of AV block, and can be paroxysmal or sustained. For sustained tachycardia with evidence of hydrops, first-line treatment is maternal oral digoxin, monitoring maternal serum digoxin, and tolerance for nausea. When second-line medications such as sotalol, flecainide or amiodarone are initiated, maternal hospitalization for 2–3 days is required. This allows for monitoring of maternal QTc interval, serial ultrasound, and nonstress tests to quantify fetal tachycardia response to therapy.

Fetal bradycardia (FHR <100) is usually due to congenital heart block found in left atrial isomerism, AV discordance, or anti-Ro and anti-La antibodies. Rarely, fetal bradycardia may be due to functional second-degree AV block in a fetus with long QT syndrome. Mothers with lupus antibodies are usually asymptomatic in pregnancy. Treating fetal AV block may include giving the mother steroids and β-mimetics to prevent progression of autoantibody interference of AV conduction.[12] In pregnancies with anti-Ro or anti-La antibodies, weekly echo assessment of fetal PR interval allows for steroid intervention when PR prolongs. Although duration of weekly fetal monitoring is unclear, the period of highest risk for maternal antibodies crossing the placenta is between 18 weeks and 24 weeks; many pediatric cardiologists follow mothers between 18 weeks and 32 weeks of gestation. Prospective studies on fetal-maternal treatment options hope to improve outcomes.[13] Risk factors for fetal demise include FHR <55, structural heart defects, and hydrops.

Nonsustained irregularity in the FHR during the late third trimester is often caused by premature atrial contractions, typically in the late third trimester, with normal cardiac anatomy, FHR, and FHR variation. Ectopic beats decrease in frequency in the first month of life and require no treatment. Parents and obstetricians may be reassured that no special delivery precautions are necessary.

## ■ NORMAL NEWBORN TRANSITION

For transition from fetal to newborn circulation, three important changes must occur at birth. The lungs expand for air exchange, effectively increasing pulmonary blood flow (PBF) up to 20-fold. Secondly, the central shunts must close or reverse direction to enable the right and left sides of the heart to pump in series. Lastly, ventricular output must increase to meet the metabolic demands of thermoregulation and breathing.

The inspired oxygen and mechanical stretch of the first breath cause a rapid drop in pulmonary vascular resistance (PVR) and increase in PBF. Chemicals such as prostacyclin, bradykinins, angiotensin II, and histamine contribute to pulmonary bed vasodilation.[14] The greatest rate of change in PVR occurs in the first days of life, with a decline to near-adult levels by 1–2 months of life.

*In utero*, highly oxygenated blood from the placenta flows into the umbilical vein and ductus venosus, streaming alongside blood from the IVC, and is directed by the Eustachian valve across the foramen ovale and into the left atrium (LA). About one-third of the combined venous return flows right-to-left across the foramen ovale to the left heart and into the coronaries and head and neck vessels. At birth, the ductus venosus functionally closes, but is still accessible for a short while thereafter to place umbilical venous catheters. As the PBF increases, blood return to the LA increases and pushes the flap of the foramen ovale towards the right atrium, reversing the atrial shunt direction. A small shunt across a stretched patent foramen ovale (PFO) is present in normal newborns and spontaneously resolves in about 75% of all children by age two.

*In utero*, the fetal DA is as large as the ascending aorta, shunting right-to-left and diverting blood away from the MPA and into the descending aorta. Once the newborn takes his/her first breath, the ductus begins to close in the first 12–28 hours after birth, especially in term infants. Ductal constriction is altered by oxygen, bradykinin, catecholamines, and arachidonic acid metabolites. Ductal constriction occurs from the proximal left PA toward the isthmus of the aorta. As the DA, venosus, and PFO shunts change, newborn circulation between right and left heart, lungs, and systemic circulation become in series.

The fetus is right-heart dominant as it pumps out 65% of combined ventricular output. At birth, the PVR drops and systemic vascular resistance (SVR) increases as oxygen causes vascular beds in the brain and myocardium to constrict. With the shift to a higher afterload and slightly higher preload from PVs, the left ventricle (LV) becomes the dominant chamber in the first week of life.

In order to meet metabolic demands of life, the newborn heart must increase output threefold. As PBF rises with an exponential decrease in PVR, central shunts constrict or reverse directions, combined ventricular output and oxygen consumption triple, and then newborn transition is stable.

## NEWBORNS WITH SUSPECTED CONGENITAL HEART DEFECT

As PVR decreases and the patent ductus arteriosus (PDA) gets smaller, serial physical examinations are important. All newborns should have their respiratory rate counted and brachial and femoral pulses checked at each visit. Infants with dysmorphic features, known trisomy or chromosomal abnormalities or other midline defects warrant a pediatric cardiology evaluation with echocardiogram, even if there is no murmur on examination.

Symptoms of CHD in the neonate should be approached in a systematic fashion:
- *Cyanosis*: Due to decreased PBF or parallel circulation
- *Pallor and poor pulses*: Due to decreased systemic output, left heart lesions or pump failure
- *Tachypnea, respiratory distress, and retractions*: Due to increased PBF

**TABLE 2:** CHD with decreased pulmonary blood flow.

| Anatomic level | Lesion |
| --- | --- |
| Tricuspid valve | Ebstein's anomaly |
| | Tricuspid valve regurgitation, stenosis, or atresia |
| Right ventricle | Hypoplastic right ventricle complexes |
| | TOF with subpulmonic VSD |
| Pulmonary valve | Absent pulmonary valve |
| | Pulmonary valve stenosis or atresia with VSD |
| | Pulmonary valve stenosis or atresia with intact ventricular septum [TOF/PA/major aortopulmonary collateral arteries (MAPCAs), or with a single ventricle physiology and malposed aorta] |
| Pulmonary artery | Supravalvar or branch PA stenosis |
| Great arteries | D-TGA (parallel circulation) |

(CHD: congenital heart defect; D-TGA: dextro-transposition of the great arteries; PA: pulmonary artery; TOF: tetralogy of Fallot; VSD: ventricular septal defect).

- *Murmur:* Due to turbulent forward or backward flow across a valve, narrow vessel, or VSD
- *Arrhythmia:* Too fast (>200) or too slow (<70), without variability during sleep and various states of arousal
- *Dysmorphology* and chromosomal syndromes.

*Profound cyanosis* at birth may be due to CHD with decreased PBF **(Table 2)** or with parallel circulations, as in D-TGA. With D-TGA, the pregnancy history is typically unremarkable and the newborn is a term male. CHD affecting the tricuspid valve, right ventricle (RV), pulmonary valve, and PA impede effective forward blood flow to the lungs for oxygenation, and therefore right-to-left shunting occurs at the atrial or ventricular level. CHD with ductal-dependent PBF have progressive cyanosis as the ductus closes and PBF decreases. Newborns with cyanotic CHD often have silent tachypnea to increase oxygenation, but rarely demonstrate respiratory distress. The varying details and pathophysiology of right heart lesions will not be discussed in this chapter, but is easily found in other sources.[4,14,15]

Acrocyanosis of newborn hands and feet may be due to immaturity and vasoconstriction of distal peripheral beds. Central cyanosis; however, is seen on the face, oral mucosa, lips, and tongue. Infants with small ASDs (including PFOs) can appear transiently dusky when crying due to a small right-to-left shunt enhanced by increased intrathoracic pressure, but are pink and have normal oxygen saturations ($SpO_2$) when calm and feeding. Cyanosis is hard to detect visually until arterial saturation <85%, and is even more challenging in the presence of anemia or in dark-skinned

**TABLE 3:** Congenital heart defect with decreased systemic output.

| Anatomic level | Lesion |
|---|---|
| Pulmonary veins | Pulmonary vein stenosis, total or partial anomalous pulmonary venous return |
| Left atrium | Restrictive atrial septum (right-to-left shunt in HLHS), atrial tumor |
| Supramitral area | Cor triatriatum, supravalvar mitral ring |
| Mitral valve | Mitral stenosis, parachute mitral valve, mitral valve atresia |
| Left ventricle | Hypoplastic LV, dilated LV, LV noncompaction, hypertrophic cardiomyopathy, tumor |
| LVOT obstruction | Diabetic cardiomyopathy, tumor, subaortic ridge |
| Coronary arteries | Anomalous left coronary artery from the pulmonary artery (ALCAPA), intramural course or ostial stenosis |
| Aortic valve | Aortic valve atresia or severe stenosis |
| Aortic arch | *CoA*: Discrete posterior shelf or tubular hypoplasia, interruption of the AA (IAA) |
| Other | SVT, large pericardial effusion or epicardial tumor impinging on LVOT structures |

(AA: aortic arch; CoA: coarctation of the aorta; HLHS: hypoplastic left heart syndrome; IAA: interrupted aortic arch; LV: left ventricular; LVOT: left ventricular outflow tract; PA: pulmonary artery; SVT: supraventricular tachycardia).

babies. A pulse oximeter sensor should be placed on the right hand and any foot for continuous monitoring when a newborn appears dusky. Most pulse oximeters are accurate ~2–3% in the >91% saturation range, and ~5% in the lower oxygen saturation range of 76–90%.[16] Persistent pulmonary hypertension of the newborn and parenchymal lung diseases are differential diagnoses of mild cyanosis in the newborn, and present with respiratory distress and tachypnea. Chest X-rays provide cardiothymic silhouette and size, quality of lung fields, and any intrapulmonary abnormalities.

*Congenital heart defect with decreased systemic output* **(Table 3)** may mimic sepsis when an infant presents in shock. Ductal-dependent lesions such as critical coarctation of the aorta (CoA) or HLHS present within the first 1–2 weeks of life when the PDA closes. The infant demonstrates poor feeding, low urine output, tachypnea, and lethargy. Poor cardiac output results in accumulation of lactate, and tachypnea occurs to facilitate excretion of carbon dioxide. Prompt recognition of these symptoms is crucial to optimizing the baby's outcome. Initiation of intravenous (IV) PGE1, intubation, and avoiding hypothermic stress in the newborn may be necessary immediate steps, especially if CHD is suspected and femoral pulses are weak or absent. It may be easier to titrate PGE up or down than to reverse organ damage due to low cardiac output and delay starting PGE.

Poor perfusion may be due to cardiomyopathy, or pump failure. Dilated cardiomyopathy, incessant arrhythmias, anomalous coronary arteries, LV noncompaction syndromes, and inborn errors of metabolism present in decreasing order of frequency as etiologies for cardiomyopathy in the newborn.

*Tachypnea* is a common newborn symptom with many etiologies. As PVR declines after birth, PBF increases 20-fold. Infants with large ASDs, VSDs or AV canal defects present with failure to thrive and increased work of breathing between 1 month and 3 months of life, at the nadir of physiologic anemia. Unlike adults, who develop low output failure from a weakened, dilated heart, infants with these lesions develop high-output cardiac failure and have hyperdynamic precordia and high-normal ejection fractions. Infant typically become symptomatic when the volume of PBF to systemic blood flow (Qp:Qs) >2.5. Premature or otherwise sick infants may manifest symptoms of tachypnea and poor weight gain with a smaller Qp:Qs. Medical and/or surgical intervention in the latter subgroup of infants is required earlier to optimize catch-up growth.

Caloric requirements may be increased in the presence of CHD. Compared to the 80–120 kcal/kg/day requirement of a healthy term newborn, an infant with a large VSD may require 140–180 kcal/kg/day just to achieve normal growth velocity. High PBF may increase lymphatic flow and interstitial fluid that stiffen the lungs. Clinically, the infant may display head bobbing, suprasternal, abdominal and/or subcostal retractions, tachypnea at rest, and hepatomegaly. The liver engorges as a reservoir for the increased blood flow, but peripheral edema is not seen since venous pressures are not elevated. Tachycardia and forehead sweating during feeding may occur as a result of higher adrenergic drive and increased cardiac output. The increased caloric expenditure and work of breathing may present as an infant with a hearty appetite but poor weight gain.

Left-to-right shunts can occur at the atrial, ventricular, AV, arterial, and arteriovenous levels. With large ASDs, sinus venosus ASDs, or partial anomalous pulmonary venous return (PAPVR), newborns rarely become symptomatic because RV thickness and compliance are relatively high in the first few months. Atrial level shunts are dependent on compliance of the RV and occur in diastole. Large ventricular shunts occur in systole and are significant just after the newborn period during the nadir of the hematocrit and PVR, when the shunt volume is maximized. Infants with AV canals and LV-to-RA shunts or severe mitral regurgitation may develop tachypnea shortly after birth

**TABLE 4:** Cardiac defects with higher pulmonary blood flow (PBF) (Qp>Qs).

| Lesion | Intracardiac right-to-left mixing? |
|---|---|
| Aortopulmonary (AP) window | No |
| Atrial septal defect (ASD): Primum, secundum, sinus venosus | None if small |
| ASD: Common atrium | Yes |
| Arteriovenous (AV) malformation | No |
| Complete AV canal | Usually |
| Partial pulmonary venous return | No |
| Patent ductus arteriosus (PDA) | No |
| Total anomalous pulmonary venous return (TAPVR), unobstructed | Yes |
| Truncus arteriosus (TA)/conotruncal defect | Yes |
| Ventricular septal defects (VSDs): Perimembranous, inlet, muscular, outlet | None if small; yes if large |
| VSDs with single ventricle physiology | Yes |

because the atrium is always lower in pressure compared to the ventricle; thus the shunt is obligatory, or independent of the distal vascular bed resistance. Another obligatory shunt is the AV malformation. The degree of output failure depends on the size of the vascular malformation. Arterial shunts such as PDAs and aortopulmonary (AP) windows transmit flow during systole and diastole, thus causing high output failure at an earlier age. **Table 4** shows CHD with an increase in PBF and occurrence of cyanosis.

*Murmurs* are produced by turbulent blood flow through newborn heart structures or blood vessels, and are distinct from normal sounds produced by closure of heart valves. They may be benign, indicate a dysfunctional valve, outflow tract obstruction, a narrow vessel, or a pressure gradient across a septal defect. Murmurs are graded on a 1–6 scale: 1 is "soft," 2 "average," 3 "loud," and 4–6 indicates a palpable thrill is present, which is never benign. Thrills are caused by a high velocity jet of a pressure-restrictive VSD hitting the anterior wall of the sternum and transmitting kinetic energy, or from a surgically-placed conduit with severe stenosis. Murmurs 5–6 out of 6 are said to be "heard without a stethoscope" and are not often encountered in the developed world. Transient systolic murmurs are heard in >80% of normal newborns 24–48 hours of life due to tricuspid regurgitation or a closing ductus. Harsh systolic murmurs immediately after birth suggest aortic or pulmonic stenosis, or a common truncal valve. A "to-and-fro" murmur over the upper sternum in a newborn suggests TOF with absent pulmonary valve, or a common truncal valve with severe stenosis and insufficiency. If "too many heart sounds" are heard, and S1 and S2 are hard to discern, it is likely Ebstein's tricuspid valve. Small muscular VSDs typically present as soft, high-pitched or "squeaky" murmurs after 24 hours of life after the PVR has dropped. Large VSDs may not present with any murmur if there is little pressure difference between the ventricles.

*Arrhythmias* may be paroxysmal or sustained. It is important to know if the newborn heart rate (HR) is <100 or >180, or is variable with sleep and arousal, and if there are other coexisting factors (suspected sepsis or fetal exposure to drugs). Newborns demonstrate high vagal tone in the first few weeks of life, showing HR variability with tactile stimulation and an HR trend that decreases with time. Sinus tachycardia (HR >180–220) is also acceptable in newborns, provided the underlying cause is understood.[17] Rarely, occult newborn fractures may explain sinus tachycardia.

Newborns with fetal arrhythmias warrant a complete echocardiogram and 12-lead electrocardiogram (ECG) shortly after birth to evaluate and assess recurrence. Newborns with normal pregnancy and birth history may present with arrhythmia. Treatment options include doing nothing, medications (e.g. propranolol or digoxin), or cardioversion if the infant is hemodynamically unstable. In ill neonates, confirm catheter tip placement if they have central lines and perform vagal maneuvers, which include gag reflex, rectal stimulation, or placing an ice pack over the eyes and bridge of the nose. SVT in a neonate with a structurally normal heart is usually treated with oral propranolol for the first year of life and the arrhythmia typically resolves after the first birthday. If oral medication is used, parents can be taught to readjust the dose with weight gain, with a goal of being medication-free shortly after the first birthday. Periodically a 24-hour Holter monitor may be used to screen for occult tachyarrhythmias. Treatment of neonatal atrial flutter is usually successful with a one-time external cardioversion or overdrive pacing with an internally placed esophageal pacing catheter.

Dysmorphic newborns or those with confirmed abnormalities in genetic testing should be screened for other organ abnormalities. Head, renal, and cardiac ultrasounds are three noninvasive studies that are useful. Down syndrome has >40% chance of CHD (AV canal defect, CoA, ASD, VSD, and TOF with AV canal) detection. Trisomy 18 and trisomy 13 have higher CHD prevalence of >90% and 80–85%, respectively **(Table 5)**.[14,15]

## ANCILLARY TESTING AND VITAL SIGNS

Since 2011, most US states have adopted the universal screening of all newborns at 24 hours of life with pulse oximetry. Newborns require retesting and evaluation if pulse oximetry reading is <90%, below 95% in both

**TABLE 5:** Congenital cardiac defects commonly associated with syndromes and genetic defects.

| Chromosomal defect | Estimated % with CHD | Associated heart defects |
|---|---|---|
| Alagille syndrome (JAG1) | 94% | PPS |
| CHARGE association | 50–70% | TOF, DORV, TA, arch anomalies, ASD, VSD, PDA, AVC |
| Deletion 5p- (Cri-du-chat) | 20–30% | ASD, VSD |
| DiGeorge syndrome (22q11-) | 75–80% | TA, IAA (type B), VSD, right AA |
| Ehlers-Danlos | Variable with age | Arteriopathy, MVP, aortic root dilation |
| Ellis-van Creveld | 50% | ASD > PDA, L-SVC, CoA, TAPVR, t |
| Fetal alcohol syndrome | Variable | ASD, VSD, TOF |
| Goldenhar syndrome | 15–50% | TOF, VSD, ASD, conotruncal defects |
| Holt-Oram (12p, TBX5) | 50% | ASD > VSD |
| Marfan syndrome (fibrillin gene) | Variable with age | MVP, aortic root dilation, PV dilation, diffuse arteriopathy |
| Noonan syndrome (PTPN11) | 50% | ASD and hypertrophic cardiomyopathy (HCM) |
| TAR syndrome (thrombocytopenia, absent radius) | 30% | ASD, TOF |
| Trisomy 13 Patau | 80–85% | ASD, VSD, TOF, PDA, dextrocardia |
| Trisomy 18 Edwards | 99% | DORV, TOF, VSD, AV canal |
| Trisomy 21 Downs | 40% | ASD, VSD, AVC, TOF, PDA |
| Turner syndrome XO | 25% | AS, BAV, CoA |
| William syndrome | 50% | Pulmonary valve stenosis (PS) and peripheral pulmonary artery stenosis (PPS) |
| VACTERLS association | 50% | TOF, VSD |

(AS: aortic stenosis; AVC: atrioventricular canal; BAV: bicuspid aortic valve; CoA: coarctation of the aorta; DORV: double outlet right ventricle; HLHS: hypoplastic left heart syndrome; IAA: interrupted aortic arch; L-SVC: left superior vena cava; MVP: mitral valve prolapse; PDA: patent ductus arteriosus; PPS: peripheral pulmonary stenosis; PV: pulmonary valve; TA: truncus arteriosus; TAPVR: total anomalous pulmonary venous return; TOF: tetralogy of Fallot).

extremities after three measurements, or if there is more than 3% difference between arm and leg. If femoral pulses are weak, a simultaneous arm and leg blood pressure are needed to look for a gradient suspicious for CoA.

## HYPEROXIA TEST

Newborns who appear dusky, are tachypneic with or without distress, and have pulse oximetry readings <92% on room air require prompt evaluation. The hyperoxia test is an invasive method of determining whether cyanosis is due to pulmonary or CHD. An arterial blood gas is obtained after the patient receives 100% oxygen for 5 minutes via an oxyhood, or endotracheal tube if already intubated. Patients with cyanotic CHD rarely exceed a $PaO_2$ of 150 mm Hg after oxygen administration.

## ROLE OF NEONATAL ELECTROCARDIOGRAM

12-lead ECG aids in the evaluation of arrhythmias as well as newborns with suspected CHD. Although many hemodynamically significant CHDs have normal ECGs (such as D-TGA), abnormal cardiac axis can help narrow down the types of CHD prior to getting the echocardiogram (Fig. 9). The QTc interval should be calculated ($QT/\sqrt{RR}$) and followed serially if >480 ms within the first 30 days of life. If hypomagnesemia or hypocalcemia are present, QTc can be prolonged and reassessed once electrolyte abnormalities are corrected. Genetic testing for long QT syndrome with close cardiology follow-up recommended if QTc exceeds 480 ms in the absence of maternal/infant medications (e.g. ondansetron) or infant electrolyte abnormalities. A detailed family history and baseline ECGs of first-degree relatives is indicated. If the newborn is found to have hypocalcemia, dysmorphic features, and suspected CHD, a diagnosis of DiGeorge syndrome should be confirmed by sending a fluorescence in situ hybridization (FISH) for 22q11.2 aberration. ECG in neonatal bradycardia helps distinguish between complete heart block and sinus bradycardia.

## ECHOCARDIOGRAMS

Transthoracic two-dimensional (2D) echocardiogram with color and Doppler interrogation are vital in CHD assessment. Several well-known pediatric cardiology textbooks provide intricate physics of 2D, Doppler, color Doppler, M-mode, and 3D echo.[3,15,19]

# CHAPTER 24: Assessment and Treatment Options for Neonates with Congenital Heart Disease

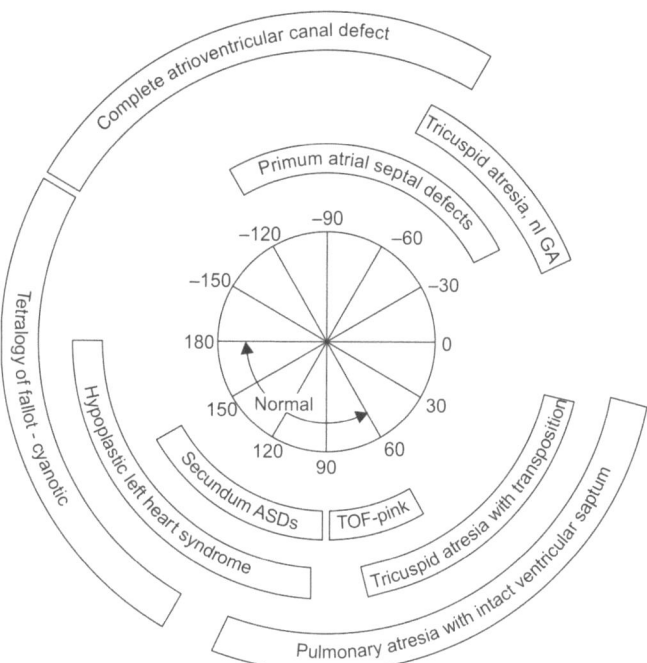

**Fig. 9:** Stanger electrocardiogram wheel. Numbers refer to QRS axis and correlating congenital heart defect.
*Courtesy:* Paul Stanger, MD, University of California, San Francisco. Revised with permission by C Sheridan, MD, 2014.

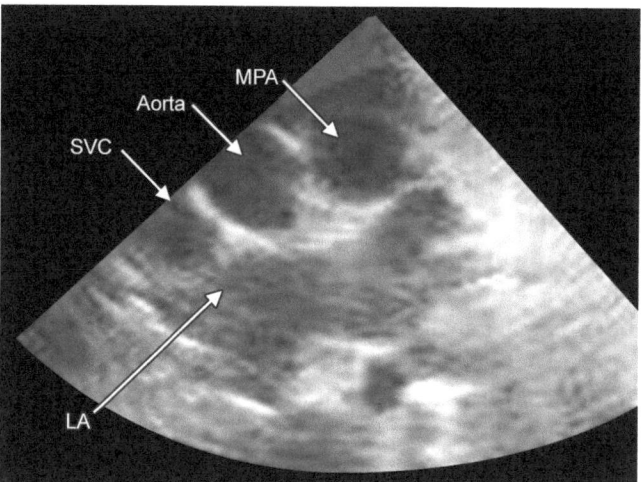

**Fig. 10:** High left suprasternal view. From the three-vessel view, posterior tilt of the transducer in the high parasternal short axis shows the superior vena cava (SVC), aorta, main pulmonary artery (MPA), pulmonary veins, and left atrium (LA).

Below is a guide for obtaining thorough detail in a newborn echocardiogram:
- Use the smallest probe with the highest frequency (12, 8 or 7 MHz)
- Capture two to three beats per image due to the higher HR
- Obtain views with 2D, color, and Doppler interrogation:
  - Parasternal long
  - *Parasternal short*: M-mode at the level of aortic valve and mitral valve papillary muscles
  - Apical four-chamber view, sweeping up to show outflow tracts
  - *Subcostal coronal and subcostal sagittal views:* It include sweep of liver diaphragm region until you see atrial septum to document situs
  - High left suprasternal, aka "crab view" **(Fig. 10)**; to see branch PAs and PV flow into LA
  - Suprasternal notch view to assess AA.

## ■ TIMING OF SURGICAL REPAIR

High-risk delivery at a tertiary care hospital allows for prompt confirmation of the cardiac anatomy, and stabilization with PGE1, intubation, etc. as indicated. This minimizes duration of profound cyanosis, potential end-organ damage, and risk of neurologic insult. Parents should be at bedside during important decision-making. Long- and short-term outcome depends on several factors, including CHD type and infant neurologic status at time of surgery. Serial brain MRI shows that newborns with CHD have baseline white matter brain changes prior to catheter or surgical intervention.[20,21]

Children who present later in life with unrepaired complex CHD are often assessed with ECG, transthoracic echo, and then considered for cardiac catheterization and/or cardiac MRI or CT scans. Elevated PVR and presence of acquired collateral vessels influence the timing and repair approach. Variation exists between institutions; each child is considered individually.

## Congenital Heart Defect with Decreased Pulmonary Blood Flow or Parallel Circulation

### D-Transposition of the Great Arteries

Newborns with D-TGA are cyanotic even with a small VSD or PDA open. The mixing occurs at the level of the atrium. Atrial septostomy is required either at bedside with echo guidance, or in the catheterization laboratory. An arterial switch operation is then performed in the first week of life to correct the anatomy. Residual mild pulmonary stenosis and peripheral pulmonary stenosis are expected surgical complications, typically not requiring intervention.

### Tetralogy of Fallot

The timing and approach to palliation and repair depends on the anatomical variation of the patient. Typical, acyanotic or "pink tets" have minimal obstruction in the right ventricular outflow tract (RVOT) region. The optimal repair age is 4-6 months, with some centers advocating early repair at 2-3 months to prevent right ventricular hypertension and potential for tet spells.[15] Some treat the infant with oral propranolol to reduce spasticity of the RVOT until surgery.

Cyanotic infants undergo primary repair as soon as possible. Surgical repair involves patch closure of the VSD, relief of the RVOT obstruction (transannular patch and/or infundibular resection), PDA ligation, and sometimes leaving a small ASD. When the PAs are hypoplastic or discontinuous, a stable source of PBF (either from the RV or from a modified Blalock–Taussig (BT) or central shunt) is needed to promote vessel growth. A modified BT shunt is a small Gore-Tex tube (2.5-4 mm in diameter), surgically placed between the proximal subclavian artery to the ipsilateral proximal branch PA. The goal is to supplement forward flow to the PAs to achieve a saturation of 75-85% on room air.[14] When the infant undergoes complete repair a few months later, patch augmentation of the main and proximal branch PAs is often needed.

Infants with *TOF and absent pulmonary valve syndrome* require a different approach. These infants do not have a DA and typically have massively dilated branch PAs that compress the bronchi. These newborns are best ventilated prone, to relieve compression of the upper airways. Primary repair consists of closing the VSD, placement of a monocusp valve in the pulmonic position, and reduction of the branch PA diameters. There are rare cases of less symptomatic children who are repaired later.

*Tetralogy of Fallot with pulmonary atresia and MAPCAs* is a unique lesion and difficult to repair. These infants require cardiac catheterization in the first few weeks of life to determine the exact number, location, and terminal route of the MAPCAs. Any collateral supplied by the ductus requires placement of either stent or BT shunt to maintain patency and flow to that lung segment. Primary repair of the intracardiac anatomy is often done at 2-4 months if the infant is acyanotic. Staged unifocalization of the MAPCAs is determined by distribution, size, and number of MAPCAs assessed by serial cardiac catheterization angiograms. Long-term care of these children requires additional cardiac catheterizations for rehabilitation of stenotic vessels, lung perfusion scans, and/or pulmonary valve replacement. Native MAPCAs are typically tortuous, tending to develop segmental stenosis over time, and impairing segmental flow to distal lung fields.

Beyond infantile TOF repair, many children will require a secondary procedure in their early teens or adulthood to revise the RVOT due to progressive RV dilation. Progressive pulmonary valve insufficiency, rather than pulmonary stenosis, becomes a greater factor over time in causing RV dilation. Several heart centers are becoming more familiar with the transcatheter placement of the Medtronic Melody® valve, therefore avoiding open heart surgery[22] for a pulmonary valve replacement. Later in life, patients need to be monitored for ventricular arrhythmias if their QRS duration approaches or exceeds 180 ms, and may require implantable cardioverter-fibrillator placement to prevent sudden death.

*Tricuspid valve abnormalities* (including Ebstein's anomaly, tricuspid atresia, stenosis, or significant regurgitation) have a range of clinical presentations and urgency of surgical intervention. With severe tricuspid valve regurgitation, initial efforts include using oxygen and/or inhaled nitric oxide (iNO) to lower PVR to promote forward flow to the PAs. Surgery is reserved for severely symptomatic infants. For severe Ebstein's anomaly, cone repair technique[23] is an option, combined with right atrial plication or reduction. Long-term results are variable and tachyarrhythmia prevalence is high. Severe Ebstein's anomaly benefits from a bidirectional Glenn shunt to effectively have a 1.5 ventricle physiology as a second stage surgery in early childhood.

## Congenital Heart Defect causing Decreased Systemic Output

*Hypoplastic left heart, interrupted aortic arch (IAA) variants, and critical CoA* present with decreased systemic output within the first week(s) of life as the ductus closes. If not detected prenatally, these newborns present without murmur and in shock with poor distal pulses. PGE1 should be started immediately. Critical aortic stenosis and some IAA types also have harsh murmurs of the VSD or stenotic valve. LVOT obstruction requires immediate stabilization of the infant and surgery to restore forward flow once acidosis and end-organ damage have improved. For HLHS, the stage 1 Norwood palliation is performed in the first few days of life and consists of anastomosing the hypoplastic aorta to the pulmonary root to create a neoaorta with patch augmentation of the arch. The atrial septum is resected and either a modified BT shunt or an RV-PA conduit is connected to supply PBF. Some centers have been performing a hybrid stage 1 palliation involving both an interventional pediatric cardiologist and cardiothoracic surgeon. In a 2010 review[9] the hybrid approach is described as yielding equivalent (but not superior) stage 1 survival rates and pre-Glenn hemodynamics leading up to stage 2. The hybrid procedure involves placement of a ductal stent and bilateral PA bands, without cardiopulmonary bypass, deep hypothermic cardiac arrest, and extensive intracardiac surgery. Improved postoperative recovery and reduced risk for neurologic insult are due to the lower inflammatory response. The disadvantages; however, involve the fragility of the hypoplastic AA, the atrial septum becoming restrictive, and the PA bands migrating and causing distortion in the interstage period. The stage 1 hybrid procedure continues to evolve, even since the writing of this chapter.

*Critical CoA and IAA* are repaired as soon as diagnosed in the newborn period, with end-to-side grafting of the transverse to isthmus and descending aorta. The associated VSD is then closed with a patch or via Rastelli–Norwood approach, depending on the anatomy. If a Norwood–Rastelli is performed, the RV-PA conduit will need replacing in 3–5 years due to progressive calcifications and stenosis. The arch needs lifelong assessment to monitor for recoarctation.

*Cardiomyopathy* in neonates requires comprehensive anatomic, infectious, and metabolic work-up. Dilated LVs mandate that coronary arteries are identified and verified with flow patterns to rule out anomalies. Incessant tachyarrhythmias must also be ruled out and treated if present. Carnitine supplementation can be started while awaiting metabolic laboratories. If a treatable cause cannot be found, therapy is supportive, maximizing the infant's caloric intake and oral medications. Medications depend on degree of ventricular dysfunction and dilation, with diuretics, digoxin, afterload reduction, and α- and β-blockade medications titrated up gradually. If ventricular dysfunction is moderate to severe, consultation with a heart failure center with transplant services is advisable.

*Obstructed total anomalous pulmonary venous return (TAPVR)* can present with a severely cyanotic neonate in respiratory distress due to pulmonary edema. If the atrial connection is restrictive, left-sided output is also decreased, resulting in poor perfusion. Surgical correction is performed immediately upon diagnosis, using echo and/or angiogram. If the PV is not obstructed, the child may only be mildly cyanotic, asymptomatic, and present later in childhood with a murmur of RV volume overload and right heart enlargement. Surgical correction is required.

## Congenital Heart Defects causing High Pulmonary Blood Flow

*Large ASDs, VSDs, AV canals, AP windows, and TA* are CHD causing high PBF. Many centers repair AP windows and TA lesions in the newborn period. For large ASDs, VSDs, and AV canals, close follow-up every 2–4 weeks in early infancy is important to monitor for congestive heart failure or volume overload to the lungs, manifested by slow weight gain, tachycardia, tachypnea, and sweating with feeds. Since early repair (2–6 months) is the goal, symptomatic infants can first be treated with diuretics and fortified feeds. Treatment with digoxin has become more of a practice style, and infants who undergo early repair before 6 months of age do well without it. Common feeding strategies include fortifying breast milk or formula to 22–26 kcal/oz by mouth or with a nasogastric tube. When mothers prefer to mainly breastfeed during the day, infants can be given oral milk after nursing or at night via a nasogastric tube. Postsurgery, these infants continue to have hearty appetites and they usually gain weight rapidly.

*Partial anomalous pulmonary venous return* with or without an ASD is a CHD where one or more PV connects abnormally to the right atrium, IVC, or SVC. Ideally, this is repaired when the child is of early school age or when the right heart enlarges significantly.

## INDICATIONS FOR CARDIAC CATHETERIZATION IN THE NEONATE

There are a few CHD in which cardiac catheterization provides vital diagnostic information and therapeutic intervention:

- *Balloon atrial septostomy for D-TGA*
- *Hybrid procedure for HLHS*: PDA stent placement
- *Critical pulmonary valve stenosis*: When the pulmonary valve appears plate-like on echo and amenable to radiofrequency ablation and balloon dilation of the annulus
- *Critical aortic stenosis*: Balloon angioplasty
- *Pulmonary atresia with intact ventricular septum*: To assess the RV sinusoids and coronary artery distribution and flow
- *TOF with pulmonary atresia and MAPCAs*: Initial roadmap to show the MAPCA connections and distributions.

## CONCLUSION

Advanced surgical and catheter techniques continue to improve in pediatric cardiology, with healthcare professionals sharing knowledge with one another. One such internet forum used internationally is *pediheart.net*. This free group allows members to inquire about local cardiologists for patients moving to other states or countries and to discuss challenging cases.

## ACKNOWLEDGMENTS

Dedicated to the memory of Dr Paul Woolf, a wise program director and a kind and patient mentor who encouraged me to study pediatric cardiology. Thank you, Dr Andrew Maxwell, Dr Claude Rogé, and Dr Paul Stanger for mentoring me all these years and editing my chapter based on their own practical experiences. My love to my dear husband Robbie and daughters Liana and Julianne for their patience as I wrote this chapter and for all of my long nights away on call. Thank you, Mom and Dad, for supporting us during my fellowship years and beyond.

## REFERENCES

1. Nicholaides KH, Heath V, Cicero S. Increased fetal nuchal translucency at 11-14 weeks. Prenatal Diagnosis. 2002;22(308):308-15.
2. Opinion C. Noninvasive prenatal testing for fetal aneuploidy. Committee Opinion, No. 545. American College of Obstetricians and Gynecologists. Obstet Gynecol. 2012;545(120):1532-4.
3. Chiappa EM, Cook AC, Botta G, et al. Echocardiographic Anatomy in the Fetus. Italy: Springer; 2009.
4. Rudolph AM. Congenital Diseases of the Heart: Clinical-Physiological Considerations, 2nd edition. New York: Futura Publishing Company, Inc; 2001.
5. Parameterz. Z-Scores and Reference Values for Pediatric Echocardiography. [online] Available from: www.parameterz.com [Last accessed September, 2019].
6. Tworetzky W, Wilkins-Haug L, Jennings RW, et al. Balloon dilation of severe aortic stenosis in the fetus. Circulation. 2004;110:2125-31.
7. Tabatabaei H, Boutin C, Nykanen DG, et al. Morphologic and hemodynamic consequences after percutaneous balloon valvotomy for neonatal pulmonary stenosis: medium-term follow-up. J Am Coll Cardiol. 1996;27(2):473-8.
8. Kothari SS, Sharma SK, Naik N. Radiofrequency perforation for pulmonary atresia and intact ventricular septum. Indian Heart J. 2004;56:50-3.
9. Honjo O, Calderon C. Hybrid palliation for neonates with hypoplastic left heart syndrome: current strategies and outcomes. Korean Circ J. 2010;40(3):103-11.
10. Maeno Y, Hirose A, Kanbe T, et al. Fetal arrhythmia: prenatal diagnosis and perinatal management. J Obstet Gynaecol Res. 2009;35(4):623-9.
11. Srinivasan S, Strasburger J. Overview of fetal arrhythmias. Curr Opin Pediatr. 2008;20(5):522-31.
12. Friedman DM, Duncanson LJ, Buyon JP. A review of congenital heart block. Images Paediatr Cardiol. 2003;5(3):36-48.
13. Buyon Lab. (2014). Congenital Heart Block in Neonatal Lupus. [online] Available from: http://www.med.nyu.edu/medicine/labs/buyonlab/research/heart.html [Last accessed September, 2019].
14. Artman M, Mahony L, Teitel DF. Neonatal Cardiology. New York: McGraw-Hill; 2002.
15. Keane JF, Lock JE, Fyler DC. Nada's Pediatric Cardiology, 2nd edition. Philadelphia: W.B. Saunders; 2006.
16. Ross PA, Newth CJ, Khemani RG. Accuracy of pulse oximetry in children. Pediatrics. 2014;133(1):22-9.
17. Montague TJ, Taylor PG, Stockton R, et al. Spectrum of cardiac rate and rhythm in normal newborns. Pediatr Cardiol. 1982;2(1):33-8.
18. Jones KL. Smith's Recognizable Patterns of Human Malformation, 5th edition. Philadelphia: W.B. Saunders; 1997.
19. Eidem BW, O'Leary PW. Echocardiography in Pediatric and Adult Congenital Heart Disease. Philadelphia: Lippincott Williams & Wilkins; 2010.
20. McQuillen PS, Barkovich AJ, Hamrick SE, et al. Temporal and anatomic risk profile of brain injury with neonatal repair of congenital heart defects. Stroke. 2007;38:736-41.
21. Miller SP, McQuillen PS, Hamrick SE, et al. Abnormal brain development in newborns with congenital heart disease. N Eng J Med. 2007;357(19):1928-38.
22. Medtronic. (2016). Transcathether Pulmonary Valves. [online] Available from: http://www.medtronic.com [Last accessed September, 2019].
23. Dearani JA, Bacha M, da Silva JP. Cone reconstruction of the tricuspid valve for Ebstein's anomaly: anatomic repair. Oper Tech Thorac Cardiovasc Surg. 2008;13(2):109-25.

# CHAPTER 25

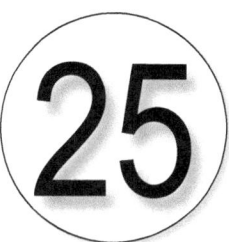

# Pulmonary Hypertension in the Neonatal Intensive Care Unit Setting

*Yueh-Tze Lan*

## ABSTRACT

Pulmonary hypertension (PH) can present at any age from birth to adulthood, with the distribution of etiologies in childhood being different than in adults. The majority of childhood PH is associated with developmental abnormalities and genetic syndrome. In the neonates, persistent pulmonary hypertension of the newborn (PPHN) is the most common type of PH and has a distinct presentation and unique time course compared to other types of PH. PH due to chronic lung disease (CLD), including bronchopulmonary dysplasia (BPD) and congenital diaphragmatic hernia (CDH), is a leading cause of infant PH and has long-term consequences due to its effect on lung growth and pulmonary vascular development. Although PH in congenital heart disease (CHD) is well known, pulmonary arterial hypertension (PAH) due to CHD is uncommon in neonates. Drug-induced PAH and heritable causes of PAH are rare in newborns but should be considered when no other cause of PH is apparent. Acute treatment of PPHN focuses on treating the underlying cause and providing supportive care. Newer pharmacological agent use in adult PAH is increasing, with off-label use in neonates reporting some success. Without established therapy for treatment of PH outside of PPHN, treatment decisions for PH in the neonatal intensive care unit (NICU) remain challenging. We review etiologies and available therapies for PH as seen in the NICU.

## INTRODUCTION

Pulmonary hypertension is associated with significant morbidity and mortality in neonates. The majority of neonatal PH is due to persistent pulmonary hypertension of the newborn (PPHN), caused primarily by meconium aspiration, sepsis, or birth asphyxia, and resolves without long-term sequelae once the underlying pathology is treated. In addition to PPHN, other well-known causes of PH in the NICU setting include BPD, CDH, CHD, surfactant deficiency, alveolar capillary hypoplasia, and heritable PH. Treatment strategies and outcomes vary based on the underlying cause of PH.

## CLASSIFICATION OF PULMONARY HYPERTENSION

Historically, PH has been classified as either primary PH (also called idiopathic pulmonary arterial hypertension, or IPAH) when the cause for PH is unknown, or as secondary PH when there is an identifiable cause. At the Second World Symposium on Pulmonary Hypertension (WSPH) held in Evian, France in 1998, a clinical classification of PH was proposed to categorize etiologies sharing similarities in pathophysiological mechanisms, clinical presentation, and therapeutic options. PH is currently classified into five groups of disorders:
- *Group 1:* Pulmonary arterial hypertension
- *Group 2:* PH due to left heart disease
- *Group 3:* PH due to CLD and/or hypoxia
- *Group 4:* Chronic thromboembolic PH
- *Group 5:* PH due to unclear multifactorial mechanisms.[1]

Updates to the classification were made after the 6th WSPH held in 2018 **(Box 1)**.[2,3] IPAH, heritable PAH,

**BOX 1:** Updated classification of pulmonary hypertension.

1. Group 1: PAH
    1.1. Idiopathic PAH
    1.2. Heritable PAH
    1.3. Drug and toxin induced
    1.4. PAH associated with:
        1.4.1. Connective tissue disease
        1.4.2. HIV infection
        1.4.3. Portal hypertension
        1.4.4 Congenital heart diseases
        1.4.5. Schistosomiasis
    1.5. PAH long-term responders to calcium channel blockers
    1.6. PAH with overt features of venous/capillaries involvement
    1.7. Persistent pulmonary hypertension of the newborn syndrome
2. Group 2: PH due to left heart disease
    2.1. Heart failure with preserved LVEF
    2.2. Heart failure with reduced LVEF
    2.3. Valvular disease
    2.4. Congenital/acquired cardiovascular conditions leading to post-capillary PH, including pulmonary vein stenosis, cor triatriatum, obstructed total anomalous pulmonary venous return, mitral/aortic stenosis, and coarctation of the aorta
3. Group 3: PH due to lung diseases and/or hypoxia
    3.1. Chronic obstructive pulmonary disease
    3.2. Restrictive lung disease
    3.3. Other pulmonary diseases with mixed restrictive and obstructive pattern
    3.4. Hypoxia without lung disease
    3.5. Developmental lung diseases, including bronchopulmonary dysplasia, congenital diaphragmatic hernia, Down syndrome, alveolar capillary dysplasia with "misalignment of veins", lung hypoplasia, surfactant protein abnormalities, pulmonary interstitial glycogenesis, pulmonary alveolar proteinosis, pulmonary lymphangiectasia
4. Group 4: PH due to pulmonary artery obstruction
    4.1 Chronic thromboembolic pulmonary hypertension
    4.2 Other pulmonary artery obstruction
5. Group 5: PH with unclear and/or multifactorial mechanisms
    5.1 Hematologic disorders: chronic hemolytic anemia, myeloproliferative disorders, splenectomy
    5.2 Systemic and metabolic disorders: sarcoidosis, pulmonary histiocytosis, lymphangioleiomyomatosis; glycogen storage disease, Gaucher disease, thyroid disorders
    5.3 Others: tumoral obstruction, fibrosing mediastinitis, chronic renal failure
    5.4 Complex congenital heart disease, including segmental PH, single ventricle and Scimitar syndrome

(PAH: pulmonary arterial hypertension; HIV: human immunodeficiency virus; LVEF: left ventricular ejection fraction; PH: pulmonary hypertension).

drug- and toxin-induced PAH, PAH associated with CHD, and PPHN remain as subgroups in Group 1 PH. Developmental lung diseases associated with PH have a Group 3 classification and include CDH, BPD, surfactant protein abnormalities, alveolar capillary dysplasia (ACD), ACD with misalignment of pulmonary veins, pulmonary hypoplasia, pulmonary interstitial glycogenesis, pulmonary alveolar proteinosis, and pulmonary lymphangiectasia.

# DIAGNOSIS OF PULMONARY HYPERTENSION

The definition of PH in children is similar to that in adults, i.e. mean pulmonary arterial pressure (mPAP) > 25 mm Hg at rest by cardiac catheterization. Due to the relatively low blood pressure of the neonate, estimated pulmonary pressure > 50% of systemic pressure defines PH in neonates and young infants. Fetal pulmonary artery pressure (PAP) is normally similar to systemic pressure, falls rapidly after birth, and reaches adult levels by age 2–3 months. Historically, pulmonary vascular resistance (PVR) has not been used to define PH; however, the most recent 6th WSPH proposed to modify the definition of PH in adults as mPAP > 20 mm Hg and to include PVR ≥ 3 Wood units (WU) to identify precapillary PH.[2] In pediatrics, especially in association with CHD, PVR indexed to body surface area (PVRi) is used to assess PH from pulmonary vascular disease (PVD), defined by PVRi ≥ 3 $WU/m^2$, and to determine suitability for CHD repair. PVR is particularly important in the management of infants with CHD when PAP may be elevated with normal PVR, as seen commonly in infants with large ventricular septal defect (VSD) or patent ductus arteriosus (PDA) before they develop PVD. When PVR is normal, infants present with respiratory distress due to pulmonary overcirculation and pulmonary edema, in contrast to patients with PH and increased PVR who may be asymptomatic without significant left-to-right shunt. The management strategy would be very different in these cases.

While cardiac catheterization is the gold standard for diagnosis of PH, echocardiogram is usually the only diagnostic tool used in the NICU. An objective measure of PH by echocardiogram is the estimate of systolic pulmonary pressure derived from tricuspid regurgitation (TR) jet peak velocity, with >3 m/s indicative of PH. Accurately estimating systolic PAP by echocardiogram depends on the presence of TR as well as the quality of the TR jet **(Figs. 1A and B)**. Assuming no right ventricular (RV) outflow obstruction, pulmonary artery (PA) systolic pressure equals RV systolic pressure. RV systolic pressure is estimated by the peak TR gradient using the formula:

RV systolic pressure = RA pressure (conventionally assumed to be 10 mm Hg) + 4 × (TR peak velocity)$^2$

Past studies have shown that the presence of adequate TR jet on echocardiogram was possible in only 31–61% of infants with CLD and suspected PH.[4-7] Other echocardiographic findings such as interventricular septal flattening, RV hypertrophy, or right atrial (RA), RV, or pulmonary artery dilatation, are qualitative measures of PH seen only in severe PH. In PH, elevated PVR is likely present when pulmonary acceleration time/ejection time

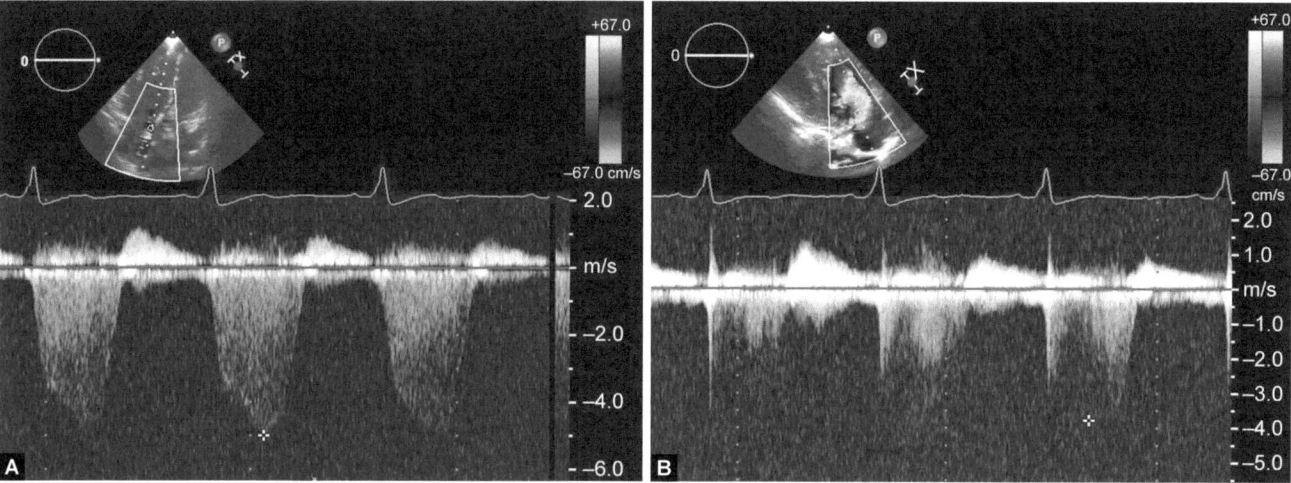

**Figs. 1A and B:** TR jet peak velocity for estimate of RV systolic pressure. (A) Clear TR jet where peak velocity is clearly visualized with calculated peak gradient of 100 mm Hg; (B) TR jet in the same patient during the same study. TR jet is indistinct and peak velocity could not be determined but was guessed and resulted in calculated peak gradient of 57 mm Hg (TR: tricuspid regurgitation; RV: right ventricular) *(For color version see Plate 4).*

ratio (AT/ET) is <0.3.[8] In addition, tricuspid annular plane systolic excursion (TAPSE) as a marker for RV function is an important prognostic marker in adults with PH[9] and also correlates with childhood PH.[10] A less common qualitative measure of pulmonary pressure is estimating pulmonary arterial end-diastolic pressure (PAEDP) by pulmonary regurgitation (PR) jet velocity **(Fig. 2)**:

PR end-diastolic gradient = 4 × (PR end-diastolic peak velocity)$^2$

PAEDP = RA pressure + PR end-diastolic gradient

The PR end-diastolic gradient > 5.0 mm Hg is diagnostically equivalent to the TR gradient > 30 mm Hg.[11]

Where PDA or VSD is present, an estimate of pulmonary arterial systolic pressure or RV systolic pressure can be obtained by subtracting peak gradient from systolic blood pressure. Although patients with severe PH often have right-to-left atrial shunt when a patent foramen ovale (PFO) or an atrial septal defect (ASD) is present, it is important to know that right-to-left atrial shunting does not necessarily mean PH, as shunting at the atrial level depends on relative atrial pressure and relative ventricular compliance. Conversely, presence of left-to-right shunt across PDA or PFO does not exclude PH.

## PERSISTENT PULMONARY HYPERTENSION OF THE NEWBORN

Contrary to other forms of PH presenting in the newborn period, PPHN is usually transient, a result of the failure of the normal post birth circulatory transition. Incidence of PPHN in term or near-term infants is 6.8/1,000 live births, and characterized by marked PH that causes hypoxemia, right-to-left intracardiac shunting, and systemic hypotension.

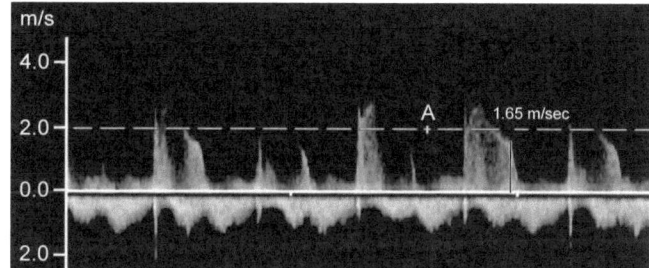

**Fig. 2:** Pulmonary insufficiency jet for estimate of PAEDP where PA velocity at end diastole is 1.65 m/s, which predicts PAEDP of 21 mm Hg (PAEDP: pulmonary arterial end-diastolic pressure; PA: pulmonary artery) *(For color version see Plate 4).*

It can present without acute perinatal distress, although often caused by meconium aspiration, birth asphyxia, or sepsis. Other conditions, such as premature intrauterine constriction of the ductus arteriosus, third trimester exposure to selective serotonin reuptake inhibitor (SSRI),[12] CHD (especially those with left-sided obstructive lesions), developmental lung disease, surfactant protein deficiencies, and alveolar capillary dysplasia are important causes of neonatal PH that bear exclusion. The latter two disorders often present with severe or lethal PH[13,14] and are important to provide appropriate prognosis and management. Although classified under Group 3.5 (PH associated with developmental lung disorder), CDH is a major congenital anomaly associated with PPHN. Advances in treatment have improved survival of neonates with isolated CDH, but overall mortality is 20–35%,[15] especially when severe PH persists beyond age 2 weeks.[16] NICU treatment of PPHN involves prevention of acidosis, hypoxemia, agitation, and pain. Despite high frequency ventilation, surfactant, inhaled nitric oxide, and extracorporeal membrane oxygenation, the mortality due to PPHN is 10-20% and is greater in resource-poor settings where these therapies are unavailable.[17]

## PULMONARY HYPERTENSION ASSOCIATED WITH DEVELOPMENTAL LUNG DISEASE

Bronchopulmonary dysplasia is the most common cause of developmental lung disease in children. The prevalence of PH in formerly premature infants with BPD is unknown, and studies [5,18-20] have shown a quarter to a third of infants with BPD develop PH. Late mortality of PH in the post-surfactant era remains high, with ~50% mortality 2 years after PH diagnosis.[20] Abnormality of developing pulmonary vasculature may not be severe enough to be clinically recognized as PH, yet may result in significant pulmonary vascular disease. Infants with BPD have impaired gas exchange requiring prolonged oxygen, diffusion abnormality, and altered pulmonary blood flow in response to stress/exercise or acute respiratory infection.

The pathogenesis of pulmonary vascular disease in BPD is multifactorial; NO-cGMP signaling is disrupted by preterm birth, lung injury, and neonatal PH.[21,22] Lung vascular growth is a dynamic process, continuing through gestation and postnatal life. Animal studies demonstrate that PH inhibits vascular growth and impairs alveolarization in the developing lung.[23] Endothelin-1 (ET-1) increases in BPD and has antiangiogenic effects in developing lungs.[24,25] Reduced alveolar numbers and intra-acinar arteries occur in premature infants with BPD and contribute to persistent PH. Increasingly, pulmonary vein stenosis (PVS) is reported in the BPD population, especially in infants with history of necrotizing enterocolitis.[26,27] Up to 26% of Spanish registry study subjects with BPD and PH undergoing cardiac catheterization had PVS.[28] PVS may develop or progress with time. Up to a median of five echocardiograms were performed prior to diagnosis of PVS.[26] Infants who have severe BPD inconsistent with their degree of prematurity may have other PH etiology. Workup to exclude chronic aspiration, airway anomalies and heritable PH is indicated.

## PULMONARY HYPERTENSION ASSOCIATED WITH DRUGS AND TOXINS

Maternal illicit drug use during pregnancy is associated with extremely low birth weight infants and more severe BPD;[29] it is unknown whether the more severe BPD is due to premature birth or due to the effect of drugs on the development of pulmonary vasculature. Although amphetamine/methamphetamine use predisposes adults to PH, and methamphetamine crosses the placenta and affects developing fetal vasculature, it is not known if maternal drug use during pregnancy increases risk of newborn PH.

Cocaine is a monoamine reuptake blocker, interfering with catecholamine and serotonin uptake. Longer periods of fetal SSRI exposure during late gestation may be associated with increased risk and severity of neonatal respiratory complications, including PPHN.[12] Accumulation of SSRIs in the lungs may result in high circulating levels of serotonin which, through its vasoconstrictive effects, increases pulmonary vascular resistance. Serotonin also exerts mitogenic and comitogenic effects on pulmonary arterial smooth muscle cells and may cause smooth muscle cell proliferation in the fetal lung.[30]

Pulmonary hypertension may occur in up to 7% of infants treated with diazoxide for hypoglycemia due to congenital hyperinsulinism, especially those with associated CHD and fluid overload. PH resolves with discontinuation of diazoxide. These infants may benefit from increased echocardiographic surveillance while on diazoxide.

## PULMONARY HYPERTENSION ASSOCIATED WITH GENETIC DISORDERS

Some neonates with PH without identifiable cause have idiopathic or heritable PH. Gene mutation associated with pathogenesis of PH have been been identified in 20-30% of pediatric sporadic PAH cases and 70-80% of familial cases.

Over 300 independent mutations in bone morphogenetic protein receptor 2 (*BMPR2*), a member of the transforming growth factor β (TGF-β) superfamily of receptors, have been identified. *BMPR2* mutations occur in 70% of familial PH, and in 10-40% of idiopathic PH.[33,34] Heritable PH due to *BMPR2* mutations is associated with earlier age of onset, more severity at diagnosis, and is less likely to respond to vasodilator testing during right heart catheterization.[35,36] Other genes in the TGF-β superfamily include *SMAD4*, *SMAD8*, *CAV1*, *ACVRL1*, and *ENG*; these are also linked to idiopathic and heritable PH.[37-43] Genetic mutations in *KCNK3* and *TBX-4* (small patella syndrome) are also found to cause PH.[44-46] *EIF2AK4* mutations were found in patients with pulmonary capillary hemangiomatosis, an autosomal recessive form of heritable PH due to pulmonary veno-occlusive disease, secondary to proliferation and invasion of capillaries into one or more of the pulmonary veins, arteries, and pulmonary interstitium.[47,48] In addition, more than 80% of all cases of hereditary hemorrhagic telangiectasia (HHT), also known as Osler-Weber-Rendu syndrome, are found to be secondary to mutations in either *ACVRL1* or *ENG*.[39,42] Of note, *ACVRL1* mutation carriers might develop both PH and HHT with PH preceding manifestations of HHT.[41]

Pediatric PH is often associated with chromosomal anomaly and genetic syndromes, in which the mechanism for PAH may be uncertain or multifactorial. Most recently, *SOX17* mutation has been found in ~3.2% of PAH-CHD and 0.7% of cases of PAH without CHD, representing a new risk gene contributing to PAH-CHD as well as idiopathic/familial PAH.[49] Several genetic syndromes, whether or not associated with CHD, have increased risk of PH. Developmental mechanisms of PH in genetic syndromes unassociated with CHD is unclear but may include upper airway obstruction and pulmonary hypoplasia in Down syndrome; upper airway obstruction, dysfunctional vascular smooth muscle cells with pulmonary vessel stenosis, and remodeling in Adams-Oliver syndrome[50,51] and neurofibromatosis type 1,[52,53] pulmonary venous obstruction in Cantu syndrome,[54] or production of diffusible hepatic factors increasing PA pressure in Gaucher disease and glycogen storage disease (GSDI and GSDIII).[55,56] Notably, patients with Gaucher disease and PH respond to treatment of the primary metabolic disorder with enzyme replacement therapy.[55]

## PULMONARY HYPERTENSION ASSOCIATED WITH CONGENITAL HEART DISEASE

Pulmonary arterial hypertension associated with CHD is classified as Group 1 PH, and PH due to left heart disease, including congenital/acquired cardiovascular condition leading to postcapillary PH, as Group 2 PH. Complex congenital heart disease, including single ventricle heart disease and Scimitar syndrome, has been reclassified to Group 5 PH.

Large VSD or PDA, aortopulmonary window, and endocardial cushion defect are common lesions causing pulmonary overcirculation. Affected neonates have elevated RV and PA pressure, but their PVR may be normal until they develop PVD from chronic elevated pressure. Obstructive total anomalous pulmonary venous return, PVS, cor triatriatum, mitral stenosis, supravalvar mitral ring, and hypoplastic left heart syndrome with restrictive ASD are well-known causes of left-sided obstructive lesions which cause pulmonary venous congestion leading to PH. Lowering PVR in neonates with large left-to-right shunting and pulmonary overcirculation may exacerbate overcirculation and congestive heart failure. Thus, in infants presenting with hypoxemia due to pulmonary overcirculation/edema, initiation of diuretics may be more appropriate than supplemental oxygen, which may worsen pulmonary overcirculation by further lowering PVR. Similarly, the use of vasodilator therapy is contraindicated for neonates with pulmonary venous obstruction, as this will increase pulmonary blood flow and worsen obstruction. Medical therapy alone is usually ineffective for most neonates with unrepaired CHD and PH. However, for neonates with Ebstein's anomaly, decreasing PVR to promote more forward pulmonary blood flow and less TR, as well as less right-to-left shunt across ASD/PFO is helpful, since cyanosis and cardiac output will improve once PVR drops.

In neonates with CHD associated with left ventricular dysfunction and elevated PA pressure, the use of milrinone (a phosphodiesterase inhibitor type 3 with both inotropic effect and pulmonary vasodilatory effect) may be efficacious. Dopamine has potential deleterious effects on PVR at higher doses, and causes more tachycardia and thus is not useful in this setting.

## TREATMENT OPTIONS FOR PULMONARY HYPERTENSION

### Inhaled Nitric Oxide and Sildenafil

Cyclic guanosine monophosphate (cGMP) reduces pulmonary vascular tone and decreases PVR. Inhaled nitric oxide (iNO) activates soluble guanylate cyclase thereby increases cGMP (**Fig. 3**) and is standard therapy for PPHN in resource-rich countries. iNO is also used for acute pulmonary hypertensive crisis associated with conditions including CDH, BPD, and CHD.[16,57-60] Because nonselective pulmonary vasodilation may lead to more ventilation/perfusion (V/Q) mismatch, treatment of patients with PH due to CLD with PAH drugs may worsen hypoxemia in patients with CLD, including BPD.[61] Nevertheless, iNO at a dose of 10-20 ppm should be initiated for acute PH crises in patients with BPD and weaned off after stabilization. Unfortunately, 30-50% of neonates with PPHN fail to respond to iNO,[62] and iNO may not be readily available in low-resource settings. In addition, many infants with CDH have PPHN refractory to conventional therapies, with only 30% of neonates responding to iNO treatment.[63] A meta-analysis of this population suggests the outcome is not improved with iNO.[64]

Sildenafil, a selective inhibitor of phosphodiesterase 5 (PDE5), decreases breakdown of cGMP (**Fig. 3**) and is available in many resource-poor countries. In addition to the pulmonary vasodilatory effect due to cGMP, sildenafil also increases matrix metalloproteinase-2 and modulates the Rho-associated kinases signaling and reduces vascular smooth muscle cell contraction and proliferation,[65,66] as well as attenuates inflammation and airway reactivity in animal models.[67] In settings where iNO and high-frequency ventilation were not available or ineffective, sildenafil has been used for the treatment of PPHN and shown to reduce mortality significantly without clinically important side effects in both term and pre-term neonates.[57,68,69]

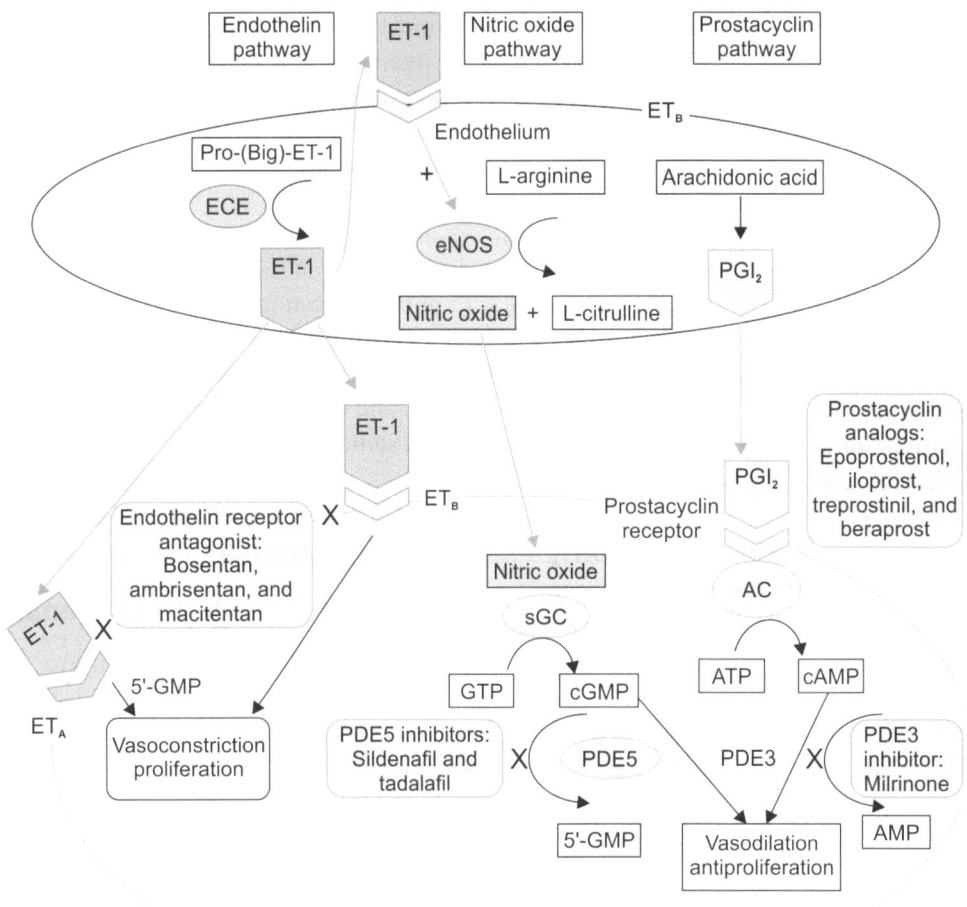

**Fig. 3:** Endothelin-1 (ET-1) is derived from cleavage of pro-ET-1 or big ET-1 by endothelin-converting enzyme (ECE) to the vasoactive peptide ET-1. ET-1 can activate endothelin receptors type A ($ET_A$) and type B ($ET_B$). While $ET_A$ is localized in vascular smooth muscle cells, $ET_B$ resides in vascular smooth muscle and endothelial cells. Activation of $ET_A$ or $ET_B$ in smooth muscle cells results in vasoconstriction and proliferation of smooth muscle cells. Activation of $ET_B$ in endothelial cells induces nitric oxide (NO) production through endothelial nitric oxide synthase (eNOS). NO is a potent vasodilator in smooth muscle cells. NO binds soluble guanylate cyclases (sGC) which then catalyzes the conversion of guanosine 5'-triphosphate (GTP) to cyclic guanosine 3',5'-monophosphate (cGMP). cGMP is a potent vasodilator and has antiproliferation effect. Cyclic GM is degrade by phosphodiesterase (PDE) 5. Prostacyclin (also known as prostaglandin $I_2$, $PGI_2$) is produced in endothelial cells from arachidonic acid metabolism. When G protein-coupled receptor (prostacyclin receptor) is activated by binding of $PGI_2$, it signals adenylyl cyclase (AC) to convert adenosine triphosphate (ATP) to cyclic adenosine monophosphate (cAMP). cAMP mediates vasodilation as well as inhibits smooth muscle proliferation.

Sildenafil also improves oxygenation independently and synergistically with iNO.[70] Sildenafil may help in weaning off iNO and preventing rebound hypoxemia during iNO withdrawal, by prolonging half-life of endogenous nitrous oxide.

Sildenafil improves alveolarization and decreases BPD-associated remodeling of pulmonary vasculature and RV hypertrophy in rodent BPD.[70,71] Several studies and case reports show improved/resolved PH in infants with BPD on chronic oral sildenafil (dose range 1.5–8 mg/kg/day).[72-74] Therefore, in infants with BPD and evidence of sustained PH, sildenafil may be indicated after treatment of underlying conditions.

Enteral sildenafil is quickly absorbed, reaching Cmax within 0.5–2.5 hours post dose, having 40% bioavailability and a half-life of ~4 hours in an adult study.[75] However, another study[76] showed no detectable sildenafil in nearly half the children undergoing acute hemodynamic testing 30 minutes after an oral dose of 0.5 mg/kg. Immature metabolism was demonstrated by a longer half-life (48–56 hours in neonates)[77] compared to 3.7 hours in adults. Because sildenafil is metabolized by cytochrome p450, plasma concentration varies with other medications, which either inhibit or induce this system. Sildenafil doses ranging from 0.5 mg/kg/dose to 2 mg/kg/dose every 6 hours have been used in various studies and conditions associated with

PH. However, because of increased mortality in a high-dose sildenafil group,[78] currently the recommended starting dose of sildenafil is 0.3-0.5 mg/kg/dose orally and titrated up to 1 mg/kg/dose q8h, with maximum dose of 10 mg/dose q8h in BPD.[79] For infants unable to tolerate oral sildenafil, an intravenous (IV) dose of 0.25-0.5 mg/kg/dose may be given over 1 hour with careful blood pressure monitoring. Sildenafil is usually well tolerated in children, including neonates. Potential side effects include hypotension, especially if given IV,[80,81] gastroesophageal reflux, irritability due to headache, bronchospasm, nasal stuffiness, fever, and priapism. Because sildenafil may increase the incidence of gastroesophageal reflux, some providers start H2 blockers concomitantly.[82] While some studies suggest increased severity of retinopathy of prematurity (ROP) in premature infants treated with sildenafil,[83,84] other studies do not.[85,86]

Inhaled/intratracheal sildenafil for treatment of PH, although not currently commercially available, has been studied in animals and shown to produce rapid decrease in mean pulmonary arterial pressure with more bioavailability than oral sildenafil. It appears to be superior to oral sildenafil by allowing for lower doses and potentially fewer systematic side effects.[60,87]

## Bosentan

Endothelin-1, a neurohormone predominantly released by vascular endothelium, is a potent vasoconstrictor. Bosentan is an ET-1 receptor antagonist, which acts on $ET_A$ and $ET_B$ receptors to affect NO and prostaglandin-independent vasodilation (see **Fig. 3**). Bosentan reverses endothelin-induced smooth muscle constriction, hypertrophy and hyperplasia, and is antifibrotic.[88,89] Because bosentan is an ET-1 antagonist and ET-1 is antiangiogenic in the developing lung and is involved in the pathogenesis of PH in CDH, bosentan may be more effective than sildenafil. Bosentan is an effective alternative treatment for PPHN in settings where iNO and ECMO are not available,[90] and as combination therapy.[91,92] It improves oxygenation and decreases duration of mechanical ventilation in infants with PH associated with CHD, CDH,[93,94] and BPD.[95] Oral bosentan starting at 0.5-1 mg/kg/dose q12h with dose increase every 2-4 weeks to a maximum of 2 mg/kg/dose, is recommended for infants with BPD complicated by PH.[79] Infants and children on bosentan must have their liver function monitored every 4 weeks due to potential liver toxicity.

## Prostacyclin

Synthetic prostacyclin (epoprostenol), prostacyclin analogs (iloprost, treprostinil, and beraprost) and selective prostacyclin receptor agonists (selexipag), act upon cyclic adenosine monophosphate (cAMP) pathway in vascular smooth muscle cells to cause NO-independent vasodilation (see **Fig. 3**). They also inhibit vascular smooth muscle cell proliferation and migration, as well as having potent anti-inflammatory, immunosuppressive, and antiaggregant effects.[96,97] Like iNO, sildenafil, and bosentan, prostanoids have been used successfully for PH in PPHN and acute pulmonary hypertensive crisis, as well as chronic therapy for PH in BPD, CDH, and CHD in outpatient settings. Owing to its short half-life, prostanoids are administered by continuous IV or subcutaneous infusion; or as continuous or q2-4h nebulization.

*Epoprostenol* is the first prostanoid approved by Food and Drug Association (FDA) for treatment of PAH in adults. It is usually given as continuous infusion via a central line for chronic treatment of PAH. However, it has been used off-label as continuous IV infusion in neonates with refractory PPHN with success.[98] Typical continuous infusion rate is initiated at 1-3 ng/kg/min, titrated up slowly every 4-6 hours. Infusion dose up to 20 ng/kg/min is recommended for infants with BPD,[79,99] although dose up to 120 ng/kg/min has been used for refractory PPHN.[98] Because IV epoprostenol is a nonselective pulmonary vasodilator, it may worsen ventilation/perfusion mismatch. It may also cause significant systemic hypotension and is associated with high risk for rebound PH with brief interruption of therapy. Inhaled epoprostenol more selectively lowers PAP and PVR than systemic epoprostenol and has been used with some success to treat PPHN and in infants with refractory PH-associated CHD at dose of 50 ng/kg/min.[100-102]

*Iloprost* is less expensive and more readily available than iNO in many developing countries. Inhaled iloprost (1-2.5 µg/kg/dose q2-4h) may be more effective than oral sildenafil (0.5-2 mg/kg/dose PO q6h) in PPHN treatment[103] as determined by time to adequate clinical response. Furthermore, inhaled iloprost may be an option when ECMO or iNO are not therapeutic options. Improved oxygenation with inhaled iloprost has been seen in preterm infants with severe respiratory distress syndrome and PH unresponsive to surfactant and conventional ventilation.[104-106] The currently recommended inhaled iloprost dose is 2.5-5 µg every 2-4 hours or 6-9 times a day with dose titration from 1-5 µg q4h to continuous inhalation.[79] Side effects include bronchospasm, hypotension, ventilator tube clogging due to crystallization, gastrointestinal (GI) disturbance, and pulmonary hemorrhage. Iloprost may also be teratogenic to caregivers. The occurrence of occasional bronchospasm may be a restricting factor in the use of inhaled prostacyclins by the BPD patients.[107] This may be preventable with bronchodilator and steroid pretreatment.

*Treprostinil* given either as continuous IV or as subcutaneous infusion has been used with success to treat PPHN due to sepsis,[108] as well as CDH-associated PH.[59,109,110] Subcutaneous infusion of treprostinil appears to be safe in infants and injection site pain may be less an issue than in adults.[109,111] Typical treprostinil dosage is 2 ng/kg/min continuous IV or subcutaneous infusion, titrated every q4-6h up to 20 ng/kg/min. Two premature neonates with sepsis and failed iNO were treated with IV treprostinil starting at 5 ng/kg/min and titrated up to 20 ng/kg/min within 3 hours with dramatic improvement and no side effects.[108] Inhaled treprostinil has longer half-life compared to iloprost and could be given 3-4 times a day instead of 6-9 times a day, and is effective in treating adult and child PAH. There are no data on inhaled treprostinil use in the NICU. Oral treprostinil was developed to avoid the complications and inconvenience associated with continuous IV and subcutaneous administration, and to allow for more drug delivery than achievable through inhalation. It was approved by the US Food and Drug Administration in late 2013 as an effective initial monotherapy treatment in adult PAH; there is limited data on its efficacy in children, and no data exists for use in neonates. Even if efficacious, its use may be limited by side effects, mostly GI.

*Beraprost* is an oral prostanoid with half-life of 35-40 minutes and has been shown to improve PH in adults, children with CHD,[112,113] and in one case series of seven neonates with PPHN treated with 1 μg/kg every 6 hours.[114]

## Prostaglandin

Prostaglandin E1 ($PGE_1$) is widely used in the NICU to maintain ductal patency for ductal-dependent CHD. In patients with severe PH and RV failure, some centers are also using $PGE_1$ to reopen ductus arteriosus, in addition to its pulmonary vasodilatory effect, to decrease RV pressure overload.[115] $PGE_1$ is also available in inhalation form and has been used to treat PPHN refractory to iNO as continuous nebulization at 150-300 ng/kg/min.[116,117]

## Milrinone

Milrinone is a phosphodiesterase 3 (PDE3) inhibitor and increases cAMP levels in cardiac muscle and vascular cells (*see* **Fig. 3**). A potent inotrope and afterload reducer, it has been used extensively in the cardiac intensive care unit, including for neonates following CHD repair. It is also a systemic and pulmonary vasodilator and has been shown to improve oxygenation as well as RV function and reduces strain and increases right and left ventricular output in infants with PPHN, including patients with CDH, CHD, and PPHN due to sepsis.[118-120] The typical dose is 0.15-0.5 μg/kg/min continuous IV infusion.

## Oxygen Therapy for BPD

Long-term supplemental oxygen therapy is considered standard treatment for BPD-associated PH.[121] Concerns for long-term complications of oxygen, however, especially for premature infants with ROP, have led to accelerated weaning of oxygen therapy. The optimal target for systemic arterial saturation in premature infants remain controversial but > 92% for infants with documented PH is recommended.[20,79]

## CONCLUSION

The majority of PH in neonates is due to PPHN, which is mostly due to meconium aspiration, sepsis, or birth asphyxia. Although PPHN is transient, mortality remains high. Other causes of PH in the neonatal period include developmental lung diseases, such as BPD, congenital diaphragmatic hernia, surfactant deficiency, alveolar capillary hypoplasia, and heritable or familial pulmonary hypertension. BPD is the leading cause of CLD in premature infants who survive the neonatal period and are at major risk for PH. For neonates with PH and uncorrected CHD, pulmonary vasodilation therapy may not be appropriate and may even be detrimental. It should be used with caution with careful consideration of the underlying cardiac defects and hemodynamics of the individual patient. Idiopathic or heritable PH accounts for a small percentage of neonates with PH, but they usually are less responsive to vasodilator therapy and more likely to progress to death or lung transplantation at a younger age. In addition to conventional therapy, inhaled nitric oxide, oral and IV sildenafil, milrinone, and prostanoids in IV, subcutaneous, and inhalation route, as well as endothelin receptor antagonist, have been shown to improve the outcome in neonates and infants with PH. iNO is used in severe newborn hypoxemic cardiorespiratory failure, but is expensive, unavailable in many resource-poor countries, not a viable option for long-term use, and is effective only half the time. Sildenafil has been found to improve PH in these settings. Milrinone infusion is used in intensive care settings, especially when PH is associated with cardiac dysfunction. Bosentan and prostanoids, although less often used and less well studied in neonates, are reasonably safe in the neonatal period for patients who have inadequate response or fail to respond to sildenafil and may be extended into outpatient setting for management of chronic PH.

## REFERENCES

1. Simonneau G, Gatzoulis MA, Adatia I. Updated clinical classification of pulmonary hypertension. J Am Coll Cardiol. 2013;62(Suppl 25):D34-41.

2. Simonneau G, Montani D, Celermajer DS, et al. Haemodynamic definitions and updated clinical classification of pulmonary hypertension. Eur Respir J. 2019;53(1). pii: 1801913.
3. Rosenzweig EB, Abman SH, Adatia I, et al. Paediatric pulmonary arterial hypertension: updates on definition, classification, diagnostics and management. Eur Respir J. 2019;53(1). pii: 1801916.
4. Mourani PM, Sontag MK, Younoszai A, et al. Clinical utility of echocardiography for the diagnosis and management of pulmonary vascular disease in young children with chronic lung disease. Pediatrics. 2008;121(2):317-25.
5. An HS, Bae EJ, Kim GB, et al. Pulmonary hypertension in preterm infants with bronchopulmonary dysplasia. Korean Circ J. 2010;40:131-6.
6. Bhat R, Salas AA, Foster C, et al. Prospective analysis of pulmonary hypertension in extremely low birth weight infants. Pediatrics. 2012;129(3):e682-9.
7. Bentar A, Clarke J, Silverman M. Pulmonary hypertension in infants with chronic lung disease: non-invasive evaluation and short term effect of oxygen treatment. Arch Dis Child Fetal Neonatal Ed. 1995;72(1):F14-9.
8. Hatle L, Angelsen B. Doppler ultrasound in cardiology, 2nd edition. Philadelphia: Lea & Febiger; 1985.
9. Hemnes AR, Forfia PR, Champion HC. Assessment of pulmonary vasculature and right heart by invasive haemodynamics and echocardiography. Int J Clin Pract Suppl. 2009;(162):4-19.
10. Singh A, Feingold B, Rivera-Lebron B, et al. Correlating objective echocardiographic parameters in patients with pulmonary hypertension due to bronchopulmonary dysplasia. J Perinatol. 2019;39(9):1282-90.
11. Ristow B, Ahmed S, Wang L, et al. Pulmonary Regurgitation End-diastolic Gradient Is a Doppler Marker of Cardiac Status: Data from the Heart and Soul Study. J Am Soc Echocardiogr. 2005;18(9): 885-91.
12. Grigoriadis S, Vonderporten EH, Mamisashvili L, et al. Prenatal exposure to antidepressants and persistent pulmonary hypertension of the newborn: systematic review and meta-analysis. BMJ. 2014;348:f6932.
13. Don M, Orsaria M, Da Dalt E, et al. Rapidly fatal "congenital lung dysplasia": a case report and review of the literature. Fetal Pediatr Pathol. 2014;33(2):109-13.
14. Andersen C, Ramsay JA, Nogee LM, et al. Recurrent familial neonatal deaths: hereditary surfactant protein B deficiency. Am J Perinatol. 2000;17(4):219-24.
15. van den Hout L, Schaible T, Cohen-Verbeek TE, et al. Actual outcome in infants with congenital diaphragmatic hernia; the role of a standardized postnatal treatment protocol. Fetal Diagn Ther. 2011;29:55-63.
16. Dillon PW, Cilley RE, Mauger D, et al. The relationship of pulmonary artery pressure and survival in congenital diaphragmatic hernia. J Pediatr Surg. 2004;39(3):307-12.
17. Walsh MC, Stork EK. Persistent pulmonary hypertension of the newborn. Clin Perinatol. 2001;28: 609-27.
18. Check J, Gotteiner N, Liu X, et al. Fetal growth restriction and pulmonary hypertension in premature infants with bronchopulmonary dysplasia. J Perinatol. 2013;33(7):553-7.
19. Kim DH, Kim HS, Choi CW, et al. Risk factors for pulmonary artery hypertension in preterm infants with moderate or severe bronchopulmonary dysplasia. Neonatology. 2011;101(1):40-6.
20. Khemani E, McElhinney DB, Rhein L, et al. Pulmonary artery hypertension in formerly premature infants with bronchopulmonary dysplasia: clinical features and outcomes in the surfactant era. Pediatrics. 2007;120(6):1260-9.
21. Afshar S, Gibson LL, Yuhanna IS, et al. Pulmonary NO synthase expression is attenuated in a fetal baboon model of chronic lung disease. Am J Physiol Lung Cell Mol Physiol. 2003;284(5):L749-58.
22. Bland RD, Ling CY, Albertine KH, et al. Pulmonary vascular dysfunction in preterm lambs with chronic lung disease. Am J Physiol Lung Cell Mol Physiol. 2003;285(1): L76-85.
23. Grover TR, Parker TA, Balasubramaniam V, et al. Pulmonary hypertension impairs alveolarization and reduces lung growth in the ovine fetus. Am J Physiol Lung Cell Mol Physiol. 2005;288(4):L648-54.
24. Gien J, Tseng N, Seedorf G, et al. Endothelin-1 impairs angiogenesis in vitro through Rho-kinase activation after chronic intrauterine pulmonary hypertension in fetal sheep. Pediatr Res. 2013;73:252-62.
25. Kambas K, Chrysanthopoulou A, Kourtzelis I, et al. Endothelin-1 signaling promotes fibrosis in vitro in a bronchopulmonary dysplasia model by activating the extrinsic coagulation cascade. J Immunol. 2011;186(11):6568-75.
26. Mahgoub L, Kaddoura T, Kameny AR, et al. Pulmonary vein stenosis of ex-premature infants with pulmonary hypertension and bronchopulmonary dysplasia, epidemiology, and survival from a multicenter cohort. Pediatr Pulmonol. 2017;52(8):1063-70.
27. Heching HJ, Turner M, Farkouh-Karoleski C, et al. Pulmonary vein stenosis and necrotising enterocolitis: is there a possible link with necrotising enterocolitis? Arch Dis Child Fetal Neonatal Ed. 2014;99(4):F282-5.
28. del Cerro MJ, Sabaté Rotés A, Cartón A, et al. Pulmonary hypertension in bronchopulmonary dysplasia: clinical findings, cardiovascular anomalies and outcomes. Pediatr Pulmonol. 2014;49(1):49-59.
29. Waruingi W, Mhanna MJ. Pulmonary hypertension in extremely low birth weight infants: characteristics and outcomes. World J Pediatr. 2014;10(1):46-52.
30. Eddahibi S, Raffestin B, Hamon M, et al. Is the serotonin transporter involved in the pathogenesis of pulmonary hypertension? J Lab Clin Med. 2002;139(4):194-201.
31. Timlin MR, Black AB, Delaney HM, et al. Development of Pulmonary Hypertension During Treatment with Diazoxide: A Case Series and Literature Review. Pediatr Cardiol 2017;38(6):1247-50.
32. Chen SC, Dastamani A, Pintus D, et al. Diazoxide-induced pulmonary hypertension in hyperinsulinaemic hypoglycaemia: Recommendations from a multicentre study in the United Kingdom. Clin Endocrinol (Oxf). 2019;91(6):770-5.
33. Ma L, Chung WK. The genetic basis of pulmonary arterial hypertension. Hum Genet. 2014;133(5):471-9.
34. Soubrier F, Chung WK, Machado R, et al. Genetics and genomics of pulmonary arterial hypertension. J Am Coll Cardiol. 2013;62(Suppl 25):D13-21.
35. Sztrymf B, Coulet F, Girerd B, et al. Clinical outcomes of pulmonary arterial hypertension in carriers of BMPR2 mutation. Am J Respir Crit Care Med. 2008;177(12):1377-83.

36. Rosenzweig EB, Morse JH, Knowles JA, et al. Clinical implications of determining BMPR2 mutation status in a large cohort of children and adults with pulmonary arterial hypertension. J Heart Lung Transplant. 2008;27(6):668-74.
37. Austin ED, Ma L, LeDuc C, et al. Whole exome sequencing to identify a novel gene (caveolin-1) associated with human pulmonary arterial hypertension. Circ Cardiovasc Genet. 2012;5(3):336-43.
38. Shintani M, Yagi H, Nakayama T, et al. A new nonsense mutation of SMAD8 associated with pulmonary arterial hypertension. J Med Genet. 2009;46(5):331-7.
39. Harrison RE, Flanagan JA, Sankelo M, et al. Molecular and functional analysis identifies ALK-1 as the predominant cause of pulmonary hypertension related to hereditary haemorrhagic telangiectasia. J Med Genet. 2003;40(12):865-71.
40. Trembath RC, Thomson JR, Machado RD, et al. Clinical and molecular genetic features of pulmonary hypertension in patients with hereditary hemorrhagic telangiectasia. N Engl J. Med. 2001;345(5):325-34.
41. Girerd B, Montani D, Coulet F, et al. Clinical outcomes of pulmonary arterial hypertension in patients carrying an ACVRL1 (ALK1) mutation. Am J Respir Crit Care Med. 2010;181(8):851-61.
42. Chaouat A, Coulet F, Favre C, et al. Endoglin germline mutation in a patient with hereditary haemorrhagic telangiectasia and dexfenfluramine associated pulmonary arterial hypertension. Thorax. 2004;59(5):446-8.
43. Nasim MT, Ogo T, Ahmed M, et al. Molecular genetic characterization of SMAD signaling molecules in pulmonary arterial hypertension. Hum Mutat. 2011;32(12):1385-9.
44. Ma L, Roman-Campos D, Austin ED, et al. A novel channelopathy in pulmonary arterial hypertension. N Engl J Med. 2013;369:351-61.
45. Nimmakayalu M, Major H, Sheffield V, et al. Microdeletion of 17q22q23.2 encompassing TBX2 and TBX4 in a patient with congenital microcephaly, thyroid duct cyst, sensorineural hearing loss, and pulmonary hypertension. Am J Med Genet A. 2011;155A(2):418-23.
46. Kerstjens-Frederikse WS, Bongers EM, Roofthooft MT, et al. TBX4 mutations (small patella syndrome) are associated with childhood onset pulmonary arterial hypertension. J Med Genet. 2013;50(8):500-6.
47. Best DH, Sumner KL, Austin ED, et al. EIF2AK4 mutations in pulmonary capillary hemangiomatosis. Chest. 2014;145(2):231-6.
48. Eyries M, Montani D, Girerd B, et al. EIF2AK4 mutations cause pulmonary veno-occlusive disease, a recessive form of pulmonary hypertension. Nat Genet. 2014;46(1):65-9.
49. Zhu N, Welch CL, Wang J, et al. Rare variants in SOX17 are associated with pulmonary arterial hypertension with congenital heart disease. Genome Med. 2018;10(1):56.
50. Patel MS, Taylor GP, Bharya S, et al. Abnormal pericyte recruitment as a cause for pulmonary hypertension in Adams-Oliver syndrome. Am J Med Genet A. 2004;129A(3):294-9.
51. Piazza AJ, Blackston D, Sola A. A case of Adams-Oliver syndrome with associated brain and pulmonary involvement: further evidence of vascular pathology? Am J Med Genet A. 2004;130A(2):172-5.
52. Montani D, Coulet F, Girerd B, et al. Pulmonary hypertension in patients with neurofibromatosis type I. Medicine (Baltimore). 2011;90:201-11.
53. Stewart DR, Cogan JD, Kramer MR, et al. Is pulmonary arterial hypertension in neurofibromatosis type 1 secondary to a plexogenic arteriopathy? Chest. 2007;132:798-808.
54. Kobayashi D, Cook AL, Williams DA. Pulmonary hypertension secondary to partial pulmonary venous obstruction in a child with Cantu syndrome. Pediatr Pulmonol. 2010;45(7):727-9.
55. Lo SM, Liu J, Chen F, et al. Pulmonary vascular disease in Gaucher disease: clinical spectrum, determinants of phenotype and long-term outcomes of therapy. J Inherit Metab Dis. 2011;34:643-50.
56. Lee TM, Berman-Rosenzweig ES, Slonim AE, et al. Two cases of pulmonary hypertension associated with type III glycogen storage disease. JIMD Rep. 2011;1:79-82.
57. Shah PS, Ohlsson A. Sildenafil for pulmonary hypertension in neonates. Cochrane Database Syst Rev. 2011;(8):CD0054594.
58. Mourani PM, Ivy DD, Gao D, et al. Pulmonary vascular effects of inhaled nitric oxide and oxygen tension in bronchopulmonary dysplasia. Am J Respir Crit Care Med. 2004;170:1006-13.
59. Lawrence KM, Hedrick HL, Monk HM, et al. Treprostinil Improves Persistent Pulmonary Hypertension Associated with Congenital Diaphragmatic Hernia. J Pediatr. 2018;200:44-49.
60. Rashid J, Patel B, Nozik-Grayck E, et al. Inhaled sildenafil as an alternative to oral sildenafil in the treatment of pulmonary arterial hypertension (PAH). J Control Release. 2017;250:96-106.
61. Hoeper MM, Andreas S, Bastian A, et al. Pulmonary hypertension due to chronic lung disease: updated Recommendations of the Cologne Consensus Conference 2011. Int J Cardiol. 2011;154 Suppl 1:S45-53.
62. Goldman AP, Tasker RC, Haworth SG, et al. Four patterns of response to inhaled nitric oxide for persistent pulmonary hypertension of the newborn. Pediatrics. 1996;98 (4 Pt 1):706-13.
63. Deprest JA, Gratacos E, Nicolaides K, et al. Changing perspectives on the perinatal management of isolated congenital diaphragmatic hernia in Europe. Clin Perinatol. 2009;36(2):329-47.
64. Finer NN, Barrington KJ. Nitric oxide for respiratory failure in infants born at or near term. Cochrane Database Syst Rev. 2006;(4): CD000399.
65. Sun XZ, Li ZF, Liu Y, et al. Inhibition of cGMP phosphodiesterase 5 suppresses matrix metalloproteinase-2 production in pulmonary artery smooth muscle cells. Clin Exp Pharmacol Physiol. 2010;37(3):362-7.
66. Broughton BR, Walker BR, Resta TC. Chronic hypoxia induces Rho kinase-dependent myogenic tone in small pulmonary arteries. Am J Physiol Lung Cell Mol Physiol. 2008;294(4):L797-806.
67. de Visser YP, Walther FJ, Laghmani el H, et al. Sildenafil attenuates pulmonary inflammation and fibrin deposition, mortality and right ventricular hypertrophy in neonatal hyperoxic lung injury. Respir Res. 2009;10:30.
68. Baquero H, Soliz A, Neira F, et al. Oral sildenafil in infants with persistent pulmonary hypertension of the newborn: a pilot randomized blinded study. Pediatrics. 2006;177:1077-83.
69. Juliana AE, Abbad FC. Severe persistent pulmonary hypertension of the newborn in a setting where limited resources exclude the use of inhaled nitric oxide: successful treatment with sildenafil. Eur J Pediatr. 2005;164(10):626-9.

70. Khorana M, Yookaseam T, Layangool T, et al. Outcome of oral sildenafil therapy on persistent pulmonary hypertension of the newborn at Queen Sirikit National Institute of Child Health. J Med Assoc Thai. 2011;94(Suppl 3):S64-73.
71. Ladha F, Bonnet S, Eaton F, et al. Sildenafil improves alveolar growth and pulmonary hypertension in hyperoxia-induced lung injury. Am J Respir Crit Care Med. 2005;172:750-6.
72. Caputo S, Furcolo G, Rabuano R, et al. Severe pulmonary arterial hypertension in a very premature baby with bronchopulmonary dysplasia: normalization with long-term sildenafil. J Cardiovasc Med (Hagerstown). 2010;11(9):704-6.
73. Mourani PM, Sontag MK, Ivy DD, et al. Effects of long-term sildenafil treatment for pulmonary hypertension in infants with chronic lung disease. J Pediatr. 2009;154(3):379-84.
74. Nyp M, Sandritter T, Poppinga N, et al. Sildenafil citrate, bronchopulmonary dysplasia and disordered pulmonary gas exchange: any benefits? J Perinatol. 2012;32(1):64-9.
75. Nichols DJ, Muirhead GJ, Harness JA. Pharmacokinetics of sildenafil after single oral doses in healthy male subjects: absolute bioavailability, food effects and dose proportionality. Br J Clin Pharmacol. 2002;53(Suppl 1):5S-12S.
76. Apitz C, Reyes JT, Holtby H, et al. Pharmacokinetic and hemodynamic responses to oral sildenafil during invasive testing in children with pulmonary hypertension. J Am Coll Cardiol. 2010;55(14):1456-62.
77. Mukherjee A, Dombi T, Wittke B, et al. Population pharmacokinetics of sildenafil in term neonates: evidence of rapid maturation of metabolic clearance in the early postnatal period. Clin Pharmacol Ther. 2009;85(1):56-63.
78. Barst RJ, Ivy DD, Gaitan G, et al. A randomized, double-blind, placebo-controlled, dose-ranging study of oral sildenafil citrate in treatment-naive children with pulmonary arterial hypertension. Circulation. 2012;125(2):324-34.
79. Krishnan U, Feinstein JA, Adatia I, et al. Evaluation and Management of Pulmonary Hypertension in Children with Bronchopulmonary Dysplasia. J Pediatr. 2017;188:24-34.
80. Steinhorn RH, Kinsella JP, Pierce C, et al. Intravenous sildenafil in the treatment of neonates with persistent pulmonary hypertension. J Pediatr. 2009;155(6):841-7.
81. Stultz JS, Puthoff T, Backes C Jr, et al. Intermittent intravenous sildenafil for pulmonary hypertension management in neonates and infants. Am J Health Syst Pharm. 2013;70(5):407-13.
82. Siehr SL, McCarthy EK, Ogawa MT, et al. Reported sildenafil side effects in the pediatric pulmonary hypertension patients. Front Pediatr. 2015;3:12.
83. Marsh CS, Marden B, Newsom R. Severe retinopathy of prematurity (ROP) in a premature baby treated with sildenafil acetate (Viagra) for pulmonary hypertension. Br J Ophthalmol. 2004;88(2):306-7.
84. Kehat R, Bonsall DJ, North R, et al. Ocular findings of oral sildenafil use in term and near-term neonates. J AAPOS. 2010;14(2):159-62.
85. Fang AY, Guy KJ, König K. The effect of sildenafil on retinopathy of prematurity in very preterm infants. J Perinatol. 2013;33(3):218-21.
86. Pierce CM, Petros AJ, Fielder AR. No evidence for severe retinopathy of prematurity following sildenafil. British Journal of Ophthalmology 2005;89:250.
87. Martell M, Blasina F, Silvera F, et al. Intratracheal sildenafil in the newborn with pulmonary hypertension. Pediatrics. 2007;119(1):215-6.
88. Rosenzweig EB, Ivy DD, Widlitz A, et al. Effects of long-term bosentan in children with pulmonary arterial hypertension. J Am Coll Cardiol. 2005;46(4):697-704.
89. Choudhary G, Troncales F, Martin D, et al. Bosentan attenuates right ventricular hypertrophy and fibrosis in normobaric hypoxia model of pulmonary hypertension. J Heart Lung Transplant 2011;30(7):827-33.
90. Nakwan N, Choksuchat D, Saksawad R, et al. Successful treatment of persistent pulmonary hypertension of the newborn with bosentan. Acta Paediatr. 2009;98(10):1683-5.
91. Radicioni M, Bruni A, Camerini P. Combination therapy for life-threatening pulmonary hypertension in a premature infant: first report on bosentan use. Eur J Pediatr. 2011;170(8):1075-8.
92. Fatima N, Arshad S, Quddusi AI, et al. Comparison Of The Efficacy Of Sildenafil Alone Versus Sildenafil Plus Bosentan In Newborns With Persistent Pulmonary Hypertension. J Ayub Med Coll Abbottabad. 2018;30(3):333-6.
93. Mohamed WA, Ismail M. A randomized, double-blind, placebo-controlled, prospective study of bosentan for the treatment of persistent pulmonary hypertension of the newborn. J Perinatol. 2012;32(8):608-13.
94. Bagby M, Zussman M, Hirsch R. Bosentan Use is Safe in Neonates and Infants with Congenital Diaphragmatic Hernia and Severe Pulmonary Hypertension. Abstract presentation at the 2011 PH Professional Network Symposium.
95. Rugolotto S, Errico G, Beghini R, et a. Weaning of epoprostenol in a small infant receiving concomitant bosentan for severe pulmonary arterial hypertension secondary to bronchopulmonary dysplasia. Minerva Pediatr. 2006;58(5):491-4.
96. Gessler T, Seeger W, Schmehl T. Inhaled prostanoids in the therapy of pulmonary hypertension. J Aerosol Med Pulm Drug Deliv. 2008;21(1):1-12.
97. Fetalvero KM, Martin KA, Hwa J. Cardioprotective prostacyclin signaling in vascular smooth muscle. Prostaglandins Other Lipid Mediat. 2007;82(1-4):109-18.
98. Eronen M, Pohjavuri M, Andersson S, et al. Prostacyclin treatment for persistent pulmonary hypertension of the newborn. Pediatr Cardiol. 1997;18(1):3-7.
99. Zaidi AN, Dettorre MD, Ceneviva GD, et al. Epoprostenol and home mechanical ventilation for pulmonary hypertension associated with chronic lung disease. Pediatr Pulmonol. 2005;40(3):265-9.
100. Brown AT, Gillespie JV, Miquel-Verges F, et al. Inhaled epoprostenol therapy for pulmonary hypertension: Improves oxygenation index more consistently in neonates than in older children. Pulm Circ. 2012;2(1):61-6.
101. Kelly LK, Porta NF, Goodman DM, et al. Inhaled prostacyclin for term infants with persistent pulmonary hypertension refractory to inhaled nitric oxide. J Pediatr. 2002;141(6):830-2.
102. Kovach J, Ibsen L, Womack M, et al. Treatment of refractory pulmonary arterial hypertension with inhaled epoprostenol in an infant with congenital heart disease. Congenit Heart Dis. 2007; 2(3):194-8.
103. Kahveci H, Yilmaz O, Avsar UZ, et al. Oral sildenafil and inhaled iloprost in the treatment of pulmonary hypertension of the newborn. Pediatr Pulmonol. 2014;49(12):1205-13.
104. Yilmaz O, Kahveci H, Zeybek C, et al. Inhaled iloprost in preterm infants with severe respiratory distress syndrome and pulmonary hypertension. Am J Perinatol. 2014;31(4):321-6.

105. Hwang SK, O YC, Kim NS, et al. Use of inhaled Iloprost in an infant with bronchopulmonary dysplasia and pulmonary artery hypertension. Korean Circ J. 2009;39(8):343-5.
106. Piastra M, De Luca D, De Carolis MP, et al. Nebulized iloprost and noninvasive respiratory support for impending hypoxaemic respiratory failure in formerly preterm infants: a case series. Pediatr Pulmonol. 2012;47(8):757-62.
107. Ivy DD, Doran AK, Smith KJ, et al. Short- and long-term effects of inhaled iloprost therapy in children with pulmonary arterial hypertension. J Am Coll Cardiol. 2008;51:161-9.
108. Park BY, Chung SH. Treprostinil for persistent pulmonary hypertension of the newborn, with early onset sepsis in preterm infant: 2 Case reports. Medicine (Baltimore). 2017;96(26):e7303.
109. Carpentier E, Mur S, Aubry E, et al. Safety and tolerability of subcutaneous treprostinil in newborns with congenital diaphragmatic hernia and life-threatening pulmonary hypertension. J Pediatr Surg. 2017;52(9):1480-3.
110. Olson E, Lusk LA, Fineman JR, et al. Short-term treprostinil use in infants with congenital diaphragmatic hernia following repairs. J Pediatr. 2015;167(3):762-4.
111. Ferdman DJ, Rosenzweig EB, Zuckerman WA, et al. Subcutaneous treprostinil for pulmonary hypertension in chronic lung disease of infancy. Pediatrics. 2014;134(1):e274-8.
112. Suzuki H, Sato S, Tanabe S, et al. Beraprost sodium for pulmonary hypertension with congenital heart disease. Pediatr Int. 2002;44(5):528-9.
113. Limsuwan A, Pienvichit P, Khowsathit P. Beraprost therapy in children with pulmonary hypertension secondary to congenital heart disease. Pediatric cardiology. 2005;26(6):787-91.
114. Nakwan N, Nakwan N, Wannaro J. Persistent pulmonary hypertension of the newborn successfully treated with beraprost sodium: a retrospective chart review. Neonatology. 2011;99(1):32-7.
115. Mohseni-Bod H, Bohn D. Pulmonary hypertension in congenital diaphragmatic hernia. Semin Pediatr Surg. 2007;16(2):126-33.
116. Sood BG, Delaney-Black V, Aranda JV, et al. Aerosolized PGE1: a selective pulmonary vasodilator in neonatal hypoxemic respiratory failure results of a Phase l/ll open label clinical trial. Pediatric Res. 2004;56(4):579-85.
117. Sood BG, Keszler M, Garg M, et al. Inhaled PGE1 in neonates with hypoxemic respiratory failure: two pilot feasibility randomized clinical trials. Trials. 2014;15:486.
118. James AT, Corcoran JD, McNamara PJ, et al. The effect of milrinone on right and left ventricular function when used as a rescue therapy for term infants with pulmonary hypertension. Cardiol Young. 2016;26(1):90-9.
119. McNamara PJ, Laique F, Muang-in S, et al. Milrinone improves oxygenation in neonates with severe persistent pulmonary hypertension of the newborn. J Crit Care. 2006;21(2):217-22.
120. Patel N. Use of milrinone to treat cardiac dysfunction in infants with pulmonary hypertension secondary to congenital diaphragmatic hernia: a review of six patients. Neonatology. 2012;102(2):130-6.
121. Stenmark KR, Abman SH. Lung vascular development: implications for the pathogenesis of bronchopulmonary dysplasia. Annu Rev Physiol. 2005;67:623-61.

CHAPTER

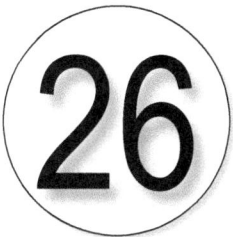

# Patent Ductus Arteriosus

*Priya Jegatheesan, Balaji Govindaswami*

## ABSTRACT

Patent ductus arteriosus (PDA) is a negative prognostic factor in severely ill preterm infants which is associated with significant neonatal morbidity. Aggressive medical and surgical treatment to close the PDA has been successful, but cumulative evidence of PDA treatment does not show benefit. This suggests that PDA is likely a marker of immaturity and not the cause of morbidities in preterm infants. Recent studies have shown that >90% of PDAs close spontaneously without treatment; however, the most immature infants [<26 weeks gestational age (GA)] ductal closure may not occur until several weeks after birth. If and when PDA treatment is indicated in the highest risk infants with a hemodynamically significant duct, choosing treatment options with minimal adverse effects is essential to optimize neonatal outcomes. Oral ibuprofen is efficacious in closing the PDA with minimal renal and gastrointestinal (GI) side effects compared to indomethacin and should be the first choice. When there is a contraindication for use of ibuprofen, acetaminophen should be considered as next option. If medical treatment has failed or is contraindicated, then minimally invasive procedures such as device closure of PDA via cardiac catheterization would be preferred over surgical ligation to minimize long-term adverse neurodevelopment outcomes. Future studies should focus on the highest risk infants to identify clinical parameters, biomarkers, timing, and choice of treatment for PDA closure. A standardized approach to evaluation and treatment of PDA inclusive of interdisciplinary discussion (e.g. pediatric surgery, cardiology, and neonatology); and monitoring outcomes including adverse effects of treatment and postdischarge PDA outcomes are essential for clinical teams to improve quality of care for preterm infants.

## INTRODUCTION: NATURAL HISTORY AND HISTORICAL PERSPECTIVE OF APPROACHES TO PATENT DUCTUS ARTERIOSUS

It is known that ductal areteriosus (DA) patency is often not associated with early clinical disease, but it is a negative prognostic factor in the severely ill neonate with respiratory distress.[1] It was also appreciated in infants <1,200 g that, despite a maturing tracheal aspirate phospholipid pattern associated with resolving respiratory distress syndrome (RDS), early development of left-to-right PDA shunt and worsening clinical status improved following ablation of the shunt.[2] While long established[3] that no deaths due to hyaline membrane disease or intraventricular hemorrhage (IVH) occurred in infants of mothers receiving betamethasone for at least 24 hours before birth, it was later found that infants not exposed to antenatal steroids (ANS) had a sevenfold PDA risk compared to infants who received ANS.[4]

The advent of surfactant replacement therapy altered the clinical course of infant RDS and the natural history and clinical course of PDA.[5]

Medical treatment of the PDA has occurred with nonsteroidal anti-inflammatory drugs (NSAIDs), and most recently, acetaminophen.[6] Other novel drug targets are being proposed to prevent ineffective therapy and inappropriate/unnecessary drug exposure.[7] Historically, the drug most used for medical closure has been indomethacin,[8] although our recent experience suggests that elimination of indomethacin use in very preterm infants is not associated with increased risk of surgical ligation.[9] A current noninferiority trial seeks to enroll 196 very preterm infants <32 weeks to oral paracetamol or oral ibuprofen for closure of hemodynamically significant ductus.[6]

A trial of indomethacin prophylaxis for prevention of IVH incidentally found that PDA closure is greater in very low birth weight (VLBW) infants randomized to indomethacin.[10] Subsequent follow-up of these infants showed no differences in long-term neurodevelopmental outcome.[11]

Although the PDA was initially ligated in an adult in 1938 by Gross,[12] it was first ligated in a preterm infant in 1963.[13] The debate on efficacy of PDA ligation[14] on infant respiratory distress is decades old.

Earlier proposals for surgical ligation as first-line therapy in very small premature infants at risk for failure of medical therapy[15] have been replaced by a more conservative approach[16] as it was recognized that while mortality was higher in infants with persistent PDA, other morbidities were not significantly different.[17] Almost two decades ago, it was suggested that the indications and timing for PDA closure were unclear, and improvement postprocedure uncertain.[18] Furthermore, surgical closure of the PDA is not without risk of significant morbidity.[19]

A small randomized controlled trial (RCT) (n = 84) of prophylactic ligation of the PDA in infants <1,000 g at birth (n = 40) showed a similar frequency of death, bronchopulmonary dysplasia (BPD), retinopathy of prematurity (ROP), and IVH in both groups. However, infants fed within 14 days of birth and whose PDA was ligated for medical reasons within 5 days of birth had a lower incidence of necrotizing enterocolitis (NEC) than those whose ductus was ligated later or not at all (2 of 10, i.e. 20%, versus 11 of 14 or 79%: p = 0.004).[20]

A meta-analysis indicates that the cumulative evidence of PDA treatment does not show benefit,[21] suggesting that PDA, while a marker of severity of illness, may not be the cause of morbidity in preterm infants.

Patent ductus arteriosus has been associated with multiple preterm neonatal morbidities, including pulmonary hemorrhage, BPD, NEC, renal impairment, IVH, and death.

The goal of this chapter is to summarize the evidence of PDA treatment briefly and provide a framework for a pragmatic and conservative approach to PDA management in preterm infants.

## EMBRYOLOGY

The DA is a large blood vessel that is present in the fetus, connecting the descending aorta and the main pulmonary artery trunk. It develops from the distal portion of the left sixth branchial arch and in the fetus is about the same size of the descending aorta. Morphologically, the DA is different from the aorta and the main pulmonary artery in that its medial layer largely consists of both longitudinally and spirally arranged smooth muscles within loose elastic tissue, rather than concentric layers of elastic fibers. The intima of the DA has the endothelial cells with smooth muscles, referred to as neointimal cushions.[22]

## PHYSIOLOGY OF DUCTAL CLOSURE

The low in utero oxygen tension and abundant circulating prostaglandins due to increased placental production and decreased clearance from the lungs are responsible for the fetal ductal patency. Postbirth, the smooth muscles in the intimal layer of the DA undergo constriction, followed by narrowing of the lumen and subsequent anatomic remodeling of the vessel. The constriction of the smooth muscles is triggered by the sudden increase in oxygen tension after birth that inhibits the voltage-dependent potassium channels, and leads to influx of calcium. The endothelial cells release vasoactive substances that are potent vasoconstrictors. The constriction and contraction of the smooth muscles lead to a "hypoxic zone" that causes cell death, releasing hypoxia-induced growth factors (e.g. vascular endothelial growth factor) that result in vascular remodeling and anatomic closure of the DA. Platelet adhesion and aggregation also play an important role in ductal closure after the initial constriction.[23]

## CLINICAL RISK FACTORS OF PATENT DUCTUS ARTERIOSUS

### Perinatal Factors

Antenatal glucocorticoids have been associated with lower incidence of PDA.[4] As little as a single dose of ANS has been associated with lower incidence of PDA in 25–27-week GA in preterm infants. Although indomethacin is used for treatment of PDA, antenatal exposure of indomethacin used for tocolysis is associated with increase in incidence and severity of PDA,[24] higher failure of medical treatment, and need for surgical closure.[25] Antenatal magnesium use has been associated with increase in PDA in some studies,[26,27] but not in others.[28] Maternal chorioamnionitis was associated with higher risk of PDA; however, a recent meta-analysis shows that this effect is not seen after adjusting for confounders such as GA and birth weight.[29] A meta-analysis including 996 infants ≤28 weeks gestation did not show effect of delayed cord clamping on PDA.[30] With increasing global embrace of delayed cord clamping in the VLBW population, the effects on PDA prevalence and natural history may be attenuated. This will require further study.

## Neonatal Factors

Lower GA and birth weight are some of the risk factors that are inversely related to the incidence of PDA. Severe lung disease, RDS, mechanical ventilation, and surfactant administration are associated with higher incidence of PDA.[6,31,32] Restricted fluid intake in preterm infants is associated with improved outcomes, including reduced PDA and NEC.[33] A systematic review and meta-analysis studying the association between chorioamnionitis and PDA showed no association for clinical chorioamnionitis, but an association with PDA with histological evidence of chorioamnionitis or histological and clinical evidence of chorioamnionitis.[34] Other risk factors at birth increasing PDA incidence include genetic predisposition, high altitude, and fetal infection. Ductal arterial sensitivity to prostaglandin E2 (PGE2), and high circulating PGE2 contributes to increased PDA frequency in preterm infants.[35] PGE2 is an abundant prostaglandin and plays a key role in inflammatory processes.[36,37]

## Biomarkers

High levels of brain/B-type natriuretic peptide (BNP), interleukins 6, 8, 10, and 12 erythropoietin, and low level of platelet-derived growth factor were associated with higher incidence of PDA.[38] Thrombocytopenia (<100,000) is shown to be associated with delayed closure of PDA in some studies,[39,40] but not in others.[41-43] A systematic review and meta-analysis[44] concluded that BNP values may need to be gestational and chronological age-specific, and combined with clinical metrics to improve generalizability and accuracy of diagnosing significant PDA. BNP has not been widely used in clinical practice.

## ■ EPIDEMIOLOGY

Overall incidence of PDA in <2,500 g infants was 21%, with GA and birth weight inversely related to the incidence of PDA.[45] About 77% of infants GA 28-30 weeks, 44% of GA 31-33 weeks, and 21% of GA 34-36 weeks showed PDA by clinical examination on days 3 and 7 of life.

A recent European study described the natural course of PDA in VLBW infants using serial echocardiograms.[46] GA and birth weight were the only significant predictors of PDA closure. The median age of closure was 71, 13, 8, and 6 days in those born at <26, 26-27, 28-29, and ≥30 weeks GA, respectively and 48, 22, 9, and 8 days in those with birth weight <750, 750-999, 1,000-1,249, and ≥1,250 grams, respectively. Overall, 93% of preterm infants' PDAs spontaneously closed without treatment, 85% closing before discharge and 8% after discharge.

In a recent prospective cohort study of 195 GA <29 weeks infants who underwent noninterventional conservative management, the incidence of PDA was 57% after the first week of life, and 95% of those infants had spontaneous closure prior to discharge from the neonatal intensive care unit (NICU).[47] Of the six infants who were discharged with an open PDA, four closed by follow-up and two required device closure. They did not show any difference in morbidity or mortality compared to those who had a hemodynamically significant PDA. Of note, the fluid management of infants in this study was restricted to <120 cc/kg/day for the first 4 weeks of life.

## ■ CLINICAL PRACTICE VARIABILITY AND PATENCY OF DUCTUS ARTERIOSUS

The epidemiology and incidence of PDA may be affected by different practices in neonatal and perinatal medicine.

Higher use of ANS, delayed cord clamping in the delivery room leading to improved cardiovascular stability, less invasive ventilatory methods, less intubation and surfactant use, lower NEC rate due to higher use of mother's breast milk and standardized feeding advance regimen, early enteral feeding approaches, and decreased central line days may all have a positive impact in the overall hemodynamic stability of the infant and thereby a lower incidence of hemodynamically significant PDA. In our single center experience in preterm infants (<33 weeks GA) with a very high antenatal steroid rate (>93%), delayed cord clamping (>85%), and increasing antenatal magnesium use from 2008 to 2018, we have shown a significant reduction in the incidence of symptomatic PDA and treatment of PDA in an era of much less invasive ventilation.[9] During this time despite elimination of use of indomethacin for PDA treatment, we showed no increase in PDA ligation.

## ■ DIAGNOSIS OF PATENT DUCTUS ARTERIOSUS

Clinical assessment of PDA (systolic murmur, precordial pulsations, wide pulse pressure, low diastolic blood pressure, and bounding femoral pulses) is neither sensitive nor specific, and often underestimates the actual incidence of PDA. A comprehensive clinical scoring system including tachycardia, metabolic acidosis, apnea/mechanical ventilation, hepatomegaly, and pulmonary deterioration was evaluated,[48] resulting in a final model that includes precordial pulsation, bounding femoral pulses, apnea/mechanical ventilation, and metabolic acidosis. This model was noted to have >80% sensitivity and specificity for hemodynamically significant PDA.

Echocardiogram provides objective structural and functional evaluation of the PDA. A standardized examination includes measuring PDA diameter at the pulmonary end (>1.5 m = moderate size), direction of flow across PDA, magnitude of left-to-right shunt using left atrium/aorta ratio >1.5, PDA diameter/left pulmonary artery ratio, antegrade diastolic flow of left pulmonary artery, and evidence of systemic steal by evaluating for absent or reversed end-diastolic flow in celiac axis, descending aorta, and middle cerebral artery.

The diagnosis of a hemodynamically significant duct by echocardiogram along with clinical instability due to effect of the left-to-right shunt is reason for ductal intervention. A proposed staging system to determine hemodynamic significance of the duct[49] incorporates signs and symptoms of pulmonary overcirculation leading to respiratory deterioration and systemic steal, i.e. hypoperfusion affecting renal and gut perfusion, and causing systemic hypotension.

## TREATMENT OPTIONS FOR PATENT DUCTUS ARTERIOSUS CLOSURE

Patent ductus arteriosus ligation was performed in the 1960s in a preterm infant with severe respiratory distress. Subsequently, many ligations were performed in larger preterm infants who showed clinical improvement. In the late 1970s, the understanding of prostaglandins role in maintaining ductal patency and observing the constriction of PDA with indomethacin in a ductal dependent lesion led to use of indomethacin for pharmacological closure of PDA.

### Medical Treatment for Patent Ductus Arteriosus Closure

*Conservative Treatment*

A pragmatic approach to manage the at-risk and symptomatic preterm infant includes fluid restriction (<130 cc/kg/day after day 3 of life) and respiratory support with higher positive end-expiratory pressure (PEEP) to prevent/treat pulmonary edema. Management of heart failure using diuretics and digoxin has also been attempted.

*Prostaglandin Synthetase Inhibitors*

Since prostaglandins play a significant role in fetal ductal patency, prostaglandin synthetase inhibitors have been used as medical treatment for PDA closure for more than four decades. Prostaglandin H2 synthase has two active sites. NSAIDs such as indomethacin and ibuprofen act on the cycooxygenase site and acetaminophen acts on the peroxidase region.

Indomethacin and ibuprofen (24 RCTs, n = 1,590 infants) have similar efficacy in PDA closure;[50,51] however, ibuprofen has lower risk of NEC and renal side effects.[52] Oral ibuprofen (5 studies, n = 406) has a lower risk of failure in PDA closure compared to intravenous (IV) ibuprofen.

Acetaminophen and ibuprofen (5 RCTs, n = 559) have similar efficacy in PDA closure; however, acetaminophen has a lower risk of gastrointestinal bleed, hyperbilirubinemia, and lower creatinine levels. Acetaminophen and indomethacin (2 RCTs, n = 277) have similar efficacy in PDA closure, and acetaminophen has lower creatinine levels, higher platelet count, and higher urine output.[52] The recent TOLERATE trial showed that Tylenol alone was only effective in constricting the PDA in 27%, compared to 62% for indomethacin.[53]

Network meta-analysis evaluating efficacy of all pharmacological treatments (14 variations of indomethacin, ibuprofen or acetaminophen, involving dose, route of administration, bolus vs. continuous, and concomitant treatment) to close a hemodynamically significant PDA showed that high-dose oral ibuprofen (20 mg/kg loading) followed by 7–10 mg/kg daily maintenance is most efficacious for PDA closure, compared to IV ibuprofen or indomethacin.[54] This analysis also showed that continuous IV ibuprofen had the lowest risk of NEC and oliguria; placebo or conservative management of PDA was not associated with worse mortality or morbidity. Preliminary evidence suggests that IV or oral paracetamol/acetaminophen is as effective in ductal closure as IV or oral ibuprofen and IV indomethacin. However, study of long-term neurodevelopmental outcomes with paracetamol is necessary before altering current clinical practice.[52,55,56]

### Surgical/Interventional Treatment for Patent Ductus Arteriosus Closure

*Surgical Ligation*

A RCT evaluating prophylactic ligation of PDA versus early ligation of symptomatic PDA (<5 days) showed a decrease in the risk of NEC.[20] However, meta-analysis of three observational studies shows that PDA ligation is associated with higher risk of BPD, severe ROP, and worse neurodevelopmental outcome.[57]

*Video-assisted Thoracoscopic Surgery for Patent Ductus Arteriosus Closure*

Initial reports of minimally invasive thoracoscopy suggested that video-assisted thoracoscopic surgery (VATS) was safe and effective.[58]

While VATS PDA ligation promised efficacy similar to traditional thoracotomy with shorter operative and recovery times and reduced hospitalization, there were more complications, especially vocal cord injuries reported in some studies.[59] Reduced cost of care is the general consensus from a large current review.[60]

Minimizing medical treatment for PDA in preterm infants in California has been accompanied by a slight increase in surgical ligation during the same period.[61] The combination of a conservative approach to intervention for PDA in the NICU and the embrace of deferred intervention (either later during hospitalization or postdischarge) has led to more interest in minimally invasive approaches such as interventional catheterization closure.

### Interventional Catheterization for Patent Ductus Arteriosus Closure

Much experience has been gained in the last decades by interventional catheterization[62] in low weight infants (<6 kg)[63] and variation in practice of PDA device closure, safety, and longer term cardiovascular outcomes are now reported.[64,65] The lack of a smaller size catheter had limited the ability to perform transcatheter device closure in extremely preterm infants. This year, following the Amplatzer duct occluder II (ADO II) clinical trial,[66] the Food and Drug Administration (FDA) has approved a smaller device[67] that can allow for performing these closures even in extremely low birth weight infants.

## Timing of Patent Ductus Arteriosus Treatment

### Prophylactic Treatment of Patent Ductus Arteriosus

Prophylactic indomethacin has been shown to decrease the incidence of symptomatic PDA and surgical ligation by 50% and severe IVH by 30%. However, there is no decrease in mortality, short-term morbidity, or long-term neurodevelopmental outcome at 18–36 months, but there is increased incidence of oliguria.[67] Similarly, prophylactic ibuprofen decreases incidence of symptomatic PDA, reduces the need for further treatment with cyclooxygenase inhibitors or ligation without improvement in other short-term morbidity, but increases risk of gastrointestinal bleed and renal function impairment.[68] This review also noted that the rate of PDA closure was 58% in the control group, suggesting that prophylactic treatment exposes infants unnecessarily to renal and gastrointestinal side effects, and thus prophylaxis is not recommended.

### Early Asymptomatic Patent Ductus Arteriosus Treatment

Early treatment of asymptomatic PDA is associated with lower incidence of symptomatic PDA and shorter duration of supplemental oxygen, without effect on mortality or other morbidities like BPD, IVH, and ROP. Similar to prophylactic treatment, this approach would also expose more infants to the side effects of treatment without significant benefit in mortality or short-term morbidity.[69]

### TOLERATE Trial

This RCT evaluated a conservative approach versus early routine pharmacological treatment of a moderate PDA after a child's first week (7-14 days) of life. In this study, 48% of preterm infants <28 weeks GA had a moderate to large PDA after the first week of life. There was no reduction in surgical ligations or discharge with an open PDA with early routine treatment, and in fact there was a delay in reaching full enteral feeds and an increase in sepsis and mortality in ≥26 weeks GA infants in the early routine treatment arm.[70]

## Effect of Patent Ductus Arteriosus Treatment on Neonatal Outcomes: Mortality and Morbidity

Despite the large number of trials that have shown successful closure of PDA in the treatment arm, a meta-analysis of all RCTs suggests that there is no significant benefit in other preterm outcomes.[71] Summary estimate of all studies of prophylaxis or treatment of symptomatic PDA fail to show any improvement in neonatal short-term or long-term outcomes except for reduction of severe IVH in the prophylaxis studies. A pooled estimate of subgroups of studies including only <29 weeks GA or those studies performed after 1989 (postsurfactant era) or rescue treatment after 6 days of life also did not show any benefits. The most recent TOLERATE study evaluating early routine treatment of a moderate to large PDA (7-14 days) compared to conservative management with predefined rescue treatment criteria further showed no difference in neonatal outcomes despite a reduction in ductal patency.

## Controversies about Patent Ductus Arteriosus Treatment

The rationale for treating PDA is to prevent the effect of ductal steal on the cerebrovascular, mesenteric and renal flow, and to decrease pulmonary overcirculation, thereby reducing neonatal morbidity and mortality. However, many RCTs and meta-analyses have failed to see any improvement in mortality or morbidity despite an increase in the rate of PDA closure.[21] Lower GA, not PDA treatment or echo score, was associated with the adverse outcome of death or BPD.[71] Surgical ligation has been associated with worse neurodevelopmental outcomes and BPD. The rationale for not treating PDA is the adverse effect associated with medical and surgical treatments.[72] There is also a concern about the change in physiology with premature closure of the duct causing a strain on the right ventricle leading to worse clinical outcome. The majority (93–95%) of PDAs close prior to discharge without treatment. Of those that remain open at discharge, very few receive transcatheter PDA closure while others spontaneously close within the first year of life.

Based on the lack of benefit in improving outcomes, most preterm infants >28 weeks GA do not need PDA treatment. In the most recent TOLERATE trial, infants ≥26 GA weeks in the early routine treatment group had higher rate of sepsis and mortality in addition to delayed full enteral feeds. This increase in sepsis may be related to interruption of enteral feeds during pharmacological treatment of PDA, leading to prolonged central line days, suggesting that the risk of treatment outweighs any benefit of treating PDAs.

A subset of highest risk premature infants that may potentially benefit from PDA closure are the most immature infants, <26 weeks GA, who have a hemodynamically significant PDA (clinically and by echocardiogram) after the first week of life. Based on the efficacy and adverse effects of pharmacological agents, the medical treatment of choice is oral ibuprofen. Contraindications for use of ibuprofen include thrombocytopenia, oliguria or elevated creatinine >1 mg/dL. In the presence of contraindications for NSAIDs, the next choice would be acetaminophen. Ideally the infants are on at least half enteral feeds to be able to tolerate oral medications. Using exclusive human milk feeding following a standardized feeding protocol is independently associated with lower risk of NEC and should be followed during treatment of PDA. Judicious management of fluids in the presence of a PDA may be necessary to optimize conservative management to optimize hemodynamic status of the infant.

A standardized approach for evaluation of PDA in preterm infants along with a process for expectant management of an open PDA with or without medical treatment is necessary for quality improvement efforts to optimize preterm care. Follow-up of the adverse effects related to the medical treatment of PDA (renal or hepatic insufficiency), postdischarge follow-up of the open PDA, and long-term outcomes are also essential to inform the optimal care of these infants in future.

## CONCLUSION

In an era of high antenatal steroid use, delayed cord clamping, and decreasing invasive ventilation, most preterm infants do not require treatment for PDA. However, timely identification and treatment of PDA may benefit a small subset of extremely preterm infants with hemodynamically significant PDA. In these high-risk infants, choosing treatment options with minimal adverse effects is essential for optimal outcomes. Future research should focus on identifying high-risk infants based on a combination of clinical characteristics and biomarkers, and the risk-benefit profile of different therapeutic strategies.

## REFERENCES

1. Dudell GG, Gersony WM. Patent ductus arteriosus in neonates with severe respiratory disease. J Pediatr. 1984;4(6):915-20.
2. Jacob J, Gluck L, DiSessa T, et al. The contribution of PDA in the neonate with severe RDS. J Pediatr. 1980;96(1):79-87.
3. Liggins GC, Howie RN. A controlled trial of antepartum glucocorticoid treatment for prevention of the respiratory distress syndrome in premature infants. Pediatrics. 1972;50(4):515-25.
4. Waffarn F, Siassi B, Cabal LA, et al. Effect of antenatal glucocorticoids on clinical closure of the ductus arteriosus. Am J Dis Child. 1983;137:336-8.
5. Clyman RI, Jobe A, Heymann M, et al. Increased shunt through the patent ductus arteriosus after surfactant replacement therapy. J Pediatr. 1982;100(1):101-7.
6. Kumar A, Sundaram V, Yadav R, et al. Oral paracetamol versus oral ibuprofen for closure of haemodynamically significant patent ductus arteriosus in preterm neonates (<32 weeks): a blinded, randomised, active-controlled, non-inferiority trial. BMJ Paediatr Open. 2017;1:e000143.
7. Shelton EL, Singh GK, Nichols CG. Novel drug targets for ductus arteriosus manipulation: looking beyond prostaglandins. Semin Perinatol. 2018;42(4):221-7.
8. Mehta SK, Younoszai A, Pietz J, et al. Pharmacological closure of the patent ductus arteriosus. Images Paediatr Cardiol. 2003;5(1):1-15.
9. Jegatheesan P, Huang A, Nudelman M, et al. Changing trends and risk factors for diagnosis and treatment of PDA in very preterm infants. Memphis, Tennessee: Abstract presentation at Second Annual International PDA Symposium; 2019.
10. Ment LR, Ehrenkranz RA, Duncan GC, et al. Low-dose indomethacin and prevention of intraventricular hemorrhage: a multicenter randomized trial. Pediatrics. 1994;93(4):543-50.
11. Ment LR, Vohr B, Allan W, et al. Outcome of children in the indomethacin intraventricular hemorrhage prevention trial. Pediatrics. 2000;105(3):485-91.
12. Alexi-Meskishvili, Vladimir V, Böttcher W. The first closure of the persistent ductus arteriosus. Ann Thorac Surg. 2010;90:349-56.
13. Powell ML. Patent ductus arteriosus in premature infants. Med J Aus. 1963;2:58.
14. Williams WH, Gelband H, Bancalai E, et al. The ductus debate: ligation in prematurity? Ann Thorac Surg. 1976;22(2):151-6.
15. Perez CA, Bustorff-Silva JM, Villasenor E, et al. Surgical ligation of patent ductus arteriosus in very low birth weight infants: is it safe? Am Surg. 1998;64(10):1007-9.
16. Bose CL, Laughon MM. Patent ductus arteriosus: lack of evidence for common treatments. Arch Dis Child Fetal Neonatal Ed. 2007;92:F498-502.
17. Brooks JM, Travadi JN, Patole SK, et al. Is surgical ligation of patent ductus arteriosus necessary? The Western Australian

experience of conservative management. Arch Dis Child Fetal Neonatal Ed. 2005;90:F235-9.
18. Van Woerkom R, Govindaswami B, Cleary J, et al. Patent ductus arteriosus ligation in very low birthweight infants: is there benefit? Pediatr Res. 2001:A32.
19. Benjamin JR, Smith PB, Cotten CM, et al. Long-term morbidities associated with vocal cord paralysis after surgical closure of a patent ductus arteriosus in extremely low birth weight infants. J Perinatol. 2010;30(6):408-13.
20. Cassady G, Crouse OT, Kirklin JW, et al. A randomized, controlled trial of very early prophylactic ligation of the ductus arteriosus in babies who weighed 1000 g or less at birth. N Eng J Med. 1989;320:1511-6.
21. Benitz WE. Treatment of persistent patent ductus arteriosus in preterm infants: time to accept the null hypothesis? J Perinatol. 2010;30(4):241-52.
22. Schneider DJ, Moore JW. Patent ductus arteriosus. Circulation. 2006;114:1873-82.
23. Echtler K, Stark K, Lorenz M, et al. Platelets contribute to postnatal occlusion of the ductus arteriosus. Nat Med. 2010;16(1):75-82.
24. Hammerman C, Glaser J, Kaplan M, et al. Indomethacin tocolysis increases postnatal patent ductus arteriosus severity. Pediatrics. 1998;102(5):E56.
25. Soraisham AS, Dalgleish S, Singhal N. Antenatal indomethacin tocolysis is associated with an increased need for surgical ligation of patent ductus arteriosus in preterm infants. J Obstet Gynaecol Can. 2010;32(5):435-42.
26. del moral T, Gonzalez-Quintero VH, Claure N, et al. Antenatal exposure to magnesium sulfate and the incidence of patent ductus arteriosus in extremely low birth weight infants. J Perinatol. 2007;27(3):154-7.
27. Basu SK, Chickajajur V, Lopez V, et al. Immediate clinical outcomes in preterm neonates receiving antenatal magnesium for neuroprotection. J Perinat Med. 2011;40(2):185-9.
28. Shimada E, Ogawa M, Matsuda Y, et al. Umbilical artery pH may be a possible confounder for neonatal adverse outcomes in preterm infants exposed to antenatal magnesium. J Matern Fetal Neonatal Med. 2013;26(3):270-4.
29. Behbodi E, Villamar-Martinez E, Degraeuwe P, et al. Chorioamnionitis appears not to be a Risk Factor for Patent Ductus Arteriosus in Preterm Infants: A Systematic Review and Meta-Analysis. Sci Rep. 2016;6:37967.
30. Fogarty M, Osborn DA, Askie L, et al. Delayed vs early umbilical cord clamping for preterm infants: a systematic review and meta-analysis. Am J Obstet Gynecol. 2018;218(1):1-18.
31. Harkin P, Marttila R, Pokka T, et al. Morbidities associated with patent ductus arteriosus in preterm infants. Nationwide cohort study. J Matern Fetal Neonatal Med. 2018;31(19):2576-83.
32. Lee HC, Durand DJ, Danielsen B, et al. Hospital variation in medical and surgical treatment of patent ductus arteriosus. Amer J Perinatol. 2015;32(4):379-86.
33. Bell EF, Acarregui MJ. Restricted versus liberal water intake for preventing morbidity and mortality in preterm infants. Cochrane Database Syst Rev. 2014;(1):CD000503.
34. Park HW, Choi YS, Kim KS, et al. Chorioamnionitis and Patent Ductus Arteriosus: A Systematic Review and Meta-Analysis. PLoS One. 2015;10(9): e0138114.
35. Dice JE, Bhatia J. Patent Ductus Arteriosus: An Overview. J Pediatr Pharmacol Ther. 2007;12(3):138-46.
36. Ricciotti E, FitzGerald GA. Prostaglandins and inflammation. Arterioscler Thromb Vasc Biol. 2011;31(5):986-1000.
37. Reese J, O'Mara PW, Poole SD, et al. Regulation of the fetal mouse ductus arteriosus is dependent on interaction of nitric oxide and COX enzymes in the ductal wall. Prostaglandins Other Lipid Medial. 2009;88(3-4):89-96.
38. Olsson KW, Larsson A, Jonzon A, et al. Exploration of potential biochemical markers for persistence of patent ductus arteriosus in preterm infants at 22-27 weeks' gestation. Pediatr Res. 2019;86(3):333-8.
39. Kulkarni VV, Dutta S, Sundaram V, et al. Preterm Thrombocytopenia and Delay of Ductus Arteriosus Closure. Pediatrics. 2016;138(4). pii:e20161627.
40. Dani C, Poggi C, Fontanelli G. Relationship between platelet count and volume and spontaneous and pharmacological closure of ductus arteriosus in preterm infants. Am J Perinatol. 2013;30(5):359-64.
41. Bas-Suarez M, Gonzalez-Luis G, Saavedra P, et al. Platelet counts in the first seven days of life and patent ductus arteriosus in preterm very low-birth-weight infants. Neonatology. 2014;106:188-94.
42. Sallmon H, Weber SC, Heming B, et al. Thrombocytopenia in the first 24 hours after birth and incidence of patent ductus arteriosus. Pediatrics. 2012;130(3):e623-30.
43. Alyamac Dizdar E, Ozdemir R, Sari FN, et al. Low platelet count is associated with ductus arteriosus patency in preterm newborns. Early Hum Dev. 2012;88(10):813-6.
44. Kulkarni M, Gokulakrishnan G, Price J, et al. Diagnosing significant PDA using natriuretic peptides in preterm neonates: a systematic review. Pediatrics. 2015;135(2):e510-25.
45. Siassi B, Blanco C, Cabal LA, et al. Incidence and clinical features of patent ductus arteriosus in low-birthweight infants: a prospective analysis of 150 consecutively born infants. Pediatrics. 1976;57(3):347-51.
46. Semberova J, Sirc J, Miletin J, et al. Spontaneous Closure of Patent Ductus Arteriosus in Infants ≤1500 g. Pediatrics. 2017;140(2). pii:e20164258.
47. Sung SI, Chang YS, Kim J, et al. Natural evolution of ductus arteriosus with noninterventional conservative management in extremely preterm infants born at 23-28 weeks of gestation. PLoS One. 2019;14(2):e0212256.
48. Kindler A, Seipolt B, Heilmann A, et al. Development of a Diagnostic Clinical Score for Hemodynamically Significant Patent Ductus Arteriosus. Front Pediatr. 2017;5:280.
49. McNamara PJ, Sehgal A. Towards rational management of the patent ductus arteriosus: the need for disease. Arch Dis Child Fetal Neonatal Ed. 2007;92(6):F424-7.
50. Gulack BC, Laughon MM, Clark RH, et al. Comparative effectiveness and safety of indomethacin versus ibuprofen for the treatment of patent ductus arteriosus. Early Hum Dev. 2015;91(12):725-9.
51. Ohlsson A, Walia R, Shah SS. Ibuprofen for the treatment of patent ductus arteriosus in preterm or low birth weight (or both) infants. Cochrane Database Syst Rev. 2018;(2):CD003481.
52. Ohlsson A, Shah PS. Paracetamol (acetaminophen) for patent ductus arteriosus in preterm or low birth weight infants. Cochrane Database Syst Rev. 2018;4(4):CD010061.
53. Liebowitz M, Kaempf J, Erdeve O, et al. Comparative effectiveness of drugs used to constrict the patent ductus arteriosus: a secondary analysis of the PDA-TOLERATE trial (NCT01958320). J Perinatol. 2019;39(5):599-607.

54. Mitra S, Florez ID, Tamayo ME, et al. Association of Placebo, Indomethacin, Ibuprofen, and Acetaminophen with Closure of Hemodynamically Significant Patent Ductus Arteriosus in Preterm Infants: A Systematic Review and Meta-analysis. JAMA. 2018;319(12):1221-38.
55. Buck ML. (2018). Update on the use of acetaminophen for patent ductus arteriosus closure. [online] Available from https://med.virginia.edu/pediatrics/wp-content/uploads/sites/237/2018/05/May18_Acetaminophen-PDA_PedPharmaco.pdf [Last accessed October, 2019].
56. Luecke CM, Liviskie CJ, Zeller BN, et al. Acetaminophen for Patent Ductus Arteriosus in Extremely Low-Birth-Weight Neonates. J Pediatr Pharmacol Ther. 2017;22(6):461-6.
57. Malviya MN, Ohlsson A, Shah SS. Surgical versus medical treatment with cyclooxygenase inhibitors for symptomatic patent ductus arteriosus in preterm infants. Cochrane Database Syst Rev. 2013;(3):CD003951.
58. Burke RP, Jacobs JP, Cheng W, et al. Video-assisted thoracoscopic surgery for patent ductus arteriosus in low birth weight neonates and infants. Pediatrics. 1999;104(2):227-30.
59. Vanamo K, Berg E, Kokki H, et al. Video-assisted thoracoscopic versus open surgery for persistent ductus arteriosus. J Pediatr Surg. 2006;;41(7):1226-9.
60. Stankowski T, Aboul-Hassan SS, Marczak J, et al. Is thoracoscopic patent ductus arteriosus closure superior to conventional surgery? Interact Cardiovasc Thorac Surg. 2015;21(4):532-8.
61. Ngo S, Profit J, Gould J, et al. Trends in patent ductus arteriosus diagnosis and management for very low birth weight infants. Pediatrics. 2017;139(4):e20162390.
62. Zahn E, Peck D, Phillips A, et al. Transcatheter Closure of Patent Ductus Arteriosus in Extremely Premature Newborns: Early Results and Midterm Follow-Up. JACC Cardiovasc Interv. 2016;9(23):2429-37.
63. Backes CH, Kennedy KF, Locke M, et al. Transcatheter occlusion of the patent ductus arteriosus in 747 infants <6 kg. JACC Cardiovasc Interv. 2017;10(17):1729-37.
64. O'Byrne ML, Kennedy KF, Rome JJ, et al. Variation in practice patterns in device closure of atrial septal defects and patent ductus arteriosus: An analysis of data from the IMproving Pediatric and Adult Congenital Treatment (IMPACT) registry. Am Heart J. 2018;196:119-30.
65. Nealon E, Stiver C, Cua C, et al. Transcatheter patent ductus arteriosus (PDA) closure in lower weight infants (<6kg): mid- and long-term follow-up. J Am Coll Cardiol. 2018;71(11 Supplement):A577.
66. NIH. (2013). AMPLATZER Duct Occluder II Clinical Study (ADO II). [online] Available from https://clinicaltrials.gov/ct2/show/NCT00713700 [Last accessed October, 2019].
67. PR Newswire. (2019). FDA Approves World's First Device for Treatment of Premature Babies and Newborns with an Opening in Their Hearts (a Common Congenital Defect). [online] Available from https://www.prnewswire.com/news-releases/fda-approves-worlds-first-device-for-treatment-of-premature-babies-and-newborns-with-an-opening-in-their-hearts-a-common-congenital-defect-300777303.html [Last accessed October, 2019].
68. Ohlsson A, Shah SS. Ibuprofen for the prevention of patent ductus arteriosus in preterm and/or low birth weight infants. Cochrane Database Syst Rev. 2019;(7):CD004213.
69. Cooke L, Steer PA, Woodgate PG. Indomethacin for asymptomatic patent ductus arteriosus in preterm infants. Cochrane Database Syst Rev. 2003;(2):CD003745.
70. Clyman R, Liebowitz M, Kaempf J, et al. PDA-TOLERATE Trial: An Exploratory Randomized Controlled Trial of Treatment of Moderate-to-Large Patent Ductus Arteriosus at 1 Week of Age. J Pediatr. 2019;205:41-8.e6.
71. Chock VY, Punn R, Oza A, et al. Predictors of brochopulmonary dysplasia or death in premature infants with a patent ductus arteriosus. Pediatr Res. 2014;75(4):570-5.
72. Mosalli R, Alfaleh K. Prophylactic surgical ligation of patent ductus arteriosus for prevention of mortality and morbidity in extremely low birth weight infants. Cochrane Database Syst Rev. 2008;(1):CD006181.

# CHAPTER 27

# Common Cardiorespiratory Disorders at Birth

*Kamakshi Devarajan, Balaji Govindaswami*

## ABSTRACT

This chapter describes causes of respiratory distress in the newborn. Discussion of fetal and transitional neonatal circulation will help provide context and promote improved understanding of the pathogenesis of conditions such as transient tachypnea of the newborn (TTN), infant respiratory distress syndrome (IRDS), meconium aspiration, and pulmonary hypertension. Clinical presentation, diagnostic approach, differential diagnosis, and treatment of the most common conditions in the neonate are addressed, as well as the pathogenesis of IRDS including lung mechanics and properties and composition of surfactant. Advances in neonatal respiratory care, i.e. noninvasive ventilation, nitric oxide, and less invasive surfactant administration (LISA) are also discussed. Current perinatal approaches to standardized definitions for chorioamnionitis, serial clinical observation of asymptomatic infants pretreated for chorioamnionitis, and universal screening for early-onset pathogens [e.g. group B *Streptococcus* (GBS)] provide opportunity for optimal antibiotics stewardship.

## INTRODUCTION

Respiratory distress is frequently seen in the immediate newborn period due to abnormal transition from fetal to extrauterine life. Although most infants make this transition successfully, ~7% of infants[1] have difficulty[2] and require respiratory assistance. Transitional difficulties may arise from factors such as airway obstruction, lung immaturity, infection, aspiration, excess lung fluid, and pulmonary hypertension.

This review will focus on common conditions associated with abnormal transition, such as TTN, IRDS, and meconium aspiration syndrome (MAS). Persistent pulmonary hypertension of the newborn (PPHN) is beyond the scope of this chapter, but covered elsewhere in a different context. Infectious causes of early respiratory distress are briefly mentioned, but are beyond the scope of this chapter.

## PHYSIOLOGIC TRANSITION FROM INTRAUTERINE TO EXTRAUTERINE LIFE

In fetal circulation (**Fig. 1**), blood from the placenta travels through the umbilical vein, ductus venosus (DV), then foramen ovale (FO) directly to the left atrium and left ventricle. Systemic venous return from the vena cavae flows through the right atrium to the right ventricle (RV), the systemic ventricle of the fetus. Almost 90% of this RV output gets passed across the ductus arteriosus (DA) to the descending aorta to the umbilical artery and back into the placenta.

There are three shunts in the fetal circulation: (1) DV, (2) FO, and (3) DA.

These are right-to-left shunts that result from low-resistance placental circulation and high-pulmonary vascular resistance (PVR) from fluid-filled lungs. After birth, initiation of breathing promotes lung expansion with clearing of alveolar fluid resulting in decrease in PVR, and umbilical cord clamping increases the systemic vascular resistance (SVR). The fall in the PVR and the rise in SVR results in closure of the right-to-left shunts across the FO and DA, effectively eliminating fetal circulatory patterns.

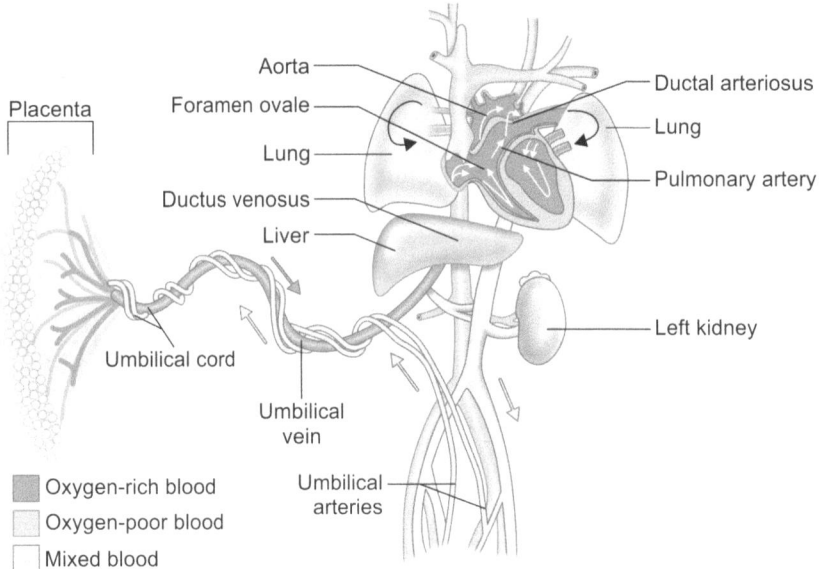

**Fig. 1:** Fetal circulation.

At birth, alveoli gas exchange occurs with initiation of breathing; the resulting decline in PVR leads to 12-fold increase in pulmonic blood flow.

## CARDIORESPIRATORY DISORDERS

### Transient Tachypnea of the Newborn

Transient tachypnea of the newborn is a common cause of respiratory distress[3,4] that arises from delayed and impaired alveolar lung fluid clearance with resulting pulmonary edema.

*Pathophysiology*

With a frequency of ~5.7/1,000 births, TTN occurs in full-term and preterm infants delivered by cesarean section before the initiation of labor. The process of lung fluid clearance begins several days prior to delivery. The catecholamine surge occurring in late gestation alters lung epithelial function from secreting chloride and water into the alveolar spaces to actively reabsorbing sodium and fluid from the airspaces. During delivery, this process is accelerated due to increased gene expression of sodium channels in the epithelial cells and an increase in oxygen tension. Oncotic pressure differential between airspaces, interstitium, and blood vessels further promote water absorption from the alveoli after birth through aquaporin water channels.

Delayed absorption results in decreased lung compliance; increased interstitial pressure causes increased airway resistance. Continued perfusion of collapsed alveoli results in ventilation perfusion mismatch (intrapulmonary shunt) that produces hypoxemia and hypercapnia.

*Risk Factors*

Elective cesarean section births (3.1%) versus vaginal (1.1%), small for gestational age (SGA), large for gestational age (LGA), male, and infants of diabetic mothers.

*Clinical Presentation*

Transient tachypnea of the newborn usually presents in the first few hours of life with respiratory rate >60 breaths per minute, with increased work of breathing. Can persist for 12–24 hours, up to 72 hours.

*Diagnosis*

Roentgenographic findings consistent with increased lung volumes and flat diaphragms, prominent vascular markings in sunburst pattern from the hilum and fluid in interlobar fissures. Arterial blood gas reveals moderate hypercapnia and hypoxemia with respiratory acidosis with normal hemogram and differential. Differentials include neonatal pneumonia, congenital heart disease, and IRDS.

*Supportive Treatment*

As TTN is a self-limiting disease with resolution in most cases by 72–96 hours, treatment is supportive, maintaining neutral thermal environment and oxygen treatment via nasal cannula or hood if needed. Rarely requires >40% $O_2$ to keep saturations >90%. If respiratory rate is >60–80 breaths per minute, feedings are orogastric with necessary intravenous supplementation. If tachypnea persists >4 hours, may need to obtain blood culture and start empiric coverage with antibiotics. Furosemide does not affect clinical course.[5] Fluid restriction may be beneficial in the management of severe TTN.[6]

## Infant Respiratory Distress Syndrome[7]

Infant respiratory distress syndrome, formerly known as hyaline membrane disease, is due to surfactant deficiency in premature infants. The disease is also seen in late preterm and some term infants due to functional/qualitative surfactant deficiency, e.g. infants born to diabetic mothers.

Surfactant deficiency results in increased surface tension within the alveoli resulting in atelectasis, edema, and cell injury. There has been significant progress made in the last two decades in prevention by antenatal steroid administration to accelerate lung maturity, postnatal surfactant treatment, and advances in neonatal respiratory care.

Knowledge of fetal lung development is essential to understand IRDS pathophysiology.

Fetal lung development occurs in four stages: embryonic (up to day 36), pseudoglandular (7–16th week), canalicular (16–25th week), and saccular (>24 weeks).

*Embryonic:* At day ~26, the fetal lung appears as a protrusion of the foregut with initial branching of the lungs and formation of the main bronchi occurring by 33 days.

*Pseudoglandular (7–16th week):* About 15–20 generations of airway branching starting from main segmental bronchi and ending as terminal bronchioles lined by morphologically undifferentiated epithelial cells. Airways are surrounded by loose mesenchyme with few blood vessels.

*Canalicular (16–25th week):* This is the phase where the respiratory bronchioles and alveolar ducts involved in gas exchange are being formed. The mesenchyme becomes more vascular and consolidates around airways with fusion of epithelial basement membranes and capillary basement membranes. At 20 weeks the cuboidal epithelial cells differentiate into alveolar type II cells and lamellar bodies. Surfactant production is first noted at 20 weeks with appearance of lamellar bodies.

*Saccular (>24 weeks):* Around 24 weeks, alveolization occurs with primitive forms of future alveoli visible with growth of septae that subdivide the terminal saccules into functional alveoli. The alveoli multiply from 0 at 32 weeks, to 50–150 million at 40 weeks, and 300 million in an adult.

The fetal lung is a solid fluid-filled organ with no ventilatory function until birth. In preparation for extrauterine life, surfactant is produced in the third trimester to promote lung expansion and prevent alveolar collapse and atelectasis. Surfactant production is developmentally regulated with production increasing with gestational age (GA).

Surfactant is composed of 90% lipids and 10% proteins. About 70% of the lipids are phosphatidylcholine (60% desaturated palmitoyl phosphatidylcholine). There are four proteins, the hydrophobic proteins surfactant protein B and C (SP-B and SP-C) and hydrophilic proteins SP-A and SP-D. SP-A regulates lung inflation and is an innate host defense protein. It promotes phagocytosis of pathogens and airway clearance of macrophages. Deficiency of SP-A has not been identified and mice that lack SP-A have normal function. SP-A is not present in currently available surfactants. SP-B; however, is a major contributor to the surface tension lowering ability of surfactant by facilitating surface absorption and spreading of phospholipids. Antibodies to SP-B result in respiratory failure; homozygous SP-B deficiency is rare and lethal. SP-C deficiency does not result in respiratory distress at birth, but patients develop progressive interstitial fibrosis in early childhood. SP-B and SP-C are present in commercial surfactant preparations. SP-D belongs to the collectin family and, like SP-A, facilitates airway clearance.

Surfactant is produced within alveolar type II cells with phospholipids synthesized in the endoplasmic reticulum and passed through to the lamellar bodies where they combine with SP-B and SP-C to form lipoprotein complex. Lamellar bodies localize to the apical side of the type II cells and release the lipoprotein complex into the alveoli by exocytosis. Tubular myelin, a lipoprotein array, forms a film within the alveoli and reduces surface tension. There is reabsorption from the air space back to the type II cells by an endocytic process. Endogenous and exogenous recycling are important contributors of the surfactant pool.

In premature infants there is both qualitative and quantitative surfactant deficiency. Antenatal steroid promotes lung maturity by stimulating phospholipid synthesis, release of surfactant, and changing lung architecture.

### Pathophysiology

Laplace's Law ($P = 2T/R$) states that the pressure (P) required to keep a sphere open is directly proportional to the surface tension (T) of the sphere and indirectly proportional to its radius (R). In surfactant deficiency, alveolar collapse occurs at end-expiration, because insufficient pressures (P) are generated in the midst of high surface tension (T) to keep the small alveoli (R) open.

Alveolar collapse due to atelectasis from surfactant deficiency causes injury to respiratory epithelium and alveolar capillary endothelium, both of which trigger lung inflammation and pulmonary edema, impeding gas exchange with resultant intrapulmonary shunting. Low lung compliance and low lung volume results in decreased functional residual capacity (FRC) and increased airway resistance.

## Incidence

Infant respiratory distress syndrome increases with decreasing GA, with an incidence of 1% in infants born at >38 weeks gestation. IRDS is male and Caucasian preponderant.

## Clinical Features

Infant respiratory distress syndrome presents within the first few minutes of life with worsening clinical course over the next 48 hours. Symptoms include tachypnea, nasal flaring, grunting (exhalation from partly closed glottis to prevent end expiratory alveolar collapse), intercostal and subcostal retractions (due to highly compliant chest wall encasing the lungs that are poorly compliant), and cyanosis. Urine output is low in the first 24–48 hours with diuresis preceding improvement.

## Diagnosis

Diagnosis is based on history, clinical examination, and radiographic findings of air bronchograms (due to alveolar atelectasis with aerated airways) and generalized ground-glass appearance of lung fields. Blood gas demonstrates hypoxemia and hypercapnia. Hyponatremia from water retention improves with diuresis and fluid restriction.

## Differential Diagnosis

- *Transient tachypnea of the newborn*: Seen more commonly in mature infant with milder symptoms and improves quickly in the first 24 hours.
- Pneumonia.
- Air leaks.
- *Congenital heart disease*: Characterized by less respiratory distress, lack of significant hypercapnia as well as X-ray findings consistent with respiratory distress syndrome (RDS).

## Management

Management can be divided into preventative care and therapeutic care. The best intervention is to prevent premature births[8] since IRDS is largely a result of lung immaturity. However, if premature birth cannot be avoided, specific interventions to prevent and/or decrease the severity of IRDS include administration of antenatal corticosteroids, treatment with exogenous surfactant, and/or provision of assisted ventilation.[9]

*Antenatal steroid therapy:* Pregnant women who are at increased risk of preterm delivery between 23 weeks and 34 weeks within the next 7 days should receive antenatal steroid therapy (ANS). A recent study suggests that ANS is also indicated for late preterm infants (34–36 weeks).[10] Furthermore, ANS is advocated for <23 weeks gestation infants.[11]

*Surfactant therapy:* Exogenous surfactant replacement therapy is effective in reducing IRDS mortality and morbidity in preterm infants, especially in infants <30 weeks. Trials comparing surfactant therapy with placebo demonstrates lower incidence and severity of IRDS and mortality, and a decreased rate of complications, i.e. pulmonary interstitial emphysema and pneumothorax. When surfactant therapy is used, the type of surfactant (natural or synthetic), indication and timing, and the technical aspects of administration need to be considered.

Natural surfactants have been shown to be superior in clinical trials compared to synthetic preparations, with lower IRDS complications in preterm infants and decreased mortality. Natural surfactants are obtained by either animal lung lavage or by mincing animal lung tissue, and purified by lipid extraction that removes hydrophilic components, including hydrophilic SP-A and SP-D. The remaining purified lipid preparation contains SP-B and SP-C, neutral lipids, and phospholipid dipalmitoylphosphatidylcholine (DPPC), the primary surface active lipid responsible for surface tension lowering property of surfactant.

In a meta-analysis published in 2011 of trials that compared poractant alfa (Curosurf/porcine surfactant) with beractant (Survanta/bovine surfactant) to treat preterm infants with IRDS, there was no difference in primary outcome of bronchopulmonary dysplasia (BPD) (defined as oxygen dependence at a postmenstrual age of 36 weeks) between the two different surfactant types (31.5 vs 29.9%).[12]

*Surfactant administration:* Early nasal continuous positive airway pressure (nCPAP) is just as effective in preventing and treating IRDS in very premature infants as intubation and early or prophylactic surfactant therapy.[13] Subsequently, international neonatal resuscitation experts recommend initiating nCPAP to all preterm infants with RDS with selective use of intubation and surfactant therapy.[14,15] The indications for intubation and administration of surfactant therapy are relative. Surfactant is often considered for preterm infants who fail nCPAP alone [defined as requiring a fraction of inspired oxygen ($FiO_2$) of 40% or higher to maintain oxygen saturation above 90%, respiratory acidosis arterial pH <7.2, and a partial pressure of carbon dioxide ($PaCO_2$) >60 mm Hg on CPAP]. Intubation may be required for infants with significant apnea, unresponsive to medical therapy, and/or requiring nasal intermittent positive pressure ventilation (NIPPV). Caffeine therapy has been a very important adjuvant therapy for apnea of prematurity.[16-20] In fact, LISA was initially described in infants who almost exclusively received caffeine.[21,22] In current era IRDS, additional doses of surfactant are seldom necessary.

*Surfactant administration techniques:* Endotracheal intubation has been the prevalent technique of surfactant administration, and may be complicated by transient airway obstruction or inadvertent instillation into only the right main stem bronchus if the endotracheal tube is advanced too far in the airway. Other complications associated with intubation and mechanical ventilation include pulmonary injury due to volutrauma and barotrauma associated with intermittent positive pressure ventilation, pulmonary air leak, and airway injury due to intubation. LISA is among many noninvasive techniques used in preterm infants with IRDS. Others include aerosolized surfactant preparations, laryngeal mask airway-aided delivery of surfactant, pharyngeal instillation, and the use of thin intratracheal catheters.[23] Systematic review and meta-analyses have reported that noninvasive surfactant administration via a thin catheter in spontaneously breathing infants may improve outcome compared with the treatment of intubation and surfactant administration.[24,25]

*Assisted ventilation techniques:* In patients with IRDS that require intubation and mechanical ventilation, while supplemental oxygen and mean airway pressures are used to improve arterial oxygenation, these interventions also contribute to the development of BPD/chronic lung disease (CLD).

Less invasive modes of ventilation, i.e. nCPAP and NIPPV have been evaluated as alternatives to mechanical ventilation that would treat the pathophysiology associated with IRDS at the same time decreasing the evolution of chronic lung inflammation and BPD from volutrauma, barotrauma, and oxygen toxicity mediated by ventilator support.

Continuous positive airway pressure can be administered via nasal prongs, nasopharyngeal tube or mask using water bubbling system [bubble continuous positive airway pressure (BCPAP)] or a ventilator. Although operator preference for bubble or ventilator CPAP is common, advantages of one form of nCPAP over the other are debatable. NIPPV does not confer any additional benefit over nCPAP.[26]

The Surfactant Positive Pressure and Pulse Oximetry Randomized Trial (SUPPORT)[27] compared 1,310 infants 24-27 weeks either on nCPAP initiated immediately after birth or given prophylactic surfactant and ventilation started within 60 minutes of birth. Overall, the death rate/BPD was lower in CPAP compared to the surfactant group (48% vs. 51%), as well as in the 24-25 weeks of GA subset [20% vs. 29%; relative risk (RR), 0.68; 95% confidence interval (CI), 0.5-0.92]. Subsequent individual patient data meta-analysis[28] has confirmed higher risk of mortality and necrotizing enterocolitis (NEC) in very preterm infants maintained at lower oxygen saturation ranges (85-89%), and higher risk of retinopathy of prematurity (ROP) for those targeted at higher (91-95%) oxygen saturation ranges.

*High flow nasal cannula:* Heated, humidified high flow nasal cannula is sometimes used to provide positive distending pressure with or without oxygen instead of traditional nCPAP devices.[29]

## Supportive Care

The following general supportive measures are provided in all preterm infants to optimize infant cardiorespiratory and metabolic status.

*Thermoregulation:* Infants should be maintained in a thermal neutral environment to minimize heat loss and maintain the core body temperature in a normal range 36.5-37°C (anterior abdominal wall) in order to reduce oxygen consumption and caloric needs. Rectal temperatures should be avoided due to risk of perforation.

*Fluid management:* Fluid management strategy is controversial in preterm infants due to limited concentrating abilities of the immature kidneys along with increased insensible loss that is exacerbated under phototherapy and radiant warmer. Excessive fluid intake may increase the risk of patent ductus arteriosus (PDA), NEC, and BPD, and therefore relative fluid restriction[30] to achieve a slightly negative water balance is recommended, especially in the first few days of the disease process. Optimal nutrition with early and prompt initiation of standard total parenteral nutrition to meet the metabolic needs of the preterm with IRDS is important.

*Cardiovascular management:* Systemic hypotension that may occur in the early stages of IRDS may be treated with vasopressor support, cautious use of normal saline for intravascular expansion, and, in refractory cases, stress doses of hydrocortisone. PDA is common in preterm infants with IRDS which may contribute to difficulty in weaning from mechanical ventilation.

*Blood gas monitoring and target oxygen saturations:* In the presence of respiratory failure, or need for supplemental oxygen >60%, an indwelling arterial line (e.g. umbilical arterial catheter) is optimal for blood gas monitoring; venous or capillary samples, while not useful for estimating partial pressure of oxygen ($PaO_2$), can be used to monitor $PaCO_2$. Permissive hypercapnia, targeting $CO_2$ levels 45-60 mm Hg is common clinical practice, although an optimal target for $PaCO_2$ is not established. Since clinical trials comparing target oxygen saturation levels demonstrate poor outcomes in premature infants with values below 89% and above 95%, maintaining oxygen saturation at 90–95% to avoid both hypoxia and hyperoxia is preferable.

### Complications

While morbidities and mortality from IRDS have improved significantly with antenatal steroids and/or surfactant therapy, there remains significant opportunity for further improvement. To optimize neonatal short- and long-term outcomes, it is essential to avoid complications related to endotracheal intubation, mechanical ventilation, subglottic stenosis, and postextubation atelectasis, and rarely esophageal and pharyngeal perforations.

## Meconium Aspiration Syndrome

Approaches to birthing,[31] especially global embrace of delayed umbilical cord clamping,[14,15] have altered in recent years. Approach to delivery via insignificant compared to significant (thick, tenacious, black, dark green, and particulate/lumpy) meconium has also changed.[32] The prevalence of MAS varies 1–2/1,000 live births. Current comprehensive reviews of MAS are readily available.[33,34]

## PULMONARY HYPERTENSION

Persistent pulmonary hypertension of the newborn occurs in 1–2/1,000 live births. Its incidence has been reported as 1.9 per 1,000 live births (0.4–6.8 per 1,000 live births) in the United States and 0.43 to 6 per 1,000 live births in the United Kingdom.[35] Neonates with severe pulmonary parenchymal disease, perinatal asphyxia, space-occupying lesions in the chest (e.g. congenital diaphragmatic hernia, pulmonary sequestration, congenital cystic adenomatoid malformation, etc.) and congenital heart disease are at high risk of sustained elevation in pulmonary artery (PA) pressure (usually defined as >50–75% systemic blood pressure). Infants with syndromic and genetic abnormalities (e.g. Down syndrome and other trisomies) have a higher frequency of PPHN due to underlying disease. Several recent comprehensive reviews are available.[36-38]

Inhaled nitric oxide (iNO) has been used for severe hypoxemic cardiorespiratory failure in newborns >34 weeks gestation.[39] Sildenafil therapy may be safe and efficacious in low-resource settings.[40] PPHN occurs in very preterm infants, particularly those with severe BDP/CLD. Early use of iNO to prevent BPD in this population has produced mixed results.[41-44] Despite the National Institutes of Health (NIH) consensus[45] recommending against using iNO either as early routine, early rescue, or later rescue in infants <34 weeks gestation, iNO use remains prevalent in neonatal intensive care units (NICUs).[46] African American infants <34 weeks GA at birth, at high risk for CLD/BPD, may merit special consideration for iNO therapy.[47]

## PNEUMONIA AND EARLY-ONSET SEPSIS

Early onset respiratory distress may be infectious in origin,[48,49] often accompanied by sepsis and with pathogens distinct from those implicated in late onset sepsis.[50] The most common early-onset pathogens include GBS, enteric coliforms (*Escherichia coli, Klebsiella*, and others), and *Listeria*. Universal antenatal GBS screening and appropriate penicillin/ampicillin prophylaxis for GBS+ women screened close to delivery has reduced burden of early onset GBS disease by 80% between 1996 and 2006 in the US.[51] There is much opportunity for further global reductions in early onset GBS disease by replicating the success in the developing world, including Asia and Africa. *Listeria* is a unique Gram-positive rod with interesting epidemiology. History of intake of fresh unpasteurized cheeses or contaminated food, including salads, may be present. Luckily the organism is exquisitely sensitive to ampicillin and readily treated if correctly diagnosed.[52-55] Gram-negative rods can be significant contributors to neonatal morbidity and mortality from early onset sepsis.[56]

Less frequently, pathogens such as *Clostridium tetani, Treponema pallidum* (syphilis), gonorrhea, and chlamydia may also be implicated. While in the past, these infections were seemingly less common in the industrialized world, the current epidemic of homelessness and substance use has led to their resurgence in high-risk populations.[57-59]

Good antibiotic jurisprudence involves elimination/minimal antibiotic use when treatable disease is absent. However, one must be prudent not to miss treatable clinical disease if antibiotics are indicated for sepsis. Current strategies include improved definitions of chorioamnionitis,[60] clinical pathways for close observation of infants pretreated for maternal chorioamnionitis,[61] and prompt initiation of antibiotics of those infants thought to have antibiotic-treatable disease.

A variety of neonatal pathogens are prevalent across the world,[62] and while the global burden of disease is enormous,[63] targeted interventions have permitted encouraging reductions in infection rates and mortality across high-risk pediatric age groups.[64] There remains much room for further reduction in infectious disease worldwide.[65]

## CONCLUSION

Successful transition of the fetus to a neonate is dependent on several factors: the gestational age of the infant, maturity of the lung parenchyma, adequacy of lung fluid clearance, in utero hypoxia, and infection which can result in pulmonary hypertension, as well as presence of anatomical abnormalities. Significant advances have been made in the understanding of these conditions in the last 25 years, permitting improved perinatal and neonatal care. Minimizing neonatal comorbidities and complications have greatly reduced the risk of prolonged invasive ventilation, leading to reduced respiratory morbidities in both preterm and term infants. Standardized definitions of chorioamnionitis and universal screening for early-onset pathogens (e.g. GBS) have much potential for prevention of early onset sepsis. Serial observations of asymptomatic infants whose mothers have been treated for chorioamnionitis reduce unnecessary postnatal antibiotic exposure. Appropriate antibiotic jurisprudence in perinatal and neonatal medicine (i.e. minimizing antibiotic utilization rate and reducing antibiotic exposure rate, while not avoiding or delaying antibiotic use when indicated) remains critical in an era of increased antibiotic resistance.

## REFERENCES

1. Reuter S, Moser C, Baack M. Respiratory distress in the newborn. Pediatr Rev. 2014;35(10):417-29.
2. Lattari Balest A. Overview of Perinatal Respiratory Disorders. [online] Available from https://www.merckmanuals.com/professional/pediatrics/respiratory-problems-in-neonates/overview-of-perinatal-respiratory-disorders [Last accessed October, 2019].
3. Jha K, Makker K. (2019). Transient Tachypnea of the Newborn. [online] Available from https://www.ncbi.nlm.nih.gov/books/NBK537354/ [Last accessed October, 2019].
4. Johnson KE, Garcia-Prats JA, Kim SM. (2018). Transient Tachypnea of the Newborn. [online] Available from https://www.uptodate.com/contents/transient-tachypnea-of-the-newborn [Last accessed October, 2019].
5. Kassab M, Khriesat WM, Anabrees J. Diuretics for transient tachypnoea of the newborn. Cochrane Database Syst Rev. 2015;(11):CD003064.
6. Stroustrup A, Trasande L, Holzman IR. Randomized controlled trial of restrictive fluid management in transient tachypnea of the newborn. J Pediatr. 2012;160(1):38-43.e1.
7. Martin R, Garcia-Prats J, Kim M. (2019). Prevention and Treatment of Respiratory Distress Syndrome in Preterm Infants.. [online] Available from https://www.uptodate.com/contents/prevention-and-treatment-of-respiratory-distress-syndrome-in-preterm-infants [Last accessed October, 2019].
8. Govindaswami B, Jegatheesan P, Nudelman M, et al. Prevention of Prematurity: Advances and Opportunities. Clin. Perinatology. 2018;45(3):579-95.
9. Govindaswami B, Nudelman M, Narasimhan S, et al. Eliminating Risk of Intubation in Very Preterm Infants with Noninvasive Cardiorespiratory Support in the Delivery Room and Neonatal Intensive Care Unit. Bio Med Res Int. 2019;2019:5984305.
10. Gyamfi-Bannerman C, Thom EA, Blackwell S, et al. Antenatal Betamethasone for Women at Risk for Late Preterm Delivery. N Engl J Med. 2016;374:1311-20.
11. Raju T, Mercer B, Burchfield D, et al. Periviable birth: executive summary of a Joint Workshop by the Eunice Kennedy Shriver National Institute of Child Health and Human Development, Society for Maternal-Fetal Medicine, American Academy of Pediatrics, and American College of Obstetricians and Gynecologists. J Perinatology. 2014;34:333-42.
12. Singh N, Hawley K, Viswanathan K. Efficacy of porcine versus bovine surfactants for preterm newborns with respiratory distress syndrome: systematic review and meta-analysis. Pediatrics. 2011;128(6):e1588-95.
13. Morley C, Davis PG, Doyle LN, et al. Nasal CPAP or intubation at birth for very preterm infants. N Engl J Med. 2008;358:700-8.
14. Wyllie J, Bruinenberg J, Roehr C, et al. European Resuscitation Council Guidelines for Resuscitation 2015: Section 7. Resuscitation and support of transition of babies at birth. Resuscitation. 2015:249-63.
15. Manley B, Owen L, Hooper S, et al. Towards evidence-based resuscitation of the newborn infant. Lancet. 2017;389(10079):22-8.
16. Schmidt B, Roberts RS, Davis P, et al. Caffeine therapy for apnea of prematurity. N Engl J Med. 2006;354:2112-21.
17. Kreutzer K, Bassler D. Caffeine for apnea of prematurity: a neonatal success story. Neonatology. 2014;105:332-6.
18. Schmidt B, Roberts RS, Anderson PJ, et al. Academic Performance, Motor Function, and Behavior 11 Years After Neonatal Caffeine Citrate Therapy for Apnea of Prematurity: An 11-Year Follow-up of the CAP Randomized Clinical Trial. JAMA Pediatr. 2017;171(6):564-72.
19. Schmidt B, Anderson PJ, Doyle LW, et al. Survival without disability to age 5 years after neonatal caffeine therapy for apnea of prematurity. JAMA. 2012;307(3):275-82.
20. Schmidt B, Davis PG, Roberts RS, et al. Timing of caffeine therapy in very low birth weight infants. J Pediatr. 2014;164(5):957-8.
21. Kribs A, Roll C, Göpel W, et al. Nonintubated Surfactant Application vs Conventional Therapy in Extremely Preterm Infants: A Randomized Clinical Trial. JAMA Pediatr. 2015;169(8):723-30.
22. Härtel C, Paul P, Hanke K, et al. Less invasive surfactant administration and complications of preterm birth. Sci Rep. 2018;8(1):8333.
23. Berneau P, Nguyen Phuc Thu T, Pladys P, et al. Impact of surfactant administration through a thin catheter in the delivery room: A quality control chart analysis coupled with a propensity score matched cohort study in preterm infants. PLoS One. 2018;13(12):e0208252.
24. Isayama T, Chai-Adisaksopha C, McDonald SD. Noninvasive Ventilation With vs Without Early Surfactant to Prevent Chronic Lung Disease in Preterm Infants: A Systematic Review and Meta-analysis. JAMA Pediatr. 2015;169:731-9.
25. Aldana-Aguirre JC, Pinto M, Featherstone RM, et al. Less invasive surfactant administration versus intubation for surfactant delivery in preterm infants with respiratory

distress syndrome: a systematic review and meta-analysis. Arch Dis Childhood Fetal Neonatal Ed. 2017;102:F17-23.
26. Kirpalani H, Millar D, Lemyre B, et al. A trial comparing noninvasive ventilation strategies in preterm infants. N Engl J Med. 2013;369:611-20.
27. SUPPORT Study Group of the Eunice Kennedy Shriver NICHD Neonatal Research Network, Finer N, Carlo W, et al. Early CPAP versus surfactant in extremely preterm infants. N Engl J Med. 2010;362:1970-9.
28. Askie L, Darlow B, Finer N, et al. neonatal Oxygenation Prospective Meta-analysis (NeOProM) Collaboration. Association between Oxygen Saturation Targeting and Death or Disability in Extremely Preterm Infants in the Neonatal Oxygenation Prospective Meta-analysis Collaboration. JAMA. 2018;319(21):2190-201.
29. Yoder BA, Stoddard RA, Li M, et al. Heated, humidified high-flow nasal cannula versus nasal CPAP for respiratory support in neonates. Pediatrics. 2013;131(5):e1482-90.
30. Barrington KJ, Fortin-Pellerin E, Pennaforte T. Fluid restriction for treatment of preterm infants with chronic lung disease. Cochrane Database Syst Rev. 2017;(2):CD005389.
31. National Institute for Healthcare Excellence (NICE). (2014). Intrapartum Care for Healthy Women and Babies. [online] Available from https://www.nice.org.uk/guidance/cg190/resources/intrapartum-care-for-healthy-women-and-babies-pdf-35109866447557 [Last accessed October, 2019].
32. Dyke M. (2017). Trust Guideline for the Management of Newborn Babies Born to Mothers with Meconium Stained Liquor. [online] Available from http://www.nnuh.nhs.uk/publication/download/newborn-babies-born-to-mothers-with-meconium-stained-liquor-io17-v2/ [Last accessed October, 2019].
33. Santhalingam T, Ali K, Greenough A. G473(P) Outcomes of infants born through meconium stained amniotic fluid (MSAF) according to grade of meconium. Arch Dis Child. 2017;102:A186-7.
34. Garcia-Prats J. (2019). Prevention and management of meconium aspiration syndrome. [online] Available from https://www.uptodate.com/contents/prevention-and-management-of-meconium-aspiration-syndrome [Last accessed October, 2019].
35. Lakshminrusimha S, Keszler M. Persistent pulmonary hypertension of the newborn. NeoReviews. 2015;16(12):e680-92.
36. Nair J, Lakshminrusimha S. Update on PPHN: mechanisms and treatment. Semin Perinatol. 2014;38(2):78-91.
37. Steinhorn RH. Neonatal pulmonary hypertension. Pediatr Crit Care Med. 2010;11(2 Suppl):S79-S84.
38. Stark A, Eichenwald E. (2019). Persistent Pulmonary Hypertension of the Newborn. [online] Available from https://www.uptodate.com/contents/persistent-pulmonary-hypertension-of-the-newborn [Last accessed October, 2019].
39. The Neonatal Inhaled Nitric Oxide Study Group. Inhaled nitric oxide in full-term and nearly full-term infants with hypoxic respiratory failure. N Engl J Med. 1997;336:597-604.
40. Kelly LE, Ohlsson A, Shah PS. Sildenafil for pulmonary hypertension in neonates. Cochrane Database Syst Rev. 2017;(8):CD005494.
41. Schreiber MD, Gin-Mestan K, Marks JD, et al. Inhaled nitric oxide in premature infants with the respiratory distress syndrome. N Engl J Med. 2003;349:2099-107.
42. Ballard RA, Truog WE, Cnaan A, et al. Inhaled nitric oxide in perterm infants undergoing mechanical ventilation. N Engl J Med. 2006;355:343-53.
43. Van Meurs KP, Wright LL, Ehrenkranz RA, et al. Inhaled nitric oxide for premature infants with severe respiratory failure. N Engl J Med. 2005;353:13-22.
44. Barrington KJ, Finer N. Inhaled nitric oxide for respiratory failure in preterm infants. Cochrane Database Syst Rev. 2010;(12):CD000509.
45. Cole FS, Alleyne C, Barks JD, et al. NIH Consensus Development Conference statement: inhaled nitric oxide therapy for premature infants. Pediatrics. 2011;127(2):363-9.
46. Handley SC, Steinhorn RH, Hopper AO, et al. Inhaled nitric oxide use in preterm infants in California neonatal intensive care units. J Perinatol. 2016;36(8):635-9.
47. Askie LM, Davies L, Schreiber M, et al. Race effects of inhaled nitric oxide in preterm infants: an individual participant data meta-analysis. J Pediatr. 2018;193:34-9.e2.
48. Tesini BL. Neonatal Pneumonia. [online] Available from https://www.merckmanuals.com/professional/pediatrics/infections-in-neonates/neonatal-pneumonia [Last accessed October, 2019].
49. Speer ME, Garcia-Prats JA, Edwards MS. (2019). Neonatal Pneumonia. [online] Available from https://www.uptodate.com/contents/neonatal-pneumonia [Last accessed October, 2019].
50. Gollehon N. (2019). Neonatal Sepsis. [online] Available from https://emedicine.medscape.com/article/978352-overview [Last accessed October, 2019].
51. Committee on Infectious Diseases and Committee on Fetus and Newborn. Recommendations for the Prevention of Perinatal Group B Streptococcal (GBS) Disease. Pediatrics. 2011;128(3):611-6.
52. Lamont RF, Sobel J, Mazaki-Tovi S, et al. Listeriosis in human pregnancy: a systematic review. J Perinat Med. 2011;39(3):227-36.
53. National Organization of Rare Disorders. (2018). Rare Disease Database: Listeriosis. [online] Available from https://rarediseases.org/rare-diseases/listeriosis/ [Last accessed October, 2019].
54. Salama M, Amitai Z, Ezemitchi AV, et al. Surveillance of listeriosis in the Tel Aviv District, Israel, 2010–2015. Epidemiol Infect. 2018;146(3):283-90.
55. Fouks Y, Amit S, Many A, et al. Listeriosis in pregnancy: under-diagnosis despite over-treatment. J Perinatology. 2018;38:26-30.
56. Cohen-Wolkowiez M, Moran C, Benjamin DK, et al. Early and late onset sepsis in late preterm infants. Pediatr Infect Dis J. 2009;28(12):1052-6.
57. Cooper JM, Michelow IC, Wozniak PS, et al. In time: the persistence of congenital syphilis in Brazil—More progress needed! Rev Paul Pediatr. 2016;34(3):251-3.
58. Murali MV, Nirmala C, Rao JV. Symptomatic early congenital syphilis: a common but forgotten disease. Case Rep Pediatr. 2012;2012:934634.

59. Govindaswami B. (2019). 2019 CAN—Antibiotics. [online] Available from https://www.researchgate.net/publication/335527315_2019_CAN_-_Antibiotics [Last accessed October, 2019].
60. Committee on Obstetric Practice. Committee Opinion No. 712: Intrapartum management of intraamniotic infection. Obstet Gynecol. 2017;130:e95-101.
61. Joshi NS, Gupta A, Allan JM, et al. Management of chorioamnionitis-exposed infants in the newborn nursery using a clinical examination–based approach. Hosp Pediatr. 2019;9(4):227-33.
62. Webber S, Wilkinson AR, Lindsell D, et al. Neonatal pneumonia. Arch Dis Child. 1990;65(2):207-11.
63. Duke T. Neonatal pneumonia in developing countries. Arch Dis Child Fetal Neonatal Ed. 2005;90:F211-9.
64. Ginsburg AS, Meulen AS, Klugman KP. Prevention of neonatal pneumonia and sepsis via maternal immunisation. Lancet Glob Health. 2014;2(12):e679-80.
65. Wang H, Liddell CA, Coates MM, et al. Global, regional, and national levels of neonatal, infant, and under-5 mortality during 1990-2013: a systematic analysis for the Global Burden of Disease Study 2013. Lancet. 2014;384(9947):956-79.

# SECTION 7

# Fetal and Neonatal Brain Development, and Neurodevelopmental Follow-up

- Feeding and Brain Development in Preterm Infants: Central Pattern Generation and Suck Dynamics
  *Steven M Barlow, Austin O Rosner, Dongli Song*

- Feeding and Brain Development in Preterm Infants: Role of Sensory Stimulation
  *Steven M Barlow, Austin O Rosner, Dongli Song*

- The Gut-Microbiota-Brain Axis: Implications for Neonatal Neurodevelopment
  *Dongli Song, Laishuan Wang*

- Neonatal Seizures
  *John Sum*

- Newborn Populations at Risk for Adverse Neurodevelopmental Outcomes
  *Ira Adams-Chapman*

- Late Preterm Infants, Cerebral Palsy, and Hypoxic-Ischemic Encephalopathy
  *Ira Adams-Chapman*

# CHAPTER 28

# Feeding and Brain Development in Preterm Infants: Central Pattern Generation and Suck Dynamics

*Steven M Barlow, Austin O Rosner, Dongli Song*

## ABSTRACT

The biological complexities of oral feeding have made it the most advanced neurological milestone of the newborn.

Fortunately, the brainstem is endowed with premotor internuncial circuits known as central pattern generators whose activity is apparent in the fetus and modulated by somatosensory feedback to support ororythmogenesis during nonnutritive and nutritive suck in preterm infants.

## BUILDING BLOCKS FOR OROMOTOR PATTERN GENERATION

Bilateral and reciprocally linked internuncial circuitries known as central pattern generators, reside in the brainstem and function as premotor inputs to lower motor neurons in the pons and medulla of the brainstem to modulate motor activity among orofacial muscles, including the lips, buccal walls, tongue, mandible, oropharynx, and hypopharynx.

## SUCK CENTRAL PATTERN GENERATOR

The mammalian suck is regulated, in part, by neuronal networks in the pontomedullary reticular formation known as the suck central pattern generator (sCPG). The sCPG consists of bilateral networks of interneurons that output to hypoglossal (XII), facial (VII), and trigeminal (V) lower motoneurons to produce rhythmic suck activity.[1,2] Katakura et al.[3] provided one of the first in vitro isolated brainstem preparations for the study of the perinatal rhythmical motor patterns in cranial nerves (CNs). During resting state, neonatal rats manifested rhythmical activity from V, VII, and XII motoneurons correlated to respiration.[3,4] However, when the glutamate agonist N-methyl-DL-aspartate (NMDA) is added to the bath, a second much faster rhythm became evident.[3-7] It was hypothesized that these rhythmic and nonrespiratory-related oromotor patterns are related to suckling given mastication does not appear in young rats before P12.[8]

Reduced brainstem preparations in neonatal rats have revealed that trigeminal, facial, and hypoglossal lower motoneurons are capable of producing the suck rhythm when surgically isolated from one another.[9] Trigeminal rhythmogenesis is also apparent following hemisection of the pons.[2] These findings suggest the presence of at least six functionally separate ororhythmic generators (two each among V, VII, and XII) that are coupled together to coordinate suckling at birth. This scenario is supported by a recent study using a modified monosynaptic rabies virus-based transsynaptic tracing method, which identified the existence of collateral premotor neurons to (1) link homonymous CPG circuitry with bilaterally projecting neurons and (2) shared collateral premotor neurons which unilaterally link V, VII, and XII motoneurons for feeding in a mouse model.[10] Suckling movements in humans have been observed in utero using fetal magnetometry and are highly coordinated in preterm infants by 32 weeks gestational age.[11] The components of the oral rhythmogenic network in the rodent model expressed through hypoglossal lower motoneurons is dominant at birth, since the trigeminal pair is inhibited by the caudal brainstem.[2] Brainstem circuits involved in oral rhythmogenesis are also modulated by descending inputs from the cortical "sucking area".[12,13] Oromotor rhythmic activities depend on the activation of NMDA receptors. The sCPG is highly responsive to sensory inputs including somatosensory, olfactory, gustatory, and auditory, and adapts to changes in task dynamics and local environment.[14-18]

## ■ MINIMAL NEURAL CIRCUITRY TO SUPPORT NON-NUTRITIVE SUCKING

The schematic shown in **Figure 1** illustrates putative brainstem nuclei and networks that support the production of non-nutritive sucking (NNS) in human neonates. Multiple CPG networks, composed of premotor interneuron circuits, are represented as yellow-filled oval elements within a hemirepresentation of the brainstem central gray. These internuncial rhythm producing networks include sCPG, dorsal swallowing groups (DSGs), ventral swallowing groups (VSGs), and the respiratory central pattern generator (rCPG). The chief sensory nucleus of the trigeminal system along with its rostral extension [mesencephalic nucleus of trigeminal complex (MES V)] and its caudal extension [spinal nucleus of trigeminal (spinal V)] which descends through the brainstem to the level of C3 in the spinal cord are shown in green. Other essential CN nuclei [motor V, VII, nucleus ambiguus (NA) IX, X, and XII] include α-motoneurons which are modulated by sensory inputs, are indicated in pink. Target muscle subsystems involved in NNS are listed in the offset panel. For NNS, somatosensory inputs are encoded by the chief sensory nucleus of V, IX, and X, while gustatory, olfactory, and auditory inputs are presumed to influence the sCPG through more complex pathways acting on the brainstem. Finally, an emergent descending cortical input is included, which is thought to exert more influence on the suck patterning with maturation and experience. Swallowing and respiratory CPGs operate quasi-independently of NNS, at least early on in an infant's experience with this form of sucking. This appears to change with experience. Recent evidence[19] suggests that as the infant gains experience and skill at NNS, dependence between suck-swallow and the phase of respiration begins to emerge, perhaps as a precursory motor skill to meet the increased demands of airway protection required for safe swallows during nutritive feeding.

## ■ NUTRITIVE SUCK-SWALLOW CENTRAL PATTERN GENERATION

Nutritive suck-swallow is a complex sensorimotor function, characterized by a coordinated bilateral sequence of activation and inhibition among more than two dozen pairs of muscles in the mouth, pharynx, larynx, and esophagus.[20-22] The development of a safe swallow involves airway protection for all newborns learning to feed orally. An important milestone in the neonatal intensive care unit (NICU) for preterm infants is the transition to independent oral feeds. It is common for infants less than 32 weeks postmenstrual age (PMA) to be tube fed until they have matured and developed the necessary sensorimotor skills to take nutrient directly from the breast/bottle.[23] In the NICU, NNS is often paired with gavage feeding to provide the infant with satiation, to provide positive association between sucking and feeding, and to facilitate the transition to independent oral feeds.[16-18] Regular NNS activity also serves to develop the timing and coordination of swallow at the correct phase of the respiratory cycle to reduce the risk of aspiration.[19]

Practiced in the womb and performed hundreds of times each day postnatally, the pharyngeal swallow is regulated by two main groups of interneurons located in the medullary dorsal and ventral reticular formation. The DSG includes the nucleus tractus solitarius (NTS) which contains the generator neurons for triggering, shaping, and timing the rhythmic swallowing pattern.[24] The VSG consists of switching neurons that distributes the swallowing drive to

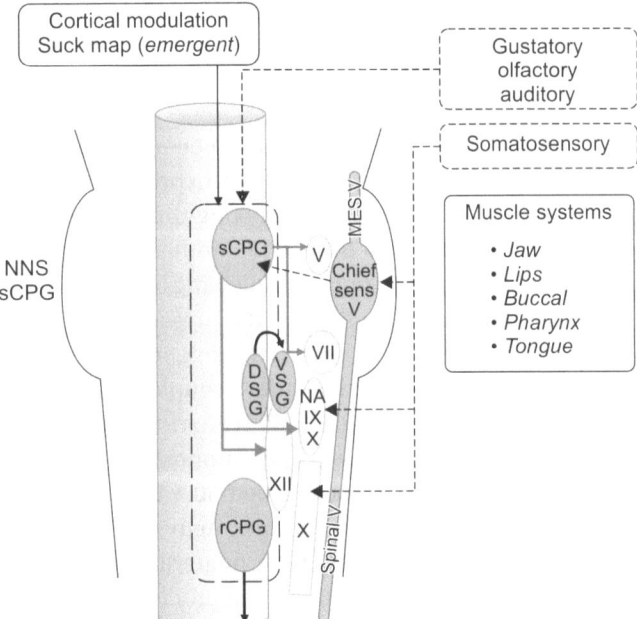

**Fig. 1:** Schematic of putative premotor, lower motoneuron pools, and sensory nuclei involved in non-nutritive sucking. [DSG: dorsal swallowing group; NA: nucleus ambiguus; cranial nuclei V (trigeminal), VII (facial), IX (glossopharyngeal), X (vagus), and XII (hypoglossal); MES V: mesencephalic nucleus of trigeminal complex; rCPG: respiratory central pattern generator; sCPG: suck central pattern generator; Spinal V: spinal nucleus of trigeminal; VSG: ventral swallowing group; chief sens V: chief sensory nucleus of trigeminal; NNS: non-nutritive sucking]

lower motoneurons in the pons and medulla. Collectively, the DSG and VSG form the swallow central pattern generator (swCPG) which produces sequential bursts of output to select cranial motoneurons to close the airway and propagate a contraction pattern (peristalsis) which propels the nutrient bolus through the muscular pharyngeal tube and esophagus. The swallowing sequence has two phases known as the oropharyngeal phase and esophageal phase, which can be initiated by stimulating the internal branch of the superior laryngeal nerve (SLN).

Another crucial function of the swCPG is to regulate interactions between relevant sensory and motor nuclei. Sensory input involved in the initiation of a swallow is derived from CNs V, VII, IX, and X. The first detectable motor action of the swCPG is contraction of the mylohyoid muscle. A swallow is regarded as a relatively stereotyped sequential motor pattern; however, the swCPG may be shaped by sensory features related to the size and physical properties (viscosity, texture, and compliance) of the bolus. Thus, the swCPG depends not only on the pattern of intrinsic connections and membrane properties of swallowing neurons, but also on descending and afferent inputs.[24] For example, changes in bolus volume produce the largest systematic changes in the oropharyngeal swallow motor pattern. As bolus volume increases, the pattern shifts from predominantly sequential (oral > pharyngeal > esophageal) for small volume swallows (saliva, formula, and breast milk) towards simultaneous oral and pharyngeal phase activation to safely clear a larger bolus from the oral and pharyngeal cavities to the esophagus. Increasing the viscosity of the nutrient results in a slower swallowing transit time owing to increased strength and force of constriction. Valve functions [e.g. velopharyngeal closure, upper esophageal sphincter (UES) dilatation, and laryngeal closure] also increase slightly in duration and are thought to generate a heightened sensory experience. Some proprioceptive cues related to the execution of a swallow are presumed to be encoded by muscle spindle primary afferents in the tongue and conveyed along CN XII. Putative sensory fields which modulate the swCPG include the posterior tongue and velopharynx (CN IX), mucosa of the valleculae and pyriform recesses (CN X), and salivary glands (CN VII). These receptive fields transmit information to the NTS which contains sensory neurons associated with CN VII, IX, and X. The NTS also receives descending input from the swallowing cortex which has been localized bilaterally to supplemental motor area (Brodmann area 6), and lies immediately anterior to the primary motor cortex (precentral gyrus, Brodmann area 4). NTS outputs to the NA located in the ventral medulla for motor sequence execution. The NA contains motoneuron cell bodies of CN IX and X, and connects with motor nuclei of CN V, VII, and XII to orchestrate sequential motor activity among striated muscles of the mouth/lower face/buccal wall, jaw, tongue, pharynx, larynx, and upper esophagus. The ventral regions (NA) of the swCPG rely on input from the dorsal regions (NTS) in the medulla to complete the swallow.

## MINIMAL NEURAL CIRCUITRY TO SUPPORT NUTRITIVE SUCKING

The schematic for the nutritive suck-swallow brainstem nuclei has added complexity, including functional connections between the pontine sCPG, DSGs, and VSGs in the rostral medulla, and the rCPG centered in the pre-Bötzinger complex in the ventral-caudal medulla oblongata **(Fig. 2)**.

A commensurate increase in multisensory feedback pathways from taste, smell, and auditory inputs afford the neonatal feeding apparatus more refined adaptation to variations in bolus size and sensory features. A vestibular input pathway has been added in view of recent evidence which demonstrated that chest wall movements in preterm infants could be modulated in the presence of linear accelerations.[25] Vagal motoneuron pools are expanded beyond the NNS model to reflect airway protection (epiglottis and intrinsic larynx) and upper esophageal motility. This is essential to protect the airway during

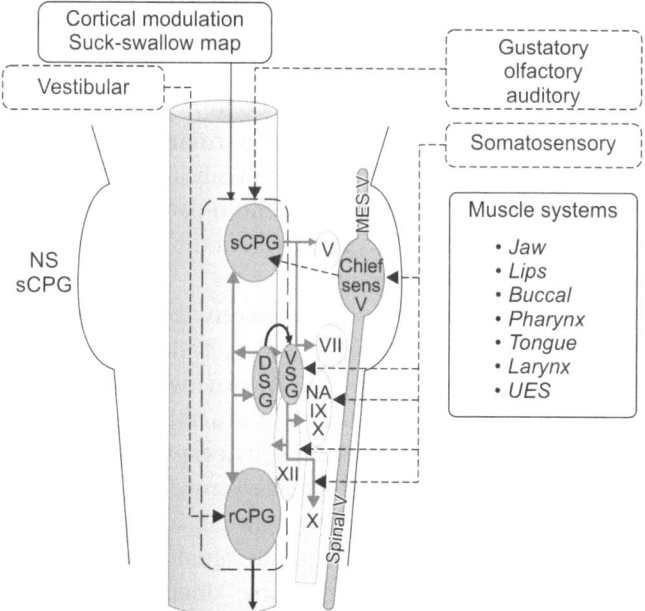

**Fig. 2:** Schematic of putative premotor, lower motoneuron, and sensory nuclei involved in nutritive sucking. [Chief sens V: chief sensory nucleus of trigeminal; DSG: dorsal swallowing group; NA: nucleus ambiguus; cranial nuclei V (trigeminal), VII (facial), IX (glossopharyngeal), X (vagus), and XII (hypoglossal); MES V: mesencephalic nucleus of trigeminal complex; rCPG: respiratory central pattern generator; sCPG: suck central pattern generator; Spinal V: spinal nucleus of trigeminal; UES: upper esophageal sphincter; VSG: ventral swallowing group; NS: nutritive sucking].

swallows and permit passage of the nutrient bolus through the pharynx and the upper esophageal segment.

A heterarchical control model consisting of the cerebral cortex, forebrain, cerebellum, and brainstem loci has been proposed to support deglutition.[26,27] Functional magnetic resonance imaging (fMRI) techniques used during reflexive swallows reveal a bilateral cortical network localized to the lateral primary somatosensory (SI) and motor (MI) cortices. In contrast, voluntary swallows show a more elaborate bilateral activation in the insula, prefrontal, anterior cingulate, parieto-occipital, SI, and MI areas.[28] The expanded representation during voluntary swallows is presumably related to motor planning and the perceived urge to swallow when presented a small water bolus. A cortical swallowing area encompassing frontoparietal cortical activation has been identified in infants at 45 weeks PMA using near infrared spectroscopy (NIRS) and pharyngoesophageal manometry.[29] This cortical representation is presumed to modulate the nutritive suck-swallow central pattern generation (NS-swCPG) during oral feeding.

## MASTICATORY CENTRAL PATTERN GENERATION

By the 6th month postnatally, most infants transition from liquid nutrient to semisolid and solid foods concurrent with the emergence of the lower incisors and chewing. Mastication involves the coordination of over 20 orofacial muscles in the ongoing stream of breathing and swallowing.[30,31] Mastication continues to develop in parallel with the eruption of the permanent dentition.[1] Similar to sucking, mastication is initially under the control of a pontine CPG [masticatory central pattern generation (mCPG)] which is later complemented by a masticatory cortical area in motor cortex.

Chewing and sucking share some basic kinematic features, including cyclic opening and closing of the mandible. The power stroke for nutritive sucking (NS) occurs during jaw opening to produce a high negative intraoral pressure to facilitate nutrient expression from the breast or bottle, whereas the power stroke for mastication occurs during the generation of jaw closing forces to tear or break food parcels into a manageable bolus size.[30] Mastication also involves additional kinematic degrees of freedom, to permit asymmetric movement patterns (lateral and rotational) to accommodate varying types of food boli.

## EMERGENT ORORHYTHMIC MOTOR BEHAVIORS

Two distinct types of sucking are apparent in infants, including NNS and NS. NNS is characterized as a repetitive

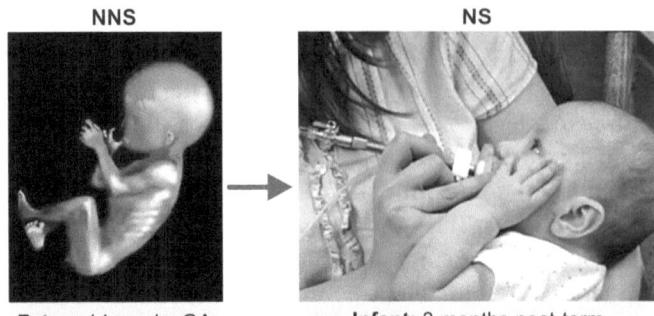

**Fig. 3:** Progression from non-nutritive sucking (NNS) to nutritive sucking (NS) (GA: gestational age) *(For color version see Plate 4)*. *Source:* Communication Neuroscience Laboratories, Lincoln NE USA.

mouthing action on a finger or pacifier nipple in the absence of a liquid stimulus,[32] whereas NS involves cyclic ororhythmic activity to express a nutrient bolus from a bottle or breast followed by a safe swallow. There are anatomic, functional, and developmental differences between NNS and NS in infants. Around the 8th week of fetal life, the nasolabial, maxillary, and midline nasal processes undergo elaborate morphological transformation with tissue translation and fusion to form the upper lip, alveolar process, and primary and secondary palate. These midface structures complement the lower lip and lingual-mandibular complex to form an oral cavity capable of rudimentary sucking. By 13 weeks, the fetus exhibits perioral reflex sensitivity and progressively more complex oromotor activities. NNS continues to develop in utero and typically precedes NS which is recruited shortly after birth **(Fig. 3)**. A new set of challenges arises for the newborn who is preterm and faced with the prospect of attaining independent oral feeding skills in the NICU due to an underdeveloped brain and feeding mechanism.

## KEY FEATURES OF NON-NUTRITIVE SUCKING

The NNS is an observable and accessible motor behavior which is often used by the care team to make inferences about brain development and prefeeding skills in preterm and term infants.[33] NNS is observable in utero as early as 12–18 weeks gestational age (GA)[34] with bursts composed of 2–13 suck cycles occurring at a modal cycle rate of approximately 2 Hz, and separated by pause periods of 2–5 seconds to accommodate respiration.[11,32,35,36] NNS as a motor skill is attained by preterm infants at 30–32 weeks PMA depending on sex and health status of the infant. NNS can be modulated by various sensory inputs, including cutaneous (trigeminal inputs),[16-18,37-44] olfactory,[45-47] and auditory.[48] The NNS is not dependent on respiratory phase; however, recent work suggests continued experience with

NNS facilitates the timing of swallows at "safe" points in the respiratory cycle (e.g. end of inspiration or expiration).[19] This may serve a preparatory function for coordinative demands associated with nutritive feeding and safe swallows.

Closer examination of NNS burst structure reveals frequency modulation (FM) of suck cycles, which is dependent on pulmonary health status in the preterm infant.[49] A typical NNS burst in a healthy infant at 32 weeks PMA consists of six to seven suck compression cycles at mean frequency of 2 Hz, and a mean peak compression pressure of 17 cm $H_2O$.[32,50,51] At 34 weeks PMA, neurotypical NNS compression cycles show significant FM with an initial suck period frequency of 2.2 Hz that decays exponentially to approximately 1.6 Hz by cycle period number 13 **(Fig. 4)**.

This stable pattern of NNS FM among healthy preterm controls at 34 weeks PMA was significantly degraded for preterm respiratory distress syndrome (RDS) infants who endured more than a month of $O_2$ supplementation therapy (mean = 34.2 days). The RDS profile shows greater variability during FM, with NNS cycling initiated at a lower frequency compared to healthy preterm, with shorter and more variable NNS bursts **(Fig. 5)**. Knowledge of the FM-structure during NNS production has been programmed into our orosensory entrainment therapy for preterm infants in the NICU.[52]

The truncated NNS burst structure characteristic of preterm infants with lung disease may be related to an altered and maladaptive sensorimotor milieu during a critical period of development of oromotor skills to support oral feeding. Prematurity significantly alters developmental processes, as interruption of these critical periods of nervous system development can disrupt central neural representations of motor and sensory systems.[53] Preterm infants are routinely subjected to unnatural or potentially aversive procedures, including intubation, continuous positive airway pressure (CPAP), nasal cannulation, or placement of feeding tubes.[44] The attachment of tubing and tape to the neonate's lower face alters the sensory milieu and restricts oral movements and limits experiences with the hands and fingers. This represents a form of sensory deprivation or maladaptive stimulation during a critical period of development which may interfere with the attainment of independent oral feedings and lengthen hospitalization.[16] Nasogastric (NG) gavage tubes (size 4–10 French) may negatively impact oral feeding development.[54] Furthermore, failure to successfully transition to oral feeding can persist into early childhood,[55,56] and are correlated with delays in babbling and speech-language acquisition.[33,57] Collectively, these factors underscore the need for physiological assessment and individualized therapeutics to facilitate the development of oromotor skills.[38,44,58,59]

## BENEFITS OF NON-NUTRITIVE SUCKING

Preterm infants who engage in NNS show enhanced growth, maturation, and gastric motility;[60] decreased stress levels;[60-62] improved prefeed state control[61,63,64] and oral feeds;[16,41,58,62,64-67] and decreased length of hospital stay.[23,68] The central patterning of NNS production is correlated to a reduction of time spent on NG tube feeding.[37,69-71] For example, preterm infants (24–34 weeks GA) with more stable NNS scores manifest a shorter transition to full oral feeds compared to infants with disorganized NNS.[72]

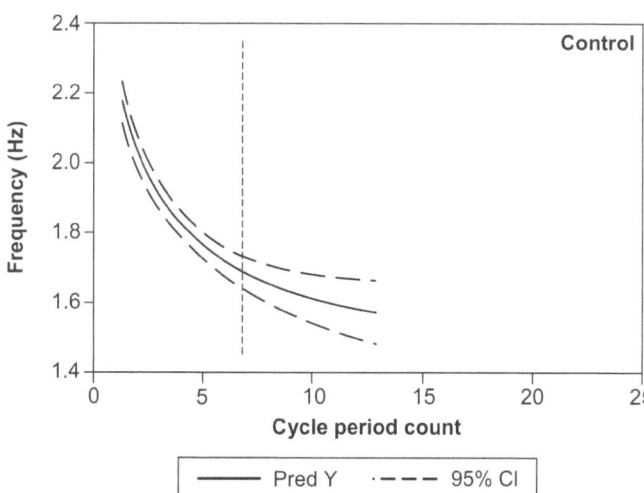

**Fig. 4:** Frequency modulation of non-nutritive sucking (NNS) cycle period count based on 17 healthy preterm infants.[49] The dotted vertical line at 5.67 compression cycles represents the mean length of NNS bursts.

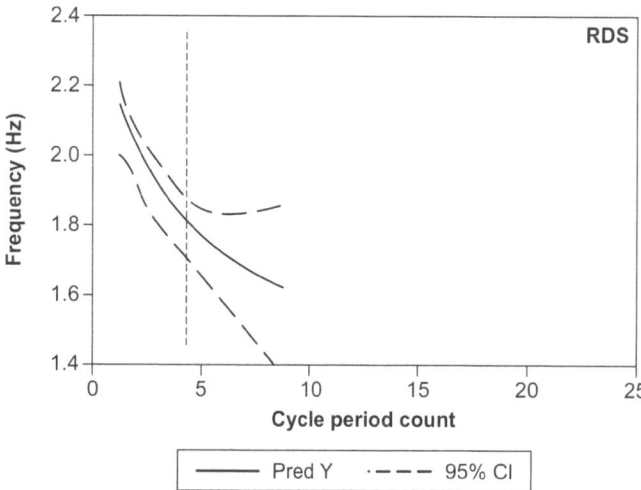

**Fig. 5:** Frequency modulation of non-nutritive sucking (NNS) cycle period count based on 17 preterm infants with respiratory distress syndrome (RDS).[49] The dotted vertical line at 3.87 compression cycles represents the mean length of NNS bursts.

A report from the National Institute of Child Health and Human Development (NICHD) Neonatal Research Network (NRN) indicated that at 18 months corrected age, premature infants with a history of feeding difficulties are more likely to exhibit language delay. Neuromotor impairment and days on mechanical ventilation are also important risk factors associated with these outcomes.[56]

# KEY FEATURES OF THE NUTRITIVE SUCKING

Contrary to NNS production, NS consists of relatively long trains of suck cycles organized as a continuous motor stream.[73,74] An NS cycle is more dynamic with compound force trajectories, including a suction phase followed approximately 100 milliseconds later by an expression phase during which the tip of the tongue blade makes an anterior-to-posterior stripping motion along the length of the breast teat or bottle nipple to express nutrient. Nutritive suckling also involves jaw closing and opening movements. These compound dynamics require activation of the intrinsic tongue muscles via the hypoglossal nerve, jaw muscles via trigeminal motor (V3), and perioral muscles via facial nerve.[75] The power stroke for the suction phase is provided by the jaw depressors during suckling. The NS train occurs at a modal frequency of approximately 1 Hz and may include more than 40 suck cycles without a pause period depending on feeding skill. NS train also lack FM characteristic of NNS activity. A comparison of compression pressure dynamics for NNS (pacifier) and NS (feeding nipple) is shown in **Figure 6**. Unlike NNS, a bolus is necessary to evoke tongue movements during NS, and trigger oropharyngeal-laryngeal-esophageal reflexive motor patterns to protect the airway for safe swallow and efficient bolus transport into the esophagus.

Safe swallows are typically performed at points in the respiratory cycle where the risk for aspiration is the least

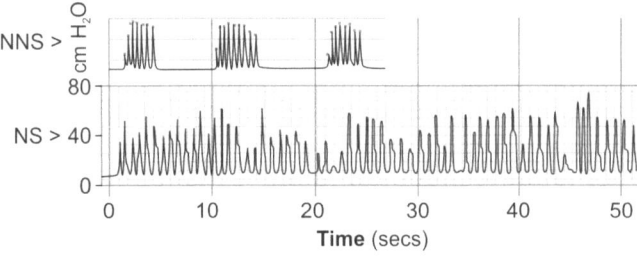

**Fig. 6:** Intraluminal pressure (inside silicone nipple) during compressions associated with non-nutritive sucking (NNS) and nutritive sucking (NS) production by infants. NNS shows the classic "burst-pause" frequency modulation (FM) structure with cycle rate within burst approximately 2 Hz, whereas the NS is characterized by a relatively long burst with individual compression cycles produced at approximately 1 Hz.
*Source:* Communication Neuroscience Laboratories, Lincoln NE USA.

(i.e. transition from inspiratory to expiratory translaryngeal airflow). Sensory modulation via trigeminal and vagal afferents is essential to coordinate pharyngeal and laryngeal muscle systems for airway protection.[29] Nutritive oral feeds are highly dependent on respiratory phase. NS experience improves coordination and timing of the suck-swallow-breathe pattern.[55,56,75,76] Coordination of suck-swallow-breathe is attained when the infant can consistently demonstrate a ratio of 1:1:1 or 2:2:1, respectively. In neurotypical preterm infants, the NS skill is usually attained by 34–37 weeks PMA, depending on GA and other factors (health, respiratory and neurologic status, etc.). Failure to achieve coordination of the suck-swallow-breathe pattern will lead to aspiration and other serious health issues.[75] Since the suck-swallow-breathe pattern is regulated by CPG premotor networks in the pons and medulla oblongata, dysfunction can occur at any phase of the sequence, making diagnosis and treatment problematic for healthcare providers in the absence of physiological and imaging tools.

Prematurity presents significant challenges in neuromotor control of the aerodigestive tract to safely coordinate the suck-swallow-breathe pattern without the risk of aspiration.[77] The transition from tube to independent oral feeding is a major developmental hurdle facing the preterm infant and their caretakers. Important factors to consider in the prospects for feeding success include neurodevelopmental status related to behavioral regulation, cardiac respiratory function, and the ability to produce a coordinated suck-swallow-breathe pattern with proper timing in the respiratory cycle to minimize the chances of aspiration.[78] Suck-swallow coordination is typically manifest shortly after introducing oral feeding, while the more challenging swallow-breathe coordination evolves more slowly with oral feeding progression.[79] Swallow-related closure of the airway is best initiated at times of zero translaryngeal airflow (i.e. end of inspiration or expiration) rather than midinspiration where air volume velocities through the glottis are relatively high. Infants who exhibit safe swallows show a stable and relatively constant relation between the timing of the pharyngoesophageal reflexive swallow and breathing.[80]

# SUMMARY

The apparent linkages between multiple CPGs which populate the brainstem, via sensory modulation and entrainment, and descending inputs provides clinicians and neuroscientists many new opportunities for exploring cross-modal and cross-CPG facilitation for the development of new therapeutic interventions for prohabilitation of the late gestation preterm infant who is learning to coordinate suck, swallow, and respiration to attain safe oral feeds.[1]

## ACKNOWLEDGMENTS

The work was supported in part by the National Institutes of Health R01 DC003311 (Barlow-PI), R01 HD086088 (Barlow and Maron-MPDs), and the Barkley Trust.

## REFERENCES

1. Barlow SM, Lund JP, Estep M, et al. Central pattern generators for speech and orofacial activity. In: Brudzynski SM (Ed). Handbook of Mammalian Vocalization. Oxford: Elsevier; 2010. pp. 351-70.
2. Tanaka S, Kogo M, Chandler SH, et al. Localization of oral-motor rhythmogenic circuits in the isolated rat brainstem preparation. Brain Res. 1999;821:190-9.
3. Katakura N, Jia L, Nakamura Y. NMDA-induced rhythmical activity in XII nerve of isolated CNS from newborn rats. Neuro Report. 1995;6:601-4.
4. Koizumi H, Ishihama K, Nomura K, et al. Differential discharge patterns of rhythmical activity in trigeminal motorneurons during fictive mastication and respiration in vitro. Brain Res Bulletin. 2002;58:129-33.
5. Kogo M, Funk GD, Chandler SH. Rhythmical oral-motor activity recorded in an in vitro brainstem preparation. Somatosensory Motor Res. 1996;13:39-48.
6. Kogo M, Tanaka S, Chandler SH, et al. Examination of the relationships between jaw opener and closer rhythmical muscle activity in an in vitro brainstem jaw-attached preparation. Somatosensory Motor Res. 1998;15:200-10.
7. Enomoto E, Kogo M, Koizumi, K, et al. Localization of premotoneurons for an NMDA-induced repetitive rhythmical activity to TMNs. Neuro Report. 2002;13:2303-7.
8. Westneat MW, Hall WG. Ontogeny of feeding motor patterns in infant rats: an electromyographic analysis of suckling and chewing. Behav Neurosci. 1992;106(3):539-54.
9. Nakamura Y, Katakura N, Nakajima M, et al. Rhythm generation for food-ingestive movements. Prog Brain Res. 2004;143:97-103.
10. Stanek E, Cheng S, Takatoh J, et al. Monosynaptic premotor circuit tracing reveals neural substrates for oro-motor coordination. Elife. 2014;3:e02511.
11. Popescu EA, Popescu M, Wang J, et al. Non-nutritive sucking recorded in utero via fetal magnetography. Physiol Meas. 2008;29:127-39.
12. Nozaki S, Iriki A, Nakamura Y. Localization of central rhythm generator involved in cortically induced rhythmical masticatory jaw-opening movement in the guinea pig. J Neurophysiol. 1986;55(4):806-25.
13. Iriki A, Nozaki S, Nakamura Y. Feeding behavior in mammals: corticobulbar projection is reorganized during conversion from sucking to chewing. Dev Brain Res. 1988;44:189-96.
14. Zimmerman E, Barlow SM. Pacifier Stiffness Alters the Dynamics of the Suck Central Pattern Generator. J Neonatal Nurs. 2008;14(3):79-86.
15. Oder AL, Stalling DL, Barlow SM. Short-Term Effects of Pacifier Texture on NNS in Neurotypical Infants. Int J Pediatr. 2013;2013:168459.
16. Barlow SM, Finan DS, Chu S, et al. Patterns for the premature brain: Synthetic orocutaneous stimulation entrains preterm infants with feeding difficulties to suck. J Perinatol. 2008;28:541-48.
17. Barlow SM, Lee J, Wang J, et al. Frequency-Modulated Orocutaneous Stimulation Promotes Non-nutritive Suck Development in Preterm Infants with Respiratory Distress Syndrome or Chronic Lung Disease. J Perinatol. 2014;34(2):136-42.
18. Barlow SM, Lee J, Wang J, et al. Effects of oral stimulus frequency spectra on the development of non-nutritive suck in preterm infants with respiratory distress syndrome or chronic lung disease, and preterm infants of diabetic mothers, J Neonatal Nursing. 2014;20:178-88.
19. Reynolds E, Grider D, Caldwell R, et al. Swallow-Breath interaction and Phase of Respiration with Swallow during Non-nutritive Suck among low-risk preterm infants. Am J Perinatol. 2010;10:831-40.
20. Jean A. Brain stem control of swallowing: neuronal network and cellular mechanisms. Physiol Rev. 2001;81:929-69.
21. Jean A, Dallaporta M. (2006). Electrophysiologic characterization of the swallowing pattern generator in the brainstem. [online] Available from https://www.nature.com/gimo/contents/pt1/full/gimo9.html [Last accessed October, 2019].
22. Humbert IA, German RZ. New directions for understanding neural control in swallowing: The potential and promise of motor learning. Dysphagia. 2013;28:1-10.
23. Pinelli J, Symington A. Non-nutritive sucking for promoting physiologic stability and nutrition in preterm infants. Cochrane Database Syst Rev. 2005;(4):CD001071.
24. Jean A, Dallaporta, M. Brainstem control of deglutition: swallowing pattern generator. In: Shaker R, Belafsky PC, Postma GN, Easterling C (Eds). Principles of Deglutition: A Multidisciplinary Text for Swallowing and its Disorders. New York: Springer; 2012. pp. 67-87.
25. Zimmerman E, Barlow SM. The effects of vestibular stimulation rate and magnitude of acceleration on central pattern generation for chest wall kinematics in preterm infants. J Perinatol. 2012;32:614-20.
26. Michou E, Hamdy S. Cortical input in control of swallowing. Curr Opin Otolaryngol Head Neck Surg. 2009;17(3):166-71.
27. Mosier K, Bereznaya I. Parallel cortical networks for volitional control of swallowing in humans. Exp Brain Res. 2001;140(3):280-9.
28. Kern MK, Jaradeh S, Arndorfer RC, et al. Cerebral cortical representation of reflexive and volitional swallowing in humans. Am J Physiol Gastrointest Liver Physiol. 2001;280:G354-60.
29. Jadcherla SR, Pakiraih JF, Hasenstab KA, et al. Esophageal reflexes modulate fronto-parietal response in neonates: novel application of concurrent NIRS and provocative esophageal manometry. Am J Physiol Gastrointest Liver Physiol. 2014;307(1):G41-9.
30. Kolta A, Morquette P, Lavoie R, et al. Modulation of rhythmogenic properties of trigeminal neurons contributing to the masticatory CPG. Prog Brain Res. 2010;187:137-47.
31. Lund JP. Mastication and its control by the brain stem. Crit Rev Oral Biol Med. 1991;2:33-64.
32. Wolff PH. The serial organization of sucking in the young infant. Pediatrics. 1968;42(6):943-56.
33. Mizuno K, Ueda A. Neonatal feeding performance as a predictor of neurodevelopmental outcome at 18 months. Dev Med Child Neurol. 2005;47(5):299-304.

34. Miller JL, Sonies BC, Macedonia C. Emergence of oropharyngeal, laryngeal and swallowing activity in the developing fetal upper aerodigestive tract: an ultrasound evaluation. Early Hum Dev. 2003;71(1):61-87.
35. Finan DS, Barlow SM. The actifier: a device for neurophysiological studies of orofacial control in human infants. J Speech Hear Res. 1996;39(4):833-8.
36. Hack M, Estabrook MM, Robertson SS. Development of sucking rhythm in preterm infants, Early Hum Dev. 1985;11(2):133-40.
37. Rocha AD, Moreira ME, Pimenta HP, et al. A randomized study of the efficacy of sensory-motor-oral stimulation and non-nutritive sucking in very low birthweight infant. Early Hum Dev. 2007;83(6):385-8.
38. Fucile S, Gisel E, Lau C. Effect of an oral stimulation program on sucking skill maturation of preterm infants. Dev Med Child Neurol. 2005;47:158-62.
39. Fucile S, Gisel E, McFarland DH, et al. Oral and non-oral sensorimotor interventions enhance oral feeding performance in preterm infants. Dev Med Child Neurol. 2011;53(9):829-35.
40. Fucile S, McFarland DH, Gisel EG, et al. Oral and non-oral sensorimotor interventions facilitate suck-swallow-respiration functions and their coordination in preterm infants. Early Hum Dev. 2012;88:345-50.
41. Poore M, Barlow SM, Wang J, et al. Respiratory distress Syndrome history predicts suck spatiotemporal index in preterm infants. J Neonatal Nurs. 2008;14:185-92.
42. Finan DS, Barlow SM. Mechanosensory modulation of non-nutritive sucking in human infants. Early Hum Dev. 1998;52(2):181-97.
43. Pimenta HP, Moreira ME, Rocha AD, et al. Effects of non-nutritive sucking and oral stimulation on breastfeeding rates for preterm, low birth weight infants: a randomized clinical trial. J Pediatr (Rio J). 2008;84(5):423-7.
44. Fucile S, Gisel E, Lau C. Oral stimulation accelerates the transition from tube to oral feeding in preterm infants. J Pediatrics. 2002;141(2):230-6.
45. Bingham PM, Abassi S, Sivieri E. A pilot study of milk odor effect on nonnutritive sucking by premature newborns. Arch Pediatr Adolesc Med. 2003;157:72-5.
46. Bingham PM, Churchill D, Ashikaga T. Breast milk odor via olfactometer for tube-fed premature infants. Behav Res Methods. 2007;39(3):630-4.
47. Schaal B. Mammary odor cues and pheromones: mammalian infant-directed communication about maternal state, mammae, and milk. Vitam Horm. 2010;83:83-136.
48. Standley JM, Cassidy J, Grant R, et al. The effect of music reinforcement for non-nutritive sucking on nipple feeding of premature infants. Pediatr Nurs. 2010;36(3):138-45.
49. Barlow SM, Urish M, Venkatesan L, et al. Frequency Modulation and Spatiotemporal Stability of the sCPG in Preterm Infants with RDS. Int J Pediatr. 2012;2012:581538.
50. Stumm S, Barlow SM, Estep M, et al. The relation between respiratory distress syndrome and the fine structure of the non-nutritive suck in preterm infants. J Neonatal Nurs. 2008;14(1):9-16.
51. Estep M, Barlow SM, Vantipalli R, et al. Non-nutritive suck burst parametrics in preterm infants with RDS and oral feeding complications. J Neonatal Nursing. 2008;14(1):28-34.
52. Barlow SM, Maron JL, Alterovitz G, et al. Somatosensory Modulation of Salivary Gene Expression and Oral Feeding in Preterm Infants: Randomized Controlled Trial. JMIR Res Protoc. 2017;6(6):e113.
53. Bosma JF. Prologue to the symposium. In: Bosma JF (Ed). Fourth Symposium on Oral Sensation and Perception. Bethesda: Charles C Thomas Publisher; 1973. p. 7.
54. Shiao SY, Youngblut JM, Anderson GC, et al. Nasogastric tube placement: effects on breathing and sucking in very-low-birth-weight infants. Nurs Res. 1995;44(2):82-8.
55. Barlow SM. Central pattern generation involved in oral and respiratory control for feeding in the term infant. Curr Opin Otolaryngol Head Neck Surg. 2009;17:187-93.
56. Barlow SM. Oral and respiratory control for preterm feeding. Curr Opin Otolaryngol Head Neck Surg. 2009;17:179-86.
57. Adams-Chapman I, Bann CM, Vaucher YE, et al. Association between feeding difficulties and language delay in preterm infants using Bayley Scales of Infant Development-Third Edition. J Pediatrics. 2013;163(3):680-5.
58. Lau C, Hurst N. Oral feeding in infants. Curr Probl Pediatr Adolesc Health Care. 1999;29:105-24.
59. da Costa SP, van den Engel-Hoek L, Bos AF. Sucking and swallowing in infants and diagnostic tools. J Perinatol. 2008;28:247-57.
60. Pickler RH, Higgins KE, Crummette BD. The effect of nonnutritive sucking on bottle-feeding stress in preterm infants. J Obstet Gynecol Neonatal Nurs. 1993;22:230-4.
61. DiPietro JA, Cusson RM, Caughy MO, et al. Behavioral and physiologic effects of nonnutritive sucking during gavage feeding in preterm infants. Pediatr Res. 1994;36:207-14.
62. Field T. Sucking for stress reduction, growth and development during infancy. Pediatric Basics. 1993;64:13-6.
63. Gill NE, Behnke M, Conlon M, et al. Nonnutritive sucking modulates behavioral state for preterm infants before feeding. Scand J Caring Sci. 1992;6:3-7.
64. Pickler RH, Frankel HB, Walsh KM, et al. Effects of nonnutritive sucking on behavioral organization and feeding performance in preterm infants. Nurs Res. 1996;45:132-5.
65. Abbasi S, Sivieri E, Samuel-Collins N, et al. Effect of non-nutritive sucking on gastric motility of preterm infants. Honolulu, Hawaii: The Meeting of the Pediatric Academic Society; 2008.
66. McCain GC. Promotion of preterm infant nipple feeding with nonnutritive sucking. J Pediatr Nurs. 1995;10:3-8.
67. Woodson R, Drinkwin J, Hamilton C. Effects of nonnutritive sucking on state and activity: Term-preterm comparisons. Infant Behav Dev. 1985;8:435-41.
68. Song D, Jegatheesan P, Nafday S, et al. Patterned Frequency-modulated oral stimulation in preterm infants: A multicenter randomized controlled trial PLoS One. 2019; 14(2): e0212675.
69. Boiron M, Da Nobrega L, Roux S, et al. Effects of oral stimulation and oral support on non-nutritive sucking and feeding performance in preterm infants. Dev Med Child Neurol. 2007;49:439-44.
70. Harding C. An evaluation of the benefits of non-nutritive sucking for premature infants as described in the literature. Arch Dis Child. 2009;94:636-40.
71. Pickler RH, Reyna BA. Effects of non-nutritive sucking on nutritive sucking, breathing, and behavior during bottle feedings of preterm infants. Adv Neonatal Care. 2004;4:226-34.

72. Bingham PM, Ashikaga T, Abbasi S. Prospective study of non-nutritive sucking and feeding skills in premature infants. Arch Dis Child Fetal Neonatal Ed. 2010;95:F194-200.
73. Gewolb IH, Vice FL, Schwietzer-Kenney EL, et al. Developmental patterns of rhythmic suck and swallow in preterm infants. Dev Med Child Neurol. 2001;43(1):22-7.
74. Lau C, Schanler RJ. Oral motor function in the neonate. Clin Perinatol. 1996;23(2):161-78.
75. Lau C. Oral feeding in the preterm infant. Neo Reviews. 2006;7(1):e19-27.
76. Medoff-Cooper B. Nutritive sucking research: from clinical questions to research answers. J Perinat Neonatal Nurs. 2005;19(3):265-72.
77. Barlow SM, Rosner AO. Oral sensorimotor development: research and treatment. In: Bahr RH, Silliman ER (Eds). Handbook of Communication Disorders. London: Routledge; 2015. pp. 103-13.
78. Delaney AL, Arvedson JC. Development of swallowing and feeding: prenatal through first year of life. Dev Disabil Res Rev. 2008;14(2):105-17.
79. Lau C, Smith EO, Schanler RJ. Coordination of suck-swallow and swallow respiration in preterm infants. Acta Peadiatr. 2003;92(6):721-7.
80. Bamford O, Taciak V, Gewolb IH. The relationship between rhythmic swallowing and breathing during suckle feeding in term neonates. Pediatr Res. 1992;31(6):619-24.

# CHAPTER 29

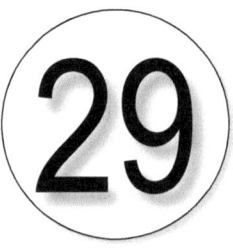

# Feeding and Brain Development in Preterm Infants: Role of Sensory Stimulation

*Steven M Barlow, Austin O Rosner, Dongli Song*

## ABSTRACT

The orofacial sensorium, includes massive afferent projections from trigeminal, facial, and olfactory receptors which encode tactile and motion sense, taste, and odorants, respectively. This stream of neural activity is relayed along modality-specific brainstem and thalamocortical pathways to an elaborate cerebral network to support the development of oral feeding through activity- and experience-dependent mechanisms which shape associated networks in the infant's 'feeding brain.' Unimodal and multimodal sensory therapies show great promise in preterm infants to stabilize behavioral state and cardiorespiratory function, modulate brain activity, promote ororhythmic sucking activity, reduce the time to attain independent oral feeding skills, and promote weight gain. The high salience of oral tactile inputs and odorants related to mother's breast milk improve sucking behavior and feeding. Recent findings indicate a critical period for somatosensory stimulation to promote oral feeding in preterm infants. The effects of sensory stimulation in newborns can be safely monitored using noninvasive biomechanical, electrophysiological, and cerebral hemodynamic methods.

## DRIVING BRAIN DEVELOPMENT

The infant brain is initially formed through activity-independent mechanisms and subsequently refined over the lifespan by experience- and activity-dependent mechanisms.[1,2] The activity-independent mechanisms (genetic instruction) occur early in fetal life and involve *"molecular sensing"* for axon outgrowth, pathfinding, and target selection. The refinement of initially diffuse connections within targets requires neuronal activity. For the orofacial neuromotor system, this process of refinement spans a protracted period of development that begins *in utero* around 7.5 weeks postmenstrual age (PMA) with the appearance of touch sensitivity.[3] Continued development and stability of synaptic connections in the nervous system are influenced by the pattern of electrical activity and competitive interaction between adjacent nerve terminals.[4] Neuronal activity affords the postnatal organism with a mechanism for adaptation, i.e. the maturing nervous system can be modified further by experience itself (adaptability). Adaptation is a hallmark feature of the orofacial system with its unique performance anatomy to support sucking, smiling, drinking and eating, hand-to-mouth coordination, cooing, babbling, and speech.[5] Thus, activity-dependent neuronal selection is a potent mechanism of normal development, and may be utilized as a neurotherapeutic to assist preterm infants at risk for neurodevelopmental sequelae.

For the premature infant, extrauterine life presents a significant challenge for the developing brain.[6] Prematurity diminishes the thalamocortical system and represents a major component of preterm brain injury that negatively impacts neurodevelopmental outcomes, including intellectual, sensory (e.g. hearing, vision), motor, feeding, and speech-language development.[7,8] Diffusion tensor tractography reveals that connections between the thalamus and the frontal cortices, supplementary motor areas, occipital lobe and temporal gyri are significantly diminished in preterm infants. Thalamocortical afferents provide a key source of input to layer IV of the developing neocortex. Methods aimed at increasing the salience and flow of sensory input to the brain is one approach being tested in animal and human models to mitigate the effects of prematurity.

## NEUROPROTECTION AND SENSORY STIMULATION

Agents of neuroprotection during the neonatal period may take the form of brain cooling, pharmacologic intervention (e.g. erythropoietin), or sensory stimulation to spare developing white matter and young neurons engaged in network formation. Very low birth weight (VLBW) preterm newborns are susceptible to chronic hypoxic injury as a consequence of abnormal lung development [i.e. chronic lung disease (CLD)], cardiac insufficiency, intraventricular hemorrhage, or neurobiological anomalies associated with hyperglycemia during gestation [i.e. infants of diabetic mothers (IDMs)]. These conditions often lead to grave neurological and behavioral consequences that may persist into adulthood. Longitudinal studies of sociodemographic factors examined among VLBW cohorts suggest that early environmental experiences have a substantial impact on neurological and behavioral outcomes.[9] A recent study using a mouse model of perinatal hypoxia, demonstrated that sensory enrichment resulted in a robust increase in neurogenesis and the number of neurons that reach maturity.[9] Using a genetic fate-mapping model in mice, the Vaccarino laboratory demonstrated that environmental enrichment (sensorimotor stimulation) following hypoxic injury, resulting from an 8-day exposure to 10% $O_2$, increases the proportion of astroglial cells that attain a neuronal fate. Environmental enrichment is a form of neuroprotection that served to increase the stem cell pool by increasing stem cell proliferation and survival into functional neural networks. In mice subjected to hypoxia and subsequent enrichment, there is an additive effect of both conditions on hippocampal neurogenesis from astroglia, resulting in a robust increase in the number of neurons arising from glial fibrillary acid protein (GFAP+) cells by the time these mice attain adulthood.

Sensory enrichment plays an important role in brain development and neurodevelopmental outcome.[10] The effects of individualized newborn care (light dimming, rest periods, supportive positioning, skin-to-skin contact) was examined for its effect on neurobehavioral, electrophysiological and neurostructural development of thirty preterm infants with severe intrauterine growth restriction (IUGR) randomized to control and enriched individualized care.[11] These infants were healthier, showed significantly improved brain development (i.e. more cortical gray matter) and better development of long tracts coursing through the internal capsule, corpus callosum, and occipital lobe as determined by diffusion MRI. The positive anatomical findings were consistent with enhanced association cortex connectivities as reflected in electroencephalographic (EEG) coherence analyses, and better neurobehavioral outcomes.

## SOMATOSENSORY "EXPERIENCE" PROMOTES STRUCTURAL CHANGES IN BRAIN CIRCUITRY AND NEUROPROTECTION: LESSONS FROM ANIMAL MODELS

The neonatal somatosensory cortex possesses considerable plasticity in its organization in response to manipulations of the sensory periphery.[12-14] In rodents, removal of a row of whiskers in the neonatal period results in shrinkage of the cortical areas known as "barrels" assigned to each extirpated whisker, while the cortex assigned to adjacent intact whiskers expands.[15] These results demonstrate activity- and experience-dependent rearrangement of the receptive field to compensate for loss of whisker input. This effect is far more robust in the neonatal period than at later ages, suggesting a critical sensory period during which sensory stimulation is potent for shaping neural networks. Numerous studies have shown activity-dependent changes in somatosensory cortical maps in rodents, primates, and other species.[16] In rodent cerebral cortex, somatosensory experience drives the continuous sprouting and retraction of synapses located on dendritic spines to remodel neural circuits.[17] Repetitive somatosensory stimulation, or changes in the frequency and strength of activation across synapses can result in long-term potentiation (LTP) or long-term depression (LTD) of neurotransmission.[18] Release of brain-derived neuronal growth factor (BDNF) from electrically active neurons enhances the formation of LTP and is associated with an enlargement of dendritic spines.[19] LTP is enhanced in the immature brain as compared to the adult brain.[20] Both LTP and LTD are essential for activity-dependent reorganization and stabilization of developing neuronal networks in sensorimotor cortex.[14] Maladaptive stimulation or somatosensory deprivation in the neonatal period will negatively impact orofacial map formation in trigeminal sensory nuclei, and ultimately impact the integrity of thalamocortical projections from the ventroposteromedial nucleus to the orofacial representations in sensorimotor cortex,[21] which could delay the development of oromotor and feeding skills.

A remarkable set of experiments have shown that low-dose repetitive somatosensory stimulation (2.15 min of 5 Hz stim/h) is highly neuroprotective if initiated within a critical time period following unilateral permanent MCA occlusion (pMCAO) in rat.[22-27] Even mild somatosensory stimulation [5 Hz sinusoidal displacement of a single vibrissa (trigeminal primary afferent)] provides 100% neuroprotection of cerebral hemisphere in pMCAO if initiated in the acute phase.[25] The model presumably works due to collateral blood flow into MCA distribution from the anterior cerebral artery (ACA)—blood flows in reverse through interarterial collaterals,[23] possibly via modulation of downstream vessel resistance in pial collaterals and other sources. Parallel studies in human have demonstrated that pulsed pneumotactile stimulation evokes a significant increase in blood flow velocity through the MCA and effects decreases in the pulsatility index to promote collateral blood flow and may offer exciting opportunities for neurotherapeutic applications in brain stroke across the lifespan.[28,29]

## BENCH-TO-BEDSIDE

An excellent opportunity in translational neuroscience exists to explore the neuroprotective value of salient somatosensory stimulation in preterm infants on brain maturation as reflected in electrocortical activity, neurovascular hemodynamics, neuroanatomy, and oromotor skill building leading to the attainment of safe oral feeds. Somatosensory stimulation strategies have proven beneficial in developing oral feeding skills in premature infants.[30] Brief tactile-motion stimulation (15 mins, 2x/day) applied to the face-mouth and body before tube feedings among 75 clinically stable preterm infants beginning at 32.3 weeks PMA (26–32 weeks GA) led to the attainment of independent oral feeding approximately 10 days earlier than infants who did not receive the stimulation.[31] This form of somatosensory stimulation also improves the dynamics of swallow-respiration coordination.[32] Pacifiers and pneumatically-motorized versions also play an important role in oromotor development, as they are often the most readily available form of oral stimulation for infants at the hospital and at home.[33] Pacifiers can facilitate and strengthen the skills necessary for transitioning to oral feeding. The mechanical properties of pacifiers, including geometry and stiffness[34] and texture,[35] significantly affect oromotor activity during infancy and should be considered when choosing age-appropriate oral stimulation devices.

A highly specialized somatosensory delivery system was developed in our laboratory >20 years ago which transforms a silicone pacifier into a dynamically pressurized orotactile stimulator, known as the NTrainer System®.[36,37] Approved for use in human preterm infants by the FDA (2008), this device has demonstrated utility in promoting the development of non-nutritive suck (NNS) and oromotor skills in respiratory distress syndrome (RDS) and CLD infants.[37-39] Orocutaneous pulse trains resembling NNS bursts generated by the NTrainer System® activate volleys of trigeminal afferent flow which influence electrocortical dynamics in preterm infants[40,41] and neuromagnetic activation fields in the sensorimotor cortex of young adults.[5] For preterm infants, this form of active oral somatosensory stimulation serves to modulate and reorganize high-amplitude EEG activity sampled over frontoparietal cortices into mid-range voltages. The CNS among preterm infants with CLD and IDM is vulnerable.[42-44] Given the stabilizing effect that orosensory entrainment has on cortical EEG, it follows that introduction of a progressive pulsed orocutaneous intervention well before NNS stabilization (30 weeks PMA) is likely to provide VLBW newborns with a trophic input to promote physiological stability and brain health, and optimize neural development in a way that positively impacts feeding behaviors, length of hospitalization, and neurodevelopmental outcome.

*Promoting ororhythmic patterning associated with NNS is dependent on the* spectral characteristics of the somatosensory entrainment stimulus. In a recent study involving 214 preterm infants, a pulsatile high-velocity orosensory entrainment stimulus was found to be significantly more effective than either a pulsed low-velocity orosensory entrainment stimulus or a sham "non-instrumented" pacifier to facilitate development of the NNS.[39] In a related randomized controlled trial (RCT) involving 160 preterm neonates, frequency-modulated (FM) pulsed *high-velocity* orocutaneous stimuli delivered through a silicone pacifier promoted NNS burst development in tube-fed RDS and CLD preterm infants.[38] This orosensory entrainment therapy was administered during tube feedings 3x/day up to 10 days while infants were in a quiet-alert to drowsy state in a developmentally supportive position (**Fig. 1**). Three blocks of 3-minute orosensory stimulation epochs were delivered during a 25-minute NG feed. Each stimulation block consisted of 34 frequency-modulated 6-cycle bursts, producing a total stimulus dose of 102 pneumotactile bursts/NG feed. Oromotor performance measures of NNS were automatically extracted from daily 3-minute digitized records of oral compression dynamics using waveform discrimination algorithms. A sample of the pulsed oral pneumotactile pulse train structure is shown in **Figure 2**. The high-velocity stimuli (right column) show a sequence of three 6-cycle bursts (top-right panel) characterized by (1) short rise times (~31 ms), (2) sharp pressure peaks

# CHAPTER 29: Feeding and Brain Development in Preterm Infants: Role of Sensory Stimulation

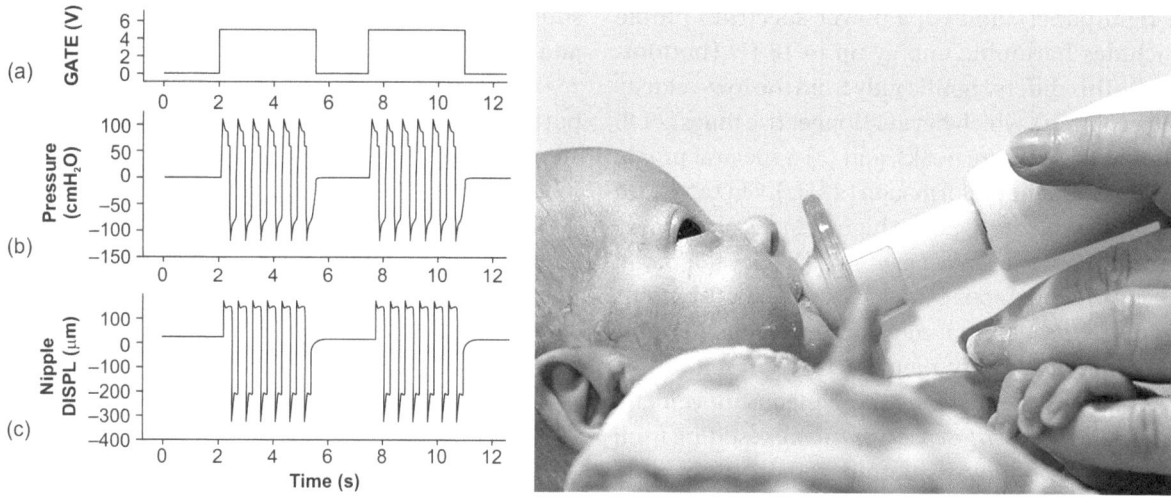

**Fig. 1:** Preterm infant receiving pulsed orocutaneous therapy. Synthesized burst-pause stimulus features delivered as frequency-modulated pneumotactile pulse trains through the pacifier nipple (left panel), (a) voltage-controlled gate signal, (b) pressure inside the nipple, and (c) mechanical displacement of the nipple cylinder wall *(For color version see Plate 4)*.
*Courtesy:* Innara Health, Inc., Olathe, Kansas USA.

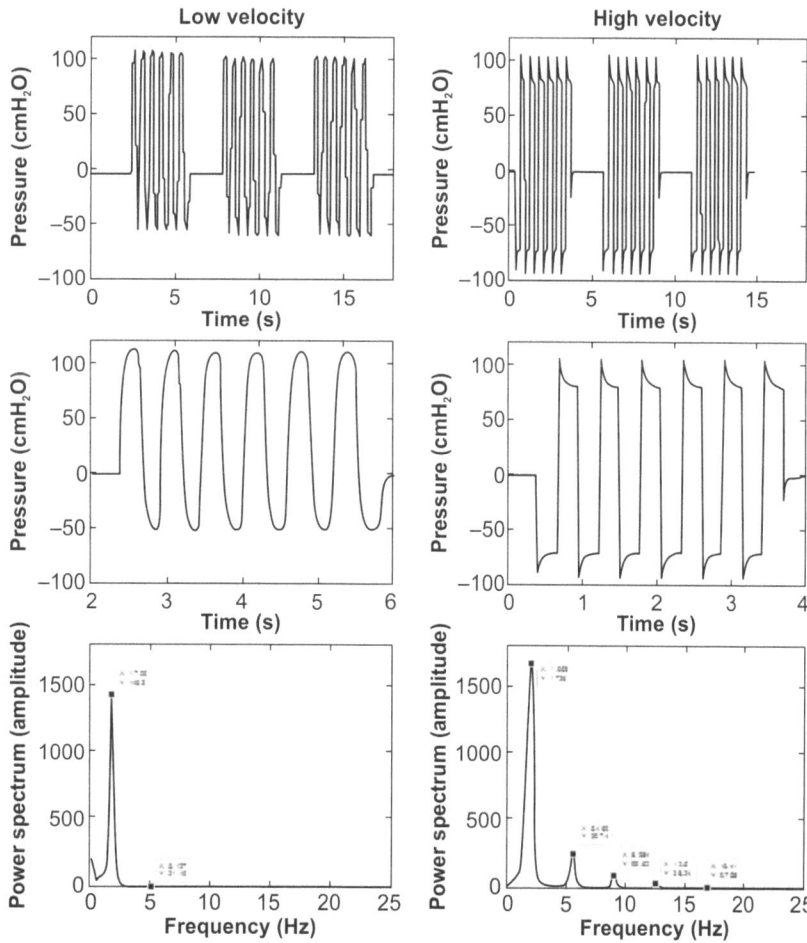

**Fig. 2:** Comparison of low and high-velocity pulsed pneumotactile stimuli when coupled to a green Soothie silicone pacifier and associated power spectra. Three stimulus bursts (top row). Expanded view of a single burst (middle row) reveal low velocity stimuli have relatively long rise time apparent in the pressure signal (left column, ~145 ms) compared to the shorter rise time for the high-velocity stimulus (right column, ~31 ms). The power spectrum (bottom row) is enhanced for the high-velocity stimulus with a fundamental peak at 1.95 Hz and harmonic energy up to 16.4 Hz.
*Source:* Adapted from Barlow SM, Lee J, Wang J, et al. Effects of oral stimulus frequency spectra on the development of non-nutritive suck in preterm infants with respiratory distress syndrome or chronic lung disease, and preterm infants of diabetic mothers. J Neonatal Nursing. 2014;20:178-88

(middle-right panel), and (3) a power spectrum profile which includes harmonic energy up to 16 Hz (bottom-right panel). This differs significantly from the low-velocity stimuli (left column), which have (1) longer rise times (~145 ms), (2) rounded pressure peaks, and (3) a spectral profile limited to low frequency information (≤2 Hz). CLD and IDM preterm infants who received the high-velocity orosensory experience showed the largest gains in NNS development. Low-velocity orocutaneous inputs lack sufficient stimulus salience to drive trigeminal mechanoreceptive afferents above background levels of neural activity present in the preterm orofacial system during spontaneous movement. This is likely due to *somatosensory masking* resulting from competition with ongoing afferent activity associated with slow postural adjustments of the lower face, mouth, and tongue produced by the infant, including attempts to suck. In essence, the infant's self-generated motor activity is sufficient to mask low-velocity orocutaneous inputs. Conversely, the high-velocity pulsed orocutaneous stimulus, with its broader spectral profile, provides the neonate with an enhanced orosensory experience to entrain the maxillary and mandibular divisions of the trigeminal system to promote and reinforce NNS motor patterns. Candidate mechanoreceptors in the infant's face include Meissner corpuscles and Merkel cell-neurites, which possess the appropriate frequency and amplitude sensitivities to encode the high-velocity orosensory stimulus. Meissner corpuscles are classified as rapidly adapting, especially sensitive to skin vibrations less than 50 Hz, and well matched to encode the dynamic features of the high-velocity oral entrainment stimulus. The Merkel ending is a slow-adapting (SA) mechanoreceptor with small receptive fields (1–8 mm) on the face (2 mechanoreceptors/mm$^2$), sensitive to low frequency micron-level vibration (~5–15 Hz), and well suited for encoding form and texture of objects contacted or manipulated in the mouth. These mechanoreceptors transmit somatosensory cues to the VPm at high conduction velocities (33–75 m/sec) by 1 year of age.[45] The salience of our high-velocity pulsed orocutaneous stimulus is consistent with experimental evidence on the mechanosensitivity of the human orofacial system.[46] Thus, pulsed oral somatosensory entrainment therapies to promote NNS motor patterns and feeding readiness should incorporate a frequency-modulated (FM), high-velocity burst-pattern stimulus profile with a spectral profile extending to 16 Hz to maximize NNS development. Current work is focusing on (1) improving the dynamics and temporal features of pneumotactile stimulus control systems in order to extend the spectral profile to include higher frequency content to the oral sensorium,[47] and (2) high data throughput for NNS digital signal processing to support neonatal intensive care units (NICUs) in the US and world-wide.[48]

A recent RCT designed to evaluate the effect of patterned, frequency-modulated oral somatosensory stimulation on time-to-full oral feeds (TOF) in 210 preterm infants (GA = 26–30 weeks, stratified among two groups: 26–28 and 29–30 weeks GA) randomized to NTrainer pulsed somatosensory stimulation versus sham (nonpulsatile pacifier) found that the experimental group manifest a significant reduction in TOF compared to the sham group (–4.1 days).[49] In the 29–30 weeks GA subgroup, infants in the experimental group manifest a 10 day reduction in time to discharge. This difference was not observed in the 26–28 weeks GA subgroup. Patterned, frequency-modulated oral somatosensory stimulation improves feeding development in premature infants and reduces their length of hospitalization.[49]

## ROLE OF SENSORY STIMULATION ON BRAIN MATURATION

Thalamocortical and corticocortical development is diminished in prematurity and correlated to EEG progression.[7] The fetal subplate zone is the origin of thalamocortical and corticocortical afferents and contributes to the evolution of EEG activity directly and indirectly via cortical connectivity.[50] Thus, defining normality of electrocortical activity represents a significant challenge in the NICU.[51] Reduced-montage dual-channel EEG is one method currently used to routinely monitor and map features of brain maturation[52-54] and assess neurological status in preterm infants.[55]

## MONITORING THE NEWBORN BRAIN WITH aEEG AND NEAR-INFRARED SPECTROSCOPY

Amplitude-integrated electroencephalography (aEEG) permits time-compressed, continuous bedside electrocortical monitoring in newborns at all maturational levels, including extremely preterm infants and the recording montage may be left in position for hours or days.[56] Typically, the aEEG is recorded from two pairs of surface electrodes (F3-P3 and F4-P4) situated over the frontoparietal cortices, which is proximal to face sensorimotor cortex. Main features extracted from the aEEG include (1) type of background activity (discontinuous/continuous), (2) estimate of interburst intervals or burst rate, (3) cyclic variation in the background activity corresponding to sleep-wake cycling (SWC), (4) amplitude band analysis, (5) spectral edge frequency (SEF), and (6) the presence of seizure patterns.

*Spectral edge frequency* defined as the frequency below which 95% of the power in a spectrum resides, provides a single estimate of the frequency content of the EEG which is thought to reflect cerebral maturation. Application of the SEF measure in healthy newborns revealed a significant positive correlation with GA ($r = 0.83$) and varied with behavioral state and brain loci.[57] Between approximately 30 and 40 weeks GA, whole brain SEF values increased from 5.4 Hz to 12 Hz. Closer inspection of the SEF over the first 3 days of life in normal preterm infants (median 29 weeks GA) using a slightly different power spectrum algorithm (90% power) revealed a decrease in SEF from 10.7 Hz on day 1 to 9.9 Hz on day 3.[58] The observed decrease in SEF reflects a possible low-grade hypoxic-ischemic event that may occur over a long period in most infants admitted to the NICU, or the response of the infant adapting to the stress of delivery and the extrauterine environment. SEF is also used to identify pathology and has been negatively correlated to the degree of white matter injury in premature infants (median GA 27 weeks).[59]

Amplitude-integrated electroencephalography monitoring has been increasingly used in neonates[55,60] to improve early diagnosis of unilateral lesions and improve seizure detection.[61,62] Results of aEEG are highly predictive of short- and long-term outcome in full-term infants with perinatal asphyxia.[63,64] Background aEEG activity is concordant with the neurological examination and with background patterns on full-scale EEG.[65] However, routine aEEG may fail to detect brief seizure patterns, which are difficult to differentiate from artifacts.[65] The aEEG and evoked potentials have the best predictive value for selecting infants for early intervention to prevent long-term sequelae.[66]

Clinical investigations utilizing aEEG have contributed important normative data on brain maturation in preterm infants at different GA and PMA.[51,53-55,67,68] aEEG characteristics, including voltage, continuity, and SWC, mature with increasing GA and PMA. For example, with greater GA the relative amount of continuous activity (aEEG > 5 μV and maximal amplitude between 20 μV and 40 μV) tends to increase while discontinuous patterns decrease. The number of bursts per hour tends to decrease with advancing GA. Sleep state differentiation appears in neurologically normal infants at 27–29 weeks PMA,[54,69] but is absent in most infants with severe IVH.[70] Sleep state differentiation in the aEEG is strongly associated with good long-term prognosis. Long-term outcome can be predicted by aEEG and EEG with 75–80% accuracy at 24 postnatal hours in very preterm infants (28–32 weeks GA), and in infants with no early indication of brain injury.[71] The aEEG upper and lower margins,[51,53,68] range-EEG amplitude bands,[54,72] and EEG spectral power are highly predictive of brain maturation ($R^2 \sim 0.90$).

Compared to aEEG, the range-EEG (rEEG) represents a less conservative estimate of peak-to-peak amplitude derived from raw EEG. The rEEG provides a more precise estimate of peak-to-peak amplitude based on the raw EEG tracing when compared with aEEG, correlates strongly with PMA,[54] and may serve as a biomarker for brain maturation and quantification of EEG suppression in brain injury.

Recent studies advocate near-infrared spectroscopy (NIRS) in preterm infants[73] to better understand the dynamics of neurovascular coupling and the effect of extrauterine life. NIRS is gaining popularity for use in newborns and infants, though there is still little information regarding brain metabolism and functional activation in these young populations compared to adults.[74] With the advancement of continuous-wave NIRS technology and miniaturized probe designs using LED sources, monitoring and imaging the preterm brain with fNIRS is gaining traction in the NICU among healthy[75] and sick[76] preterm infants.

## EEG Correlates and Hemodynamic Indicators of Pulsed Pneumatic Orocutaneous Stimulation in Preterm Infants

Nearly all studies of preterm brain cortical activity using aEEG and rEEG have been designed to map developmental features of maturation (continuity, amplitude margins, amplitude bands, etc.) and/or pathologic brain activity (e.g. seizures, discontinuity) during resting or quiescent states. However, stimulation of the nervous system also plays an important role in brain development and neurodevelopmental outcome.[11] Studies aimed at mapping the relations between sensory stimulation and modulation of the aEEG and EEG are limited in preterm infants. Orosensory stimulation presented during tube feedings begun at 32 weeks PMA exerts a significant modulatory effect on electrocortical and brain hemodynamic activity in preterm infants. In the electrocortical domain, numerous short- (seconds) and longer-term (minutes) effects of orocutaneous stimulation have been reported in the aEEG and range-EEG (rEEG) amplitude bands,[41] and shifts in the spectral edge frequency (SEF-90).[40] Short-term changes in the aEEG and rEEG were found during the 3-minute stimulation periods, while longer-term changes across stimulus epochs were noted by the persistence or "after-effects" in the EEG parameters in the minutes following stimulus removal. This is evidence of neural adaptation, a form of plasticity along the thalamocortical projection. Presentation of 3-minute pulsed orocutaneous stimulation epochs significantly enhanced band C (25–50 μV) rEEG activity while suppressing higher voltage band E (>100 μV) rEEG activity. Preterm infants exposed to the pulsed orocutaneous stimulation yielded a greater proportion of band C activity throughout the 23-minute sampling period that followed the first stimulus block when compared to infants who were given an ordinary pacifier. O'Reilly and colleagues[54] reported that the percentages of the high voltage band (band E), and low voltage band (band A), decreased with advancing PMA, while the percentage of the middle band voltage (band C) increased. These changes were correlated with the increase in the lower margin and decrease in the upper margin of the rEEG, and bandwidth narrowing. The rEEG values become less variable and concentrated in band C (25-50 μV) during orocutaneous stimulation, a characteristic of the maturing infant. Thus, low-dose pulsed orocutaneous stimulation appears to promote a more "mature" state of electrocortical dynamics in preterm infants which persists after the somatosensory stimulus is removed.

Application of patterned, low-dose pneumatic orocutaneous stimulation of the preterm infant at 30-32 weeks PMA achieves synchronous activation of trigeminal mechanosensitive afferents which drive thalamocortical afferents to prime the orofacial sensorimotor cortex. The effects on electrocortical dynamics are multiple, including modulation of the upper and lower margins of the aEEG, and a robust reorganization of rEEG with shifts in the proportion of voltages from amplitude bands D and E to band C. Cortical asymmetry also was apparent in both aEEG and rEEG amplitude measures.[41]

These results illustrate how practitioners can apply a functional somatosensory stimulation regimen with aEEG and rEEG for monitoring electrocortical activity and brain maturation in the NICU. Several features of this approach are parsimonious with this form of brain monitoring in preterm infants. First, human infants are precocial for trigeminal somatic sensation[45] which benefits sucking, facial expression, communication (crying, cooing, and babble), feeding, airway protection, and physiological state control. Perioral skin, oral mucosa, and anterior tongue dorsum contain a high density of mechanoreceptors associated with rapidly-conducting Aβ axons, which are responsive to subtle mechanical deformation applied to their receptive fields.[46] Second, the high innervation density and representation of Aβ rapidly conducting mechanoreceptor types in the lips, tongue, oral mucosa, and/or mandible are associated with high cortical magnification factors which is defined as the ratio between the area of representation in the primary somatosensory cortex (S1) to the area of the skin.[77] Facial skin, lip vermilion, mouth, and buccal mucosa are predominantly populated with slow-adapting (SA) mechanoreceptors with well-defined receptive fields (2-3 mm) which encode facial movements, whereas the tongue tip is dominated by fast-adapting (FA) mechanoreceptors with very small receptive fields (~1 mm).[78] These mechanoreceptive afferents are distinguished by their adaptation profile, best frequency, and receptive field size. Serendipitously, the dual-channel EEG recording montage used routinely by many NICUs world-wide is placed over the infant's lateral cerebral convexity (e.g. proximal to the face cortex) to sample brain activity correlated with trigeminal mechanosensory events. Third, the pneumatic orocutaneous stimulation provided by the NTrainer system is a midline input to the infant's mouth and anterior tongue, two highly sensitive cutaneous surfaces, rivaled only by the glabrous skin of the hand.

Multimodal monitoring of brain function in preterm, including EEG, regional cerebral tissue oxygenation r-cSO$_2$, and continuous wave near-infrared spectroscopy (cw-NIRS) will likely enhance our understanding of the dynamic influences of sensory stimulation (tactile, olfactory, and auditory) on neural activity and neurovascular coupling. The sample shown in **Figure 3** includes the relative proportion of EEG spectra by frequency band [β (16-31 Hz), α (8-15 Hz), θ (4-7 Hz), and Δ (<4Hz)], SEF-90, and rSO$_2$ during one session in a stable preterm infant ($28^{2/7}$ weeks GA) who received pulsed orocutaneous stimulation in a series of 3-min blocks at $32^{1/7}$ weeks PMA. EEG frequency band modulation is apparent with adaptation in evoked activity apparent between the 1st, 2nd, and 3rd pulsed orocutaneous stimulation blocks (black filled bars) for δ and β waves, in contrast to minimal adaptation of α waves. Beta wave modulation apparent during the initial block of stimulation is absent during stimulation blocks 2 and 3. Modulation of SEF with progressive adaptation in latter stimulation blocks is apparent in the upper-right plot panel. The regional cerebral O$_2$ modulation obtained from NIRS sensors placed over C3 shows progressively delayed increases in r-cSO$_2$% for the latter two stimulus blocks as the infant drifts into a sleep cycle.

## EARLY INTERVENTION

Sensory stimulation is used widely as a therapeutic intervention in preterm infants to stabilize behavioral state and cardiorespiratory function, promote ororhythmic sucking activity, reduce the time to attain independent oral feeding skills, and promote weight gain. The high salience of oral tactile inputs and odorants related to mother's breast milk improve sucking behavior and feeding.[79-82] Changes in infant posture and orientation attributable to movements of the caretaker serve to stimulate the infant's vestibular system, however, lengthy stays in the NICU means this important sensory system is often understimulated for

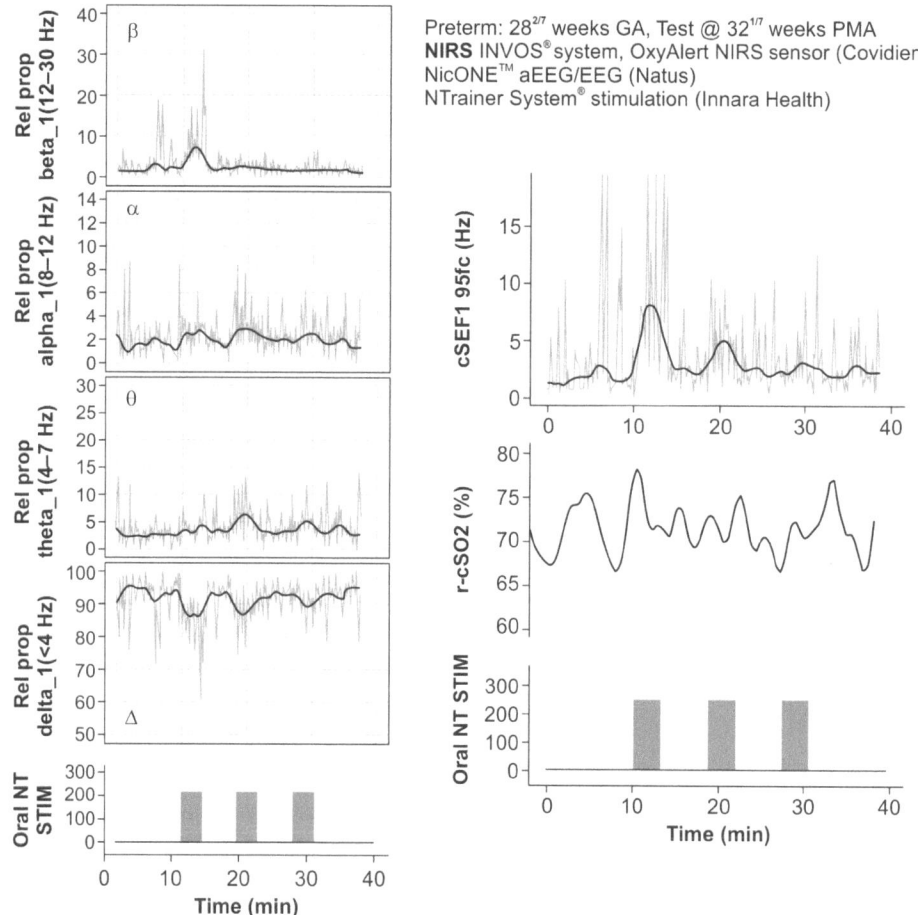

**Fig. 3:** Evoked electrophysiologic and hemodynamic activity in a preterm infant to a series of 3-minutes orocutaneous stimulation epochs (black bars). β, α, Θ, Δ relative proportion of EEG band activity (*left column*). Spectral edge frequency (SEF) and regional cerebral oxygen (L-frontoparietal, over C3) (*right column*).

extended periods of time. Exposure to vestibular stimulation by daily rocking and gliding can reduce the frequency of apneic attacks, modulate respiratory rates, and decrease the need for respiratory therapies.[83,84] Auditory stimulation in the form of lullabies,[85] live music,[86] and biological maternal sounds[87-89] has been shown to improve vital signs, NNS activity levels, oral feeding, and sleep in infants.

Multimodal sensory therapies show great promise. The combination of tactile, auditory, visual and vestibular (ATVV) leads to enhanced arousal state control and physiological stability,[90] improved neuromotor function,[91] decreased length of hospital stay, and a reduction in time-to-full oral feeds.[90] Direct skin-to-skin contact between an infant and their parent, known as Kangaroo Care, provides a rich source of tactile, auditory, kinesthetic, olfactory, and movement-related vestibular stimulation to the infant. The result is improved regulation of body temperature, reduced apnea and bradycardia events with commensurate increases in $O_2$ saturation, more periods of quiet sleep, reduced length of hospitalization, promotes breastfeeding,[92] and enhanced brain maturation.[93]

## SUMMARY

Oral sensorimotor development is necessary to support life-sustaining functions, such as sucking and swallowing. Close examination of feeding skill in the preterm infant provides a window into the integrity and development brainstem and suprabulbar pathways. Translational research continues on the role of patterned somatosensory stimulation of the orofacial sensorium and multimodal stimulation to inform new therapeutic strategies for individualized care to promote development of safe feeding in preterm infants.[94]

## ACKNOWLEDGMENTS

Supported in part by NIH R01 DC003311 (SM Barlow-PI), R01 HD086088 (SM Barlow and J Maron, MPDs), and the Barkley Trust.

## REFERENCES

1. Catalano SM, Shatz CJ. Activity-dependent cortical target selection by thalamic axons. Science. 1998;281:559-62.

2. Penn AA, Shatz CJ. Brain waves and brain wiring: the role of endogenous and sensory-driven neural activity in development. Pediatr Res. 1999;45:447-58.
3. Fitzgerald GE, Windle WF. Some observations on early human fetal movements. J Comp Neurol. 1942;76:159-67.
4. Garraghty PE, Kaas JH, Florence SL. Plasticity of sensory and motor maps in adult and developing mammals. In: Casagrande VA, Shinkman PG (Eds). Advances in Neural and Behavioral Development. Norwood, NJ: Ablex Publishing Corporation; 1994. pp. 1-36.
5. Venkatesan L, Barlow SM, Popescu M, et al. Adaptation in the human somatosensory cortical network following repetitive hand and face stimulation. Exp Brain Res. 2014;232:3545-54.
6. Limperopoulos C, Gauvreau KK, O'Leary H, et al. Cerebral hemodynamic changes during intensive care of preterm infants. Pediatrics. 2008;122:e1009-13.
7. Ball G, Boardman JP, Aljabar P, et al. The influence of preterm birth on the developing thalamocortical connectome. Cortex. 2013;49:1711-21.
8. Volpe JJ. Brain injury in premature infants: a complex amalgam of destructive and developmental disturbances. Lancet Neurol. 2009;8:110-24.
9. Salmaso N, Silbereis J, Komitova M, et al. Environmental enrichment increases the GFAP+ stem cell pool and reverses hypoxia-induced cognitive deficits in juvenile mice. J Neurosci. 2012;32:8930-39.
10. Als H, Duffy FH, McAnulty GB, et al. Early experience alters brain function and structure. Pediatrics. 2004;113:846-57.
11. Als H, Duffy FH, McAnulty GB, et al. NIDCAP improves brain function and structure in preterm infants with severe intrauterine growth restriction. J Perinatol. 2012;32:797-803.
12. Erzurumlu RS, Gaspar P. Development and critical period plasticity of the barrel cortex. Eur J Neurosci. 2012;35:1540-53.
13. Belford GR, Killackey HP. The sensitive period in the development of the trigeminal system of the neonatal rat. J Comp Neurol. 1980;193:335-50.
14. Feldman DE, Nicoll RA, Malenka RC. Synaptic plasticity at thalamocortical synapses in developing rat somatosensory cortex: LTP, LTD, and silent synapses. J Neurobiol. 1999;41:92-101.
15. Inan M, Crair MC. Development of cortical maps: perspectives from the barrel cortex. Neuroscientist. 2007;13:49-61.
16. Buonomano DV, Merzenich MM. Cortical plasticity: from synapses to maps. Annu Rev Neurosci. 1998;21:149-86.
17. Trachtenberg JT, Chen BE, Knott GW, et al. Long-term in vivo imaging of experience-dependent synaptic plasticity in adult cortex. Nature. 2002;420:788-94.
18. Citri A, Malenka RC. Synaptic plasticity: multiple forms, functions, and mechanisms. Neuropsychopharmacology. 2008;33:18-41.
19. Hartmann M, Heumann R, Lessmann V. Synaptic secretion of BDNF after high-frequency stimulation of glutamatergic synapses. EMBO J. 2001;20:5887-97.
20. Crair MC, Malenka RC. A critical period for long-term potentiation at thalamocortical synapses. Nature. 1995;375:325-28.
21. Fox K, Wong RO. A comparison of experience-dependent plasticity in the visual and somatosensory systems. Neuron. 2005;48:465-77.
22. Davis MF, Lay CC, Chen-Bee CH, et al. Amount but not pattern of protective sensory stimulation alters recovery after permanent middle cerebral artery occlusion. Stroke. 2011;42:792-8.
23. Lay CC, Davis MF, Chen-Bee CH, et al. Mild sensory stimulation completely protects the adult rodent cortex from ischemic stroke. PLoS One. 2010;5:e11270.
24. Lay CC, Davis MF, Chen-Bee CH, et al. Mild sensory stimulation reestablishes cortical function during the acute phase of ischemia. J Neurosci. 2011;31:11495-504.
25. Lay CC, Davis MF, Chen-Bee CH, et al. Mild sensory stimulation protects the aged rodent from cortical ischemic stroke after permanent middle cerebral artery occlusion. J Am Heart Assoc. 2012;1:e001255.
26. Lay CC, Frostig RD. Complete protection from impending stroke following permanent middle cerebral artery occlusion in awake, behaving rats. Eur J Neurosci. 2014;40:3413-21.
27. Lay CC, Jacobs N, Hancock AM, et al. Early stimulation treatment provides complete sensory-induced protection from ischemic stroke under isoflurane anesthesia. Eur J Neurosci. 2013;38:2445-52.
28. Hage B, Way E, Barlow SM, et al. Cerebral hemodynamic response to tactile somatosensory stimulation. J Neuroimaging. 2018;28:615-20.
29. Barlow SM, Bashford GR, Singh S. (2019). Neuroprotection in acute MCA stroke by somatosensory-induced collateral blood flow. R01 NS117741-01 proposal to NINDS.
30. Fucile S, Gisel E, Lau C. Effect of an oral stimulation program on sucking skill maturation of preterm infants. Dev Med Child Neurol. 2005;47:158-62.
31. Fucile S, Gisel E, McFarland DH, et al. Oral and non-oral sensorimotor interventions enhance oral feeding performance in preterm infants. Dev Med Child Neurol. 2011;53:829-35.
32. Fucile S, McFarland DH, Gisel EG, et al. Oral and nonoral sensorimotor interventions facilitate suck-swallow-respiration functions and their coordination in preterm infants. Early Hum Dev. 2012;88:345-50.
33. Barlow SM, Rosner AO. Oral sensorimotor development: research and treatment. In: Bahr RH, Silliman ER (Eds). Handbook of Communication Disorders. London: Routledge; 2015. pp. 103-13.
34. Zimmerman E, Barlow SM. Pacifier stiffness alters the dynamics of the suck central pattern generator. J Neonatal Nurs. 2008;14:79-86.
35. Oder AL, Stalling DL, Barlow SM. Short-term effects of pacifier texture on NNS in neurotypical infants. Int J Pediatr. 2013;2013:168459.
36. Finan DS, Barlow SM. Mechanosensory modulation of non-nutritive sucking in human infants. Early Hum Dev. 1998;52:181-97.
37. Barlow SM, Finan DS, Chu S, et al. Patterns for the premature brain: Synthetic orocutaneous stimulation entrains preterm infants with feeding difficulties to suck. J Perinatol. 2008;28:541-8.
38. Barlow SM, Lee J, Wang J, et al. Frequency-modulated orocutaneous stimulation promotes non-nutritive suck development in preterm infants with respiratory distress syndrome or chronic lung disease. J Perinatol. 2014;34:136-42.
39. Barlow SM, Lee J, Wang J, et al. Effects of oral stimulus frequency spectra on the development of non-nutritive suck in preterm infants with respiratory distress syndrome

or chronic lung disease, and preterm infants of diabetic mothers. J Neonatal Nursing. 2014;20:178-88.
40. Song D, Jegatheesan P, Weiss S, et al. Modulation of EEG spectral edge frequency during patterned pneumatic oral stimulation in preterm infants. Pediatr Res. 2014;75:85-92.
41. Barlow SM, Jegatheesan P, Weiss S, et al. Amplitude integrated EEG and range-EEG modulation associated with pneumatic orocutaneous stimulation in preterm infants. J Perinatol. 2014;32:213-9.
42. Khaksar Z, Jelodar G, Hematian H. Cerebrum malformation in offspring of diabetic mothers. Comp Clin Pathol. 2012;21:699-703.
43. Nelson CA, Wewerka S, Thomas KM, et al. Neurocognitive sequelae of infants of diabetic mothers. Behav Neurosci. 2000;114:950-6.
44. Nold JL, Georgieff MK. Infants of diabetic mothers. Pediatr Clin North Am. 2004;51:619-37.
45. Barlow SM, Dusick A, Finan DS, et al. Mechanically evoked perioral reflexes in premature and term human infants. Brain Res. 2001;899:251-4.
46. Trulsson M, Essick GK. Mechanosensation. In: Miles TS, Nauntofte B, Svensson P (EDS). Clinical Oral Physiology. Copenhagen: Quintessence Books; 2004. pp. 165-97.
47. Greenwood J, Barlow SM. pTACS: A New Platform for Neurotherapeutics and Neuroprotection in Large Vessel Ischemic Stroke. Santa Barbara, CA: Motor Speech Conference; 2020.
48. Liao C, Rosner AO, Maron JL, et al. Automatic non-nutritive suck waveform discrimination and feature extraction in preterm infants. Comput Math Methods Med. 2019; 7496591.
49. Song D, Jegatheesan P, Nafday S, et al. Patterned frequency-modulated oral stimulation in preterm infants: A multicenter randomized controlled trial. PloS One. 2019;14:e0212675.
50. Kostovic I, Jovanov-Milosevic N. The development of cerebral connections during the first 20-45 weeks' gestation. Semin Fetal Neonatal Med. 2006;11:415-22.
51. Griesmaier E, Enot DP, Bachmann M, et al. Systematic characterization of amplitude-integrated EEG signals for monitoring the preterm brain. Pediatr Res. 2013;73:226-35.
52. Niemarkt HJ, Andriessen P, Peters CH, et al. Quantitative analysis of amplitude-integrated electroencephalogram patterns in stable preterm infants, with normal neurological development at one year. Neonatology. 2010;97:175-82.
53. Niemarkt HJ, Jennekens W, Pasman JW, et al. Maturational changes in automated EEG spectral power analysis in preterm infants. Clin Neurophysiol. 2011;70:2139-53.
54. O'Reilly D, Navakatikyan MA, Filip M, et al. Peak-to-peak amplitude in neonatal brain monitoring of premature infants. Clin Neurophysiol. 2012;123:2139-53.
55. Hellström-Westas L, de Vries LS, Rosén I. Atlas of Amplitude-Integrated EEGs in the Newborn, 2nd edition. United Kingdom: Informa Healthcare; 2008. pp. 1-187.
56. Maynard DE. EEG analysis using an analogue frequency analyser and a digital computer. Electroencephalogr Clin Neurophysiol. 1967;23:487.
57. Bell AH, McClure BG, McCullagh PJ, et al. Variation in power spectral analysis of the EEG with gestational age. J Clin Neurophysiol. 1991;8:312-9.
58. West CR, Harding JE, Williams CE, et al. Quantitative electroencephalographic patterns in normal preterm infants over the first week after birth. Early Hum Dev. 2006;82:43-51.
59. Inder TE, Buckland L, Williams CE, et al. Lowered electroencephalographic spectral edge frequency predicts the presence of cerebral white matter injury in premature infants. Pediatrics. 2003;111:27-33.
60. Verma UL, Archbald F, Tejani NA, et al. Cerebral function monitor in the neonate. I: normal patterns. Dev Med Child Neurol. 1984;26:154-61.
61. Shah DK, de Vries LS, Hellström-Westas L, et al. Amplitude-integrated electroencephalography in the newborn: a valuable tool. Pediatrics. 2008;122:863-65.
62. van Rooij LG, de Vries LS, van Huffelen AC, et al. Additional value of two-channel amplitude integrated EEG recording in full-term infants with unilateral brain injury. Arch Dis Child Fetal Neonatal Ed. 2010;95:F160-8.
63. Shalak LF, Laptook AR, Velaphi SC, et al. Amplitude-integrated electroencephalography coupled with an early neurologic examination enhances prediction of term infants at risk for persistent encephalopathy. Pediatrics. 2003;111:351-7.
64. Groenendaal F, de Vries LS. Selection of babies for intervention after birth asphyxia. Semin Neonatol. 2000;5:17-32.
65. Toet MC, van der Meij W, de Vries LS, et al. Comparison between simultaneously recorded amplitude-integrated electroencephalogram (cerebral function monitor) and standard electroencephalogram in neonates. Pediatrics. 2002;109:772-9.
66. Pike AA, Marlow N. The role of cortical evoked responses in predicting neuromotor outcome in very preterm infants. Early Hum Dev. 2000;57:123-35.
67. Olischar M, Klebermass K, Kuhle S, et al. Reference values for amplitude integrated electroencephalographic activity in preterm infants younger than 30 weeks' gestational age. Pediatrics. 2004;113:e61-6.
68. Zhang D, Liu Y, Hou X, et al. Reference values for amplitude-integrated EEGs in infants from preterm to 3.5 months of age. Pediatrics. 2011;e1280-7.
69. Curzi-Dascalova L, Figueroa JM, Eiselt M, et al. Sleep state organization in premature infants of less than 35 weeks' gestational age. Pediatr Res. 1993;34:624-8.
70. Hellström-Westas L, Klette H, Thorngren-Jerneck K, Rosén I. Early prediction of outcome with aEEG in preterm infants with large intraventricular hemorrhages. Neuropediatrics. 2001;32:319-24.
71. Wikström S, Pupp IH, Rosén I, et al. Early single-channel aEEG/EEG predicts outcome in very preterm infants. Acta Paediatr. 2012;101:719-26.
72. Navakatikyan M. Peak-to-peak amplitude of EEG for the monitoring of brain function. In: Proceedings of 8th World Congress of Perinatal Medicine; 2007; Florence. Florence, Italy: Medimond; 2007.p. 643-7.
73. Greisen G, Leun T, Wolf M. Has the time come to use near-infrared spectroscopy as a routine clinical tool in preterm infants undergoing intensive care? Phil Trans R Soc. 2011;369:4440-51.
74. Roche-Labarbe N, Fenoglio A, Radhakrishnan H, et al. Somatosensory evoked changes in cerebral oxygen consumption measured non-invasively in premature infants. NeuroImage. 2014;85:279-86.
75. Franceschini MA, Thaker S, Themelis G, et al. Assessment of infant brain development with frequency-domain near-infrared spectroscopy. Pediatr Res. 2007;61:546-51.

76. Roche-Labarbe N, Fenoglio A, Aggarwal A, et al. Near-infrared spectroscopy assessment of cerebral oxygen metabolism in the developing premature brain. J Cereb Blood Flow Metab. 2012;32:481-8.
77. Toda T, Taoka M. Converging patterns of inputs from oral structures in the postcentral somatosensory cortex of conscious macaque monkeys. Exp Brain Res. 2004;158:43-9.
78. Trulsson M, Johansson RS. Orofacial mechanoreceptors in humans: encoding characteristics and responses during natural orofacial behaviors. Behav Brain Res. 2002;135:27-33.
79. Schaal B. Mammary odor cues and pheromones: Mammalian infant-directed communication about maternal state, mammae, and milk. Vitam Horm. 2010;83:83-136.
80. Varendi H, Porter RH, Winberg J. Does the newborn baby find the nipple by smell? Lancet. 1994;344:989-90.
81. Raimbault C, Saliba E, Porter RH. The effect of the odour of mother's milk on breastfeeding behavior of premature neonates. Acta Peadiatr. 2007;96:368-71.
82. Yildiz A, Arikan D, Gözüm S, et al. The effect of the odor of breast milk on the time needed for transition from gavage to total oral feeding in preterm infants. J Nurs Scholarsh. 2011;43:256-73.
83. Tuck SJ, Monin P, Duvivier C, et al. Effect of a rocking bed on apnoea of prematurity. Arch Dis Child. 1982;57:475-7.
84. Zimmerman E, Barlow SM. The effects of vestibular stimulation rate and magnitude of acceleration on central pattern generation for chest wall kinematics in preterm infants. J Perinatol. 2012;32:614-20.
85. Standley JM, Cassidy J, Grant R, et al. The effect of music reinforcement for non-nutritive sucking on nipple feeding of premature infants. Pediatr Nurs. 2010;36:138-45.
86. Loewy J, Stewart K, Dassler AM, et al. The effects of music therapy on vital signs, feeding, and sleep in premature infants. Pediatrics. 2013;131:902-18.
87. Chorna OD, Slaughter JC, Wang L, et al. A pacifier-activated music player with mother's voice improves oral feeding in preterm infants. Pediatrics. 2014;133:462-8.
88. Filippa M, Devouche E, Arioni C, et al. Live maternal speech and singing have beneficial effects on hospitalized preterm infants. Acta Peadiatr. 2013;102:1017-20.
89. Zimmerman EA, Keunen K, Norton M, et al. Weight gain velocity in very low-birth-weight infants: effects of exposure to biological maternal sounds. Am J Perinatol. 2013;30:863-70.
90. White-Traut RC, Nelson MN, Silvestri JM, et al. Effect of auditory, tactile, visual, and vestibular intervention on length of stay, alertness, and feeding progression in preterm infants. Dev Med Child Neurol. 2002;44:91-7.
91. Kanagasabai PS, Mohan K, Lewis LE, et al. Effect of multisensory stimulation on neuromotor development in preterm infants. Indian J Pediatr. 2013;80:460-4.
92. Bauer J, Sontheimer D, Fisher C, et al. Metabolic rate and energy balance in very low birthweight infants during kangaroo holding by their mothers and fathers. J Pediatrics. 1996;129:608-11.
93. Scher MS, Ludington-Hoe S, Kaffashi F, et al. Neurophysiologic assessment of brain maturation after an 8-week trial of skin-to-skin contact on preterm infants. Clin Neurophysiol. 2009;120:1812-8.
94. Barlow SM, Maron JL, Alterovitz G, et al. Somatosensory Modulation of Salivary Gene Expression and Oral Feeding in Preterm Infants. JMIR Res Protoc. 2017;6:e113.

CHAPTER

# The Gut-Microbiota-Brain Axis: Implications for Neonatal Neurodevelopment

*Dongli Song, Laishuan Wang*

## ABSTRACT

Symbiotic rapport between microbiota and their hosts is established early in life and influences multiple physiological processes. Recent animal experiments and human clinical studies reveal intriguing communications between the gut, microbiota, and brain—the gut-microbiota-brain axis plays a critical role in neurodevelopment and behavior regulation. Multiple perinatal factors affect the newborn microbiome and gut dysbiosis is common in preterm infants. Perturbations of the developing gut microbiota in this vulnerable population may alter gut-brain signaling, increase risk of brain injury, modify brain development trajectories, and lead to long-term neurological impairments such as cerebral palsy, poor cognitive function, and behavior disorders.

## INTRODUCTION

Survival for preterm infants has improved significantly in past decades. However, long-term neurological impairment remains an important challenge in perinatal-neonatal medicine. While brain injuries such as intraventricular hemorrhage (IVH) and white matter injury (periventricular leukomalacia or PVL) have long been recognized and well characterized in very premature infants, many infants who exhibit long-term impairment have no identifiable brain injuries on head ultrasound (HUS) and/or brain MRI taken before neonatal intensive care unit (NICU) discharge,[1] highlighting abnormal brain maturation as a major contributor to poor long-term neurodevelopmental outcomes.

The human body shares an intimate and lifelong partnership with a myriad of resident microbial species including bacteria, viruses, protozoa, and fungi, collectively referred to as the microbiota. While microbes colonize all surfaces in and on the human body, the largest microbial component of the human microbiota is located in the gut. The normal gut microbiota consists of approximately 100 trillion microorganisms, 10 times the total number of cells in the human body, and at least 100 times as many genes as the human genome.[2,3] The human host establishes its symbiotic rapport with microbes and relies on them to develop and maintain physiological homeostasis. Growing numbers of studies demonstrate gut-microbiota-brain signaling involvement in early neurodevelopmental programming and pathogenesis of behavior and emotional disorders such as autism spectrum disorders (ASD), attention deficit hyperactivity disorder (ADHD), and anxiety.[4-6] Premature birth and subsequent NICU stay lead to gut microbiota dysbiosis (an unbalanced state of microbiota), which is an underlying contributor to abnormal brain development. Improving preterm gut microbial colonization represents a new research avenue for developing neuroprotective strategies and therapeutic interventions.

This chapter reviews the establishment of neonatal gut microbiota in term and preterm infants, gut-microbiota-brain axis signaling and its implication in healthy brain development, and prevention of long-term neurodevelopmental impairment.

## THE GUT-MICROBIOTA-BRAIN AXIS

The gut-microbiota-brain axis represents a complex network of communications between the gastrointestinal tract, its resident microbiota, and the brain, which regulates digestive and metabolic processes, immunity, as well as emotional response to endogenous (e.g., visceral) and exogenous environmental stimuli.

### Experimental Data from Animal Microbiota Studies

Most direct evidence linking gut microbiota, brain function, and behavior comes from animal studies using germ-free (GF) mice (born and raised in completely sterile conditions), in combination with gut microbiota manipulation using fecal transplant, antibiotics or probiotics. It was first demonstrated that GF mice displayed an exaggerated response to restraint stress, compared to mice raised with normal gut flora.[7] This behavior was mediated by the hypothalamic-pituitary-adrenal (HPA) axis, as GF mice have high levels of corticosterone. Remarkably, fecal transplant from normal mice to GF mice at an early developmental stage successfully restored the stress response to basal levels, although the same procedure was not as efficacious at a later age, suggesting that the influence of gut microbes on neuronal circuits and plasticity has a critical developmental window. Another example of gut microbiota affecting host behavior comes from a probiotic study—mice receiving 28-day *Lactobacillus* probiotic supplement displayed decreased anxiety-like behavior in elevated plus maze and open-field tests.[8] This effect was abolished by vagotomy, suggesting that microbes can directly activate the enteric nervous system (ENS) and transmit ENS input to the brain through the vagus nerve. Similar experimental animal studies have demonstrated that alterations in gut microbiota affect a range of host animal behaviors that resemble human conditions of anxiety, depression, social impairment, and autism.[5,9,10]

### Evidence from Human Microbiota Studies

Human studies testing whether microbiota have similar effects on neurological function using functional magnetic resonance imaging (fMRI) have analyzed brain response to emotional stimuli in healthy women who consumed a fermented, probiotic milk product for 4 weeks.[11,12] Subsequent fMRI measuring response to a standardized emotional faces attention task showed that brain regions involved in emotional processing, including the primary interoceptive and somatosensory regions, were less activated following emotional stimulation. Two other studies of probiotic consumption showed decreased self-reported feelings of sadness, aggressive thoughts, anxiety, and reduced cortisol levels in urine.[13] In a study of young children, fecal samples collected from 89 healthy 1-year-olds were assigned to three groups based on their fecal bacterial composition by cluster analysis.[14] Remarkably, the cognitive performances of these three groups at the age of 2 years were significantly different. The human studies, while the sample size is small, represent an essential first step in translational research.

### Microbiota-Gut-Brain Signaling Pathways

The mechanistic insight into how gut microbiota affect brain function is under study. Animal studies have investigated complex signaling pathways connecting the gut microbiota and brain.[5,15] In addition to the above-mentioned ENS/vagus nerve and HPA pathways, ongoing research demonstrates that microbiota-gut-brain communications are also mediated through the immune system/cytokines and neurotransmitters/metabolites generated by the gut and microbes **(Table 1)**.

The neuroimmune system is a key communication route between gut microbiota and brain.[16] The gastrointestinal tract represents the largest surface area exposed to external environmental microbes and contains 70–80% of the body's immune cells. Balanced gut microbiota

| TABLE 1: Factors affecting gut-microbiota-brain axis. | |
| --- | --- |
| Neurodevelopmental outcomes | • Brain injury (e.g., white matter injury) and abnormal functional connection<br>• Developmental delay, cerebral palsy, autism, and learning disorders |
| Brain development | • Blood-brain barrier formation and integrity<br>• Neurogenesis; glial cells—pre-oligodendrocyte maturation and myelination production, microglia maturation and ramification<br>• Expression of neurotropins and neurotransmitters and their receptors<br>• Synaptogenesis/synaptic formation and connectivity |
| *Gut-brain signaling pathways* | • Hypothalamic-pituitary-adrenal axis<br>• Enteric nervous system<br>• Immune system/cytokines<br>• Neurotransmitters (e.g., serotonin) and metabolites (e.g., short-chain fatty acids) |

*Contd...*

*Contd...*

| | |
|---|---|
| Intestinal tract | • Enteric development, integrity, and function<br>• Immune system maturation and balanced response to microbes |
| Gut microbiota | • Progression and diversity of microbiota colonization |
| Prematurity-related | • Preterm rupture of membranes, maternal infection, C-section, exposure to pathogenic and resistant hospital microbes<br>• Lack of close maternal-infant contact<br>• Perinatal and postnatal antibiotic exposure<br>• Decreased colostrum and breast milk/breastfeeding, delayed enteral feeding<br>• Low gastric pH, $H_2$-blocker use, and poor gut motility |

colonization early in life is fundamental to ensure that the naive immune system develops homeostatic tolerance to the host to prevent aberrant inflammation and yet mounts appropriate responses to protect its host from pathogenic attacks. Microbial-associated pattern molecules, such as lipopolysaccharide, bacterial lipoprotein, flagellin, and CpG DNA, activate various lymphocytes and innate immune cells such as macrophages, neutrophils, and dendritic cells located in the gastrointestinal tract. Activation of these cells produces numerous pro-inflammatory (i.e., IL-1a, IL-1b, TNFα, and IL-6) and anti-inflammatory (i.e., IGF-1 and IL-10) cytokines. In the periphery, these cytokines are capable of acting on receptors in afferent nerves, relaying their signals to the brain. Alternatively, these cytokines can reach the brain by crossing the blood-brain barrier (BBB) via both diffusion and cytokine transporters. These cytokines act on receptors expressed by neurons and glial cells, particularly microglia (brain-resident, innate immune phagocytes), altering their activation status.

Gut dysbiosis may trigger aberrant activation of the immune system and exaggerate inflammatory response, leading to localized intestinal tissue damage and long-term alteration of brain function. Abnormal microbiota-gut-brain signaling has been proposed as the main underlying mechanism of bowel destruction and brain white matter injury observed in necrotizing enterocolitis (NEC) in preterm infants.[17]

A well-established physiological function of the microbiota is generation of metabolites, such as vitamins and other cofactors, which are essential for host physiology. One group of such metabolites is short-chain fatty acids (SCFAs) (i.e., acetate, butyrate, and propionate), which are produced by gut microbiota from fermentation of complex carbohydrates. While SCFAs are capable of crossing the BBB and serve as an important energy source for the brain, their ability to regulate the BBB has attracted recent research interest. Studies from GF mice displayed decreased expression of key brain endothelial tight junction proteins and thus significantly increased BBB permeability.[18] Supplementing GF mice with butyrate was sufficient to restore BBB integrity. Similarly, colonization of GF mice with SCFA-producing bacteria (*Clostridium tyrobutyricum* or *Bacteroidesthetaiotaomicron*) increased production of tight junction expression and restored BBB integrity. These animal studies suggest that BBB permeability may be actively regulated by metabolic signals from gut microbiota during physiological and pathological conditions. These findings have significant implications in that the status of the microbiota influences the abilities of various macromolecules in the blood circulation to reach the brain parenchyma, thereby affecting brain structural and functional integrity.

Neurotransmitters derived both from the brain and gastrointestinal tract have been shown to participate in the bidirectional communication between gut microbiota and brain. While the brain plays a major role in regulating gut homeostasis, motility, and secretion, the proportion of total body levels of various neurotransmitters is greater in the gut than in the brain. Interestingly, gut bacteria are capable of producing neurotransmitters such as serotonin (5-hydroxytryptamine or 5-HT), dopamine, norepinephrine, epinephrine, gamma-aminobutyric acid (GABA), and acetylcholine.[19] Evidence from *in vitro* and *in vivo* animal studies suggests that gut microbes can control the concentration of various neurotransmitters, both in the brain and in the periphery. Serotonin, a major neurotransmitter regulating emotion, is the most studied neurotransmitter.[20] The vast majority of 5-HT in the body (>90%) is produced by gut enterochromaffin cells. The production of 5-HT in the gut can be regulated by gut microbial-derived metabolites (e.g., SCFAs). Although 5-HT is not known to cross the BBB, gut microbiota-produced tryptophan and the central 5-HT precursor are capable of crossing the BBB to participate in 5-HT synthesis in the brain.[6,20] GF mice have lower levels of 5-HT and specific 5-HT receptors in brain regions such as the amygdala and hippocampus. Intriguingly, colonization with a defined cocktail of spore-forming gut bacteria in GF mice restored their 5-HT levels in the gut and normalized their anxiety-like behavior.

## THE NEONATAL GUT MICROBIOTA

Vertical transmission of maternal microbiota before, during, and after birth is the first and most important step in gut microbiota colonization in the perinatal period.[21] While the profile of gut microbiota follows a general pattern in healthy neonates delivered vaginally, infant microbiota composition is unstable and may be altered in diversity and/or composition by feeding type, infection, and antibiotic treatment, as well as other environmental factors. Premature birth disrupts the natural ecological colonization process and gut dysbiosis may lead to neonatal complications (NEC and PVL) and long-term developmental disorders such as ASD.

### Does Microbiota Colonization occur in Utero?

The traditional belief that the womb is sterile is now challenged by findings that microbes and their DNA are present in amniotic fluid, umbilical cord blood, fetal membranes, and the placenta of healthy term pregnancies after both vaginal and C-section deliveries.[22-24] Furthermore, the placental microbiome has been shown to be similar to the mother's oral cavity.[22] Although how oral bacteria make their way to the placenta is not clear, one possibility is that they travel through the bloodstream. This raises the possibility that maternal oral hygiene may influence the microbiota of the fetoplacental unit. These findings are controversial and many researchers remain deeply skeptical.[25,26] A recent study suggests that identified traces of placental microbes may represent contaminants from DNA-extraction kits used in the research.[27]

### Postnatal Gut Microbiota Colonization in Term Infants

Regardless of intrauterine exposure, the most dramatic change in composition of infant gut microbiota occurs at birth and during early postnatal life with exposure to maternal microbes in vagina, feces, skin, and oral cavity (via kisses).[28] During vaginal delivery, newborns are colonized by large numbers of *Enterobacter, Staphylococcus,* and *Streptococcus*. These facultative anaerobic bacteria produce anaerobic environs in the first few days after birth that allow subsequent establishment of strict anaerobes like *Bacteroides, Bifidobacterium,* and *Clostridium* by 4–7 days of life. In the subsequent weeks, gut anaerobic colonization proceeds rapidly through breastfeeding. The infant gut colonization profile follows a progression from organisms facilitating lactate utilization during lactation to anaerobes facilitating utilization of nutrients after introduction of solid food.[29] By age 2-3 years, the gut microbiome is more diversified and complex, similar to that of adults.[30,31]

### Gut Microbiota Dysbiosis in Preterm Infants

Preterm birth and subsequent NICU hospitalization disrupt every aspect of the critical initial phase of microbiota colonization. The list of risk factors is long,[32] including preterm rupture of membranes, maternal infection, increased incidence of C-section delivery, perinatal and postnatal broad-spectrum antibiotic exposure, lack of close maternal-infant contact, exposure to pathogenic and resistant hospital microbes, decreased colostrum and breast milk/breastfeeding, exposure to formula and bovine protein-based fortifier, delayed enteral feeding, periods of fasting, low gastric pH, $H_2$ blocker use, and poor gut motility.

A number of studies[33,34] have characterized gut microbiota development in very premature preterm infants (born <33 weeks gestation). Not surprisingly, compared to term infants, preterm infants' gut microbiota display a distinct different pattern of progress; in early life, bacilli and Gram-positive cocci such as *Staphylococci* and *Streptococci* predominate in gut bacterial content. Bacilli are soon overtaken by Gram-negative facultative organisms (a diversity of genera and species within the Gamma proteobacteria class), which is counterbalanced by a gradually increasing abundance of *Clostridia* (many genera and species) and *Negativicutes* (predominantly *Veillonella* and *Enterococci*). As very preterm infants approach 33–36 weeks postmenstrual age (PMA) the gut is well colonized by anaerobes. Gestational age (GA) of the infants, vaginal versus C-section birth, type of feeding, and antibiotic use all influence progression of colonization. Overall, the preterm infant gut ends up with reduced diversity, very low abundance of anaerobes, and increased pathogenic colonization (Coagulase-negative *Staphylococci, Enterococci, Enterobacteriaceae),* as well as increased yeasts and viral diversity.[35] The early dysbiosis of gut microbiota affects the developing gut and immune system and influences the immature brain, which normally develops *in utero,* an environment with almost no microbes. Gut dysbiosis may cause NEC, neonatal late-onset sepsis during the neonatal period, and atopic diseases, obesity, metabolic syndrome, as well as neurodevelopmental disorders later in life.[17,36,37]

### Factors affecting Gut Colonization

*Maternal Microbiota Changes during Pregnancy*

Compared with nonpregnant women, pregnant women have lower vaginal bacterial diversity, with dominance of *Lactobacilli, Clostridiales, Bacteroidales,* and *Actinomycetales.*[22,38-40] The increasing presence of *Lactobacilli* during gestation maintains a low vaginal pH, reducing bacterial diversity and preventing ascending bacterial infection. The role of microorganisms in preterm birth has shifted toward a more holistic viewpoint.[41-43] Higher microbial diversity in the vagina, rather than the presence of discrete and identifiable pathogens, is a risk factor for preterm birth. Disruption of normal bacterial balance is thought to be involved in either rendering susceptibility to or promoting early onset of labor. Premature birth, in turn, adversely affects gut colonization.

## Maternal Stress during Pregnancy

Many prospective studies show that maternal depression, anxiety, or stress during pregnancy increases the risk of a wide range of adverse outcomes for the children, including emotional problems, ADHD, or impaired cognitive development.[44] The gut microbiota is suggested as one of the mechanisms linking maternal psychological stress during pregnancy and adverse neurodevelopmental outcomes of the offspring.[45] Subjecting pregnant mice to stress lowers the abundance of vaginal *Lactobacillus*, which is associated with lower levels of *Lactobacilli* and *Bifidobacteria* gut colonization in their offspring.[46,47] A similar finding was observed in a human epidemiological study in the Netherlands.[44] Infants of mothers with high cumulative stress (i.e., high reported stress and high cortisol concentrations) during pregnancy had more pathogenic bacterial species (related to *Escherichia*, *Serratia*, and *Enterobacter*) and fewer beneficial bacterial species (lactic acid bacteria and *Bifidobacteria*).

## Mode of Delivery

The initial gut microbiota colonization depends on birth delivery mode.[48] Infants born vaginally have gut colonization reflective of maternal fecal and vaginal flora such as *Lactobacillus* and *Prevotella* species. In contrast, infants born by C-section harbor bacterial species found in human skin and hospital environments; they have a deficiency or delayed colonization of anaerobes like *Bacteroides* and *Bifidobacterium* but are more colonized by *C. difficile*.[49] While some studies report that the pattern of colonization after C-section delivery may persist for months or even years after birth,[50] a recent review indicates that previously observed significant differences disappear after 6 months of life.[48]

## Type of Feeding

During the first days of life, breastfeeding promotes colonization and maturation of the developing gut microbiota.[51] Human milk contains bacteria that are shown to be predominated by a few genera including *Staphylococcus*, *Streptococcus*, *Serratia*, *Pseudomonas*, *Corynebacterium*, *Ralstonia*, *Propionibacterium*, *Sphingomonas*, and *Bradyrhizobiaceae*, as well as *Bifidobacterium* and *Lactobacillus* species.[52] However, the origin of these microbes and their complex maternal-infant exchange remains poorly understood.

Human milk contains abundant prebiotic oligosaccharides that promotes the growth of beneficial bacterial species like *Bifidobacterium*.[53] These anaerobes inhibit the growth of pathogenic organisms, support mucosal barrier function, and modulate immunological and inflammatory responses.[54] The gut microbiota of formula-fed infants, compared to exclusively breastfed infants, shows increased bacterial diversity and contains higher abundance of potentially pathogenic bacteria such as *C. difficile* and *Escherichia coli*.[55] Introduction of formula may perturb neonatal intestinal microbiota colonization, thereby reducing the benefits of breastfeeding.[56-58]

Preterm infants are fed based on their nutrition requirements and availability of mother's own milk (MOM) or donor human milk (DHM). Bovine protein-based products including formula, human milk fortifier, and protein supplements are almost universally introduced to very premature infants during their NICU stay to meet their high caloric, protein, and mineral requirements. MOM feeding protects preterm infants from multiple dysbiosis risk factors and helps them establish a balanced microbial community pattern.[59] Infants fed with at least 70% MOM had high abundance of *Clostridiales*, *Lactobacillales*, and *Bacillales*, whereas infants fed primarily DHM or formula had an abundance of *Enterobacteriales*. The protected effect with MOM feeding was observed in preterm infants regardless of their gestation age, birth weight, postnatal age, or nutrition status; each of these factors can affect gut microbiota.[60] When MOM is not available, DHM is increasingly used in the NICU for the preterm population. However, pasteurization and freezing/thawing kill the live cells and microbes normally present in fresh MOM, thus reducing some of its protective effect. Direct breastfeeding, as compared to MOM or DHM bottle-feeding, may provide additional benefits by direct microbial exchange between mother and infant. Currently there is limited microbiota research specifically related to this topic.

## Antibiotic Exposure

Given the instability of the newborn gut microbiota, early life antibiotic administration interferes significantly with the initial phase of gut colonization, leading to an overall reduction in bacterial diversity and alters composition. Forty-eight hours of parenteral ampicillin and gentamicin given to term newborns significantly reduced gut *Bifidobacterium* and *Lactobacillus*, which were replaced by *Proteobacteria* (including *Enterobacteriaceae*), and these changes persisted for at least 8 weeks after treatment.[61]

Perinatal antibiotic use, including intrapartum antibiotic prophylaxis for group B streptococcal infection, and neonatal empiric and therapeutic antibiotic administration, is a common practice which has long been considered "safe." While proper antibiotic therapy is critical for treating infection and saving lives, growing evidence shows that unnecessary antibiotic exposure may have profound adverse effects. Many epidemiological studies have shown that early life antibiotic use may lead to long-lasting alterations in the composition and metabolic activity of the gut microbiota, resulting in adult-onset obesity.[62] A recent Canadian Neonatal Network study found that antibiotic use in very low-birth weight infants without culture-proven sepsis or without NEC is associated with increased neonatal mortality and severe morbidity.[17] These observations underscore the importance of improved antibiotic jurisprudence.

### NICU Environment

Many preterm infants, in particular very preterm infants, are cared for in the NICU for weeks or even months. They are exposed to a myriad of hospital microbial sources, including healthcare providers' skin and equipment and workspace surfaces.[63] Infant microbiota colonization is also affected by intubation, feeding tube placement, incubator temperatures, and humidity. Reducing colonization of NICU environmental bacteria on provider skin, work surfaces, and equipment as well as protection of the infant's epidermal barrier are important measures to prevent exposure to pathological organisms and have been shown to significantly decrease neonatal infection. Research has begun to examine the influence of maternal-infant contact on preterm infant colonization. A recent skin-to-skin care study showed that contact between the infant and mother is associated with an increased pace of oral microbe composition maturity.[64]

## GUT MICROBIOTA AND PRETERM INFANT BRAIN DEVELOPMENT AND INJURY

Neurodevelopment is a complex process controlled by both intrinsic and extrinsic signals. It is particularly sensitive to environmental inputs during preferred windows of opportunity called critical periods.[65] Remarkably, gut microbiota colonization occurs in parallel with neurodevelopment and they share similar critical developmental windows.[6,66] Preterm birth results in precocious gut colonization. Dysbiosis, common in preterm infants, disrupts the dynamic microbiota-host interaction during a critical period, which leads to brain injury and/or abnormal neuro-programming early in life and poor long-term neurodevelopmental outcome.

Commonly described brain injuries in preterm infants include white matter injury (PVL on ultrasound), IVH, and cerebellar hemorrhage.[67,68] Brain MRI also detects brain volume reduction, in particular in the gray matter, cerebrum, basal ganglia, and limbic system.[1,69,70] These neonatal brain abnormalities are associated with cerebral palsy (CP), and cognitive and behavioral deficits (i.e., autism and ADHD) later in life.[10,71] It is important to note that many preterm infants who have poor cognitive function and behavior problems, in fact, do not have identifiable lesions on their brain MRI prior to NICU discharge. The "invisible" brain injury may be attributed to abnormal neuronal network and conductivity reflecting axon and dendritic development, synaptogenesis, and synaptic transmission. All these processes are sensitive to environmental influences.

The etiology underlying brain injury is complex and remains not fully understood.[72,73] The microbiota–gut–brain axis is emerging as a key factor in neurodevelopment. Gut microbiota is linked to multiple neurodevelopmental processes, including BBB formation and integrity,[18] neurogenesis,[74] microglia maturation and ramification,[75,76] myelination and expression of neurotrophins,[77] synaptogenesis/synaptic connectivity,[78] neurotransmitters[20] and their respective receptors. Importantly, in many cases, the efficacy of the gut microbiota depends on the timing of when gut microbes' signals interact with the specific neurodevelopmental process.

The identification of the gut–microbiota–brain axis is opening new research avenues. For example, regulation of brain epithelium tight junctions by gut microbiota raises the possibility of their role in IVH and white matter injury. Gut microbes alter BBB permeability, allowing harmful micromolecules to reach the brain and cause damage to brain parenchymal tissue. Gut dysbiosis is a major risk factor for NEC, which is known to cause white matter injury in the developing brain. In this case, gut-initiated inflammation prevents pre-oligodendrocytes from developing into mature oligodendrocytes, affecting their ability to produce myelin, which leads to CP later in life. Recent studies have discovered many more diversified functions of pre-oligodendrocytes, including modulating synaptic transmission, supporting BBB, promoting angiogenesis, and maintaining neuronal function.[79,80] Thus, damage to pre-oligodendrocytes not only leads to decreased myelination but also affects neuro-programming and plasticity. This may explain why preterm infants with CP often show cognitive and behavior abnormalities. Microglia brain macrophages are critical for protecting neural tissue from infection. Recent studies found that microglia control brain synaptic density and neuronal network homeostasis.[75,81] Consistent with this finding, microglial dysfunction is associated with several developmental disorders.[82] Interestingly, gut microbiota-generated SCFAs have been shown to regulate microglial development and function. Investigating how gut dysbiosis affects these newly discovered functions of pre-oligodendrocytes and microglia may shed light on the molecular and neurobiochemical mechanisms underlying injury in the developing preterm brain.

## CONCLUSION

Over the last two decades, a growing number of microbiota studies have been conducted by basic science researchers and clinical investigators in different fields. The studies were initiated from microbiology and gastroenterology, then rapidly branched into immunology, neuroscience, neurodevelopmental biology, psychiatrics, and most recently obstetrics and neonatology. This remarkable transdisciplinary research effort has unraveled an unexpectedly complex network of communications between gut microbiota and the brain. The concept of parallel and interacting microbial-neural critical windows underscores the importance of perinatal symbiosis as a crucial step for optimizing brain development and mental health later in life. While studies have begun to characterize gut microbiota colonization in preterm infants, little is known about the impact of gut dysbiosis on brain development and neuro-programming in the unique NICU environment. The new avenue of microbiota research in perinatology will undoubtedly advance our understanding of the etiology of preterm brain injury and developing novel microbiota modulation based neuroprotective strategies and interventions.

## REFERENCES

1. Inder TE, Warfield SK, Wang H, et al. Abnormal cerebral structure is present at term in premature infants. Pediatrics. 2005;115(2):286-94.
2. Gill SR, Pop M, Deboy RT, et al. Metagenomic analysis of the human distal gut microbiome. Science. 2006;312(5778):1355-9.
3. Eckburg PB, Bik EM, Bernstein CN, et al. Diversity of the human intestinal microbial flora. Science. 2005;308(5728):1635-8.
4. Tamburini S, Shen N, Wu HC, et al. The microbiome in early life: implications for health outcomes. Nat Med. 2016;22(7):713-22.
5. Dinan TG, Stilling RM, Stanton C, et al. Collective unconscious: how gut microbes shape human behavior. J Psychiatr Res.2015;63:1-9.
6. Sharon G, Sampson TR, Geschwind DH, et al. The central nervous system and the gut microbiome. Cell. 2016;167(4):915-32.
7. Sudo N, Chida Y, Aiba Y, et al. Postnatal microbial colonization programs the hypothalamic-pituitary-adrenal system for stress response in mice. J Physiol. 2004;558(Pt 1):263-75.
8. Bravo JA, Forsythe P, Chew MV, et al. Ingestion of Lactobacillus strain regulates emotional behavior and central GABA receptor expression in a mouse via the vagus nerve. Proc Natl Acad Sci USA. 2011;108(38):16050-5.
9. Sampson TR, Mazmanian SK. Control of brain development, function, and behavior by the microbiome. Cell Host Microbe. 2015;17(5):565-76.
10. Li Q, Han Y, Dy ABC, et al. The gut microbiota and autism spectrum disorders. Front Cell Neurosci.2017;11:120.
11. Tillisch K, Labus J, Kilpatrick L, et al. Consumption of fermented milk product with probiotic modulates brain activity. Gastroenterology. 2013;144(7):1394-401, 1401.e1-4.
12. Tillisch K, Mayer EA, Gupta A, et al. Brain structure and response to emotional stimuli as related to gut microbial profiles in healthy women. Psychosom Med. 2017;79(8):905-13.
13. Steenbergen L, Sellaro R, van Hemert S, et al. A randomized controlled trial to test the effect of multispecies probiotics on cognitive reactivity to sad mood. Brain Behav Immun 2015;48:258-64.
14. Carlson AL, Xia K, Azcarate-Peril MA, et al. Infant gut microbiome associated with cognitive development. Biol Psychiatry. 2018;83(2):148-59.
15. Lerner A, Neidhöfer S, Matthias T. The gut microbiome feelings of the brain: a perspective for non-microbiologists. Microorganisms. 2017;5(4).pii: E66.
16. Veiga-Fernandes H, Pachnis V. Neuroimmune regulation during intestinal development and homeostasis. Nat Immunol. 2017;18(2):116-22.
17. Neu J, Pammi M. Pathogenesis of NEC: Impact of an altered intestinal microbiome. Semin Perinatol 2017;41(1):29-35.
18. Braniste V, Al-Asmakh M, Kowal C, et al. The gut microbiota influences blood-brain barrier permeability in mice. Sci Transl Med. 2014;6(263):263ra158.
19. Wall R, Cryan JF, Ross RP, et al. Bacterial neuroactive compounds produced by psychobiotics. Adv Exp Med Biol.2014;817:221-39.
20. O'Mahony SM, Clarke G, Borre YE, et al. Serotonin, tryptophan metabolism and the brain-gut-microbiome axis. Behav Brain Res.2015;277:32-48.
21. Stinson LF, Payne MS, Keelan JA. Planting the seed: Origins, composition, and postnatal health significance of the fetal gastrointestinal microbiota. Crit Rev Microbiol. 2017;43(3):352-69.
22. Aagaard K, Ma J, Antony KM, et al. The placenta harbors a unique microbiome. Sci Transl Med. 2014;6(237):237ra65.
23. Stout MJ, Conlon B, Landeau M, et al. Identification of intracellular bacteria in the basal plate of the human placenta in term and preterm gestations. Am J Obstet Gynecol. 2013;208(3):226.e1-7.
24. Walker RW, Clemente JC, Peter I, et al. The prenatal gut microbiome: are we colonized with bacteria in utero? Pediatr Obes. 2017;12(Suppl 1):3-17.
25. Perez-Muñoz ME, Arrieta MC, Ramer-Tait AE, et al. A critical assessment of the "sterile womb" and "in utero colonization" hypotheses: implications for research on the pioneer infant microbiome. Microbiome. 2017;5(1):48.
26. Willyard C. When drugs unintentionally affect gut bugs. Nat Rev Drug Discov. 2018;17(6):383-4.
27. Lauder AP, Roche AM, Sherrill-Mix S, et al. Comparison of placenta samples with contamination controls does not provide evidence for a distinct placenta microbiota. Microbiome. 2016;4(1):29.

28. Mueller NT, Bakacs E, Combellick J, et al. The infant microbiome development: mom matters. Trends Mol Med. 2015;21(2):109-17.
29. Koenig JE, Spor A, Scalfone N, et al. Succession of microbial consortia in the developing infant gut microbiome. Proc Natl Acad Sci USA. 2011;108(Suppl 1):4578-85.
30. Palmer C, Bik EM, DiGiulio DB, et al. Development of the human infant intestinal microbiota. PLoS Biol. 2007;5(7):e177.
31. Yatsunenko T, Rey FE, Manary MJ, et al. Human gut microbiome viewed across age and geography. Nature. 2012;486(7402):222-7.
32. Unger S, Stintzi A, Shah P, et al. Gut microbiota of the very-low-birth-weight infant. Pediatr Res. 2015;77(1-2):205-13.
33. La Rosa PS, Warner BB, Zhou Y, et al. Patterned progression of bacterial populations in the premature infant gut. Proc Natl Acad Sci USA. 2014;111(34):12522-7.
34. Warner BB, Tarr PI. Necrotizing enterocolitis and preterm infant gut bacteria. Semin Fetal Neonatal Med. 2016;21(6):394-9.
35. Adlerberth I, Wold AE. Establishment of the gut microbiota in Western infants. Acta Paediatr. 2009;98(2):229-38.
36. Warner BB, Deych E, Zhou Y, et al. Gut bacteria dysbiosis and necrotising enterocolitis in very low birthweight infants: a prospective case-control study. Lancet. 2016;387(10031):1928-36.
37. Underwood MA, Sohn K. The microbiota of the extremely preterm infant. Clin Perinatol. 2017;44(2):407-27.
38. Aagaard K, Riehle K, Ma J, et al. A metagenomic approach to characterization of the vaginal microbiome signature in pregnancy. PloSOne. 2012;7(6):e36466.
39. Romero R, Hassan SS, Gajer P, et al. The composition and stability of the vaginal microbiota of normal pregnant women is different from that of non-pregnant women. Microbiome. 2014;2(1):4.
40. Koren O, Goodrich JK, Cullender TC, et al. Host remodeling of the gut microbiome and metabolic changes during pregnancy. Cell. 2012;150(3):470-80.
41. DiGiulio DB, Romero R, Amogan HP, et al. Microbial prevalence, diversity and abundance in amniotic fluid during preterm labor: a molecular and culture-based investigation. PloSOne. 2008;3(8):e3056.
42. Mysorekar IU, Cao B. Microbiome in parturition and preterm birth. SeminReprod Med. 2014;32(1):50-5.
43. Vinturache AE, Gyamfi-Bannerman C, Hwang J, et al. Maternal microbiome—A pathway to preterm birth. Semin Fetal Neonatal Med. 2016;21(2):94-9.
44. Zijlmans MA, Korpela K, Riksen-Walraven JM, et al. Maternal prenatal stress is associated with the infant intestinal microbiota. Psychoneuroendocrinology. 2015;53:233-45.
45. O'Mahony SM, Clarke G, Dinan TG, et al. Early-life adversity and brain development: Is the microbiome a missing piece of the puzzle? Neuroscience. 2017;342:37-54.
46. Bailey MT, Lubach GR, Coe CL. Prenatal stress alters bacterial colonization of the gut in infant monkeys. J Pediatr Gastroenterol Nutr. 2004;38(4):414-21.
47. Jašarević E, Howerton CL, Howard CD, et al. Alterations in the vaginal microbiome by maternal stress are associated with metabolic reprogramming of the offspring gut and brain. Endocrinology. 2015;156(9):3265-76.
48. Rutayisire E, Huang K, Liu Y, et al. The mode of delivery affects the diversity and colonization pattern of the gut microbiota during the first year of infants' life: a systematic review. BMC Gastroenterol. 2016;16(1):86.
49. Jakobsson HE, Abrahamsson TR, Jenmalm MC, et al. Decreased gut microbiota diversity, delayed Bacteroidetes colonisation and reduced Th1 responses in infants delivered by caesarean section. Gut. 2014;63(4):559-66.
50. Salminen S, Gibson GR, McCartney AL, et al. Influence of mode of delivery on gut microbiota composition in seven year old children. Gut. 2004;53(9):1388-9.
51. O'Sullivan A, Farver M, Smilowitz JT. The influence of early infant-feeding practices on the intestinal microbiome and body composition in infants. NutrMetab Insights. 2015;8(Suppl 1):1-9.
52. Hunt KM, Foster JA, Forney LJ, et al. Characterization of the diversity and temporal stability of bacterial communities in human milk. PLoS One. 2011;6(6):e21313.
53. Barile D, Rastall RA. Human milk and related oligosaccharides as prebiotics. Curr Opin Biotechnol. 2013;24(2):214-9.
54. Sudo N, Sawamura S, Tanaka K, et al. The requirement of intestinal bacterial flora for the development of an IgE production system fully susceptible to oral tolerance induction. J Immunol. 1997;159(4):1739-45.
55. Penders J, Vink C, Driessen C, et al. Quantification of Bifidobacterium spp., *Escherichia coli* and *Clostridium difficile* in faecal samples of breast-fed and formula-fed infants by real-time PCR. FEMS Microbiol Lett. 2005;243(1):141-7.
56. Palmer C, Bik EM, DiGiulio DB, et al. Development of the human infant intestinal microbiota. PLoS Biol. 2007;5(7):e177.
57. Madan JC, Salari RC, Saxena D, et al. Gut microbial colonisation in premature neonates predicts neonatal sepsis. Arch Dis Child FetalNeonatalEd. 2012;97(6):F456-62.
58. Xu W, Judge MP, Maas K, et al. Systematic review of the effect of enteral feeding on gut microbiota in preterm infants. J Obstet Gynecol Neonatal Nurs. 2018;47(3):451-63.
59. Cong X, Judge M, Xu W, et al. Influence of feeding type on gut microbiome development in hospitalized preterm infants. Nurs Res. 2017;66(2):123-33.
60. Gregory KE, Samuel BS, Houghteling P, et al. Influence of maternal breast milk ingestion on acquisition of the intestinal microbiome in preterm infants. Microbiome. 2016;4(1):68.
61. Fouhy F, Guinane CM, Hussey S, et al. High-throughput sequencing reveals the incomplete, short-term recovery of infant gut microbiota following parenteral antibiotic treatment with ampicillin and gentamicin. Antimicrob Agents Chemother. 2012;56(11):5811-20.
62. Cox LM, Blaser MJ. Antibiotics in early life and obesity. Nat Rev Endocrinol. 2015;11(3):182-90.
63. Hartz LE, Bradshaw W, Brandon DH. Potential NICU environmental influences on the neonate's microbiome: a systematic review. Adv Neonatal Care. 2015;15(5):324-35.
64. Hendricks-Muñoz KD, Xu J, Parikh HI, et al. Skin-to-skin care and the development of the preterm infant oral microbiome. Am J Perinatol. 2015;32(13):1205-16.
65. Berardi N, Pizzorusso T, Maffei L. Critical periods during sensory development. Curr Opin Neurobiol. 2000;10(1):138-45.
66. Borre YE, O'Keeffe GW, Clarke G, et al. Microbiota and neurodevelopmental windows: implications for brain disorders. Trends Mol Med. 2014;20(9):509-18.

67. Inder TE, Wells SJ, Mogridge NB, et al. Defining the nature of the cerebral abnormalities in the premature infant: a qualitative magnetic resonance imaging study. J Pediatr.2003;143(2):171-9.
68. Miller SP, Ferriero DM. From selective vulnerability to connectivity: insights from newborn brain imaging. Trends Neurosci. 2009;32(9):496-505.
69. Peterson BS, Vohr B, Staib LH, et al. Regional brain volume abnormalities and long-term cognitive outcome in preterm infants. JAMA. 2000;284(15):1939-47.
70. Kidokoro H, Anderson PJ, Doyle LW, et al. Brain injury and altered brain growth inpreterminfants: predictors and prognosis.Pediatrics. 2014;134(2):e444-53.
71. Robertson CM, Watt MJ, Yasui Y. Changes in the prevalence of cerebral palsy for children born very prematurely within a population-based program over 30 years. JAMA. 2007;297(24):2733-40.
72. Volpe JJ. The encephalopathy of prematurity—brain injury and impaired brain development inextricably intertwined. Semin Pediatr Neurol.2009;16(4):167-78.
73. Volpe JJ. Brain injury in premature infants: a complex amalgam of destructive and developmental disturbances. Lancet Neurol.2009;8(1):110-24.
74. Ogbonnaya ES, Clarke G, Shanahan F, et al. Adult hippocampal neurogenesis is regulated by the microbiome. Biol Psychiatry. 2015;78(4):e7-9.
75. Erny D, Hrabě de Angelis AL, Jaitin D, et al. Host microbiota constantly control maturation and function of microglia in the CNS. Nat Neurosci. 2015;18(7):965-77.
76. Erny D, Hrabě de Angelis AL, Prinz M. Communicating systems in the body: how microbiota and microglia cooperate. Immunology. 2017;150(1):7-15.
77. Hoban AE, Stilling RM, Ryan FJ, et al. Regulation of prefrontal cortex myelination by the microbiota. Transl Psychiatry. 2016;6:e774.
78. Werneburg S, Feinberg PA, Johnson KM, et al. A microglia-cytokine axis to modulate synaptic connectivity and function. Curr Opin Neurobiol.2017;47:138-45.
79. Birey F, Kokkosis AG, Aguirre A. Oligodendroglia-lineage cells in brain plasticity, homeostasis and psychiatric disorders. Curr Opin Neurobiol.2017;47:93-103.
80. Ntranos A, Casaccia P. The microbiome-gut-behavior axis: crosstalk between the gut microbiome and oligodendrocytes modulates behavioral responses. Neurotherapeutics. 2018;15(1):31-5.
81. Derecki NC, Katzmarski N, Kipnis J, et al. Microglia as a critical player in both developmental and late-life CNS pathologies. Acta Neuropathol. 2014;128(3):333-45.
82. Prinz M, Priller J. Microglia and brain macrophages in the molecular age: from origin to neuropsychiatric disease. Nat Rev Neurosci. 2014;15(5):300-12.

CHAPTER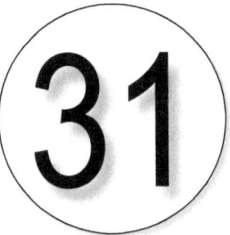

# Neonatal Seizures

*John Sum*

## ABSTRACT

Neonatal seizures represent one of the most significant and common neurological problems in the newborn period. Despite this, there remains much controversy regarding the diagnosis, treatment, and overall management of these children. While there are many very good retrospective studies looking at neonatal seizures, there has been a scarcity of well-designed, prospective, and controlled randomized studies in the treatment of the newborn with seizures. This has led to a lack of consensus on a variety of topics such as the best pharmacologic treatment strategy for these children, the question of the role of maturation of the newborn brain in treatment decisions, the risk versus benefit of aggressive treatment of subclinical seizures, the use of different types of electroencephalogram (EEG) monitoring, and the effects of hypothermia on management. That being said, we continue to learn a lot about the etiology, semiology, and biology of neonatal seizures even though our treatment of neonatal seizures has not significantly changed in the last decade or more.

## SCOPE OF THE PROBLEM

Neonatal seizures represent a significant problem in the newborn nursery. It is estimated that neonatal seizures occur in 0.1-0.5% of all newborn infants.[1] The incidence rates do vary depending on the presence of various risk factors. In the preterm infant, the rates are significantly higher, affecting up to 4.4-64 per 1,000 live births depending on birth weight. In the term infant, however, the rate is closer to 1-3 per 1,000 live births.[2-6] As technology has changed over the years, there has been both better management of neonates and improved recognition of neonatal seizures as well.[7] As such, neonatal seizures represent not only one of the most common causes for neurological consultation in the neonatal intensive care unit (NICU), but also a changing and evolving clinical problem.[8]

As a major problem in the NICU, the recognition of neonatal seizures is of paramount importance. Neonatal seizures are an indication of significant neurological dysfunction or injury that requires immediate diagnosis and treatment. It is well known that seizures themselves can result in medical instability complicating general management of the child. Further, a delay in recognition and treatment may lead to further secondary injury of the developing brain. Underlying illnesses that are readily treatable could also be missed, leading to increased morbidity and mortality.[9,10]

## ETIOLOGY OF NEONATAL SEIZURES

Neonatal seizures are those seizures that occur from birth up to 28 days post-term, or a conceptual age of 44 weeks. Within this time frame, the etiology of neonatal seizures depends not only on the time of seizure onset, but to a large extent on the child's gestational age, be it term or preterm. Most neonatal seizures occur within the first couple of days of life, with the majority occurring by 7 days of life.[8,10]

By far the most common cause of neonatal seizures is hypoxic-ischemic encephalopathy (HIE) both in the term and the preterm infant. In particular, a 5-minute Apgar score <5, cord pH <7.0, and need for intubation in the delivery room, all correlate with the presence of clinical neonatal seizures. Most of these seizures occur within the first 24 hours of life, and often within the first 12 hours after birth.[8,11]

Intracranial hemorrhage is the second most common cause of neonatal seizures, especially in the preterm infant. In the preterm, germinal matrix hemorrhage, with or without periventricular hemorrhagic infarction, is a major cause of seizures in the 1st week of life. Subarachnoid hemorrhage is a less common cause of seizures in term infants. Subdural hemorrhage from trauma also causes neonatal seizures.[11,12]

Intracranial infection can be from either bacterial or viral causes and represents a significant cause of neonatal seizures. Bacterial infections are mostly from Group B *Streptococcus* or *E. coli*, and present late in the 1st week of life. Nonbacterial causes include toxoplasmosis, herpes, coxsackie, rubella, and *cytomegalovirus* (CMV). Time of presentation will depend upon the timing of the infection, whether pre- or postnatal.[11] Infectious causes most likely lead to 5-10% of cases of neonatal seizures.[12]

Some of the most important etiologies to diagnose are the metabolic causes, as often they are readily treatable. Hypoglycemia, hypocalcemia, hypomagnesemia, or electrolyte abnormalities should all be checked urgently and treated. Hyperammonemia and acidosis may indicate an inborn error of metabolism. Pyridoxine and folinic acid-related seizures must also be considered in refractory seizures, as they too can be easily treated with high doses of vitamins. Failure to recognize these causes and to treat them promptly may lead to adverse developmental outcomes.[8]

Other central nervous system (CNS) structural lesions may also cause seizures, such as focal cerebral infarction. The increased use of magnetic resonance imaging (MRI) has led to stroke becoming recognized as a significant cause of neonatal seizures, estimated to occur in as many as 1 in 1,600–5,000 live births.[13] Congenital malformation of the brain, possibly from a genetic cause, may also cause seizures later in the neonatal period.[8] There are also several both benign and severe neonatal syndromes that must be considered, such as benign familial neonatal seizures.[11] In the case of more refractory seizures, severe syndromes such as Ohtahara syndrome should be considered.[14]

## RECOGNITION OF NEONATAL SEIZURES

The clinical semiology of seizures in the neonatal period is very different from those seen in older infants and children. The differences occur due to the immature nature of the neonatal brain, both anatomically and neurophysiologically.[11,15] These differences also lead to the clinical fact that many seizures in the neonatal period are unaccompanied by an EEG correlate; in fact, electrographic seizures often occur with no clinical signs whatsoever. Seizure recognition is further complicated by the fact that many seizures in the newborn are very subtle, can mimic normal behavior, and that they rarely, if ever, present as obvious generalized tonic-clonic seizures. As a result, neonatal seizures are often overlooked by caregivers unless they are vigilant.

Because of the problem of both false positives and false negatives in detection of neonatal seizures by employing observation alone, electrographic and other monitoring is required. Heart rate or respiratory changes and response to stimulation can be used to help in the differential diagnosis of neonatal seizures. Continuous EEG monitoring with amplitude-integrated EEG (aEEG) or traditional video EEG greatly aids in diagnosis as well.[16,17]

There are four main types of neonatal seizures that are generally recognized—subtle, tonic, clonic, and myoclonic.[11,17,18] Subtle seizures include phenomena such as tonic eye deviation, staring, blinking, repetitive oral/buccal/lingual movements, boxing/swimming/progressive movements, or apnea/autonomic instability. Clonic movements involve 0.5–3 Hz repetitive jerking of the limbs and may be focal, multifocal, or fragmentary. Tonic seizures involve tonic extension or posturing of one limb or more parts of the body. These may also be focal or generalized. Myoclonic seizures are characterized by rapid jerking of one or more parts of the body and may be focal, multifocal, or generalized. Complicating matters, the same infant may manifest multiple seizure types.[19,20]

Focal and multifocal clonic seizures are the most common type of seizure that is associated with time-synchronized ictal EEG-documented seizures. These seizures are also often correlated with the presence of a focal structural CNS lesion. Focal tonic seizures are also consistently associated with ictal EEG discharges. Interestingly, generalized clonic seizures are almost never seen in the newborn. Tonic horizontal eye deviation has also been found to be consistently associated with electrographic EEG discharges. Some (Mizrahi and Kellaway) have also categorized such seizures as a form of focal clonic seizure, while others classify this type of seizure as a subtle neonatal seizure (Volpe). In addition, generalized myoclonic seizures are also often associated with EEG ictal electrographic phenomena. These types of generalized myoclonic seizures clinically mimic the infantile spasm type of seizures seen in older infants.[19]

The other manifestations of clinical neonatal seizures are only inconsistently associated with ictal EEG phenomena, and so represent an active area of controversy. Such seizures include many subtle seizures, generalized tonic seizures, and focal or multifocal myoclonic seizures. Many of these phenomena are seen in neonates with very severe injury, and often mimic reflex automatisms. Some have deemed these brainstem release phenomena and possibly not epileptic.[20] Many of these phenomena are also stimulus sensitive and can be stopped by gentle restraint, thus arguing for the nonepileptic nature of many of these seizures. However, animal studies do find electrical discharges in deep structures of the brain (such as the inferior colliculus) during such clinical activity, indicating that some of these phenomena may still be epileptic, though too deep to be detected by surface EEG.[11] Subtle seizures are particularly difficult to diagnose as these phenomena, such as sustained eye opening, pedaling movements, or chewing, can be associated with EEG ictal discharges, particularly in preterm infants. Other phenomena, such as tonic eye deviation, or apnea, more commonly have an EEG correlate in term newborns primarily. Autonomic phenomena are rarely the only manifestation of neonatal seizures, and should be considered in the context of other clinical seizure activity.[11]

## DIFFERENTIAL DIAGNOSIS

There are many normal infant behaviors that one must consider in the differential of neonatal seizures in order to avoid over diagnosis. Jitteriness is a common movement disorder seen in neonates, and it is often seen in the same contexts as one might observe seizures, such as mild HIE. Jitteriness, however, is usually characterized by more of a tremor, and is very sensitive to stimulation or holding of the body. There are also no other autonomic, or subtle activities seen with jitteriness such as might occur with epileptic seizures.[12,21]

Other activity that is often confused with seizures includes normal neonatal body movements, such as benign neonatal sleep myoclonus. Normal baby sucking, puckering, or roving eye movements can all be considered normal neonatal activity. Opisthotonus or posturing may also be a manifestation of severe brain injury, and yet not be epileptic. Rare neurological disorders such as hyperekplexia (familial startle disease) must also be kept in mind. It is therefore, very important to be very careful in evaluating an infant for neonatal seizures and use both clinical and electrographic criteria in establishing a diagnosis.[21]

## INVESTIGATION

The investigation of an infant for possible neonatal seizures involves a good clinical assessment, laboratory testing, brain imaging, and EEG testing. A high degree of suspicion is required by nursing staff and physicians regarding any child at risk for neonatal seizures, such as newborns who underwent a difficult delivery or who are likely to have HIE. Laboratory testing should include a stat blood glucose level, serum electrolytes, arterial blood gas, calcium and magnesium, complete blood panel (CBC), blood culture, liver function tests, creatinine, and ammonia. If the child is stable and infection is considered a possibility, a lumbar puncture should be done for microscopy and culture. If no etiology is found, then tests for serum amino acids and urine organic acids should be considered along with cerebrospinal fluid (CSF) lactate, pyruvate, amino acids, and neurotransmitters to look for rarer metabolic causes of seizures.[14,22]

Neuroimaging should be done as soon as possible, with either head ultrasound, X-ray, computed tomography (CT), and/or MRI scan. Cranial ultrasound is the easiest test to obtain at the bedside and readily reveals hemorrhage, hydrocephalus, cystic or larger mass lesions, and at times ischemic lesions. Large malformations can also be seen on ultrasound. It is also ideal for the premature infants who are very fragile and prone to intraventricular hemorrhage (IVH). When the ultrasound is unrevealing, a CT or MRI should be done; preferably the MRI, though it requires the child be stable enough to tolerate the test, and to be very still. However, MRI is very sensitive in detecting hemorrhage, cerebral malformation, strokes, mass lesions, infection, and trauma. If MRI cannot readily be obtained, CT is a rapid test that can accurately detect hemorrhage, strokes, more obvious malformations, hydrocephalus, calcifications, and gross pathological conditions. Unfortunately, CT also exposes the child to ionizing radiation, though the risk is considered to be small.[9,16,22]

Electroencephalogram monitoring with video should be done in any child suspected of having neonatal seizures. This is the best test for detecting seizures in neonates. Amplitude-integrated EEG is now routinely used in the NICU to detect the background cerebral activity and function of neonates. It also is capable of detecting some seizures in newborns, though its sensitivity and specificity is only 50–60%. Part of the problem is that aEEG uses a very limited number of electrodes, so its spatial detection is somewhat impaired. That being said, even for routine EEG, only up to 10% of neonates with suspected seizures will have EEG confirmation of seizure activity.[23] The EEG pattern of neonatal seizures can also be highly variable, but generally consists of spikes, sharp waves, or sinusoidal waves that occur repetitively from slow to fast frequencies. The amplitude of the EEG discharges is also highly variable, may present as focal or multifocal, and may be synchronous or asynchronous between the two hemispheres. The seizure discharges may build up or be abrupt in onset or offset, and their morphology may change even within the same seizure.[18,24]

Probably more consistent is the background EEG pattern. The background gives a relatively accurate depiction of the child's brain function at that particular time. A flat or burst suppression background is an extreme EEG pattern that indicates a very severe injury and bodes poorly for long-term good outcome. A normal background, on the other hand is an excellent prognostic indicator.[9,11,18]

Electroclinical dissociation is a major problem in the assessment for neonatal seizures. Clinical seizures occur with EEG-associated electrical discharges, or they can occur in the absence of EEG phenomena. In addition, electrographic seizures often occur in the absence of clinical seizure activity, especially after treatment with antiepileptic drugs (AEDs). What this means for treatment and ultimate prognosis is not yet defined. There is some evidence, however, that treating subclinical seizures in the neonate may reduce future brain injury[25,26] and so further research in this area is needed.

## TREATMENT

The proper management of neonatal seizures first requires the accurate diagnosis of seizures using both clinical and electrographic criteria, while promptly ensuring adequate ventilatory and cardiovascular support. Once seizures are suspected, a rapid assessment of blood glucose, calcium, magnesium, and electrolytes should be performed and corrections should be performed immediately. The child should also immediately be evaluated for infection/meningitis as a potentially devastating but treatable cause of neonatal seizures.[22] As noted above, accurate diagnosis generally requires the use of EEG monitoring with either standard conventional video EEG or aEEG.[25] Once a diagnosis of seizure is firmly established, then a decision regarding treatment with antiepileptic medication must be made. Treatment should be initiated without delay if the seizures are affecting cardiovascular or respiratory function, or if the child is having repetitive or prolonged seizures.[17] Treatment generally should be started as soon as possible as seizure burden is felt to peak within the first 6 hours of seizure onset, especially in cases of suspected HIE.[27]

It should be remembered that treatment is not necessarily benign. AEDs have significant side effects such as hypotension or respiratory depression, and can potentially cause neuronal apoptosis.[28] In addition, the issue of electroclinical dissociation of seizures and the evidence that neonatal seizures themselves may cause brain injury raise the question of how aggressive one should be in treating neonatal seizures.[26] It is generally felt that even electrographic seizures may cause secondary neuronal injury through energy depletion, release of excitatory amino acids, or disturbances of cerebral blood flow. Such factors would lead one to be more aggressive about treatment of neonatal seizures. Still, there is no evidence that conclusively shows that treatment with AEDs alters the ultimate outcome and neurological prognosis, beyond what we can glean from the etiology of the seizures alone.[11,29] Nevertheless, there are still no evidence-based guidelines for the treatment of neonatal seizures.[22,30] Currently, traditional drugs such as phenobarbital and phenytoin are the standard first-line treatment for neonatal seizures. Now, as newer drugs such as levetiracetam or topiramate have become available for use in the NICU, these drugs have started to become more widely accepted as second- or third-line therapy.[30,31] These newer drugs, it is hoped, might be more effective and at the same time offer a better benefit-risk profile to the newborn.[32]

### Phenobarbital

Phenobarbital is considered to be the drug of first choice in treating neonatal seizures, as it has been around the longest, and we have the most extensive experience in using it. Generally, a loading dose of 15–20 mg/kg is administered over 10–15 minutes as an intravenous (IV) bolus. Infusion should be slowed if there are cardiovascular/respiratory side effects. Unfortunately, with this therapy, still less than 50% efficacy is often obtained. Further rapid loading doses of 5–10 mg/kg can be given if seizures persist, up to as high as 40 mg/kg if clinically tolerated. With this treatment, up to 77% efficacy can be achieved.[33] Phenobarbital levels of 15–40 mcg/mL are considered therapeutic, but often levels as high as 60 mcg/mL are required to stop the seizure activity, and even with this increased dosage, a second agent is often needed.[11,17] The half-life of phenobarbital in the newborn is highly variable and often very prolonged due to immaturity of the liver and poor metabolism of the phenobarbital. This is particularly true for the premature infant. The half-life of phenobarbital may range from 40 hours to 200 hours, and hypothermia may prolong the half-life even further. Thus, high therapeutic levels are often sustained even 48–72 hours after a loading dose. Therefore, maintenance is often not required immediately after administration. If maintenance is needed, however, a maintenance dose of 4–5 mg/kg/day can be given (divided, twice daily) once a steady state level has been achieved after the bolus.[9]

Phenobarbital is thought to work mostly through potentiating and activation of gamma-aminobutyric acid type A ($GABA_A$) receptors. This results in an increase in chloride influx into the cells and subsequent hyperpolarization and decreased neuronal excitation. In neonates, however, there is some controversy, as $GABA_A$ excitation in the newborn may lead to neuronal excitation rather than inhibition. This is due to differential overexpression of the sodium/potassium/chloride cotransporter isoform 1 (NKCC1) and underexpression of the potassium/chloride cotransporter (KCC2) in the newborn, which results in a reversal of the chloride gradient.[34] Whether or how these neurodevelopmental changes affect the treatment of neonatal seizures is still an active area of investigation. Some suggest bumetanide may be the next best treatment for neonatal seizures as a consequence by blocking NKCC1 and preventing intracellular chloride buildup.[35]

## Phenytoin

Phenytoin is considered a second-line drug for controlling neonatal seizures, should phenobarbital be ineffective. As a water-soluble prodrug of phenytoin, fosphenytoin is favored over the older phenytoin medicine as it has fewer side effects, has a neutral pH, is less caustic to veins and tissues, and does not cause the same cardiovascular side effects as phenytoin. A loading dose of 15-20 mg/kg phenytoin equivalents is generally given with trough levels measured 48 hours later, again due to poor metabolism in the newborn infant. If necessary, maintenance dosing with 4-5 mg/kg/day (divided, twice daily) can be started. The advantage of phenytoin is that it is less sedating than phenobarbital, but it has many more drug-drug interactions due to high protein binding, and transition to oral maintenance is problematic due to poor oral absorption. As with phenobarbital, the half-life can be variable, ranging from 8 hours up to 75 hours depending on gestational age. Phenytoin also has a saturable metabolism that results in wide variations in blood concentrations with even small dose changes, making accurate dosing more difficult.[9,11] In neonates, competitive binding with bilirubin is also a consideration because of possible concerns over kernicterus risk.[36]

Phenytoin works via inhibiting voltage-gated sodium channel and so operates through a different mechanism than phenobarbital. Therefore, it makes sense to use these two drugs as complementary medications in the treatment of neonatal seizures.[35]

## Benzodiazepines

Benzodiazepines, such as midazolam or lorazepam, have been used as second-line medicines for neonatal seizures also. Their effectiveness, however, seems to be variable. Lorazepam has been used in doses of 0.05-0.1 mg/kg in repeated IV pushes to achieve seizure control. Midazolam has a very short half-life and is used more as a continuous drip in cases of status epilepticus. A loading dose of 0.15 mg/kg is given, followed by a continuous infusion of 0.1-0.4 mg/kg/hr. Success rates of anywhere from 50% to 100% have been reported in the literature.[9,35] In several small studies, IV midazolam was able to control seizures despite failure of both phenobarbital and phosphenytoin.[32] This is despite the fact that the benzodiazepines are also thought to act on the immature GABA receptor system.[35]

## Levetiracetam

Levetiracetam has been available since 1999, though it was not approved by the Food and Drug Administration (FDA) for use in children and infants as young as 1 month until 2012. Levetiracetam is thought to work by effects on synaptic vesicle 2A (SV2A) and calcium channels, though its precise mechanism in neonates, is unknown. In children, its safety and pharmacokinetic profile have been quite favorable, making it an attractive potential treatment for neonatal seizures.[34,35] Because it is metabolized by type-B esterases to inactive metabolites and has minimal hepatic metabolism, there are few drug-drug interactions. It also has low-protein binding and is eliminated primarily in urine (66%). As a result, its clearance is dependent on good kidney function and not hepatic metabolism.[36] Perhaps related to decreased glomerular filtration rate (GFR) in the newborn, the half-life is somewhat longer (closer to 9 hours) in neonates than compared to older children.[37] In addition, there is evidence that unlike phenobarbital, levetiracetam does not seem to cause neuronal apoptosis in animal models. There is even some evidence that it may be neuroprotective.[22]

Despite these positive aspects of levetiracetam, its use in the NICU has been limited. It has mostly been used as a second- or third-line treatment for neonatal seizures. Although dosing has not been clearly defined, there have been reports of it being used to treat neonatal seizures in doses of 10-20 mg/kg as an IV load, with some using doses as high as 50-60 mg/kg.[36] Seizures have been reported to stop in up to 35-64% within 24 hours of administration and up to 52-100% of patients within 72 hours. Maintenance dosing of 10-80 mg/kg/day (divided, twice daily) has been used following acute IV loading.[36] There are still no published placebo-controlled studies for levetiracetam as a first-line treatment for neonatal seizures, though there are several studies that are now in progress.[38]

## Lidocaine

Lidocaine has been used in the past as a third-line treatment in refractory neonatal seizures. It works through inhibition of voltage-gated sodium channels. It is given as an IV initial load of 2 mg/kg followed by a continuous infusion initially of 6 mg/kg/hr and then in a gradually reducing dose every

12 hours as the seizures are controlled. Levels can be obtained and are maintained in the 2.8–10.5 mg/mL range. There have been several studies that have shown lidocaine to be effective in treating both premature and term infants with intractable neonatal seizures.[32,34] Unfortunately, there is a very narrow safety index for lidocaine, which can cause cardiac arrhythmias, and at high levels can also be pro-convulsant. In particular, lidocaine should not be used in children with cardiac anomalies, or in children on phenytoin who have a higher risk of arrhythmias and cardiac toxicity. Lidocaine levels are also increased during hypothermia due to decreased clearance, and so dosing should be adjusted. All children undergoing IV lidocaine treatment need continuous cardiac monitoring and it is generally thought that levels should be maintained below 9 mg/L.[35]

## Topiramate

Topiramate has been used in limited trials to treat neonatal seizures. Its use is somewhat restricted due to the lack of an intravenous formulation in addition to very limited pharmacokinetic data in neonates.[31] Topiramate has multiple mechanisms of action, including sodium channel blockade, $GABA_A$ receptor agonist, glutamate receptor antagonist, and carbonic anhydrase inhibition. All of these mechanisms make its potential use promising for refractory neonatal seizures.[35] However, there is limited information on use of topiramate in neonates. Doses of topiramate have been given in the range of 10 mg/kg as a loading dose, with some positive results and generally few side effects.[39] Currently, there are mostly just small case reports, though studies are ongoing looking at use of Topamax in neonates.[40]

## ■ MANAGEMENT

Despite a relative lack of randomized controlled trials for neonatal seizures, there are suggested protocols for treatment of neonatal seizures.[15,18,30] First, metabolic disturbances such as hypoglycemia or hypocalcemia must be corrected. Infectious causes must also be investigated and treated expeditiously. When treatment is started with antiseizure medicines, generally, phenobarbital is considered first-line treatment for neonatal seizures, with repeated doses up to a maximum of 40 mg/kg total. Phenytoin, levetiracetam, and lidocaine are all considered effective second-line treatments after phenobarbital has failed to completely control seizures. Phenytoin is usually given as a bolus up to 20 mg/kg, while lidocaine is given as described above as a continuous infusion. Keppra can also be given as a second-line medication in doses of 40–50 mg/kg as an initial bolus. By this time, intubation and ventilation are often needed, and continuous video EEG monitoring should be instituted. Also, vitamin B6 100 mg IV and folinic acid 5 mg should be tried at this point if the seizures have not abated.[18] Midazolam has then been used as a third-line agent for treating neonatal seizures, if seizures persist after the first- and second-line medicines have failed to totally control the seizures. A bolus of 0.15–0.2 mg/kg is given followed by an infusion of 0.5–18 mcg/kg/min.[9] Beyond this, Topamax can be added in combination with one or more of the above-mentioned medications if seizures remain uncontrolled.[34]

Unfortunately, much more study is needed in the area of treatment, with many unanswered questions regarding efficacy and potential side effects of treatment. As was alluded to earlier, there is evidence that neonates preferentially express the NKCCl cotransporter isoform over the KCC2 isoform, which would lead to neuronal depolarization, rather than hyperpolarization. It is thought that a switch to the more mature ion transporter subtype does occur around the time of birth; however, the timing of this change is not precisely known. As a result, excitation of neuronal activity rather than inhibition may occur with phenobarbital use.[35] This raises the question of whether preterm neonates should be treated any differently from full-term babies with seizures. After all, as noted above, different seizure types and etiologies of seizures are seen in the preterm versus the full-term infant. There is also a concern that some of these medicines we use to treat neonatal seizures may potentially cause neuronal injury and apoptosis. N-methyl D-aspartate (NMDA) receptor antagonists, GABA agonists, and sodium channel blockers have all been shown to cause neuronal injury in animal models.[36] The long-term safety and efficacy of all of these medicines, especially the newer AEDs such as topiramate and levetiracetam are thought to be better, but are still unknown.[35] In fact, there are reports that topiramate may exacerbate apoptosis when added to phenytoin. The combined effects of hypothermia with these medicines and their interaction are also unknown. Further study of the pharmacokinetics and pharmacodynamics of antiepileptic drugs in the hypothermic infant is needed.[31] Whether newer medicines such as bumetanide may be better options also is wide open for study with randomized controlled trials.[35]

One of the major topics that also remains largely unexplored is the treatment of electrographic seizures that have no clinical accompaniment. Generally, neonatal seizures are treated to eliminate at least most or nearly all clinically apparent seizures. While it is believed that seizures can injure the brain and that there is a relationship between poorly controlled seizures and poor outcome, it is also true that the more severe the underlying cause, the harder the seizures are to control. Prognosis may be more related to the etiology than the effectiveness of therapy.[10,11] It is also true that the natural history of neonatal seizures, especially those caused by HIE, is that they will usually abate over time, as the encephalopathy itself clears. Thus, treatment of refractory seizures may often become easier over time, even without aggressive intervention. It may be the case that the complete elimination of all electrographic seizures may not necessarily be the ultimate goal of therapy. Rather, it is more of a balance between the elimination of prolonged and frequent seizures, including electrographic, and the potential side effects of the medication. Long-term, multicenter trials will be needed to answer the question of how neonatal seizures affect outcome apart from etiology of the seizures themselves.[9,34]

## PROGNOSIS

Overall prognosis of neonates who experience seizures has improved a great deal over the last several decades, mostly as a result of excellent obstetrical and neonatal ICU care. Mortality is estimated to have decreased from 40% to only 20% of all cases of neonatal seizures. The incidence of adverse neurological outcome, however, has been relatively unchanged. It is estimated that between 35% and 60% of infants with neonatal seizures suffer some neurological long-term abnormalities, such as cerebral palsy, cognitive delay, or epilepsy.[11] In general, however, the ultimate prognosis depends greatly on the etiology of the seizures in the first place. Hypocalcemia or hypomagnesemia, for example, bodes for a good prognosis. Severe cerebral malformations or injury portend a poor prognosis. Those with mild hypoxia, small focal strokes, or CNS infections have an intermediate prognosis. Clinically, an abnormal examination or extreme prematurity also predict a poor outcome. The EEG also can give some prognostic information. A normal EEG background will often predict a more normal outcome. A severely abnormal background that remains persistently abnormal even on follow-up EEG often predicts a poor outcome neurologically. Overall, term infants also fare better than premature infants,[18] and up to a third of all children will develop postnatal epilepsy.[15]

## FUTURE DIRECTIONS

Neonatal seizures are a major clinical problem and there remain many unanswered questions surrounding pathophysiology, diagnosis, and treatment. A better understanding of the underlying mechanism of neonatal seizures is needed to guide future research into more effective therapies. We also need to explore the mechanism and prognosis of electrographic and subclinical seizure activity. On a practical level, we need to develop better diagnostic methods and tests to determine the presence of neonatal seizures. Further, treatment protocols need to be developed that look for differences between the premature and full-term infant, and take into account the biology of the newborn brain with a view to improving neurological outcome. Fortunately, there are ongoing trials to look at new medications and address the major gaps of our knowledge in treatment of newborns with seizures. The long-term effects of brain cooling on treatment and prognosis must also be studied in addition to other newer therapeutic and diagnostic interventions.

## CONCLUSION

Neonatal seizures represent a major cause of morbidity and mortality in the NICU. It is critical to be vigilant in detecting neonatal seizures and rapidly institute diagnostic studies and interventions to prevent neurological injury. Prolonged video EEG is critical in the diagnosis and treatment of such infants. Treatment should be tailored to the individual patient, with an eye to mitigating secondary injury while avoiding doing any further harm. Still, there are many questions about neonatal seizures that remain to be answered.

## REFERENCES

1. Olson DM. Neonatal seizures. NeoRev. 2012:13(4):e213-23.
2. van Zeben-van der Aa DM, Verloove-Vanhorick SP, den Ouden L, et al. Neonatal seizures in the very preterm and very low birthweight infants: mortality and handicaps at two years of age in a nationwide cohort. Neuropediatrics. 1990;21(2):62-5.
3. Kohelet D, Shochat R, Lusky A, et al. Israel Neonatal Network. Risk factors for neonatal seizures in very low birthweight infants: population-based survery. J Child Neurol. 2004;19(2):123-8.
4. Rennie JM. Neurological problems of the neonate: assessment of the neonatal neurological system. In: Rennie JM, Robertson NR (Eds). Robertson's Textbook of Neonatology, 4th edition. Edinburgh, United Kingdom: Elsevier Health Sciences; 2005. pp. 1093-105.
5. Ronen GM, Buckley D, Penney S, et al. Long-term prognosis in children with neonatal seizures: a population-based study. Neurology. 2007;69(19):1816-22.
6. Davis AS, Hintz SR, Van Meurs KP, et al. Eunice Kennedy Shriver National Institute of Child Health and Human Development Neonatal Research Network. Seizures in extremely low birth weight infants are associated with adverse outcome. J Pediatr. 2010;157(5):720-5.e1-2.
7. West CR, Harding JE, Williams CE, et al. Cot-side electroencephalography for outcome prediction in preterm infants: observational study. Arch Dis Child Fetal Neonatal Ed. 2011;96(2):F108-13.
8. Vasudeven C, Levene M. Epidemiology and aetiology of neonatal seizures. Semin Fetal Neonatal Med. 2013;18(4): 185-91.

9. Glass HC, Sullivan JE. Neonatal seizures. Curr Treat Options Neurol. 2009;11(6):405-13.
10. Thibeault-Eybalin MP, Lortie A, Carmant L. Neonatal Seizures: Do they damage the brain? Pediatr Neurol. 2009;40(3):175-80.
11. Volpe JJ. Neonatal seizures. In: Volpe JJ (Ed). Neurology of the Newborn, 5th edition. Philadelphia: Saunders; 2008. pp. 203-45.
12. Sheth RD, Hobbs GR, Mullett M. Neonatal seizures: incidence, onset, and etiology by gestational age. J Perinatol. 1999;19(1):40-3.
13. Lynch JK. Epidemiology and classification of perinatal stroke. Semin Fetal Neonatal Med. 2009;14(5):245-9.
14. Yamamoto H, Okumura A, Fukuda M. Epilepsies and epileptic syndromes starting in the neonatal period. Brain Dev. 2011;33(3):213-20.
15. Kanhere S. Recent advances in neonatal seizures. Indian J Pedtiatr. 2014;81(9):917-25.
16. Hallberg B, Blennow M. Investigations for neonatal seizures. Semin Fetal Neonatal Med. 2013;18(4):196-201.
17. Evans D, Levene M. Neonatal seizures. Arch Dis Child Fetal Neonatal Ed. 1998;78(1):F70-5.
18. Sivaswamy L. Approach to neonatal seizures. Clin Pediatr (Phila). 2012;51(5):415-25.
19. Mizrahi EM. Pediatric electroencephalographic video monitoring. J Clin Neurophysiol. 1999;16(2):100-10.
20. Mizrahi EM, Kellaway P. Characterization and classification of neonatal seizures. Neurology. 1987;37(12):1837-44.
21. Plouin P, Kaminska A. Neonatal seizures. In: Dulac O, Lassonde M, Sarnat HB (Eds). Handbook of Clinical Neurology. Vol. 111. Amsterdam: Elsevier; 2013. pp. 467-76.
22. Glass HC. Neonatal seizures: advances in mechanisms and management. Clin Perinatol. 2014;4(1):177-90.
23. Scher MS, Painter MJ, Bergman I, et al. EEG diagnoses of neonatal seizures: clinical correlations and outcome. Pediatr Neurol. 1989;5(1):17-24.
24. Rakshasbhuvankar A, Paul S, Nagarajan L, et al. Amplitude-integrated EEG for detection of neonatal seizures: a systemic review. Seizure. 2015;33:90-8.
25. van Rooij LG, Toet MC, van Huffelen AC, et al. Effect of treatment of subclinical neonatal seizures detected with aEEG: randomized, controlled trial. Pediatrics. 2010;125(2):e358-66.
26. Bourez-Swart MD, van Rooij L, Rizzo C, et al. Detection of subclinical electroencephalographic seizure patterns with multichannel amplitude-integrated EEG in full-term neonates. Clin Neurophysiol. 2009;120(11):1916-22.
27. Lynch NE, Stevenson NJ, Livingstone V, et al. The temporal evolution of elctrographic seizure burden in neonatal hypoxic ischemic encephalopathy. Epilepsia. 2012;53(3):549-57.
28. Bittigau P, Sifringer M, Genz K, et al. Antiepileptic drugs and apoptotic neurodegeneration in the developing brain. Proc Natl Acad Sci USA. 2002;9(23):15089-94.
29. van Rooij LG, Hellström-Westas L, de Vries LS. Treatment of neonatal seizures. Semin Fetal Neonatal Med. 2013;18(4):209-15.
30. Slaughter LA, Patel AD, Slaughter JL. Pharmacological treatment of neonatal seizures: a systematic review. J Child Neurol. 2013;28(3):351-64.
31. Spagnoli C, Pavlidis E, Pisani F. Neonatal seizures therapy: we are still looking for the efficacious drug. Ital J Pediatr. 2013;39:37.
32. Zeller B, Giebe J. Pharmacologic management of neonatal seizures. Neonatal Netw. 2015;34(4):239-44.
33. Gilman JT, Gal P, Duchowny MS, et al. Rapid sequential phenobarbital treatment of neonatal seizures. Pediatrics. 1989;83(5):674-8.
34. Vesoulis ZA, Mathur AM. Advances in management of neonatal seizures. Indian J Pediatr. 2014;81(6):592-8.
35. Donovan MD, Griffin BT, Kharoshankaya L, et al. Pharmacotherapy for neonatal seizures: current knowledge and future perspectives. Drugs. 2016;76(6):647-61.
36. Mruk AL, Garlitz KL, Leung NR. Levetiracetam in neonatal seizures: a review. J Pediatr Pharmacol Ther. 2015;20(2):76-89.
37. Merhar SL, Schibler KR, Sherwin CM, et al. Pharmacokinetics of levetiracetam in neonates with seizures. J Pediatr. 2011;159(1):152-4.e3.
38. Clinicaltrials.gov website. [online] Available from: https://clinicaltrials.gov/ct2/show/NCT01720667?term=neonate+levetiracetam&rank=1. [Last accessed Sep., 2019].
39. Glass HC, Poulin C, Shevell MI. Topiramate for the treatment of neonatal seizures. Pediatr Neurol. 2011;44(6):439-42.
40. Clinicaltrials.gov website. [online] Available from: https://clinicaltrials.gov/ct2/show/NCT01765218?term=neonate+topiramate&rank=2. [Last accessed Sep., 2019].

CHAPTER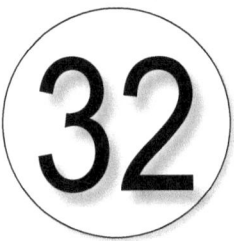

# Newborn Populations at Risk for Adverse Neurodevelopmental Outcomes

Ira Adams-Chapman

## ABSTRACT

Innovations in perinatal and neonatal medicine have improved neurodevelopmental (ND) outcomes in surviving infants. Changes in management of maternal and neonatal diseases associated with adverse ND outcomes have impacted morbidity and mortality. In this two-part chapter, we will review contemporary ND outcome data of infants cared for in the neonatal intensive care setting in the context of medical morbidity associated with care, including chronic lung disease, necrotizing enterocolitis, sepsis, intraventricular hemorrhage, and periventricular leukomalacia. We will emphasize the maturational vulnerability of the developing preterm brain.

## INTRODUCTION

Historically, most neonatal intensive care focused on increasing survival in preterm infants. Modern obstetrics and perinatal-neonatal practice have reduced morbidity and mortality attributable to preterm birth. Compared to a bygone era when many neonatal clinical trials focused on short-term outcomes, most current clinical trials are designed to ensure that short-term neonatal outcome is met while preventing adverse neurodevelopmental (ND) outcomes among those exposed. In a thought-provoking meta-analysis by Keith Barrington on the use of postnatal steroids in the preterm population, he demonstrates that focus on short-term respiratory outcomes without adequate evaluation of long-term outcomes resulted in the exposure of thousands of preterm infants to steroids before retrospective studies showed that postnatal steroid use was associated with increased risk for adverse cognitive and motor outcomes.[1] Clinical trials should evaluate both short-term outcomes and long-term ND outcomes before widespread use of unproven therapies.

Large cohort studies have allowed us to better understand outcomes in the preterm population, but site-specific outcomes are very important as well because there are wide variations between centers in the frequency of various morbidities and ND outcomes.

This section focuses on ND outcome of high-risk populations, including neonates with sepsis, prematurity, and intraventricular hemorrhage (IVH). Neuroimaging to better understand brain development and injury is discussed.

## POPULATIONS AT RISK FOR ADVERSE NEURODEVELOPMENTAL OUTCOMES

Several potential modifiable causes of global neonatal mortality exist, including preterm birth, neonatal infections, and hypoxic-ischemic encephalopathy (HIE). Survivors of any of these complications are at high risk for adverse ND outcome. Regional programs devised to address each of these areas should result in decreased neonatal mortality and potentially improve ND outcomes in survivors (Fig. 1).

## NEONATAL SEPSIS AND NEURODEVELOPMENTAL OUTCOME

The United Nation's Millennium Development Goal 4 was to decrease childhood mortality by two-thirds between

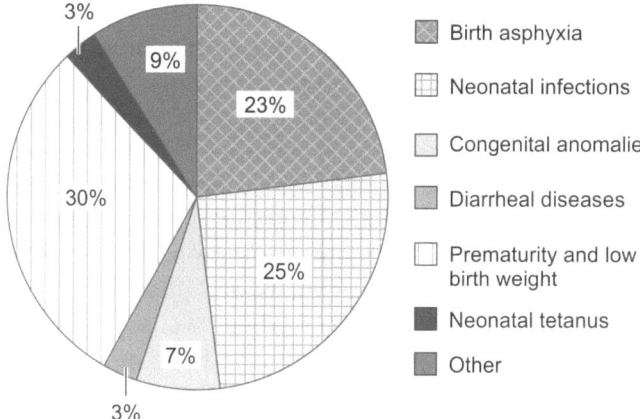

Fig. 1: Causes of neonatal death worldwide.[2]

1990 and 2015.[3] Examination of the global burden of under-five mortality between 1990 and 2013 showed that neonatal deaths (0–6 days) accounted for 41.6% of deaths in 2013 compared to 37.4% in 1990.[4] Worldwide, one-third of neonatal deaths are attributed to neonatal sepsis and infection, the majority occurring in the first 24 hours of life. Ninety percent of these infection-related deaths occur in resource-limited areas with a heavy burden of disease in sub-Saharan Africa. Since most deliveries in resource-limited regions occur at home, in 2009 the WHO formed a collaborative project entitled "Saving Newborn Lives," examining best practice principles for home delivery practitioners. Their recommendations included using skilled delivery attendants and providing additional training for community healthcare workers, who are typically the first responders to a sick newborn. Standards for in-home delivery and cord care were established. Wide regional variability in pathogen distribution responsible for neonatal sepsis exists, thus prevention strategies must be environmentally specific and therapies should be targeted. Novel strategies to increase access to unit dose antibiotics and coordinated regionalized care are required. Short-term data are available on ND outcome of surviving infants in these regions. However, a longer-term impact of neonatal infection is primary or secondary injury to the developing brain, resulting in increased risk for abnormal ND outcome.

In 2006, the Centers for Disease Control (CDC) reported that infection was the eighth leading cause of neonatal death in the United States.[5] Premature newborns are susceptible to infections in the perinatal period, immediately following delivery, and later during hospitalization (nosocomial infection). In addition to higher attributable mortality, there is increased risk of adverse ND outcome in infection survivors, due to both primary injury to the developing brain and secondary cytokine-mediated injury.

## Chorioamnionitis and Neurodevelopmental Outcome

Intrauterine infection is associated with preterm delivery. The diagnosis of chorioamnionitis is debatable, often lacking histological evidence of chorioamnionitis in mothers with clinical signs and symptoms of chorioamnionitis (such as maternal fever and uterine tenderness). Preterm labor and premature rupture of membranes (PROM) are frequently associated with chorioamnionitis. The relationship between premature labor, PROM, and their relationship to latency in pregnancy has been previously described.[6] Pregnancies affected by preterm labor and/or PROM are more likely to have not only elevated amniotic fluid cytokines, but also shorter latency periods. Furthermore, the fetus is capable of generating a cytokine response, as evidenced by elevated cytokine levels in umbilical cord blood. Elevated levels of interleukin (IL)-6 and IL-8 in amniotic fluid result in cystic periventricular leukomalacia (PVL) in animal brain.[7] Similar associations between elevated cord blood levels of IL-6 with PVL have been demonstrated in preterm newborns. These early studies provided biologic plausibility to cytokine exposure in the developing fetus and subsequent neurologic injury.

Although neonates born to mothers with suspected chorioamnionitis are more likely to have evidence of early onset sepsis (EOS) than their unexposed peers, a strong association between maternal chorioamnionitis and adverse ND outcome in surviving newborns is not shown. In 2,390 infants born <27 weeks of gestation participating in the National Institute of Child Health and Human Development (NICHD) Neonatal Research Network (NRN), outcomes were compared between those with no history of chorioamnionitis, those with histological chorioamnionitis, and those with both clinical and histological chorioamnionitis.[8] Neonates exposed to chorioamnionitis were of lower gestational age (GA) and had higher rates of EOS and severe IVH compared to unexposed neonates. However, the association between chorioamnionitis and ND outcome at age of 2 years was largely mediated by differences in GA at birth. Similarly, others evaluating fetal exposure to inflammation and neurocognitive outcomes at age of 6 years and found that differences in outcome were primarily mediated by GA.[9] Exposure to elevated inflammatory markers or clinical/histologic chorioamnionitis was not associated with lower intelligence quotient (IQ), after adjustment for GA at birth. Most published trials fail to show statistically significant differences in ND outcome in preterm children exposed to chorioamnionitis. In a meta-analysis evaluating the relationship between perinatal infection and ND outcome, chorioamnionitis did not affect mental or motor outcomes.[10]

Variables affecting ND outcome are multifactorial. It is possible that even though exposure to perinatal infection contributes to adverse outcomes, it is outweighed by other morbidities associated with prematurity, including GA, which appears to have a more profound impact. Further research is needed in this area.

## Group B *Streptococcus*

Group B Streptococcal (GBS) infection in the neonate is a leading cause of global neonatal morbidity and mortality with wide variability by country and region. A systematic review of worldwide cases in high-income countries found a European incidence of 0.53 per 1,000 live births compared to 0.67 in North America and 0.0 (0.00–0.44) in Australia.[11] A systematic review in low income countries found an incidence of 0–3.06 per 1,000 live births, with wide variation between geographic regions.[12] Epidemiologists are monitoring frequency of GBS EOS after peripartum implementation of either universal screening or risk-based screening for GBS.

Systematic interventions designed to identify at-risk pregnancies have led to a dramatic decrease in the rates of GBS EOS in the US.[13] Consensus guidelines initially established in 1996 by the CDC and subsequently adopted by the American Academy of Pediatrics and the American College of Obstetricians and Gynecologists[14] were further refined in 2002 to recommend universal third trimester screening in all pregnancies. While rates of GBS EOS have decreased 80% after implementation of these guidelines, prevalence of late onset GBS remains unchanged **(Fig. 2)**.[13,15]

Between 1990 and 2005, 1,726 GBS cases were accompanied by a case fatality rate of 4.3%.[15] Black infants and those born <37 weeks of gestation were more likely to be affected. Meningitis was the presenting clinical sign in 24%. Incidence of GBS EOS was three times higher than late onset sepsis (LOS) prior to consensus guidelines. In contrast, after consensus statement guidelines were adopted, rates were similar, decreasing to 0.34 cases per 1,000 live births annually. For GBS LOS, the risk of death varied by site of involvement. The case-fatality ratios for those with bacteremia, meningitis, and pneumonia were 3%, 6%, and 12%, respectively.[15] While 7% of neonates with GBS EOS have evidence of meningitis, it is more common among those presenting with GBS LOS and is associated with worse neurologic outcomes. In a review of 90 neonates with GBS meningitis, 5 died prior to the 3-year assessment; of the 43 survivors available for developmental assessment, 56% were normal, 25% had mild to moderate delays, and 19% were severely developmentally delayed. Hearing loss was identified in four (9.3%) of the children evaluated.[16]

## Early Onset Sepsis and Neurodevelopmental Outcome

Early onset sepsis incidence in the US very low birth weight (VLBW) population is ~15–19 per 1,000 live births.[17] VLBW sepsis has a US incidence of 2%, essentially unchanged over two recent decades.[18] Several times higher than the sepsis rate among term infants, EOS incidence in VLBWs varies inversely with GA. Due to the decrease in GBS EOS, *Escherichia coli* is now a more frequent pathogen, particularly among very preterm infants (VPI) born <33 weeks of GA. It is crucial to monitor GBS epidemiology, antibiotic resistance due to widespread use, and the distribution of pathogens over time.

A cohort of 2,665 French VPI were evaluated at 5 years of age.[19] These children, born 22–32 weeks GA, had a comprehensive neuropsychological battery performed at follow-up. NICU infection was as follows: 159 (5%) had EOS, 752 (28%) had LOS, and 64 (2%) had both EOS and LOS. Overall impairment rates for the cohort at age of 5 years included 9% cerebral palsy (CP) and 12% cognitive impairment. The frequency of CP was higher in infants with isolated EOS {odds ratio (OR): 1.70 [95% confidence interval (CI): 0.84–3.45]} or isolated LOS [OR: 1.71 (95% CI: 1.14–2.56)] than in uninfected infants, and this risk was even higher in cases of combined EOS and LOS [OR: 2.33 (95% CI: 1.02–5.33)]. There was no association between neonatal infection and cognitive impairment in this cohort.

## Late Onset Sepsis and Prematurity

Late onset sepsis is defined as a documented bloodstream infection at ≥3 days of age. Many more preterm infants receive treatment for clinical sepsis, which is defined as

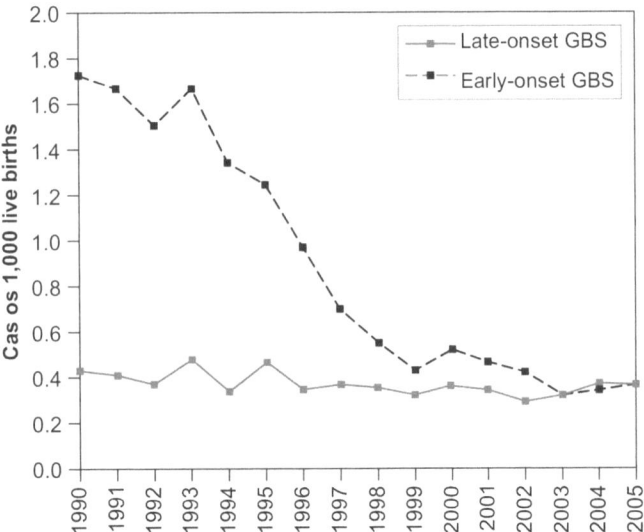

**Fig. 2:** Incidence of early- and late-onset invasive group B streptococcal (GBS) disease—Active Bacterial Core surveillance areas, 1990–2005.[15]

clinical symptoms suggestive of a bacterial infection, but with negative cultures. Preterm infants are at risk for LOS, as reported by the NICHD NRN in 2004, reporting that 65% of extremely low birth weight (ELBW) infants weighing <1,000 g in their cohort had either clinical sepsis (35%), culture positive sepsis (32%), necrotizing enterocolitis (NEC) plus sepsis (5%), or meningitis (3%).[20] Compared to uninfected children, those in any infection group were more likely to have CP, lower Bayley Scale of Infant Development (BSID)-II Mental Developmental Index (MDI) and Psychomotor Developmental Index (PDI) scores, and more likely to have visual impairment, consistent with other published studies. The relationship between any LOS and increased risk for adverse ND outcome is evident in **Figures 3 and 4**.

Abnormal ND outcome in children with LOS is etiologically multifactorial. The cascade of physiologic responses to a systemic infection is a combination of direct and indirect cytotoxic injuries to current and developing neuronal tissues.[22,23] Cytokinemia in the face of ischemia may be even more damaging to the neonatal brain than LOS; white matter injury (WMI) in the preterm brain has also been described in response to cytokinemia. Cytokines cross the immature blood-brain barrier in the preterm neonate, resulting in neuronal cell death. They also activate other cytopathic pathways that result in injury to developing oligodendrocytes in the white matter, eventually manifesting in survivors as adverse neurologic outcomes.

## PREMATURITY

Premature birth increases risk of death and adverse ND outcomes among survivors. This risk is inversely related to GA due to a combination of maturational vulnerability of the developing brain and increased risk of associated morbidities known to be associated with central nervous system (CNS) injury, including sepsis, NEC, chronic lung disease, IVH, and WMI.

## INTRAVENTRICULAR HEMORRHAGE

### Epidemiology

Intraventricular hemorrhage is a serious complication of preterm birth associated with both short- and long-term sequelae. Up to 25% of VLBW neonates have evidence of IVH.[24] The long-term burden of disability and chronic health impact is evident in data published from the NICHD and the CDC; in the US, there are over 3,600 new cases of long-term cognitive disability attributable to IVH each year. The lifetime care cost for these children exceeds 3.6 billion dollars.[25]

In general, IVH frequency has decreased over time, particularly severe grade 3-4 IVH. The NICHD NRN has published data on cohorts of VLBW infants in various epochs over time. Rates of IVH in two published studies are outlined in **Table 1**. Trends over 20 years and rates of various

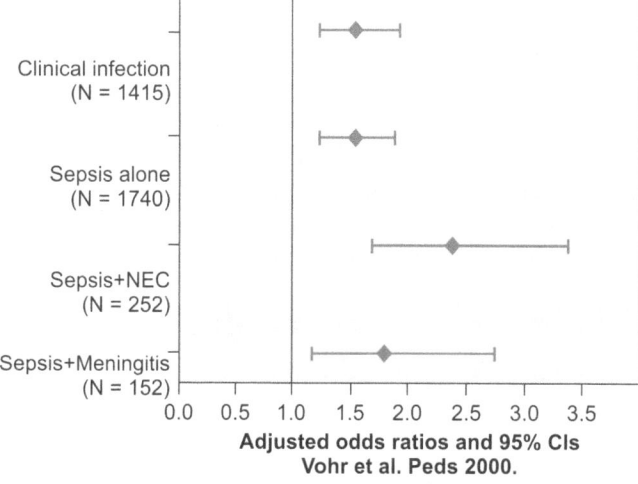

**Fig. 3:** Relationship between LOS and PDI.[21]
Adjusted odds ratio and 95% confidence intervals for LOS and PDI on the BSID-II. Clinical infection defined as culture negative but treated with antibiotics >5 days; sepsis alone defined as positive blood culture; sepsis + NEC defined as positive blood culture and ≥ Bells Stage 2 disease; sepsis + meningitis defined as positive blood culture and positive cerebrospinal fluid culture.
(BSID-II: Bayley Scale of Infant Development-II; LOS: late onset sepsis; ND: neurodevelopmental; NEC: necrotizing enterocolitis; PDI: psychomotor developmental index).

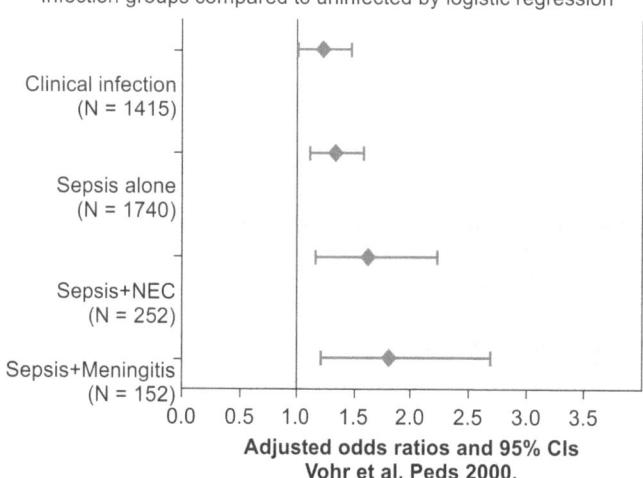

**Fig. 4:** Relationship between LOS and MDI.[21]
Adjusted odds ratio and 95% confidence intervals for LOS and PDI on the BSID-II. Clinical infection defined as culture negative but treated with antibiotics >5 days; sepsis alone defined as positive blood culture; sepsis + NEC defined as positive blood culture and ≥ Bells Stage 2 disease; sepsis + meningitis defined as positive blood culture and positive CSF culture.
(BSID-II: Bayley Scale of Infant Development-II; LOS: late onset sepsis; MDI: mental developmental index; ND: neurodevelopmental; NEC: necrotizing enterocolitis; PDI: psychomotor developmental index).

grades of IVH are reported (**Table 2**). Rates of severe IVH decreased for infants with GA 26–28 weeks, but there was no significant decrease for those 22–25 weeks GA.[18] Similarly, PVL rates decreased from 8% to 4% for infants 26–28 weeks GA.

In addition to GA-mediated risk, recent data suggest that there are genetic polymorphisms that modify risk for a variety of factors contributing to IVH, CNS injury, response to inflammation, angiogenesis, thrombosis, and oxidative pathways.[24,28-30] How these genetic modifiers affect outcome is unknown.

## Risk Factors for Intraventricular Hemorrhage

Intraventricular hemorrhage risk varies inversely with GA and birthweight; thus the most effective prevention strategy is to prevent preterm delivery. A variety of strategies are now in place to prolong gestation latency in the absence of maternal indicators that necessitate premature delivery of the infant, resulting in dramatic decline in the rate of preterm delivery over the past decade in the US and Europe.

The CNS in premature newborns has an immature germinal matrix surrounded by a microvasculature which lacks a basement membrane or tight junctions, resulting in increased vulnerability to alterations in cerebral blood flow.[24] Blood flow in the preterm CNS is affected by hypotension, hypoxemia, hypercapnia, and acidosis, all of which increase IVH risk.

Brain development is a maturation-dependent process that continues throughout gestation. Early neuronal progenitor cells are present in the first few weeks of gestation and this process of proliferation and migration continues to term gestation and beyond. The highly vascular germinal matrix is the originating site of early CNS development, but is also a region at risk for injury and hemorrhage. The supporting vascular and surrounding soft tissue network is fragile and vulnerable to hemodynamic shifts and cytotoxic injury. Various modulators of cerebral blood flow have been identified in the developing brain, including the cyclooxygenase-2 (COX-2) system and prostaglandins. COX-2 expression is induced by hypoxia, hypotension, epidermal growth factor receptor, transforming growth factor β, and inflammatory modulators including IL-6, IL-1β, tumor necrosis factor α (TNF-α), and NFkappaB.[24] This cascade results in an increase release of vascular endothelial growth factor (VEGF) potent in angiogenic effects. These immunomodulators also disrupt tight junctions, increasing permeability of the blood-brain barrier and activating microglia in developing white matter. Activated microglia release reactive oxygen species (ROS) which increase the risk of endothelial damage and alter hemostasis.[31] ROS are also released as a downstream response to activation of the COX-2 system. The premature brain appears more sensitive to ROS than the mature brain, contributing to IVH pathogenesis.

Given that 90% of IVH occurs within the first week of life, prevention strategies have emphasized improved stability and early optimization of care. A quality improvement strategy designed to reduce rates of IVH in preterm infants focused on delivery room and NICU care in the first week of life, reporting 10.5% decreased incidence of any IVH,

**TABLE 1:** Rates of IVH over time in NICHD Neonatal Research Network.

|  | NICHD 2004[26] N = 7,693 | NICHD 2010[27] N = 9,575 |
|---|---|---|
| Normal | 67% | 64% |
| Grade 1 | 13% | 10% |
| Grade 2 | 7% | 6% |
| Grade 3 | 7% | 7% |
| Grade 4 | 6% | 2% |

(IVH: intraventricular hemorrhage; NICHD: National Institute of Child Health and Human Development).

**TABLE 2:** Rates of IVH by GA from NICHD NRN.

| Weeks GA → | 22 | 23 | 24 | 25 | 26 | 27 | 28 | Total |
|---|---|---|---|---|---|---|---|---|
| Normal | 32 | 41 | 57 | 65 | 70 | 77 | 77 | 64 |
| Grade 1 | 13 | 9 | 11 | 9 | 11 | 10 | 10 | 10 |
| Grade 2 | 13 | 9 | 9 | 8 | 5 | 5 | 4 | 6 |
| Grade 3 | 8 | 15 | 12 | 8 | 7 | 6 | 4 | 7 |
| Grade 4 | 30 | 21 | 14 | 13 | 7 | 5 | 3 | 9 |
| Ventriculomegaly without IVH | 4 | 3 | 3 | 3 | 2 | 2 | 1 | 2 |
| PVL | 6 | 4 | 3 | 4 | 3 | 2 | 2 | 3 |

Modified from Stoll, et al. 2010 from NICHD NRN reporting outcomes of neonates cared for in NRN centers between January 1, 2003 and December 31, 2007 and survives >12 hours.[27]
(GA: gestational age; IVH: intraventricular hemorrhage; NICHD: National Institute of Child Health and Human Development; NRN: Neonatal Research Network; PVL: periventricular leukomalacia).

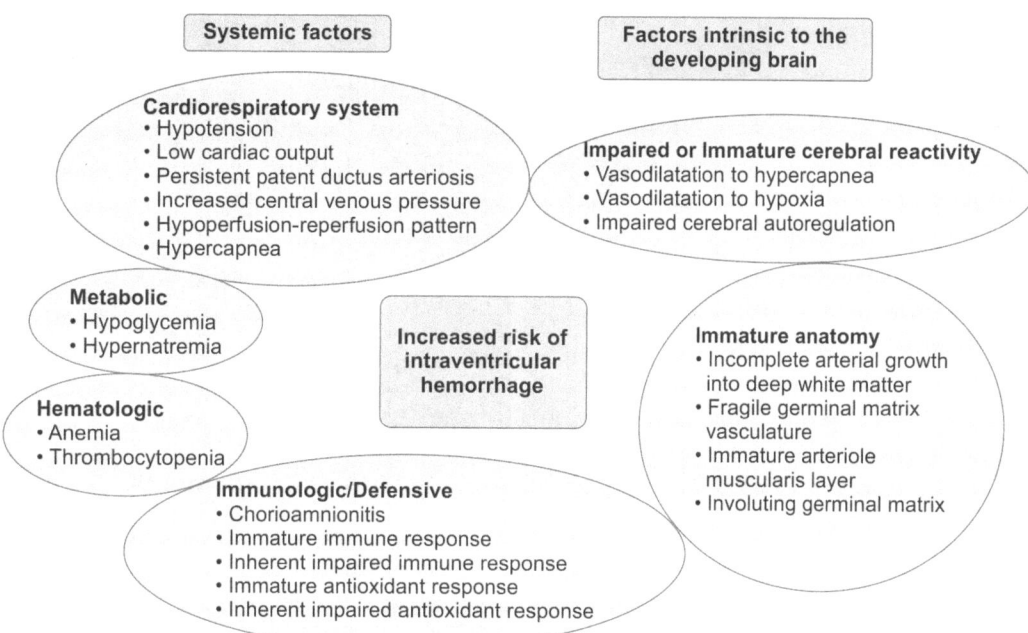

**Fig. 5:** Factors modifying IVH risk in the preterm neonate.
(CNS: central nervous system; IVH: intraventricular hemorrhage).
*Courtesy:* Reprinted with permission. Diagram illustrates numerous systemic and intrinsic CNS factors likely contribution to increase IVH risk. Many of these interrelated factors contribute to other comorbidities of prematurity.[33]

3.7% decrease in incidence of severe IVH, and increased probability of survival without IVH.[32]

Various other neonatal complications and morbidities have been associated with an increased risk for IVH, including hypotension, sepsis, hypoxemia, hypercapnia, pneumothorax, and pulmonary hemorrhage **(Fig. 5)**. With improved care, these complications are less frequent.

| TABLE 3: "Papile" criteria for grading of IVH. | |
|---|---|
| Grade 1 IVH | Subependymal hemorrhage |
| Grade 2 IVH | Bleeding into the ventricle but no dilatation |
| Grade 3 IVH | Bleeding into the ventricle with ventricular dilatation |
| Grade 4 IVH | Parenchymal hemorrhage |
| (IVH: intraventricular hemorrhage). | |

## Diagnosis of Intraventricular Hemorrhage

Cranial ultrasonography (CUS) is the commonly used modality to evaluate a preterm infant for IVH. It is portable, reproducible, and can be performed on even the most unstable patient. CUS is excellent for evaluating evidence of bleeding and monitoring ventricular size in those at risk for developing posthemorrhagic hydrocephalus (PHH). Images obtained through the mastoid window are more likely to identify cerebellar hemorrhage. Magnetic resonance imaging (MRI) is also an excellent imaging modality to evaluate CNS injury; however, in most clinical settings the patient is transported, sometimes sedated, and requires expert interpretation. MRI is a superior modality for cerebellar imaging and is capable of quantitative measurements.[34] MRI is better than CUS in diagnosing WMI and PVL.[34-38] CT scan is limited as a neuroimaging modality in preterm infants.

Preterm IVH originates in the germinal matrix and subependymal region. Larger hemorrhages extend into the ventricles. Increased particulate circulation of proteinaceous material in the cerebrospinal fluid (CSF) can result in an obliterative or obstructive hydrocephalus, or PHH. Obstruction to venous circulation in the trigone results in hemorrhagic venous infarction in a fan-like appearance that extends into the surrounding parenchyma, the most common location being the angle of the lateral ventricle.

The majority of data regarding timing of IVH is derived from 1980s studies.[39-41] Routine screening of high-risk premature infants was developed from these data. Outcomes from a series of 105 infants with IVH diagnosed by ultrasonography showed that 50% of IVH occurs within the first postnatal day, 25% by the second day, and an additional 15% by the third day of life.[42] The vast majority of IVH in the preterm infant is evident within the first week of life.

Various classification systems exist; however, common criteria are based on the evolution of IVH noted on serial CT scans of 36 consecutively born low birth weight infants <1,500 g.[43] Grading is based on location of the bleeding and associated degree of ventricular dilatation as outlined in **Table 3**. Images of each grade of IVH are provided in **Figure 6**.

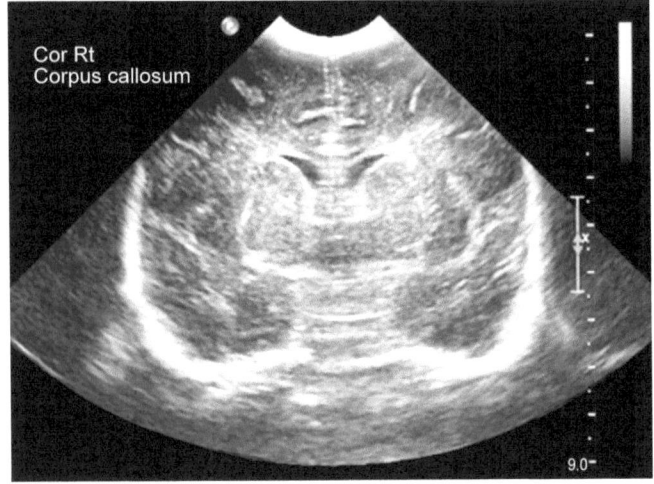

Normal CUS

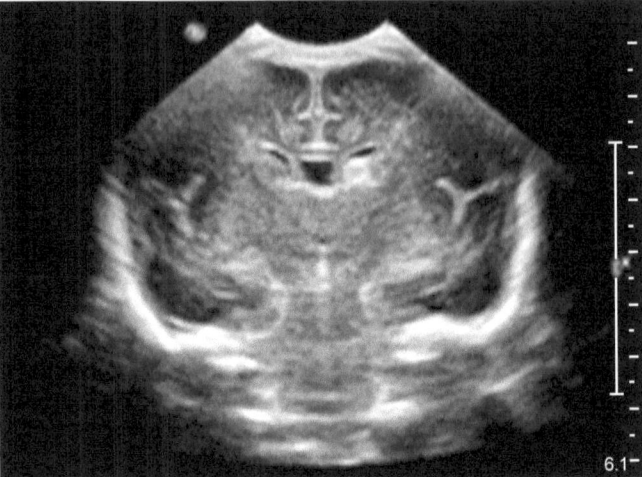

Grade 1 IVH
Small amount of blood in the left subependymal region.

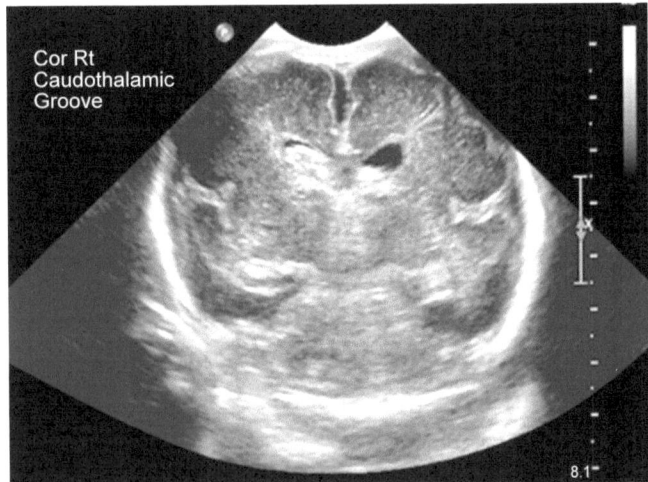

Grade 2 IVH
Echogenic material in right ventricle. Ventricle size within normal limits.

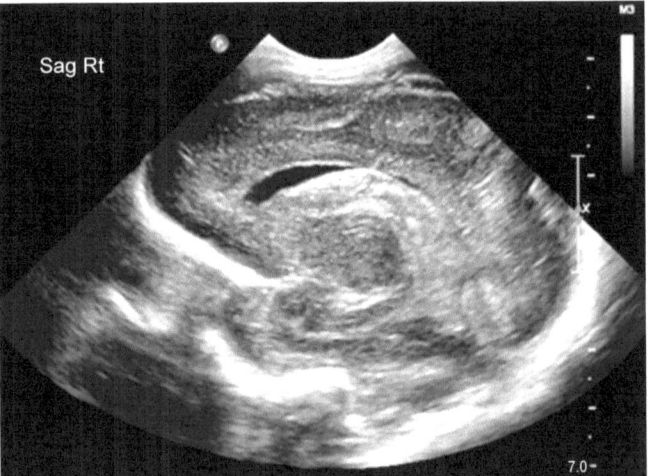

Sagittal view of Grade 2 IVH. Blood filling the ventricle.

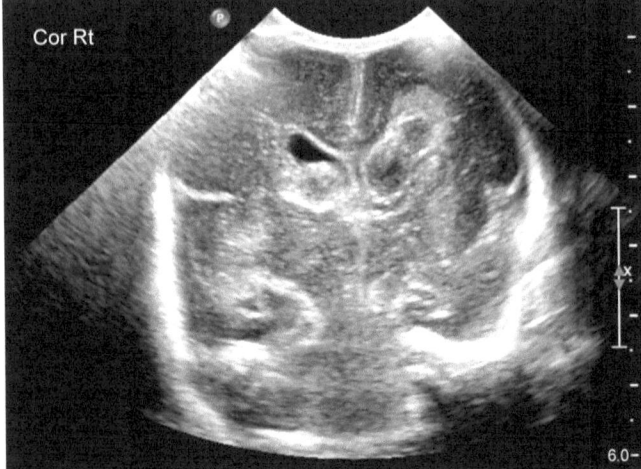

Grade 3 IVH
Intraventricular blood on both sides. Grade 3 IVH (right) and Grade 4 IVH (left).

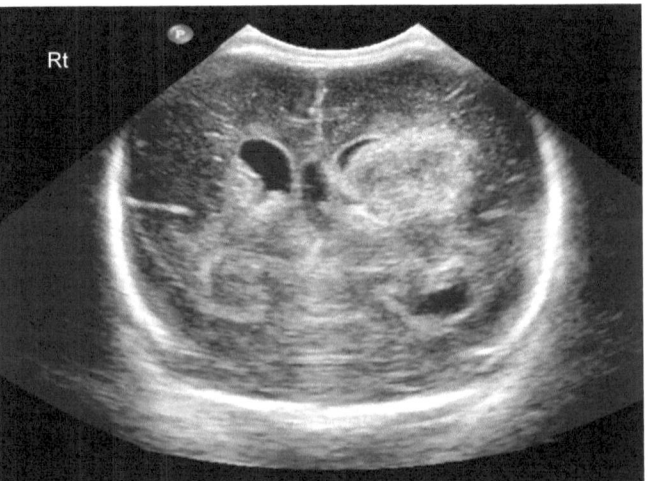

Grade 4 IVH
Grade 4 IVH (left). Patient also has a Grade 3 IVH (right).

**Fig. 6:** *Continued...*

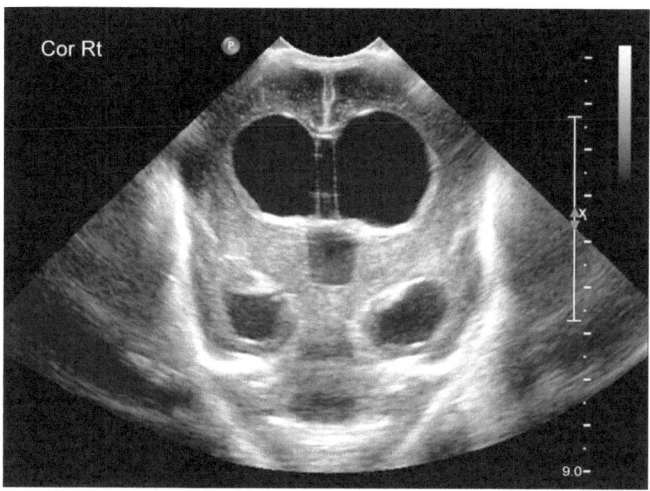

Posthemorrhagic Hydrocephalus.

**Fig. 6:** Examples of grades of IVH.
(CUS: cranial ultrasonography; IVH: intraventricular hemorrhage).
*Courtesy:* Images reprinted with permission from author—Ira Adams Chapman, MD Emory University.

## Prevention Studies

Effective IVH prevention strategies prevent premature birth. Various therapies have been studied, hoping to modify IVH risk. Intercenter variation in IVH prevalence suggests that modifiable factors exist and, if better understood, may result in development of "best practice" measures. Of the pharmacologic agents proposed, none has proven conclusively to decrease IVH risk.

Phenobarbital at one time was considered as an available agent to prevent IVH by stabilizing blood pressure and decreasing free radical-induced injury. A systematic review of published data concluded that phenobarbital does not decrease IVH in preterm infants and therefore is not appropriate for the prevention of IVH in clinical practice.[44]

Indomethacin, a nonspecific COX inhibitor, results in decreased production of prostaglandin synthesis and is thought to prevent IVH by stabilizing blood pressure and promoting microvasculature maturation. Recent evidence suggests that indomethacin may indeed be pathologic because it blocks COX activity, resulting in decreased production of prostaglandin E2, known to be neuroprotective.[24,45] In contrast, other studies have shown that indomethacin may be neuroprotective both by preventing the upregulation of genes linked to oxidative stress and also by downregulating the production of various inflammatory mediators known to be damaging to the developing CNS, including IL-6 and TNF-α.[46] To further complicate the role of this agent in neuroprotection, there are two different genetic polymorphisms that regulate COX-2 activity, therefore individual medication response may be modified by genetic predisposition.[45] It is unclear why decreased risk of IVH has not translated to improved ND outcome in preterm infants exposed to indomethacin.[47] Analysis of data from early indomethacin trials found

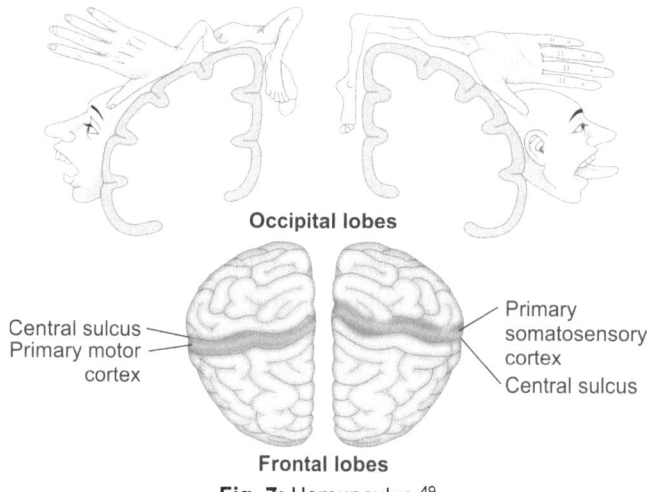

**Fig. 7:** Homunculus.[49]

that males exposed to indomethacin had a lower rate of neonatal IVH, and at school age they performed better on the Peabody Picture Vocabulary Test-R at age of 3, 4, 6, and 8 years;[48] thus gender is important in the complex paradigm related to indomethacin exposure, IVH, and ND outcome.

## Intraventricular Hemorrhage and Neurodevelopmental Outcome

Preterm IVH has long been recognized as a risk factor for adverse ND outcome; this risk varies inversely with GA and birthweight. Severity of hemorrhage is associated with worse outcomes. The topography of structural injury to the brain, particularly seen with severe grades 3 and 4 IVH, typically correlates with abnormal findings on clinical examination. The homunculus pictorially represents localization of function in the human brain (**Fig. 7**). Injury to vulnerable regions in the motor and somatosensory stripes is consistent with patterns of described neurologic

**TABLE 4:** Neurodevelopmental outcomes by grade of IVH and shunt status.

|  | No IVH/No Shunt N = 5163 | Grade 3 IVH/No Shunt N = 459 | Grade 3 IVH/Shunt N = 103 | Grade 4 IVH/No Shunt N = 311 | Grade 4 IVH/Shunt N = 125 |
|---|---|---|---|---|---|
| Median MDI | 82 | 75 | 61 | 72 | 50 |
| Median PDI | 87 | 82 | 51 | 75 | 49 |
| CP | 10% | 23% | 57% | 37% | 80% |
| NDI | 35% | 55% | 78% | 63% | 92% |

Neurodevelopmental outcomes of ELBW infants in the NRN evaluated at 18 months adjusted age using the BSID-II. All outcomes were statistically significantly different between grade 3 with or without shunt compared to No IVH/No Shunt and also between grade 4 with or without shunt compared to No IVH/No Shunt.[26]
(CP: cerebral palsy; IVH: intraventricular hemorrhage; MDI: mental developmental index; NDI: neurodevelopmental impairment; PDI: psychomotor developmental index; ELBW: extremely low birth weight; BSID-II: Bayley Scale of Infant Development; NRN: Neonatal Research Network).

abnormalities in extremely low gestational age newborns (ELGANs) (<29 weeks), including spasticity often involving the lower extremities (diplegia) and abnormal sensory responsiveness and hypersensitivity.

Historically, clinicians assumed that lower grades of IVH were not associated with adverse ND outcomes. Recently, data have shown that the risk for adverse outcome is increased by the presence of even a low-grade IVH.

Infants with severe grade 3 or 4 IVH have the highest risk for adverse ND outcome. Comparing those with severe grade 3 and 4 IVH with and without shunt insertion to those with no IVH **(Table 4)**, follow-up evaluation used the BSID-II administered at 2 years adjusted age. With each increasing grade of severity of CNS injury, there was a comparable decrease in the BSID-II score, with the worst outcome for those with grade 4 IVH requiring a shunt. Interestingly, a small but significant percentage (12%) of those with severe IVH (with or without shunt) tested within normal limits on the Bayley assessment at 18 months adjusted age. Those with normal outcomes were more likely to be female, have no evidence of PVL on CUS and have normal growth parameters at the 18-month follow-up visit.[26]

Serial measurements of head circumference and ventricle size using CUS are recommended to identify children with severe IVH who progress to develop PHH. Of those who develop hydrocephalus early in the process, 20–30% have arrest of dilatation and never require shunt insertion. The need and timing for a ventricular diversion should be discussed in consultation with a pediatric neurosurgeon. The neurosurgical community is actively researching various alternatives for PHH management.

In an Austrian cohort of ELGANs (<29 weeks) born 23–28 weeks of GA, outcomes were evaluated at 2–3 years of age in relationship to abnormalities noted on CUS.[50] Those with grade 3–4 IVH had highest risk of adverse outcome and neurodevelopmental impairment (NDI). Those with Grade 1–2 IVH had a higher rate of neurosensory impairment compared to those without IVH [neurosensory impairment (22% vs. 12.1%), developmental delay (7.8% vs. 3.4%), CP (10.4% vs. 6.5%), and deafness (6.0% vs. 2.3%)]. These differences persisted after excluding those with CUS evidence of PVL. Newborns with Grade 1–2 IVH had a higher rate of adverse ND outcome compared to those without IVH, this risk being modified inversely with GA.[51]

A multicenter collaborative evaluation of outcomes of a cohort of ELGANs reported ND outcomes:[52] 1,064 ELGANs born 2002–2004 who survived to the age of 2 years were evaluated using a standardized neurologic examination and the BSID-II. Severe IVH was strongly correlated with WMI, as 41% of those with IVH also had WMI. Adverse outcomes were most closely associated with WMI rather than IVH alone. The extent of WMI using MRI was not available for this cohort.

A US study with both early and late CUS and an MRI near term reported ND outcomes at 2 years from 480 ELGANs.[34] Subjects had an early CUS performed day of life 4–14, a late CUS performed 35–42 weeks postmenstrual age (PMA) and MRI performed 35–42 weeks PMA. In addition, a standardized neurological examination was performed and the cognitive scales of the BSID-III were administered by certified investigators. Approximately 10% of the cohort had severe grade 3–4 IVH or cystic PVL on the early CUS and 5.8% had significant abnormalities noted on the late CUS. In contrast, 19.3% had some evidence of white matter abnormalities (WMA) on the near-term MRI. MRI detected cerebellar injury in 16.2%, higher than the CUS detection rate. In multivariable models, both late CUS and MRI, but not early CUS, were independently associated with NDI or death [MRI cerebellar lesions: OR, 3.0 (95% CI: 1.3–6.8); late CUS: OR, 9.8 (95% CI: 2.8–35)]. Those with abnormalities on late CUS or WMA were at increased risk for significant gross motor impairment. While medical decision-making is often based on severe abnormalities noted on early CUS, these findings have limited positive predictive value for

**TABLE 5:** Neurodevelopmental outcomes by MRI findings of NRN NEURO cohort.[34]

| ND Outcome at 18–22 months | Mild WMA N = 261 | Moderate WMA N = 68 | Severe WMA N = 18 | P value |
|---|---|---|---|---|
| Cognitive score Mean ± SD | 92.6 (13.1) | 89.9 (15.3) | 77.7 (14.5) | <0.05 |
| Cognitive score <70 | 4.3% | 10.5% | 22.2% | 0.011 |
| Any CP | 5.5% | 5.9% | 61.1% | <0.05 |
| Mod/Severe CP | 1.2% | 1.5% | 50% | <0.05 |
| Death/NDI | 9.4% | 15.5% | 65% | <0.05 |

(CP: cerebral palsy; MRI: magnetic resonance imaging; NDI: neurodevelopmental impairment; WMA: white matter abnormalities; SD: standard deviation; NRN: Neonatal Research Network).

risk of death or adverse outcome at age of 2 years. These data should be interpreted cautiously because outcomes may have been biased by the study design which required antenatal consent; therefore, some high-risk patients with CNS injury may have been excluded from the analysis. However, among those enrolled, only late CUS or abnormalities on a near-term MRI predicted outcome at age of 2 years, noting that 74% of the prediction in these multivariate models was contributed by neonatal and perinatal variables. Thus, the relative value of preterm birth prevention in improving neonatal outcomes is underscored. ND outcomes at 2 years are presented in **Table 5**. Although prediction improves with the use of MRI, the presence of abnormalities on MRI is not always associated with adverse outcomes. Among those with moderate WMA on MRI, only 5.9% had any CP and 1.5% had moderate or severe CP. Only severe WMA was more strongly correlated with adverse outcomes at age of 2 years.

## NEUROIMAGING

While CUS is clearly advantageous, recent evidence shows that CUS alone underestimates both cerebellar injury and WMI, particularly noncystic WMI. CUS remains the standard of care for routine screening of preterm CNS injury. As we continue to better understand the differential predictive value on long-term ND outcome associated with MRI findings, these guidelines are subject to change. All studies to date have examined the relationship between near-term MRI abnormalities and long-term ND outcome. It is unclear how these findings would correlate with MRI studies obtained at earlier GAs when the information could assist decision-making and goals of care.

## WHITE MATTER INJURY/PERIVENTRICULAR LEUKOMALACIA

Advanced neuroimaging, including MRI of the brain, has improved our understanding of newborn brain development while enhancing our ability to identify WMI. Traditional CUS has limited ability to detect small cystic areas in the periventricular white matter and is unable to identify noncystic diffuse WMI. In contrast, MRI detects and quantifies WMI, even in the very premature brain. Macrostructural injury, including IVH and cerebellar hemorrhage, is readily identified by MRI. Volumetric measurements in various regions of the brain (including the white matter), while possible with MRI, are not widely available.

## White Matter Injury and Magnetic Resonance Imaging

Preterm WMI can be the result of infection, inflammation or ischemia.[22] Classic cystic PVL represents cystic degeneration of both glial and axonal cell lines. These cysts are typically >1 mm. In contrast, microcystic (<1 mm) necrosis is more common in preterm WMI (*see* **Fig. 7**). These microcystic lesions, while not evident on CUS, are visualized on neuropathology. It is unclear how microcystic lesions contribute to long-term neurologic outcome in preterm infants. Diffuse WMI is the form of CNS injury most commonly encountered in contemporary cohorts and is typically associated with injury to the preoligodendroglia with relative sparing of the axons.[22] These lesions are readily seen on MRI of the brain and are reported in up to one-third of preterm infants. It is speculated that these structural abnormalities are further compounded by microstructural disruption in brain development (i.e. abnormal fractional anisotropy) (**Figs. 8A and B**).

Magnetic resonance imaging studies were performed in 89 preterm infants at median age 32 weeks adjusted age and repeated near-term in a subset of this cohort. The BSID-II was administered at 18 months adjusted age. Abnormal outcome was associated with increasing severity of WMI, ventriculomegaly, and IVH on MRI, as well as moderate/severe abnormalities on the first [relative risk (RR) = 5.6; P = 0.002] and second MRI studies (RR = 5.3; P = 0.03).[53]

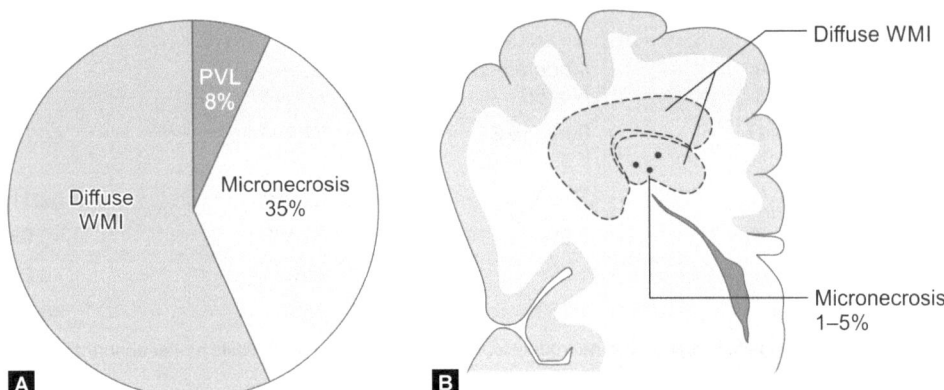

**Figs. 8A and B:** Types of WMI in preterm neonates. (A) Pie chart showing the approximate relative percentages of human diffuse WMI, cystic periventricular leukomalacia (PVL), and microscopic necrosis. (B) Schematic diagram showing the relative burden of human microcysts (dots) relative to diffuse WMI (within dotted lines), which typically comprises >80% of the total burden of WMI. Modified and adapted from Back and Miller.[22]
(WMI: white matter injury).

An evaluation of 167 preterm infants using MRI at term equivalent and ND evaluations at age of 2 years[54] identified moderate/severe WMA in 21% of this cohort, findings correlated with an increased risk of CP at 2 years. These investigators also evaluated neurocognitive performance at 4 years and 6 years in a preterm cohort.[35] There were no differences in outcomes between preterms with a normal MRI and term controls. However, abnormalities in the white matter correlated with abnormalities in neurocognitive performance and executive functioning at both 4 years and 6 years of age.

## Cerebellar Injury and Magnetic Resonance Imaging

Cerebellar injury is more readily identified by MRI than CUS.[34] In the NRN evaluation of 445 preterm infants who had neuroimaging with both CUS and MRI near term, only 7 infants had evidence of cerebellar lesions on early or late CUS compared to 72 (16%) infants identified with cerebellar lesions on MRI.[54] Visualization through a mastoid window improves imaging of the posterior fossa when using CUS. This study found that at age of 2 years significant cerebellar lesions independently predicted the composite outcome of death and/or NDI; or death and/or significant gross motor impairment. Another study[55] evaluated ND outcomes of a preterm cohort at 32 months adjusted age that had evidence of either isolated cerebellar hemorrhage and/or cerebellar hemorrhage associated with IVH, to children in a control group with normal imaging. Neurologic abnormalities were noted in 62% of those with isolated cerebellar hemorrhage compared to 5% in the control group. Affected children had lower scores in all domains evaluated including gross motor, cognitive, language, and functional skills. Interestingly, these children were more likely to have abnormalities on the Modified Checklist for Autism in Toddlers (M-CHAT) and also were more likely to demonstrate internalizing behaviors. Hypotonia with severe gross motor impairment was a common neurologic finding in this population. The cerebellum is known to be important for coordination and recent studies have suggested that it may also be important in cognitive function, language development, and social skills. The impact of cerebellar injury on long-term ND outcome of preterm children is unclear but likely critical. In other studies, investigators have also shown that cerebellar volumes are lower in preterm infants compared to term controls.[56,57] These differences are magnified when cerebellar hemorrhage accompanies IVH.

## REFERENCES

1. Barrington KJ. The adverse neuro-developmental effects of postnatal steroids in the preterm infant: a systematic review of RCTs. BMC Pediatr. 2001;1:1.
2. Lopez AD, Mathers CD, Ezzati M, et al. Measuring the global burden of disease and risk factors, 1990–2001. In: Lopez AD, Mathers CD, Ezzati M, Jamison DT, Murray CJ (Eds). Global Burden of Disease and Risk Factors. Washington (DC): The International Bank for Reconstruction and Development/The World Bank; New York: Oxford University Press; 2006.
3. Millennium Development Goals. 2016. [online] Available from: http://www.un.org/millenniumgoals/. [Last accessed September, 2019].
4. Wang H, Liddell CA, Coates MM, et al. Global, regional, and national levels of neonatal, infant, and under-5 mortality during 1990–2013: a systematic analysis for the Global Burden of Disease Study 2013. Lancet. 2014;384(9947):957-79.
5. Anderson RN. Deaths: leading causes for 1999. Natl Vital Stat Rep. 2001;49(11):1-87.
6. Romero R, Gomez R, Ghezzi F, et al. A fetal systemic inflammatory response is followed by the spontaneous onset of preterm parturition. Am J Obstet Gynecol. 1998;179(1):186-93.

7. Yoon BH, Park CW, Chaiworapongsa T. Intrauterine infection and the development of cerebral palsy. BJOG. 2003;110(Suppl 20):124-7.
8. Pappas A, Kendrick DE, Shankaran S, et al. Eunice Kennedy Shriver National Institute of Child Health and Human Development Neonatal Research Network. Chorioamnionitis and early childhood outcomes among extremely low-gestational-age neonates. JAMA Pediatr. 2014;168(2):137-47.
9. Andrews WW, Cliver SP, Biasini F, et al. Early preterm birth: association between in utero exposure to acute inflammation and severe neurodevelopmental disability at 6 years of age. Am J Obstet Gynecol. 2008;198(4):466.e1-466.e11.
10. van Vliet EO, de Kieviet JF, Oosterlaan J, et al. Perinatal infections and neurodevelopmental outcome in very preterm and very low-birth-weight infants: A meta-analysis. JAMA Pediatr. 2013;167(7):662-8.
11. Edmond KM, Kortsalioudaki C, Scott S, et al. Group B streptococcal disease in infants aged younger than 3 months: systematic review and meta-analysis. Lancet. 2012;379(9815):547-56.
12. Dagnew AF, Cunnington MC, Dube Q, et al. Variation in reported neonatal group B streptococcal disease incidence in developing countries. Clin Infect Dis. 2012;55(1):91-102.
13. Centers for Disease Control and Prevention. 2016. [online] Available from: https://www.cdc.gov/. [Last accessed September, 2019].
14. Group B Streptococcal Infections. In: Larry KP (Ed.). Red Book. Illinois: American Academy of Pediatrics; 2012. pp. 680-5.
15. Jordan HT, Farley MM, Craig A, et al. Active Bacterial Core Surveillance (ABCs)/Emerging Infections Program Network, CDC. Revisiting the need for vaccine prevention of late-onset neonatal group B streptococcal disease: a multistate, population-based analysis. Pediatr Infect Dis J. 2008;27(12):1057-64.
16. Libster R, Edwards KM, Levent F, et al. Long-term outcomes of group B streptococcal meningitis. Pediatrics. 2012;130(1):e8-15.
17. Stoll BJ, Hansen NI, Sanchez PJ, et al. Eunice Kennedy Shriver National Institute of Child Health and Human Development Neonatal Research Network. Early onset neonatal sepsis: the burden of group B Streptococcal and E. coli disease continues. Pediatrics. 2011;127(5):817-26.
18. Stoll BJ, Hansen NI, Bell EF, et al. Eunice Kennedy Shriver National Institute of Child Health and Human Development Neonatal Research Network. Trends in care practices, morbidity, and mortality of extremely preterm neonates, 1993-2012. JAMA. 2015;314(10):1039-51.
19. Mitha A, Foix-L'Hélias L, Arnaud C, et al. EPIPAGE Study Group. Neonatal infection and 5-year neurodevelopmental outcome of very preterm infants. Pediatrics. 2013;132(2):e372-80.
20. Stoll BJ, Hansen NI, Adams-Chapman I, et al. National Institute of Child Health and Human Development Neonatal Research Network. Neurodevelopmental and growth impairment among extremely low-birth-weight infants with neonatal infection. JAMA. 2004;292(19):2357-65.
21. Vohr BR, Wright LL, Dusick AM, et al. Neurodevelopmental and functional outcomes of extremely low birth weight infants in the National Institute of Child Health and Human Development Neonatal Research Network, 1993-1994. Pediatrics. 2000;105(6):1216-26.
22. Back SA. Cerebral white and gray matter injury in newborns: new insights into pathophysiology and management. Clin Perinatol. 2014;41(1):1-24.
23. Back SA, Rosenberg PA. Pathophysiology of glia in perinatal white matter injury. Glia. 2014;62(11):1790-815.
24. McCrea HJ, Ment LR. The diagnosis, management and postnatal prevention of intraventricular hemorrhage in the preterm neonate. Clin Perinatol. 2008;35(4):777-92, vii.
25. Centers for Disease Control and Prevention (CDC). Economic costs associated with mental retardation, cerebral palsy, hearing loss, and vision impairment—United States, 2003. MMWR Morb Mortal Wkly Rep. 2004;53(3):57-9.
26. Adams-Chapman I, Hansen NI, Stoll BJ, et al. NICHD Research Network. Neurodevelopmental outcome of extremely low birth weight infants with posthemorrhagic hydrocephalus requiring shunt insertion. Pediatrics. 2008;121(5):e1167-77.
27. Stoll BJ, Hansen NI, Bell EF, et al. Eunice Kennedy Shriver National Institute of Child Health and Human Development Neonatal Research Network. Neonatal outcomes of extremely preterm infants from the NICHD Neonatal Research Network. Pediatrics. 2010;126(3):443-56.
28. Gopel W, Gortner L, Kohlmann T, et al. Low prevalence of large intraventricular haemorrhage in very low birthweight infants carrying the factor V Leiden or prothrombin G20210A mutation. Acta Paediatr. 2001;90(9):1021-4.
29. Harding DR, Dhamrait S, Whitelaw A, et al. Does interleukin-6 genotype influence cerebral injury or developmental progress after preterm birth? Pediatrics. 2004;114(4):941-7.
30. Harding D, Brull D, Humphries SE, et al. Variation in the interleukin-6 gene is associated with impaired cognitive development in children born prematurely: a preliminary study. Pediatr Res. 2005;58(1):117-20.
31. Chao CC, Hu S, Molitor TW, et al. Activated microglia mediate neuronal cell injury via a nitric oxide mechanism. J Immunol. 1992;149(8):2736-41.
32. Schmid MB, Reister F, Mayer B, et al. Prospective risk factor monitoring reduces intracranial hemorrhage rates in preterm infants. Dtsch Arztebl Int. 2013;110(29-30):489-96.
33. Robinson S. Neonatal posthemorrhagic hydrocephalus from prematurity: pathophysiology and current treatment concepts. J Neurosurg Pediatr. 2012;9(3):242-58.
34. Hintz SR, Barnes PD, Bulas D, et al. SUPPORT Study Group of the Eunice Kennedy Shriver National Institute of Child Health and Human Development Neonatal Research Network. Neuroimaging and neurodevelopmental outcome in extremely preterm infants. Pediatrics. 2015;135(1):e32-42.
35. Woodward LJ, Clark CA, Bora S, et al. Neonatal white matter abnormalities an important predictor of neurocognitive outcome for very preterm children. PloS one. 2012;7(12):e51879.
36. Limperopoulos C, Chilingaryan G, Sullivan N, et al. Injury to the premature cerebellum: outcome is related to remote cortical development. Cereb Cortex. 2014;24(3):728-36.
37. Limperopoulos C, Benson CB, Bassan H, et al. Cerebellar hemorrhage in the preterm infant: ultrasonographic findings and risk factors. Pediatrics. 2005;116(3):717-24.
38. Dyet LE, Kennea N, Counsell SJ, et al. Natural history of brain lesions in extremely preterm infants studied with serial magnetic resonance imaging from birth

and neurodevelopmental assessment. Pediatrics. 2006;118(2):536-48.
39. Perlman JM, Volpe JJ. Intraventricular hemorrhage in extremely small premature infants. Am J Dis Child. 1986;140(11):1122-4.
40. Perlman JM, Volpe JJ. Cerebral blood flow velocity in relation to intraventricular hemorrhage in the premature newborn infant. J Pediatr. 1982;100(6):956-9.
41. Leviton A, Pagano M, Kuban KC, et al. The epidemiology of germinal matrix hemorrhage during the first half-day of life. Dev Med Child Neurol. 1991;33(2):138-45.
42. Volpe JJ. Neurology of the Newborn, 5th edition. Philadephia, PA: WB Saunders; 2008.
43. Papile LA, Burstein J, Burstein R, et al. Incidence and evolution of subependymal and intraventricular hemorrhage: a study of infants with birth weights less than 1,500 gm. J Pediatr. 1978;92(4):529-34.
44. Whitelaw A, Odd D. Postnatal phenobarbital for the prevention of intraventricular hemorrhage in preterm infants. Cochrane Database Syst Rev. 2007;(4):CD001691.
45. Harding DR, Humphries SE, Whitelaw A, et al. Cognitive outcome and cyclo-oxygenase-2 gene (-765 G/C) variation in the preterm infant. Arch Dis Child Fetal Neonatal Ed. 2007;92(2):F108-12.
46. Monje ML, Toda H, Palmer TD. Inflammatory blockade restores adult hippocampal neurogenesis. Science. 2003;302(5651):1760-5.
47. Fowlie PW, Davis PG. Prophylactic indomethacin for preterm infants: a systematic review and meta-analysis. Arch Dis Child Fetal Neonatal Ed. 2003;88(6):F464-6.
48. Ment LR, Vohr BR, Makuch RW, et al. Prevention of intraventricular hemorrhage by indomethacin in male preterm infants. J Pediatr. 2004;145(6):832-4.
49. Porter R. Merck Manual Professional Version (Known as the Merck Manual in US and Canada and the MSD, NJ: Merck Sharp & Dohme Corp.; 2016. Manual in the Rest of the World), Kenilworth. Available from: https://www.merckmanuals.com/professional/neurologic-disorders/function-and-dysfunction-of-the-cerebral-lobes/overview-of-cerebral-function. [Last accessed September, 2019].
50. Bolisetty S, Dhawan A, Abdel-Latif M, et al. New South Wales and Australian Capital Territory Neonatal Intensive Care Units' Data Collection. Intraventricular hemorrhage and neurodevelopmental outcomes in extreme preterm infants. Pediatrics. 2014;133(1):55-62.
51. Klebermass-Schrehof K, Czaba C, Olischar M, et al. Impact of low-grade intraventricular hemorrhage on long-term neurodevelopmental outcome in preterm infants. Childs Nerv Syst. 2012;28(12):2085-92.
52. O'Shea TM, Allred EN, Kuban KC, et al. ELGAN Study Investigators. Intraventricular hemorrhage and developmental outcomes at 24 months of age in extremely preterm infants. J Child Neurol. 2012;27(1):22-9.
53. Miller SP, Ferriero DM, Leonard C, et al. Early brain injury in premature newborns detected with magnetic resonance imaging is associated with adverse early neurodevelopmental outcome. J Pediatr. 2005;147(5):609-16.
54. Woodward LJ, Anderson PJ, Austin NC, et al. Neonatal MRI to predict neurodevelopmental outcomes in preterm infants. N Engl J Med. 2006;355(7):685-94.
55. Limperopoulos C, Bassan H, Gauvreau K, et al. Does cerebellar injury in premature infants contribute to the high prevalence of long-term cognitive, learning, and behavioral disability in survivors? Pediatrics. 2007;120(3):584-93.
56. Limperopoulos C, Soul JS, Haidar H, et al. Impaired trophic interactions between the cerebellum and the cerebrum among preterm infants. Pediatrics. 2005;116(4):844-50.
57. Limperopoulos C, Soul JS, Gauvreau K, et al. Late gestation cerebellar growth is rapid and impeded by premature birth. Pediatrics. 2005;115(3):688-95.

# CHAPTER 33

# Late Preterm Infants, Cerebral Palsy, and Hypoxic-Ischemic Encephalopathy

Ira Adams-Chapman

## ABSTRACT

Specific neonatal conditions are associated with an increased risk of adverse long term outcomes. This section reviews neurodevelopmental outcomes in the late preterm. We will also present the neurologic outcomes of term newborns with cerebral palsy and hypoxic-ischemic encephalopathy. Developmental evaluations and early intervention are discussed.

## LATE PRETERM INFANTS

Late preterm infants (LPIs) (34 0/7-36 6/7 weeks gestational age, or GA) are a population at risk for adverse neurodevelopment. Human brain development is an active and dynamic process that continues throughout gestation. Half of cortical volume increase occurs between 34 weeks and 40 weeks GA.[1] Animal studies defining which cell lineages are present at specific points in the developing central nervous system (CNS) have improved understanding of the maturational vulnerability of the developing brain even in the LPI.

Subcortical neurons are present as early as 10 weeks gestation and cell number peaks at 22-35 weeks gestation. Neuronal proliferation continues until 24 weeks and remains incomplete prior to term gestation. Brain weight and volume increase in a linear fashion throughout gestation. At 34 weeks, brain weight is ~65% of that at term.[1-3] Dendritic connections become more complex and extend into the deeper layers of the brain with increasing GA. Disruption to any of these developing pathways can result in disruption in neuronal connectivity. Although growth is somewhat linear, brain development and maturation is nonlinear and many critical processes occur during the last 6 weeks of gestation. Gyral and sulcal formation are incomplete in the LPI (**Fig. 1**).

Unmyelinated white matter fibers predominate in early gestation.[4] By mid-gestation, there are equal amounts of myelinated and unmyelinated fibers. These

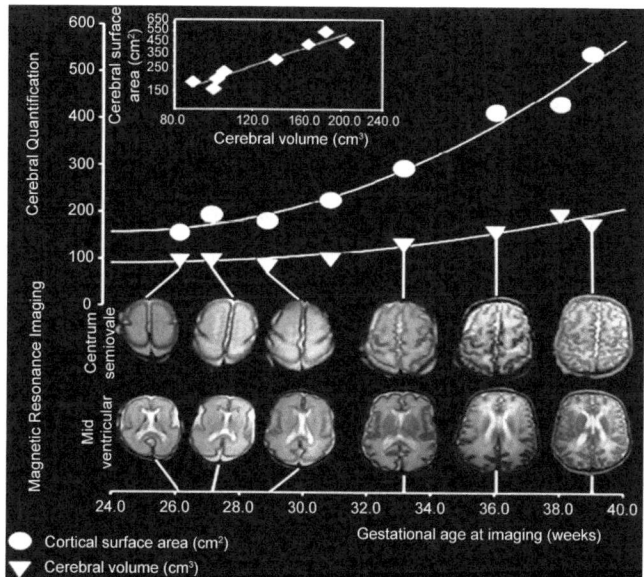

**Fig. 1:** Maturational changes in brain volumes and complexity with increasing GA. Reprinted with permission. Changes in brain volume and maturation with increasing GA.[3]
(GA: gestational age).

preoligodendrocytes are uniquely vulnerable to cytotoxic injury secondary to infection or ischemia. Myelinated white matter increases fivefold between 30 weeks and 40 weeks gestation; the very active nature of white matter development creates a zone of vulnerability for injury during this GA. Historically, cystic periventricular leukomalacia (PVL) was the most common type of white matter injury (WMI), but in contemporary preterm cohorts diffuse microcystic WMI is the most common form of injury.[5] Current evidence suggests that microstructural injury to developing preterm white and gray matter results in disruption of glial progenitor cells and neurons,[5] initiating a cascade of aberrant repair and regeneration that produces a glial pool that fails to differentiate and myelinate normally. This apparent "arrested development" creates dysmature preterm neuronal cells, with altered response to subsequent hypoxic or inflammatory insult.

Late preterm infants account for 74% of all preterm infants.[6] Since the majority of these neonates are asymptomatic, it was assumed that they were at low risk for neurologic complications. Thus, this population was not systematically evaluated over time for risk of intraventricular hemorrhage (IVH) or long-term neurodevelopmental difficulties. Statewide school readiness evaluations indicate that late preterm children are more likely to require special needs services at school entry.[7-9] Since these early reports, numerous studies report increased neurocognitive risk, behavior problems, and need for special education services in LPI compared to term controls.[7,8,10] Kugelman equates the effect as a "disruption of the maturational trajectory of the system" during a critical window in brain development **(Table 1)**.[10]

The overwhelming majority of LPI is not followed in neurodevelopmental follow-up programs, thus providers should have a lower index of suspicion and refer at-risk patients with any concerns of delayed developmental milestones or difficulty with school performance. The parents of LPI should be appropriately counseled regarding future risks of developmental delay. Similarly, educators should be aware of the current literature and risk for difficulties with school performance and behavior in these children as they approach school age. Registry and surveillance data regarding school performance should enhance understanding of developmental delay in this population. From a public health perspective, the magnitude of the impact is huge given that LPI represents a large proportion of live births.

# CEREBRAL PALSY

Cerebral palsy (CP) is defined as a nonprogressive neurologic disorder associated with abnormalities in tone and/or posture affecting motor function. CP is the most common cause of motor disability in children worldwide, affecting 2-3 per 1,000 live births.[18-20] Overall rates have remained somewhat stable over time. The absolute risk of CP is higher among at-risk populations, including children with birth defects, history of premature birth, or birth asphyxia **(Fig. 2)**. There is a strong inverse relationship

**TABLE 1:** Long-term neurodevelopmental outcomes of LPI.

| Reference | Study design | Participants | Main outcomes |
|---|---|---|---|
| Chyi et al.[11] | Retrospective | 767 LPI/13,671 term | Increased risk for below-average reading competence at all grade levels, increased need for individualized education program at early school ages and increased need for special education |
| Gray et al.[12] | Prospective | 260 LPI/General population | Increased rate of behavior problems at age of 8 years |
| Huddy et al.[13] | Retrospective | 83 LPI | Increased rate of hyperactivity, behavioral or emotional problems |
| Woythaler et al.[14] | Prospective | 1,200 LPI/6,300 term | Increased risk of mental or physical developmental delay at 24 months |
| Morse et al.[8] | Retrospective | 7,152 LPI/152,661 term | Increased risk for developmental delay or school-related problems through age of 5 years |
| Lipkind et al.[15] | Retrospective | 13,207 LPI/199,599 term | Increased need for special education and lower adjusted Math and English scores at school age. Linear association between GA and test scores through 39 weeks |
| Quigley et al.[7] | Retrospective | 537 LPI/6,159 term | Increased risk of poorer educational achievement at 5 years |
| Talge et al.[16] | Retrospective | 168 LPI/168 term | Increased risk of behavior problems and lower IQ at 6 years |
| Gurka et al.[17] | Prospective | 55 LPI/1,245 term | No difference in cognitive, achievement, behavior, and social and emotional development in early childhood |

Summary of published outcomes of LPI. Revised and reprinted with permission.[10]
(GA: gestational age; IQ: intelligence quotient; LPI: late preterm infants).

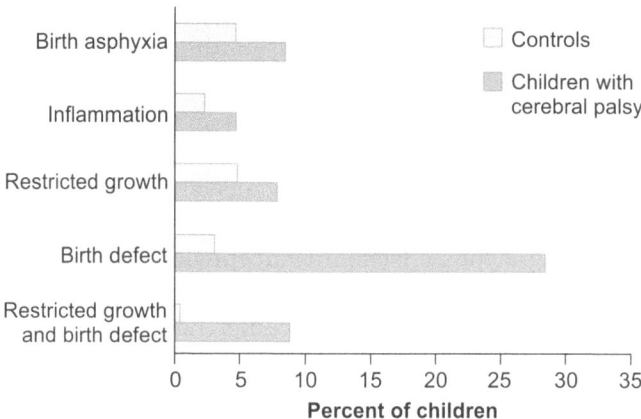

**Fig. 2:** Distribution of four major risk factors in singleton children with CP born at GA of at least 35 weeks, 1980–1995.
(CP: cerebral palsy; GA: gestational age).
*Source:* Reprinted with permission. Data are from a study of 496 children with CP and 508 controls. The four risk factors were a potentially asphyxiating intrapartum event, evidence of inflammation, fetal growth restriction (defined as birth weight >2 standard deviations below the optimal weight for gestation, sex, maternal height, and parity, or a neonatal diagnosis of fetal growth restriction), and a major birth defect. One or more of these risk factors exists in at least 2% of children with CP or controls. Major birth defects were the most frequently occurring risk factor in children with CP, and when combined with fetal growth restriction, they were associated with the highest risk ratio (RR).[21]

between GA and CP. Improved neonatal care has led to slight decreases in CP rates among preterm children; however, their absolute risk remains significantly higher than term infants. Prematurity is responsible for ~35% of CP.

While CP is 40 times more prevalent in preterm infants compared to term, two-thirds of children with CP are born >37 weeks GA.[21] Although emergency and elective cesarean delivery rates have increased exponentially over the past decade, in large part in response to fetal heart rate abnormality detection and concern for asphyxia, the prevalence rate for CP has remained unchanged in term infants. Despite concern that many cases of CP were secondary to perinatal events or asphyxia, more recent evidence suggests that most causes are due to other prenatal factors **(Fig. 2)**. The most common antecedents to CP in singleton term infants are disordered developmental processes, including birth defects, placental abnormalities, intrauterine growth restriction, and genetic mutations.[21] Advanced genetic testing, including whole exome sequencing, now permits identification of various genetic point mutations and polymorphisms associated with increased CP risk. The role of prenatal inflammation remains unclear but likely contributory. Understanding the causal pathway is further compounded by the knowledge that children with CNS abnormalities and birth defects have increased asphyxia risk. The Perinatal Collaborative Project reported that 35% of children with birth asphyxia had a major malformation and 12% had neonatal seizures.[22]

While CP is defined by motor dysfunction, many affected patients also exhibit intellectual disability, visual impairment, and language delay.[23] In the review from Surveillance of Cerebral Palsy in Europe (SCPE), 30% were nonambulatory, 31% had severe intellectual impairment, 11% had severe visual impairment, and 20% had an active seizure disorder.[18] Although there is often congruence between severity of motor and mental disability, children with CP may have relative sparing of cognition. At 2.5 years of age, 35% of children had more delayed motor function than mental function based on performance on the Bayley Scale of Infant Development (BSID)-II Mental Developmental Index (MDI).[24]

Cerebral palsy classification can be challenging, particularly at very young ages. In the first year of life, many children exhibit significant motor dysfunction which improves over time, leading to recommendations to delay a formal diagnosis of CP until age of 2 years, particularly in those with mild motor dysfunction. There are a variety of systems that can be used to classify the type and severity of CP. These include systems based on severity of CP (mild, moderate or severe); topography/site of involvement (i.e. quadriplegia or hemiplegia), and motor tone (spastic or nonspastic). There are various subtypes for each form of CP. The classification system used by the SCPE is outlined in **Flowchart 1**.

Functional impairment of motor performance can be quantified using a Gross Motor Function Classification Score (GMFCS).[26] **Table 2** describes the recommended algorithm before and after age of 2 years.[27] For clinical trials, CP severity is often stratified based on the GMFCS, with Levels 2 and 3 considered moderate and ≥ Level 4 severe. This highlights the importance of a thorough evaluation of all developmental domains so that cognition is not underestimated in this population.

Tenacious and timely evaluation of epidemiologic trends in CP prevalence rates is necessary as neonatal care improves. The risk profile is likely to shift over time and it is essential to understand which neonatal morbidities are contributing disproportionately to CP. Large collaborative networks across centers are important to avoid ascertainment bias toward children cared for in larger centers.

## DEVELOPMENTAL EVALUATION

Developmental milestones appear in a very predictable pattern over time. Various standardized developmental assessment tools allow healthcare providers to evaluate childhood developmental trajectory **(Table 3)**. Childhood developmental progression mirrors CNS maturation over time. Commercially available developmental screening instruments vary in complexity from self-administered parent questionnaires to formal assessments administered by an advanced level trained professional. Each instrument has advantages and limitations, and thus selection should be tailored to the appropriate clinical setting. Neuropsychological testing can be performed by trained examiners that will assess intelligence quotient (IQ), executive function, and other behavioral measures. Examples include The Wechsler Intelligence Scale for Children (WISC), which is an intelligence test for children between the ages of 6 years and 16 years; The Stanford-Binet Intelligence Scale, an intelligence test for ages of 2 years through adulthood; and the Neuropsychological Assessment (NEPSY), frequently used to evaluate executive function. The Movement Assessment Battery for Children (Movement ABC) identifies motor impairment in children aged 3–16 years and is useful in diagnosing Developmental Coordination Disorder.

The child's development should be evaluated in all domains to allow thorough assessment of functional status. Disturbance in appropriate developmental progression may be the result of focal injury (e.g. CNS infarction) or global insult (e.g. hypoxic-ischemic encephalopathy or HIE). Children may exhibit abnormalities in one or all domains of developmental functioning. A comprehensive evaluation must include cognition, gross and fine motor function, language, and personal/social skills. Developmental performance may betray underlying neuropathology. While a quantitative assessment of developmental progress compared to age-expected norms is important, it is equally important to evaluate the quality and manner in which the child performs the various tasks.

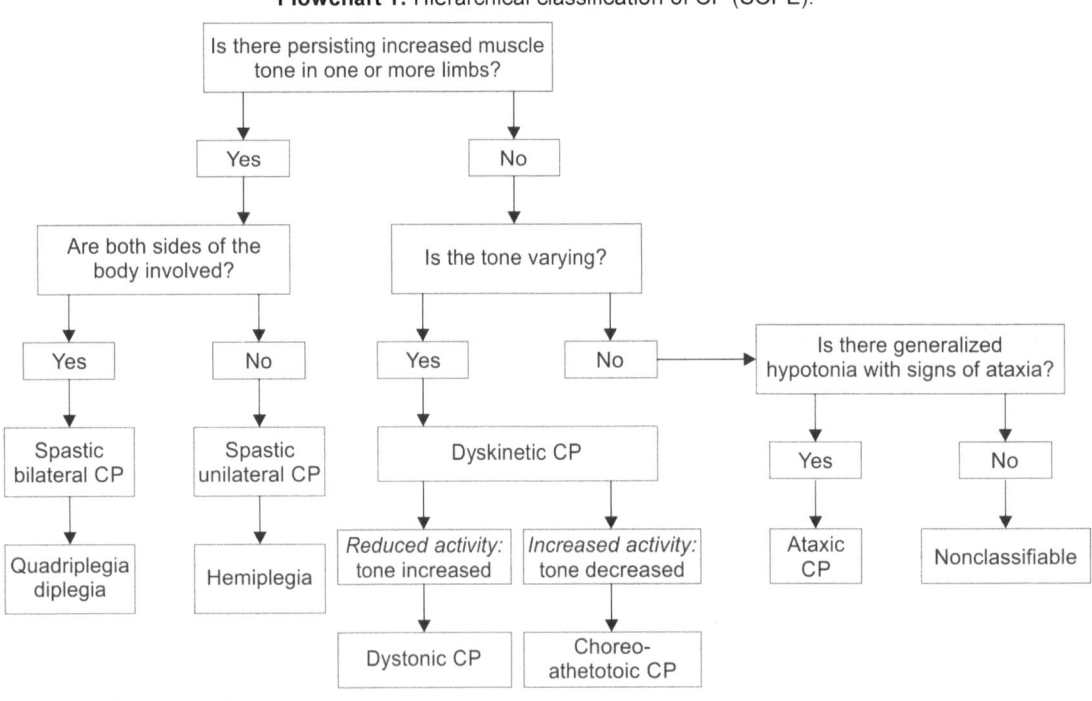

**Flowchart 1:** Hierarchical classification of CP (SCPE).

(CP: cerebral palsy; SCPE: surveillance of cerebral palsy in Europe).
*Source:* Reprinted with permission.[25]

| | **TABLE 2:** GMFCS criteria before and after the age of 2 years. | |
|---|---|---|
| Table II: Age-specific age band of the gross motor function classification system levels I to V | | |
| | *Before 2nd birthday* | *Between 2nd and 4th birthday* |
| Level I | Infants move in and out of sitting and floor sit with both hands free to manipulate objects. Infants crawl on hands and knees, pull to stand, and take steps holding on to furniture. Infants walk between 18 months and 2 years of age without the need for any assistive mobility device. | Children floor sit with both hands free to manipulate objects. Movements in and out floor sit are performed without adult assistance. Children walk as the preferred method of mobility without the need for any assistive mobility device. |

*Contd...*

*Contd...*

*Table II: Age-specific age band of the gross motor function classification system levels I to V*

| | Before 2nd birthday | Between 2nd and 4th birthday |
|---|---|---|
| Level II | Infants maintain floor sitting but may need to use their hands for support to maintain balance. Infants creep on their stomach or crawl on hands and knees. Infants may pull to stand and take steps holding on to furniture. | Children floor sit but may have difficulty with balance when both hands are free to manipulate objects. Movements in and out of sitting are performed without adult assistance. Children pull to stand on a stable surface. Children crawl on hands and knees with a reciprocal pattern, cruise holding onto furniture and walk using an assistive mobility device as preferred method of mobility. |
| Level III | Infants maintain floor sitting when the low back is supported. Infants roll and creep forward on their stomachs. | Children maintain floor sitting often by 'W-sitting' (sitting between flexed and internally rotated hips and knees) and may require adult assistance to assume sitting. Children creep on their stomach or crawl on hands and knees (often without reciprocal leg movements) as their primary methods of self-mobility. Children may pull to stand on a stable surface and cruise short distances. Children may walk short distances indoors using an assistive mobility device and adult assistance for steering and turning. |
| Level IV | Infants have head control but trunk support is required for floor sitting. Infants can roll to supine and may roll to prone. | Children floor sit when placed, but are unable to maintain alignment and balance without use of their hands for support. Children frequently require adaptive equipment for sitting and standing. Selfmobility for short distances (within a room) is achieved through rolling, creeping on stomach, or crawling on hands and knees without reciprocal leg movement. |
| Level V | Physical impairments limit voluntary control of movement. Infants ate unable to maintain antigravity head and trunk postures in prone and sitting. Infants require adult assistance to roll. | Physical impairments restrict voluntary control of movement and the ability to maintain antigravity head and trunk postures. All areas of motor function are limited. Functional limitations in sitting and standing are not fully compensated for through the use of adaptive equipment and assistive technology. At Level V, children have no means of independent mobility and are transported. Some children achieve self-mobility using a power wheelchair with extensive adaptations. |

(GMFCS: gross motor function classification score).
*Source:* Reprinted with permission.[27]

**TABLE 3:** Developmental screening tools.

| Developmental screening tool | Age range | Administration | Items | Advantages/Disadvantages |
|---|---|---|---|---|
| Ages and stages Questionnaire (ASQ 3rd edition) | 4–60 months | 10–15 minutes Parent report English/Spanish/French | 30 | • 0.70–0.90 sensitivity; 0.76–0.9 specificity<br>• Easy to score<br>• Normed in 2008 on diverse ethnic and SES background<br>• Risk categorization in five domains to indicate need for further screening |
| Battelle Developmental Inventory Screening Tool (BDI-ST) | 1–95 months | 10–15 minutes < 3 years old or 20–30 minutes > 3 years old Some special training required | 100 | • Sensitivity 0.72–0.94; specificity 0.72–0.93<br>• Normed in 2,500 children based on demographic from census<br>• Scores in five domains<br>• Provides pass/fail score and age equivalents<br>• Designed for use by various providers |
| Child Developmental Inventory (CDI) | 18 months–6 years | 30–50 minutes | 300 | • 0.80–1.00 sensitivity; 0.94–0.96 specificity<br>• Parent Questionnaire to evaluate social, self-help, language, and general developmental skills<br>• Provides developmental quotients and age equivalents<br>• Normative sample included 568 children from MN from working class families and 43 high risk children |

*Contd...*

*Contd...*

| Developmental screening tool | Age range | Administration | Items | Advantages/Disadvantages |
|---|---|---|---|---|
| Denver Developmental Screening Tests (DDST) | 2 weeks–6 years | 10–20 minutes No special training required | 125 | • 0.56–0.83 sensitivity; 0.43–0.80 specificity<br>• Normed on 2096 term children from Colorado from diverse SES profile<br>• Risk categorization classifies children as normal, suspect or delayed |
| BSID Screener (BINS) | 3–24 months | 15–25 minutes to administer Special training required | 11–13 | • 0.75–0.86 sensitivity; 0.75–0.86 specificity<br>• Normed on 1,700 children matching demographic from 2,000 census<br>• Risk categorization grading children as low, moderate or high risk in each of 4 domains |
| BSID-III Revision | 1–42 months | 50–90 minutes to administer Special training required | Varies depending on age and ceiling | • Five domains evaluated are cognitive, gross motor, fine motor, receptive language, and expressive language<br>• Age equivalents available<br>• Some concern that scores higher in current version of BSID compared to previous versions but strongly correlated with other instruments |
| Parent's Evaluation of Developmental Status (PEDS) | 0–8 years | 5–10 minutes to administer and score No special training required | 10 | • 0.74–0.79 sensitivity; 0.70–0.80 specificity overall but lower sensitivity and specificity in preterm populations<br>• Questions designed as a high-level screen for developmental delay<br>• Limited utility in high risk population<br>• Normed on population of 771 children from diverse ethnic and SES backgrounds<br>• More detailed instrument to confirm abnormal findings<br>• Risk categorization as low, medium or high risk |
| Modified Checklist for Autism in Toddlers (MCHAT) | 16–30 months | 5–10 minutes | 23–29 | • Sensitivity 0.85–0.97; specificity 0.93–0.99<br>• Easy to use parent questionnaire<br>• May overidentify children with language delay and developmental delay<br>• Risk categorization to determine need for further evaluation<br>• Standardized and validated instrument |

(BINS: Bayley infant neurodevelopment screen; BSID: Bayley scale for infant development; MN: Minnesota; SES: Socioeconomic status).
*Source:* Reprinted with permission.[28] All tests available in English and Spanish.

# NEURODEVELOPMENTAL OUTCOMES AND PREMATURITY

Improvements in the neurodevelopmental outcome of surviving LPI have occurred in an era of concern for increased survival with disability in extremely immature infants. A single center study of 1,178 infants born <1,000 g between 1982 and 1998 studied outcomes in two epochs, 1982-1989 and 1990-1998, reporting increased survival from 49% to 67% with increased neurodevelopmental impairment from 26% to 36% among survivors,[29] a 2.3× increased survival with impairment between the two time periods. Fortunately, these findings were not confirmed when evaluated in larger cohorts. The Victorian Infant Collaborative Study Group, utilizing a population-based cohort to evaluate outcomes of preterm children born 1979-2005, reported significantly lower rates of neurosensory impairment and severe developmental delay over time.[30] Similarly, the National Institutes of Child Health and Human Development (NICHD) Neonatal Research Network (NRN) reported increasing survival from 1993 to 1999, but no difference in rates of CP, BSID-II Psychomotor Developmental Index (PDI) <70, or overall neurodevelopmental impairment.[31] However, they did note an increase in children with BSID-II MDI <70 from 40% to 47%. Reporting outcomes at school age and young adult life for preterm children and monitoring the developmental trajectory of these populations over time is critical as neonatology evolves.

## Early Childhood

Neurodevelopmental outcome studies of extremely low gestational age newborns (ELGANs) have largely focused on the first 2 years of life. While these early childhood outcomes are not absolute predictors of school age or adult outcomes, early studies have value as they allow us to evaluate short-term impact of new therapies or intervention strategies permitting practice modification, and avoidance of therapies deemed harmful or producing adverse early outcomes.

Risk factors are associated with adverse cognitive and motor outcomes **(Figs. 3 and 4)** and have remained relatively consistent over time in cohorts in the US and Europe. These morbidities are often benchmarked for NICU quality improvement because of the link to neurodevelopmental outcome.

Reports of neurodevelopmental outcome vary worldwide. The Surfactant, Positive Pressure and Pulse Oximetry Randomized Trial (SUPPORT) Study[33] and the ELGAN Study represent published literature of a contemporary cohort.[34]

SUPPORT was a randomized clinical trial (RCT) designed to evaluate respiratory support in the delivery room and pulse oximetry target range on neurodevelopmental outcome at 2 years of age. Using a 2 × 2 design, 1,316 neonates 24–27 weeks GA were enrolled. Standardized neurosensory examination and the BSID-III were administered at follow-up. There were no differences in the composite outcome of neurodevelopmental impairment based on mode of delivery room ventilation. However, children randomized to the lower saturation group had lower risk of retinopathy of prematurity but higher risk of death. Death before discharge occurred more frequently in the low oxygen saturation group compared to the high [19.9% of infants vs. 16.2%; risk ratio (RR), 1.27; 95% confidence interval (CI), 1.01–1.60; P = 0.04]. Neurodevelopmental outcomes **(Table 4)** allow comparison between the two randomization groups, also showing baseline occurrence of these outcomes for this group of ELGANs.

Extremely low GA newborns investigators evaluated the neurodevelopmental outcome of 949 infants born <28 weeks GA by comparing outcomes based on BSID-II and a standardized neurosensory examination. The prevalence of WMI was 19% in this cohort, higher than that typically reported in extremely low birth weight infants [<1,000 g, extremely low birth weight (ELBW)]. There was a strong correlation between IVH and PVL in this study. Approximately 12% had CP, 27% had MDI <70, and 31% had PDI <70.[34] PVL presence was the strongest predictor of neurodevelopmental outcome in this cohort.

## School Age

The Epidémiologique sur les Petits Ages Gestationnels (EPIPAGE) Study performed longitudinal follow-up on a cohort of French (very premature infants) VPI children (<33 weeks GA) up to 8 years old. Of 90% of the original cohort evaluated, major motor deficits occurred in 14% and

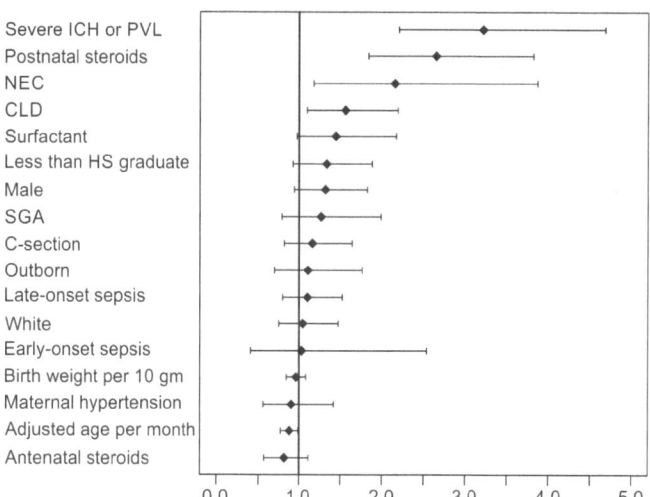

**Fig. 3:** Risk factors associated with PDI <70.
Infants evaluated using BSID-II. Adjusted risk factors for PDI <70 (OR and 95% CI) from cohort in NICHD NRN.[32]
(CLD: chronic lung disease; ICH: intracranial hemorrhage; NEC: necrotizing enterocolitis; NICHD NRN: National Institute of Child Health and Human Development Neonatal Research Network; PDI: psychomotor developmental index; PVL: periventricular leukomalacia; SGA: small for gestational age; OR: odds ratio; CI: confidence interval; BSID: Bayley scale for infant development).

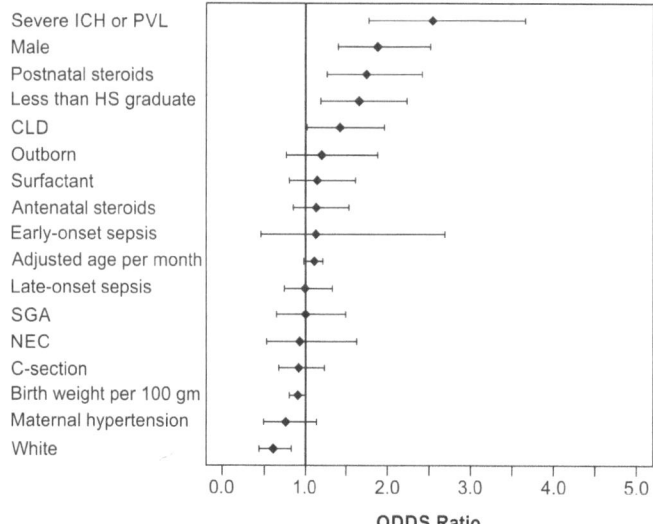

**Fig. 4:** Risk factors associated with risk MDI <70.
Infants evaluated using BSID-II. Adjusted risk factors for MDI <70 (OR and 95% CI) from cohort in NICHD NRN.[32]
(CLD: chronic lung disease; ICH: intracranial hemorrhage; MDI: mental developmental index; NEC: necrotizing enterocolitis; NICHD NRN: National Institute of Child Health and Human Development Neonatal Research Network; PVL: periventricular leukomalacia; SGA: small for gestational age; NEC: necrotizing enterocolitis; BSID: Bayley scale for infant development; OR: odds ratio; CI: confidence interval).

major cognitive deficits in 31%.[35] The risk for impairment was inversely related to GA and highest among those with severe WMI. Interestingly, among those without CNS injury on cranial sonogram, isolated cognitive deficits were the

**TABLE 4:** Neurodevelopmental outcomes from SUPPORT study group.[33]

| Variable | CPAP | Surfactant | ARR | p |
|---|---|---|---|---|
| NDI[†] | 10.9% | 9.1% | 1.16 (0.79–1.71) | 0.44 |
| BSID-III cognitive <70 | 7.2% | 7.6% | 0.95 (0.61–1.50) | 0.84 |
| GMFCS ≥2 | 5.1% | 4.8% | 0.98 (0.57–1.69) | 0.95 |
| Mod/Severe CP | 4.1% | 4% | 0.93 (0.51–1.72) | 0.82 |
| Bilateral blindness | 0.8% | 1.5% | 0.53 (0.16–1.78) | 0.31 |
| Hearing Impairment | 3.3% | 1.5% | 2.27 (0.96–5.37) | 0.06 |

Outcomes randomized by randomization group for initial respiratory management.
[†]NDI defined as a composite outcome of BSID-III Cognitive <70, BSID-III Psychomotor <70, Moderate to severe CP with GMFCS ≥2, bilateral blindness or hearing impairment that interferes with communication with or without amplification. GMFCS based on Palisano definition.[26]
(ARR: adjusted risk ratio; BSID: Bayley scale for infant development; CP: cerebral palsy; CPAP: continuous positive airway pressure; GMFCS: gross motor function classification score; NDI: neurodevelopmental impairment; SUPPORT: surfactant, positive pressure and pulse oximetry randomized trial).

most common abnormality. Isolated motor deficiency occurred in 6%, isolated cognitive deficiency in 23%, and both occurred in 8% of children. The high utilization rate of rehabilitation services and special education required by children who had been VPI as they approach school age was also emphasized. At 5 years of age, 41% of those born 24–28 weeks GA (compared to 15% born at term) received outpatient rehabilitation services. Among children with cognitive impairment, special services were required by 37% at age of 5 years, increasing to 63% at age of 8 years.[36] Compared to term peers, those born preterm were more likely to have hyperactivity and/or behavior problems. Awareness of school age cognitive impairment and behavioral difficulties with attention, hyperactivity, and executive functioning in preterm children is essential to optimize planning for learning disability.

## Adult Outcomes

Neurocognitive outcomes of the prematurely born surviving to adulthood is a growing area of research to understand the impact of early birth across a lifespan. Advanced neuroimaging demonstrates that structural alterations in regional gray and white matter volumes persist into adulthood. A cohort of 68 young adults aged 19–20 years born VPI had brain magnetic resonance imaging (MRI) and neurocognitive testing and outcomes compared to a control group of 71.[37] Lower GA was associated with smaller subcortical white matter and gray matter volumes, particularly in the temporal, parietal, and occipital regions, and lower scores for executive functioning, nonverbal memory, and IQ. Subcortical white matter volumes in the left inferior frontal gyrus accounted for 14% of the variance in lower full scale IQ scores in those born preterm. Lower white matter volumes in the posterior corpus callosum, thalamus, and fornix, and gray matter volumes in the temporal gyri accounted for 21% of variance in executive functioning. Additional data regarding neurocognitive and behavioral outcomes in young adulthood are few but concerning. A cohort of very low birth weight (VLBW) adults at age of 20 years using two subtests from the Wechsler Adult Intelligence Scale-Revised (WAIS-R) and found that preterm adults scored lower than term controls and differences were most striking in males.[38] Longitudinal neuropsychological testing performed on a United Kingdom cohort of 94 VPI and 44 term controls at 15 years and 19 years of age;[39] at both ages evaluated, VPI had lower full scale, verbal and performance IQ, and also lower phonological verbal fluency. When comparing outcomes between the two assessments, verbal fluency increased in the term subjects with increased age, but not in VPI. Males had decreasing verbal IQ between ages 15 years and 19 years. Other researchers have shown that adults born VPI have difficulty with executive functioning, hyperactivity, and inattention.[40] Of equal concern, low birth weight children have more psychiatric disorders in adulthood. Several population-based registries in Europe show higher prevalence of schizophrenia compared to adults born at term.[40] In one such Swedish cohort, premature birth was associated with increased psychiatric hospital admission from age 8 years to 29 years, with 5.2% of adults born 24–28 weeks GA having at least one psychiatric hospitalization.[40,41]

## HYPOXIC-ISCHEMIC ENCEPHALOPATHY

Hypoxic-ischemic encephalopathy is responsible for >20% of neonatal deaths globally. Survivors are at increased risk for long-term neurologic sequelae due to global neonatal brain injury secondary to low perfusion and hypoxemia. The initial insult is followed by a cascade of inflammatory responses that lead to secondary glutamate-induced brain injury. Hypothermia downregulates the inflammatory cascade and suppresses the cytotoxic response after an initial insult.

The use of hypothermia was extensively evaluated in US and European clinical trials prior to widespread application to ensure that this therapy was indeed beneficial. The use of hypothermia as a potentially neuroprotective strategy was studied in RCTs, most using similar inclusion criteria including: GA ≥36 weeks, history of perinatal event and/or perinatal depression, clinical evidence of moderate or severe encephalopathy, and initiating hypothermia within age of 6 hours. Similar protocols included achieving target temperature of 33-35° for 72 hours by using whole body cooling or selective head cooling. Some studies required infant electroencephalography (EEG) abnormalities to qualify for inclusion.

The first large RCT to evaluate hypothermia efficacy was the 2005 Cool Cap Trial, utilizing selective head cooling for 72 hours. Enrolled patients had clinical seizures or abnormal EEG at baseline. Death or severe disability was noted in 59 of 108 (55%) cooled infants versus 73 of 110 (66%) control-group infants, odds ratio (OR) 0.61 (95% CI 0.34-1.09); with mortality rates of 33% versus 38%, OR 0.81 (0.47-1.41) and severe disability in 14 of 72 (19%) versus 21 of 68 (31%), OR 0.54 (0.25-1.17) in the cooled and control groups, respectively. While differences were not statistically significant, a lower percentage of cooled infants had a Bayley MDI <70 compared to control infants (30% vs. 39%; p = ns).[42] The Total Body Hypothermia for Neonatal Encephalopathy Trial (TOBY Trial) was the largest RCT evaluating outcomes of children with HIE enrolled at multiple European centers evaluating 325 children and reported outcomes at 2 years of age. Abnormal baseline EEG in addition to the inclusion criteria above were required to be enrolled in TOBY. No significant difference was found for the composite outcome of death or severe disability between hypothermia and control patients. However, survivors who received hypothermia had less CP compared to controls (28% vs. 41%, p <0.05) and were less likely to have multiple disabilities at follow-up.[43] The largest US RCT evaluated outcomes of 208 children reported at age of 2 years (**Table 5**); survival benefit is evident from the Kaplan-Meier curve in **Figure 5** showing that the majority of deaths occurred early. 91% of children enrolled in this clinical trial of hypothermia were evaluated at age of 6-7 years.[44] Death after discharge was similar in both hypothermia and control groups. At school age, all survivors had similar IQ scores on neurocognitive testing with the Wechsler Scales of Intelligence without difference in the composite outcome of death or IQ <70. However, survivors who received hypothermia were less likely to have moderate/severe disability. Children who received hypothermia were less likely to die during the study period.[44] TOBY reported similar rates of death by school age for hypothermia and control patients at age of 6 years (29% vs. 30%, p = ns);[45] treated survivors had more survival without severe disability, less CP, and improved gross motor function. Full scale IQ scores were similar between the two groups.

**TABLE 5:** Neurodevelopmental outcomes of children at 2 years from the NICHD NRN hypothermia study.

| | Hypothermia N = 102 | Control N = 106 | RR (95% CI) |
|---|---|---|---|
| Death | 24% | 37% | RR = 0.68 95% CI 0.44–1.05, p = ns |
| CP | 19% | 30% | RR = 0.68 95% CI 0.38–1.22, p = ns |
| Death or moderate/ Severe disability | 44% | 62% | RR = 0.72 95% CI 0.54 – 0.95, p < 0.05 |

(CI: confidence interval; CP: cerebral palsy; NICHD: National Institutes of Child Health and Human Development; NRN: neonatal research network; RR: risk ratio).

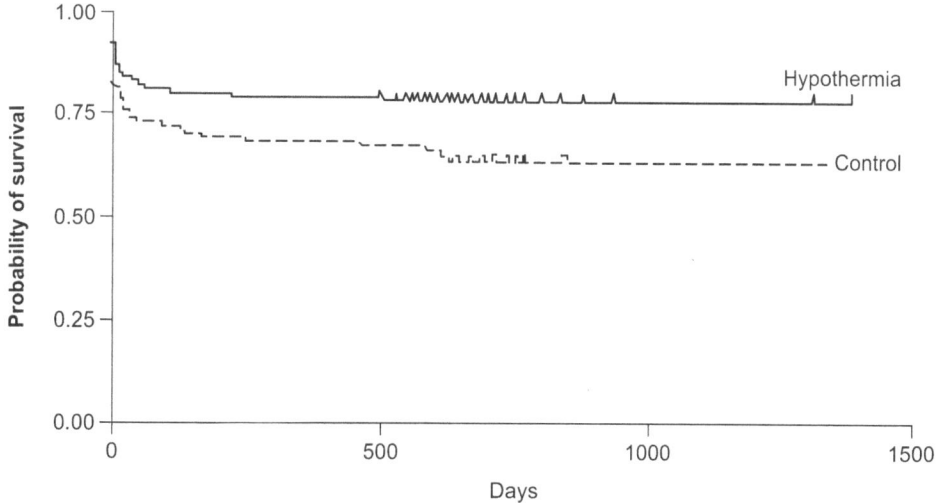

**Fig. 5:** Kaplan–Meier curve comparing survival for hypothermia-treated children compared to control.[44]

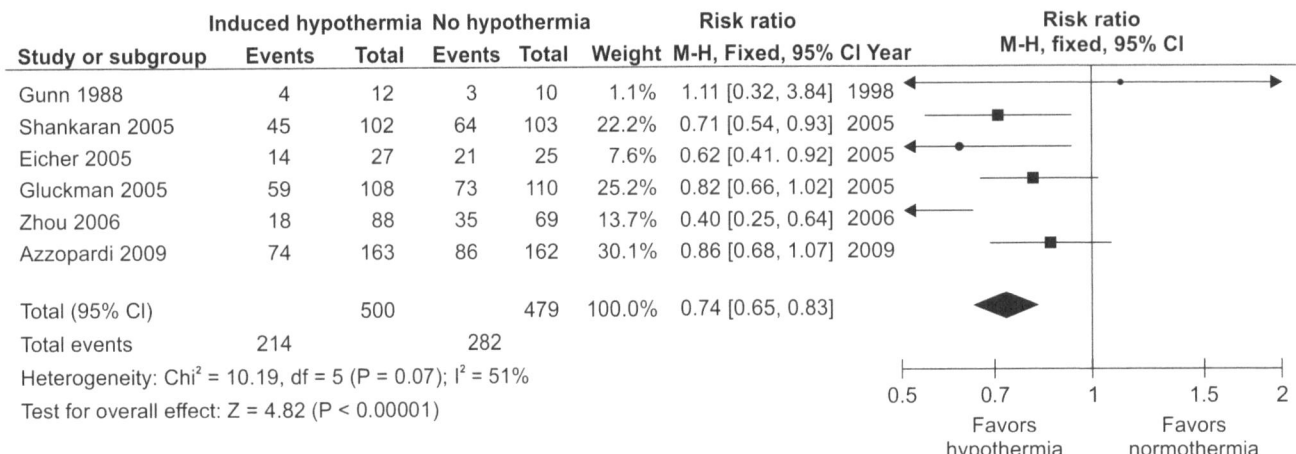

**Fig. 6:** Meta-analysis of neurodevelopmental outcome of hypothermia RCTs for neonatal HIE.
(CI: confidence interval; HIE: hypoxic-ischemic encephalopathy; RCT: randomized controlled trial).
*Source:* Reprinted with permission. Forest plot of primary outcome of death or moderate-severe neurodevelopmental disability in survivors.[47]

A meta-analysis of US and European trials **(Fig. 6)** with published neurodevelopmental outcomes at age of 2 years found that hypothermia treatment in term neonates with moderate-severe encephalopathy is beneficial with a RR of 0.74 (0.65–.83) when hypothermia is initiated within the first 6 hours of life.[46] Survivors remain at risk for neurologic and developmental difficulties, including epilepsy (12%), cognitive and learning difficulties (45%), CP (29%), and visual impairment (26%).[47]

In summary, whole body or selective head cooling administered to term infants within 6 hours of age decreases risk for the composite outcome of death and/or moderate-severe neurologic impairment among survivors at age of 2 years. At school age, survivors who received hypothermia have a lower risk of death or severe disability and similar IQ to untreated survivors. The benefit of therapy is clearest for those with moderate encephalopathy; selective hypothermia initiated within 6 hours of birth is now standard of care for newborns with moderate encephalopathy.

Data are limited for the efficacy of hypothermia in resource-limited countries. In a meta-analysis of seven RCTs evaluating outcomes in low-middle income countries including 567 infants, there was no improvement in neonatal mortality with use of hypothermia.[49] These data are likely confounded by the lack of other supportive therapies, including mechanical ventilation, and/or poor quality of cooling devices utilized. There were insufficient data to evaluate impact on neurologic outcome. Additional studies are needed to better understand the role of hypothermia in this population/setting.

Studies are ongoing in the US and Europe to explore the utility of hypothermia in preterm children < 36 weeks gestational age; caution should be exercised in the use of this therapy in preterm infants until these studies are complete.

# EARLY INTERVENTION

## Historical Perspective

US Federal Legislation (1975) supported educational services for all people, including those with disabilities. Public Law 94–142, the Individual with Disabilities Education Act (IDEA), ensures the right to public education for all school aged children with disabilities. In 1986, Part C of IDEA extended early intervention to infants and toddlers < age of 3 years, equipping families to meet the special needs of their disabled children, enhancing development, reducing future disability, and reducing remediation and special needs services.

Part C of IDEA applies to all 50 states. States receive federal funds to operationalize these programs, but the specific nuances for each program are state-regulated and controlled. Approximately 340,000 children < 3 years of age receive developmental therapies through this program annually in the US.

While providers involved in neurodevelopmental outcomes research can attest to the perceived benefit of early intervention services (EIS) for developmentally disabled children, these benefits have been difficult to demonstrate in RCTs. A meta-analysis of studies evaluating short- and long-term benefit of EIS showed improved cognition during infancy and at preschool, albeit unsustained at school age.[50] Furthermore, there was no improvement in motor outcomes. As many preterm children referred for services have structural CNS injury, therapy is unlikely to completely ameliorate these deficits. The qualitative and incremental

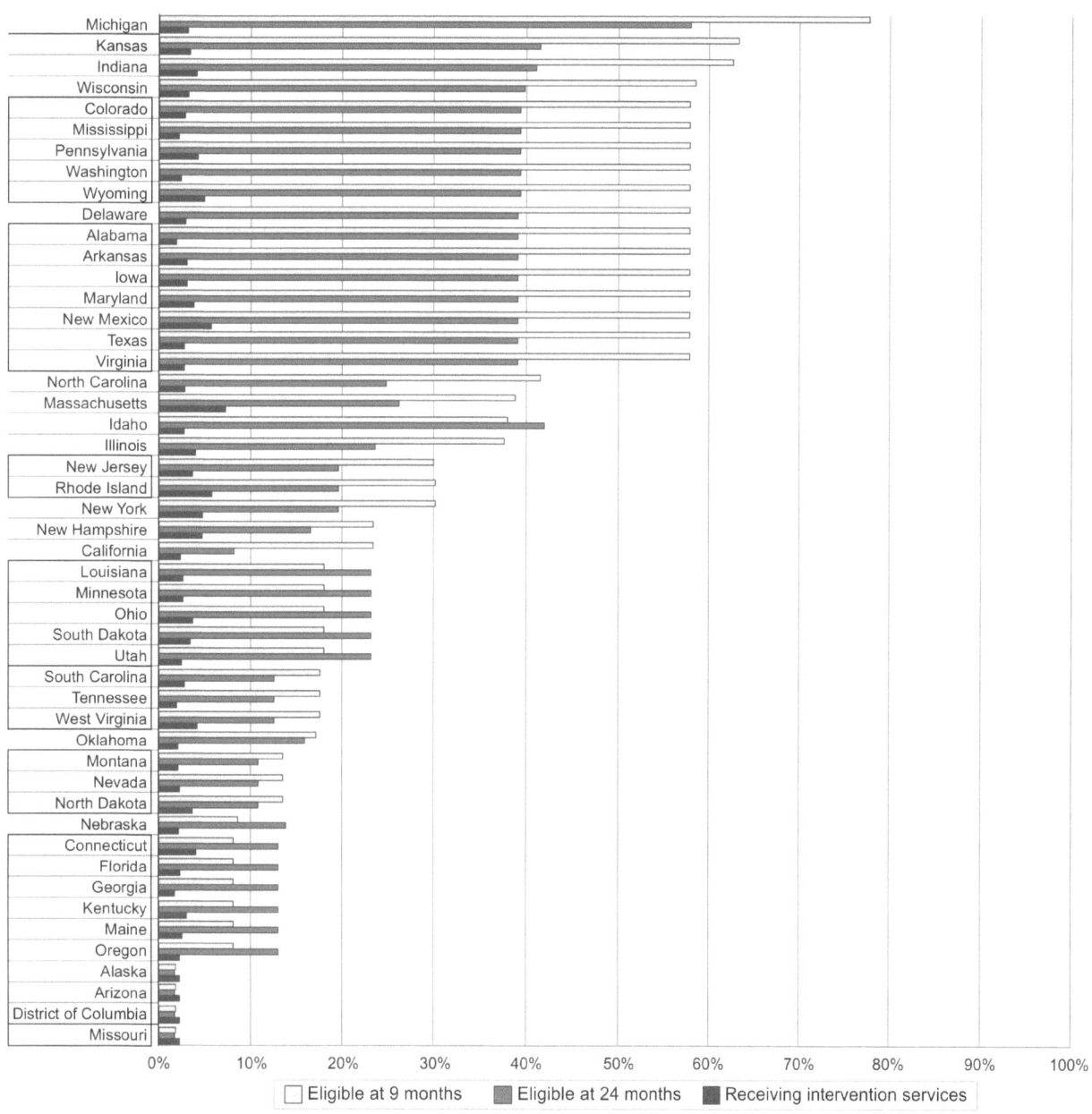

**Fig. 7:** Variability in eligibility for early intervention by state in US. Estimated rates of eligibility for EIS based on developmental delay. States sharing the same numerical eligibility criteria are grouped within boxes.
(EIS: early intervention services).

benefit in improved function, while difficult to quantify, may be as important as eliminating the underlying abnormality. More qualitative measures to evaluate the benefit of EIS may be preferable to expecting elimination of the downstream effects of structural CNS injury.

Early intervention services for children vary widely across states, regions, and countries. The World Health Organization categorizes the different programs into three groups—primary prevention of disability, secondary prevention of additional impairment, and tertiary prevention to minimize impact of disability.[51] There is wide regional variability in the types of early intervention providers available. Other than Part C of IDEA requiring that services be provided in the child's natural environment and that affected children have a service coordinator, states have latitude in deciding their program structure and eligibility criteria. Some states' criteria for eligibility are quite restrictive, while others are liberal,[52] proportion of eligible children enrolled ranging from 1.48% in Georgia to 6.96% in Massachusetts. Liberal eligibility states like Michigan and Washington identified 26 times more eligible children than those receiving services, suggesting that the capacity of systems is maximized and that states only provide services to a defined number of children (**Fig. 7**).

In Canada, educational systems are governed by the provinces, there being no federal requirement that EIS be provided; thus services are widely available but created based on organizational initiatives and funded by programs that improve outcomes for women and children. Due to the variability in funding and scope, the distribution of services may not reflect the distribution of disability in the community. For example, EIS review in Ontario showed the majority of services were for children with autism and communication disorders even though other developmental disability types were more common.[49]

Despite its variability, the goal of EIS is maximizing functional potential, services being provided by trained providers at home or a center. Physical therapists address gross motor function and tonal abnormalities. Occupational therapists address fine motor delay, and sensory and behavioral problems. Speech therapists address expressive or receptive language difficulties. While these therapies are most frequently utilized, other rehabilitation services including aquatic therapy, hippotherapy, and vision and feeding therapy may be helpful.

Early intervention services are costly. Between July 1999 and June 2000, Massachusetts had total program costs of $66 billion per year with a mean cost per survivor of $857 per year, noting significant variability in cost by GA, the highest cost attributed to the preterm.[53] Mean annual costs for preterm children 24–31 weeks GA were twice the cost of term children ($1578 vs. $725, annually), and costs were higher for multiples compared to singletons.

Public health and downstream impact related to resource utilization and allocation needs critical evaluation as ELBW survival increases. While neurodevelopmental outcomes have improved, increasing demand for EIS will occur as the ELGAN population rises. As these children utilize disproportionate healthcare and educational resources, prudent strategies, and guidelines outlining best practice initiatives will determine which services are most cost-effective and most beneficial in maximizing childhood and adult functional outcomes.

## CONCLUSION

Clinicians should be aware of at-risk populations and understand the appropriate tools that can be used to evaluate their developmental status. Early intervention strategies are help address many of the problems that present in early childhood.

## REFERENCES

1. Adams-Chapman I. Neurodevelopmental outcome of the late preterm infant. Clin Perinatol. 2006;33(4):947-64; abstract xi.
2. Huppi PS, Warfield S, Kikinis R, et al. Quantitative magnetic resonance imaging of brain development in premature and mature newborns. Ann Neurol. 1998;43(2):224-35.
3. Kapellou O, Counsell SJ, Kennea N, et al. Abnormal cortical development after premature birth shown by altered allometric scaling of brain growth. PLoS Med. 2006;3(8):e265.
4. Back SA, Luo NL, Borenstein NS, et al. Late oligodendrocyte progenitors coincide with the developmental window of vulnerability for human perinatal white matter injury. J Neurosci. 2001;21(4):1302-12.
5. Back SA. Cerebral white and gray matter injury in newborns: New insights into pathophysiology and management. Clin Perinatol. 2014;41(1):1-24.
6. Honein MA, Kirby RS, Meyer RE, et al. National Birth Defects Prevention Network. The association between major birth defects and preterm birth. Matern Child Health J. 2009;13(2):164-75.
7. Quigley MA, Poulsen G, Boyle E, et al. Early term and late preterm birth are associated with poorer school performance at age 5 years: a cohort study. Arch Dis Child Fetal Neonatal Ed. 2012;97(3):F167-73.
8. Morse SB, Zheng H, Tang Y, et al. Early school-age outcomes of late preterm infants. Pediatrics. 2009;123(4):e622-9.
9. McGowan JE, Alderdice FA, Holmes VA, et al. Early childhood development of late-preterm infants: a systematic review. Pediatrics. 2011;127(6):1111-24.
10. Kugelman A, Colin AA. Late preterm infants: near term but still in a critical developmental time period. Pediatrics. 2013;132(4):741-51.
11. Chyi LJ, Lee HC, Hintz SR, et al. School outcomes of late preterm infants: special needs and challenges for infants born at 32 to 36 weeks gestation. J Pediatr. 2008;153(1):25-31.
12. Gray RF, Indurkhya A, McCormick MC. Prevalence, stability, and predictors of clinically significant behavior problems in low birth weight children at 3, 5, and 8 years of age. Pediatrics. 2004;114(3):736-43.
13. Huddy CL, Johnson A, Hope PL. Educational and behavioural problems in babies of 32-35 weeks gestation. Arch Dis Child Fetal Neonatal Ed. 2001;85(1):F23-8.
14. Woythaler MA, McCormick MC, Smith VC. Late preterm infants have worse 24-month neurodevelopmental outcomes than term infants. Pediatrics. 2011;127(3):e622-9.
15. Lipkind HS, Slopen ME, Pfeiffer MR, et al. School-age outcomes of late preterm infants in New York city. Am J Obstet Gynecol. 2012;206(3):222.e1-6.
16. Talge NM, Holzman C, Wang J, et al. Late-preterm birth and its association with cognitive and socioemotional outcomes at 6 years of age. Pediatrics. 2010;126(6):1124-31.
17. Gurka MJ, LoCasale-Crouch J, Blackman JA. Long-term cognition, achievement, socioemotional, and behavioral development of healthy late-preterm infants. Arch Pediatr Adolesc Med. 2010;164(6):525-32.
18. Prevalence and characteristics of children with cerebral palsy in Europe. Dev Med Child Neurol. 2002;44(9):633-40.
19. MacLennan AH, Thompson SC, Gecz J. Cerebral palsy: causes, pathways, and the role of genetic variants. Am J Obstet Gynecol. 2015;213(6):779-88.
20. Maenner MJ, Blumberg SJ, Kogan MD, et al. Prevalence of cerebral palsy and intellectual disability among children identified in two U.S. National Surveys, 2011-2013. Ann Epidemiol. 2016;26(3):222-6.

21. Nelson KB, Blair E. Prenatal factors in singletons with cerebral palsy born at or near term. N Engl J Med. 2015;373(10):946-53.
22. Montenegro MA, Cendes F, Saito H, et al. Intrapartum complications associated with malformations of cortical development. J Child Neurol. 2005;20(8):675-8.
23. Sewell MD, Eastwood DM, Wimalasundera N. Managing common symptoms of cerebral palsy in children. BMJ. 2014;349:g5474.
24. Enkelaar L, Ketelaar M, Gorter JW. Association between motor and mental functioning in toddlers with cerebral palsy. Dev Neurorehabil. 2008;11(4):276-82.
25. Surveillance of Cerebral Palsy in Europe. Surveillance of cerebral palsy in Europe: a collaboration of cerebral palsy surveys and registers. Surveillance of Cerebral Palsy in Europe (SCPE). Dev Med Child Neurol. 2000;42(12):816-24.
26. Palisano R, Rosenbaum P, Walter S, et al. Development and reliability of a system to classify gross motor function in children with cerebral palsy. Dev Med Child Neurol. 1997;39(4):214-23.
27. Gorter JW, Ketelaar M, Rosenbaum P, et al. Use of the GMFCS in infants with CP: the need for reclassification at age 2 years or older. Dev Med Child Neurol. 2009;51(1):46-52.
28. Council on Children With Disabilities; Section on Developmental Behavioral Pediatrics; Bright Futures Steering Committee; Medical Home Initiatives for Children With Special Needs Project Advisory Committee. Identifying infants and young children with developmental disorders in the medical home: an algorithm for developmental surveillance and screening. Pediatrics. 2006;118(1):405-20.
29. Wilson-Costello D, Friedman H, Minich N, et al. Improved survival rates with increased neurodevelopmental disability for extremely low birth weight infants in the 1990s. Pediatrics. 2005;115(4):997-1003.
30. Doyle LW, Roberts G, Anderson PJ. Victorian Infant Collaborative Study Group. Changing long-term outcomes for infants 500-999 g birth weight in Victoria, 1979-2005. Arch Dis Child Fetal Neonatal Ed. 2011;96(6):F443-7.
31. Hintz SR, Kendrick DE, Vohr BR, et al. National Institute of Child Health and Human Development Neonatal Research Network. Changes in neurodevelopmental outcomes at 18 to 22 months' corrected age among infants of less than 25 weeks' gestational age born in 1993-1999. Pediatrics. 2005;115(6):1645-51.
32. Vohr BR, Wright LL, Dusick AM, et al. Neurodevelopmental and functional outcomes of extremely low birth weight infants in the National Institute of Child Health and Human Development Neonatal Research Network, 1993-1994. Pediatrics. 2000;105(6):1216-26.
33. Vaucher YE, Peralta-Carcelen M, Finer NN, et al. SUPPORT Study Group of the Eunice Kennedy Shriver NICHD Neonatal Research Network. Neurodevelopmental outcomes in the early CPAP and pulse oximetry trial. N Engl J Med. 2012;367(26):2495-504.
34. O'Shea TM, Allred EN, Kuban KC, et al. ELGAN Study Investigators. Intraventricular hemorrhage and developmental outcomes at 24 months of age in extremely preterm infants. J Child Neurol. 2012;27(1):22-9.
35. Marret S, Marchand-Martin L, Picaud JC, et al. EPIPAGE Study Group. Brain injury in very preterm children and neurosensory and cognitive disabilities during childhood: The EPIPAGE cohort study. PloS One. 2013;8(5):e62683.
36. Delobel-Ayoub M, Arnaud C, White-Koning M, et al. EPIPAGE Study Group. Behavioral problems and cognitive performance at 5 years of age after very preterm birth: the EPIPAGE Study. Pediatrics. 2009;123(6):1485-92.
37. Nosarti C, Nam KW, Walshe M, et al. Preterm birth and structural brain alterations in early adulthood. Neuroimage Clin. 2014;6:180-91.
38. Hack M, Flannery DJ, Schluchter M, et al. Outcomes in young adulthood for very-low-birth-weight infants. N Engl J Med. 2002;346(3):149-57.
39. Allin M, Walshe M, Fern A, et al. Cognitive maturation in preterm and term born adolescents. J Neurol Neurosurg Psychiatry. 2008;79(4):381-6.
40. Doyle LW, Anderson PJ. Adult outcome of extremely preterm infants. Pediatrics. 2010;126(2):342-51.
41. Lindstrom K, Lindblad F, Hjern A. Psychiatric morbidity in adolescents and young adults born preterm: a Swedish national cohort study. Pediatrics. 2009;123(1):e47-53.
42. Gluckman PD, Wyatt JS, Azzopardi D, et al. Selective head cooling with mild systemic hypothermia after neonatal encephalopathy: multicentre randomised trial. Lancet. 2005;365(9460):663-70.
43. Azzopardi DV, Strohm B, Edwards AD, et al. TOBY Study Group. Moderate hypothermia to treat perinatal asphyxial encephalopathy. N Engl J Med. 2009;361(14):1349-58.
44. Shankaran S, Laptook AR, Ehrenkranz RA, et al. National Institute of Child Health and Human Development Neonatal Research Network. Whole-body hypothermia for neonates with hypoxic-ischemic encephalopathy. N Engl J Med. 2005;353(15):1574-84.
45. Shankaran S, Pappas A, McDonald SA, et al. Eunice Kennedy Shriver NICHD Neonatal Research Network. Childhood outcomes after hypothermia for neonatal encephalopathy. N Engl J Med. 2012;366(22):2085-92.
46. Azzopardi D, Strohm B, Marlow N, et al. TOBY Study Group. Effects of hypothermia for perinatal asphyxia on childhood outcomes. N Engl J Med. 2014;371(2):140-9.
47. Shah PS. Hypothermia: a systematic review and meta-analysis of clinical trials. Semin Fetal Neonatal Med. 2010;15(5):238-46.
48. Shankaran S, Laptook AR, Tyson JE, et al. Eunice Kennedy Shriver National Institute of Child Health and Human Development Neonatal Research Network. Evolution of encephalopathy during whole body hypothermia for neonatal hypoxic-ischemic encephalopathy. J Pediatr. 2012;160(4):567-72.e3.
49. Pauliah SS, Shankaran S, Wade A, et al. Therapeutic hypothermia for neonatal encephalopathy in low- and middle-income countries: a systematic review and meta-analysis. PloS One. 2013;8(3):e58834.
50. Spittle AJ, Orton J, Doyle LW, et al. Early developmental intervention programs post hospital discharge to prevent motor and cognitive impairments in preterm infants. Cochrane Database Syst Rev. 2007;(2):CD005495.
51. Underwood K. Mapping the early intervention system in Ontario, Canda. Int J Spec Educ. 2012;27(2):125-34.
52. Rosenberg SA, Robinson CC, Shaw EF, et al. Part C early intervention for infants and toddlers: percentage eligible versus served. Pediatrics. 2013;131(1):38-46.
53. Clements KM, Barfield WD, Ayadi MF, et al. Preterm birth-associated cost of early intervention services: an analysis by gestational age. Pediatrics. 2007;119(4):e866-74.

# SECTION 8

# Growth, Lactation and Nutrition

- Body Composition and Electrolytes
  *Sonya Misra*
- Macronutrients and Micronutrients
  *Sonya Misra*
- Stages of Nutritional Support
  *Sonya Misra*
- Human Milk Composition and Lactation
  *Sudha Rani Narasimhan, Alganesh G Kifle*
- Necrotizing Enterocolitis
  *Arwin Valencia, Antoine Soliman*

# CHAPTER 34

# Body Composition and Electrolytes

*Sonya Misra*

## ABSTRACT

Understanding and prioritizing growth and nutrition in neonatal care is essential to achieving maximal physical, mental, and developmental goals. The second and third-trimester fetus undergoes growth when many specific factors such as phosphorus, protein, and fat-soluble vitamins are rapidly accumulated. Optimal infant feeding is mother's own milk, which is influenced by maternal nutrition. Specific deficiency states, such as anemia of prematurity and osteopenia, should be prevented, monitored and treated.

Throughout the next three chapters, we will discuss safe feeding practices I developmental barriers and growth challenges in the preterm infant.

## GOALS AND CHALLENGES

The goal of nutrition in the preterm neonate is to maintain homeostasis and attempt to mimic fetal growth. Providers should aim to supply energy, protein, and other substrates to maintain an anabolic state and increase lean body mass.[1] This is crucial to optimize physical and developmental outcomes. Children who are better grown or appropriate for gestational age (AGA) at the time of discharge from the neonatal intensive care unit (NICU) have better neurological outcomes at follow-up.[2-4] Better head growth is associated with improved developmental outcomes; and better bone mineralization results in improved skeletal growth.[5] Studies show large inter-site variations in weight growth velocities of extremely low-birth weight (ELBW) infants.[6] Changing clinical practices can improve growth outcomes.[7] Although the universal goal is age-appropriate nutritional support, achievement of this goal is often hindered by a fragile, sick infant with an immature gut, liver, lungs, and kidneys, at risk for iatrogenic problems, necrotizing enterocolitis (NEC), and infection.

The major challenge to feeding is the developmental immaturity of the gut. The immature gut mucosa has diminished cell mass, motility, and enzyme activity.[8] Furthermore, transition of the gut from fetal to neonatal life post-birth leads to abnormal microbiota with less complex bacterial patterns and an increased representation of hospital bacteria. These factors may predispose the infant to developing NEC.

Gut development continues through the last trimester of pregnancy.

*Relevant developmental milestones are as follows:*
- Intestinal length almost doubles and surface area increases.
- Some hormonal/enzyme patterns mature during this time, e.g. fatty acid absorption occurs at 24 weeks and enterokinase (the enzyme that catalyzes activation of trypsinogen to trypsin) is expressed by 26 weeks.
- Mouth-only suck/swallow patterns have been noted by 28 weeks and mature suck/swallow patterns are seen by 33–36 weeks.[9]
- Mature suck, swallow, and breathing coordination may occur as late as 37 weeks.
- Gastrointestinal motility, a complex process requiring coordination between the central nervous system

enteric neurons, enteric motor neurons, myogenic control networks, and smooth muscle cells, matures by 32–36 weeks; so gastric emptying time at these gestational ages (GAs) is similar to that of term infants.[10]

The gut slowly accelerates development after birth with stimulation by food. For example, the enzyme lactase is induced when the intestine is exposed to lactose. Exposure to medication may also accelerate gut development, e.g. antenatal steroid exposure prior to birth has been associated with reduced NEC [RR = 0.46 (95% confidence interval (CI), 0.29–0.74)].[11]

One of the greatest barriers to establishing feeding is reduced motility in the first few days after birth. Factors found to improve motility in preterm infants are higher adjusted GA, increasing feed intervals, higher postnatal age, larger volume of bolus feeds, higher volume of daily feeds, and greater length of time receiving enteral feeds.[12]

During the third trimester, multiple micronutrients are transferred to the fetus. These nutrients include the majority of iron, long-chain polyunsaturated fatty acids (>18 carbons), vitamins, calcium, and phosphorus. As preterm infants miss part of their fetal development, they begin life with nutritional deficits. These deficits can manifest with growth failure, anemia, osteopenia, and long-term neurological impairment.

Factors other than inadequate nutrition may affect growth, such as endocrine imbalance. Hypothyroidism, both transient and permanent, can present in the preterm infant. Examples include transient hypothyroxinemia of prematurity, sick euthyroid syndrome, and iodine deficiency or excess.[13] Chronic inflammation may affect growth hormone/insulin-like growth factor-1 (IGF-1) axis and lead to shorter body lengths.[14] Chronic hypoxia may lead to growth failure, e.g. infants with cyanotic heart disease. Children in Tibet living at altitudes above 4,000 m show reduced growth compared to children living at lower altitudes.[15]

Adequately nourished infants are not guaranteed to grow and thrive. Infants in the NICU may be sensory-deprived, stressed, often experience pain, and have elevated sympathetic tone. Examination of sick preterm infants has revealed an overriding sympathetic response or an impaired parasympathetic response to feeding.[16]

### Interventions to Improve Parasympathetic Tone Multiple factors adversely affecting infant growth are summarized below:

Studies have shown that human touch (including skin-to-skin) or infant massage is associated with weight gain, attributable to an increase in vagal activity leading to increased IGF-1 production and increased gastric motility.[17] Separately, elevated parasympathetic tone is related to increased skeletal mass accrual.[18] In a randomized controlled trial, preterm infants who experienced skin-to-skin (holding the naked child against a parent's skin without clothes or blankets) versus traditional holding had significantly greater head growth.[19] Increasing parental visitation also provides many benefits to the child. Children who were visited more, demonstrated less arousal, less excitability, and better sleep.[20] While weight gain and growth parameters were not reported in this study, other studies have shown that better sleep enhances growth. Interestingly, prone positioning is reported to reduce sympathetic tone, but is not linked to weight gain.[21]

- *Nutritional factors:*
  – Inadequate calories
  – Inadequate protein
  – Electrolyte imbalances, e.g. hyponatremia
  – Specific micronutrient deficits, e.g. anemia and osteopenia.
- *Non-nutritional factors:*
  – Physiologic stress, e.g. severe illness
  – Inflammation
  – Endocrine factors, e.g. hypothyroidism
  – Infection
  – Medications, e.g. corticosteroids
  – Chronic hypoxia
  – Pain and sensory deprivation
  – Altered microbiota.

## GROWTH EVALUATION

### Anthropometric Measurements

Performing measurements at birth is important to assess fetal growth **(Boxes 1 and 2)**. Serial weekly measurements are necessary to identify growth patterns.[22]

Children who are between 10th percentiles and 90th percentiles on a growth chart are considered AGA.

---

**BOX 1:** Occipital frontal circumference (OFC) measurement.

Occipital frontal circumference is measured over the most prominent part on the back of the head (occiput) and just above the eyebrows (supraorbital ridges). This is thought to be the largest head circumference.

*Procedure for measuring OFC:*
- Position tape just above the eyebrows, above the ears, and around the biggest part of the back of the head
- Pull tape snugly to compress the hair
- Read measurement to the nearest 0.1 cm
- Write measurement on the chart
- Reposition tape measure and take a second measurement (repeat steps 1 through 4)

*Notes:*
The two measurements should agree within 0.2 cm.
If the difference is > 0.2 cm, repeat the measurement a third time and take the average of the two measurements in closest agreement and record.

> **BOX 2: Length board measurements.**
>
> *Procedure for measuring length using a length board:*
> - Accurate length measurements require two measurers
> - One person holds the infant's head against the headboard (the infant should be looking up)
> - The second person ensures that the infant's legs are fully extended and toes are pointing upward with feet flat against the foot piece
> - Legs should be straightened (if knees are flexed, gently press them down on the table). The second person slides the footboard up against the soles of the feet
> - Record the length to the nearest 0.1 cm
> - Reposition infant and take a second measurement (repeat steps 1 through 6)
>
> *Notes:*
> Length measurements should be done twice.
> The difference between measurements should be within 0.5 cm.
> If the difference is > 0.5 cm, repeat the measurement a third time and take the average of the two measurements in closest agreement, and record.

**TABLE 1:** Extrauterine growth requirements to mimic intrauterine growth velocity.

| Infant weight | Fetal weight gain g/kg/day |
|---|---|
| 500–700 g | 21 |
| 701–900 g | 20 |
| 901–1,200 g | 19 |
| 1,201–1,500 g | 18 |
| 1,501–1,800 g | 16 |
| 1,801–2,200 g | 14 |

Those above the 90th percentile are considered large for gestational age (LGA) or overgrown and those below the 10th percentile are considered small for gestational age (SGA) or undergrown.[23]

The more commonly used growth metrics in preterm neonates are the Fenton Growth Chart[24] and the Ehrenkranz curves. Currently the most widely used growth curve in the US is the Fenton's because it has incorporated more international data, Olsen data, and has been modified to fit World Health Organization (WHO) growth curves.

Fetal growth curves are best for measuring a preterm infant's growth, even as this approach remains debated as standard of care.[25] Fetal growth is sigmoidal rather than linear. Currently, suggested average targets using fetal growth data are 18–20 g/kg/day for weight; 1.1–1.4 cm/week for length; and 0.9–1.1 cm/week for head circumference.[26] More specific guidelines are suggested in **Table 1**.

World Health Organization curves are recommended for measuring growth after a preterm infant has reached term gestation and after discharge, and are considered superior to other childhood growth charts, as they were created from a large database of culturally diverse populations of children with nonsmoking mothers who planned to breastfeed.[27] Preterm infants should be plotted using adjusted age until they reach 2–3 years old. For example, a child of 32 weeks' gestation born 4 months prior to the observation date should be plotted at 2 months and not at 4 months on the chart.

## Growth Velocity

Growth velocity has been measured in several different ways. Some studies have used only the days after the child has regained birth weight. The currently recommended equation[28] is the two-point model shown below:

$$GV = \frac{[1000 * (W_n - W_1)]}{\left\{(D_n - D_1) * \left[\frac{W_n - W_1}{2}\right]\right\}}$$

The most accurate model is the exponential (Patel) model:[29]

$$GV = \frac{1000 * \ln\left(\frac{W_n}{W_1}\right)}{D_n - D_1}$$

GV = growth velocity
$W_n$ = weight in grams on day $n$
$D_n$ = day of time interval
$n = 1$ = beginning of time interval
$n$ = end of time interval in days

## Small for Gestational Age and Intrauterine Growth Restriction

Children born preterm are more likely to have experienced complicated pregnancies and thus suffered fetal growth restriction.[30] Sometimes these complications result in a weight of <10th percentile, or an SGA infant.[31] Factors leading to SGA or intrauterine growth restriction (IUGR) include placental insufficiency, TORCH (toxoplasmosis, other, rubella, cytomegalovirus, and herpes) infections, and chromosomal anomalies. Maternal factors affecting intrauterine growth include smoking, hypertension, preeclampsia, diabetes, and repeated courses of antenatal steroids.[32] Outcomes of both SGA and IUGR preterm infants are worse than the outcomes of those who grew appropriately.[33,34] SGA infants are considered at risk for metabolic syndrome in adulthood, possibly mediated by obesity, with higher risk of cardiovascular disease, dyslipidemia, insulin resistance, and type II diabetes. A recent study suggests that fetal exposure to preeclampsia rather than SGA status may be important.[35] Growth restriction in preterm infants, both fetal and postnatal, is associated with renal impairment, manifested by lower childhood glomerular filtration rate.[36] The severity of growth restriction is related to neonatal morbidities[37] and lower intellectual performance,[38] regardless of the cause. Infants born SGA who remain SGA by 8 months of age have worse cognitive and motor outcomes than infants who become AGA.[39]

### Extrauterine Growth Restriction

Extrauterine growth restriction is common in preterm infants in the NICU; the postnatal growth failure, and nutritional deficits start immediately after birth and accumulate over time. It is a significant problem. A large 2003 US study[40] of preterm infants born <34 weeks showed that 28%, 34%, and 16% have a weight, length, and head circumference under the 10th percentile, respectively on discharge. Growth restriction may begin at any time during the hospital stay, or may manifest later in childhood. A slow transition to optimal parenteral nutrition (PN) and oral feeds, along with inadequate calorie consumption, may lead to further deficits. Fluid restriction may restrict caloric intake in growing, enterally fed preterm infants. Independent risk factors for EUGR include male gender, need for assisted ventilation on first day of life, need for respiratory support at 28 days, and exposure to postnatal steroids.

### Overgrown Infants

Large for GA infants of diabetic mothers or of obese mothers are at risk for metabolic syndrome. AGA infants of diabetic and nondiabetic mothers, on the other hand, have less risk.[41] AGA infants of diabetic mothers have a higher percentage of body fat as compared to control infants, and this increased adiposity is seen as early as 30 weeks' GA.[42]

### Body Proportionality

Body proportionality, measured by weight as compared to height/length, is important to consider because it is a crude measure of adiposity. Other body proportionality indices are the Ponderal Index (PI) mass in kg/(height in m)$^3$ and body mass index (BMI) in mass/height$^2$, both of which are mathematical relationships between height and weight, and represent estimates of adiposity or leanness.

Before term, PI is preferred as it better identifies infants who will be very short or very tall. After term gestation, BMI is more useful but still lacks accuracy, as it misses symmetric growth restriction and does not distinguish between fat mass and fat-free mass provided by body composition analysis.[43] Comparison of BMI to air displacement plethysmography (ADP) in infants <36 weeks showed that all proportionality indices poorly predicted percent body fat. Albeit the best predictor, BMI explained only 27% of variance of body fat.[44] Therefore, BMI is not optimal for assessment of preterm adiposity.

### Body Composition Analysis

Air displacement plethysmography, a noninvasive method, measures the body composition of infants directly and allows a clear measure of fat mass and fat-free mass. Fat mass represents adipose tissue/fat, and fat-free mass represents the body cell mass, extracellular mass including bone, metabolic tissue, and total body water (TBW). Another technology is dual-energy X-ray absorptiometry (DEXA or DXA) scans that use X-rays to measure body composition.

Analyses in preterm infants at term-equivalent age have higher percentages of body fat/fat mass and lower amounts of fat-free mass than term infants.[45] Much of this fat is abdominal and linked to risk of diabetes and cardiovascular disease in adults. The lower amounts of fat-free mass represent a reduction in muscle mass and bone density often seen in growing preterm infants with shorter lengths. Reduction in fat-free mass is linked to inflammation and lower protein intake.

Body weight represents almost entirely fat-free mass until ~29–30 weeks gestation, when fat mass accumulation begins.[46] Measuring skinfold thickness, mid-arm circumference, and abdominal circumference provides an estimation of the amount of adiposity or fat mass in infants. Mid-arm circumference in growing preterm infants may show up to 60% of the variance in adiposity compared to fat mass measured by ADP, and is easily done in the absence of ADP.[47]

### Specific Nutritional Deficits Evaluation

It is important to look beyond anthropometrics and be vigilant for evidence of specific nutritional deficits. Two common deficits that require monitoring are anemia and osteopenia. Anemia can be identified by clinical examination and by monitoring hemoglobin and ferritin levels. Osteopenia is monitored with calcium and phosphorus levels and by observing trends of alkaline phosphatase. The most accurate way to diagnose osteopenia is to use DEXA to track bone density changes, a technology not prevalent in clinical practice. Osteopenic radiographic changes may only be appreciated in severe cases.

### Endocrine Imbalances

Screening for hypothyroidism should be considered in growth failure. Repeat universal screening for hypothyroidism at 1 month of age in preterm infants is currently standard of care in several states in the US.[48,49]

## FLUIDS

### Composition of Body Fluids and Solids

*Body Fluids*

Body fluid composition changes throughout gestation and alters rapidly after delivery as the baby adjusts from being surrounded by fluid to air. In early fetal life, >85% of body mass is comprised of TBW. Two-thirds of TBW is in the extracellular space and a third is intracellular. Early fetal life is characterized by a large number of small cells, with less fluid in the cells. By term, the infant body mass is only 75% water, of which half is in the extracellular space and the other half is in the intracellular space.[50] This shift to more intracellular fluid is because the number and size of individual cells has grown. The trend continues until 3 months of age, when only 60% of body mass is water, very similar to that of adults.

**Figure 1** illustrates that sodium is the predominant extracellular cation, and chloride and bicarbonate are the major anions. Potassium is the predominant intracellular cation, while phosphate and sulfates are the major anions. Routine clinical practice measures the extracellular compartment (plasma), thus resultant fluid therapies adjust extracellular electrolytes like sodium and calcium. Growth and development require increase of intracellular fluid that consists of a majority of potassium, magnesium and phosphates; and while intracellular levels of these substances are not directly measured, maintaining normal to high-normal levels, which is thought to provide enough for the intracellular environment.

*Body Solids*

Body solids are 15–30% fat, 12% protein, and 3% minerals. The most variable solid throughout life is body fat. In contrast, the fetus at 27 weeks is 86% water, 12% fat-free dry solids, and only 2% fat.[51] Fat deposition happens mainly in the third trimester, and by term, the proportion of body solids is up to 24%, mostly due to fat. Fat mass variation explains ~46% of observed variance in birth weight. ADP shows that the mean fat in term babies in the US is 15%. In AGA preterm infants, the weight loss following birth is likely a reduction in TBW, primarily due to reduction of extracellular water.[52]

In SGA/IUGR-preterm infants, there is often a reduction in protein and mineral deposition, reflecting nutritional deprivation.[53] As the fat and protein content is lower, the TBW percentage is higher.

### Fluid Administration

Preterm infants receive a combination of parenteral and enteral nutrition. Fluid volumes have been described from 50–100 mL/kg/day started at birth, with a gradual increase of 20 mL/kg/day to a usual maximum of 140–150 mL/kg/day. Fluid volumes >170 mL/kg/day have been associated with the outcome of patent ductus arteriosus (PDA).[54] The neonate handles enteral and parenteral fluids differently and is able to tolerate higher volumes enterally, up to 180 mL/kg/day, without causing significant fluid overload. The very premature infant experiences tremendous losses of fluids and electrolytes through skin or immature kidneys, which leads to the need for higher volume administrations. Infants with prenatal steroid protection have more mature skin, reduced transepithelial loss, and thus have lower fluid needs and incidence of hypernatremia.[55]

In a Cochrane meta-analysis[56] of restricted fluids versus liberal fluids, fluid restriction was found to be protective against PDA and NEC with a trend toward excessive weight loss, reduced chronic lung disease (CLD), and intraventricular hemorrhage. Researchers studying infants <72 hours of age restricted fluids for 3, 5, 7, 28 and up to

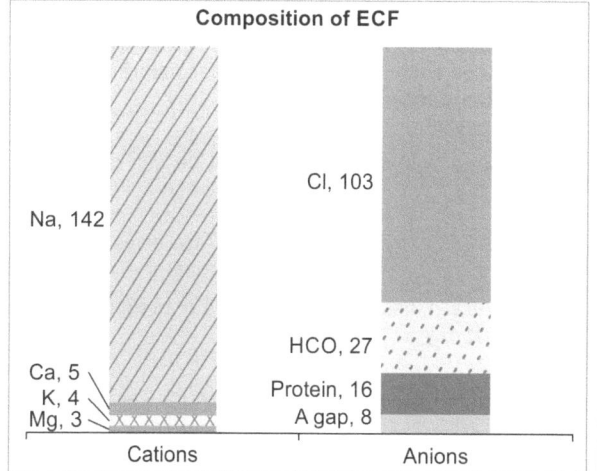 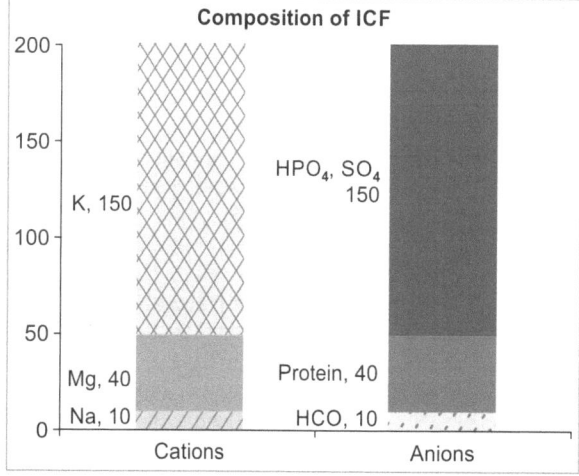

**Fig. 1:** Electrolytes in the extracellular fluid and intracellular fluid (ECF: extracellular fluid; ICF: intracellular fluid).

30 days. No children <750 grams birth weight were included in any studies and the mean GA at birth was 31 weeks (15% weight loss was accepted). The studies were carried out in the 1980s and 1990s in a different era of newborn care.

### Development of Epidermal Skin Barrier in the Preterm Infant

Full histological epidermal development usually occurs by 34 weeks and functionally increased transcutaneous losses usually end by ~30–32 weeks. Most preterm infants regardless of GA are believed to undergo rapid maturation of their skin epithelial integrity by 2 weeks of age.[57] However, those born <26 weeks may not develop epithelial integrity until 3–4 weeks of age or later.[58]

### Techniques to Reduce Transcutaneous Water Loss

Administering high volumes of fluids may increase risk of pulmonary edema and future CLD. Thus, significant effort to prevent transcutaneous water loss and reduce infused fluid volume must be made in early life. A secondary benefit of these efforts is reduction of solute load problems caused by excess sodium or glucose.

Different techniques **(Table 2)** have been used to reduce water loss and minimize fluid administration in the ELBW infant (<1,000 g).

### Evaluation of Water Balance

Be vigilant for signs of under- and overhydration by checking the following:

- *Daily weights:* Increased weight is an early sensitive sign of overhydration.
- Plasma sodium levels.
- Creatinine concentration.
- Urine output.
- Urine specific gravity.
- Urinary fractional excretion of sodium helps distinguish prerenal from renal failure.
- Clinical evaluation. Dry mucous membranes and depressed fontanels are late findings of underhydration.

### Fluids Provided = Parenteral + Enteral Nutrition

After birth, it is important to provide protein and carbohydrate to the neonate as soon as possible to maintain euglycemia and positive nitrogen balance, which prevents

**TABLE 2:** Techniques to reduce transcutaneous water loss in the ELBW infant.

| Technique | Reduction of water loss | Negative effects | Current recommendations |
| --- | --- | --- | --- |
| Humidification[59] | Reduction of ½–two-thirds transcutaneous losses | Increased cultures with gram-negative organisms, e.g. *Escherichia coli* and *Klebsiella*, not *Pseudomonas* | • Under 80% humidity in modern isolettes. Move to isolettes as soon as possible<br>• Humidity protocol example for infants <28 weeks, 1,000 g or less, with gelatinous skin.<br>• Starts at 85% humidity for 1 week, then weans by 5% humidity Q 12 hours x2, then 5% Q 24 hours till down to 40%, then D/C |
| Aquaphor[60] (Petroleum ointment) | Improved skin | • Higher incidence of Candida[61]<br>• Increased coagulase-negative staphylococci infections[62] | Not currently recommended due to higher risk of nosocomial infection |
| Plastic shields—thin plastic wrap | 24–48 hours after birth will reduce water loss with radiant warmers | Hard to keep closed | • Use with radiant warmers or when out of isolette in first few days of life<br>• Also helps maintain temperature |
| Plastic shields—Polyurethane cover—2 patches of 3 cm × 3 cm[63] | Used for first 5 days leads to two-thirds reduction in water loss | Minimal keratin loss when removed at day 5 | Try not to remove if placed |
| Plastic shields—polyurethane cover all over body[64,65] | When used in first 2 weeks of life, reduced water loss, weight loss and CLD | Skin loss if polyurethane is removed | Try not to remove if placed |

(CLD: chronic lung disease; ELBW: extremely low birth weight).

the effects of starvation or catabolism. This is provided by parenteral and/or enteral nutrition.

Parenteral nutrition is necessary to support the infant when full enteral or oral feeding support is not an option. It is frequently used in preterm infants <34 weeks GA while transitioning to feeds, for postoperative periods, and in infants who have short gut or NEC. The aim of PN is to provide enough nutrition to maintain growth. PN intravenous (IV) solutions are made of combinations of electrolytes, carbohydrate, fat, protein micronutrients, and vitamins. Until central venous access is established, peripheral parenteral fluids and nutrition can be administered through a peripheral IV. The increased risk of thrombophlebitis prevents use of more than 12.5% dextrose and 3.5% amino acids in PN solutions.

Enteral nutrition refers to food and nutrients provided by alimentary canal. Food given by this route needs to be digested and absorbed, and may not be fully utilized by the body. The combination of carbohydrates, fats, protein, vitamins, and minerals is more varied and complex than that provided by the parenteral route. Thus functional immaturity of hepatic and intestinal enzyme systems is relevant to optimal enteral nutrition.

## ELECTROLYTES

Electrolytes are minerals in the body fluids and bloodstream that carry an electrical charge. They affect the amount of water in the body, blood acidity, muscle, neuronal function, and cell membrane function. Imbalances lead to multiple problems; severe depletion or excess may result

**TABLE 3:** Electrolytes.

| Ion<br>Mean first week level<br>Urinary concentration | Serum level/Abnormality<br>Problems associated | Causes in preterm neonates | Parenteral supplementation |
|---|---|---|---|
| Sodium ($Na^+$)<br>Main extracellular cation<br>Controls body fluids<br>Essential for growth<br>Mean first week level<br>139.6 (133–146) mEq/L[66] | *Hyponatremia*<br><135 mEq/L<br>Severe levels<br><125 mEq/L<br>Hearing loss[68,69]<br>Cerebral palsy[70] | *Dilutional*<br>Excess free water administration—most common cause in first week of life<br>Syndrome of inappropriate diuretic hormone<br>Renal failure<br>*Urinary losses*<br>Reduced renal $Na^+$ concentrating ability—most common cause after first week of life.<br>Inadequate intake | As there often is increased extracellular fluid volume with high Na at birth, no early intake if possible<br>Restriction of Na in first few days of life reduces CLD<br><br>*Maintenance*<br>3–5 mEq/kg/day<br>Infants supplemented with [$Na^+$] from day 4 to day 14 have better growth and developmental outcomes[71,72] |
| Typical urinary concentrations are 20–40 mmol/L[67] | *Hypernatremia*<br>>145 mEq/L | *Excess free water losses*<br>Immature skin<br>Lack of urinary concentration<br>Osmotic diuresis—glycosuria<br>Exogenous Na administration<br>Saline flushes and boluses<br>Antibiotics<br>Sodium bicarbonate | |
| Potassium ($K^+$)<br>Main intracellular cation<br><br>Mean first week level 5.6 (4.6–6.7) mEq/L[67] | *Hypokalemia*<br><3.5 mEq/L<br>Decreased bowel motility | *Inadequate supplementation*<br>Loop and thiazide diuretics<br>May lead to urinary losses<br>Aggressive nutrition regimens[73]<br>Alkalosis | *Maintenance*<br>1–3 mEq/kg/day |
| | Hyperkalemia<br>> 6.5 mEq/L in ELBW without cardiac electrical changes | *Nonoliguric hyperkalemia*<br>2–4th day of life<br>Reflects renal inability to secrete $K^+$ from the distal tubule<br>Diminished if given antenatal steroids, which suggests it is caused by destabilization of the cell membrane<br>Na/K-ATPase leading to leaking of $K^+$ out of the cell[74]<br>Spurious—Hemolysis, e.g. heel stick<br>Renal failure | |
| Typical urinary concentrations 10–30 mmol/L[68] | | | |

*Contd...*

*Contd...*

| Ion<br>Mean first week level<br>Urinary concentration | Serum level/Abnormality<br>Problems associated | Causes in preterm neonates | Parentral supplementation |
|---|---|---|---|
| Calcium ($Ca^{++}$)<br>Bone and multiple enzyme reactions<br>Ionized Ca is 1.2–1.4 mmol/L<br>Mean first week level<br>9.2 (6.1–11.6) mg/dL[67] | Hypocalcemia<br><9 mg/dL | Hyperphosphatemia<br>Metabolic alkalosis<br>Hypoparathyroidism<br>Vitamin D deficiency<br>Renal tubular disease | *Maintenance*<br>Elemental calcium<br>120–200 mg/kg/day[75]<br>AAP 2013 – 150–220 mg/kg/day<br>Diminished in low albumin states<br>Normal dip in serum levels on first day of life. |
| | Hypercalcemia<br>>10.5 mg/dL | Overtreatment with Vitamin D<br>Phosphate deficiency<br>Calcium infusions without phosphate | |
| Magnesium ($Mg^{++}$) | Hypomagnesemia<br><0.8 mmol/L or 1.6 mEq/L | *Renal losses*<br>Increased bone deposition<br>Accompany low Ca levels | *Maintenance*<br>0.3–0.5 mg/kg/day<br>May need extra if diabetic mother is on insulin<br>Hold for hypermagnesemia |
| | Hypermagnesemia >1.1 mmol/L or >2.2 mEq/L | *Exogenous administration*<br>Maternal Mg therapy | |
| Chloride ($Cl^-$)<br>Mean first week level<br>108.2 (100–117) mEq/L[67] | Hypochloremia<br><95 mEq/L | Inadequate supplementation<br>Hypochloremic metabolic alkalosis<br>After diuretic use, e.g. furosemide | Metabolism seems to follow [$Na^+$] |
| | Hyperchloremia<br>>105 mEq/L | Large saline infusions | |
| Bicarbonate ($HCO_3^-$)<br>Major buffer<br>$CO_2$ mean first week level 20.3 (13.8–27.1) mg/dL[67] | Low levels <23 | Inability to conserve $HCO_3$ by immature kidney<br>Sepsis | *Maintenance*<br>0.5–3 mEq kg/day<br>Supplemented as acetate in fluids |
| | High levels >28 | Metabolic compensation for chronic respiratory acidemia | |
| Phosphate ($PO_4$)<br>Essential for energy ATP, intracellular anion cell membrane and DNA functions<br>Mean first week level<br>7.6 (5.4–10.9) mg/dL[67] | Hypophosphatemia<br>5 mg/dL (1.6 mmol/L) | *Inadequate supplementation*<br>Need to start as soon as able | *Maintenance*<br>60–140 mg/kg/day[76]<br>ESPGHAN 2010 60–90 mg/kg/day<br>AAP 2013<br>75–140 mg/kg/day<br>Monitor closely in SGA/IUGR babies |
| | Hyperphosphatemia | Exogenous administration of phosphate without adequate calcium | |

(AAP: American Academy of Pediatrics; ATP: adenosine triphosphate; CLD: chronic lung disease; DNA: deoxyribonucleic acid; ESPGHAN: European Society of Paediatric Gastroenterology, Hepatology and Nutrition; SGA: small for gestational age; IUGR: intrauterine growth restriction; ATP: adenosine triphosphate).

in exhaustion, poor growth, and cardiac arrhythmias. Imbalances are common in the first few days of life while the preterm infant's kidney function matures and the immature gut is unable to support full feeds. Optimizing electrolyte levels is dependent upon careful monitoring and supplementation through IV fluids and PN adjustments **(Table 3)**. Electrolytes may be positively charged cations or negatively charged anions. They are mainly present in the lean body mass of the infant. Balance between these two groups maintains electrical neutrality.

*Frequently used mg to mmol/mEq conversions:*

- Phosphorus 31 mg = 1 mmol
- Magnesium 24 mg = 1 mmol = 2 mEq
- Sodium 23 mg = 1 mmol = 1 mEq
- Potassium 39 mg = 1 mol = 1 mEq
- Calcium 40 mg = 1 mmol = 2 mEq.

# REFERENCES

1. Ziegler EE. Meeting the nutritional needs of the low-birth-weight infant. Ann Nutr Metab. 2011;58(Suppl 1):8-18.
2. Hack M, Breslau N, Weissman B, et al. Effect of very low birth weight and subnormal head size on cognitive abilities at school age. N Engl J Med. 1991;325(4):231-7.
3. Ehrenkranz RA, Dusick AM, Vohr BR, et al. Growth in the neonatal intensive care unit influences neurodevelopmental and growth outcomes of extremely low birth weight infants. Pediatrics. 2006;117(4):1253-61.

4. Franz AR, Pohlandt F, Bode H, et al. Intrauterine, early neonatal, and postdischarge growth and neurodevelopmental outcome at 5.4 years in extremely preterm infants after intensive neonatal nutritional support. Pediatrics. 2009;123(1):e101-9.
5. Bishop NJ, Dahlenburg SL, Fewtrell MS, et al. Early diet of preterm infants and bone mineralization at age five years. Acta Paediatr. 1996;85(2):230-6.
6. Olsen IE, Richardson DK, Schmid CH, et al. Intersite differences in weight growth velocity of extremely premature infants. Pediatrics. 2002;110(6):1125-32.
7. Bloom BT, Mulligan J, Arnold C, et al. Improving growth of very low birth weight infants `in the first 28 days. Pediatrics. 2003;112(1 Pt 1):8-14.
8. Walker A. Breast milk as the gold standard for protective nutrients. J Pediatr. 2010;156(Suppl 2):S3-7.
9. Lebenthal A, Lebenthal E. The ontogeny of the small intestinal epithelium. JPEN J Parenter Enteral Nutr. 1999;23(Suppl 5):S3-6.
10. Neu J. Gastrointestinal development and meeting the nutritional needs of premature infants. Am J Clin Nutr. 2007;85(2):629S-34S.
11. Roberts D, Dalziel S. Antenatal corticosteroids for accelerating fetal lung maturation for women at risk of preterm birth. Cochrane Database Syst Rev. 2006;(3):CD004454.
12. Bisset WM, Watt J, Rivers RP, et al. Postprandial motor response of the small intestine to enteral feeds in preterm infants. Arch Dis Child. 1989;64(10 Spec No):1356-61.
13. Fisher DA. Hypothyroxinemia in premature infants: is thyroxine treatment necessary? Thyroid. 1999;9(7):715-20.
14. Gardelis JG, Hatzis TD, Stamogiannou LN, et al. Activity of the growth hormone/insulin-like growth factor-I axis in critically ill children. J Pediatr Endocrinol Metab. 2005;18(4):363-72.
15. Dang S, Yan H, Yamamoto S. High altitude and early childhood growth retardation: new evidence from Tibet. Eur J Clin Nutr. 2008;62(3):342-8.
16. Smith SL, Doig AK, Dudley WN. Impaired parasympathetic response to feeding in ventilated preterm babies. Arch Dis Child Fetal Neonatal Ed. 2005;90(6):F505-8.
17. Field T, Diego M, Hernandez-Reif M. Potential underlying mechanisms for greater weight gain in massaged preterm infants. Infant Behav Dev. 2011;34(3):383-9.
18. Bajayo A, Bar A, Denes A, et al. Skeletal parasympathetic innervation communicates central IL-1 signals regulating bone mass accrual. Proc Natl Acad Sci U S A. 2012;109(38):15455-60.
19. Rojas MA, Kaplan M, Quevedo M, et al. Somatic growth of preterm infants during skin-to-skin care versus traditional holding: a randomized, controlled trial. J Dev Behav Pediatr. 2003;24(3):163-8.
20. Reynolds LC, Duncan MM, Smith GC, et al. Parental presence and holding in the neonatal intensive care unit and associations with early neurobehavior. J Perinatol. 2013;33(8):636-41.
21. Jean-Louis M, Anwar M, Rosen H, et al. Power spectral analysis of heart rate in relation to sleep position. Biol Neonate. 2004;86(2):81-4.
22. Ehrenkranz RA, Younes N, Lemons JA, et al. Longitudinal growth of hospitalized very low birth weight infants. Pediatrics. 1999;104(2 Pt 1):280-9.
23. Lubchenco LO, Searls DT, Brazie JV. Neonatal mortality rate: relationship to birth weight and gestational age. J Pediatr. 1972;81(4):814-22.
24. University of Calgary. Fenton Preterm Growth Chart Web Page. [online] Available from: http://www.ucalgary.ca/fenton/2013chart. [Last accessed September, 2019].
25. Merialdi M, Widmer M, Gülmezoglu AM, et al. WHO multicentre study for the development of growth standards from fetal life to childhood: the fetal component. BMC Pregnancy Childbirth. 2014;14:157.
26. Brenner WE, Edelman DA, Hendricks CH. A standard of fetal growth for the United States of America. Am J Obstet Gynecol. 1976;126(5):555-64.
27. Fenton TR, Kim JH. A systematic review and meta-analysis to revise the Fenton growth chart for preterm infants. BMC Pediatr. 2013;13:59.
28. Prince A, Groh-Wargo S. Nutrition management for the promotion of growth in very low birth weight premature infants. Nutr Clin Pract. 2013;28(6):659-68.
29. Patel AL, Engstrom JL, Meier PP, et al. Calculating postnatal growth velocity in very low birth weight (VLBW) premature infants. J Perinatol. 2009;29(9):618-22.
30. Ott WJ. Intrauterine growth retardation and preterm delivery. Am J Obstet Gynecol. 1993;168(6 Pt 1):1710-7.
31. Zaw W, Gagnon R, da Silva O. The risks of adverse neonatal outcome among preterm small for gestational age infants according to neonatal versus fetal growth standards. Pediatrics. 2003;111(6 Pt 1):1273-7.
32. Lausman A, Kingdom J; Maternal Fetal Medicine Committee. Intrauterine growth restriction: screening, diagnosis, and management. J Obstet Gynaecol Can. 2013;35(8):741-8.
33. Garite TJ, Clark R, Thorp JA. Intrauterine growth restriction increases morbidity and mortality among premature neonates. Am J Obstet Gynecol. 2004;191(2):481-7.
34. de Bie HM, Oostrom KJ, Delemarre-van de Waal HA. Brain development, intelligence and cognitive outcome in children born small for gestational age. Horm Res Paediatr. 2010;73(1):6-14.
35. Al-Nasiry S, Ghossein-Doha C, Polman SE, et al. Metabolic syndrome after pregnancies complicated by pre-eclampsia or small-for-gestational-age: a retrospective cohort. BJOG. 2015;122(13):1818-23.
36. Bacchetta J, Harambat J, Dubourg L, et al. Both extrauterine and intrauterine growth restriction impair renal function in children born very preterm. Kidney Int. 2009;76(4):445-52.
37. Kramer MS, Olivier M, McLean FH, et al. Impact of intrauterine growth retardation and body proportionality on fetal and neonatal outcome. Pediatrics. 1990;86(5):707-13.
38. Bergvall N, Iliadou A, Johansson S, et al. Risks for low intellectual performance related to being born small for gestational age are modified by gestational age. Pediatrics. 2006;117(3):e460-7.
39. Latal-Hajnal B, von Siebenthal K, Kovari H, et al. Postnatal growth in VLBW infants: significant association with neurodevelopmental outcome. J Pediatr. 2003;143(2):163-70.
40. Clark RH, Thomas P, Peabody J. Extrauterine growth restriction remains a serious problem in prematurely born neonates. Pediatrics. 2003;111(5 Pt 1):986-90.
41. Boney CM, Verma A, Tucker R, et al. Metabolic syndrome in childhood: association with birth weight, maternal obesity, and gestational diabetes mellitus. Pediatrics. 2005;115(3):e290-6.

42. Demerath E, Davern B, Misra S, Anderson C, Gray H, Ramel SE. Maternal Diabetes is Associated with Higher Percent Body Fat as Early as 30-36 Weeks Gestation. PAS Poster No. 3807. 170. 2014.
43. Cole TJ, Henson GL, Tremble JM, et al. Birthweight for length: ponderal index, body mass index or Benn index? Ann Hum Biol. 1997;24(4):289-98.
44. Ramel SE, Zhang L, Misra S, et al. Do anthropometric measures accurately reflect body composition in preterm infants? Pediatr Obes. 2017;12(Supp 1):72-7.
45. Ramel SE, Gray HL, Ode KL, et al. Body composition changes in preterm infants following hospital discharge: comparison with term infants. J Pediatr Gastroenterol Nutr. 2011;53(3):333-8.
46. Misra S, Jegatheesan P, Song D, et al. Effect of Antibiotics around Delivery on Body Composition of Preterms < 34 Weeks Close to Discharge. Researchgate. 2015. [online] Available from: https://www.researchgate.net/publication/288671296_Effect_of_Antibiotics_Around_Delivery_on_Body_Composition_of_Preterms_34_Weeks_Close_To_Discharge. [Last accessed September, 2019].
47. Daly-Wolfe KM, Jordan KC, Slater H, et al. Mid-arm circumference is a reliable method to estimate adiposity in preterm and term infants. Pediatr Res. 2015;78(3):336-41.
48. LaFranchi SH. Screening preterm infants for congenital hypothyroidism: better the second time around. J Pediatr. 2014;164(6):1259-61.
49. Vigone MC, Caiulo S, Di Frenna M, et al. Evolution of thyroid function in preterm infants detected by screening for congenital hypothyroidism. J Pediatr. 2014;164(6):1296-302.
50. Friis-Hansen B. Body water compartments in children: changes during growth and related changes in body composition. Pediatrics. 1961:28:169-81.
51. Ziegler EE, O'Donnell AM, Nelson SE, et al. Body composition of the reference fetus. Growth. 1976;40(4):329-41.
52. Bauer K. Body Fluid compartments in the fetus and newborn infant with growth considerations. In: Oh W, Guignard J, Baumgart S (Eds). Nephrology and Fluid/Electrolyte Physiology: Neonatal Questions and Controversies. Philadelphia: Saunders; 2008. p. 156.
53. Padoan A, Rigano S, Ferrazzi E, et al. Differences in fat and lean mass proportions in normal and growth-restricted fetuses. Am J Obstet Gynecol. 2004;191(4):1459-64.
54. Stephens BE, Gargus RA, Walden RV, et al. Fluid regimens in the first week of life may increase risk of patent ductus arteriosus in extremely low birth weight infants. J Perinatol. 2008;28(2):123-8.
55. Omar SA, DeCristofaro JD, Agarwal BI, et al. Effects of prenatal steroids on water and sodium homeostasis in extremely low birth weight neonates. Pediatrics. 1999;104(3 Pt 1):482-8.
56. Bell EF, Acarregui MJ. Restricted versus liberal water intake for preventing morbidity and mortality in preterm infants. Cochrane Database Syst Rev. 2014;12:CD000503.
57. Evans NJ, Rutter N. Development of the epidermis in the newborn. Biol Neonate. 1986;49(2):74-80.
58. Kalia YN, Nonato LB, Lund CH, et al. Development of skin barrier function in premature infants. J Invest Dermatol. 1998;111(2):320-6.
59. Gaylord MS, Wright K, Lorch K, et al. Improved fluid management utilizing humidified incubators in extremely low birth weight infants. J Perinatol. 2001;21(7):438-43.
60. Nopper AJ, Horii KA, Sookdeo-Drost S, et al. Topical ointment therapy benefits premature infants. J Pediatr. 1996;128(5 Pt 1):660-9.
61. Campbell JR, Zaccaria E, Baker CJ. Systemic candidiasis in extremely low birth weight infants receiving topical petrolatum ointment for skin care: a case-control study. Pediatrics. 2000;105(5):1041-5.
62. Conner JM, Soll RF, Edwards WH. Topical ointment for preventing infection in preterm infants. Cochrane Database Syst Rev. 2004;(1):CD001150.
63. Knauth A, Gordin M, McNelis W, et al. Semipermeable polyurethane membrane as an artificial skin for the premature neonate. Pediatrics. 1989;83(6):945-50.
64. Bhandari V, Brodsky N, Porat R. Improved outcome of extremely low birth weight infants with Tegaderm application to skin. J Perinatol. 2005;25(4):276-81.
65. Donahue ML, Phelps DL, Richter SE, et al. A semipermeable skin dressing for extremely low birth weight infants. J Perinatol. 1996;16(1):20-6.
66. Klaus MH, Fanaroff AA. Care of the High-Risk Neonate, 3rd edition. Philadelphia: WB Saunders; 1988.
67. Fusch C, Jochum F. Water, sodium, potassium and chloride. In: Koletzko B, Poindexter B, Uauy R (Eds). Nutritional Care of Preterm Infants: Scientific Basis and Practical Guidelines. Vol. 110. Basel: Karger; 2014. p. 105.
68. Ertl T, Hadzsiev K, Vincze O, et al. Hyponatremia and sensorineural hearing loss in preterm infants. Biol Neonate. 2001;79(2):109-12.
69. Leslie GI, Kalaw MB, Bowen JR, et al. Risk factors for sensorineural hearing loss in extremely premature infants. J Paediatr Child Health. 1995;31(4):312-6.
70. Bhatty SB, Tsirka A, Bigini-Quinn P, et al. Rapid correction of hyponatremia in extremely low birth weight (ELBW) premature infants is associated with long term developmental delay. Pediatr Res. 1997;41:140A-3.
71. Al-Dahhan J, Jannoun L, Haycock GB. Effect of salt supplementation of newborn premature infants on neurodevelopmental outcome at 10-13 years of age. Arch Dis Child Fetal Neonatal Ed. 2002;86(2):F120-3.
72. Ayisi RK, Mbiti MJ, Musoke RN, et al. Sodium supplementation in very low birth weight infants fed on their own mothers milk I: Effects on sodium homeostasis. East Afr Med J. 1992;69(10):591-5.
73. Moltu SJ, Strømmen K, Blakstad EW, et al. Enhanced feeding in very-low-birth-weight infants may cause electrolyte disturbances and septicemia--a randomized, controlled trial. Clin Nutr. 2013;32(2):207-12.
74. Omar SA, DeCristofaro JD, Agarwal BI, et al. Effect of prenatal steroids on potassium balance in extremely low birth weight neonates. Pediatrics. 2000;106(3):561-7.
75. Mimouni F, Mandel D, Lubetzky R, et al. Calcium, phosphorus, magnesium and vitamin D requirements of preterm infants. In: Koletzko B, Poindexter B, Uauy R (Eds). Nutritional Care of Preterm Infants, Scientific Basis and Practical Guidelines. Vol. 110. Basel: Karger; 2014. p. 142.
76. Agostoni C, Buonocore G, Carnielli VP, et al.; ESPGHAN Committee on Nutrition. Enteral nutrient supply for preterm infants: commentary from the European Society of Paediatric Gastroenterology, Hepatology and Nutrition Committee on Nutrition. J Pediatr Gastroenterol Nutr. 2010;50(1):85-91.

CHAPTER

# Macronutrients and Micronutrients

*Sonya Misra*

## ABSTRACT

Our greatest challenge in the preterm infant is to prevent malnutrition and avoid morbidities that may be worsened or caused by nutritional deficiencies. To avoid malnutrition an understanding of the components, functions, and needs of the building blocks of nutrition or nutrients provided is essential. Nutrients are digested differently if provided enterally versus parenterally thus needs may be different.

## MACRONUTRIENTS

Major dietary energy and growth sources include carbohydrates, fat, and protein. To maintain basal metabolism, ~30–40 calories/kg/day and 1.5 g/kg/day of protein are required. Optimal growth requires more calories and protein **(Table 1)**.

Protein/energy (P:E) ratio is the proportion of protein to calories. Each gram of protein requires energy for optimization. Excess glucose might lead to hyperglycemia, resultant hyperinsulinemia, and fatty deposition; excess protein might increase underutilized amino acids (AAs) in blood. Growing infants need ~3.6 g/kg/day protein with ~115–130 cal/kg/day. Excess calories may increase infant fat; additional protein does not add lean body mass **(Tables 2 and 3)**.[1,2]

## Carbohydrates

Carbohydrates are converted to glucose, then stored as glycogen. Glucose is the primary source of energy for brain and heart, as alternative fuels are scarce, and long-chain fatty acid oxidation is immature in the infant heart.[3]

**TABLE 1:** Caloric requirements (kcal/kg/day).

| Activity | Enterally fed | Intravenously fed |
|---|---|---|
| Basal metabolic rate | 50 | 50 |
| Movement | 0–15 | 0–5 |
| Thermostasis | 5.0–10.0 | 0–5 |
| Energy used for synthesis | 10 | 10 |
| Fecal energy loss | 10 | 0 |
| Growth | 25–35 | 25 |
| Total | 100–130 | 85–95 |

**TABLE 2:** Macronutrient caloric intake.

| Parenteral macronutrients | % of total calories | kcal/g |
|---|---|---|
| Carbohydrates | 35–60 | 3.4 |
| Fat | 30–50 | 9 |
| Protein | 7–15 | 4 |

**TABLE 3:** Protein and energy estimates to achieve fetal growth.

| Fetal weight (g) | 500–1,500 | 1,500–1,800 | 1,500–1,800 |
|---|---|---|---|
| *Protein intake (g/kg/d)* | | | |
| Parenteral | 3.5 | 3.2 | 3.0 |
| Enteral | 4.0 | 3.6 | 3.4 |
| *Energy (kcal/kg)* | | | |
| Parenteral | 89–101 | 109 | 111 |
| Enteral | 105 (<700 g)–127 (>1,200 g) | 129 | 131 |

## Parenteral Carbohydrates

*Form:* Parenteral carbohydrates are provided as dextrose or D-glucose, a plant monosaccharide. D5%–D25% are used (D5% = 5 g dextrose/100 mL water). Peripheral veins are irritated by >D12.5%, and intravascular hemolysis occurs with <D5%. Concentrations as low as D3.5% may be used with added protein to improve osmolality.

Glucose tolerance is monitored by following blood glucose. Glucose infusion rate (GIR) is adjusted to maintain euglycemia (80–140 mg/dL) and ~160 mg/dL is tolerated without glucosuria. Insulin is not recommended in the very preterm.

Monitoring GIR is indicated when fluid volumes or dextrose concentrations change.

$$\text{GIR} = \frac{(\text{Dextrose concentration, g/100 mL}) \times (\text{Infusion rate, mL/hr}) \times 1{,}000 \text{ (mg/g)}}{(\text{Weight, kg}) \times 60 \text{ min/hr}}$$

GIR range is 4–6 mg/kg/min to 12 mg/kg/min.

## Enteral Carbohydrates

*Form:* Lactose is the predominant human milk (HM) carbohydrate. Enteral (intestinal wall) lactase converts lactose to glucose and galactose. With hepatic first-pass, galactose is absorbed by the liver and converted to glucose. Very preterm intestinal lactase may be ~30% of activity at term.[4] Lactase is inducible with substrate exposure.

*Human milk oligosaccharides (HMOs) and carbohydrates:* HM contains a variety of carbohydrates, including inositol, which is involved in surfactant production and reduces risk of retinopathy of prematurity (ROP).[5] HM also contains >150 HMOs, nourishing bacteria[6] that use specific enzymes (e.g. sialidases and fucosidases). These HMOs and bacteria support an appropriate gut microbiome and augment the intestinal lining with anti-adhesive properties, reducing bacterial invasion. HMOs are not heat sensitive, thus are functional in pasteurized HM.

## Fats

Fats provide caloric density. They help absorb (fat-soluble) vitamins and have other essential functions, including cell membrane phospholipid presence, membrane fluidity, cell signaling, and protein regulation/expression for immune and inflammatory responses. Essential fatty acid deficiency manifests as dermatitis, thrombocytopenia, infection risk, and failure to thrive.[7]

### Energy Storage

Adiposal triglycerides (TGs) undergo mitochondrial beta-oxidation creating energy. Acylcarnitines assist transport and mitochondrial metabolism. Fatty acids entering the Krebs cycle as acetyl coenzyme A (CoA) are converted to adenosine triphosphate (ATP) for energy; e.g. one palmitate molecule becomes 106 ATP molecules.

### Structure

Fatty acids have an acetyl-CoA primer and exist as saturated (no double bonds), monounsaturated, and polyunsaturated (≥2 double bonds). They are named by the position of the first double bond (e.g. ω-3 or n-3) in the 3 carbon location. Double bonds change functionality of the fatty acid. At the double bond, a cis or a trans isomerism occurs—cis allows the fatty acid to bend and enhance membrane fluidity, while trans leads to a flat or unfolded shape, impairing ability to bend. When trans (saturated) fats are in cell membranes, there is altered membrane fluidity and receptor function.

### Essential Fatty Acids

Humans cannot synthesize n-3 and n-6 fatty acids. Essential precursor fatty acids are α-linolenic acid (18:3 n-3) and linoleic acid (18:2 n-6), respectively, metabolized to make long-chain polyunsaturated fatty acids (LCPUFAs).[8]

Linoleic acid (n-6) constitutes ~8–20% of milk fat and is a precursor of arachidonic acid (ARA); deficiency results in poor growth and scaly skin. Derivatives of ARA are proinflammatory eicosanoid versions of prostaglandins, leukotrienes, and thromboxanes.[9]

α-linolenic acid (n-3) constitutes 0.5–1% of dietary fat, and deficiency is associated with visual and neurological abnormalities.[10] α-linolenic acid is a precursor for eicosanoids and docosanoids, and is less inflammatory than those produced by the n-6 series. Another n-3, eicosapentaenoic acid, creates anti-inflammatory products, such as resolvins.

Fatty acids of the n-3, n-6, and n-9 types compete for the same enzymes; thus a larger percentage of one fatty acid makes less enzyme available for others n-3 fatty acids, which are preferentially catabolized when compared to n-6 and n-9.[11] The ratio of these long-chain unsaturated fatty acids changes the balance of pro- and anti-inflammatory products. Changes in n-6:n-3 ratio in preterm infants affect neonatal morbidities.[12]

### Long-chain Polyunsaturated Fatty Acid

Long-chain polyunsaturated fatty acids have 18 minimum C-atoms, plus two or more double bonds, and are synthesized in humans from precursor essential fatty acids (linoleic acid n-6 and α-linolenic acid n-3). Endogenous production of some neural LCPUFAs[13] like ARA (20:4 n-6), derived from linoleic acid, and docosahexaenoic acid (DHA) (22:6 n-3), derived from α-linolenic acid, may be inadequate in preterm and term infants.[14] DHA and ARA supplementation in maternal and infant diet shows increased infant blood levels and beneficial effects on visual acuity/visual evoked potentials at 2, 4, and 12 months,[15] but has no effect on neurodevelopment in term[16] and preterm infants.[17] Prenatal fish oil supplementation is associated with a less allergenic infant;[18] decreased atopic eczema,[19] decreased frequency of egg sensitization,[20] and asthma reduction in adolescence.[21] Supplementation in children <1,250 g may reduce chronic lung disease (CLD) in boys, and reduces hay fever at 12-18 months.[22] No negative effect of LCPUFA supplementation (up to 1% of dietary fat) on preterm infant growth is known.

## Intravenous Lipids

*Form:* Intralipid (IL) solution contains 20% soybean oil, 1.2% egg yolk phospholipids, 2.25% glycerine, water, and sodium hydroxide to bring pH to 8. IL provides essential fatty acids—linoleic acid and α-linolenic acid. Soybean oil phytocholesterols inhibit liver bile salt uptake and cause cholestasis.[23] Optimal n-6/n-3 ratio is not provided in most intravenous (IV) lipids. Fish oil (Omegaven) is used but not ideal. Currently SMOF (safflower, medium-chain triglycerides [MCT], olive oil, fish oil) is used as an alternative lipid solution.[24]

*Requirements:* IL 0.5-3 g/kg/day or SMOF 1.5-3 g/kg/day is recommended.

*Tolerance measure:* Lipids are measured using serum TG; ~200-250 mg/dL is tolerated.[25] IL 20% infused over 24 hours is preferred to 10% as it minimizes volume infused and is less likely to elevate blood TGs.[26]

## Enteral Fat

*Form:* The majority of dietary fats are TGs, cholesterol, and phospholipids. Human breast milk (HM) fat is 98% triacylglycerol, 1% phospholipids, and 0.5%[27] cholesterol/cholesterol esters. Maternal diet affects HM fatty acid profile. Before 2002, 12-18% of HM was trans fat (US and Canada); subsequently, the percent trans in HM has decreased. Trans fat presence in HM is problematic in countries where partially hydrogenated oils exist in food.[28]

*Requirements:* About 15-30% of dietary calories should be from fat.

*Enteral fat absorption:* Preterm infants have reduced fat absorption. Enteral fat absorption depends upon lipase (lingual and gastric) and bile salts. Nasogastric feeds limit salivary digestion. Discarded gastric residuals waste beneficial enzymes and reduce bile salts. Unpasteurized HM contains heat-sensitive and bile salt-stimulated lipases that digest fat. Pasteurizing HM reduces enzymes and fat absorption, resulting in slower growth.[29] Bolus feeds result in less fat absorbed (~6% reduction) versus continuous feeds (~40-50% reduction).[30] Blood fat travels in chylomicrons and metabolized by tissue lipoprotein lipase, which is deficient in preterm and small for gestational age (SGA) infants.[31] MCTs are easily absorbed without digestion.

## Protein

Proteins are alpha AA chains which exist in complex 3-D arrangements, allowing great functional diversity. Protein is the major structural and functional component of cells. Inadequate protein intake causes growth restriction. Proteins are integral to glutathione (a major antioxidant), hormones, heme, creatinine, nitric oxide, bile acids, neurotransmitters such as glutamate, enzymes, transporters, and other essential cellular activity.

### Essential Amino Acids

Essential AAs are not synthesized in the human body. In the preterm infant, functional immaturity of certain enzymes requires some nonessential AAs to be provided. These enzymes usually mature by term, when AA supplementation is unnecessary **(Table 4)**.

### Parenteral Protein

*Form:* Intravenous protein is composed of AAs.

*Requirements:* Protein required to maintain positive nitrogen balance is 1.3-1.5 g/kg/day and >3.5-4 g/kg/day of protein is required to achieve optimal growth. Very sick and catabolic infants, especially those <26 weeks' gestation, are unable to anabolize excess AAs which accumulate, leading to metabolic acidosis, hyperammonemia, and azotemia. Initiating 3-4 g/kg/day protein proximate to birth promotes anabolism. Safety is unknown in infants <26 weeks' gestation/weighing <1,000 g. A randomized

**TABLE 4:** Essential amino acids in preterm and term infants.

| Indispensable/Essential amino acids | Conditionally essential in neonates | Nonessential amino acids |
|---|---|---|
| Leucine | Arginine | Alanine |
| Isoleucine | Glutamine | Aspartic acid |
| Valine | Proline | Asparagine |
| Threonine | Glycine | Serine |
| Methionine | Cysteine | Glutamic acid |
| Phenylalanine | Tyrosine | |
| Tryptophan | | |
| Lysine | *Possibly taurine* | |
| Histidine | *Possibly carnitine* | |

control trial (RCT) of <1,000 g infants comparing "low" protein (0.5 g/kg/day, advancing by 0.5 g/kg/day) versus "high" protein (2 g/kg/day, advancing by 1 g/kg/day until reaching 4 g/kg/day) shows several AAs (phenylalanine, tyrosine, and methionine) abnormally elevated in cord blood and in breastfed infants given high protein, especially at 3 days of age.[32] Infants <26 weeks' gestation given ≥3 g/kg/day of AAs are more likely positive for phenylketonuria and maple syrup urine disease on blood AA analysis by day 3 of life, but profiles normalize by 5–7 days.[33]

### Enteral Protein

*Form:* Enteral proteins (more complex) require digestion for absorption. Two classes of milk protein are whey (acid-soluble) and casein (acid-precipitable). HM whey is predominantly α-lactoglobulin and then lactoferrin, whereas cow's milk whey is predominantly lactoferrin and then β-1 lactoglobulin.[34] HM protein is ideal as its whey:casein ratio matures as lactation progresses. Human colostrum has whey:casein = 90:10, while mature HM is 60:40.[35] When formula is necessary, a whey formula is recommended; bovine milk protein is widely used, although soy and protein hydrolysate formulas are available.

Enteral protein is digestible by enzymes like enterokinase. While these enzymes' functions appear immature in the preterm, digestion and absorption of proteins occur. Digestive enzymes are inducible, thus early minimum enteral nutrition (MEN) enhances digestion and absorption.

*Requirements:* Protein requirements are higher in enteral feeds than in parenteral, as some protein is lost in the stool or used by the gut. Providing infants 3.5–4.5 g/kg/day optimizes preterm growth,[36] while 2.5 g/kg/day is sufficient at term.[37] Adverse neurological sequelae do not occur at this protein intake. Protein <2.5 g/kg/day (even with adequate caloric intake) results in postnatal growth failure and worse neurological outcomes.[2] Preterm protein >6–7.2 g/kg/day may result in lethargy, poor feeding, and lower IQ scores at 5–6 years.[38,39]

*Human milk and protein intake:* Human milk protein is easily digested and contains specific bioactive glycoproteins that protect against infection and necrotizing enterocolitis (NEC)[40] (e.g. lactoferrin, lysozyme, secretory IgA, haptocorrin, lactoperoxidase, α-lactalbumin, bile salt-stimulated lipase, and tumor growth factor β). Breast milk protein decreases in the first few days of lactation—colostrum has 2.5 g/dL,[41] preterm milk ~1.4 g/dL, and after 2 weeks of lactation, term milk provides ~0.9 g/dL of protein. Low protein limits growth of lean body mass. Several supplementary strategies exist to provide adequate dietary protein. HM fortifiers, available in powder and/or liquid, supply protein, calcium, phosphorus, sodium, and vitamins. Powders have solubility issues and are less bioavailable, while liquid fortifiers reduce HM volume and some increase metabolic acidosis.[42] Whey protein powder or liquid protein may be necessary. In resource-poor environments with commercial formulations unavailable, added skim milk powder 2.5 g/100 mL mother's own milk (MOM) has been used.

*Formula and protein intake:*
- **Cow protein formula:** Bovine protein is available, inexpensive, and mammalian. Sensitivity to cow's milk protein occurs in preterm infants, with hematochezia within a week of adding bovine protein to the diet.[43] These bloody stools may be confused with/be a precursor to NEC. Preterm formula uses a bovine 60:40 whey-casein with higher protein, phosphorus, calcium, and vitamin supplements based on preterm needs. Formula is used only when HM is unavailable.
- **Soy protein formula:** Soy formula is suboptimal for preterm infants because of plant origin, aluminum, and cross-reactivity with bovine protein. Soy phytates bind to calcium, making it less bioavailable. Soy contains high isoflavone with adverse endocrine effects. Soy is recommended by the European Society for Paediatric Gastroenterology, Hepatology and Nutrition (ESPGHAN) only for severe lactose intolerance, galactosemia, or vegan lifestyle.[44]
- **Partially-hydrolyzed whey formula:** Being expensive and highly osmolar, it is inadequate for preterms due to insufficient protein, caloric density, and vitamins. A meta-analysis of 15 studies showed allergy prevention in children with family history of atopy.[45] It was hoped that extensively hydrolyzed formula would prevent insulin-dependent diabetes in those with first-degree Type I diabetic relatives by reducing autoantibodies.[46] However, "TRIGR" (Trial to Reduce Insulin-dependent diabetes mellitus in the Genetically at Risk), a large multicenter, double-blind, RCT of 2,159 infants, did not reduce beta islet cell-associated autoantibodies in children followed for 7 years.[47]

## CALCIUM, PHOSPHORUS, AND MAGNESIUM

Calcium (Ca), phosphorus/phosphate (P), and magnesium (Mg) represent ~3% of body weight and are important for bone mineralization, muscle contractility, and nerve excitability/function.

Serum levels do not reflect body content, minerals being actively transferred to the fetus, mostly in the third trimester.

These minerals are essential to critical function (**Table 5**), including:
- *Calcium:* Clotting, nitric oxide production, second messenger for hormones, and cell death/pro-apoptosis

- *Phosphorus/phosphate:* Major intracellular anion, component of nucleic acids, and cell energy (adenosine tri-/diphosphate)
- *Magnesium:* Important intracellular cation, part of multiple intracellular enzymes, important role in transmembrane transport of ions (Na/K-ATPase pump); anti-apoptosis; calcium antagonist; modulates vascular tone, heart rhythms, platelet-activated thrombosis, and role in insulin and parathyroid secretions.

Mineral needs are estimated by fetal accretion rates, adjusting for reduced absorption once on enteral feeds. Fetal accretion of calcium is 100–130 mkd and phosphorus

**TABLE 5:** Calcium, phosphorus, and magnesium disorders—risk factors, symptoms, and management.

| Mineral | Risk factors | | Infant symptoms/Treatment | |
|---|---|---|---|---|
| Calcium (Ca) | *Early hypocalcemia birth—72 hours* | | Symptoms | |
| | Maternal diabetes and hypomagnesemia | | Often asymptomatic early in life | |
| | Maternal hyperparathyroidism | | Jitteriness | Seizures (rare) |
| | Placental dysfunction | | High-pitched cry | Irritability |
| | Perinatal depression | | Tetany | Muscle twitching |
| | IUGR | | Poor feeding | Lethargy |
| | *Late hypocalcemia* | | Treatment | |
| | Hypoparathyroidism | | Supplemental calcium | |
| | Hypomagnesemia | | Hypoparathyroidism—calcitriol | |
| | Vitamin D deficiency | | If parathyroid function normal—ergocalciferol | |
| | Renal insufficiency | | | |
| | High phosphate intake | | Treat underlying cause, if possible | |
| | DiGeorge syndrome | | | |
| | *Hypercalcemia* | | Symptoms | |
| | Maternal hypoparathyroidism | | Poor feeding | Emesis |
| | Maternal high vitamin D | | Lethargy | Polyuria |
| | Infant hyperparathyroidism | | Constipation | |
| | Excessive Ca or vitamin D intake | | | |
| | Hypophosphatemia | | Treatment | |
| | Infantile hypophosphatasia | | Saline and furosemide | |
| | Induced by thiazide diuretics | | Low-calcium formula | |
| | Subcutaneous fat necrosis | | Reduce vitamin D access | |
| | Williams syndrome | | Treat underlying cause, if possible | |
| Phosphorus | *Hypophosphatemia* | | Symptoms | |
| | Maternal illness leading to: | | Hypercalcemia | Poor growth |
| | Placental dysfunction | | Fatigue/energy failure | |
| | Inadequate intake | IUGR | Rickets of prematurity—shorter babies | |
| | Renal tubular disorder | | Elevated alkaline phosphatase and parathormone | |
| | Refeeding syndrome in very infant | IUGR | Reversible respiratory failure | |
| | High protein load soon after birth in very immature infants | | Impairment of cardiac contractility | |
| | | | Treatment | |
| | | | IV/IM/oral supplementation | |
| | *Hyperphosphatemia* | | Symptoms | |
| | Very low calcium levels | | Tetany | Muscle cramps |
| | | | Perioral numbness or tingling | |
| | | | Treatment | |
| | | | Calcium infusions | |

*Contd...*

*Contd...*

| Mineral | Risk factors | | Infant symptoms/Treatment |
| --- | --- | --- | --- |
| Magnesium | *Hypomagnesemia* | | *Symptoms* |
| | Maternal illness leading to: | | Tremors |
| | Placental dysfunction | | Irritability |
| | Inadequate intake | IUGR | Seizures |
| | Renal tubular disorder | | Muscle weakness |
| | After medication, e.g. amphotericin B | | Prolonged QT interval |
| | Hypoparathyroidism | | |
| | Perinatal depression | | *Treatment* |
| | | | IV/IM or oral supplementation |
| | *Hypermagnesemia* | | *Symptoms* |
| | Excess maternal supplementation: | | Majority asymptomatic |
| | Used for neuroprotection | | May have decreased respiratory effort |
| | Preterm labor | | Hypotonia   Flaccidity |
| | Pre-eclampsia | | Urinary retention + reduced bowel motility |
| | | | Reduced deep tendon reflexes |
| | | | *Treatment* |
| | | | Hydrate and provide loop diuretics |
| | | | Possible calcium supplementation |

(IUGR: intrauterine growth restriction; IV/IM: intravenous/intramuscular).

is 60–70 mkd. Bone (hydroxyapatite [$Ca_{10}(PO_4)_6(OH)_2$]) deposition requires a combination of calcium, phosphorus, and magnesium, and its mineral content provides an estimate of ossification density.

## Parenteral

Intravenous Ca delivery is limited by Ca-P precipitation and high osmolarity is injurious to peripheral veins. Central lines can deliver higher mineral concentrations **(Table 6)**.

## Enteral

Diet affects mineral intake. Preterm infants on unsupplemented HM (lower in phosphorus) have higher incidence of rickets.[48] Thus, breastfed preterms require mineral fortification, while those on preterm formula do not. For enteral feeds, high protein and molar elemental Ca:P ratio 1.5:1 is recommended.[49,50] Absorption affects availability; Ca intake of 120–230 mkd provides only 60–90 mkd for bone mineralization as calcium absorption rate is 50–65%. Phosphate absorption is more efficient at 80–90%. Magnesium absorption is only ~40%.[51]

## ■ IRON (Fe)

Infant iron is 75–80% hemoglobin, 10% tissue iron-containing proteins (myoglobin and cytochromes), and 10% storage (ferritin and hemosiderin).[52] About 60% of newborn Fe is transferred in the third trimester, dependent on mother's iron status, and placental function. The body prioritizes fetal hemoglobin over other iron-containing proteins. Normal hematocrit occurs with low storage or tissue forms. Cord ferritin levels used to evaluate newborn iron stores[53] defined deficiency at term as <60 mcg/L. Severe deficiency (cord ferritin <35 mcg/L) was associated with 70% reduction in liver iron and lower brain iron.[54] Newborn iron status is affected by placental transfusion; delayed cord clamping (>2–3 minutes in term, >1 minute in preterm) allows newborns an additional 10–35 cc/kg, raising infant iron considerably. Blood conservation, erythropoietin, type of feeding, and iron supplementation all affect infant iron status.

**TABLE 6:** Recommended parenteral calcium, phosphorus, and magnesium intake.

| Mineral | First day of life/TPN | Goal |
| --- | --- | --- |
| Elemental Ca | 25–40 mkd (1 mmol/kg/day) | 65–100 mkd (1.6–2.5 mmol/kg/day) |
| P | 18–30 mkd (1 mmol/kg/day) | 50–80 mkd (1.6–2.5 mmol/kg/day) |
| Mg | 0–3 mkd (0–0.12 mmol/kg/day) | 7–10 mkd (0.3–0.4 mmol/kg/day) |

*Note:* 100 mg calcium gluconate = 9 mg elemental calcium
(TPN: total parenteral nutrition).

Worldwide, mothers have malnutrition and/or iron deficiency. Anemic mothers have lower fetal iron transfer. Maternal hemoglobin <6 g/dL resulted in very low infant cord ferritin of 29 mcg/L (±11.8); maternal Hb between 6.1 g/dL and 8.5 g/dL had marginal mean cord ferritin of 58 mcg/dL.[55] Maternal diabetes,[54] smoking,[56] preeclampsia, and intrauterine growth restriction[57] result in adequate infant hematocrits but lower tissue, storage, and brain Fe.

Critical to brain development, first-year iron deficiency interferes with hippocampal development, leading to long-term neurological, processing speed, effect, learning, and memory deficits.[58] Early childhood iron deficiency impairs mental, social, motor, and emotional functions later in life.[59]

Iron excess is toxic, associated with oxygen free radicals and oxidant stress. In neonatal hemochromatosis, infant ferritin ~800 mcg/L is often fatal. Multiple transfusions in preterms may produce ferritin levels ~500 mcg/L[60] and high liver iron storage.[61] Oral iron, while neither well-studied nor neurotoxic in humans, induces adverse brain changes in mice. Oral iron alters gut flora, increases biodiversity,[62] encourages *Escherichia coli*/pathogenic bacteria, and discourages Bifido bacillus/helpful bacteria.[63]

Perinatal iron deficiency is managed by maternal screening, treatment, and early supplementation.

*Parenteral iron:* Intravenous iron is used in infants nil per os (NPO) for >4-6 weeks. Parenteral iron anaphylaxis can occur. Low doses of 200–300 mcg$^{-1}$ mg are recommended. Iron-sucrose 2 mg/kg IV enhances erythropoiesis in patients on Epogen.[64]

## MICRONUTRIENTS

### Vitamins

Vitamins are essential to metabolism. Vitamins A, E, and C are antioxidants[1] placentally transferred in fetal life and through MOM. Maternal deficiency may manifest in the infant. Pregnancy, lactation, and multiple gestations increase maternal vitamin requirements.

### Requirements

Breastfed term infants of vitamin-replete mothers do not require supplementation, except vitamin D in regions of deficiency (e.g. the USA). Formula-fed term infants receive adequate vitamins from formula at 750 mL/day, an intake that they may not achieve till long after discharge.

Preterm infants have less placental transfer, thus have higher vitamin needs.[65] They may be sick, incur urinary losses, and absorb fat-soluble vitamins poorly due to immature digestion. Rapid growth necessitates supplementation.

Pasteurization, freezing, and light exposure of feeds inactivate or reduce vitamins. Pasteurization degrades vitamin C, thiamine, pyridoxine, folate, and reduces vitamin A.[66] Freezing reduces biotin, vitamin E, and inactivates vitamin C.[67] Light exposure on parenteral nutrition (PN) reduces vitamin C, riboflavin, pyridoxine, folate, and vitamins A and E.[68]

Vitamins are water-soluble or fat-soluble **(Table 7)**: Water-soluble vitamins (not synthesized/stored by humans) include vitamins C and B group. They require daily intake and do not accumulate, thus is less likely toxic. They cross by active transport from placenta to fetus.

Fat-soluble vitamins A, D, E, and K are synthesized from precursors and are stored in fat. Daily intake of fat-soluble vitamins is unnecessary, and excess consumption toxic. They cross from placenta to fetus by simple, facilitated diffusion, and mostly transferred in the third trimester.

### Maternal Vitamin D

Maternal poor calcium intake and/or severe vitamin D deficiency may result in neonatal severe hypocalcemia, neonatal seizures, and heart failure. Mid-pregnancy vitamin D deficiency is associated with preeclampsia,[73] shorter gestational length, shorter fetal knee-to-heel length,[74] and reduced fetal femur and humerus length with low intake <1,050 mg/day.

**TABLE 7:** Vitamins, role and deficiency in the preterm neonate.

| Vitamins | Functions | | Neonatal symptoms | |
|---|---|---|---|---|
| Fat-soluble | | | | |
| A | Epithelial tissues integrity, especially respiratory | | *Deficiency* = Plasma <200 µg/L(0.70 µmol/L) | |
|  | Bone | Immune function | Possible CLD risk factor[67] | Osteopenia |
|  | Visual acuity | Growth regulation | Generalized scaling | Failure to thrive |
|  | Cell differentiation | | *Excess* | |
|  | Antioxidant | | Vomiting | Skin changes |
|  | Surfactant and pneumocyte differentiation | | Higher intracranial pressure | |
|  | Inactivated by light exposure of TPN | | Not reported in preterms | |

*Contd...*

*Contd...*

| Vitamins | Functions | Neonatal symptoms | |
|---|---|---|---|
| D | Maintains serum calcium via intestine and bone | *Deficiency* | |
| | | Rickets | Osteomalacia |
| | Increases phosphate absorption | *Excess* | |
| | | Nephrocalcinosis | Hypercalcemia |
| E | Antioxidant properties | *Deficiency* | |
| | Free radical scavenger | Hemolytic anemia | Edema |
| | Stabilizes cell membranes | Thrombocytopenia | |
| | Prevents unsaturated fatty acid peroxidation | Spinocerebellar degeneration | |
| | Important for retina, nervous and skeletal systems | 50–200 mg/kg IV reduced intracranial hemorrhage, ROP, and blindness, but increased sepsis [68] | |
| | | *Excess* = >35 mg/L | Increased sepsis risk |
| K | Blood coagulation factors II, VII, IX, X | *Deficiency* | |
| | Proteins C, S, and Z | Hemorrhagic disease of the newborn (HDN) | |
| | Cell cycle regulation    Cell adhesion[69] | Adequate HDN prophylaxis: | |
| | Bone metabolism through osteocalcin in osteoblasts | 0.5 mg IM (0.2 mg for <1 kg) | |
| | | *Excess:* Hemolysis in G6PD-deficient | |
| *Water-soluble* | | | |
| C | Antioxidant properties | *Deficiency* | |
| | Collagen biosynthesis | Diarrhea | |
| | Proline and lysine hydroxylation | Frank hemorrhage | |
| | Dopamine/carnitine synthesis | Scurvy | |
| | Tyrosine catabolism    Iron absorption | Fatigue | |
| | Transient tyrosinemia | Muscle weakness | |
| B1 | Impaired carbohydrate metabolism | *Deficiency* | |
| | If pyruvate dehydrogenase deficient | Beriberi | |
| | Neurotransmitter function | Fatigue | Irritability |
| | Maple syrup urine disease association | Constipation | Heart failure |
| | | Consider deficiency if pyruvate/lactate accumulation | |
| | | Deficiency seen in alcoholics | |
| B2 | Mitochondrial oxidation | Deficiency rare, most preterms have high levels | |
| | Cofactor for NADPH, xanthine oxidase | | |
| | Associated with glutaric aciduria type I | Failure to thrive | |
| B3 | Component of coenzyme I (NAD) and coenzyme II (NADP), many others | Deficiency rare | |
| | | Pellagra | Diahrrhea |
| | Oxidative phosphorylation and fatty acid metabolism | Dermatitis | Dementia |
| B6 | Cofactor for transaminases | *Deficiency* | |
| | and decarboxylases | Dermatitis | Irritability |
| | Pivotal role in brain function/development, brain amino acid and neurotransmitter metabolism[70] | Seizures | Depression |
| | | Microcytic anemia | |
| | Associated with homocystinuria | | |
| Pantothenic acid | Component of CoA, tricarboxylate cycle | *Deficiency (rare)* | |
| | Lipid synthesis | Depression | Fatigue |
| | Other enzymatic reactions | Hypotension | Muscle weakness |
| | | Abdominal pain | |

*Contd...*

*Contd...*

| Vitamins | Functions | Neonatal symptoms | |
|---|---|---|---|
| Biotin | Coenzyme of carboxylases, e.g. acetyl CoA carboxylase | Deficiency | Increased cholesterol |
| | | Anorexia | Pallor |
| | Glucogenesis    Leucine catabolism | Alopecia | Seborrheic dermatitis |
| | Fatty acid metabolism | Severe deficiency | |
| | Synthesized by intestinal bacteria | Seizures | Hypotonia |
| | Associated with biotinidase deficiency | Lactic acidosis | Organic acid urea[71] |
| B12 | Red cell membrane maturation | Deficiency | |
| | CNS metabolism | Pernicious anemia | Megaloblastic anemia |
| | Methylmalonyl-CoA mutase | Neurological deterioration | |
| | Metabolism of methionine | Methylmalonic acidemia | |
| Folate | Action as tetrahydrofolate synthesis of purine and pyrimidines or DNA methylation reactions | Deficiency | |
| | | Reduced DNA in cell division | |
| | | Megaloblastic anemia | |
| | Essential in cell division | Impaired cellular immunity | |
| | Interacts with choline and methionine to modulate epigenetic phenomena[72] | If mother deficient: | |
| | | Neural tube defects | Cleft palate |

(CLD: chronic lung disease; CNS: central nervous system; DNA: deoxyribonucleic acid; ROP: retinopathy of prematurity; NADPH: nicotinamide adenine dinucleotide phosphate; CoA: coenzyme A).

**TABLE 8:** Microminerals—functions, deficiency, and features.

| Element | Functions | Deficiency | Special features |
|---|---|---|---|
| Chromium[75] | Insulin metabolism<br>Enhances insulin | Impaired glucose utilization | Preterms have higher level than term infants[76] |
| Enteral intake 0.03–2.25 mcg | | | TPN contaminant |
| Copper (Cu)[75] | Component of electron transport chain | Sideroblastic anemia<br>Thrombocytopenia | Levels inversely proportional to Zn intake |
| Fetal accretion = 30 mcg/kg/day | Neuropeptide synthesis | Neutropenia<br>Osteoporosis | If Zn supplemented at 2 mg, Cu 210 mcg/kg/day required |
| Deficiency: Plasma Cu <35 mcg/dL<br>Ceruloplasmin deficient plasma <15 mg/dL | Metalloproteins, e.g. antioxidant enzymes superoxide dismutase (CuZn SOD) | Poor weight gain<br>Depigmented hair<br>Apnea | If Zn supplemented at 2.3 mg, Cu 232 mcg/kg/day required |
| Enteral intake: 150–230 mcg/kg/day | Hemoglobin and RBC formation | | Toxicity from water in copper pipes or utensils |
| | Iron absorption | | |
| | Connective tissue (e.g. collagen) biosynthesis | | Liver, kidney, and CNS |
| | | | Indian childhood cirrhosis |
| Manganese (Mn)[77] | Key component of Mn-SOD, Superoxide Dismutase 2 | Short stature | Manganism (neurological toxicity) |
| Enteral Intake 1–15 mcg | Protection from free radicals | Brittle bones | Basal ganglia deposition in adults on long-term TPN |
| Measure level of Mn in | Bone structure/formation<br>Carbohydrate metabolism | Scaly dermatitis in adults | Cognitive impairment in children |
| White blood or RBC | Polysaccharide and glycoprotein synthesis | | Increased retention if poor bile secretion |
| Selenium (Se)[75] | Cofactor for glutathione peroxidase | CLD in the neonate[78] | Less need to supplement in MOM fed infants |

*Contd...*

*Contd...*

| Element | Functions | Deficiency | Special features |
|---|---|---|---|
| Measured by serum selenium level | Antioxidant enzymes prevent free radical formation and oxygen toxicity | Oxidative injury ROP White matter injury | |
| Cannot use glutathione level in preterm infants | | Cardiomyopathy (Keshan's disease) | Check if formula contains Selenium |
| | Deiodinase-Thyroid hormone metabolism | Alopecia | |
| Enteral Intake, 5–10 mcg or 2 mcg/kg | | Pseudo albinism | |
| | | Erythrocyte Macrocytosis | |
| | | Muscle weakness | |
| Zinc (Zn)[75] | Cellular growth and differentiation | Acrodermatitis Enteropathica with skin rash | When on TPN, give up to 400 mcg/kg/day |
| Fetal accretion rate unknown | Nucleic acid and protein metabolism | Stunted growth | High supplementation may reduce Cu |
| Measure: Plasma Zn | Over 300 enzymatic reactions | Failure to thrive | IUGR preterm infants and those with enterostomies have increased losses, require supplementation beyond 400 mg/kg/day[79] |
| Enteral intake 1.4–2.5 mg/kg/day ensures Zn retention of 400 mcg/kg/day | | Alopecia | |
| | | Increased infection risk | |
| AAP recommends 1–3 mg/kg/day | | Neurodevelopment effect unclear | |
| Iodine (I)[75] | Thyroid hormone T3 and T4 regulate metabolism, thermoregulation, growth and development | MOM-fed infants of deficient mothers | Iodine is absorbed through preterm infant skin if iodine-containing topical antiseptics used |
| Measure: Urinary iodine levels or newborn TSH | | | |
| | | Goiter | |
| Enteral intake 10–55 mcg/kg/day | | Mild to moderate impaired mental function and delayed development | Most preventable cause of brain damage worldwide[80] |
| Parenteral intake of 10 mcg/kg/d may decrease to 1 mcg/kg/day if using iodine topical disinfectants | | Severe (Cretinism) | |
| | | Poor growth | |
| | | Increased mortality | |
| Molybdenum[75] | Redox-enzymes, e.g. xanthine oxidase | Deficiency not reported in children | Only necessary if long-term PN needed |
| Enteral intake 0.3–5 mcg | | | |
| | Sulfite oxidase | | |
| | Aldehyde oxidase | | |

(AAP: American Academy of Pediatrics; CLD: chronic lung disease; CNS: central nervous system; IUGR: intrauterine growth restriction; RBC: red blood cell; ROP: retinopathy of prematurity; TSH: thyroid stimulating hormone; TPN: total parenteral nutrition; MOM: mother's own milk).

*Infant vitamin D:* Optimal preterm vitamin D levels are not established, but <50 nmol/L 25(OH) D3 is deficient. Maternal vitamin D deficiency is common, thus 400 IU vitamin D is recommended daily for breastfed infants in the first 6 months. For preterm infants, ESPGHAN 2010 recommends 800–1,000 IU vitamin D. If born to a vitamin D-deficient mother, supplementation increases to 800–1,500 IU/day.[51]

**TABLE 9:** Commercially available trace elements with reference guidelines.

| Parenteral dose | Chromium | Copper | Manganese | Molybdenum | Selenium | Zinc |
|---|---|---|---|---|---|---|
| Trace elements[a] µg/kg | 0.17–0.2 | 20 | 5 | 0 | 0 | 100–300 |
| Guidelines[b] µg/kg/day | 0.05–0.3 | 20<br>40[75] | 1.0 | 0.25 | 1.5–4.5<br>5–7[75] | Preterm: 400<br>Term (<3 months old): 250 |

[a]Based on dose of 0.2 mL/kg
[b]For stable growing preterms[36]

**TABLE 10:** Enteral micronutrient intake for preterm infants.

| Enteral intake recommendations in /kg/day | < 1800 g | < 1000 g/kg | 1,000–1,500 g |
|---|---|---|---|
| Substance | ESPGHAN 2010 | TSANG 2005 | TSANG 2005 |
| Fluids, mL | 135–200 | 160–220 | 135–190 |
| Energy, kcal | 110–135 | 130–150 | 110–130 |
| Protein, <1 kg body weight in g | 4.0–4.5 | 3.8–4.4 | |
| Protein, 1–1.8 kg body weight in g | 3.5–4 | | 3.4–4.2 |
| Lipids, g | 4.8–6.6 | 6.2–8.4 | 5.3–7.2 |
| Linolenic acid, mg | 385–1,540 | | |
| α-linoleic acid, mg | >55 (0.9% of fat) | 700–1,680 | 600–1,440 |
| DHA, mg | 12.0–30.0 | | |
| Arachadonic acid, mg | 18–42 | ≥28 | ≥24 |
| carbohydrate, g | 11.6–13.2 | 9.0–20.0 | 7.0–17 |
| Sodium, mg | 69–115 | 69–115 | 69–115 |
| Potassium, mg | 66–132 | 78–117 | 78–117 |
| Cloride, mg | 105–177 | 107–249 | 107–249 |
| Calcium, mg | 120–140 | 100–220 | 100–220 |
| Phosphate, mg | 60–90 | 60–140 | 60–140 |
| Magnesium, mg | 8.0–15.0 | 7.9–15 | 7.9–15 |
| Iron, mg | 2.0–3.0 | 2.0–4.0 | 2.0–4.0 |
| Zinc, mg | 1.1–2.0 | 1.0–3.0 | 1.0–3.0 |
| Copper, mcg | 100–132 | 120–150 | 120–150 |
| Selenium, mcg | 5.0–10.0 | 1.3–4.5 | 1.3–4.5 |
| Manganese, mcg | <27.5 | 0.7–7.75 | 0.7–7.75 |
| Flouride, mcg | 1.5–60 | | |
| Iodine, mcg | 11.0–55.0 | 10.0–60.0 | 10.0–60.0 |
| Chromium, mcg | 30–1,230 | 0.1–2.25 | 0.1–2.25 |
| Molybdenum, mcg | 0.3–5 | 0.3 | 0.3 |
| Thiamine, mcg | 140–300 | 180–240 | 180–240 |
| Riboflavin, mcg | 200–400 | 250–360 | 250–360 |
| Niacin, mg | 0.380–5.5 | 3.6–4.8 | 3.6–4.8 |
| Pantothenic acid, mg | 0.33–2.1 | 1.2–1.7 | 1.2–1.7 |
| Pyridoxine, mcg | 45–300 | 150–210 | 150–210 |
| Cobalamine/Vitamin B12, mcg | 0.1–0.77 | 0.3 | 0.3 |
| Folic acid, mcg | 35–100 | 25–50 | 25–50 |
| L-Ascorbic acid/Ascorbate, mg | 11.0–46.0 | 18–24 | 18–24 |
| Biotin, mcg | 1.7–16.5 | 3.6–6 | 3.6–6 |

*Contd...*

*Contd...*

| Enteral intake recommendations in /kg/day | <1800 g | <1000 g/kg | 1000–1500 g |
|---|---|---|---|
| Vitamin A, mcg RE, 1 mcg = 3.33 IU | 400–1,000 | 700–1,500 IU | 700–1,500 IU |
| Vitamin E, mcg RE, (alpha-tocopherol equivalents) | 2.2–11 | 6–12 IU | 6–12 IU |
| Vitamin K1, mcg | 4.4–28 | 8.0–10.0 | 8.0–10.0 |
| Nucleotides, mg | <5 | | |
| Choline, mg | 8.0–55.0 | 14.4–28 | 14.4–28 |
| Inositol, mg | 4.4–53 | 32–81 | 32–81 |
| Taurine, mg | | 4.5–9.0 | 4.5–9.0 |
| Carnitine, mg | | ~2.9 | ~2.9 |

(ESPGHAN: European Society for Paediatric Gastroenterology Hepatology and Nutrition equivalents; DHA: docosahexaenoic acid).

## Microminerals

Trace elements comprise <0.01% of body weight. Chromium, copper, manganese, zinc, selenium, and molybdenum are essential trace elements in humans, transferred to the fetus mostly during the third trimester. Deficiencies develop in fast-growing infants because of low fetal stores, increased growth demand, and inadequate intake. Human milk reflects maternal micronutrient status; deficient mothers have produced infants with iodine and zinc deficiency. Formula has fixed micronutrients; enterally fed preterm infants require more micronutrients. Functions, features, and deficiencies are listed in **Table 8**.

In preterms, fed IV, it is important to add PN micronutrients. Different trace elements are available PN. For preterms, 0.2 mL/kg is usually added. Available supplements lack selenium, molybdenum, and have inadequate zinc, but more than adequate manganese[77] **(Table 9)**.

**Table 10** summarizes enteral requirements/recommendations for various ages and sizes of infants.

## REFERENCES

1. Kashyap S, Forsyth M, Zucker C, et al. Effects of varying protein and energy intakes on growth and metabolic response in low birth weight infants. J Pediatr. 1986;108(6):955-63.
2. Ziegler EE. Meeting the nutritional needs of the low-birth-weight infant. Ann Nutr Metab. 2011;58(Suppl 1):8-18.
3. Hay W, Brown L, Denne S. Energy and carbohydrates. In: Koletzko B, Poindexter B, Uauy R (Eds). Nutritional Care of Preterm Infants: Scientific Basis and Practical Guidelines. Vol. 110. Basel: Karger; 2014. pp. 64-81.
4. Antonowicz I, Lebenthal E. Developmental pattern of small intestinal enterokinase and disaccharidase activities in the human fetus. Gastroenterology. 1977;72(6):1299-303.
5. Fang JL, Sorita A, Carey WA, et al. Interventions To Prevent Retinopathy of Prematurity: A Meta-analysis. Pediatrics. 2016;137(4). pii: e20153387.
6. Marcobal A, Southwick AM, Earle KA, et al. A refined palate: bacterial consumption of host glycans in the gut. Glycobiology. 2013;23(9):1038-46.
7. Paulsrud JR, Pensler L, Whitten CF, et al. Essential fatty acid deficiency in infants induced by fat-free intravenous feeding. Am J Clin Nutr. 1972;25(9):897-904.
8. Innis SM. Essential fatty acids in growth and development. Prog Lipid Res. 1991;30(1):39-103.
9. Calder PC. Immunomodulation by omega-3 fatty acids. Prostaglandins Leukot Essent Fatty Acids. 2007;77(5-6):327-35.
10. Wheeler TG, Benolken RM, Anderson RE. Visual membranes: specificity of fatty acid precursors for the electrical response to illumination. Science. 1975;188(4195):1312-4.
11. Holman RT. Nutritional and biochemical evidences of acyl interaction with respect to essential polyunsaturated fatty acids. Prog Lipid Res. 1986;25(1-4):29-39.
12. Martin CR, Dasilva DA, Cluette-Brown JE, et al. Decreased postnatal docosahexaenoic and arachidonic acid blood levels in premature infants are associated with neonatal morbidities. J Pediatr. 2011;159(5):743-9.e1-2.
13. Martinez M. Tissue levels of polyunsaturated fatty acids during early human development. J Pediatr. 1992;120(4 Pt 2):S129-38.
14. Makrides M, Uauy R. LCPUFAs as conditionally essential nutrients for very low birth weight and low birth weight infants: metabolic, functional, and clinical outcomes-how much is enough? Clin Perinatol. 2014;41(2):451-61.
15. Qawasmi A, Landeros-Weisenberger A, Bloch MH. Meta-analysis of LCPUFA supplementation of infant formula and visual acuity. Pediatrics. 2013;131(1):e262-72.
16. Simmer K, Patole SK, Rao SC. Long-chain polyunsaturated fatty acid supplementation in infants born at term. Cochrane Database Syst Rev. 2011;(12):CD000376.
17. Schulzke SM, Patole SK, Simmer K. Long-chain polyunsaturated fatty acid supplementation in preterm infants. Cochrane Database Syst Rev. 2011;(2):CD000375.
18. Dunstan JA, Mori TA, Barden A, et al. Fish oil supplementation in pregnancy modifies neonatal allergen-specific immune responses and clinical outcomes in infants at high risk of atopy: a randomized, controlled trial. J Allergy Clin Immunol. 2003;112(6):1178-84.
19. Furuhjelm C, Warstedt K, Larsson J, et al. Fish oil supplementation in pregnancy and lactation may decrease the risk of infant allergy. Acta Paediatr. 2009;98(9):1461-7.
20. Palmer DJ, Sullivan T, Gold MS, et al. Effect of n-3 long chain polyunsaturated fatty acid supplementation in pregnancy on infants' allergies in first year of life: randomised controlled trial. BMJ. 2012;344:e184.

21. Olsen SF, Østerdal ML, Salvig JD, et al. Fish oil intake compared with olive oil intake in late pregnancy and asthma in the offspring: 16 y of registry-based follow-up from a randomized controlled trial. Am J Clin Nutr. 2008;88(1):167-75.
22. Manley BJ, Makrides M, Collins CT, et al.; DINO Steering Committee. High-dose docosahexaenoic acid supplementation of preterm infants: respiratory and allergy outcomes. Pediatrics. 2011;128(1):e71-7.
23. Carter BA, Taylor OA, Prendergast DR, et al. Stigmasterol, a soy lipid-derived phytosterol, is an antagonist of the bile acid nuclear receptor FXR. Pediatr Res. 2007;62(3):301-6.
24. Fell GL, Nandivada P, Gura KM, et al. Intravenous Lipid Emulsions in Parenteral Nutrition. Adv Nutr. 2015;6(5):600-10.
25. Adamkin DH, Gelke KN, Andrews BF. Fat emulsions and hypertriglyceridemia. JPEN J Parenter Enteral Nutr. 1984;8(5):563-7.
26. Haumont D, Richelle M, Deckelbaum RJ, et al. Effect of liposomal content of lipid emulsions on plasma lipid concentrations in low birth weight infants receiving parenteral nutrition. J Pediatr. 1992;121(5 Pt 1):759-63.
27. Innis SM. Impact of maternal diet on human milk composition and neurological development of infants. Am J Clin Nutr. 2014;99(3):734S-41S.
28. Mosley EE, Wright AL, McGuire MK, et al. trans Fatty acids in milk produced by women in the United States. Am J Clin Nutr. 2005;82(6):1292-7.
29. Casper C, Carnielli VP, Hascoet JM, et al. rhBSSL improves growth and LCPUFA absorption in preterm infants fed formula or pasteurized breast milk. J Pediatr Gastroenterol Nutr. 2014;59(1):61-9.
30. Rogers SP, Hicks PD, Hamzo M, et al. Continuous feedings of fortified human milk lead to nutrient losses of fat, calcium and phosphorous. Nutrients. 2010;2(3):230-40.
31. Griffin EA, Bryan MH, Angel A. Variations in intralipid tolerance in newborn infants. Pediatr Res. 1983;17(6):478-81.
32. Blanco CL, Gong AK, Green BK, et al. Early changes in plasma amino acid concentrations during aggressive nutritional therapy in extremely low birth weight infants. J Pediatr. 2011;158(4):543-8.e1.
33. Misra S, Song D. Amino Acid Abnormalities increase in Newborn Screen of NICU Patients in an Era of Early Aggressive Protein Use. Pediatric Academic Societies; 2012.
34. Heine WE, Klein PD, Reeds PJ. The importance of alpha-lactalbumin in infant nutrition. J Nutr. 1991;121(3):277-83.
35. Kunz C, Lönnerdal B. Re-evaluation of the whey protein/casein ratio of human milk. Acta Paediatr. 1992;81(2):107-12.
36. Tsang RC, Uauy R, Koletzko B, et al. Nutrition of the Preterm Infant: Scientific Basis and Practical Guidelines, 2nd edition. Cincinnati, Ohio: Digital Educational Publishing Inc.; 2005.
37. Lapillonne A, O'Connor DL, Wang D, et al. Nutritional recommendations for the late-preterm infant and the preterm infant after hospital discharge. J Pediatr. 2013;162(Suppl 3):S90-100.
38. Goldman HI, Freudenthal R, Holland B, et al. Clinical effects of two different levels of protein intake on low-birth-weight infants. J Pediatr. 1969;74(6):881-9.
39. Goldman HI, Goldman J, Kaufman I, et al. Late effects of early dietary protein intake on low-birth-weight infants. J Pediatr. 1974;85(6):764-9.
40. van Goudoever JB, Vlaardingerbroek H, van den Akker CH, et al. Amino acids and proteins. In: Koletzko B, Poindexter B, Uauy R (Eds). Nutritional Care of Preterm Infants: Scientific Basis and Practical Guidelines. Basel: Karger. 2014;(110):49-63.
41. Wu ZC, Chijang CC, Lau BH, et al. Crude protein content and amino acid composition in Taiwanese human milk. J Nutr Sci Vitaminol (Tokyo). 2000;46(5):246-51.
42. Cibulskis CC, Armbrecht ES. Association of metabolic acidosis with bovine milk-based human milk fortifiers. J Perinatol. 2015;35(2):115-9.
43. Vlieghe V, Des Roches A, Payot A, et al. Human milk fortifier in preterm babies: source of cow's milk protein sensitization? Allergy. 2009;64(11):1690-1.
44. Agostoni C, Axelsson I, Goulet O, et al.; ESPGHAN Committee on Nutrition. Soy protein infant formulae and follow-on formulae: a commentary by the ESPGHAN Committee on Nutrition. J Pediatr Gastroenterol Nutr. 2006;42(4):352-61.
45. Szajewska H, Horvath A. Meta-analysis of the evidence for a partially hydrolyzed 100% whey formula for the prevention of allergic diseases. Curr Med Res Opin. 2010;26(2):423-37.
46. Knip M, Virtanen SM, Seppä K, et al.; Finnish TRIGR Study Group. Dietary intervention in infancy and later signs of beta-cell autoimmunity. N Engl J Med. 2010;363(20):1900-8.
47. Knip M, Åkerblom HK, Becker D, et al.; TRIGR Study Group. Hydrolyzed infant formula and early β-cell autoimmunity: a randomized clinical trial. JAMA. 2014;311(22):2279-87.
48. Koo WW, Sherman R, Succop P, et al. Sequential bone mineral content in small preterm infants with and without fractures and rickets. J Bone Miner Res. 1988;3(2):193-7.
49. Rigo J, Pieltain C, Salle B, et al. Enteral calcium, phosphate and vitamin D requirements and bone mineralization in preterm infants. Acta Paediatr. 2007;96(7):969-74.
50. Agostoni C, Buonocore G, Carnielli VP, et al.; ESPGHAN Committee on Nutrition. Enteral nutrient supply for preterm infants: commentary from the European Society of Paediatric Gastroenterology, Hepatology and Nutrition Committee on Nutrition. J Pediatr Gastroenterol Nutr. 2010;50(1):85-91.
51. Bhatia J, Griffin I, Anderson D, et al. Selected macro/micronutrient needs of the routine preterm infant. J Pediatr. 2013;162(Suppl 3):S48-55.
52. Rao R, Georgieff MK. Iron in fetal and neonatal nutrition. Semin Fetal Neonatal Med. 2007;12(1):54-63.
53. Saarinen UM, Siimes MA. Iron absorption from breast milk, cow's milk, and iron-supplemented formula: an opportunistic use of changes in total body iron determined by hemoglobin, ferritin, and body weight in 132 infants. Pediatr Res. 1979;13(3):143-7.
54. Petry CD, Eaton MA, Wobken JD, et al. Iron deficiency of liver, heart, and brain in newborn infants of diabetic mothers. J Pediatr. 1992;121(1):109-14.
55. Singla PN, Tyagi M, Shankar R, et al. Fetal iron status in maternal anemia. Acta Paediatr. 1996;85(11):1327-30.
56. Chełchowska M, Laskowska-Klita T. Effect of maternal smoking on some markers of iron status in umbilical cord blood. Rocz Akad Med Bialymst. 2002;47:235-40.
57. Georgieff MK, Mills MM, Gordon K, et al. Reduced neonatal liver iron concentrations after uteroplacental insufficiency. J Pediatr. 1995;127(2):308-4.
58. Fretham SJ, Carlson ES, Georgieff MK. The role of iron in learning and memory. Adv Nutr. 2011;2(2):112-21.
59. Lozoff B, Beard J, Connor J, et al. Long-lasting neural and behavioral effects of iron deficiency in infancy. Nutr Rev. 2006;64(5 Pt 2):S34-43; discussion S72-91.

60. Cooke RW, Drury JA, Yoxall CW, et al. Blood transfusion and chronic lung disease in preterm infants. Eur J Pediatr. 1997;156(1):47-50.
61. Ng PC, Lam CW, Lee CH, et al. Hepatic iron storage in very low birthweight infants after multiple blood transfusions. Arch Dis Child Fetal Neonatal Ed. 2001;84(2):F101-5.
62. Krebs NF, Sherlock LG, Westcott J, et al. Effects of different complementary feeding regimens on iron status and enteric microbiota in breastfed infants. J Pediatr. 2013;163(2):416-23.
63. Zimmermann MB, Chassard C, Rohner F, et al. The effects of iron fortification on the gut microbiota in African children: a randomized controlled trial in Cote d'Ivoire. Am J Clin Nutr. 2010;92(6):1406-15.
64. Pollak A, Hayde M, Hayn M, et al. Effect of intravenous iron supplementation on erythropoiesis in erythropoietin-treated premature infants. Pediatrics. 2001;107(1):78-85.
65. Burris HH, Van Marter LJ, McElrath TF, et al. Vitamin D status among preterm and full-term infants at birth. Pediatr Res. 2014;75(1-1):75-80.
66. Leaf A, Lansdowne Z. Vitamins-conventional uses and new insights. In: Koletzko B, Poindexter B, Uauy R (Eds). Nutritional Care of Preterm Infants: Scientific Basis and Practical Guidelines. Vol. 110. Basel: Karger; 2014. pp. 152-66.
67. Darlow B, Graham P, Rosas-Reyes MX. Vitamin A supplementation to prevent mortality and short- and long-term morbidity in very low birth weight infants. Cochrane Neonatal Rev. 2016;(8):CD000501.
68. Brion LP, Bell EF, Raghuveer TS. Vitamin E supplementation for prevention of morbidity and mortality in preterm infants. Cochrane Database Syst Rev. 2003;(4):CD003665.
69. Costakos DT, Greer FR, Love LA, et al. Vitamin K prophylaxis for premature infants: 1 mg versus 0.5 mg. Am J Perinatol. 2003;20(8):485-90.
70. Albersen M, Groenendaal F, van der Ham M, et al. Vitamin B6 vitamin concentrations in cerebrospinal fluid differ between preterm and term newborn infants. Pediatrics. 2012;130(1):e191-8.
71. Tokuriki S, Hayashi H, Okuno T, et al. Biotin and carnitine profiles in preterm infants in Japan. Pediatr Int. 2013;55(3):342-5.
72. Zeisel SH. Choline: critical role during fetal development and dietary requirements in adults. Annu Rev Nutr. 2006;26:229-50.
73. Wei SQ, Audibert F, Hidiroglou N, et al. Longitudinal vitamin D status in pregnancy and the risk of pre-eclampsia. BJOG. 2012;119(7):832-9.
74. Morley R, Carlin JB, Pasco JA, et al. Maternal 25-hydroxyvitamin D and parathyroid hormone concentrations and offspring birth size. J Clin Endocrinol Metab. 2006;91(3):906-12.
75. Domellöf M. Nutritional care of premature infants: microminerals. World Rev Nutr Diet. 2014;110:121-39.
76. Bougle D, Bureau F, Voirin J, et al. Chromium status of full-term and preterm newborns. Biol Trace Elem Res. 1992;32:47-51.
77. Burjonrappa SC, Miller M. Role of trace elements in parenteral nutrition support of the surgical neonate. J Pediatr Surg. 2012;47(4):760-71.
78. Darlow BA, Inder TE, Graham PJ, et al. The relationship of selenium status to respiratory outcome in the very low birth weight infant. Pediatrics. 1995;96(2 Pt 1):314-9.
79. Barbarot S, Chantier E, Kuster A, et al. Symptomatic acquired zinc deficiency in at-risk premature infants: high dose preventive supplementation is necessary. Pediatr Dermatol. 2010;27(4):380-3.
80. Ghirri P, Lunardi S, Boldrini A. Iodine supplementation in the newborn. Nutrients. 2014;6(1):382-90.

# CHAPTER 36

# Stages of Nutritional Support

*Sonya Misra*

## ABSTRACT

With the use of human milk, and better preparation with antenatal steroids, the practice of nutrition is evolving safely towards more and earlier enteral nutrition. A focus on optimal protein and calorie intake, avoiding an accumulation of nutritional component deficits can provide optimal outcomes.

There are four stages of nutritional support in a preterm infant <34 weeks gestational age (GA).
*Stage 1:* Total parenteral nutrition (TPN) with minimal enteral nutrition (MEN).
*Stage 2:* Graduated transition to enteral feeds and a slow reduction in support by TPN.
*Stage 3:* Enteral nutrition.
*Stage 4:* Postdischarge nutrition.

A conceptual general description of the transition and stages of feeding is illustrated in **Figure 1**.

## STAGE 1: TOTAL PARENTERAL NUTRITION WITH MINIMAL ENTERAL NUTRITION

### Total Parenteral Nutrition

Total parenteral nutrition provides early nutritional support and maintains positive nitrogen balance, facilitating growth until complete enteral feeds are tolerated. Ideally,

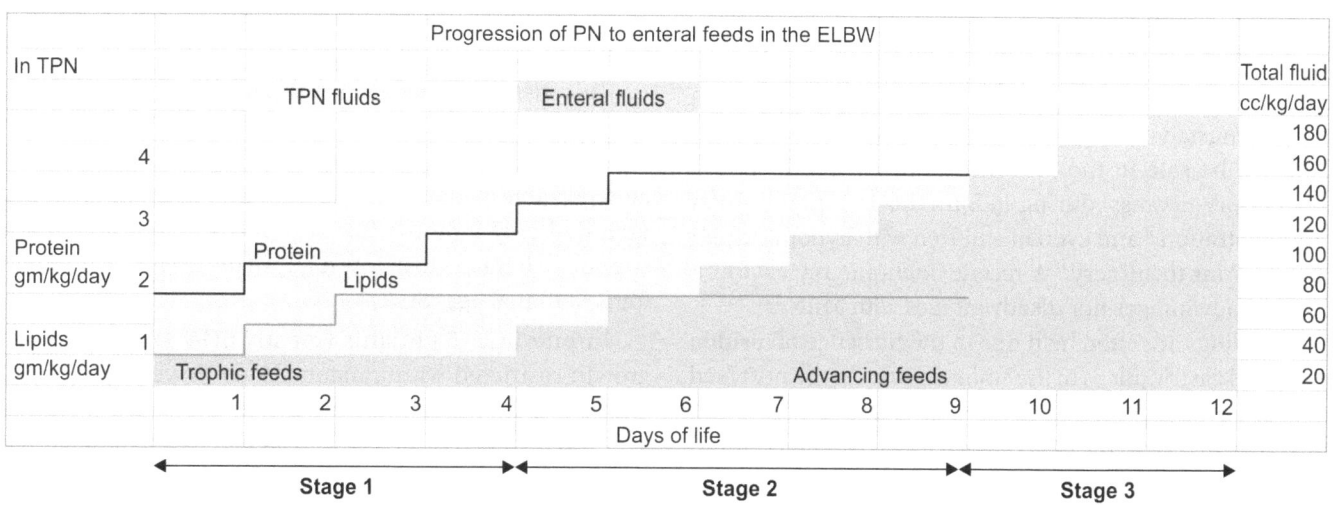

**Fig. 1:** Progression of PN to enteral feeds in the extremely low birthweight (ELBW) infant.
(PN: parenteral nutrition; TPN: total parenteral nutrition).

parenteral nutrition (PN) should commence as proximate as possible to the birth of a preterm infant. A dextrose solution containing amino acids should be started <4 hours of life. Common stock solutions are available, with 2-3% amino acid solution mixed in 10% dextrose with 300 mg of calcium gluconate/100 mL. If such solutions are not available, a solution of 5-10% dextrose can be used temporarily.

## Minimal Enteral Nutrition

Minimal enteral nutrition or *trophic feeding*, is the process of providing constant, small volume (usually <25 mL/kg/day) enteral feeds for stimulation of the alimentary canal, usually lasting 2-10 days. MEN should be started as soon as possible with undiluted food. Colostrum or human milk (HM), preferably maternal, is optimal, well-tolerated, provides immunological support, and supports optimal microbial colonization. In the absence of mother's own milk (MOM), donor human milk (DHM) is superior to preterm formula in prevention of necrotizing enterocolitis (NEC).[1] If DHM is unavailable, preterm infant formula is used.

Minimal enteral nutrition stimulates the immature gut. A cumulative volume of <96 mL of feeds induces maturation of the motor response in preterm infants.[2] MEN is associated with a reduction in time to full feeds and reduction in length of hospital stay, without increase in complications. Lack of feeding is associated with gut atrophy and delayed gut maturation.[3,4] A randomized control trial (RCT) compared infants fed PN and supplemented with formula vs. water in the first 2-10 days of life and found that the formula-fed children achieved the following milestones:[5]

- Full feeds—12 days sooner
- Nipple feeds—20 days sooner
- Birth weight—9 days sooner
- Discharge—20 days sooner.

Trophic feeding of preterm infants should not be delayed because of fear of NEC. While 90% of infants with NEC receive enteral feeds, there is no clear evidence that enteral feeds cause NEC. A meta-analysis found that fasting vs. feeding had no effect on NEC rates.[6] Other studies show MEN to be safe in the presence of umbilical lines[7] and respiratory distress, during indomethacin and ibuprofen administration,[8] and even in children with hypoplastic left hearts prior to surgery.[9] A recent Cochrane review found neither advantages nor disadvantages with MEN.[10]

Feedings are often held due to the presence of residual milk and gastric juices in the stomach prior to the next feed. This phenomenon reflects reduced motility of the bowel and gastric emptying in the first 5 days of life, as residual volumes (percentage of feeds) are normally higher than at any later time, reaching as high as 150% of feeds in the first few days.[11] While an infant is on MEN, gastric aspirates may be greenish-yellow, which may not be an indicator of "intolerance" or gut pathology, but rather reflects the immaturity of the preterm gut and dysmotility. On the other hand, in units where there is low frequency of NEC, bloody residuals have been associated with NEC.[12] Despite the presence of residuals, trophic feeds may be continued for a few days.

## ■ STAGE 2: GRADUATED TRANSITION TO ENTERAL FEEDS AND A SLOW REDUCTION IN TOTAL PARENTERAL NUTRITION

The volume and quality of enteral feeds in the first week of life predict neurological outcomes.[13] Over the years, criteria including residuals, frequency of feeding, respiratory stability, presence of umbilical lines, and use of vasopressors have been used to decide if and when to advance feeds. The fear of NEC has also led to cautious advances in feeds. This fear needs to be balanced with maintaining optimal nourishment for the infant and the increased risk of sepsis caused by prolonged parenteral access.

Mother's own milk is the gold standard for this stage in the preterm infant's life. Advancing feeds while using HM has been shown to reduce NEC in several studies. Decreased NEC is also associated with the use of a standardized protocol/guideline for feeding advancements.[14-16] Studies that compared feeding advances using a standardized feeding protocol found lower NEC frequency in their control group compared to their historical NEC rate.

A 2013 Cochrane analysis of five RCTs (n = 588) comparing feeding advances from a slow rate at 15-20 mL/kg/day to a fast rate at 30-35 mL/kg/day in babies <1,500 g found no significant difference in NEC incidence [relative risk (RR) = 0.97, confidence interval (CI) 0.54-1.74] or mortality (RR = 1.41, CI = 0.81-2.74).[17] Infants who advanced feeds more slowly took 2-5 days longer to establish full feeds and regain birth weight. There was a trend toward shorter time in the hospital for the faster feeding group.

This meta-analysis had several limitations—only 38 of 536 infants weighed <1,000 g and the majority of infants were >28 weeks' gestation.[18,19] Thus, these results are not generalizable to infants <1,000 g or <28 weeks. Some studies included only infants who did not need $O_2$ or ventilator support.[20] It is not clear how many of the infants were small for gestational age (SGA).

In one RCT, 53 infants (mostly SGA or intrauterine growth restricted with a mean GA of 33 weeks) received trophic exclusive HM, after which the rapid advance group reached 180 mL/kg/day feeds 5 days sooner than the slow advance group. There were two cases of NEC and three of sepsis in the rapid advance group, and 10 cases of sepsis in the slower advance group.[21] Without optimal

PN availability and/or with high sepsis prevalence, rapid feeding advancement may confer a better benefit:risk profile.

A Turkish RCT with trophic feeds (mostly HM) in smaller children (mean birth weight of ~1,000 g) showed the faster feeding advance group and the slower group was no different in the time taken to reach 80 mL/kg/day, which was ~15 days of age.[20] The time to attain full feeds, however, was statistically significantly different at 19 (rapid group) versus 22 days (slow group).[20] This may suggest feasibility of feeding smaller babies faster once they tolerate 80 mL/kg/day.

Feeds were withheld in these studies when residuals were >30% of feeding volume or 3 mL (whichever was greater), with an abnormal abdominal examination, bilious or bloody residuals, and abdominal girth increase of 2 cm.

Sample feeding guidelines for adding HM fortifier to HM are shown in **Table 1**.

**Table 2** shows formula feeding guidelines and **Table 3** includes residual treatment guidelines for preterm infants.

Signs of pathological residuals may include one or more of the following:
- Dark bile or bloodstained gastric aspirate ≥1 mL
- Vomiting
- Abdominal distension, discoloration or tenderness
- Visible bowel loops
- Bloody stool
- Abdominal X-ray showing signs of intestinal dilatation
- Metabolic acidosis or new thrombocytopenia
- Evidence that the child is not well—apnea (new onset or increasing frequency), respiratory distress, lethargy, poor perfusion, temperature instability, etc.

## STAGE 3: ENTERAL NUTRITION

The optimal enteral nutrition for all infants is MOM, best administered with standardized feeding guidelines.

### Human Milk

#### Mother's Milk

Mother's own milk provides immunological support for the infant, creates the correct microbiome in the infant gut,[22] reduces atopy,[23] prevents NEC, reduces days on TPN,[24] and may improve cardiovascular outcomes.[25,26] However, MOM does not meet all preterm infant needs; deficiencies of protein, calcium, phosphorus, and sodium develop if the milk is not fortified. The quality of MOM varies by gestation. MOM progresses from colostrum to preterm

**TABLE 1:** Sample feeding guidelines using HM fortifier to supplement HM, in mL/kg/day.

| Day of feeding HM | Birthweight: 401–700 g<br>GA: 23–25 weeks | 701–1,000 g<br>26–28 weeks | 1,001–1,250 g<br>29–30 weeks | 1,250–1,500 g<br>31–32 weeks |
|---|---|---|---|---|
| 1 | 20 | 20 | 20 | 20 |
| 2 | 20 | 20 | 20 | 40–50 |
| 3 | 20 | 20 | 40–50 | 60–80 |
| 4 | 20 | 30 | 60–80 | 80–110 |
| 5 | 20 | 45 | 80–110 | 100–140 Concentrate TPN 100/kg |
| 6 | 30 | 60‡ | 100–140 Concentrate TPN 100/kg | 120* + HMF–170 |
| 7 | 45 | 80 | 120* + HMF–170 | 140†–180* |
| 8 | 60‡ | 100 Concentrate TPN 100/kg | 140†–180* | 160–180† |
| 9 | 80 | 120§ | 160–180† | 180 |
| 10 | 100 Concentrate TPN 100/kg | 140 | 180 | |
| 11 | 120 | 160 | | |
| 12 | 140 | 180 | | |
| 13 | 160 | | | |

\* = Fortifying to 22 calories
† = Fortifying to 24 calories
‡ = Fortifying to 24 calories with HM-based fortifier
§ = Fortifying to 26 calories with HM-based fortifier
Italicized numbers above indicate a faster rate deemed acceptable by meta-analysis of 25–30 cc/kg/day advances in children >1,000 g on HM. This is useful in areas with high infection risk.
(GA: gestational age; HM: human milk; TPN: total parenteral nutrition).

**TABLE 2:** Very preterm and/or VLBW formula feeding guidelines, in mL/kg/day.

| Day of preterm formula feeding | Birthweight: 401–700 g GA: 23–25 weeks | 701–1,000 g 26–28 weeks | 1,001–1,250 g 29–30 weeks | 1,250–1,500 g 31–32 weeks |
|---|---|---|---|---|
| 1 | 15 | 15 | 15 | 15 |
| 2 | 15 | 15 | 15 | 30 |
| 3 | 15 | 15 | 30 | 45 |
| 4 | 15 | 30 | 45 | 60 |
| 5 | 15 | 45 | 60 | 80 |
| 6 | 30 | 60 | 80 | 100 |
| 7 | 45 | 80 | 100 | 120 |
| 8 | 60 | 100 | 120 | 140 |
| 9 | 80 | 120 | 140 | 160 |
| 10 | 100 | 140 | 160 | 180 |
| 11 | 120 | 160 | 180 | |
| 12 | 140 | 180 | | |
| 13 | 160 | | | |
| 14 | 180 | | | |

(GA: gestational age; VLBW: very low birth weight).

**TABLE 3:** Residual treatment guidelines for preterm infants.

| Signs of feeding intolerance | | Management considerations: |
|---|---|---|
| Gastric aspirate prior to feeding* | Other signs of feeding intolerance† (see below signs of pathological residuals) | • Check feeding tube placement<br>• Position infant prone, right side down<br>• Consider glycerine suppository, if no stools in 18–24 hours<br>• If recurrent episodes occur after a recent feed advance or fortification, consider returning to the previously tolerated feeding volume/concentration |
| *No feeding intolerance* | | |
| A. If ≤2 mL | None | Refeed aspirate and continue the ordered feeding amount |
| B. If >2 mL but <1/3 of previous feed volume | None | Check infant, refeed aspirate, and continue the ordered feeding amount |
| *Possible feeding intolerance* | | |
| C. If >2 mL and >1/3 of previous feed volume | None | Notify doctor<br>Stop feeding and recheck gastric aspirate in 3 hours<br>Resume feeding when conditions revert to A or B above |
| D. No gastric aspirate, but other signs of feeding intolerance | Present | Notify doctor<br>Stop feeding, evaluate appropriately, resume feeding when stable and conditions revert to A or B above |

*Some units choose not to follow residuals in the first few days. The safety of this practice is unknown.
†Evaluating significant feeding intolerance should be done by the primary clinical team according to standard procedure at institution (physical examination, abdominal roentgenograph, complete blood count, blood culture, etc.).

to term variably, but is assumed to transition at 14 days to term/mature milk. There is considerable inter-mother variation of HM. Maternal nutritional status affects some factors; vitamin A, vitamin $B_6$, vitamin $B_{12}$, folate, selenium, iodine, vitamin D, ratios of fatty acids, and long-chain polyunsaturated fatty acid content can all vary based on maternal levels, intake, and supplementation. Interestingly, maternal dietary lipid intake is the most important factor contributing to the variability in lipid profiles of MOM. MOM does not have an adequate content of zinc and iron and should not be considered a primary source of these micronutrients.[27]

Lactating mothers have higher nutritional needs than nonpregnant women. They need 500 additional calories/day, with increased requirements above the nonpregnant of 54% protein; 60% vitamin C; 20-50% vitamin B's; 25 mcg folate; 85% vitamin A; 26% vitamin E; 93% iodine; and 27% selenium. Mothers who avoid dairy require vitamin D and calcium supplements, while those following a vegan diet without eggs or dairy should take vitamin $B_{12}$ throughout lactation.

## Donor Human Milk

In areas or times where MOM may not be available, DHM can be used. DHM is pooled and pasteurized, usually by heat flash pasteurization, making the milk microbiologically safe to use.[28] The composition of DHM is similar to that of mature HM, with a mean energy of 65 ± 11 kcal/dL. The macronutrient composition varies considerably—protein has been found to be 1.16% ± 0.25%; fat 3.22% ± 1%; and lactose 7.8% ± 0.88%.[29] Due to pasteurization, heat-sensitive components of the milk are reduced.[30] The 150 + HM oligosaccharides are not affected by heat, thus providing prebiotics for development of an optimal infant gut microbiome.[23]

Growth goals ~0.5 Z- (standard deviation from mean) score below the birth Z-score for optimal weight gain in infants appropriate for gestational age (AGA) at birth, and under the 90th percentile for those infants born large for gestational age (LGA). For a child that is SGA, the aim is to get the infant's size above the 10th percentile.

Infants who are SGA or postnatally growth restricted require supplemental protein and calories to help gain optimal lean body mass. Protein intake, calculated by factorial method to ensure catch-up growth by term equivalent in a child at an adjusted GA of 34 weeks, requires 5.1 g/kg/day of protein with an additional 8 calories/kg/day. To achieve half of catch-up growth requires 4.2 g/kg/day of protein and 4 extra calories/kg/day. This suggests a much higher protein:energy requirement to achieve catch-up growth.[31] Dropping caloric and protein intake to match fetal growth (Table 4) in this subgroup is not beneficial, as it does not allow recovery from deficits.

## Practical Nutritional Critical Periods in the Infant Fed Human Milk

There are recognizable milestones during the neonatal intensive care unit (NICU) stay when very low birth weight (VLBW) infants may falter in intake. These include:
- The first week after birth
- When weaning off TPN
- The feeder/grower phase.

### Critical Issues in First Week after Birth

The bulk of protein intake being parenteral, institution of standardized feeding, including trophic feeds, is important. In addition to increasing parenteral protein, total protein is improved with enteral maternal colostrum and milk for feeds. **Table 5** illustrates the importance of DHM and MOM. Once enteral feeds are included in total fluids at 6 days, protein intake falls, even with 4% protein in TPN. The required intake of 4 g/kg/day of protein is unachievable without fortified feeds in the first 10 days of life.

### Transitioning from Total Parenteral Nutrition

Early fortification of HM is necessary to achieve adequate protein intake even prior to stopping TPN. As part of bloodstream infection reduction, it is recommended that central lines be discontinued at 120 cc/kg/day of feeding. Thus, without fortification of HM or TPN, delivery of calories, protein, calcium, and phosphorus is suboptimal **(Table 6)**. Providing 300-600 mg/kg of calcium gluconate is only 27.9-55.8 mg elemental calcium, which is inadequate. HM-fed infants experience less NEC and so there is less concern about early fortification when using predominantly MOM and DHM.

Despite fortification at 100 cc/kg/day, PN supplements may need to be continued and total fluids maintained at a higher level.

| TABLE 4: Adjustment of feeds based on intrauterine growth velocity. | | | | | |
|---|---|---|---|---|---|
| GA in weeks | <33 | 34–36 | 37–38* | Preterm SGA[†] | Postdischarge VLBW[†] |
| Weight gain g/kg/day | 18 (15–21) | 12–14 | 11 | | |
| Protein g/kg/day | 3.5–4.5 | 3.1 | 2.5 | | 2.8–3.2 |
| Energy calories/kg/day | 125–140 | 110–130 | 115 | | 105–125 |
| Calcium mg/kg/day[†] | 120–140 | 120–140 | 70–120 | 120–160 | 70–140 |
| Phosphorus mg/kg/day[†] | 60–90 | 60–90 | 35–75 | 60–90 | 35–90 |

Adapted from *Tsang 2005,[32] [†]Fenton 2013,[33] Uauy 2013[34]
(GA: gestational age; SGA: small for gestational age; VLBW: very low birth weight).

**SECTION 8:** Growth, Lactation and Nutrition

**TABLE 5:** Nutritional breakdown of following feeding guidelines described in Figure 1 and Table 1 at 24-week infant in the first 10 days of life (starting IV plus PO feeding for total fluids at day 6 when feeding advances start).

| Day of life | 1 | 2 | 3 | 4 | 5 | 6 | 7 | 8 | 9 | 10 |
|---|---|---|---|---|---|---|---|---|---|---|
| TPN protein g/kg/day | 1.6 | 2.5 | 2.5 | 3 | 3.5 | 3.1 | 2.7 | 3 | 2.2 | 1.6 |
| Lipids g/kg/day | 0 | 1 | 2 | 3 | 3 | 3 | 3 | 3 | 3 | 2 |
| Volume by lipids cc/kg/day | 0 | 5 | 10 | 15 | 15 | 15 | 15 | 15 | 15 | 10 |
| Fluids total cc/kg/day | 95 | * | * | * | * | 150 | 150 | 150 | 150 | 150 |
| Feeds cc/kg/day | 15 | 15 | 15 | 15 | 15 | 30 | 45 | 60 | 80 | 100 |
| Calories by feeds/kg/day | 10 | 10 | 10 | 10 | 10 | 20 | 30 | 40 | 50 | 60 |
| DHM protein/kg/day (0.95–1 g/dL) | 0.15 | 0.15 | 0.15 | 0.15 | 0.15 | 0.3 | 0.45 | 0.6 | 0.75 | 0.95 |
| Preterm MOM protein/kg/day (1.5 g/dL) | 0.23 | 0.23 | 0.23 | 0.23 | 0.23 | 0.46 | 0.69 | 0.92 | 1.15 | 1.38 |
| Total protein intake DHM g/kg/day | 1.75 | 2.65 | 2.65 | 3.15 | 3.65 | 3.4 | 3.15 | 3.6 | 2.95 | 2.55 |
| Total protein intake PT MOM g/kg/day | 1.89 | 2.73 | 2.73 | 3.23 | 3.73 | 3.56 | 3.39 | 3.92 | 3.35 | 2.98 |

*As deemed necessary by free fluid requirements
(DHM: donor human milk; MOM: mother's own milk; TPN: total parenteral nutrition; IV: intravenous; PT: preterm; PO: enteral).

**TABLE 6:** Calorie-protein-mineral content and osmolality of enteral feeds at 100 mL/kg/day (and parenteral feeds at 50 mL/kg/day).

| Type of milk at 100 mL/kg/day | DHM/Mature MOM | DHM + powdered fortifier = 22 calories | DHM + powdered fortifier = 24 calories | + Additional D10 TPN, fat 1 g/kg/day, protein 2 g/kg/day |
|---|---|---|---|---|
| | | | | At 50 mL/kg/day |
| Calories/kg | 66 | 73 | 80 | 38 |
| Protein g/kg/day | 0.8–1 | 1.5 | 2 | 2 |
| Calcium mg | 27.9 | 70 | 114 | varies |
| Phosphorus mg | 14.3 | 38 | 62 | varies |
| Osmolality | 286 | 308 | 325 | No extra but need IV access |

All these numbers vary by formulation and are used for illustration.
(DHM: donor human milk; MOM: mother's own milk; TPN: total parenteral nutrition; IV: intravenous).

**TABLE 7:** Nutrient intakes at 150 mL/kg/day.

| 150 mL/kg/day of feeds | Mature milk + Postdischarge formula powder to provide 27 calories/oz | Mature milk + powdered fortifier to provide 26 calories/oz | Recommended requirements for infants <29 weeks |
|---|---|---|---|
| Calories kg/day | 137 | 128 | 120–140 |
| Protein g/kg/day | 2.8 | 3.6–4 | 3.5–4.5 |
| Calcium mg/kg/day | 86 | 286 | 120–140/100–220 |
| Phosphorus mg/kg/day | 44 | 161 | 60–90/ 60–140 |
| Osmolality | ~347 | ~345–420 | |

Approximate numbers for illustration and vary by supplemental formulation.

### Feeder/Grower Phase: Maintaining Growth in the HM-fed VLBW Infant When Fluid is Restricted

It is unreasonable to fortify HM with postdischarge formula as it provides inadequate protein, calcium, and phosphorus for a preterm infant prior to term **(Tables 7 and 8)**. Currently, manufacturers do not recommend more than 24-calorie fortification; however, increased fortification with calories or protein beyond this level may be needed for growth if the blood urea nitrogen (BUN) level is under 9.[35] Keeping the infant at 180 mL/kg/day when on routinely fortified enteral HM feeds provides the best balanced diet. In fact, a high-volume strategy of 180–200 mL/kg/day enterally in a MOM-fed child may be preferable to a strategy of lower volume and more fortification, as the benefits of more MOM accrue to the child.

| TABLE 8: Calorie-protein-mineral content in mature milk. | | | |
|---|---|---|---|
| | Mature milk with powdered fortifier to reach 24 calories at 160 mL/kg/day of feeds | Mature milk with powdered fortifier to reach 24 calories at 180 mL/kg/day of feeds | Recommended requirements for <29 week infants |
| Calories/kg/day | 128 | 144 | 120–140 |
| Protein g/kg/day | 3.2–3.4 | 3.6–3.8 | 3.5–4.5 |
| Calcium mg/kg/day | 184–231 | 206–259 | 120–140/100–220 |
| Phosphorus mg/kg/day | 100–129 | 113–146 | 60–90/60–140 |

## Special Nutritional Considerations in the Very Preterm

### Osteopenia of Prematurity

Optimal ossification of bones requires adequate calcium/phosphorus accrual and metabolism.

Infants at risk for osteopenia, a lack of appropriate ossification, are:
- <1,500 g or <29 weeks at birth
- On TPN for >1 month
- Those requiring diuretics or steroids.

The standard for osteopenia diagnosis is a dual-energy X-ray absorptiometry (DEXA) scan, an expensive and not readily available test. Noninvasive studies such as quantitative ultrasound (US) are still being evaluated. Bone mineral content is usually reduced by at least 30–40% prior to roentgenographic detection.[36]

Regular interval screening of at-risk patients for blood phosphorus, calcium, Ca:P ratio, and alkaline phosphatase should be considered. Once the levels are reassuring/improved, the test frequency can be reduced. Phosphorus <1.8 mmol/L is associated with rickets. Elevated newborn blood phosphorus values are accepted as they are due to hyperparathormonemia, in which case supplemental P should not be stopped. Alkaline phosphatase >3× normal values (~500 IU) with a low P are suggestive of osteopenia.[37] The mainstay of treatment is prevention, focused on:
- Maximize balanced calcium and phosphorus intake in the TPN
- Early oral/enteral feedings in all at-risk children
- Adequate intake in the diet, especially early and adequate fortification of HM with protein and minerals
- Adequate vitamin D supplementation of the diet (800–1,000 IU/day)
- Avoid therapies reducing of bone mineralization
- Avoid limiting infant movement
- Passive stretching exercises and gentle massage regimen
- Monitor at-risk patients.

*Phosphorus supplementation:* Strategies to increase supplemental P include replacing one of three breast milk feeds with preterm formula, especially if the infant is on banked breast milk, and increasing daily vitamin D to 800–1,000 IU.

Adequate P supplementation can be followed by measuring renal tubular reabsorption of phosphate (TRP).

$$TRP\% = \left[1 - \left(\frac{\text{Urine phosphate}}{\text{Urine creatinine}} \times \frac{\text{Plasma creatinine}}{\text{Plasma phosphate}}\right)\right] \times 100$$

If TRP >95%, P supplementation is inadequate.

### Anemia of Prematurity

Delayed cord clamping (DCC) should be an integral part of the birthing process and is the simplest method to increase iron endowment at birth. The World Health Organization currently recommends 1–3 minutes of DCC at birth.[38] Term infants of normal iron status mothers that are breastfed[39] or receive DCC[40] do not need supplemental Fe for 6–8 months. Risk-based screening for iron deficiency should be done. In high-risk mothers, serum ferritin levels close to birth may be examined. Preterm infants have only enough stores till they double their birth weight (1–2 months of age, or earlier if excess phlebotomy losses) and will need supplements. It is unclear how DCC in preterm infants affects iron supplementation needs. One approach may include evaluating ferritin prior to starting supplemental Fe. Elemental iron prophylaxis starts at 2–6 weeks of age for infants 1,500–2,500 g at 2 mkd, and for the VLBW <1,500 g at 2 weeks. The late preterm infant with DCC needs elemental Fe supplements of 2 mkd from 6 weeks till 6 months of age if breastfed, and will need to be reassessed at 6 months with the introduction of complementary feeds. In areas with endemic maternal Fe deficiency/low dietary iron, supplementation may be continued for 1–2 years. Higher doses (6 mkd) may be associated with high oxidative stress and are best not used routinely. Recently transfused infants may not require oral supplements as they retain less oral iron as parenteral iron infused.

## Feeding the Infant with Birth Defects

Children with cardiac defects may become undernourished for many reasons.[41] Their growth can be improved by optimal nutrition.[42] Growth restriction is associated with increased length of hospital stay.[41] At birth, DCC should be performed, especially if the infant has a known cardiac defect. Enteral feeds are initiated if possible while awaiting surgery. Colostrum and MEN with breast milk is tolerated in these situations, and should be encouraged even if the infant is on vasopressors. TPN should be started early and an effort should be made to provide enough nutrition, even with the very small fluid volumes available for nutrition perioperatively. Sufficient protein must be provided to keep the infants anabolic at all times. Many vasopressors can be mixed in dextrose concentrations instead of saline to increase caloric intake. Careful attention is paid to the potassium, calcium, phosphorus, and magnesium intakes and balance. An imbalance can affect cardiac function, as low stores of calcium and the diuretics given in cardiac disease may affect micronutrient/mineral balance by increasing urinary losses. These issues are amplified in preterm infants with cardiac disease, who may require medical stabilization prior to surgery. It is important to monitor and identify residual postoperative problems, such as trauma to the recurrent laryngeal nerve[43] and chylothorax. Children with a left recurrent laryngeal nerve injury may delay transition to oral feeds, with aspiration and difficulty swallowing possibly complicating optimal feeding. Children with a chylothorax may have delayed feeding. New formulas with lipid fraction of medium chain triglycerides are now available, allowing infants to feed enterally while recovering from this major problem.[44] Nonspecialized feeds can be started 1 week after the resolution of the chylothorax; currently these formulas are not designed for the preterm infant. In areas where these formulas are not available, a skimmed milk diet has been used.[45] Many infants with cardiac disease are very sick and separated from their families. Mothers should be encouraged to breastfeed, parental skin-to-skin contact optimized, and parental visitation maximized to prevent nonorganic failure to thrive.

### Infants of Mothers Who have had Bariatric Surgery

Multiple nutritional deficiencies have been noted in obese mothers prior to surgery and may worsen after bariatric surgery. There is higher incidence of lower birth weight, NICU admissions, preterm birth, and maternal anemia.[46] Following surgery, lack of intake and changes in absorption are the main reasons for these deficiencies. Pregnant mothers (especially those who have had bariatric surgery) have special vitamin and nutritional needs. Studies have reported deficiencies of vitamins such as folic acid, vitamin D, vitamin A, vitamin $B_1$ and $B_{12}$, and vitamin C. During pregnancy, these women are also at risk for deficiencies in micronutrients such as iron, copper, selenium, and zinc, many of which are absorbed in the stomach, duodenum, and proximal jejunum. In one study, the prevalence of postoperative deficiencies of copper was 0–5%, selenium 11–15%, and zinc 7–15%.[47] Close monitoring of breastfeeding infants with iron and vitamin supplementation for a few months, while not currently recommended by studies, is probably prudent.

## STAGE 4: FEEDING AFTER DISCHARGE

Preterm infants discharge from the NICU with a unique growth history. This history is a sum of GA, nutrition, and growth trajectories complicated by lung disease and inflammation, modified by parental time investment. Some infants begin life SGA; some become SGA. Some are fed with HM; others are formula fed. Some are good feeders; others are marginal. Other relevant questions are: Were maternal nutrition and uteroplacental perfusion optimal? Did the infant receive DCC? Was protein delivery optimized? Most preterm infants have some anemia of prematurity, protein debt, and osteopenia. It is difficult with such a diverse group to have a single discharge feeding strategy. The aim of treatment, however, is very clear—help the infant recover from deficits while supporting breastfeeding and a normal AGA growth pattern. Excessive supplements after recovery from deficits are not recommended. Pediatricians and high-risk infant follow-up clinics need to monitor patients' nutritional needs and adequacy.[48]

Optimal weight attainment in infants AGA at birth is 0.5 Z-score below the birth Z-score and under the 90th percentile for those infants born LGA. For an SGA infant, the goal is >10th percentile.

The need for extra protein, calcium, and phosphorus continues; monitoring length of the infant and alkaline phosphatase can be a guide to treatment duration. Many preterm infants are sent home prior to term and may need to be fed as preterm until term. Close monitoring of weight, length, and head circumference after discharge is recommended, especially if the infant's diet changed close to discharge. If intake volumes are limited, caloric fortification may be necessary.

Postdischarge fortification is best done with preterm formula or fortifiers, which may not be readily available. Consider discontinuing or reducing fortification when the child shows good growth, at least over the 10th percentile for head circumference, length, and weight.

Strong support of breastfeeding is necessary. Consider outpatient monitoring for specific deficiencies and BUN, ferritin, vitamin D levels, and alkaline phosphatase.

*Iron:* Iron supplements are recommended; ferritin levels may guide duration of therapy. The late preterm infant who receives DCC will need a Fe supplement of 2 mg/kg until 6 months of age if breastfed and will need to be reassessed at

6 months with the introduction of complementary feeds. In areas where mothers are deficient, diets are low in iron, or DCC is not done, supplementation up to 6 mg/kg/day and continued for 1-2 years.

## Vitamins

Formula-fed infants require vitamin supplementation till intake exceeds ~750 mL/day.

## CONCLUSION

Growth and nutrition of the preterm infant is a subject much studied and largely poorly understood. Special medical conditions in the preterm infant (e.g. severe cardiopulmonary disease and hormonal deficiencies) may result in suboptimal growth. At the same time, certain genetic conditions limit growth potential, and neurological disorders that lead to inactivity may decrease an infant's basal metabolic needs. All components of nutrition should be considered, including water, macronutrients, and micronutrients. Growth velocity varies with gestation and postnatally with neonatal course and complications.

Changes in neonatal practice will inevitably affect nutritional practice and growth patterns. Much of the variation in practice patterns and growth velocity requires further study. Maternal malnutrition and contributions of maternal disease to infant growth failure needs to be better understood in order to optimize infant growth.

## REFERENCES

1. Boyd CA, Quigley ML, Brocklehurst P. Donor breast milk versus infant formula for preterm infants: systematic review and meta-analysis. Arch Dis Child Fetal Neonatal Ed. 2007;92(3):F169-75.
2. Bisset WM, Watt J, Rivers RP, et al. Postprandial motor response of the small intestine to enteral feeds in preterm infants. Arch Dis Child. 1989;64(10 Spec No):1356-61.
3. Hughes CA, Dowling RH. Dowling RH. Speed of onset of adaptive mucosal hypoplasia and hypofunction in the intestine of parenterally fed rats. Clin Sci (Lond). 1980;59(5):317-27.
4. Berseth CL. Effect of early feeding on maturation of the preterm infant's small intestine. J Pediatr. 1992;120(6):947-53.
5. Berseth CL, Nordyke C. Enteral nutrients promote postnatal maturation of intestinal motor activity in preterm infants. Am J Physiol. 1993;264(6 Pt 1):G1046-51.
6. Bombell S, McGuire W. Delayed introduction of progressive enteral feeds to prevent necrotising enterocolitis in very low birth weight infants. Cochrane Database Syst Rev. 2008;(2) CD001970.
7. Davey AM, Wagner CL, Cox C, et al. Feeding premature infants while low umbilical artery catheters are in place: a prospective, randomized trial. J Pediatr. 1994;124(5 Pt 1):795-9.
8. Clyman R, Wickremasinghe A, Jhaveri N, et al.; Ductus Arteriosus Feed or Fast with Indomethacin or Ibuprofen (DAFFII) Investigators. Enteral feeding during indomethacin and ibuprofen treatment of a patent ductus arteriosus. J Pediatr. 2013;163(2):406-11.
9. Toms R, Jackson KW, Dabal RJ, et al. Preoperative trophic feeds in neonates with hypoplastic left heart syndrome. Congenit Heart Dis. 2015;10(1):36-42.
10. Morgan J, Bombell S, McGuire W. Early trophic feeding versus enteral fasting for very preterm or very low birth weight infants. Cochrane Database Syst Rev. 2013;3:CD000504.
11. Cormack BE, Bloomfield FH. Audit of feeding practices in babies <1200 g or 30 weeks gestation during the first month of life. J Paediatr Child Health. 2006;42(7-8):458-63.
12. Bertino E, Giulian F, Pandi G, et al. Necrotizing enterocolitis: risk factor analysis and role of gastric residuals in very low birth weight infants. J Pediatr gastroenterol Nutr. 2009;48(4):437-42.
13. Cormack BE, Bloomfield FH, Dezoete A, et al. Does more protein in the first week of life change outcomes for very low birthweight babies? J Paediatr Child Health. 2011;47(12): 898-903.
14. Gephart SM, McGrath JM, Effken JA, et al. Necrotizing enterocolitis risk: state of the science. Adv Neonatal Care. 2012;12(2):77-87.
15. Patole SK, de Klerk N. Impact of standardised feeding regimens on incidence of neonatal necrotizing enterocolitis: a systematic review and meta-analysis of observational studies. Arch Dis Child Fetal Neonatal Ed. 2005;90(2):F147-51.
16. Krishnamurthy S. Gupta P, Debnath S, et al. Slow versus rapid enteral feeding advancement in preterm infants 1000-1499 g: a randomized controlled trial. Acta Paediatr. 2010;99(1):42-6.
17. Morgan J, Young L, McGuire W. Slow advancement of enteral feed volumes to prevent necrotising enterocolitis in very low birth weight infants. Cochrane Database Syst Rev. 2013;(3):CD001241.
18. Rayyis SF, Ambalavanan N, Wright L, et al. Randomized trial of "slow" versus "fast" feeding advancement on the incidence of necrotizing enterocolitis in very low birth weight infants. J Pediatr. 1999;134(3):293-7.
19. Caple J, Armentrout D, Huseby V, et al. Randomized, controlled trial of slow versus rapid feeding volume advancement in preterm infants. Pediatrics. 2004;114(6):1597-600.
20. Karagol BS, Zenciroglu A, Okumus N, et al. Randomized controlled trial of slow versus rapid enteral feeding advancements on the clinical outcome of preterm infants with birth weight 750-1250 g. JPEN J Parenter Enteral Nutr. 2013;37(2):223-8.
21. Salhotra A, Ramji S. Slow versus fast enteral feed advancement in very low birth weight infants: a randomized control trial. Indian Pediatr. 2004;41(5):435-41.
22. De Leoz ML Kalanetra KM, Bokulich NA, et al. Human milk glycomics and gut microbial genomics in infant feces show a correlation between human milk oligosaccharides and gut microbiota: a proof-of-concept study. J Proteome Res. 2015;14(1):491-502.
23. Orivuori L, Loss G, Roduit C, et al.; PASTURE Study Group. Soluble immunoglobulin A in breast milk is inversely associated with atopic dermatitis at early age: the PASTURE cohort study. Clin Exp Allergy. 2014;44(1):102-12.

24. Cristofalo EA, Schanler RJ, Blanco CL, et al. Randomized trial of exclusive human milk versus preterm formula diets in extremely premature infants. J Pediatr. 2013;163(6):1592-5.e1.
25. Singhal A, Cole TJ, Fewtrell M, et al. Breastmilk feeding and lipoprotein profile in adolescents born preterm: follow-up of a prospective randomised study. Lancet. 2004;363(9421):1571-8.
26. Martin RM, Patel R, Kramer MS, et al. Effects of promoting longer-term and exclusive breastfeeding on cardiometabolic risk factors at age 11.5 years: a cluster-randomized, controlled trial. Circulation. 2014;129(3):321-9.
27. Innis SM. Impact of maternal diet on human milk composition and neurological development of infants. Am J Clin Nutr. 2014;99(3):734S-41S.
28. Arslanoglu S, Corpeleijn W, Moro G, et al.; ESPGHAN Committee on Nutrition. Donor human milk for preterm infants: current evidence and research directions. J Pediatr Gastroenterol Nutr. 2013;57(4):535-42.
29. Wojcik KY, Rechtman DJ, Lee ML, et al. Macronutrient analysis of a nationwide sample of donor breast milk. J Am Diet Assoc. 2009;109(1):137-40.
30. Akinbi H, Meinzen-Derr J, Auer C, et al. Alterations in the host defense properties of human milk following prolonged storage or pasteurization. J Pediatr Gastroenterol Nutr. 2010;51(3):347-52.
31. Ziegler EE. Nutrient needs for catch-up growth in low-birthweight infants. Nestle Nutr Inst Workshop Ser. 2015;81:135-43.
32. Tsang RC, Uauy R, Koletzko B, et al. Nutrition of the Preterm Infant: Scientific Basis and Practical Guidelines, 2nd edition. Cincinnati, OH: Digital Educational Publishing Inc.; 2005.
33. Fenton TR, Kim JH. A systematic review and meta-analysis to revise the Fenton growth chart for preterm infants. BMC Pediatr. 2013;13:59.
34. Proceedings of the Global Neonatal Consensus Symposium: Feeding the Preterm Infant, October 13-15, 2010, Chicago, Illinois. J Pediatr. 2013;162(Suppl 3):S1-116.
35. Arslanoglu S, Moro GE, Ziegler EE, The Wapm Working Group On Nutrition. Optimization of human milk fortification for preterm infants: new concepts and recommendations. J Perinat Med. 2010;38(3):233-8.
36. Mazess RB, Peppler WW, Chesney RW, et al. Does bone measurement on the radius indicate skeletal status? Concise communication. J Nucl Med. 1984;25(3):281-8.
37. Harrison CM, Gibson AT. Osteopenia in preterm infants. Arch Dis Child Fetal Neonatal Ed. 2013;98(3):F272-5.
38. Abalos E. Effect of Timing of Umbilical Cord Clamping of Term Infants on Maternal and Neonatal Outcomes: RHL Commentary. Geneva: The WHO Reproductive Health Library; 2009.
39. Saarinen UM, Siimes MA. Iron absorption from breast milk, cow's milk, and iron-supplemented formula: an opportunistic use of changes in total body iron determined by hemoglobin, ferritin, and body weight in 132 infants. Pediatr Res. 1979;13(3):143-7.
40. Dewey KG, Chaparro CM. Session 4: Mineral metabolism and body composition iron status of breast-fed infants. Proc Nutr Soc. 2007;66(3):412-22.
41. Costello C, Gellatly M, Daniel J, et al. Growth restriction in infants and young children with congenital heart disease. Congenit Heart Dis. 2015;10(5):447-56.
42. Kaufman J, Vichayavilas P, Rannie M, et al. Improved nutrition delivery and nutrition status in critically ill children with heart disease. Pediatrics. 2015;135(3):e717-25.
43. Hamdan AL, Moukarbel RV, Farhat F, et al. Vocal cord paralysis after open-heart surgery. Eur J Cardiothorac Surg. 2002;21(4):671-4.
44. Biewer ES, Zürn C, Arnold R, et al. Chylothorax after surgery on congenital heart disease in newborns and infants – risk factors and efficacy of MCT-diet. J Cardiothorac Surg. 2010;5:127.
45. Gupta V, Mahendri NV, Tete P, et al. Skimmed milk preparation in management of congenital chylothorax. Indian Pediatr. 2014;51(2):146-8.
46. Galazis N, Docheva N, Simillis C, et al. Maternal and neonatal outcomes in women undergoing bariatric surgery: a systematic review and metaanalysis. Eur J Obstet Gynecol Reprod Biol. 2014;181:45-53.
47. Papamargaritis D, Aasheim ET, Sampson B, et al. Copper, selenium and zinc levels after bariatric surgery in patients recommended to take multivitamin-mineral supplementation. J Trace Elem Med Biol. 2015;31:167-72.
48. Lapillonne A. Feeding the preterm infant after discharge. World Rev Nutr Diet. 2014;110:264-77.

# CHAPTER 37

# Human Milk Composition and Lactation

Sudha Rani Narasimhan, Alganesh G Kifle

## ABSTRACT

Human milk (HM) provides the best nourishment for all infants, including premature and sick newborns. The composition of HM offers the standard for infant nutrition and is individually created for each human infant. Understanding HM composition and its developmental and geographic variability may lead to better comprehension of infant growth.

## INTRODUCTION

Human milk is nutritionally complete, containing appropriate amounts of carbohydrates, fat, and protein. In addition to macronutrients, HM contains vital micronutrients, vitamins, bioactive components, immunologic factors, and oligosaccharides; also detailed in the chapters on Growth and Nutrition in the Preterm Infant and in a recent comprehensive review.[1] In this chapter, we use current International Lactation Consultants Association terminology.[2]

## HUMAN MILK COMPOSITION

Colostrum is the initial milk produced by the mother soon after delivery. Denser than mature milk, it is rich in protein and immunoglobulins. The transition from colostrum to mature HM begins by day 3–5. HM is considered mature by day 10, with 70% whey protein and 30% casein (in contrast to bovine milk, which contains 18% whey and 82% casein). The predominant type of whey protein (41% of the whey and 28% of total protein) in HM is α-lactalbumin, whereas in bovine milk, the major protein is β-lactoglobulin and only 3% is α-lactalbumin. α-lactalbumin forms the regulatory subunit of lactose synthase, increasing lactose production, binding calcium and zinc, and possibly possessing bactericidal/antitumor properties. α-lactalbumin is rich in several amino acids critical for infant development, such as cysteine, a building block of the antioxidant glutathione, and tryptophan, a precursor to the neurotransmitter serotonin and the neurosecretory hormone melatonin.[3]

The major carbohydrate found in HM is lactose; a small portion is not absorbed, thus promoting softer stools, reducing pathogenic fecal flora, and improving mineral absorption. Oligosaccharides constitute 5–10% of total HM carbohydrates, functioning as prebiotics and enhancing favorable microorganism (bacterial and fungal) growth that contributes to infant well-being. Scientific reviews[4] of HM oligosaccharides (HMOs) are available.[5]

The most variable component in HM is fat. Infant fat absorption from HM is better than bovine milk because of lipase action on triglycerides, resulting in free fatty acids and two monoglycerides. Further reading on HM fat[6] and understanding of the milk fat globule[7] is recommended.

The HM proteome is known to contain over 970 proteins, many with immune properties. Emerging papers on the proteomics and metabolomics of HM suggest significant geographic variability and impact of lifestyles and atopy on HM composition.[8-11]

Human milk contains maternal cells, from leukocytes to epithelial cells of various developmental stages and immunological factors. It also contains stem cells, progenitor cells, lactocytes, and myoepithelial cells.[12] Scientists first observed cells in HM through microscopy in the 1600s–1700s.[13,14] Research technology advances have permitted further characterization of the cellular composition of HM, including a cellular hierarchy of stem cells.[15,16] Currently, HM cell content is thought to be 10,000–13,000,000 cells/mL.[17] Cellular content variation is attributed to factors including breast fullness, stage of lactation, maternal health, breast epithelial development, and basement membrane permeability. Colostrum and early milk are more cellular than mature HM. HM cell content and composition are dynamic throughout lactation.[18] HM cellular heterogeneity includes predominant leukocytosis (13–70%) in colostrum and epithelial predominance in mature HM. Blood-derived leukocytes are the most studied HM cells and are transported into the milk via paracellular mechanisms.[18] HM leukocytes include granulocytes and mononuclear leukocytes, including lymphocytes, macrophages, and monocytes. Macrophages are predominant in colostrum, up to 40–50% of total leukocytes. T-cells are the majority lymphocytes, conferring active infant immunity and possibly protecting maternal mammary glands from infection.[14] HM cellular content and composition is influenced by the health status of both mother and infant, with increased HM leukocytes and macrophages observed in response to infection.

Epithelial cells composing ~99% of the cellular component of mature HM are present in the structure and function of the lactating breast. These cells detach passively from ducts and alveoli during milk synthesis and milk ejection, or actively due to milk removal by infant or breast pump.[19] Alveolar lactocytes are present in mature HM.

Human milk stem cells can differentiate into mammary lineage cells that synthesize and secrete milk proteins. These pluripotent stem cells also differentiate into other lineages including cells with properties of cardiomyocytes, neurons, osteoblasts, adipocytes, and hepatocytes.[16]

In summary, HM contains an abundant variety of living cells.

## VARIATIONS IN COMPOSITION

Human milk varies dynamically in composition, differing within a feed, during the day, over the lactation period, and between mothers, adapting specifically to optimize infant growth and maturation. Lactation gradually evolves into mature milk; while initial colostrum is rich in immunological factors and protein, the volume is small. The immunologic components in colostrum include secretory immunoglobulin A (IgA), lactoferrin, leukocytes, and growth factors. Compared to mature milk, colostrum levels of sodium, chloride, and magnesium are higher and levels of lactose, potassium, and calcium are lower.

As lactogenesis progresses, tight junction closure in the mammary epithelium reduces sodium/potassium ratio and increases lactose concentration. Secretory activation and production of transitional milk increases milk production to support the infant's nutritional needs, while sharing some colostrum properties. After 2 weeks, mature milk is produced, ~600 mL/day.

Early small sample size studies of HM show both similarities and differences between preterm and term milk. More recent larger sample size studies demonstrate that fat content in hindmilk is two- to threefold of that in foremilk. Early in lactation, preterm milk contains more IgA, lactoferrin, and lysozyme.[20]

Preterm milk has higher concentrations of protein, sodium, chloride, and lower concentrations of lactose compared to term milk.[21] Some have found no differences between term and preterm milk in nonprotein nitrogen, volume, solids, total calories, lactose, fat, fatty acids, potassium or calcium, but significantly higher levels of total nitrogen, protein nitrogen, sodium, chloride, magnesium, and iron in preterm milk.[22] Concentrations of sodium and chloride are higher in preterm milk and decrease with ongoing lactation.[21] These functional differences meet the differential needs of a preterm infant.

The serial composition of HM in both term and preterm mothers is illustrated here.[23]

## COMPARISON WITH OTHER ANIMAL MILKS

Milk is specific and unique to each species. Genomic studies comparing bovine genome to other species, including human, show that milk and mammary genes are relatively more conserved and have evolved slowly compared to other genes. Highly conserved genes are those for milk fat globule membrane proteins. Highly divergent genes are those with nutritional or immunological characteristics, suggesting each species' milk has distinct differences related to growth and protection against infections.

## STUDIES OF HUMAN MILK COMPOSITION

Human milk contains several amino acids and proteins, summarized here.[24]

Several intact nonhuman proteins are transferred into HM; this may provide insight into allergy. There is growing interest in the HM metabolome as this can give insight to nutrition for optimal infant growth.[25-27]

## ADVANTAGES OF HUMAN MILK

While HM is ideal infant nutrition, other health benefits accrue to the HM-fed infant; protection from infections such as otitis media and lower respiratory tract and gastrointestinal disease. HM decreases necrotizing enterocolitis (NEC), a devastating and life-threatening disease in the preterm population.[28] HM also reduces the incidence of noninfectious disease such as juvenile diabetes, leukemia, asthma, obesity, and sudden infant death syndrome.[29,30]

## THE PRENATAL PERIOD

Lactation education should be provided as early as possible, preferably before conception. Cohesive lactation support from peers, nurses, physicians, and lactation consultants optimizes infant health and maternal well-being. Mothers thus assisted are more likely to initiate and continue lactation.[31]

Prenatal education should target a few simple messages—(1) breastfeeding is desirable and achievable, (2) professional and community support are available, and (3) exclusive breastfeeding for ≥6 months is important. Healthcare professionals should take a careful history from the mother to examine her feeding decision, obtain previous lactation history, and explore previous surgery such as breast augmentation/reduction, nipple-piercing, or trauma. Care providers, family, and friends may discuss breastfeeding/lactation experience, beliefs, and feelings.

Complex hormonal signals in pregnancy prepare the breasts for lactation. Healthcare providers should examine the breasts, discussing breast changes during pregnancy and any concerns about lactation. Physical characteristics, e.g. nipple eversion/inversion, nipple piercing, surgical scars, anomalies of the breast (such as hypoplasia), asymmetric breasts, and nipple abnormalities should be assessed. Marked discrepancy in size of breasts, leading to possible challenges with infant positioning should be communicated early in pregnancy to plan for individualized support. Parents should have a written, customized, and culturally sensitive birth and feeding plan before birth, tailored specifically to their circumstances and birthing facility, with particular attention to high-risk mothers (e.g. extremes of age, diabetic, obese, and those with other illnesses or disability).

## STRUCTURE AND FUNCTION OF THE BREAST

Mammary glands (Latin "mamma" meaning breast) are not fully developed at birth, undergoing three major phases of growth and development before pregnancy and lactation—fetal, the first 2 years of life, and puberty.

Breast tissue includes parenchyma, ductular-lobular-alveolar structures, and stroma, composed of connective tissue, fat, blood vessels, nerves, and lymphatics. Montgomery tubercles (with antibacterial secretions lubricating the nipple) contain ductal orifices of sebaceous and small lactiferous glands.

## STAGES OF LACTATION

Mammogenesis starts in the embryo; by 12 weeks' gestation, nipples, areolae, alveoli, and mammary buds are developed. At puberty, estrogen and pituitary growth factors stimulate breast growth. In pubertal menstrual cycles, estrogen induces ductal proliferation and progesterone induces alveolar development. Pregnancy accelerates mammary organogenesis and ductular sprouting and intensifies lobular-alveolar development.

Lactogenesis I, the first stage of milk production, occurs mid-pregnancy to 2 days postpartum. Breast differentiation is sufficient to secrete small quantities of specific milk components such as casein and lactose. Breasts may feel swollen due to alveolar colostrum.

Lactogenesis II, the onset of copious milk secretion, occurs on day 3 to the first week postpartum. After placental delivery and subsequent drop in progesterone, alveoli assume a full secretory role, releasing milk into the lumen and then into ductules and ducts. In this stage, the alveolar cells become tightly packed, with the milk containing increased lactose, glucose, and milk lipids and decreased protein, sodium, chloride, nitrogen, and magnesium.

Lactogenesis III or galactopoiesis, milk supply maintenance, occurs from the second week postpartum until weaning.

## HORMONES

Prolactin and oxytocin are the two major lactation hormones, with independent and separate pathways. Suckling releases both hormones, prolactin from the anterior and oxytocin from the posterior pituitary. The sudden drop in progesterone after delivery triggers a prolactin surge, which stimulates and maintains milk production. Retained placenta may cause absent milk supply.

Oxytocin releases milk (the letdown reflex) and helps myoepithelial cellular contraction around the alveoli, moving milk into ducts. Oxytocin is released in response to many stimuli—nipple stretching during feeding; seeing, touching, hearing, or smelling the infant; hearing another infant cry; massage-like motions of the infant's hand on the breast,[32] as well as chest-skin contact. Stimuli exposure at bedside assists HM expression and milk production.

Oxytocin release is behaviorally mediated and a conditioned response. Women may experience several letdowns during a single feeding as oxytocin response may be transient/intermittent. Extreme pain or stress temporarily inhibits oxytocin, reducing milk supply. Inadequate suckling diminishes prolactin, adversely affecting milk supply. Reasons for low milk volume include infrequent feedings, scheduled vs. demand feedings, and lack of night feedings. Feeding on demand increases milk supply and is developmentally supportive.

## IMMEDIATELY AFTER BIRTH

### Skin-to-skin contact

Following birth, the infant is best placed on the mother's abdomen. Birth routines that support immediate uninterrupted skin-to-skin contact between mother and infant, including postcesarean section, and breastfeeding within the first hour are critical to successful lactation. Skin-to-skin contact enhances maternal-infant bonding, increasing infant weight gain[33] and milk production. It also improves infant feeding and regulation of respiratory and arousal mechanisms, and is analgesic during painful procedures (e.g. heel sticks). Lactation duration is increased with frequent skin-to-skin contact.[34]

Labor and delivery practices have a strong impact on lactation. The ambience and comforts of a birthing suite encourage early breastfeeding, where father and family members can share the intimacy of breastfeeding and newborn bonding.

Maternal anesthesia may have a negative effect on suckling, and thus delay lactogenesis. Suctioning the infant's mouth/nose after birth also may result in adversity; suction causes nasal edema/stuffiness, and feeding success compromised until swelling subsides.[35] Infant gastric suctioning may delay rooting and suckling. If necessary, gentle bulb syringe suctioning of mouth and nares is best.

### Conditions Promoting Breastfeeding

Some birth practices are beneficial in breastfeeding success and experience.

Early and frequent breastfeeding benefits the mother, as suckling stimulates uterine contractions and aids placental expulsion, thus diminishing progesterone and avoiding delayed lactogenesis II. Frequent removal of milk (via expression or infant feeding) keeps the breasts empty and stimulates continued synthesis of HM.[36]

Rooming-in (newborn stays with mother) and on-demand feedings help the mother recognize her infant's sleep/alert state changes and feeding cues. Feeding cues include rooting, mouthing activities, hand-to-face activities, lip-smacking, and tongue extension. Crying is a late feeding cue and means that earlier cues were missed; it is more difficult to breastfeed a crying infant. Cue-fed infants are more likely to breastfeed to satiety, establish and maintain a good milk supply,[37] with optimal (not excessive) weight gain[38] and less jaundice with decreased enterohepatic recirculation of bilirubin. While controversial,[39,40] the better a mother gets to know her baby's feeding cues, the more likely is breastfeeding success. Infants breastfed on demand self-regulate milk quantity and quality. Longer suckling ensures higher fat content received in hindmilk.

Correct positioning and latch makes breastfeeding productive and enjoyable for mother and infant. Distressed mothers and infants should be calmed before feeding. Good positioning transfers sufficient milk to infant without damage to breast or nipples. Effective suckling occurs when adequate areola and breast tissue is drawn into the infant's mouth to form an airtight lock around the breast with lips flanged, creating a seal with lips, mouth, and throat to establish effective suck/swallow/breathe.

Feeding is a complicated multidimensional task with dynamic and intricate coordination between suck/swallow/breathe and the infant's behavioral state.[41] Successful feeding requires ingesting mother's milk, digesting and absorbing nutrients, and excreting metabolic waste. Understanding oral development, anatomy, and the science of suckling is integral to optimize infant feeding.

Cleft palate/lip, ankyloglossia, muscular dystrophy, cerebral palsy, and Down syndrome require extra lactation coaching.[42] Other factors leading to ineffective suckling are important to identify which mother/infant couplets may need lactation assistance/coaching.

Breast tenderness is experienced in late pregnancy and nipple sensitivity heightened with early breastfeeding, peaking 3–5 days postpartum and diminishing as milk volume increases. Infant positioning for successful feeding varies. Many thriving nursing dyads feed in unusual or uncomfortable-looking positions, yet maintain good milk transfer without maternal discomfort. Medical professionals are advised to avoid changing a mother's breastfeeding position if it works for her infant and is comfortable for her.[35]

Proper positioning and latch ensure efficient milk transfer and infant weight gain. Poor positioning and incorrect latch can cause painful nipples, discouraging the mother from infant feeding. Inadequate milk transfer resulting from bad position/latch may result in failure to thrive. Diabetic mothers, maternal overweight, or excessive pregnancy weight gain are risk factors for delayed lactogenesis II. Infant positioning may challenge an obese mother, possibly leading to early breastfeeding cessation. Consistent individualized lactation support is critical, especially at 3–5 days postpartum.[33]

Factors leading to low milk supply include insufficient glandular tissue,[43] breast surgery (reduction/augmentation), and prior chest tube placement, potentially damaging intercostal nerve pathways to areola and nipple. Breast/nipple piercings may interfere with breastfeeding, depending on size and location. The resulting hole after removal of a ring may interfere with milk flow; too large a hole permitting excessive milk flow may choke the infant. Scarring from prior infections may compromise milk duct and nipple pore patency.

### Engorgement and Milk Stasis

Breast engorgement implies any type of breast fullness, including edema or milk stasis.[35] Breast fullness in the early postpartum period is due to increased vascularity and the transition from colostrum to transitional/mature milk. Milk removal is essential to optimal production. Care plans should help the mother to breastfeed often around the clock, with feeding on demand to ensure complete emptying of the breast.

When a milk ejection reflex is compromised or slow, warmth improves engorgement by oxytocin uptake,[35] while ice pack application causes vasoconstriction. Techniques to reduce engorgement are discussed by Cotterman.[44]

A plugged duct due to infrequent breastfeeding and milk stasis often presents with a tender benign breast lump, and is managed by frequent feeding, as well as gentle local massage to move the lump toward the nipple, facilitating drainage.

### Mastitis

Mastitis prevention begins with lactation education, with mothers trained to recognize and manage problems promptly. Improper positioning with poor latch may cause skin erosion and microbial (bacterial or fungal) proliferation leading to mastitis. Breast inflammation/mastitis produces systemic flu-like symptoms, characterized by extreme tenderness, swelling, redness, and warmth in a breast region. *Staphylococcus aureus*, *Escherichia coli*, and occasionally *Streptococcus* are the usual pathogens and should be treated with antibiotics. Mothers should be advised to continue to feed and apply ice packs or warm packs to the affected area, depending on which is most comfortable. Considerable maternal pain is associated with reluctance to remove milk frequently or sufficiently.

Tools for evaluation of proper latch critical to breastfeeding success—Bristol Breastfeeding Assessment Tool[45] and LATCH Assessment Tool are given below.[46]

|  | 0 | 1 | 2 | Totals |
|---|---|---|---|---|
| Latch | Too sleepy or reluctant latch or suck achieved | • Repeated attempts for sustained latch or suck<br>• Hold nipple to mouth | • Grasps breast<br>• Tongue down<br>• Lips flanged<br>• Rhythmical sucking | |

*Contd...*

*Contd...*

|  | 0 | 1 | 2 | Totals |
|---|---|---|---|---|
| Audible swallowing | None | A few with stimulation | Spontaneous and intermittent (<24 hours old) spontaneous and frequent (>24 hours old) | |
| Type of nipple | Inverted | Flat | Everted | |
| Comfort | Engorged, cracked, bruised, and severe discomfort | Filling and reddened blisters | • Soft<br>• Nontender | |
| Hold (Positioning) | • Full assist<br>• Staff holds infant at breast | • Minimal assist<br>• Teach one side, mother does other<br>• Staff holds, then mother takes over. | • No assist from staff<br>• Mother able to hold and position infant | |

## Feeding Preterm Infants

Human milk provides optimal nutrition for preterm infants and is protective against several prematurity-related conditions.

### Colostrum

The lactation team must teach family members about colostrum's importance and take care to collect and store all colostrum. Mothers may hand express or pump colostrum into small collection containers made specifically for this purpose.[47] Early expression of colostrum optimizes colonization of the infant's gut microbiome and increases milk production.[48]

Breastfeeding and skin-to-skin contact facilitates favorable microbial colonization, protecting the infant from pathogens. Low birthweight infant methicillin-resistant *Staphylococcus aureus* (MRSA) colonization may be reduced by spreading maternal HM/colostrum on/into the infant's mouth at birth.[35,49] Oral colostrum swabs to intubated infants may prevent ventilator-associated pneumonia.

### Support

Maternal praise for providing HM for preterm infants is indicated for giving the infant the best possible start in life.

A family-centered approach is beneficial by actively involving parents in infant care. Parental confusion with changing terminology is avoided by using scripting. Support and education on maintenance of HM is imperative.[50,51]

Mothers of neonatal intensive care unit (NICU) infants need a hospital grade breast pump and information on maintenance and safe milk storage. Skilled health professionals (lactation consultants) knowledgeable about lactation management are critical to achieving maternal breastfeeding goals.[52,53] The most important factor for mothers who will be breastfeeding a preterm infant at home is maintaining a milk supply that exceeds requirements at hospital discharge.

Lactation should be initiated with latch, hand expression, or with a breast pump as early as possible following delivery. Hand expression, in addition to pumping, increases milk production in mothers of preterm infants.[54]

Infants with special needs and infants with birth trauma (forceps births and vacuum deliveries) might present with sleepiness, feeding intolerance, and inability to suckle/swallow. A fractured clavicle can affect the infant's ability to suckle due to decreased movement and challenges to positioning while breastfeeding. Lactation consultant referral and close community follow-up (public health and home visits) are recommended.

Breastfeeding is usually possible in high-risk perinatal situations, such as hypertension, severe eclampsia, and HELLP (hemolysis, elevated liver enzymes, low platelet) syndrome. With support, even sedated mothers may hold their infants skin-to-skin. Later breastfeeding may depend on maternal health and medications.

## Breastfeeding Multiples

Feeding twins at the same time develops schedule synchrony and increases milk supply. Mothers need individualized feeding plans for triplets and higher order multiples.[55]

## Jaundice

Healthcare providers should promote and support breastfeeding. Colostrum intake ensures earlier meconium passage and lowers bilirubin levels.[56] Infants not feeding are at significant risk for developing hyperbilirubinemia and should receive expressed breast milk. Breastfeeding is recommended with phototherapy treatment for hyperbilirubinemia.[57]

## Craniofacial Anomalies (Cleft Lip/Palate)

For the infant with a cleft, breastfeeding may prevent upper respiratory infections (otitis media) and encourage speech development by use of oral-facial musculature. Breastfeeding before and after surgery is recommended.[58-60]

## Establishing Full Breastfeeding

Breastfeeding is a developmental skill, successful when an infant is neurobehaviorally ready. Readiness to breastfeed depends on the individual infant's cues. Lactation should be initiated with a breast pump as early as possible; hand expression can be used effectively when mechanical expression is not possible. Pumping or manually expressing each breast at least 8 times in 24 hours should yield 800–1,000 mL by day 10. Mothers should compress each breast during expression for increased higher fat content milk.

## Methods of Milk Expression

### Relaxation and Massage

Mothers should be instructed to use all sensory means to foster relaxation and effective letdown (music, darkened room, and gentle motion of rocking chair). Gentle breast massage facilitates milk flow.

### Manual Expression

All mothers should know how to express milk by hand.[61] For many, it is faster, easier, and more cost-effective than using a pump. Steps to manual expression:
- Wash hands and massage breasts
- Place thumb and forefinger on areola
- Push back toward chest wall
- While pushing back press thumb and forefinger gently together
- Repeat gentle compression of thumb and forefinger
- When milk flow decreases to an occasional droplet, stop massage, and express other breast.

### Adapting Techniques

Introduction of the preterm infant to the breast will require continued gavage feedings of expressed HM in the beginning and subsequent cue-based feeding. Feeding frequency gradually increases. Optimal feeding positions include the football (clutch) hold, cross-cradle, and the dancer hand position with larger preterm infants and continued skin-to-skin contact. Transition to full cue-based breastfeeding depends on infant readiness, including signs of demand sucking. Lactation/nursing/therapist teams should assess infant readiness to transition to breastfeeding.

It has become common, especially in the US, to feed an infant expressed breast milk without ever putting baby to breast.[62] Women give many reasons for pumping without breastfeeding; however, this practice is associated with earlier formula use.[63] Early lactation support is critical to optimize latch and successful breastfeeding.

## Discharge Planning

A detailed plan for preterm infants after discharge should include support from the NICU and ambulatory teams. Evans et al. discuss the Academy of Breastfeeding Medicine guidelines for hospital discharge.[64]

## Contraindications of Breastfeeding are Rare[65]

Conditions in which breastfeeding is not recommended include newborn galactosemia, maternal human immunodeficiency virus (HIV), herpes lesion on breasts, active untreated tuberculosis, maternal medications that are contraindicated in breastfeeding, and active maternal substance use.[66] ABM recommendations for contraindications exist for breastfeeding in women with a history of substance use.[67]

## Embracing Maternal Social and Cultural Context

Mother's overall well-being, attitude toward lactation, and maternal/infant health are influenced by tradition, culture, economics, and historical factors. Breastfeeding programs should include traditional beliefs such as prelacteal feeding, feeding restrictions, or maternal food avoidance, as long as they are practiced safely. Cultural practices may be beneficial, harmless, or harmful:[68]

- Beneficial cultural practices include breastfeeding on demand, carrying infants constantly, and spacing pregnancies by long-term breastfeeding. Strong maternal lactation support from family and community results in better breastfeeding outcomes.
- Harmless lactation practices may include seclusion, a period after giving birth which may promote mother-infant bonding and milk supply. It may also reduce exposure of the mother and infant to infection. Seclusion may also prevent stressful life events leading to postpartum depression.
  In many cultures, maternal "hot/cold" foods must be balanced to sustain or restore health after birth.[69]
- Harmful practices include deliberately avoiding early infant feeds/colostrum. Most cultures encourage colostrum as the first food for infants. Some, however, consider colostrum "old" milk that has been in the breasts for months and discard it until the transitional milk comes. Infants are also fed depending on local practices, i.e. some are fed water with sugar, butter, or rice milk.

## Racial and Ethnic Disparities in Breastfeeding

Immigrant mothers tend to adopt the cultural practices of their new country. For newcomers to the US, this often means formula feeding.

Wet nursing, where one lactating mother feeds another's child, is a tradition in most cultures, but sometimes discouraged due to concerns of infection transmission. It is now established that racial and ethnic disparities exist for success in HM at discharge in high-risk infants.[70] Access to prenatal care, socioeconomic status, cultural influence, and postpartum breastfeeding support all influence breastfeeding rates. In the US, black women are more likely than others to "prefer bottle-feeding" (formula-feeding) to breastfeeding. They are more likely to be low-income, single, and less educated. Disparate breastfeeding rates are contributory to excess black infant mortality. Lactation promotion initiatives focused on black women should emphasize education and encourage black women to feed their infants HM.

## Family Planning

During postpartum follow-up at 6 weeks, discussion about contraception to space pregnancies is encouraged. One method of natural family planning is the Lactational Amenorrhea Method (LAM); exclusive breastfeeding and infant suckling reduce fertility hormones, causing amenorrhea and temporary inability to conceive. LAM is part of World Health Organization's (WHO) list of accepted methods of family planning, with 98% effectiveness.[71] LAM also help reduce supplemental feedings, thus reducing costs by eliminating need for formula, bottles, and other medications/contraceptive drugs. Improved lactation support by organizations embracing LAM improves breastfeeding practices among women who practice it.

Lactation Amenorrhea Method can be used under three conditions:
1. The mother's menses have not yet returned.
2. The infant breastfeeds around the clock, including nighttime feedings.
3. The infant is younger than 6 months.[42]

## Milk Sharing

Milk sharing has been part of human culture for centuries, starting from wet nursing as a form of informal milk sharing to more recent use of HM banks. Because breast milk is the best infant nutrition, mothers often seek alternate sources in times when they cannot produce enough. When done properly, with good background information on who/where the milk comes from, informal milk sharing can be safely practiced.[72,73] HM banking is most useful for the very preterm infant, since the alternative, formula, is detrimental to premature infant health by increasing risk of NEC.[74,75] The Human Milk Banking Association of North America (HMBANA) has recommendations for handling donated breast milk and for operating a milk bank.[76] This nonprofit oversees several milk banks in the US, providing pasteurized

HM nationally. Other types of milk banks exist in the US as well, many for profit.[77,78] Milk-sharing cultural beliefs must be considered as they vary widely.[79-81]

## Public Health Approaches to Optimizing Infant Nutrition and Lactation

Several breastfeeding promotion strategies have optimized implementation, the most successful and evidence-based being the Baby-Friendly Hospital Initiative from WHO.

This international effort, developed by WHO and UNICEF in 1991, promotes, protects, and supports lactation in hospitals and birth centers worldwide.[82] The ten steps to successful breastfeeding, developed by a team of global experts, consists of evidence-based practices known to increase lactation initiation and duration. Baby-friendly hospitals and birthing facilities adhere to the ten steps to receive and retain baby-friendly designation. Originally intended for term infants, a preterm version of the ten steps is currently being developed.[83]

## The Ten Steps to Successful Breastfeeding[84]

1a. Comply fully with the International Code of Marketing of Breast-milk Substitutes and relevant World Health Assembly resolutions.
1b. Have a written infant feeding policy that is routinely communicated to staff and parents.
1c. Establish ongoing monitoring and data management systems.
2. Ensure that staff has sufficient knowledge, competence, and skills to support breastfeeding.
3. Discuss the importance and management of breastfeeding with pregnant women and their families.
4. Facilitate immediate and uninterrupted skin-to-skin contact and support mothers to initiate breastfeeding as soon as possible after birth.
5. Support mothers to initiate and maintain breastfeeding and manage common difficulties.
6. Do not provide breastfed newborns any food or fluids other than breast milk, unless medically indicated.
7. Enable mothers and their infants to remain together and to practice rooming-in 24 hours a day.
8. Support mothers to recognize and respond to their infants' cues for feeding.
9. Counsel mothers on the use and risks of feeding bottles, teats, and pacifiers.
10. Coordinate discharge so that parents and their infants have timely access to ongoing support and care.

## CONCLUSION

Breastfeeding is the optimal method for feeding newborn infants and provides great value.

There are long-term benefits to human bonding, growth, neurodevelopment, health promotion, and disease prevention at minimal cost. Healthcare providers can greatly influence successful breastfeeding. Globally, with societal support and progressive parental leave policies, most families should enjoy a healthy breastfeeding experience. Some high-risk mothers and infants will need special attention, but with optimal support and encouragement, most should achieve their breastfeeding goals.

## REFERENCES

1. Ballard O, Morrow AL. Human milk composition: nutrients and bioactive factors. Pediatr Clin North Am. 2013;60(1):49-74.
2. McGrath JM, Brandon D. Why Human Milk and Not Breast Milk Among Other Changes: 2018 Author Guideline Updates. Adv Neonatal Care. 2017;17(5):325-6.
3. Heine WE, Klein PD, Reeds PJ. The importance of alpha-lactalbumin in infant nutrition. J Nutr. 1991;121(3):277-83.
4. German JB, Freeman SL, Lebrilla CB, et al. Human milk oligosaccharides: evolution, structures and bioselectivity as substrates for intestinal bacteria. Nestle Nutr Workshop Ser Pediatr Program. 2008;62:205-18; discussion 218-22.
5. Vandenplas Y, Berger B, Carnielli VP, et al. Human Milk Oligosaccharides: 2'-Fucosyllactose (2'-FL) and Lacto-N-Neotetraose (LNnT) in Infant Formula. Nutrients. 2018;10(9). pii: E1161.
6. López-López A, López-Sabater MC, Campoy-Folgoso C, et al. Fatty acid and sn-2 fatty acid composition in human milk from Granada (Spain) and in infant formulas. Eur J Clin Nutr. 2002;56(12):1242-54.
7. Gallier S, Vocking K, Post JA, et al. A novel infant milk formula concept: Mimicking the human milk fat globule structure. Colloids Surf B Biointerfaces. 2015;136:329-39.
8. van Herwijnen MJ, Zonneveld MI, Goerdayal S, et al. Comprehensive proteomic analysis of human milk-derived extracellular vesicles unveils a novel functional proteome distinct from other milk components. Mol Cell Proteomics. 2016;15(11):3412-23.
9. Williamson P, LeMay D. The Dynamic Human Milk Proteome. Splash Milk Science. 2016. [online] Available from: http://milkgenomics.org/article/dynamic-human-milk-proteome. [Last accessed September, 2019].
10. Zhu J, Garrigues L, Van den Toorn H, et al. Discovery and Quantification of Nonhuman Proteins in Human Milk. J Proteome Res. 2019;18(1):225-38.
11. Gay MC, Koleva PT, Slupsky CM, et al. Worldwide variation in human milk metabolome: indicators of breast physiology and maternal lifestyle? Nutrients. 2018;10(9): pii: 1151.
12. Witkowska-Zimny M, Kaminska-El Hassan E. Cells of human breast milk. Cell Mol Biol Lett. 2017;22:11.
13. Ho FC, Wong RL, Lawton JW. Human colostral and breast milk cells. A light and electron microscopic study. Acta Paediatri Scand. 1979;68(3):389-96.
14. Hassiotou F, Geddes DT, Hartmann PE. Cells in human milk: state of the science. J Hum Lact. 2013;(2):171-82.
15. Cregan MD, Fan Y, Appelbee A, et al. Identification of nestin-positive putative mammary stem cells in human breastmilk. Cell Tissue Res. 2007;329(1):129-36.

16. Hassiotou F, Beltran A, Chetwynd E, et al. Breastmilk is a novel source of stem cells with multilineage differentiation potential. Stem Cells. 2012;30(10):2164-74.
17. Brooker BE. The epithelial cells and cell fragments in human milk. Cell Tissue Res. 1980;210(2):321-32.
18. Hassiotou F, Geddes D. Anatomy of the human mammary gland: Current status of knowledge. Clin Anat. 2013;26(1):29-48.
19. Piper KM, Berry CA, Cregan MD. The bioactive nature of human breastmilk. Breastfeed Rev. 2007;15(3):5-10.
20. Saarela T, Kokkonen J, Koivisto M. Macronutrient and energy contents of human milk fractions during the first six months of lactation. Acta Paediatr. 2005;94(9):1176-81.
21. Gross SJ, Geller J, Tomarelli RM. Composition of breast milk from mothers of preterm infants. Pediatrics. 1981;68(4):490-3.
22. Lemons JA, Moye L, Hall D, et al. Differences in the composition of preterm and term human milk during early lactation. Pediatr Res. 1982;16(2):113-7.
23. Narang AP, Bains HS, Kansal S, et al. Serial composition of human milk in preterm and term mothers. Indian J Clin Biochem. 2006;21(1):89-94.
24. Lönnerdal B, Erdmann P, Thakkar SK, et al. Longitudinal evolution of true protein, amino acids and bioactive proteins in breast milk: a developmental perspective. J Nutr Biochem. 2017;41:1-11.
25. Cesare Marincola F, Dessì A, Corbu S, et al. Clinical impact of human breast milk metabolomics. Clin Chim Acta. 2015;451(Pt A):103-6.
26. Sundekilde UK, Larsen LB, Bertram HC. NMR-based milk metabolomics. Metabolites. 2013;3(2):204-22.
27. Narasimhan S, Kinchen J, Kifle A, et al. Metabolomic Differences Between Mothers' Own Breast Milk and Donor Breast Milk. Poster Presented at Pediatric Academic Society Annual Meeting. Baltimore, MD: Pediatric Academic Society; 2016.
28. Herrmann K, Carroll K. An exclusively human milk diet reduces necrotizing enterocolitis. Breastfeed Med. 2014;9(4):184-90.
29. Section on Breastfeeding. Breastfeeding and the use of human milk. Pediatrics. 2012;129(3):e827-41.
30. Kramer MS, Chalmers B, Hodnett ED, et al.; PROBIT Study Group (Promotion of Breastfeeding Intervention Trial). Promotion of Breastfeeding Intervention Trial (PROBIT): a randomized trial in the Republic of Belarus. JAMA. 2001;285(4):413-20.
31. Baydar N, McCann M, Williams R, et al. Final Report: WIC Infant Feeding Practices Study. Seattle, Washington: Battelle Centers for Public Health Research and Evaluation; 1997. [online] Available from: https://fns-prod.azureedge.net/sites/default/files/WICIFPS.pdf. [Last accessed September, 2019].
32. Matthiesen AS, Ransjö-Arvidson AB, Nissen E, et al. Postpartum maternal oxytocin release by newborns: effects of infant hand massage and sucking. Birth. 2001;28(1):13-9.
33. Yamauchi Y, Yamanouchi I. The relationship between rooming-in/not rooming-in and breast-feeding variables. Acta Paediatr Scand. 1990;79(11):1017-22.
34. Mikiel-Kostyra K, Mazur J, Bołtruszko I. Effect of early skin-to-skin contact after delivery on duration of breastfeeding: a prospective cohort study. Acta Paediatr. 2002;91(12):1301-6.
35. Wambach K, Riordan J. Breastfeeding and Human Lactation, 5th edition. Burlington, MA: Jones & Bartlett Learning; 2016.
36. Kent JC, Prime DK, Garbin CP. Principles for maintaining or increasing breast milk production. J Obstet Gynecol Neonatal Nurs. 2012;41(1):114-21.
37. Little EE, Legare CH, Carver LJ. Mother-Infant Physical Contact Predicts Responsive Feeding among U.S. Breast-feeding Mothers. Nutrients. 2018;10(9): pii: E1251.
38. Shloim N, Vereijken CM, Blundell P, et al. Looking for cues - infant communication of hunger and satiation during milk feeding. Appetite. 2017;108:74-82.
39. Ng CA, Ho JJ, Lee ZH. The effect of rooming-in on duration of breastfeeding: A systematic review of randomised and non-randomised prospective controlled studies. PLoS One. 2019;14(4):e0215869.
40. Jaafar SH, Ho JJ, Lee KS. Rooming-in for new mother and infant versus separate care for increasing the duration of breastfeeding. Cochrane Database Syst Rev. 2016;(8):CD006641.
41. Wolf LS, Glass RP, Carr AB. Feeding and Swallowing Disorders in Infancy: Assessment and Management, 2nd edition. Austin, Texas: The Psychological Corporation; 1992.
42. Walker M. Breastfeeding Management for the Clinician: Using the Evidence. Burlington, MA: Jones & Bartlett Learning; 2007.
43. Neifert MR, Seacat JM, Jobe WE. Lactation failure due to insufficient glandular development of the breast. Pediatrics. 1985;76(5):823-8.
44. Cotterman KJ. Reverse pressure softening: a simple tool to prepare areola for easier latching during engorgement. J Hum Lact. 2004;20(2):227-37.
45. Ingram J, Johnson D, Copeland M, et al. The development of a new breast feeding assessment tool and the relationship with breast feeding self-efficacy. Midwifery. 2015;31(1):132-7.
46. Jensen D, Wallace S, Kelsay P. LATCH: a breastfeeding charting system and documentation tool. J Obstet Gynecol Neonatal Nurs. 1994;23(1):27-32.
47. Spatz DL, Edwards TM. The Use of Human Milk and Breastfeeding in the Neonatal Intensive Care Unit: Position Statement 3065. Adv Neonatal Care. 2016;16(4):254.
48. Parker LA, Sullivan S, Krueger C, et al. Effect of early breast milk expression on milk volume and timing of lactogenesis stage II among mothers of very low birth weight infants: a pilot study. J Perinatol. 2012;32(3):205-9.
49. Kitajima H. Prevention of methicillin-resistant Staphylococcus aureus infections in neonates. Pediatr Int. 2003;45(2):238-45.
50. Cartwright J, Atz T, Newman S, et al. Integrative review of interventions to promote breastfeeding in the late preterm infant. J Obstet Gynecol Nurs. 2017;46(3):347-56.
51. Estalella I, San Millán J, Trincado MJ, et al. Evaluation of an intervention supporting breastfeeding among late-preterm infants during in-hospital stay. Women Birth. 2018. pii: S1871-5192(18)30356-1.
52. Ikonen R, Paavilainen E, Helminen M, et al. Preterm infants' mothers' initiation and frequency of breast milk expression and exclusive use of mother's breast milk in neonatal intensive care units. J Clin Nurs. 2018;27(3-4):e551-8.
53. Ikonen R, Paavilainen E, Kaunonen M. Preterm infants' mothers' experiences with milk expression and breastfeeding: an integrative review. Adv Neonatal Care. 2015;15(6):394-406.
54. Morton J, Hall JY, Wong RJ, et al. Combining hand techniques with electric pumping increases milk production in mothers of preterm infants. J Perinatol. 2009;29(11):757-64.

55. O'Rourke MP, Spatz DL. Women's Experiences with Tandem Breastfeeding. MCN Am J Matern Child Nurs. 2019;44(4):220-7.
56. Ketsuwan S, Baiya N, Maelhacharoenporn K, et al. The Association of Breastfeeding Practices with Neonatal Jaundice. J Med Assoc Thai. 2017;100(3):255-61.
57. Flaherman VJ, Maisels MJ; Academy of Breastfeeding Medicine. ABM Clinical Protocol #22: Guidelines for management of jaundice in the breastfeeding infant 35 weeks or more of gestation-revised 2017. Breastfeed Med. 2017;12(5):250-7.
58. Matsunaka E, Ueki S, Makimoto K. Impact of breastfeeding and/or bottle-feeding on surgical wound dehiscence after cleft lip repair in infants: A systematic review. J Craniomaxillofac Surg. 2019;47(4):570-7.
59. Kaye A, Cattaneo C, Huff HM, et al. A pilot study of mothers' breastfeeding experiences in infants with cleft lip and/or palate. Adv Neonatal Care. 2019;19(2):127-37.
60. Alperovich M, Frey JD, Shetye PR, et al. Breast Milk feeding rates in patients with cleft lip and palate at a North American craniofacial center. Cleft Palate Craniofac J. 2017;54(3):334-7.
61. Morton J. Stanford Medicine Newborn Nursery. Hand Expression of Breast Milk. [online] Available from: https://med.stanford.edu/newborns/professional-education/breastfeeding/hand-expressing-milk.html. [Last accessed September, 2019].
62. Loewenberg Weisband Y, Keim SA, Keder LM, et al. Early Breast Milk Pumping Intentions Among Postpartum Women. Breastfeed Med. 2017;12(1):28-32.
63. Keim SA, Boone KM, Oza-Frank R, et al. Pumping Milk Without Ever Feeding at the Breast in the Moms2Moms Study. Breastfeed Med. 2017;12(7):422-9.
64. Evans A, Marinelli KA, Taylor JS; Academy of Breastfeeding Medicine. ABM clinical protocol #2: Guidelines for hospital discharge of the breastfeeding term newborn and mother: "The Going Home Protocol," revised 2014. Breastfeed Med. 2014;9(1):3-8.
65. World Health Organization. Infant Feeding for the Prevention of Mother-to-Child Transmission of HIV. e-Library of Evidence for Nutrition Actions (eLENA), 2019. [online] Available from: https://www.who.int/elena/titles/hiv_infant_feeding/en/. [Last accessed September, 2019].
66. Centers for Disease Control and Prevention. Contraindications to Breastfeeding or Feeding Expressed Breast Milk to Infants. [online] Available from: https://www.cdc.gov/breastfeeding/breastfeeding-special-circumstances/contraindications-to-breastfeeding.html. [Last accessed September, 2019].
67. Reece-Stremtan S, Marinelli KA. ABM clinical protocol #21: guidelines for breastfeeding and substance use or substance use disorder, revised 2015. Breastfeed Med. 2015;10(3):135-41.
68. Pickett E. A Closer Look at Cultural Issues Surrounding Breastfeeding. International Lactation Consultant Association Lactation Matters Blog Archive. 2012. [online] Available from: https://lactationmatters.org/2012/10/. [Last accessed September, 2019].
69. Wambach K. The cultural context of breastfeeding. In: Wambach K, Riordan J (Eds). Breastfeeding and Human Lactation, 5th edition. Burlington, MA: Jones & Bartlett Learning; 2016.
70. Profit J, Gould JB, Bennett M, et al. Racial/ethnic disparity in NICU quality of care delivery. Pediatrics. 2017;140(3):e20170918.
71. Labbok MH, Hight-Laukaran V, Peterson AE, et al. Multicenter study of the Lactational Amenorrhea Method (LAM): I. Efficacy, duration, and implications for clinical application. Contraception. 1997;55(6):327-36.
72. Akre JE, Gribble KD, Minchin M. Milk sharing: from private practice to public pursuit. Int Breastfeed J. 2011;6:8.
73. Gribble KD, Hausman BL. Milk sharing and formula feeding: Infant feeding risks in comparative perspective? Australas Med J. 2012;5(5):275-83.
74. Cristofalo EA, Schanler RJ, Blanco CL, et al. Randomized trial of exclusive human milk versus preterm formula diets in extremely premature infants. J Pediatr. 2013;163(6):1592-5.e1.
75. Updegrove K. Necrotizing enterocolitis: the evidence for use of human milk in prevention and treatment. J Human Lact. 2004;20(3):335-9.
76. Human Milk Banking Association of North America. 2019 Best Practice for Handling Human Milk. [online] Available from: https://www.hmbana.org/. [Last accessed September, 2019].
77. Palmquist AE, Doehler K. Human milk sharing practices in the U.S. Matern Child Nutr. 2016;12(2):278-90.
78. Ruhe N. The Battle over Breast Milk: For-profit Milk Banks Versus Non-profit Milk Banks. Med City News. 2015. [online] Available from: https://medcitynews.com/2015/07/breast-milk-milk-banks/ [Last accessed September, 2019].
79. Ibarra Peso J, Mesa Vásquez S, Aguayo Gajardo K. Experiences, beliefs and attitude on donation of human milk in women of Arauco province. Rev Child Pediatr. 2018;89(5):592-9.
80. Murray L, Anggrahini SM, Woda RR, et al. Exclusive breastfeeding and the acceptability of donor breast milk for sick, hospitalized infants in Kupang, Nusa Tenggara Timur, Indonesia: a mixed-methods study. J Hum Lact. 2016;32(3):438-45.
81. El-Khuffash A, Unger S. The concept of milk Kinship in Islam: issues raised when offering preterm infants of Muslim families donor human milk. J Hum Lact. 2012;28(2):125-7.
82. UNICEF. The Baby-Friendly Hospital Initiative. [online] Available from: https://www.unicef.org/programme/breastfeeding/baby.htm. [Last accessed September, 2019].
83. UNICEF, United Kingdom. The Baby Friendly Initiative; Guidance for Neonatal Units.[online] Available from: https://www.unicef.org.uk/babyfriendly/wp-content/uploads/sites/2/2015/12/Guidance-for-neonatal-units.pdf. [Last accessed September, 2019].
84. World Health Organization. Nutrition: Ten Steps to Successful Breastfeeding (Revised 2018). [online] Available from: https://www.who.int/nutrition/bfhi/ten-steps/en/. [Last accessed September, 2019].

# CHAPTER 38

# Necrotizing Enterocolitis

*Arwin Valencia, Antoine Soliman*

## ABSTRACT

Necrotizing enterocolitis (NEC) is one of the most widely studied neonatal diseases due to its high mortality rate, frequent poor outcomes, and impact on healthcare costs. It continues to be difficult to eradicate, despite recent advancements in the understanding of the mechanisms and factors that predispose a newborn to NEC. Exclusive use of mother's own milk (MOM), availability of pasteurized human donor milk, and the use of probiotics in very low-birth weight (VLBW) infants have made a substantial impact in prevention. Current theories focus on the role of intestinal immaturity, abnormal host immunologic reaction, and excessive inflammatory response by the premature gut. Recent changes in feeding practices in preterm infants may relate to the shift in the time of occurrence, favoring an earlier presentation. Also, a bimodal age distribution has been observed. Collectively, these observations may suggest alternate pathogenesis, to be clarified by ongoing research efforts.

## INTRODUCTION

Necrotizing enterocolitis continues to be one of the most serious gastrointestinal (GI) crises in newborn infants worldwide.[1] It is characterized by inflammation of the intestines and may be difficult to differentiate from sepsis. It can later complicate into intestinal perforation (IP) and peritonitis. It is estimated that about 7-11% of VLBW premature infants are afflicted,[2,3] but extremely low-birth weight (ELBW) infants are primarily at risk.[4] NEC has very high mortality, and when surgical intervention is required its mortality rate is over 30%.[5,6] In ELBW infants, surgical NEC has very high mortality rates and significantly higher neurodevelopmental impairment in survivors.[6] The age of onset is inversely related to the postmenstrual age (PMA) at birth and the incidence rate only decreases after 34-35 weeks gestation.[7] There is a predilection for males in death risk compared to females.[3] In most cases, the etiology is unknown and multifactorial, but recent evidence has underscored the essential roles of insufficient epithelial barrier, inappropriate immune response, abnormal gut microbiome, and feeding with formula.[8] The classic histopathologic finding of NEC is hemorrhagic ischemic necrosis.[8,9] The events that generate this result appear to be set off by an excessive and dysregulated inflammatory response by an exceedingly immunoreactive intestine.[9] This reaction that at first starts locally can later spread systemically. Further compromise may result in a substantial increased risk for neurodevelopmental delays.[6]

Necrotizing enterocolitis and its subsequent morbidities continue to be one of the most expensive complications in premature infants.[1] Withholding enteral feedings for a substantial period of time leads to prolonged parenteral nutrition, an increase in central line-associated bloodstream infections (CLABSI), an increased rate of postnatal growth deficiency at the time of discharge, and an overall increased length of hospitalization.[10] Total annual cost of care in the United States due to NEC is 500 million to 1 billion dollars.[1] Infants who developed NEC were hospitalized 20 days longer for those that only required medical treatment, and

60 days longer when surgical intervention was necessary.[10,11] Total mean cost of care over a 5-year period with those with short bowel resection is 1.5 million dollars.[11]

## PATHOGENESIS OF NECROTIZING ENTEROCOLITIS

The amniotic fluid serves several important functions and is crucial for the growth and development of the gut.[12] Fetal swallowing begins between 10 weeks and 14 weeks of gestation and more than 700 mL of amniotic fluid is consumed per day in late gestation.[13] Up to 0.3 g/kg or 18% of human fetal protein requirements can be derived from this activity.[14] Amniotic fluid contains proteins, carbohydrates, and growth factors such as epidermal growth factor (EGF).[12,15] Intestinal epithelial growth is regulated by EGF.[16,17] EGF-receptors (EGF-R) are abundant in the intestinal mucosa, predominantly in the ileum.[18] Significant concentrations of EGF have been detected in amniotic fluid as early as 16 weeks of gestation and have been shown to influence fetal and neonatal GI tissue development.[19] The amniotic fluid controls and protects the fetal intestinal environment which may be the reason why NEC has not been identified in utero.[20] Amniotic fluid is also important in the maturation of the gut in that it is necessary for successful postnatal feeding.[12] Preterm infants, however, are unable to complete this developmental process, leading to compromised immune barrier and immune response. The combination of intestinal immaturity, abnormal host immunologic reaction, and excessive inflammatory response by the premature gut today are all considered to be factors initiating NEC.[20]

### Epithelial Barrier

Differentiation of the epithelium and villus formation proceeds in a cephalocaudal direction. By the 11th postconceptional week, the entire small intestine is already lined by columnar epithelium. The intestinal epithelium is arranged in villi associated with mucosal invaginations known as the crypts of Lieberkühn, the depth of which indicates intestinal maturation.[21]

The immaturity of the GI tract of preterm infants born before 28 weeks of gestation requires a period of dependence on total parenteral nutrition (TPN) before enteral feeding can be established and successfully advanced. Prolonged TPN use results in intestinal atrophy and delayed microbial colonization.[22] Intestinal motility is not mature until the third trimester and some components of the mucus lining are also deficient.[23] These factors may alter the sensitive balance maintained in the epithelium and may predispose it to injury over repair. In normal physiologic conditions, the process of healing and recovery happens instantaneously,[24] but when the barrier is compromised, enterocyte migration and proliferation is reduced, leading to further injury and enhanced bacterial translocation.[25]

### Innate Immunity

Premature infants have inappropriate immunologic responses.[26,27] Epithelial cell proliferation potential is diminished, resulting in an amplified susceptibility to intestinal diseases.[25] Because of ineffective signal transduction pathways and inefficient cortisol surge, the immature gut is unable to enhance crypt depth in response to feeding as the gut of a term infant can.[28] The increase of pro-inflammatory mediators and the upregulation of their gene expression in NEC suggest the role of inflammation in its pathogenesis.[29,30] These observations are further supported by the decrease in incidence in those who received antenatal steroids, a well-known potent anti-inflammatory agent.[31]

The intestinal epithelial cells (IEC) are exposed to microbes and their protein products called microbe-associated molecular products (MAMP).[28] Specific receptors in the IEC, named pattern recognition receptors (PRRs), allow communications between the IECs.[28] Activation of these PRRs launch regulatory pathways.[27] One of the main pathways is through the nuclear factor kappa-light-chain-enhancer of activated B cells (NF-κB).[32] Depending on how the signal is perceived, translation may be that of an inflammatory response, cytoprotection, and recovery or destruction and consequent apoptosis.[33]

Recent studies have identified a key role for a particular group of PRRs called Toll-like receptors (TLRs) in NEC—primarily, TLR4.[25] TLRs are important in the innate inflammatory cytokine production and regulation of adaptive immune response.[27,30] Activation of TLR4 inhibits enterocyte migration leading to programed cell death in the mouse model via NF-κB pathway.[25,32] Signal inhibition in the IEC, on the other hand, prevents NEC and attenuates the degree of enterocyte apoptosis in the mouse model and cell cultures.[25]

Elevated levels of TLR4 are normally expressed in utero in the developing fetus until the end of gestation without increased risk for NEC,[25,34] which may be partly due to amniotic fluid protection. In prematurely born infants, exaggerated expression is observed in the presence of abnormal bacterial colonization with pathogenic bacteria.[25] Consequently, this leads to a cascade of events that starts with barrier failure and bacterial translocation followed by the activation of systemic inflammatory response.[25,34]

### Intestinal Microbiota

The newborn gut previously had been assumed to be sterile at birth, with natural bacterial colonization beginning only on the first day of life.[20] In term breastfed infants, *Bifidobacterium* appears as early as 4 days of age.[35] By 7–10 days, most of healthy full-term breastfeeding infants are colonized with a combination of both Gram-positive and Gram-negative bacteria.[35,36] Natural gut microflora protect against invading pathogens by providing physical and immunologic barriers.[37]

The intestinal microbiota in normal circumstances has a harmless or symbiotic relationship with the host. In infants born prematurely, many factors alter this fragile balance that probably began in the early fetal stage and was sustained all throughout postnatal life. This altered balance may result in deficient diversity in preterm microbial colonization and possibly even less diversity in those infants who will later develop NEC.[36,38]

The use of polymerase chain reaction (PCR) technique to detect the presence of microorganisms in the amniotic fluid, generated 30–50% more microorganisms than previously identified by the regular culture-based method.[39] This, together with the recent findings of the presence of microbial DNA in fetal meconium, suggests that there is exposure of fetal intestine to amniotic fluid microbes.[39,40] In the developing fetus, this exposure to small quantities of TLR agonists (MAMPs) results in the overexpression of TLR4 control epithelial proliferation and differentiation.[34] Over time, these interactions may allow the intestines to develop tolerance against further inflammatory stimuli.[41] This is clearly demonstrated in the immunologic response of term infants. Premature infants, due to their early birth, are deprived of this critical period, which explains the compromised state of their intestine. Postnatally, this condition is further aggravated by the later exposure to more virulent bacteria leading to pathogenic colonization.[35] Dysbiosis results in leaky barriers and easy bacterial translocation across epithelial cell layers.[25]

Colonization of the intestine is also influenced by many postnatal factors. Those infants born via cesarean section (CS) are largely colonized by an assortment of potentially harmful bacteria—both hospital-acquired and natural skin flora from the mother.[42] The pervasive use of antibiotics in neonatal intensive care units (NICUs) may not only reduce the diversity of intestinal flora and delay colonization with beneficial bacteria, but also allow for the proliferation of pathogenic species after just three days.[43] Increasing gastric pH by the use of antacids in preterm infants promotes bacterial translocation.[44] With gastric pH <3, NEC is decreased, but with pH >4, enteric bacterial colony counts increase.[44]

### Enteral Feeding

Adequate adaptation of the GI tract is essential for survival. Preterm infants are unable to fully digest carbohydrates and proteins partly because of dysmotility,[23] and undigested carbohydrates cause production of organic acids which are harmful to the developing intestines.[45] Undigested caseins are a chemoattractant for neutrophils.[45,46] Infants fed with formula produce large amounts of butyric acid but breastfed infants produce acetic acid.[46] Butyric acid triggers interleukin-8 (IL-8) response, which is a potent chemotactic agent for neutrophils and proinflammatory cytokines.[45,46]

Aggressive feeding in premature infants is largely thought to result in stasis of milk substrates that result in intestinal dilatation and impairment of the epithelial barrier. In the presence of abnormal colonization, normal signal transduction is distorted, causing shift to excessive inflammation, apoptosis, and necrosis instead of the normal message of growth and repair of enterocytes.[47]

Human milk decreases NEC in animal and human studies.[48,49] Human milk oligosaccharides (HMO) containing a lactose core function as prebiotics promoting proliferation of normal bacterial flora, mostly *Bifidobacterium* species.[50] A multicenter study compared the outcomes of infants on a diet of human donor milk and human milk only-based diet versus infants on a combination of human and bovine milk-based products. The human milk only diet resulted in lower rates of both clinical and surgical NEC. The use of the human milk strategy alone reduced incidence of medical NEC by 50% and surgical NEC by 90%.[48] Because of these benefits, the American Academy of Pediatrics (AAP) recommends offering donor milk to all preterm infants when MOM is not available.[51]

## NECROTIZING ENTEROCOLITIS AND BLOOD TRANSFUSION

Previous reports proposed that blood transfusion for anemia of prematurity in otherwise stable growing premature infants increases the risk of late-onset NEC.[52,53] A prospective matched case-controlled investigation did not substantiate an association, however.[54] At present, many practitioners continue to adopt a cautious approach in susceptible populations, particularly in those NICUs with high NEC rates. Some will temporarily withhold oral feeds when giving transfusions, but the practice varies among different centers. There is no consensus as to the correct timing and duration for withholding feeds.[55] Lately, emphasis is directed toward preventing anemia or allowing lower hemoglobin values for as long as the patient is asymptomatic and growing. Practices like delayed cord clamping, cord milking, using cord blood for initial blood work, and minimizing blood draws have been largely accepted.

## MEDIATORS OF NECROTIZING ENTEROCOLITIS

### Nuclear Factor Kappa-Light-Chain-Enhancer of Activated B Cells

Nuclear factor kappa-light-chain-enhancer of activated B cells is a transcription factor that regulates the expression of many pro-inflammatory molecules including cytokines, chemokines, and leukocyte adhesion molecules.[30] In animal models, NF-κB is constitutively low in adult rat intestines and is activated in platelet-activating factor (PAF)-induced acute bowel injury.[56] Blocking NF-κB activation in rats protects against NEC.[57] Breastfeeding and the use of probiotics attenuate IEC NF-κB activation.[57,58]

### Toll-like Receptors

Toll-like receptors are receptors for bacterial products; currently, there are 10 TLRs identified in humans. Human and rat NEC are associated with increased intestinal expression of both TLR2 and TLR4 but decreased TLR9.[59] TLR4 is the receptor for endotoxin and has a deleterious role in NEC.[25] It is expressed significantly in animals exposed to formula feeding but is downregulated in dam-fed animals during the first 72 hours of life.[60] TLR2 has been shown to confer responsiveness to cell wall components of both Gram-positive and Gram-negative bacteria and *Mycoplasma spp.*[61] TLR9 activation has been shown to be protective; in TLR9-deficient mice, increase in NEC severity has been demonstrated.[59] Its activation by its ligand CpG-DNA inhibits lipopolysaccharide (LPS)—mediated TLR4 signaling in enterocytes and reduces severity of NEC.[59]

### Platelet-activating Factor

Platelet-activating factor (PAF) is an endogenous mediator released by many cells and is elevated in NEC.[62] It is rapidly degraded by platelet-activating factor acetyl hydrolase (PAF-AH), which is found to be deficient in those infants who develop NEC.[63,64] PAF is abundant in breast milk.[63] The ileum, which is the site of predilection of NEC, has the highest amount of PAF receptors.[65] PAF also mediates injury induced by hypoxia and reperfusion, tumor necrosis factor (TNF)-alpha, and lipopolysaccharides (LPS).[66]

### Interleukins

Interleukin-6 (a cytokine produced by macrophages, endothelial and epithelial cells) is elevated in the plasma and stools of patients with NEC[67] and correlates with the severity of the disease.[28] IL-8, a chemokine, is upregulated only in fetal enterocytes and not the mature enterocytes, which may increase susceptibility to inflammation.[68] IL-10 has been shown to be protective against NEC in the rat models by attenuating the degree of intestinal inflammation and epithelial apoptosis.[69] IL-12 is upregulated in the ileum of neonatal rats with NEC, which corresponds with tissue damage progression.[70] IL-18, a pro-inflammatory cytokine, is also upregulated in the ileum of neonatal rats with NEC.[70]

### Tumor Necrosis Factor-alpha

Tumor necrosis factor-alpha (TNF-α) is not consistently found to be higher in the plasma of infants with NEC,[29,67] but its protein is noted to be increased in resected intestinal tissues.[71] In the neonatal rat bowel injury model induced by hypoxia/reperfusion, TNF-α is found to be elevated, but not in the NEC rat model.[72,73]

### Nitric Oxide

Nitric oxide (NO), a free radical known to regulate many physiologic functions when released by activated macrophages, inhibits enterocyte migration.[74] Localized production by villus enterocytes impair proliferation and increase apoptosis.[75] NO also mediates dendritic cell apoptosis while protecting other cell type apoptosis.[76]

### Reactive Oxygen Species

Xanthine-oxidase/dehydrogenase is one of the main producers of reactive oxygen species (ROS) in the intestines, and is probably the final effector of PAF and other cytokines.[77] Xanthine oxidase (XO) and superoxide have been shown to play central roles in intestinal reperfusion injury.[78] Allopurinol, a XO inhibitor, protects against PAF-induced bowel necrosis.[79]

## NECROTIZING ENTEROCOLITIS IN FULL-TERM BABIES

In term infants, NEC is rare and occurs in a subset of neonates admitted to the NICU for some other illness or condition.[80] Features predisposing term infants to NEC include conditions leading to reduced mesenteric perfusion (perinatal asphyxia, polycythemia, and sepsis), congenital heart disease with diminished systemic cardiac output, and among infants withdrawing from maternal opioid narcotics.[81,82] It is also recognized in term babies with predisposing GI pathology who are fed higher volumes of cow's milk formula than a breastfeeding neonate would normally receive.[81]

## TIMING OF PRESENTATION

In the 1980s investigators found that NEC occurred more commonly in preterm infants between 33 weeks and

35 weeks PMA.[83] Recently, a bimodal age distribution seems apparent, appearing as early as 7 days in more mature infants <33 weeks' gestation and later (2-3 weeks) for infants born at 28 weeks or earlier gestational age (GA).[84] Compared with late-onset NEC, those infants who developed early-onset NEC had the following—lower incidence of respiratory distress syndrome, patent ductus arteriosus (PDA) treated with indomethacin, reduced use of postnatal steroids, and shortened duration of ventilation days.[83-85] Higher GA and vaginal delivery were associated with increased risk of early-onset NEC in multivariate logistic regression analysis.[84]

## CLINICAL PRESENTATION

Signs and symptoms of NEC are nonspecific, varying from insidiously developing over days to a fulminant presentation in just a few hours of GI symptoms, systemic dysfunction, disseminated intravascular coagulation (DIC), and shock.[1] Early signs are indistinguishable from those of sepsis and may include temperature and glucose instability, lethargy, apnea/bradycardia and hypotension.[2]

The pathologic features of NEC resemble those of ischemic necrosis.[8] The initial phase is an inflammatory process that leads to increased blood flow to the region, beginning in the mucosa and extending through the entire bowel wall. The distal ileum and proximal colon are the areas commonly affected.

In 1978, Bell and his associates developed the staging system for NEC to describe surgical outcomes in preterm infants.[86] They proposed the following stratification: Stage I is suspected NEC, Stage II is definite NEC, and Stage III is advanced NEC. Each stage is based on historical, clinical, and radiographic data.

The clinical signs of stage I or suspected NEC include temperature instability, apnea/bradycardia, and lethargy. GI signs include poor feeding, elevated pregavage residuals, abdominal distension, emesis (may be bilious) or blood in the stool. Abdominal radiographs may show distension with mild ileus.

In Stage II NEC, the systemic and GI signs are like Stage I, but GI signs also include persistent occult and gross intestinal bleeding, elevated pregavage residuals, and marked abdominal distention. Abdominal radiographs show significant intestinal distension with ileus, small bowel separation, edema in bowel wall or signs of ascites, unchanging or persistent bowel loops, portal vein gas, and pneumatosis intestinalis, which is manifested by small gas bubbles (produced by bacteria) in the bowel wall.

Infants with Stage III or advanced NEC are severely ill with all the signs and symptoms seen with Stage I and II, with additional deterioration of vital signs, evidence of septic shock, marked GI hemorrhage and marked distension.

Abdominal radiographs show pneumoperitoneum, significant intestinal distension, pneumatosis intestinalis, portal vein gas, and perforation. The propensity for these focal lesions to occur in the watershed areas of the terminal ileum or jejunum support the theory of arterial occlusion with embolism.[87] Histopathology demonstrates muscle wall thinning, distention, focal degeneration, and extensive remodeling of the extracellular matrix.[88,89]

## ISOLATED INTESTINAL PERFORATION (IIP)

Thought to be a clinically different entity than NEC, isolated IIP is usually not associated with feedings and the histologic findings reveal a focal perforation without inflammation.[85] It occurs during the first week of life and has been associated with early indocin use for intraventricular hemorrhage (IVH) prophylaxis or for treatment of PDA.[85] Indocin blocks prostaglandin E2 (PGE2), which is necessary for intestinal growth and function through its EGF-R influence, which then results in vasoconstriction and ischemia.[90]

Despite its benefits, several studies have demonstrated that the early use of postnatal steroids in the premature neonate is associated with an increased risk of IIP.[91,92] The neonatal ileum is uniquely primed by steroids to respond to insulin-like growth factor-I (IGF-I), which mediates intestinal growth precociously.[91] This involves volume expansion, increased bowel diameter, and stretching and thinning of the surrounding smooth muscles.[91,92] Exposure to both steroid and indomethacin may cause ischemic damage to an already thin smooth muscle, resulting in matrix degradation and perforation.[85,90-92]

## MANAGEMENT

Management of premature infants with suspected NEC requires a high level of suspicion for its presence, particularly when feeding intolerance is the only presenting symptom. For suspected NEC, withholding enteral feeds and maintaining hydration via intravenous (IV) fluids or TPN are typically used. Abdominal radiography and serial abdominal examinations are often necessary. Gastric decompression for ileus is considered. Complete workup for infection and initiation of broad-spectrum antibiotics is usually warranted. Surgical cause of abdominal distension will need to be ruled out and the patient should be observed closely for worsening of condition. If there is improvement, cautious feeding may be initiated in subsequent days.

Pediatric surgery involvement is recommended in definite and advanced stages of NEC.[1,5] Feeding is withheld for 7-10 days and nutrition and hydration is maintained by IV fluids. Because of "third spacing", patient may require intravascular fluid resuscitation to improve bowel perfusion.

Strict monitoring of input and output is important because of decreased renal perfusion that can lead to acute renal failure. Gastric decompression is performed, and serial abdominal radiographs are obtained to evaluate for possible perforation, especially during the first 12-24 hours of onset. Assisted ventilation may be required. Arterial blood pressure should be maintained with volume expanders and vasopressors if necessary.

Operative intervention is indicated for bowel perforation, evidence of necrotic bowel (fixed loop, metabolic acidosis, DIC, and shock) or progressively worsening of clinical condition despite intensive medical management. Surgical options for advanced NEC are laparotomy and primary peritoneal drainage without laparotomy, but the relative benefits of these procedures have been controversial.[93] Laparotomy is the traditional treatment for Stage III NEC and IIP. The use of peritoneal drainage became popular in the 1970s when it was used in neonates who were too critical for laparotomy; however, a recent multi-institutional cohort study showed that the outcome of the commonly used peritoneal drainage procedure was poor.[94,95] In fact, infants who underwent laparotomy were shown to be less likely to die and to have better neurodevelopmental outcome than those who underwent peritoneal drainage for NEC.[96] Regardless of the controversy concerning one procedure's superiority over the other, these studies clearly suggest that once surgery is required, there is a higher probability of a poor outcome.

The mortality rate for NEC remains high depending on the severity of illness and the amount of bowel resected. Long-term complications may include intestinal stricture with bowel obstruction, short bowel syndrome, fistula, abscess, recurrent NEC, cholestasis (if there is prolonged dependence on TPN), severe growth restriction, and neurodevelopmental delay.[97]

## PREVENTIVE OPTIONS

Because of the high mortality and poor outcome after NEC, emphasis is currently focused on finding an effective method of prevention. Advancements in our knowledge have drawn attention on the unique role of the intestinal epithelium. Studies are underway to examine preservation of the intestinal epithelium by nutritional interventions, altering the gut environment by modifying the gut microbial ecology, and pharmacologic modulation of TLR4 signal.

### Glutamine

Glutamine is the most abundant free amino acid in the human body. It is the main source of energy for intestinal tissues and has a protective role in maintaining intestinal mucosal integrity.[98] Oral administration of glutamine in rats protects endotoxemia-induced injury and improves mucosal injury.[99] It may reduce the expression of TLR2 and TLR4 and inhibits apoptosis.[100]

### Arginine

L-Arginine, through the synthesis of NO, regulates vascular perfusion. Low arginine levels in preterm infants may predispose them to NEC. Enteral L-arginine supplementation appears to reduce the incidence of Stage III NEC.[101]

### Zinc

Zinc plays a role in the maintenance of epithelial barrier function and induction of adequate immune response in experimental models of NEC.[102] A recent clinical trial demonstrates the efficacy of oral zinc supplementation in reducing NEC in preterm neonates when administered in high doses.[102]

### Erythropoietin

Erythropoietin is a component of breast milk and was previously shown to preserve intestinal barrier function.[103] Supplementation significantly decreased autophagy and apoptosis by blocking signaling pathways (Akt/mTOR, MAPK/ERK).[103]

### EGF

EGF, abundant in amniotic fluid, is important in the development of the intestinal epithelium, but the protective role was mainly shown in animal models of NEC and only in limited human trials.[104,105] Although further investigations need to be done to determine safety and efficacy in humans, the idea appears very promising.[106]

### Short-chain Fatty Acids

A by-product of bacterial metabolism of carbohydrates has a potent anti-inflammatory effect on the mucosa and helps in its maturation. It holds a great therapeutic potential for NEC, but studies remain limited.[107]

### Probiotics

The most promising and widely studied preventative intervention with the best evidence to date is probiotic supplements. The use of live microbes to alter the gut microbiome by encouraging colonization of favorable bacterial flora has been shown to be very effective in preventing NEC in multiple randomized clinical trials. These microbes promote carbohydrate fermentation and absorption, reducing gut permeability, enhancing mucus production, and releasing antibacterial substances against pathogens.[108] They may decrease the incidence of NEC (59%) and improve mortality (34%) but consistent recommendations for use in VLBW infants are still lacking. Probiotics significantly reduced the incidence of severe NEC (Stage II or more) and all-cause mortality in preterm infants.[109] There was no significant difference for nosocomial sepsis risk between those who received probiotics versus those who did not.[110] Additional studies are required to determine the optimal genus, species, and dosing combination of probiotics.

## CONCLUSION

Most NICUs have embraced standardized feeding protocols, early colostrum administration, better antibiotic stewardship, and as much exclusive human milk nutrition as possible into practice in an effort to decrease risk of NEC and IIP for our smallest babies. In the last decade, substantial progress has been made to further our understanding of the mechanisms associated with the development of NEC. However, its complex and multifactorial pathophysiology have impeded eradication of the disease. Further research is warranted. Future directions should focus on early identification, management planning, and the development of effective preventive strategies.

## REFERENCES

1. Neu J, Walker WA. Necrotizing enterocolitis. N Engl J Med. 2011;364(3):255-64.
2. Thompson AM, Bizzarro MJ. Necrotizing enterocolitis in newborns: pathogenesis, prevention and management. Drugs. 2008;68(9):1227-38.
3. Stoll BJ, Hansen NI, Bell EF, et al.; Eunice Kennedy Shriver National Institute of Child Health and Human Development Neonatal Research Network. Neonatal outcomes of extremely preterm infants from NICHD Neonatal Research Network. Pediatrics. 2010;126(3):443-56.
4. Stoll BJ, Hansen NI, Bell EF, et al.; Eunice Kennedy Shriver National Institute of Child Health and Human Development Neonatal Research Network. Trends in Care Practices, Morbidity, and Mortality of Extremely Preterm Neonates, 1993-2012. JAMA. 2015;314(10):1039-51.
5. Hull MA, Fisher JG, Gutierrez IM, et al. Mortality and management of surgical necrotizing enterocolitis in very low birth weight neonates: a prospective cohort study. J Am Coll Surg. 2014;218(6):1148-55.
6. Wadhawan R, Oh W, Hintz SR, et al. Neurodevelopmental outcomes of extremely low birth weight infants with spontaneous intestinal perforation or surgical necrotizing enterocolitis. J Perinatol. 2014;34(1):64-70.
7. Sharma R, Hudak ML, Tepas JJ 3rd, et al. Impact of gestational age on the clinical presentation and surgical outcome of necrotizing enterocolitis. J Perinatol. 2006;26(6):342-7.
8. Neu J, Mihatsch W. Recent developments in necrotizing enterocolitis. JPEN J Parenter Enteral Nutr. 2012;36(Suppl 1):30S-5S.
9. Hsueh W, Caplan MS, Qu XW, et al. Neonatal necrotizing enterocolitis: clinical considerations and pathogenic concepts. Pediatr Dev Pathol. 2003;6(1):6-23.
10. Bisquera JA, Cooper TR, Berseth CL. Impact of necrotizing enterocolitis on length of stay and hospital charges in very low birth weight infants. Pediatrics. 2002;109(3):423-8.
11. Spencer AU, Kocevich D, McKinney-Barnett M, et al. Pediatric short-bowel syndrome: the cost of comprehensive care. Am J Clin Nutr. 2008;88(6):1552-9.
12. Wagner CL. Amniotic fluid and human milk: a continuum of effect? J Pediatr Gastroenterol Nutr. 2002;34:513-4.
13. Hofmann GE, Abramowicz JS. Epidermal growth factor (EGF) concentrations in amniotic fluid and maternal urine during pregnancy. Acta Obstet Gynecol Scand. 1990;69(3):217-21.
14. Pitkin RM, Reynolds WA. Fetal ingestion and metabolism of amniotic fluid protein. AM J Obstet Gynecol. 1975;123(4):356-63.
15. M Ller HK, Fink LN, Sangild PT, et al. Colostrum and amniotic fluid from different species exhibit similar immunemodulating effects in bacterium-stimulated dendritic cells. J Interferon Cytokine Res. 2011;31(11):813-23.
16. Warner BW, Warner BB. Role of epidermal growth factor in the pathogenesis of neonatal necrotizing enterocolitis. Semin Pediatr Surg. 2005;14(3):175-80.
17. Duh G, Mouri N, Warburton D, et al. EGF regulates early embryonic mouse gut development in chemically defined organ culture. Pediatr Res. 2000;48(6):794-802.
18. Chailler P, Ménard D. Ontogeny of EGF receptors in human gut. Front Biosci. 1999;4:D87-101.
19. Wagner CL, Taylor SN, Johnson D. Host factors in amniotic fluid and breast milk that contribute to gut maturation. Clin Rev Allergy Immunol. 2008;34(2):191-204.
20. Terrin G, Scipione A, De Curtis M. Update in pathogenesis and prospective in treatment of necrotizing enterocolitis. Biomed Res Int. 2014;2014:543765.
21. Calvert R, Pothier P. Migration of fetal intestinal intervillous cells in neonatal mice. Anat Rec 1990;227:199-206.
22. Bombell S, McGuire W. Early trophic feeding for very low birth weight infants. Cochrane Database Sys Rev. 2009;(3):CD000504.
23. Berseth CL. Gut motility and the pathogenesis of necrotizing enterocolitis. Clin Perinatol. 1994;21(2):263-70.
24. Richter JM, Schanbacher BL, Huang H, et al. LPS-binding protein enables intestinal epithelial restitution despite LPS exposure. J Pediatr Gastroenterol Nutr. 2012;54(5):639-44.
25. Leaphart CL, Cavallo J, Gribar SC, et al. A critical role for TLR4 in the pathogenesis of necrotizing enterocolitis by modulating intestinal injury and repair. J Immunol. 2007;179(7):4808-20.
26. Abreu MT. The Ying and Yang of bacterial signaling in necrotizing enterocolitis. Gastroenterology. 2010;138(1):39-43.
27. Fusunyan RD, Nanthakumar NN, Baldeon ME, et al. Evidence for an innate immune response in the immature human intestine: toll-like receptors on fetal enterocytes. Pediatr Res. 2001;49(4):589-93.
28. Neu J, Chen M, Beierle E. Intestinal innate immunity: how does it relate to the pathogenesis of necrotizing enterocolitis. Semin Pediatr Surg. 2005;14(3):137-44.
29. Viscardi RM, Lyon NH, Sun CC, et al. Inflammatory cytokine mRNAs in surgical specimens of necrotizing enterocolitis

and normal newborn intestines. Pediatr Pathol Lab Med. 1997;17(4):547-59.
30. Claud EC, Lu L, Anton PM, et al. Developmentally regulated IkappaB expression in intestinal epithelium and susceptibility to flagellin-induced inflammation. Proc Natl Acad Sci USA. 2004;101(19):7404-8.
31. Israel EJ, Schiffrin EJ, Carter EA, et al. Cortisone strengthens the intestinal mucosal barrier in a rodent necrotizing enterocolitis model. Adv Exp Med Biol. 1991;310:375-80.
32. Carmody RJ, Chen YH. Nuclear factor-kappaB: activation and regulation during toll-like receptor signaling. Cell Mol Immunol. 2007;4(1):31-41.
33. Frost BL, Jilling T, Caplan MS. The importance of pro-inflammatory signaling in neonatal necrotizing enterocolitis. Semin Pathol. 2008;32(2):100-6.
34. Sodhi CP, Neal MD, Siggers R, et al. Intestinal epithelial Toll-like receptor 4 regulates goblet cell development and is required for necrotizing enterocolitis in mice. Gastroenterology. 2012;143(3):708-18.e5.
35. Claud EC, Walker WA. Hypothesis: inappropriate colonization of the premature intestine can cause necrotizing enterocolitis. FASEB J. 2001;15(8):1398-403.
36. Wang Y, Hoenig JD, Malin KJ, et al. 16S rRNA gene-based analysis of fecal microbiota from preterm infants with and without necrotizing enterocolitis. ISME J. 2009;3(8):944-54.
37. Lin PW, Stoll BJ. Necrotizing enterocolitis. Lancet. 2006;368(9543):1271-83.
38. Mai V, Young CM, Ukhanova M, et al. Fecal microbiota in premature infants prior to necrotizing enterocolitis. PLoS One. 2011;6(6):e20647.
39. DiGiulio DB, Gervasi MT, Romero R, et al. Microbial invasion of the amniotic cavity in pregnancies with small-for-gestational-age fetuses. J Perinat Med. 2010;38(5):495-502.
40. Nanthakumar NN, Fusunyan RD, Sanderson I, et al. Inflammation in the developing human intestine: a possible pathophysiologic contribution to necrotizing enterocolitis. Proc Natl Acad Sci USA. 2000;97(11):6043-8.
41. Medzhitov R, Schneider DS, Soares MP. Disease tolerance as a defense strategy. Science. 2012;335(6071):936-41.
42. Neu J, Rushing J. Cesarean versus vaginal delivery: long-term infant outcomes and hygiene hypothesis. Clin Perinatol. 2011;38(2):321-33.
43. Cotton CM, Taylor S, Stoll B, et al. Prolonged duration of initial empirical antibiotic treatment is associated with increased rates of necrotizing enterocolitis and death for extremely low birth weight infants. Pediatrics. 2009;123(1):58-66.
44. Canani RB, Terrin G. Gastric acidity inhibitors and the risk of intestinal infections. Curr Opin Gastroenterol. 2010;26(1):31-5.
45. Thymann T, Møller HK, Stoll B, et al. Carbohydrate maldigestion induces necrotizing enterocolitis in preterm pigs. Am J Physiol Gastrointest Liver Physiol. 2009;297(6):G1115-25.
46. Abdelhamid AE, Chuang SL, Hayes P, et al. Evolution of in vitro cow's milk protein-specific inflammatory and regulatory cytokines responses in preterm infants with necrotising enterocolitis. J Pediatr Gastroenterol Nutr. 2013;56(1):5-11.
47. Martin CR, Walker WA. Intestinal immune defenses and the inflammatory response in necrotizing enterocolitis. Semin Fetal Neonatal Med. 2006;11:369-77.
48. Sullivan S, Schanler RJ, Kim JH, et al. An exclusively human milk-based diet is associated with a lower rate of necrotizing enterocolitis than a diet of human milk and bovine milk-based products. J Pediatr. 2010;156(4):562-7.e1
49. Lucas A, Cole TJ. Breast milk and neonatal necrotising enterocolitis. Lancet. 1990;336(8730):1519-23.
50. Ward RE, Niñonuevo M, Mills DA, et al. In vitro fermentation of breast milk oligosaccharides by Bifidobacterium infantis and Lactobacillus gasseri. Appl Environ Microbiol. 2006;2(6):4497-9.
51. Section on Breastfeeding. Breastfeeding and the use of human milk. Pediatrics. 2012;129(3):e827-41.
52. Paul DA, Mackley A, Novitsky A, et al. Increased odds of necrotizing enterocolitis after transfusion of red blood cells in premature infants. Pediatrics. 2011;127(4):635-41.
53. Singh R, Visintainer PF, Frantz ID 3rd, et al. Association of necrotizing enterocolitis with anemia and packed red blood cell transfusions in preterm infants. J Perinatol. 2011;31(3):176-82.
54. dos Santos AM, Guinsburg R, de Almeida MF, et al.; Brazilian Network of Neonatal Research. Red blood cell transfusions are independently associated with intra-hospital mortality in very low birth weight preterm infants. J Pediatr. 2011;159(3):371-6.e1-3.
55. El-Dib M, Narang S, Lee E, et al. Red blood cell transfusion, feeding and necrotizing enterocolitis in preterm infants. J Perinatol. 2011;31(3):183-7.
56. Sampath V, Le M, Lane L, et al. The NGKB1 (g.-24519delATTG) variant is associated with necrotizing enterocolitis (NEC) in premature infants. J Surg Res. 2011;169(1):e51-7.
57. Neish AS, Gewirtz AT, Zeng H, et al. Prokaryotic regulation of epithelial responses by inhibition of IkappaB-alpha ubiquitination. Science. 2000;289(5484):1560-3.
58. Lin PW, Nasr TR, Beradinelli AJ, et al. The probiotic Lactobacillus GG may augment intestinal host defense by regulating apoptosis and promoting cytoprotective responses in developing murine gut. Pediatr Res. 2008;64(5):511-6.
59. Gribar SC, Sodhi CP, Richardson WM, et al. Reciprocal expression and signaling of TLR4 and TLR9 in the pathogenesis and treatment of necrotizing enterocolitis. J Immunol. 2009;182(1):636-46.
60. Jilling T, Simon D, Lu J, et al. The roles of bacteria and TLR4 in rat and murine models of necrotizing enterocolitis. J Immunol. 2006;177(5):3273-82.
61. Rhee SH. Basic and translational understandings of microbial recognition by toll-like receptors in the intestine. J Neurogastroenterol Motil. 2011;17(1):28-34.
62. Benveniste J, Chignard M, Le Couedic JP, et al. Biosynthesis of platelet-activating factor (PAF-ACETHER). II. Involvement of phospholipase A2 in the formation of PAF-ACETHER and lyso-PAF-ACETHER from rabbit platelets. Thromb Res. 2003;25(5):375-85.
63. Caplan MS, Lickerman M, Adler, et al. The role of recombinant platelet-activating factor acetylhydrolase in neonatal rat model of necrotizing enterocolitis. Pediatr Res. 1997;42(6):779-83.
64. Caplan M, Hsueh W, Kelly A, et al. Serum PAF acetylhydrolase increases during neonatal malnutrition. Prostaglandins. 1990;39(6):705-14.
65. Wang H, Tan X, Chang H, et al. Regulation of platelet-activating factor receptor gene expression in vivo by endotoxin, platelet-activating factor and endogenous tumour necrosis factor. Biochem J. 1997;322(Pt 2):603-8.

66. Sun XM, Hsueh W. Bowel necrosis induced by tumor necrosis factor in rats is mediated by platelet-activating factor. J Clin Invest. 1998;81(5):1328-31.
67. Morecroft JA, Spitz L, Hamilton PA, et al. Plasma cytokine levels in necrotizing enterocolitis. Acta Paediatr Suppl. 1994;396:18-20.
68. Edelson MB, Bagwell CE, Rozycki HJ. Circulating pro- and counterinflammatory cytokine levels and severity in necrotizing enterocolitis. Pediatrics. 1999;103(4 Pt 1):766-71.
69. Emami CN, Chokshi N, Wang J, et al. Role of interleukin-10 in the pathogenesis of necrotizing enterocolitis. Am J Surg. 2012;203(4):428-35.
70. Halpern MD, Holubec H, Dominguez JA, et al. Up-regulation of IL-18 and IL-12 in the ileum of neonatal rats with necrotizing enterocolitis. Pediatr Res. 2002;51(6):733-9.
71. Baregamian N, Song J, Bailey CE, et al. Tumor necrosis factor-alpha and apoptosis signal-regulating kinase 1 control reactive oxygen species release, mitochondrial autophagy, and c-Jun N-terminal kinase/p38 phosphorylation during necrotizing enterocolitis. Oxid Med Cell Longev. 2009;2(5):297-306.
72. Akisu M, Baka M, Yalaz M, et al. Supplementation with Saccharomyces boulardii ameliorates hypoxia/reoxygenation-induced necrotizing enterocolitis in young mice. Eur J Pediatr Surg. 2003;13(5):319-23.
73. Nadler EP, Dickinson E, Knisely A, et al. Expression of inducible nitric oxide synthase and interleukin-12 in experimental necrotizing enterocolitis. J Surg Res. 2000;92(1):71-7.
74. Anand RJ, Dai S, Ripel C, et al. Activated macrophages inhibit enterocyte gap junctions via the release of nitric oxide. Am J Physiol Gastrointest Liver Physiol. 2008;294(1):G109-19.
75. Potoka DA, Upperman JS, Zhang XR, et al. Peroxynitrite inhibits enterocyte proliferation and modulates Src kinase activity in vitro. Am J Physiol Gastrointest Liver Physiol. 2003;285(5):G861-9.
76. Chen Y, Stanford A, Simmons RL, et al. Nitric oxide protects thymocytes from gamma-irradiation-induced apoptosis in correlation with inhibition of p53 upregulation and mitochondrial damage. Cell Immunol. 2001;214(1):72-80.
77. Baregamian N, Song J, Papaconstantinou J, et al. Intestinal mitochondrial apoptotic signaling is activated during oxidative stress. Pediatr Surg Int. 2011;27(8):871-7.
78. Parks DA, Bulkley GB, Granger DN, et al. Ischemic injury in the cat small intestine: role of superoxide radicals. Gastroenterology. 1982;82(1):9-15.
79. Qu XW, Rozenfeld RA, Huang W, et al. The role of xanthine oxidase in platelet activating factor induced intestinal injury in the rat. Gut. 1999;44(2):203-11.
80. Polin RA, Pollack PF, Barlow B, et al. Necrotizing enterocolitis in term infants. J Pediatr. 1976;89(3):460-2.
81. Buangtrakool R, Laohapensang M, Sathornkich C, et al. Necrotizing enterocolitis: a comparison between full-term and preterm neonates. J Med Assoc Thai. 2001;84(3):323-31.
82. McElhinney DB, Hendrick HL, Bush DM, et al. Necrotizing enterocolitis in neonates with congenital heart disease: risk factors and outcomes. Pediatrics. 2000;106(5):1080-7.
83. Kliegman RM, Hack M, Jones P, et al. Epidemiological study of necrotizing enterocolitis among low-birth-weight infants. Absence of identifiable risk factors. J Pediatr. 1982;100(3):440-4.
84. Yee WH, Soraisham AS, Shah VS, et al. Incidence and timing of presentation of necrotizing enterocolitis in preterm infants. Pediatrics. 2012;129(2):e298-304.
85. Sharma R, Hudak ML, Tepas JJ 3rd, et al. Prenatal or postnatal indomethacin exposure and neonatal gut injury associated with isolated intestinal perforation and necrotizing enterocolitis. J Perinatol. 2010;30(12):786-93.
86. Bell MJ, Ternberg JL, Feigin RD, et al. Neonatal necrotizing enterocolitis: therapeutic decisions based upon clinical staging. Ann Surg. 1978;187(1):1-7.
87. Nowicki PT, Nankervis CA. The role of the circulation in the pathogenesis of necrotizing enterocolitis. Clin Perinatol. 1994;21(2):219-34.
88. Ballance WA, Dahms BB, Shenker N, et al. Pathology of neonatal necrotizing enterocolitis: a ten-year experience. J Pediatr. 1990;117(1 Pt 2):S6-13.
89. Gould SJ. The pathology of necrotizing enterocolitis. Semin Neonatol. 1994;4:239-44.
90. Gordon PV, Attridge JT. Understanding clinical literature relevant to spontaneous intestinal perforations. Am J Perinatol. 2009;26(4):309-16.
91. Stark AR, Carlo WA, Tyson JE, et al. Adverse effects of early dexamethasone treatment in extremely-low-birth-weight infants. National Institute of Child Health and Human Development Neonatal Research Network. N Engl J Med. 2001;344(2):95-101.
92. Watterberg KL, Gerdes JS, Cole CH, et al. Prophylaxis of early adrenal insufficiency to prevent bronchopulmonary dysplasia: a multicenter trial. Pediatrics. 2004;114(6):1649-57.
93. Rees CM, Eaton S, Kiely EM, et al. Peritoneal drainage or laparotomy for neonatal bowel perforation? A randomized controlled trial. Ann Surg. 2008;248(1):44-51.
94. Rees CM, Eaton S, Khoo AK, et al. Peritoneal drainage does not stabilize extremely low birth weight infants with perforated bowel: data from the NET Trial. J Pediatr Surg. 2010;45(2):324-9.
95. Sola JE, Tepas JJ 3rd, Koniaris LG. Peritoneal drainage versus laparotomy for necrotizing enterocolitis and intestinal perforation: a meta-analysis. J Surg Res. 2010;161(1):95-100.
96. Blakey ML, Tyson JE, Lally KP, et al. Laparotomy versus peritoneal drainage for necrotizing enterocolitis or isolated intestinal perforation in extremely low birth weight infants: outcomes through 18 months adjusted age. Pediatrics. 2006;117(4):e680-7.
97. Ricketts RR, Jerles ML. Neonatal necrotizing enterocolitis: experience with 100 consecutive surgical patients. World J Surg. 1990;14(5):600-5.
98. Novak F, Heyland DK, Avenell A, et al. Glutamine supplementation in serious illness: a systemic review of the evidence. Crit Care Med. 2002;30(9):2022-9.
99. Sukhotnik I, Agam M, Shamir R, et al. Oral glutamine prevents gut mucosal injury and improves mucosal recovery following lipopolysaccharide endotoxemia in a rat. J Surg Res. 2007;143(2):379-84.
100. Zhou W, Li W, Zheng XH, et al. Glutamine downregulates TLR-2 aNd TLR-4 expression and protects intestinal tract in preterm neonatal rats with necrotizing enterocolitis. J Pediatr Surg. 2014;49(7):1057-63.
101. Polycarpou E, Zachaki S, Tsolia M, et al. Enteral L-arginine supplementation for prevention of necrotizing enterocolitis

101. in very low birth weight neonates: a double-blind randomized pilot study of efficacy and safety. JPEN J Parenter Enteral Nutr. 2013;37(5):617-22.
102. Terrin R, Berni Canani R, Passariello A, et al. Zinc supplementation reduces morbidty and mortality in very low birth-weight preterm neonates: a hospital-based randomized, placebo-controlled trial in an industrialized country. Am J Clin Nutr. 2013;98(6):1468-74.
103. Yu Y, Shiou SR, Guo Y, et al. Erythropoietin protects epithelial cells from excessive autophagy and apoptosis in experimental neonatal necrotizing enterocolitis. PloS One. 2013;8(7):e69620.
104. Dvorak B, Halpern MD, Holubec H, et al. Epidermal growth factor reduces the development of necrotizing enterocolitis in a neonatal rat model. Am J Physiol Gastrointest Liver Physiol. 2002;282(1):G156-64.
105. Feng J, El-Assal ON, Besner GE. Heparin-binding epidermal growth factor-like growth factor reduces intestinal apoptosis in neonatal rats with necrotizing enterocolitis. J Pediatr Surg. 2006;41(4):742-7.
106. Sullivan PB, Lewindon PJ, Cheng C, et al. Intestinal mucosa remodeling by recombinant human epidermal growth factor (1-48) in neonates with severe necrotizing enterocolitis. J Pediatr Surg. 2007;42:462-9.
107. Canani RB, Costanzo MD, Leone L, et al. Epigenetic mechanisms elicited by nutrition in early life. Nutr Res Rev. 2011;24(2):198-205.
108. Ng SC, Hart AL, Kamm MA, et al. Mechanisms of action of probiotics: recent advances. Inflamm Bowel Dis. 2009;15(2):300-10.
109. Mihatsch WA. What is the power of evidence recommending routine probiotics for necrotizing enterocolitis prevention in preterm infants? Curr Opin Clin Nutr Metab Care. 2011;14(3):302-6.
110. Al Faleh K, Anabrees J. Probiotics for prevention of necrotizing enterocolitis in preterm infants. Cochrane Database Syst Rev. 2014;(4):CD005496.

# SECTION 9

# Pain and Addiction

- Newborn Pain: Recognition and Management
  *Matthew JR Nudelman*
- Introduction to Addiction Medicine
  *Balaji Govindaswami*

CHAPTER

# Newborn Pain: Recognition and Management

*Matthew JR Nudelman*

## ABSTRACT

Newborns are often exposed to painful procedures during hospital stay. Teaching and providing comprehensive pain assessment and management remains challenging. Under- and overtreatment of pain have deleterious short- and long-term physiological, behavioral, and cognitive effects. Site-specific neonatal pain control programs should focus on—(1) educating care providers and parents about neonatal pain, (2) performing routine pain assessments, (3) minimizing painful procedures, and (4) applying optimal analgesic methodologies. Various physiological, biochemical, and behavioral cues can be used to identify, locate, and assess pain severity. Pain assessment tools are strongly recommended and should be used when clinically appropriate. Nonpharmacological analgesic modalities can successfully reduce pain and should be utilized whenever possible. Local, topical, and systemic analgesic pharmacotherapies are frequently utilized but providers must consider their adverse effects.

## INTRODUCTION

Newborns are often exposed to painful procedures during hospital stay, and frequently if admitted to the neonatal intensive care unit (NICU). Historically, it was thought that newborns did not perceive pain to the same extent as older children and thus did not need pain assessment nor the use of pain control. Current physiological and behavioral evidence shows newborns and even fetuses as early as 25 weeks of gestational age (GA) perceive and respond to painful stimuli.[1-9] Preterm infants have unmyelinated nociceptive inhibitory pathways and a paucity of inhibitory neurotransmitters, which make them more sensitive to pain compared to mature infants.[10-16]

Preterm infants are more likely to be exposed to painful stimuli as they typically require additional procedures and extended hospital stay.[17-20] Teaching and providing comprehensive pain assessment and management continues to be challenging, despite the development and availability of recommendations and guidelines from leading pain experts/panels.[18-24]

## PAIN NEGLECT

Reasons for neglect of newborn pain are often related to a provider's lack of knowledge of—(1) an infant's ability to perceive pain, (2) which clinical practices can cause pain, (3) painless routes and methods of analgesia, and (4) reluctance to use analgesics due to fear of side effects, inclusive of opioid dependency.[9] Providers are often unaware of the range of clinical practices, which elicit painful stimuli;[9] even noninvasive procedures such as tape removal and physical therapy maneuvering cause pain **(Table 1)**. Common procedures seen in the NICU, which elicit pain, have been described along with recommended treatment modalities to mitigate the infant's pain.[6,9]

Undertreatment of pain has deleterious short- and long-term physiological, behavioral, and cognitive effects including altered pain processing, attention deficit disorder, impaired visual-perceptual ability or visual-

| TABLE 1: Common pain-inducing procedures. | |
|---|---|
| Diagnostic | Interventional |
| • Arterial puncture | • Adhesive removal |
| • Bladder catheterization | • Any surgical procedure |
| • Bronchoscopy | • Central venous line insertion/removal |
| • Endoscopy | • Chest physiotherapy |
| • Heel/finger stick | • Chest tube insertion/removal |
| • Heel lancing | • Circumcision |
| • Lumbar puncture | • Dressing change |
| • Retinopathy of prematurity eye examination | • Endotracheal intubation/extubation/suction |
| • Suprapubic bladder tap | • Gavage tube |
| • Venipuncture | • Intubation/extubation |
| | • Mechanical ventilation |
| | • Naso- and orogastric tube insertion/removal |
| | • Percutaneous arterial/venous catheter insertion |
| | • Peripheral arterial or venous cutdown |
| | • Postural drainage |
| | • Subcutaneous or intramuscular injection |
| | • Sutures |
| | • Umbilical catheter insertion |

| TABLE 2: Newborn's response to pain. | | |
|---|---|---|
| | Increased | Decreased |
| Physiological/autonomic changes | • Respiratory rate<br>• Heart rate<br>• Blood pressure<br>• Palmar sweating<br>• Mean airway pressure<br>• Muscle tone<br>• Intracranial pressure<br>• Flushing<br>• Pallor<br>• Mydriasis | • Oxygen saturation<br>• Vagal tone<br>• Peripheral blood flow |
| Biochemical changes | • Corticosteroids<br>• Epinephrine<br>• Norepinephrine<br>• Glucagon<br>• Growth hormone<br>• Renin<br>• Aldosterone<br>• Antidiuretic hormone | • Insulin<br>• Prolactin<br>• Immune response |
| Behavioral changes | • Frowning/Grimacing<br>• Nasal flaring<br>• Tongue cupping<br>• Chin quivering<br>• Finger clenching<br>• Back arching<br>• Head banging | |

motor integration,[17-19] and poor executive function,[20,21] as well as abnormal neurodevelopment, somatosensory, and stress response systems.[10,18,25-36] Overtreating pain affects growth and development adversely, prolonging mechanical ventilation, or delaying feeding.[26,27]

## NEONATAL PAIN CONTROL PROGRAMS

Several leading societies recommend the establishment of site-specific neonatal pain control programs. These programs should focus on—(1) educating care providers and parents about neonatal pain, (2) performing routine pain assessments, (3) minimizing painful procedures, and (4) applying optimal analgesic methodologies.[21,23,37]

## ASSESSMENT

The American Academy of Pediatrics (AAP) recommends validated pain assessment tools can be used before, during, and after painful procedures in order to monitor effectiveness of the pain relief intervention.[21] Unlike older children and adults, newborns are unable to self-report their pain. Instead, providers must rely on various physiological, biochemical, and behavioral cues to best identify, locate, and assess pain severity **(Table 2)**.[9,18,38] Behavioral cues are commonly used to assess pain and they are subjective with high inter-rater variability leading to inconsistent pain management.[22,39-41] Surrogate markers are best used in combination to improve accurate pain assessment.[17] Emerging modalities for pain assessment include near-infrared spectroscopy, amplitude-integrated electroencephalography, functional MRI, skin conductance, and heart rate variability assessment.[41,42]

## Physiologic Parameters

### Autonomic Markers

Autonomic markers for pain include an increase in heart rate, respiratory rate, blood pressure, intracranial pressure, muscle tone, and palmar sweating; or a decrease in transcutaneous oxygen saturation, vagal tone, and peripheral blood flow. Pain is also associated with mydriasis, nausea, vomiting, pallor, gagging, hiccoughing, diaphoresis, and dilated pupils.[43-50]

### Biochemical Markers

Biochemical markers for pain include increased catecholamines, glucagon, cortisol, renin, aldosterone, and antidiuretic hormone; and decreased prolactin, insulin, and immune responses.[9,49,51,52]

## Behavioral Responses

### Crying

Crying commonly occurs with pain and has a high sensitivity relative to other pain surrogates.[44,53-56] The duration, frequency, amplitude, and pitch of an infant's cry can be used to assess whether the infant is crying due to pain or other stimuli such as hunger or fear.[57-60] Crying patterns is used to assess pain intensity.[61] Infants with low-energy reserves such as preterm, low-birth weight, sick, or intubated infants may silently present with painful faces, also known as a "silent cry."[62]

### Facial Expressions

Facial pain expressions include grimace, agitation, squeezed eyes, pursed lips, open mouth, cupped tongue, quivering chin, furrowed, and bulged brows[63,64] and are some of the most reliable indicators of pain.[43,65-67]

### Hand and Body Movements

Body movements associated with pain include fisting, splayed fingers, muscle tensing, back arching, and squirming of the legs and arms.[68] Infants with low-energy reserves may present with flaccidity.[45]

### Muscle Tone

Infants display increased muscle tone during acute pain, which may be diminished with exhaustion.

### Sleep Patterns

Pain is associated with immature sleep–wake cycling,[45,46] longer durations of nonrapid eye movement sleep,[42] as well as increased wakefulness[43] and agitation.[44,69-73]

## Emerging Modalities

Neurophysiological and imaging techniques that measure brain activity are being used to validate pain scales.[39,74] Skin conductance, near-infrared spectroscopy, electroencephalography, and MRI are emerging technologies used to assess pain.[25] Many of these modalities are not yet clinically useful because either they require specialized equipment unavailable at the bedside or currently they do not yield real-time results.[25]

## Scales

Neither single parameter nor any combination of behavioral and physiological parameters has perfect reliability with regard to objective pain assessment for all clinical scenarios and gestational ages.[9,17,75] Neurologically compromised or preterm infants may have limited ability to express the same behavioral or physiological patterns as healthy term infants; hence, the need for several different pain scales.[11,36,76-78] The most commonly used and rigorously tested pain scales are Neonatal Facial Coding System, Premature Infant Pain Profile (PIPP), Neonatal Pain and Sedation Scale, Behavioral Infant Pain Profile, and Douleur Aiguë du Nouveau-né.[36]

Despite the challenges of reliability, pain assessment tools are strongly recommended by the AAP and international organizations.[6,21,79] Several articles and reviews provide detailed descriptions of the different pain scales and the specific clinical circumstances in which particular pain scales should be utilized.[36,80] A summary of different pain scales is provided in **Table 3**.

Pain scales are severely limited by inter-rater variability and subjectivity of assessment.[22,39,81,82] As the most likely group to undergo painful procedures, premature infants less consistently exhibit the responses to pain stated by these assessment tools.[11,62,73,83] No methods for assessment of persistent or prolonged pain in neonates (for major surgery, osteomyelitis, and necrotizing enterocolitis) have been developed or validated.[29,42,84]

## PAIN MANAGEMENT

Pain management varies, ranging from absence of pain assessment to highly standardized protocols for nonpharmacological relief to prescribed drug(s) including regimen, dose, and routes of administration.[85,86]

### Pain Prevention and Harm Reduction

Preventing pain without compromising newborn care should always be a priority.[25,87] Bedside disruptions and painful interventions should be minimized, especially during sleep cycles, by anticipating and coordinating medical procedures and other routine clinical care. When possible, an infant should be given adequate time and rest to recover from a painful event.[88] The necessity of all reoccurring laboratories and procedures should be reassessed daily. Noninvasive diagnostic and therapeutic modalities are preferred whenever available, e.g., transcutaneous monitors rather than heelsticks, or use of transdermal patches instead of invasive analgesia.[88] Environmental controls should be optimized to prevent overstimulation from light and noise, as well as for ensuring ideal temperature. A peripheral or central line should be considered for infants who receive several heelsticks per day. Venous punctures have been shown to be less painful than heelsticks, thus venous punctures should be performed when possible.[88] Venous puncture limits should be set (e.g., two attempts per provider).[88]

The AAP recommends that each institution should "have written guidelines, based on existing and emerging

**TABLE 3:** Different newborn pain scales.

| Unidimensional pain scales | Multidimensional pain scales |
|---|---|
| *Acute procedural pain* | *Acute/procedural pain* |
|    MAX—Maximally discriminative facial coding system |    NIPS—Neonatal infant pain score |
|    NFCS—Neonatal facial coding system |    NPAT—Neonatal pain assessment tool |
|    IBCS—Infant body coding system |    PIPP—Premature infant pain profile |
|    DAN—Douleur aigue du Nouvea-ne |    PIPPR—Premature infant pain profile revised |
|    BIIP—Behavioral indicator of infant pain |    DSVNI—Distress scales for ventilated newborn infants |
| *Postoperative pain* |    EVENDOL—Evaluation enfant douleur |
|    CCS—Clinical scoring system |    SUN—Scale for use in newborns |
|    LIDS—Liverpool infant distress scale |    PAIN—Pain assessment in neonates |
|    FLACC—Face, legs, activity, cry, consolability |    BPSN—Bernese pain scale for neonates |
|    UWCH—University of Wisconsin children's hospital pain scale |    FANS—Faceless acute neonatal pain scale |
|    CHIPPS—Children's and infants postoperative pain scale |    COVERS—Neonatal pain scale |
| *Prolonged pain* |    PASPI—Pain assessment scale for preterm infants |
|    BPS—Behavioral pain score | *Postoperative pain* |
|    EDIN—Echelle douleur inconfort nouveau-ne |    COMFORT |
|    COMFORTneo |    PAT—Pain assessment tool |
| |    CRIES—Crying, requires oxygen saturation, increased vital signs, expression, sleeplessness |
| |    MIPS—Modified infant pain scale |
| |    MAPS—Multidimensional assessment pain scale |
| | *Prolonged/ongoing pain* |
| |    N - PASS—Neonatal pain, agitation, and sedation scale |

evidence, for a stepwise pain prevention and treatment plan, which includes judicious use of procedures, routine assessment of pain, use of both pharmacologic and nonpharmacologic therapies for the prevention of pain associated with routine minor procedures, and effective medications to minimize pain associated with surgery and other major procedures."[36]

## Nonpharmacological Analgesia

Nonpharmacological analgesia can successfully reduce pain and should be used whenever possible;[36] these therapies are easily applied, noninvasive, do not require intensive monitoring, and have limited to no side effects. Greater analgesic efficacy occurs when these modalities are used as an adjunct therapy with other nonpharmacological and pharmacological interventions.[37] Despite their success and recommended use, nonpharmacological modalities continue to be underutilized.[89]

### Breastfeeding

Breastfeeding with effective latch and sustained sucking and swallowing for 5 minutes prior and during heel lancing, intramuscular injections, or venipuncture reduces pain.[90,91] In infants receiving heelsticks, breastfeeding while receiving skin-to-skin (STS) is more effective in pain reduction.[92] Systematic reviews show breastfeeding reduces pain responses during heel lance and venipuncture with similar efficacy as oral sucrose or glucose solutions in term neonates.[91,93]

### Non-nutritive Suck

Offering a pacifier to encourage non-nutritive suck (NNS) provides acute procedural pain relief in term and preterm infants, although the mechanism of action is not fully understood.[94] NNS has greater efficacy when used with sucrose.[95]

### Skin-to-Skin

The STS is safe and effective in reducing pain symptoms in term and preterm neonates with and without sweetener administration.[96] STS is recommended 10–15 minutes prior to the pain event.[90,96] During heelsticks in preterm infants, STS is comparable to facilitated tucking with regard to decreasing crying time, improving pain scores, and decreasing stress.[96,97] While the mechanism of action is not fully understood, it may be related to better infant self-regulation by listening to maternal heartbeat.[98,99]

### Facilitated Tucking

In this position, the provider or parent gently brings the infant's legs and arms to the middle of their body in a flexed, fetal-position tuck. Facilitated tucking provides effective procedural pain relief during endotracheal suctioning and heelsticks, although it may not be as effective as oral sucrose during repeated painful interventions.[100,101]

### Swaddling

The provider or parent uses a thin blanket or sheet to securely wrap the infant in a flexed fetal position. Swaddling in preterm infants has also been shown to provide procedural pain relief.[94]

### Rocking

The motion of rocking an infant causes cochlear-vestibular stimulation and has been shown to be comforting when performed prior to heelstick.[102]

### Sucrose/Glucose

Oral sucrose and glucose decrease pain in term and preterm infants during mild and moderately painful procedures including heelsticks, heel lances, venipuncture, retinopathy of prematurity screening, and oral gastric tube insertion.[36,62,95,101,103-105] Sweeteners provide improved pain relief when given before and after a procedure rather than in a single prior dose.[38] Pain relief is improved when used in combination with other analgesic interventions including NNS and swaddling.[106-109] Despite extensive use, the exact mechanism of action, appropriate dosage, timing, and safety of long-term oral sucrose/glucose use, is not yet fully understood and as such, it should be prescribed and regularly monitored similar to other analgesic pharmacotherapies.[36,106,110-117] Sucrose and glucose are typically ineffective after 3 months of age.[18]

### Music Therapy

There is little evidence supporting the use of music therapy for analgesic purposes. If music therapy is used, it should be limited to 15 minutes per intervention to prevent overstimulation.[118,119]

### Massage Therapy

Two-minute massage therapy has been shown to be effective prior to heelsticks.[120-122] It is believed that massage increases vagal activity and subsequently lowers cortisol and epinephrine levels.[123]

### Multisensorial Stimulation

Multisensorial combinational uses of tactile, auditory, or visual stimulation have shown to be effective in reducing pain.[124-126] Such combinations include the following:
- Sweeteners and gentle facial massage while speaking softly[125,127]
- Sweeteners and facilitated tucking[101]
- Sweeteners and breastfeeding[128]
- Sweeteners and STS.[129]

## Pharmacological Analgesia

### Local Analgesics

Local anesthetics work either by topical application or injection and can be used for procedural pain relief.

*Lidocaine:* Lidocaine works by blocking sodium channels and inhibiting axonal transmission. Lidocaine is frequently used for circumcision and has been shown to be more effective than Eutectic Mixture of Local Anesthetic (EMLA).[130,131]

*Epinephrine:* Epinephrine causes vasoconstriction and can be used in combination with other local anesthetics to increase their duration of action. There has been concern that the use of epinephrine/adrenaline in parts of body supplied by end arteries (i.e., penis, digits, and ears) can lead to necrosis. However, more contemporary studies in adults suggest that adrenaline can be used in conjunction with other local analgesics.[132] This has not yet been studied in neonates.

### Topical Analgesics

Topical analgesics have been shown to be effective for venous cannulation, lumbar puncture, venipuncture, percutaneous central venous catheter insertion, and peripheral arterial puncture.[25,133-137] Topical analgesics have not been shown to decrease pain for heelsticks.[13,138] Side effects include local irritation, allergic reactions, and methemoglobinemia especially in preterm infants.[137,139-142] Local anesthetics should not be used on wounds, broken skin, the ears, nose, eyes, mouth, the genitalia, or anus.[88]

*Eutectic mixture of local anesthetic:* EMLA, a mixture of lidocaine (2.5%) and prilocaine (2.5%), has been shown to be effective during circumcision and venipuncture.[37,88,143] EMLA analgesic duration lasts a few minutes and should be applied an hour before starting the painful intervention.[9]

*Tetracaine gel (also known as ametop gel):* Tetracaine gel should be applied half an hour prior to, but cleaned off before beginning, the painful intervention. The analgesic duration lasts several hours. Tetracaine gel causes vasodilation, which may cause transient redness of the skin.[88]

### Systemic Analgesics

*Opioids:* Opioids provide the most potent analgesic effect and are frequently used to alleviate moderate and severe pain. Morphine and fentanyl are the most commonly used opioids for neonatal analgesia.[25] Other opioids include sufentanil, alfentanil, remifentanil, and tramadol. Opioid dosing requires careful attention, as newborn hepatorenal clearance and pharmacokinetics vary greatly between patients, especially sick or preterm infants.[144-146] Opioids should be used with extreme caution, as they have several short- and long-term side effects including hypotension, bradycardia, severe intraventricular hemorrhage (IVH), impaired gut motility, and worse neurodevelopmental outcomes.[37,147] Respiratory depression is a serious side effect and can be reversed using naloxone:[148]

- *Morphine*: Morphine is the most commonly used opioid for neonatal analgesia. Morphine is frequently used to alleviate moderate-to-severe pain; however, its use for acute procedural events and in ventilated neonates is controversial.[149-151] Morphine is hepatically metabolized into morphine-6-glucuronide (M6G), which has even higher analgesic and respiratory depressant effects than morphine. M6G is eliminated by the kidneys, so great care should be taken, if an infant is renally impaired.
- *Fentanyl*: Fentanyl is a frequently used rapid-acting opioid. Compared to morphine, it causes less sedation, reduced gastrointestinal motility impairment, less urinary retention, and fewer incidents of hypotension, but can result in greater tolerance, more serious withdrawal symptoms, and increased chest wall rigidity and laryngospasm.[152-155] Slow administration of fentanyl can help to prevent the occurrence of side effects.[37] Many of fentanyl's side effects, including respiratory depression, can be rapidly reversed with naloxone.[37] Chest wall rigidity may be reversed using rocuronium, a skeletal muscle relaxant.[37] Fentanyl is less commonly used for tracheal intubation, central line placement, incision and drainage, and postoperative procedural pain. Routine use in ventilated preterm infants is controversial.[156] Fentanyl can be effectively administered intravenously. Inhaled fentanyl has been used in newborn palliative care.[157]
- *Remifentanil*: Remifentanil is a very short-acting opioid that lasts <15 minutes and has twice the analgesic effect of fentanyl.[25] It is metabolized by plasma esterases rather than by the liver and kidneys[158] and has been used during brief painful procedures such as line placement and tracheal intubation.[159,160] Remifentanil has also been used in operating room studies and may have future applications.[161-163]
- *Alfentanil*: Alfentanil is another short-acting (20-30 minutes) opioid that is more potent than morphine and commonly used during brief painful procedures such as tracheal intubation.[164,165] More studies are needed to better understand its safety and efficacy.[166]

*Acetaminophen*: Acetaminophen is one of the most studied and frequently utilized systemic analgesics. It can be safely used during mild-to-moderately painful procedures including heelsticks, fingersticks, adhesive removal, dressing changes, immunizations, circumcisions, venipuncture, arterial puncture, and wound treatment.[38,136,137,167-169] Acetaminophen works by inhibiting prostaglandin COX-2 formation and has less severe side effects compared to opioids.[170,171] For moderate-to-severe pain, such as postsurgical pain, acetaminophen is often used as an adjunct therapy with opioids, which can help to reduce the need for higher opioid dosages.[29,172,173] Acetaminophen can cause liver and renal toxicity, although those occur less frequently in newborns compared to older children and adults.[167,169,174-177] Acetaminophen can be administered orally, rectally, or intravenously.[25]

*Nonsteroidal anti-inflammatory drugs (NSAIDs):* NSAIDs have anti-inflammatory, antipyretic, and analgesic properties that work by inhibiting cyclooxygenase enzymes (COX-1 and COX-2). NSAIDs can be used to treat minor pain or can be effective as an adjunct therapy during moderately painful procedures in order to reduce the need for higher dosing of opioids.[9] Side effects include renal dysfunction, pulmonary hypertension, and platelet dysfunction.[25,178]

*Sedatives:*

- *Midazolam*: Midazolam is one of the most utilized sedatives and is often used for painful procedures and during mechanical ventilation.[179] Midazolam is a short-acting benzodiazepine that is metabolized by the liver, which may potentially inhibit bilirubin metabolism. Midazolam has a half-life of 30-60 minutes, which may vary depending on GA.[180] It has also shown to be effective for postoperative pain as well as noninvasive procedural pain such as radiological procedures.[35,181,182] However, there are concerns about the efficacy, adverse effects, and clinical outcomes of midazolam compared to opioids.[183-186] Concerns about midazolam compared to morphine include increased risk of IVH, periventricular leukomalacia, death, seizures, longer hospital stay, and benzyl alcohol exposure.
- *Lorazepam*: Lorazepam is another common sedative with a long duration (6-12 hours). Adverse effects include neuronal toxicity.[187]
- *Dexmedetomidine*: Dexmedetomidine is a selective α-2 adrenergic receptor agonist. Unlike most other sedatives, dexmedetomidine causes minimal respiratory depression. It has been used for imaging procedures and supraventricular tachyarrhythmias.[188-192] Research regarding the pharmacokinetics, safety, and efficacy of dexmedetomidine in neonates is limited and, therefore, routine use is not yet recommended.[149,188,189,193-196] Potential adverse effects include seizures, bradycardia, and hypothermia.[197-199]
- *Phenobarbital*: Phenobarbital is frequently used in combination with opioids in infants with neonatal abstinence syndrome or seizures.[200] There is limited data on its efficacy as an analgesic.[183,201]
- *Propofol*: Although not frequently used in neonates, recent studies show propofol is comparable to morphine, atropine, and suxamethonium with regard to intubation

times, higher oxygen saturations, and trauma.[202-204] Side effects include neurotoxicity, severe hypotension, and decreased oxygen saturations.[205,206]

- *Ketamine*: Ketamine is an NMDA receptor antagonist and is called a dissociative anesthetic because it provides analgesia, amnesia, and sedation. It has commonly been used in older children for procedural, operative, and postoperative analgesia and sedation, but there are limited studies evaluating its use in neonates.[207] Ketamine maintains respiratory drive and allows for bronchodilation, which improves ventilation and hemodynamic functioning.[208,209] It also increases heart rate and blood pressure.[208,209] Ketamine has been preferentially used in hypotensive infants because it does not significantly affect cerebral blood flow.[210] Due to ketamine's high potency and the lack of studies in neonates, it is advised that it should only be used for invasive procedures.[25]

## CONCLUSION

It is important to recognize that newborns are frequently exposed to painful procedures. Comprehensive pain assessment and management continues to present challenges. Providers should use pain assessment tools whenever clinically appropriate in order to avoid the deleterious effects of too little or too much treatment. Nonpharmacological analgesic modalities should be utilized whenever possible; clinicians must take into consideration the adverse effects associated with analgesic pharmacotherapies. More studies are needed to better understand the physiological mechanisms and efficacy of these current and emerging analgesic assessment tools and therapies.

## REFERENCES

1. Anand KJ, Runeson B, Jacobson B. Gastric suction at birth associated with long-term risk for functional intestinal disorders in later life. J Pediatr. 2004;144(4):449-54.
2. Bartocci M, Bergqvist LL, Lagercrantz H, Anand KJ. Pain activates cortical areas in the preterm newborn brain. Pain. 2006;122(1-2):109-17.
3. Mancuso T, Burns J. Ethical concerns in the management of pain in the neonate. Paediatr Anaesth. 2009;19(10):953-7.
4. Mather L, Mackie J. The incidence of postoperative pain in children. Pain. 1983;15(3):271-82.
5. Peters JW, Schouw R, Anand KJ, van Dijk M, Duivenvoorden HJ, Tibboel D. Does neonatal surgery lead to increased pain sensitivity in later childhood? Pain. 2005;114(3):444-54.
6. Anand KJ; International Evidence-Based Group for Neonatal Pain. Consensus statement for the prevention and management of pain in the newborn. Arch Pediatr Adolesc Med. 2001;155(2):173-80.
7. Anand KJ, Sippell WG, Aynsley-Green A. Randomised trial of fentanyl anaesthesia in preterm babies undergoing surgery: effects on the stress response. Lancet. 1987;1(8527):243-8.
8. Anand KJ. Effects of perinatal pain and stress. Prog Brain Res. 2000;122:117-29.
9. Mathew PJ, Mathew JL. Assessment and management of pain in infants. Postgrad Med J. 2003;79(934):438-43.
10. Anand KJ. Clinical importance of pain and stress in preterm neonates. Biol Neonate. 1998;73(1):1-9.
11. Johnston CC, Stevens BJ, Yang F, Horton L. Differential response to pain by very premature neonates. Pain. 1995;61(3):471-9.
12. Fitzgerald M. Developmental biology of inflammatory pain. Br J Anaesth. 1995;75(2):177-85.
13. Fitzgerald M, McIntosh N. Pain and analgesia in the newborn. Arch Dis Child. 1989;64(4 Spec No):441-3.
14. Majcher TA, Means LJ. Pain management in children. Semin Pediatr Surg. 1992;1(1):55-64.
15. Fitzgerald M, Beggs S. The neurobiology of pain: developmental aspects. Neuroscientist. 2001;7(3):246-57.
16. Larsson BA. Pain and pain relief during the neonatal period. Early pain experiences can result in negative late-effects. Lakartidningen. 2001;98(14):1656-62.
17. Cong X, McGrath JM, Cusson RM, Zhang D. Pain assessment and measurement in neonates: an updated review. Adv Neonatal Care. 2013;13(6):379-95.
18. Anand KJ, Aranda JV, Berde CB, Buckman S, Capparelli EV, Carlo W, et al. Summary proceedings from the neonatal pain-control group. Pediatrics. 2006;117(3 Pt 2):S9-S22.
19. Carbajal R, Rousset A, Danan C, Coquery S, Nolent P, Ducrocq S, et al. Epidemiology and treatment of painful procedures in neonates in intensive care units. JAMA. 2008;300(1):60-70.
20. Simons SH, van Dijk M, Anand KS, Roofthooft D, van Lingen RA, Tibboel D. Do we still hurt newborn babies? A prospective study of procedural pain and analgesia in neonates. Arch Pediatr Adolesc Med. 2003;157(11):1058-64.
21. American Academy of Pediatrics Committee on Fetus and Newborn; American Academy of Pediatrics Section on Surgery; Canadian Paediatric Society Fetus and Newborn Committee, Batton DG, Barrington KJ, Wallman C. Prevention and management of pain in the neonate: an update. Pediatrics. 2006;118(5):2231-41.
22. Ranger M, Johnston CC, Anand KJ. Current controversies regarding pain assessment in neonates. Semin Perinatol. 2007;31(5):283-8.
23. Stevens BJ, Abbott LK, Yamada J, Harrison D, Stinson J, Taddio A, et al. Epidemiology and management of painful procedures in children in Canadian hospitals. CMAJ. 2011;183(7):E403-10.
24. Karling M, Renstrom M, Ljungman G. Acute and postoperative pain in children: a Swedish nationwide survey. Acta Paediatr. 2002;91(6):660-6.
25. Hall RW, Anand KJ. Pain management in newborns. Clin Perinatol. 2014;41(4):895-924.
26. Ferguson SA, Ward WL, Paule MG, Hall RW, Anand KJ. A pilot study of preemptive morphine analgesia in preterm neonates: effects on head circumference, social behavior, and response latencies in early childhood. Neurotoxicol Teratol. 2012;34(1):47-55.

27. de Graaf J, van Lingen RA, Simons SH, Anand KJ, Duivenvoorden HJ, Weisglas-Kuperus N, et al. Long-term effects of routine morphine infusion in mechanically ventilated neonates on children's functioning: five-year follow-up of a randomized controlled trial. Pain. 2011;152(6):1391-7.
28. Grunau RE, Holsti L, Peters JW. Long-term consequences of pain in human neonates. Semin Fetal Neonatal Med. 2006;11(4):268-75.
29. Anand KJ, Palmer FB, Papanicolaou AC. Repetitive neonatal pain and neurocognitive abilities in ex-preterm children. Pain. 2013;154(10):1899-901.
30. Doesburg SM, Chau CM, Cheung TP, Moiseev A, Ribary U, Herdman AT, et al. Neonatal pain-related stress, functional cortical activity and visual-perceptual abilities in school-age children born at extremely low gestational age. Pain. 2013;154(10):1946-52.
31. Vinall J, Grunau RE. Impact of repeated procedural pain-related stress in infants born very preterm. Pediatr Res. 2014;75(5):584-7.
32. Hermann C, Hohmeister J, Demirakca S, Zohsel K, Flor H. Long-term alteration of pain sensitivity in school-aged children with early pain experiences. Pain. 2006;125(3):278-85.
33. Walker SM, Franck LS, Fitzgerald M, Myles J, Stocks J, Marlow N. Long-term impact of neonatal intensive care and surgery on somatosensory perception in children born extremely preterm. Pain. 2009;141(1-2):79-87.
34. Schmelzle-Lubiecki BM, Campbell KA, Howard RH, Franck L, Fitzgerald M. Long-term consequences of early infant injury and trauma upon somatosensory processing. Eur J Pain. 2007;11(7):799-809.
35. Ranger M, Chau CM, Garg A, Beg MF, Bjornson B, Poskitt K, et al. Neonatal pain-related stress predicts cortical thickness at age 7 years in children born very preterm. PLoS One. 2013;8(10):e76702.
36. Lim Y, Godambe S. Prevention and management of procedural pain in the neonate: an update, American Academy of Pediatrics, 2016. Arch Dis Child Educ Pract Ed. 2017;102(5):254-6.
37. Witt N, Coynor S, Edwards C, Bradshaw H. A Guide to Pain Assessment and Management in the Neonate. Curr Emerg Hosp Med Rep. 2016;4:1-10.
38. Lago P, Garetti E, Merazzi D, Pieragostini L, Ancora G, Pirelli A, et al. Guidelines for procedural pain in the newborn. Acta Paediatr. 2009;98(6):932-9.
39. Anand KJ. Pain assessment in preterm neonates. Pediatrics. 2007;119(3):605-7.
40. Guedj R, Danan C, Daoud P, Pieragostini L, Ancora G, Pirelli A, et al. Does neonatal pain management in intensive care units differ between night and day? An observational study. BMJ Open. 2014;4(2):e004086.
41. van Dijk M, Koot HM, Saad HH, Tibboel D, Passchier J. Observational visual analog scale in pediatric pain assessment: useful tool or good riddance? Clin J Pain. 2002;18(5):310-6.
42. Stevens BJ, Pillai Riddell R. Looking beyond acute pain in infancy. Pain. 2006;124(1-2):11-2.
43. Stevens B, McGrath P, Dupuis A, Gibbins S, Beyene J, Breau L, et al. Indicators of pain in neonates at risk for neurological impairment. J Adv Nurs. 2009;65(2):285-96.
44. Gibbins S, Stevens B, McGrath PJ, Yamada J, Beyene J, Breau L, et al. Comparison of pain responses in infants of different gestational ages. Neonatology. 2008;93(1):10-8.
45. Franck LS, Boyce WT, Gregory GA, Jemerin J, Levine J, Miaskowski C. Plasma norepinephrine levels, vagal tone index, and flexor reflex threshold in premature neonates receiving intravenous morphine during the postoperative period: a pilot study. Clin J Pain. 2000;16(2):95-104.
46. Johnston CC, Stevens B, Yang F, Horton L. Developmental changes in response to heelstick in preterm infants: a prospective cohort study. Dev Med Child Neurol. 1996;38(5):438-45.
47. Lindh V, Wiklund U, Hakansson S. Heel lancing in term newborn infants: an evaluation of pain by frequency domain analysis of heart rate variability. Pain. 1999;80(1-2):143-8.
48. Stevens B, Johnston C. Premature infants' response to pain. Nurs Que. 1991;11(6):82-8; 90-5.
49. Cong X, Ludington-Hoe SM, Walsh S. Randomized crossover trial of kangaroo care to reduce biobehavioral pain responses in preterm infants: a pilot study. Biol Res Nurs. 2011;13(2):204-16.
50. Stevens BJ, Franck LS. Assessment and management of pain in neonates. Paediatr Drugs. 2001;3(7):539-58.
51. Anand KJ, Carr DB. The neuroanatomy, neurophysiology, and neurochemistry of pain, stress, and analgesia in newborns and children. Pediatr Clin North Am. 1989;36(4):795-822.
52. Fitzgerald M, Walker SM. Infant pain management: a developmental neurobiological approach. Nat Clin Pract Neurol. 2009;5(1):35-50.
53. Brown L. Physiologic responses to cutaneous pain in neonates. Neonatal Netw. 1987;6(3):18-22.
54. Ludington-Hoe SM, Cong X, Hashemi F. Infant crying: nature, physiologic consequences, and select interventions. Neonatal Netw. 2002;21(2):29-36.
55. Weissman A, Aranovitch M, Blazer S, Zimmer EZ. Heel-lancing in newborns: behavioral and spectral analysis assessment of pain control methods. Pediatrics. 2009;124(5):e921-6.
56. Barr RG, Chen S, Hopkins B, Westra T. Crying patterns in preterm infants. Dev Med Child Neurol. 1996;38(4):345-55.
57. Sisto R, Bellieni CV, Perrone S, Buonocore G. Neonatal pain analyzer: development and validation. Med Biol Eng Comput. 2006;44(10):841-5.
58. Fuller BF. Acoustic discrimination of three types of infant cries. Nurs Res. 1991;40(3):156-60.
59. Fuller B. Meanings of discomfort and fussy-irritable in infant pain assessment. J Pediatr Health Care. 1996;10(6):255-63.
60. Porter FL, Porges SW, Marshall RE. Newborn pain cries and vagal tone: parallel changes in response to circumcision. Child Dev. 1988;59(2):495-505.
61. Porter FL, Miller RH, Marshall RE. Neonatal pain cries: effect of circumcision on acoustic features and perceived urgency. Child Dev. 1986;57(3):790-802.
62. Johnston CC, Stevens BJ, Franck LS, Jack A, Stremler R, Platt R. Factors explaining lack of response to heel stick in preterm newborns. J Obstet Gynecol Neonatal Nurs. 1999;28(6):587-94.
63. Franck LS, Greenberg CS, Stevens B. Pain assessment in infants and children. Pediatr Clin North Am. 2000;47(3):487-512.
64. Phillips P. Neonatal pain management: a call to action. Pediatr Nurs. 1995;21(2):195-9.

65. Grunau RV, Johnston CC, Craig KD. Neonatal facial and cry responses to invasive and non-invasive procedures. Pain. 1990;42(3):295-305.
66. Schiavenato M, von Baeyer CL. A Quantitative Examination of Extreme Facial Pain Expression in Neonates: The Primal Face of Pain across Time. Pain Res Treat. 2012;2012:251625.
67. Stevens BJ, Johnston CC. Physiological responses of premature infants to a painful stimulus. Nurs Res. 1994;43(4):226-31.
68. Holsti L, Grunau RE. Initial validation of the Behavioral Indicators of Infant Pain (BIIP). Pain. 2007;132(3):264-72.
69. Axelin A, Kirjavainen J, Salantera S, Lehtonen L. Effects of pain management on sleep in preterm infants. Eur J Pain. 2010;14(7):752-8.
70. Grunau RE, Linhares MB, Holsti L, Oberlander TF, Whitfield MF. Does prone or supine position influence pain responses in preterm infants at 32 weeks gestational age? Clin J Pain. 2004;20(2):76-82.
71. Gunnar MR, Fisch RO, Korsvik S, Donhowe JM. The effects of circumcision on serum cortisol and behavior. Psychoneuroendocrinology. 1981;6(3):269-75.
72. Olischar M, Davidson AJ, Lee KJ, Hunt RW. Effects of morphine and midazolam on sleep-wake cycling in amplitude-integrated electroencephalography in post-surgical neonates ≥32 weeks of gestational age. Neonatology. 2012;101(4):293-300.
73. Porter FL, Wolf CM, Miller JP. Procedural pain in newborn infants: the influence of intensity and development. Pediatrics. 1999;104(1):e13.
74. Holsti L, Grunau RE, Shany E. Assessing pain in preterm infants in the neonatal intensive care unit: moving to a 'brain-oriented' approach. Pain Manag. 2011;1(2):171-9.
75. Ahn Y, Jun Y. Measurement of pain-like response to various NICU stimulants for high-risk infants. Early Hum Dev. 2007;83(4):255-62.
76. Beggs S, Torsney C, Drew LJ, Fitzgerald M. The postnatal reorganization of primary afferent input and dorsal horn cell receptive fields in the rat spinal cord is an activity-dependent process. Eur J Neurosci. 2002;16(7):1249-58.
77. Hummel P, van Dijk M. Pain assessment: current status and challenges. Semin Fetal Neonatal Med. 2006;11(4):237-45.
78. Stevens B, Johnston C, Petryshen P, Taddio A. Premature Infant Pain Profile: development and initial validation. Clin J Pain. 1996;12(1):13-22.
79. Prevention and management of pain and stress in the neonate. American Academy of Pediatrics. Committee on Fetus and Newborn. Committee on Drugs. Section on Anesthesiology. Section on Surgery. Canadian Paediatric Society. Fetus and Newborn Committee. Pediatrics. 2000;105(2):454-61.
80. Beltramini A, Milojevic K, Pateron D. Pain Assessment in Newborns, Infants, and Children. Pediatr Ann. 2017;46(10):e387-95.
81. Duhn LJ, Medves JM. A systematic integrative review of infant pain assessment tools. Adv Neonatal Care. 2004;4(3):126-40.
82. Stapelkamp C, Carter B, Gordon J, Watts C. Assessment of acute pain in children: development of evidence-based guidelines. Int J Evid Based Healthc. 2011;9(1):39-50.
83. Grunau RE, Oberlander T, Holsti L, Whitfield MF. Bedside application of the Neonatal Facial Coding System in pain assessment of premature neonates. Pain. 1998;76(3):277-86.
84. van Ganzewinkel CJ, Anand KJ, Kramer BW, Andriessen P. Chronic pain in the newborn: toward a definition. Clin J Pain. 2014;30(11):970-7.
85. Debillon T, Bureau V, Savagner C, Zupan-Simunek V, Carbajal R; French National Federation of Neonatologists. Pain management in French neonatal intensive care units. Acta Paediatr. 2002;91(7):822-6.
86. Gradin M. Need for a reliable pain evaluation scale in the newborn in Sweden. Acta Anaesthesiol Scand. 2000;44(5):552-4.
87. Sharek PJ, Powers R, Koehn A, Anand KJ. Evaluation and development of potentially better practices to improve pain management of neonates. Pediatrics. 2006;118 (Suppl 2):S78-86.
88. Raeside L RK, Jackson L, O'Shea J, Patel A. (2019). Neonatal pain guideline. [online] Available from https://www.clinicalguidelines.scot.nhs.uk/ggc-paediatric-guidelines/ggc-guidelines/neonatology/neonatal-pain-guideline/. [Last accessed March, 2020].
89. Ismail AQ, Gandhi A. Non-pharmacological analgesia: effective but underused. Arch Dis Child. 2011;96(8):784-5.
90. Cignacco E, Hamers JP, Stoffel L, van Lingen RA, Gessler P, McDougall J, et al. The efficacy of non-pharmacological interventions in the management of procedural pain in preterm and term neonates. A systematic literature review. Eur J Pain. 2007;11(2):139-52.
91. Shah PS, Herbozo C, Aliwalas LL, Shah VS. Breastfeeding or breast milk for procedural pain in neonates. Cochrane Database Syst Rev. 2012;12:CD004950.
92. Marin Gabriel MA, del Rey Hurtado de Mendoza B, Jimenez Figueroa L, Medina V, Iglesias Fernández B, Vázquez Rodríguez M, et al. Analgesia with breastfeeding in addition to skin-to-skin contact during heel prick. Arch Dis Child Fetal Neonatal Ed. 2013;98(6):F499-503.
93. Shah PS, Aliwalas LI, Shah V. Breastfeeding or breast milk for procedural pain in neonates. Cochrane Database Syst Rev. 2006;(3):CD004950.
94. Pillai Riddell RR, Racine NM, Turcotte K, Uman LS, Horton RE, Din Osmun L, et al. Non-pharmacological management of infant and young child procedural pain. Cochrane Database Syst Rev. 2011;(10):CD006275.
95. Stevens B, Yamada J, Ohlsson A, Haliburton S, Shorkey A. Sucrose for analgesia in newborn infants undergoing painful procedures. Cochrane Database Syst Rev. 2016;(7):CD001069.
96. Johnston C, Campbell-Yeo M, Fernandes A, Inglis D, Streiner D, Zee R. Skin-to-skin care for procedural pain in neonates. Cochrane Database Syst Rev. 2014(1):CD008435.
97. Cong X, Cusson RM, Walsh S, Hussain N, Ludington-Hoe SM, Zhang D. Effects of skin-to-skin contact on autonomic pain responses in preterm infants. J Pain. 2012;13(7):636-45.
98. McCain GC, Ludington-Hoe SM, Swinth JY, Hadeed AJ. Heart rate variability responses of a preterm infant to kangaroo care. J Obstet Gynecol Neonatal Nurs. 2005;34(6):689-94.
99. Morelius E, Theodorsson E, Nelson N. Salivary cortisol and mood and pain profiles during skin-to-skin care for an unselected group of mothers and infants in neonatal intensive care. Pediatrics. 2005;116(5):1105-13.

100. Axelin A, Salantera S, Lehtonen L. 'Facilitated tucking by parents' in pain management of preterm infants-a randomized crossover trial. Early Hum Dev. 2006;82(4):241-7.
101. Cignacco EL, Sellam G, Stoffel L, Gerull R, Nelle M, Anand KJ, et al. Oral sucrose and "facilitated tucking" for repeated pain relief in preterms: a randomized controlled trial. Pediatrics. 2012;129(2):299-308.
102. Campos RG. Rocking and pacifiers: two comforting interventions for heelstick pain. Res Nurs Health. 1994;17(5):321-31.
103. Bueno M, Yamada J, Harrison D, Khan S, Ohlsson A, Adams-Webber T, et al. A systematic review and meta-analyses of nonsucrose sweet solutions for pain relief in neonates. Pain Res Manag. 2013;18(3):153-61.
104. Kristoffersen L, Skogvoll E, Hafstrom M. Pain reduction on insertion of a feeding tube in preterm infants: a randomized controlled trial. Pediatrics. 2011;127(6):e1449-54.
105. O'Sullivan A, O'Connor M, Brosnahan D, McCreery K, Dempsey EM. Sweeten, soother and swaddle for retinopathy of prematurity screening: a randomised placebo controlled trial. Arch Dis Child Fetal Neonatal Ed. 2010;95(6):F419-22.
106. Blass EM, Watt LB. Suckling- and sucrose-induced analgesia in human newborns. Pain. 1999;83(3):611-23.
107. Corbo MG, Mansi G, Stagni A, Romano A, van den Heuvel J, Capasso L, et al. Nonnutritive sucking during heelstick procedures decreases behavioral distress in the newborn infant. Biol Neonate. 2000;77(3):162-7.
108. Liaw JJ, Zeng WP, Yang L, Yuh YS, Yin T, Yang MH. Non-nutritive sucking and oral sucrose relieve neonatal pain during intramuscular injection of hepatitis vaccine. J Pain Symptom Manage. 2011;42(6):918-30.
109. Mitchell A, Waltman PA. Oral sucrose and pain relief for preterm infants. Pain Manag Nurs. 2003;4(2):62-9.
110. Anseloni VC, Ren K, Dubner R, Ennis M. A brainstem substrate for analgesia elicited by intraoral sucrose. Neuroscience. 2005;133(1):231-43.
111. Blass EM, Shah A. Pain-reducing properties of sucrose in human newborns. Chem Senses. 1995;20(1):29-35.
112. Fernandez M, Blass EM, Hernandez-Reif M, Field T, Diego M, Sanders C. Sucrose attenuates a negative electroencephalographic response to an aversive stimulus for newborns. J Dev Behav Pediatr. 2003;24(4):261-6.
113. Harrison D, Beggs S, Stevens B. Sucrose for procedural pain management in infants. Pediatrics. 2012;130(5):918-25.
114. Holsti L, Grunau RE. Considerations for using sucrose to reduce procedural pain in preterm infants. Pediatrics. 2010;125(5):1042-7.
115. Shide DJ, Blass EM. Opioidlike effects of intraoral infusions of corn oil and polycose on stress reactions in 10-day-old rats. Behav Neurosci. 1989;103(6):1168-75.
116. Slater R, Cornelissen L, Fabrizi L, Patten D, Yoxen J, Worley A, et al. Oral sucrose as an analgesic drug for procedural pain in newborn infants: a randomised controlled trial. Lancet. 2010;376(9748):1225-32.
117. Wilkinson DJ, Savulescu J, Slater R. Sugaring the pill: ethics and uncertainties in the use of sucrose for newborn infants. Arch Pediatr Adolesc Med. 2012;166(7):629-33.
118. Harrison D, Yamada J, Stevens B. Strategies for the prevention and management of neonatal and infant pain. Curr Pain Headache Rep. 2010;14(2):113-23.
119. Hartling L, Shaik MS, Tjosvold L, Leicht R, Liang Y, Kumar M. Music for medical indications in the neonatal period: a systematic review of randomised controlled trials. Arch Dis Child Fetal Neonatal Ed. 2009;94(5):F349-54.
120. Diego MA, Field T, Hernandez-Reif M, Deeds O, Ascencio A, Begert G. Preterm infant massage elicits consistent increases in vagal activity and gastric motility that are associated with greater weight gain. Acta Paediatr. 2007;96(11):1588-91.
121. Jain S, Kumar P, McMillan DD. Prior leg massage decreases pain responses to heel stick in preterm babies. J Paediatr Child Health. 2006;42(9):505-8.
122. Procianoy RS, Mendes EW, Silveira RC. Massage therapy improves neurodevelopment outcome at two years corrected age for very low birth weight infants. Early Hum Dev. 2010;86(1):7-11.
123. Field T, Diego M, Hernandez-Reif M. Preterm infant massage therapy research: a review. Infant Behav Dev. 2010;33(2):115-24.
124. Bellieni CV, Bagnoli F, Perrone S, Nenci A, Cordelli DM, Fusi M, et al. Effect of multisensory stimulation on analgesia in term neonates: a randomized controlled trial. Pediatr Res. 2002;51(4):460-3.
125. Bellieni CV, Tei M, Coccina F, Buonocore G. Sensorial saturation for infants' pain. J Matern Fetal Neonatal Med. 2012;25(Suppl 1):79-81.
126. Gitto E, Pellegrino S, Manfrida M, Aversa S, Trimarchi G, Barberi I, et al. Stress response and procedural pain in the preterm newborn: the role of pharmacological and non-pharmacological treatments. Eur J Pediatr. 2012;171(6):927-33.
127. Bellieni CV, Buonocore G, Nenci A, Franci N, Cordelli DM, Bagnoli F. Sensorial saturation: an effective analgesic tool for heel-prick in preterm infants: a prospective randomized trial. Biol Neonate. 2001;80(1):15-8.
128. Gradin M, Finnstrom O, Schollin J. Feeding and oral glucose—additive effects on pain reduction in newborns. Early Hum Dev. 2004;77(1-2):57-65.
129. Chermont AG, Falcao LF, de Souza Silva EH, de Cassia Xavier Balda R, Guinsburg R. Skin-to-skin contact and/or oral 25% dextrose for procedural pain relief for term newborn infants. Pediatrics. 2009;124(6):e1101-7.
130. Lander J, Brady-Fryer B, Metcalfe JB, Nazarali S, Muttitt S. Comparison of ring block, dorsal penile nerve block, and topical anesthesia for neonatal circumcision: a randomized controlled trial. JAMA. 1997;278(24):2157-62.
131. Taddio A, Katz J, Ilersich AL, Koren G. Effect of neonatal circumcision on pain response during subsequent routine vaccination. Lancet. 1997;349(9052):599-603.
132. Nielsen LJ, Lumholt P, Holmich LR. [Local anaesthesia with vasoconstrictor is safe to use in areas with end-arteries in fingers, toes, noses and ears]. Ugeskr Laeger. 2014;176(44): pii: V04140238.
133. Garcia OC, Reichberg S, Brion LP, Schulman M. Topical anesthesia for line insertion in very low birth weight infants. J Perinatol. 1997;17(6):477-80.
134. Gradin M, Eriksson M, Holmqvist G, Holstein A, Schollin J. Pain reduction at venipuncture in newborns: oral glucose compared with local anesthetic cream. Pediatrics. 2002;110(6):1053-7.

135. Kapellou O. Blood sampling in infants (reducing pain and morbidity). BMJ Clin Evid. 2009;2009:pii: 0313.
136. Kaur G, Gupta P, Kumar A. A randomized trial of eutectic mixture of local anesthetics during lumbar puncture in newborns. Arch Pediatr Adolesc Med. 2003;157(11):1065-70.
137. Taddio A, Ohlsson A, Einarson TR, Stevens B, Koren G. A systematic review of lidocaine-prilocaine cream (EMLA) in the treatment of acute pain in neonates. Pediatrics. 1998;101(2):E1.
138. Larsson BA, Norman M, Bjerring P, Egekvist H, Lagercrantz H, Olsson GL. Regional variations in skin perfusion and skin thickness may contribute to varying efficacy of topical, local anaesthetics in neonates. Paediatr Anaesth. 1996;6(2):107-10.
139. Brisman M, Ljung BM, Otterbom I, Larsson LE, Andreasson SE. Methaemoglobin formation after the use of EMLA cream in term neonates. Acta Paediatr. 1998;87(11):1191-4.
140. Essink-Tebbes CM, Wuis EW, Liem KD, van Dongen RT, Hekster YA. Safety of lidocaine-prilocaine cream application four times a day in premature neonates: a pilot study. Eur J Pediatr. 1999;158(5):421-3.
141. Frey B, Kehrer B. Toxic methaemoglobin concentrations in premature infants after application of a prilocaine-containing cream and peridural prilocaine. Eur J Pediatr. 1999;158(10):785-8.
142. Taddio A, Lee CM, Parvez B, Koren G, Shah V. Contact dermatitis and bradycardia in a preterm infant given tetracaine 4% gel. Ther Drug Monit. 2006;28(3):291-4.
143. Hui-Chen F, Hsiu-Lin C, Shun-Line C, Tai-Ling T, Li-Jung W, Hsing-I T, et al. The effect of EMLA cream on minimizing pain during venipuncture in premature infants. J Trop Pediatr. 2013;59(1):72-73.
144. Bhat R, Chari G, Gulati A, Aldana O, Velamati R, Bhargava H. Pharmacokinetics of a single dose of morphine in preterm infants during the first week of life. J Pediatr. 1990;117(3):477-81.
145. Lynn AM, Slattery JT. Morphine pharmacokinetics in early infancy. Anesthesiology. 1987;66(2):136-9.
146. Scott CS, Riggs KW, Ling EW, Fitzgerald CE, Hill ML, Grunau RV, et al. Morphine pharmacokinetics and pain assessment in premature newborns. J Pediatr. 1999;135(4):423-9.
147. Hall RW, Kronsberg SS, Barton BA, Kaiser JR, Anand KJ, Group NTI. Morphine, hypotension, and adverse outcomes among preterm neonates: who's to blame? Secondary results from the NEOPAIN trial. Pediatrics. 2005;115(5):1351-9.
148. Taddio A. Opioid analgesia for infants in the neonatal intensive care unit. Clin Perinatol. 2002;29(3):493-509.
149. Carroll CL, Krieger D, Campbell M, Fisher DG, Comeau LL, Zucker AR. Use of dexmedetomidine for sedation of children hospitalized in the intensive care unit. J Hosp Med. 2008;3(2):142-7.
150. Simons SH, van Dijk M, van Lingen RA, Roofthooft D, Duivenvoorden HJ, Jongeneel N, et al. Routine morphine infusion in preterm newborns who received ventilatory support: a randomized controlled trial. JAMA. 2003;290(18):2419-27.
151. Taddio A, Lee C, Yip A, Parvez B, McNamara PJ, Shah V. Intravenous morphine and topical tetracaine for treatment of pain in [corrected] neonates undergoing central line placement. JAMA. 2006;295(7):793-800.
152. Ancora G, Lago P, Garetti E, Pirelli A, Merazzi D, Mastrocola M, et al. Efficacy and safety of continuous infusion of fentanyl for pain control in preterm newborns on mechanical ventilation. J Pediatr. 2013;163(3):645-51.
153. Franck LS, Vilardi J, Durand D, Powers R. Opioid withdrawal in neonates after continuous infusions of morphine or fentanyl during extracorporeal membrane oxygenation. Am J Crit Care. 1998;7(5):364-9.
154. Ionides SP, Weiss MG, Angelopoulos M, Myers TF, Handa RJ. Plasma beta-endorphin concentrations and analgesia-muscle relaxation in the newborn infant supported by mechanical ventilation. J Pediatr. 1994;125(1):113-6.
155. Saarenmaa E, Huttunen P, Leppaluoto J, Meretoja O, Fellman V. Advantages of fentanyl over morphine in analgesia for ventilated newborn infants after birth: A randomized trial. J Pediatr. 1999;134(2):144-50.
156. Bellu R, de Waal K, Zanini R. Opioids for neonates receiving mechanical ventilation: a systematic review and meta-analysis. Arch Dis Child Fetal Neonatal Ed. 2010;95(4):F241-51.
157. Harlos MS, Stenekes S, Lambert D, Hohl C, Chochinov HM. Intranasal fentanyl in the palliative care of newborns and infants. J Pain Symptom Manage. 2013;46(2):265-74.
158. Welzing L, Roth B. Experience with remifentanil in newborns and infants. Drugs. 2006;66(10):1339-50.
159. Lago P, Tiozzo C, Boccuzzo G, Allegro A, Zacchello F. Remifentanil for percutaneous intravenous central catheter placement in preterm infant: a randomized controlled trial. Paediatr Anaesth. 2008;18(8):736-44.
160. Pereira e Silva Y, Gomez RS, Marcatto Jde O, Maximo TA, Barbosa RF, Simoes e Silva AC. Morphine versus remifentanil for intubating preterm neonates. Arch Dis Child Fetal Neonatal Ed. 2007;92(4):F293-4.
161. Davis PJ, Galinkin J, McGowan FX, Lynn AM, Yaster M, Rabb MF, et al. A randomized multicenter study of remifentanil compared with halothane in neonates and infants undergoing pyloromyotomy. I. Emergence and recovery profiles. Anesth Analg. 2001;93(6):1380-6, table of contents.
162. Galinkin JL, Davis PJ, McGowan FX, Lynn AM, Rabb MF, Yaster M, et al. A randomized multicenter study of remifentanil compared with halothane in neonates and infants undergoing pyloromyotomy. II. Perioperative breathing patterns in neonates and infants with pyloric stenosis. Anesth Analg. 2001;93(6):1387-92, table of contents.
163. Ross AK, Davis PJ, Dear Gd GL, Ginsberg B, McGowan FX, Stiller RD, et al. Pharmacokinetics of remifentanil in anesthetized pediatric patients undergoing elective surgery or diagnostic procedures. Anesth Analg. 2001;93(6):1393-401, table of contents.
164. Marlow N, Weindling AM, Van Peer A, Heykants J. Alfentanil pharmacokinetics in preterm infants. Arch Dis Child. 1990;65(4 Spec No):349-51.
165. Saarenmaa E, Huttunen P, Leppaluoto J, Fellman V. Alfentanil as procedural pain relief in newborn infants. Arch Dis Child Fetal Neonatal Ed. 1996;75(2):F103-107.
166. Durrmeyer X, Vutskits L, Anand KJ, Rimensberger PC. Use of analgesic and sedative drugs in the NICU: integrating clinical trials and laboratory data. Pediatr Res. 2010;67(2):117-27.
167. Howard CR, Howard FM, Weitzman ML. Acetaminophen analgesia in neonatal circumcision: the effect on pain. Pediatrics. 1994;93(4):641-6.

168. Roman-Rodriguez CF, Toussaint T, Sherlock DJ, Fogel J, Hsu CD. Pre-emptive penile ring block with sucrose analgesia reduces pain response to neonatal circumcision. Urology. 2014;83(4):893-8.
169. Shah V, Taddio A, Ohlsson A. Randomised controlled trial of paracetamol for heel prick pain in neonates. Arch Dis Child Fetal Neonatal Ed. 1998;79(3):F209-211.
170. Bhalla T, Shepherd E, Tobias JD. Neonatal pain management. Saudi J Anaesth. 2014;8(Suppl 1):S89-97.
171. Menon G, Anand KJ, McIntosh N. Practical approach to analgesia and sedation in the neonatal intensive care unit. Semin Perinatol. 1998;22(5):417-24.
172. Wong T, Stang AS, Ganshorn H, Hartling L, Maconochie IK, Thomsen AM, et al. Combined and alternating paracetamol and ibuprofen therapy for febrile children. Cochrane Database Syst Rev. 2013(10):CD009572.
173. Ceelie I, de Wildt SN, van Dijk M, van den Berg MM, van den Bosch GE, Duivenvoorden HJ, et al. Effect of intravenous paracetamol on postoperative morphine requirements in neonates and infants undergoing major noncardiac surgery: a randomized controlled trial. JAMA. 2013;309(2):149-54.
174. Allegaert K, Rayyan M, De Rijdt T, Van Beek F, Naulaers G. Hepatic tolerance of repeated intravenous paracetamol administration in neonates. Paediatr Anaesth. 2008;18(5):388-92.
175. Morris JL, Rosen DA, Rosen KR. Nonsteroidal anti-inflammatory agents in neonates. Paediatr Drugs. 2003;5(6):385-405.
176. Truog R, Anand KJ. Management of pain in the postoperative neonate. Clin Perinatol. 1989;16(1):61-78.
177. van den Anker JN, Tibboel D. Pain relief in neonates: when to use intravenous paracetamol. Arch Dis Child. 2011;96(6):573-4.
178. Allegaert K, Vanhole C, de Hoon J, Guignard JP, Tibboel D, Devlieger H, et al. Nonselective cyclo-oxygenase inhibitors and glomerular filtration rate in preterm neonates. Pediatr Nephrol. 2005;20(11):1557-61.
179. Benini F, Farina M, Capretta A, Messeri A, Cogo P. Sedoanalgesia in paediatric intensive care: a survey of 19 Italian units. Acta Paediatr. 2010;99(5):758-62.
180. Ince I, de Wildt SN, Wang C, Peeters MY, Burggraaf J, Jacqz-Aigrain E, et al. A novel maturation function for clearance of the cytochrome P450 3A substrate midazolam from preterm neonates to adults. Clin Pharmacokinet. 2013;52(7):555-65.
181. Lane RD, Schunk JE. Atomized intranasal midazolam use for minor procedures in the pediatric emergency department. Pediatr Emerg Care. 2008;24(5):300-3.
182. Mekitarian Filho E, de Carvalho WB, Gilio AE, Robinson F, Mason KP. Aerosolized intranasal midazolam for safe and effective sedation for quality computed tomography imaging in infants and children. J Pediatr. 2013;163(4):1217-9.
183. Anand KJ, Barton BA, McIntosh N, Lagercrantz H, Pelausa E, Young TE, et al. Analgesia and sedation in preterm neonates who require ventilatory support: results from the NOPAIN trial. Neonatal Outcome and Prolonged Analgesia in Neonates. Arch Pediatr Adolesc Med. 1999;153(4):331-8.
184. Arya V, Ramji S. Midazolam sedation in mechanically ventilated newborns: a double blind randomized placebo controlled trial. Indian Pediatr. 2001;38(9):967-72.
185. Chess PR, D'Angio CT. Clonic movements following lorazepam administration in full-term infants. Arch Pediatr Adolesc Med. 1998;152(1):98-99.
186. Shehab N, Lewis CL, Streetman DD, Donn SM. Exposure to the pharmaceutical excipients benzyl alcohol and propylene glycol among critically ill neonates. Pediatr Crit Care Med. 2009;10(2):256-9.
187. McDermott CA, Kowalczyk AL, Schnitzler ER, Mangurten HH, Rodvold KA, Metrick S. Pharmacokinetics of lorazepam in critically ill neonates with seizures. J Pediatr. 1992;120(3):479-83.
188. Chrysostomou C, Morell VO, Wearden P, Sanchez-de-Toledo J, Jooste EH, Beerman L. Dexmedetomidine: therapeutic use for the termination of reentrant supraventricular tachycardia. Congenit Heart Dis. 2013;8(1):48-56.
189. Chrysostomou C, Sanchez De Toledo J, Avolio T, Motoa MV, Berry D, Morell VO, et al. Dexmedetomidine use in a pediatric cardiac intensive care unit: can we use it in infants after cardiac surgery? Pediatr Crit Care Med. 2009;10(6):654-60.
190. Mason KP. Sedation trends in the 21st century: the transition to dexmedetomidine for radiological imaging studies. Paediatr Anaesth. 2010;20(3):265-72.
191. Mason KP, Zurakowski D, Zgleszewski S, Prescilla R, Fontaine PJ, Dinardo JA. Incidence and predictors of hypertension during high-dose dexmedetomidine sedation for pediatric MRI. Paediatr Anaesth. 2010;20(6):516-23.
192. Mason KP, Zurakowski D, Zgleszewski SE, Robson CD, Carrier M, Hickey PR, et al. High dose dexmedetomidine as the sole sedative for pediatric MRI. Paediatr Anaesth. 2008;18(5):403-11.
193. Barton KP, Munoz R, Morell VO, Chrysostomou C. Dexmedetomidine as the primary sedative during invasive procedures in infants and toddlers with congenital heart disease. Pediatr Crit Care Med. 2008;9(6):612-5.
194. Bejian S, Valasek C, Nigro JJ, Cleveland DC, Willis BC. Prolonged use of dexmedetomidine in the paediatric cardiothoracic intensive care unit. Cardiol Young. 2009;19(1):98-104.
195. Lam F, Bhutta AT, Tobias JD, Gossett JM, Morales L, Gupta P. Hemodynamic effects of dexmedetomidine in critically ill neonates and infants with heart disease. Pediatr Cardiol. 2012;33(7):1069-77.
196. Potts AL, Anderson BJ, Holford NH, Vu TC, Warman GR. Dexmedetomidine hemodynamics in children after cardiac surgery. Paediatr Anaesth. 2010;20(5):425-33.
197. Berkenbosch JW, Tobias JD. Development of bradycardia during sedation with dexmedetomidine in an infant concurrently receiving digoxin. Pediatr Crit Care Med. 2003;4(2):203-5.
198. Finkel JC, Quezado ZM. Hypothermia-induced bradycardia in a neonate receiving dexmedetomidine. J Clin Anesth. 2007;19(4):290-2.
199. Kubota T, Fukasawa T, Kitamura E, Magota M, Kato Y, Natsume J, et al. Epileptic seizures induced by dexmedetomidine in a neonate. Brain Dev. 2013;35(4):360-2.
200. Ebner N, Rohrmeister K, Winklbaur B, Baewert A, Jagsch R, Peternell A, et al. Management of neonatal abstinence syndrome in neonates born to opioid maintained women. Drug Alcohol Depend. 2007;87(2-3):131-8.

201. Gonzalez-Darder JM, Ortega-Alvaro A, Ruz-Franzi I, Segura-Pastor D. Antinociceptive effects of phenobarbital in "tail-flick" test and deafferentation pain. Anesth Analg. 1992;75(1):81-6.
202. Ghanta S, Abdel-Latif ME, Lui K, Ravindranathan H, Awad J, Oei J. Propofol compared with the morphine, atropine, and suxamethonium regimen as induction agents for neonatal endotracheal intubation: a randomized, controlled trial. Pediatrics. 2007;119(6):e1248-55.
203. Jenkins IA, Playfor SD, Bevan C, Davies G, Wolf AR. Current United Kingdom sedation practice in pediatric intensive care. Paediatr Anaesth. 2007;17(7):675-83.
204. Shah PS, Shah VS. Propofol for procedural sedation/anaesthesia in neonates. Cochrane Database Syst Rev. 2011;(3):CD007248.
205. Allegaert K, Peeters MY, Verbesselt R, Tibboel D, Naulaers G, de Hoon JN, et al. Inter-individual variability in propofol pharmacokinetics in preterm and term neonates. Br J Anaesth. 2007;99(6):864-870.
206. Welzing L, Kribs A, Eifinger F, Huenseler C, Oberthuer A, Roth B. Propofol as an induction agent for endotracheal intubation can cause significant arterial hypotension in preterm neonates. Paediatr Anaesth. 2010;20(7):605-11.
207. Barois J, Tourneux P. Ketamine and atropine decrease pain for preterm newborn tracheal intubation in the delivery room: an observational pilot study. Acta Paediatr. 2013;102(12):e534-8.
208. Chambliss CR, Anand KJ. Pain management in the pediatric intensive care unit. Curr Opin Pediatr. 1997;9(3):246-53.
209. Hall RW, Shbarou RM. Drugs of choice for sedation and analgesia in the neonatal ICU. Clin Perinatol. 2009;36(1):15-26.
210. Betremieux P, Carre P, Pladys P, Roze O, Lefrancois C, Malledant Y. Doppler ultrasound assessment of the effects of ketamine on neonatal cerebral circulation. Dev Pharmacol Ther. 1993;20(1-2):9-13.

# CHAPTER 40

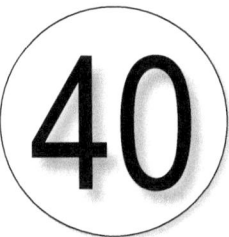

# Introduction to Addiction Medicine

*Balaji Govindaswami*

## ABSTRACT

An insight into addiction is critical to the understanding of modern newborn medicine. The evolution of traditional patterns of substance use involved many naturally occurring compounds (tobacco, alcohol, caffeine, betel nut, coca, khat), and has been a part of establishing cultural social norms, such as planting and growing crops, brewing and distilling, or using for ceremonial purposes. Our present-day ability to synthesize molecules and establish global distribution networks—both legal and illicit—has led to rapid escalation in substance use, misuse, and abuse. Furthermore, novel ways of recreationally administering drugs for acute onset and intensity of drug effect have led to unusual clinical presentations.

Scientists seek to understand the myriad neurobiological endogenous substance and receptor pathways [nicotinic, gamma-aminobutyric acid (GABA), serotonin, cannabinoid, opioid, etc.] to gain insight into mechanisms that predispose people to or result in neurobehavioral disruption/dysfunction in the world's increasingly socio-behaviorally complex and geographically isolated individuals and societies.

A range of substances has found various uses and misuse in disparate societies. Efforts to legalize previously illicit drugs are complicated by increasing concentrations of known chemicals [e.g., tetrahydrocannabinol (THC) in cannabis], multiple substance use, and temporal changes in mode of delivery (e.g., recent vaping trends in nicotine and cannabis). Deliberate addition of substances (such as Fentanyl, a synthetic opioid) to prescription narcotics, heroin, or other drugs; and unintended household or occupational contact have adversely affected users and those exposed accidentally.

The rapidly changing socio-demography of populations, including those who use and misuse substances, has implications for our gametes, reproduction, neurodevelopment/behavior, psychosocial function, and lifespan. Intergenerational consequences of early adverse childhood experiences, often complicated by substance use, have led to increasingly disenchanted, disenfranchised, and sometimes institutionalized populations. Newborns emerging in these populations face distinct disadvantages relating to prenatal disruption, further complicated by being "nurtured" in suboptimal circumstances. Public health approaches will have to inform risk attenuation and early prevention and intervention if, where, and when feasible. It is essential that trauma-informed healthcare delivery systems provide optimal care to these critically at-risk populations. Knowledge of associated disease burden [e.g., sexually transmitted diseases (STDs), suicide, hepatitis C, and human immunodeficiency virus (HIV)] will give modern healthcare providers prevention targets for decreasing morbidity and mortality in this re-emerging Dickensian world amidst populations who have so much.

## DEATHS OF DESPAIR: DEFINING MORTALITY FROM A NEW MULTIFACTORIAL PHENOMENON

The United States is the only wealthy country where life expectancy is declining.[1] Deaths of despair [mortality rates from accidental or intent-undetermined alcohol and drug poisoning, suicide, alcoholic liver disease (ALD), and cirrhosis] from 1989 to 2014 were higher in the United States for non-Hispanic whites (NHWs) compared to other groups or compared to their peers in other countries.[2] This is attributable to an epidemic of preventable deaths among the less than college educated white population.

Over a million deaths from suicide, drugs, and alcohol have occurred in the decade 2006-2015. A record 36% of all the US counties experienced natural decrease (deaths exceed live births) in 2012, compared to 28% in 2009. In 2012, for the first time in US history, deaths exceeded births in two entire states, West Virginia and then Maine.[3] Natural decrease is twice as common in rural areas as in urban. Economic and job opportunities (+ environmental degradation, danger at home, natural disaster) affect migration. Increasing geographic mobility has seen individuals migrate away from social and family support systems integral to health and well-being of society. Health was defined by the World Health Organization in 1948 as a state of complete physical, mental, and social well-being, and not merely the absence of disease and infirmity.

As deaths were increasing for NHW ages 45-54 from 1998 to 2013,[4] it was later realized that all-cause mortality is greater for women.[5] The largest relative increases in mid-life mortality have occurred in New England and the Ohio Valley. An estimated 33,307 excess the US deaths were attributed to increased mid-life mortality in 2010-2017. One-third of these deaths occurred in four Ohio Valley states (West Virginia, Ohio, Indiana, and Kentucky).[6] The state of Ohio reports that for the year 2018, the leading cause of death in children ages 10-14 and second leading cause for ages 15-19 was suicide.[7]

## DREAMLAND: UNDERSTANDING THE EPIDEMIOLOGY

A remarkable understanding of the opiate epidemic in the US is well conveyed in the book Dreamland by Sam Quinones,[8] and the evolutionary origin of substance use is clearly outlined in a review in the Harm Reduction Journal.[9] The United Nations' World Drug Report of 2004 reported that 3% of the world population (185 million people) has misused drugs in the prior 12 months with cannabis (150 million) and amphetamine-type stimulants (38 million, including 8 million ecstasy users) being the most prevalent, followed by opiates—heroin, morphine, and opium—(15 million) and cocaine (13 million). Misuse of opiates is the world's most serious drug problem, accounting for 67% of drug treatment in Asia, 61% in Europe, and 47% in Oceania. In Southeast Asia, methamphetamine (MA) use is the main problem, while cocaine is prevalent on

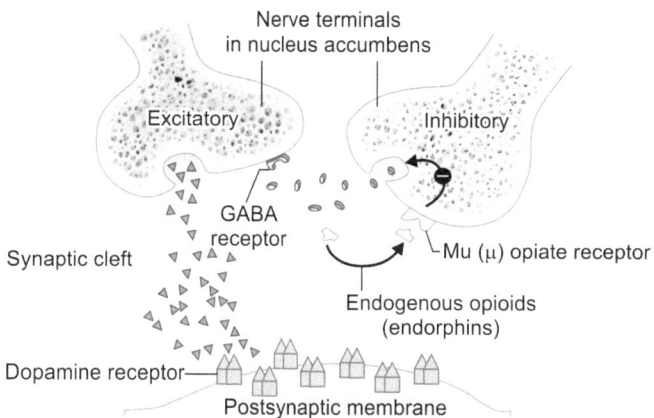

**Fig. 1:** The mu (μ) opiate receptor.

the American continent and cannabis dominates in Africa (65%).[10] Worldwide, 1.3 billion tobacco smokers account for 25 times as many lives lost (4.9 million vs 200,000 from drug abuse in the year 2000). Disability-adjusted (aka healthy) life years lost are 11.1 million from drug abuse, compared to 59.1 million from tobacco. Tobacco results in more death, but other drug use results in more healthy life years lost.

The ten most common addictions in the US today are: nicotine (> 40 million), alcohol (18 million), marijuana (4.2 million), painkillers (1.8 million), cocaine (821,000 in 2011), heroin (426,000), benzodiazepines (400,000), stimulants (329,000), inhalants (140,000), and barbiturates (78,000).[11]

The opioid crisis was declared on October 27, 2017 in the US. In that year, 16,000 US deaths were attributed to heroin, and a further 15,000 to prescription narcotics. The American Medical Association estimates that 3-19% of people taking prescription pain medications develop an addiction to them.[12] Drugs implicated in the US deaths vary by region as described in a 2017 National Vital Statistics Report.[13]

Opiate receptors and pathways are closely linked to GABA **(Fig. 1)**. GABAergic drugs such as barbiturates and benzodiazepines are known disruptors to the developing nervous system. Newer drugs such as gabapentin have found widespread use in pain management and are increasingly recognized as having addiction potential. Their impact on the developing nervous system is less well known but early reports of serious morbidity in newborns exist.[14,15]

## DEFINITION AND CONSEQUENCES OF ADDICTION

The American Psychiatric Association defines addiction as a complex brain disease, manifested by compulsive substance use despite harmful consequences.[16] These substances harm brain function; imaging studies show changes in brain areas related to judgment, decision-making, learning, memory, and behavior control. Recent studies suggest alterations in the amygdala and cingula may alter behavior and personality, and may provide mechanistic insights into long-term consequences of addiction.[17]

Studying empathy has led to better understanding of several neuropsychiatric dysfunctional states.[18] Gender-specific differences in response to neuropeptides, e.g., oxytocin, and the interactions between cannabinoid receptors and oxytocin may vary between individuals.[19] The complex interactions between neuropathophysiology and addiction are just beginning to come to light. Preserving mental hygiene and preventing relapse are challenges in addiction medicine. The overlap between mental health disorders and addiction is significant. Models exist for action plans targeting discrete substance abuse and mental health crises.[20]

Substance use disorders often are associated with prior trauma and abuse, making control and regulation of emotion difficult; which in turn increases vulnerability to substance use. Mindful awareness in body-oriented therapy (MABT) specifically teaching interoceptive awareness skills improves abstinence and emotional health in women: 187 low income women treated primarily for misuse of stimulants, alcohol and narcotics were randomly assigned to receive treatment as usual (TAU), TAU plus MABT, or TAU plus women's health education. MABT and women's health education interventions were delivered individually and weekly for 8 weeks. After 1 year, women who received MABT maintained higher levels of abstinence compared to those in the other two groups. All participants were women with low socioeconomic status who reported substantial interpersonal trauma. In addition, 75% of participants were white, factors that limit the generalizability of these findings.[21]

A recent study shows the importance of incorporating voluntary choice between drugs and social rewards. In this study, rats preferred spending time with another rat rather than access to heroin and MA, more than 90% of the time. Rats choosing abstinence showed no signs of intensification of drug craving that normally happens over time in both rat and human models who abstain from drug use. In contrast, rats forced to be abstinent sought the drug more avidly 15 and 45 days after the last dose than after the first day of abstinence. The ultimate goal of such studies is to learn how social rewards might be used to prevent and treat human addiction.[22]

## ■ IMPLICATIONS FOR PREGNANCY, THE FETUS, THE NEWBORN, CHILDHOOD, AND ADOLESCENCE

Numerous substances and medications can affect a woman preconception, as well as during pregnancy and breastfeeding.[23] Alcohol's effects on the fetus and newborn should be targeted to avoid the most common preventable cause of birth defects and mental retardation in the world.[24]

## Alcohol

The US deaths from ALD are at their highest level since 1999, and have risen every year since 2006 in almost all racial, ethnic, and age groups. It is likely that increasing alcohol use, possibly in combination with other underlying liver disease, is putting people at increased risk for ALD. 2017 ALD deaths were 13.1/100,000 in men and 5.6/100,000 in women. Compared to 1999, this represents a more than 25% increase in ALD mortality for men, and an ~70% increase for women.[25] Absolute increase in ALD mortality is particularly pronounced in Native American women and NHW men and women. Trends such as these are very concerning because of their implications for intergenerational effects in women and men of reproductive age. The global prevalence of fetal alcohol spectrum disorders (FASDs) among children and youth approximates 8 per 1,000 in the general population and exceeds 1% in 76 countries. One of every 13 women who consumed alcohol in pregnancy delivered a child with FASD.[26] The World Health Organization (WHO) European region had the highest prevalence (almost 2%), while the Eastern Mediterranean region had the lowest rate (1 per 10,000). Countries such as South Africa had a prevalence exceeding 11%, followed by Croatia more than 5% and Ireland almost 5%. FASD is a rampant developmental disability that is largely preventable. Universal public health messaging about the potential harm of prenatal alcohol exposure is required to curb endemic FASD, and routine screening protocols are needed to provide intervention if, when, and where appropriate.

Fetal alcohol spectrum disorder consists of at least four diagnostic entities:
1. Fetal alcohol syndrome (FAS)[27,28]
2. Partial FAS
3. Alcohol-related neurodevelopmental disorders
4. Alcohol-related birth defects.[29,30]

The lifetime costs for a person in North America with FASD exceeds $1,000,000. The highest pooled prevalence (between 50% and 90%) of comorbid conditions includes abnormalities in the peripheral nervous system and special senses, conduct disorder, receptive language disorder, chronic serous otitis media, and expressive language disorder.[31] It is estimated that globally 1,700 FASD infants are born every day (>600,000 annually), and FASD is more frequent in special populations such as the aboriginal population, children in care, those in the incarcerated population, and those in psychiatric care. These findings prompt an urgent call to action on perinatal approaches to prevention of FASD and related disorders.

## Nicotine

Tobacco-related effects on the fetus and newborn may be the most common preventable cause of growth restriction in utero.[32] While the number of children age 3–11 in the US who are tobacco smoke exposure (TSE) has been declining steadily since 1999, in 2014 an estimated 14 million were still exposed with variation in different sociodemographic groups. The decline in TSE for ages 3–11 was from 64.5% in 1999 to 38% in 2014. Hispanic children were twice as likely as NHW children to be exposed, and children from low-income households were greater than three times more likely to be TSE than those from the highest income households. Children living in rented homes were TSE more than twice as often as those living in family-owned homes.[33] TSE in children greater than age 11 years has not been studied.

The majority of cannabis users also use tobacco. This population is likely growing, given the 183 million cannabis users in the past year worldwide,[34] with cannabis now surpassing opiates as the primary reason for first treatment entry of all illicit drugs in Europe.[35] A growing body of evidence shows that nicotine and cannabis have interactive effects on brain structure and function, suggesting that specialized intervention is indicated for those who use both. Functional magnetic resonance imaging revealed both nicotine and cannabis users have reduced neural connectivity compared with nonusers in two networks, including one supporting salience or assigning importance to environmental stimuli. The nicotine users had reduced connectivity in seven additional networks supporting functions including vision, cognition, and bodily awareness. Users of both drugs had connectivity comparable to nonusers in all networks suggesting that nicotine cognition enhancing-effects may facilitate cannabis use by countering cannabis' negative impact on networks supporting cognition. This emerging understanding points to the necessity of considering specialized therapy for patients who use both cannabis and nicotine.[36]

## Tetrahydrocannabinol

This drug alters emotional processes, executive function, and reward function via the endocannabinoid system **(Fig. 2)**. Cannabis misuse/dependence is associated with changes in neural circuitry in brain regions related to reward processing and habit formation with resultant psychopathology.[37] Exposing adolescent rats to THC[38] disrupt normal maturation of key neurons in brain areas corresponding to the human prefrontal cortex. These disruptions provide structural differences resembling patterns observed in humans with addiction and schizophrenia.[39] Volumetric study of the brains of 110 25-year-old poor rural African-Americans found use of alcohol, tobacco, and marijuana before age 19 was associated with less gray matter volume in two brain areas. The amygdala was small in youth reporting drug use ages 12–15, while the *pars opercularis*, a subregion of the inferior frontal gyrus, was small in those who reported use at ages 16–18.[40] While this association is limited by the chicken and egg analogy (pending preadolescent longitudinal brain volumetric nomograms), it parallels staged maturation of the adolescent brain in which the more primitive and emotive limbic system (amygdala) matures prior to cognition (forebrain circuit including the *pars opercularis* which supports the ability to refrain from impulsive behaviors). Parental exposure to THC as

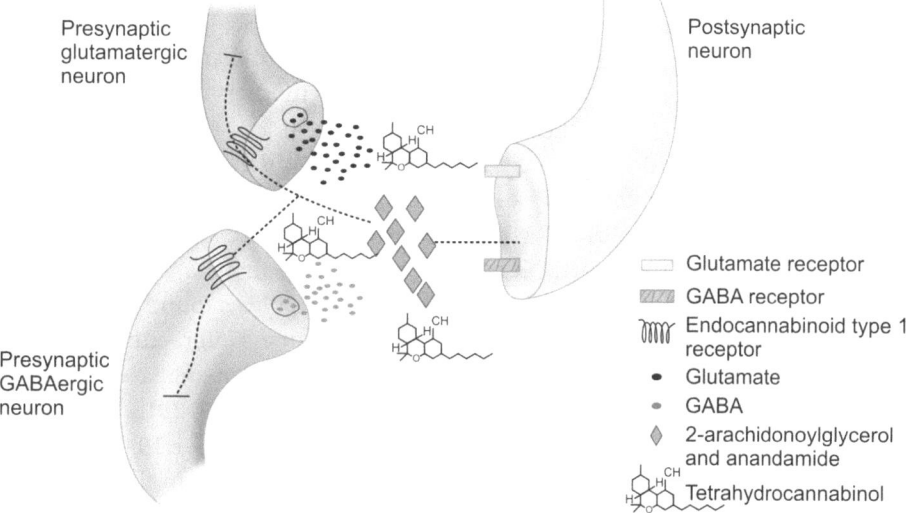

**Fig. 2:** Endocannabinoid type 1 receptor.

adolescents has also been shown to lead to compulsive heroin seeking in subsequent generation mice.[41] Although the mechanisms are not completely elucidated, they are consistent with other studies suggesting that parental drug use, even preconception, affects child brain function and behavior.

Currently more adults over age 50 use marijuana; a recent study found 9% of respondents age 50-64 and 2.9% of those more than age 65 reported using marijuana in the past year. Marijuana use is three times as prevalent in those ages 50-64 compared to those over 65 years of age. More than 80% of respondents aged 50-64 had tried marijuana by age 19, compared to slightly more than half of those over 65 years of age. Respondents reporting marijuana use prior to age 19 had a 13-fold increase in their odds of being current marijuana users.[42]

As global prevalence increases, and age at first use decreases, the likelihood of periconceptional exposure increases. Emerging evidence, albeit inconclusive, suggests that greater than weekly marijuana use may increase risk of low birth weight, postpartum depression, and decrease duration of lactation.[43-45] The US Surgeon General recommends that no one should use tobacco or marijuana around babies[46] or small children.

## Cocaine

Glucocorticoid hormones have a central role in susceptibility to relapse in times of stress. It has been postulated that an identified mechanism may potentiate cocaine-induced increased extracellular dopamine in nucleus accumbens (NAc).[47] Lasting changes in the NAc contribute to persistence of functional changes in the addicted brain. Furthermore, novel transcription factors such as *E2f3a* (described through overexpression or knockdown in mouse NAc) regulate cocaine-induced locomotor and place conditioning.[48] The ventral pallidum (VP) receives GABA input from the NAc reward center through two distinct pathways and ultimately relays it forward to the motor cortex. The relative strength of GABA in these two pathways determines if mouse motor cortical neurons will be sufficiently excited to initiate movement, suggesting that cocaine-induced serotonin increases in the VP could weaken one's ability to curb impulsive behaviors.[49] It has been proposed that serotonin-mediated loss of regulation in occipitofrontal circuitry following cocaine experience is an enduring change that plays a role in the disruption of decision-making in addiction disorders.[50]

## Methamphetamines

Long-term use of MAs is associated with cognitive dysfunction in many domains. Neuroimaging studies have shown structural and metabolic changes. There is considerable evidence for brain behavior relationship dysfunction, particularly in cognitive control and decision-making.[51] Crystal MA is one of the world's most commonly-used illicit drugs, now second only to cannabis. Methamphetamine use is an important factor for poor mental health, associated with higher odds of psychosis, violence, suicidality, and depression, while MA use disorder is associated with higher rates of psychosis, violence, and suicidality.[52]

Currently, a study aiming to assess the gaps in providing evidence for psychological treatment for MA use seeks to comprehensively review associated symptoms of mental ill health in experimental/control clinical settings.[53] Experience from the state of Washington in the US shows a quadrupling of deaths attributed to MA poisoning in the last decade. This comprehensive review of effective treatment for MA use disorder[54] provides a useful summary of 13 different mechanisms of action of nearly 40 medications examined for MA use disorders. A recent comprehensive review examining correlates of psychosis among MA users found that more frequent MA use was associated with dose-related increase in methamphetamine-associated psychosis (MAP). Polysubstance use, especially alcohol dependence and frequent use of cannabis, is also associated with MAP.[55]

A systematic review and meta-analysis of pharmacotherapy for methamphetamine/amphetamine (MA/A) use disorder examining low strength evidence from two randomized controlled trials (RCTs) (n = 34 + 54 = 88) shows that methylphenidate may reduce MA/A use. Most other medications evaluated (anticonvulsants, antipsychotics, opioid antagonists, varenicline, and atomoxetine) did not show statistically significant benefits.[56]

## Opiates

It was estimated that more than 6 per thousand US babies are born to mothers with opiate use or misuse (CDC 2014). About 50-80% of these newborns are diagnosed with neonatal abstinence syndrome (NAS), thus, based on 2014 data, ~8/1,000 US live births were diagnosed with NAS.[57] In Medicaid-financed (i.e., medically indigent) births covering costs for more than 73% of NAS-related births in 2004 and 82% in 2014, it was found that the prevalence of NAS had quintupled in the intervening decade, from 0.28 to 1.44%.[58] NAS incidence also increased notably in Canada between 2005-2006 and 2015-2016, from 0.2% to 0.5%. Maternal mortality was 1.99 per 10,000 women in the NAS group versus 0.31 per 1,000 in the comparison group; neonatal mortality and/or severe morbidity rates were 6.36% in infants with NAS versus 1.73 percent in those without.[59]

## Clinical Implications

A systematic review and meta-analysis among patients with outpatient opioid prescriptions shows that risk of opiate misuse is higher among those at a younger age, a history of current substance use or mental health diagnosis, and male gender.[60] From 1996 to 2012, a 471% increase occurred in the total quantity of prescribed opioids in the United States. The proportion of office-based prescriptions was high, increasing throughout the study, from 71% of total in 1996 to 83% in 2012. However, opioids originating in the emergency department (ED) was modest and declined throughout the study (7.4% in 1996 and 4.4% in 2012).[61] A current emergency room study is more reassuring in that only 1% of subjects suffering acute pain on ED discharge had persistent opioid use.[62] Of these 410 patients, 20% of opioid-naive patients receiving opioids at discharge filled at least two opioid prescriptions in 6 months.

One in five pregnant women insured by Medicaid filled an opioid prescription in the US between 2002 and 2007.[63] The incidence of opioid use disorders among women of reproductive age has increased significantly.[64,65] Subsequently, the population of opioid-exposed newborns (OENs) has increased from 1.20 to 3.39 per 1,000 hospital births per year nationally.[66,67] In Colorado, while the incidence of NAS at 2.9 per 1,000 live births in 2013 is less than in other parts of the US,[68] opioid overdose is nevertheless the leading cause of maternal mortality.[69] Hospital variations in OEN care have been associated with more pharmacologic treatment, longer lengths of stay, and higher healthcare costs.[70] Moreover, recent publications by Grossman et al. and Wachman et al. provide evidence for novel approaches that could be implemented within a quality improvement framework.[71,72]

A comprehensive review on neonatal drug withdrawal from the American Academy of Pediatrics is recommended reading.[73] Since this review, the epidemic of neonatal opioid exposure has continued to grow. A subsequent childhood outcomes workshop is also a good resource to understand the current state of the epidemic and solutions being generated in the US.[74] Recent data from maternal opiate exposure in an urban, low-income, multiethnic US population show significant increase in adverse short- and long-term outcomes across developmental stages. Higher rates of physical and neurodevelopmental disorders in affected children highlight the need for emergent efforts to prevent the opioid epidemic.[75]

## Approaches to Treatment of Neonatal Abstinence Syndrome

The American College of Obstetricians and Gynecologists has updated guidelines on opioid use disorder in pregnancy.[76] Numerous progressive social hospital-based approaches (such as rooming-in) have been successful in treating children born to opioid-dependent mothers.[77-79] Non-opiate treatment shows promising results with shorter length of stay.[80] Several resources exist for further education on up-to-date guidelines in the management of NAS.[81-84]

## DUAL DIAGNOSIS DISORDER (MENTAL ILLNESS AND ADDICTION)

Both mental illness and dependency have shared risk factors. Environmental triggers such as post-traumatic stress disorder (PTSD), drug exposure in critical periods of brain development including adolescence, and brain abnormalities of structure and function can coexist. Not all addicts have mental illness, but the overlap is significant enough that treatment can be jeopardized by judging abnormal behavior while under the influence. Sobriety from drug dependence is necessary to diagnose underlying mental illness, if it exists. It is generally accepted that several months of rehabilitation, including in-house care for up to 6 months, may be needed to understand and address these issues effectively. A first step in recovering from addiction is admitting that one has a problem; this can only be acknowledged by the user. There are controversial approaches to treatment, but these are beyond the scope of this book. Treatment requires the collaboration of addiction experts, mental health experts including psychiatrists and psychologists, specialists in PTSD if it is present, and mental health advocates familiar with the individual's history, life, family, and circumstances. Institutional approaches to recovery have been highly specialized, revolving around single substances or focused on in-patient facilities for dual diagnosis disorder followed by outpatient recovery programs. Programs are also specialized to specific high-risk populations, e.g., veterans and PTSD recovery, HIV-positive populations, and prison populations.[85-87] Better understanding of neurosciences and functional network connectivity[88,89] and development of novel medications[90] provide reasons for optimism for future approaches to substance use recovery.

Healthcare systems will have to collaborate with inpatient and outpatient mental health and addiction specialists to build the future superstructure that can successfully support the growing population of people with co-occurring substance use and mental health issues. Several faith-based institutions historically have been involved. Current principles of drug addiction treatment are outlined here.[91] The definition of "rehab" is not standardized and thus relapse rates are difficult to quantify. This complex subject is discussed further in a recent paper on drug rehabilitation success rates.[92] Other sources provide continually updated resources.[93]

## SUCCESSFUL NEW PARADIGMS OF CARE FOR ASSOCIATED DISEASES

It is really important to consider success stories from needle exchange programs to prevent risk of infectious disease and transmission of blood-borne particles, and outpatient programs such as perinatal substance and recovery with chronic methadone or buprenorphine therapy that have been effective in large urban centers and some rural areas. Maintaining vigilance for associated infectious diseases such as HIV, hepatitis C, and other STDs (e.g., syphilis) are all considerations when healthcare workers have access to inpatient and outpatient recovery programs. There is abundant evidence that chronic antiviral therapy is prolonging life and quality of life in HIV positive patients, and these models are now being applied to treatment of hepatitis C, which may require 3-6 months of therapy. Recurrent hepatitis C has been described in the high-risk population and may require retreatment. Staying alert for and prompt treatment of hepatitis C will prevent chronic liver disease.[94] Similar vigilance should be maintained for STDs, particularly syphilis, which is easily treatable, but if left unaddressed has serious consequences for the fetus and newborn. Reduced risk of perinatal vertical transmission of HIV and hepatitis C has been demonstrated by treatment with chronic antiviral therapy in pregnancy.

## CONCLUSION

Adverse childhood experiences associated with adult mental health issues and substance use often affects the next generation, leading to a vicious cycle of trauma, mental illness, and substance use. Addiction has a basis in genetics, with no socioeconomic or geographic boundaries. Trauma-informed care and reducing social isolation are key to optimal management of the dual disorders of mental illness and substance use.

Emerging neuroscientific evidence suggests that given the plasticity of the nervous system, substance exposure, especially in critical periods of neurodevelopment, may irreversibly alter brain structure and function, impairing impulse control, decision-making, and personality. Furthermore, severe mental health disorders including psychoses, sometimes irreversible, may be consequent to sufficient drug use.

Rapid demographic changes, substance availability, and distribution have led to the environment we have today of increasing numbers of addicted parents and exposed children who are now predisposed to become addicted themselves.

While a discussion of treatment is beyond the scope of this chapter, we have provided the context for understanding the rapidly shifting scene that faces current and future care providers in newborn medicine.

## REFERENCES

1. Brookings. (2019). Understanding the role of despair in America's opioid crisis. [online] Available from: https://www.brookings.edu/policy2020/votervital/how-can-policy-address-the-opioid-crisis-and-despair-in-america/ [Last accessed July, 2010].
2. Case A, Angus D. Mortality and morbidity in the 21st century. Brookings Pap Econ Act. 2017;2017:397-476.
3. Johnson KM. Deaths Exceed Births in Record Number of U.S. Counties. Carsey Institute, Winter 2013, Fact Sheet Number 25. Durham, NH: University of New Hampshire; 2013. pp. 1-2.
4. Case A, Deaton A. Rising morbidity and mortality in midlife among white non-Hispanic Americans in the 21st century. Proc Natl Acad Sci. 2015;112(49):15078-83.
5. Gelman A, Auerbach J. Age-aggregation bias in mortality trends. Proc Natl Acad Sci U S A. 2016;113(7):E816-7.
6. Woolf SH, Schoomaker H. Life expectancy and mortality rates in the United States, 1959-2017. JAMA. 2019;322(20):1996-2016.
7. Ohio Department of Health. (2019). Suicide Demographics and Trends, Ohio, 2018. [online] Available from: https://odh.ohio.gov/wps/wcm/connect/gov/fef3e5ee-b4c6-4e2e-a0b1-40c68e123f9f/2018_Suicide_Fact_Sheet.pdf?MOD=AJPERES&CONVERT_TO=url&CACHEID=ROOTWORKSPACE.Z18_M1HGGIK0N0JO00QO9DDDDM3000-fef3e5ee-b4c6-4e2e-a0b1-40c68e123f9f-mVCbMqs [Last accessed July, 2020].
8. Quinones S. Dreamland: The True Tale of America's Opiate Epidemic. New York, NY: Bloomsbury Press; 2017.
9. Saah T. The evolutionary origins and significance of drug addiction. Harm Reduct J. 2005;2:8.
10. UNIS. (2004). Press Release: United Nations' World Drug Report 2004 Presents An In-Depth Look into Global Drug Trends. United Nations Information Service. [online] Available from: http://www.unis.unvienna.org/unis/pressrels/2004/unisnar849.html [Last accessed July, 2020].
11. Addiction Center. (2020). 10 Most Common Addictions. [online] Available from: https://www.addictioncenter.com/addiction/10-most-common-addictions/ [Last accessed July, 2020].
12. American Psychiatric Association. (2017). Addiction and Substance Use Disorders: Opioid Use Disorder. [online] Available from: https://www.psychiatry.org/patients-families/addiction/opioid-use-disorder/opioid-use-disorder [Last accessed July 2020].
13. Hedegaard H, Bastian BA, Trinidad JP, et al. Regional differences in the drugs most frequently involved in drug overdose deaths: United States, 2017. Natl Vital Stat Rep. 2019;68(12):1-16.
14. Loudin S, Murray S, Prunty L, et al. An atypical withdrawal syndrome in neonates prenatally exposed to gabapentin and opioids. J Pediatr. 2017;181:286-8.

15. Loudin S, Haas J, Payne M, et al. Identifying co-exposure to opiates and gabapentin during pregnancy. J Pediatr. 2020;217:196-98.
16. American Psychiatric Association. Addiction and Substance Use Disorders: What is Addiction? [online] Available from: https://www.psychiatry.org/patients-families/addiction/what-is-addiction [Last accessed July, 2020].
17. Zhang X, Ge T, Yin G, et al. Stress-induced functional alterations in amygdala: implications for neuropsychiatric diseases. Front Neurosci. 2018;12:367.
18. Decety J, Moriguchi Y. The empathic brain and its dysfunction in psychiatric populations: implications for intervention across different clinical conditions. Biopsychosoc Med. 2007;1:22.
19. Herpertz SC, Bertsch K. A new perspective on the pathophysiology of borderline personality disorder: a model of the role of oxytocin. Am J Psychiatry. 2015;172(9):840-51.
20. SAMHSA. Strategic Plan, FY2019-2023. [online] Available from: https://www.samhsa.gov/sites/default/files/samhsa_strategic_plan_fy19-fy23_final-508.pdf [Last accessed July, 2020].
21. Price CJ, Thompson EA, Crowell S, et al. Longitudinal effects of interoceptive awareness training through mindful awareness in body-oriented therapy (MABT) as an adjunct to women's substance use disorder treatment: a randomized controlled trial. Drug Alcohol Depend. 2019;198:140-9.
22. Venniro M, Zhang M, Caprioli D, et al. Volitional social interaction prevents drug addiction in rat models. Nat Neurosci. 2018;21(11):1520-9.
23. WIC Works Resource System, U.S. Department of Agriculture. Substance Use and Medication Safety. [online] Available from: https://wicworks.fns.usda.gov/resources/substance-use-and-medication-safety [Last accessed July, 2020].
24. CDC. (2019). Basics About Fetal Alcohol Spectrum Disorders. [online] Available from: https://www.cdc.gov/ncbddd/fasd/facts.html [Last accessed July, 2020].
25. Moon AM, Yang JY, Barritt AS 4th, et al. Rising mortality from alcohol-associated liver disease in the United States in the 21st century. Am J Gastroenterol. 2020;115(1):79-87.
26. Lange S, Probst C, Gmel G, et al. Global prevalence of fetal alcohol spectrum disorder among children and youth: a systematic review and meta-analysis. JAMA Pediatr. 2017;171(10):948-56.
27. Jones KL, Smith DW, Ulleland CN, et al. Pattern of malformation in offspring of chronic alcoholic mothers. Lancet. 1973;301(7815):1267-71.
28. Jones KL, Smith DW. Recognition of the fetal alcohol syndrome in early infancy. Lancet. 1973;302(7836):999-1001.
29. Chudley AE, Conry J, Cook JL, et al. Fetal alcohol spectrum disorder: Canadian guidelines for diagnosis. CMAJ. 2005;172(5 Suppl):S1-S21.
30. Hoyme HE, May PA, Kalberg WO, et al. A practical clinical approach to diagnosis of fetal alcohol spectrum disorders: clarification of the 1996 institute of medicine criteria. Pediatrics. 2005;115(1):39-47.
31. Popova S, Lange S, Shield K, et al. Comorbidity of fetal alcohol spectrum disorder: a systematic review and meta-analysis. Lancet. 2016;387(10022):978-87.
32. CDC. (2020). Smoking, Pregnancy, and Babies. [online] Available from: https://www.cdc.gov/tobacco/campaign/tips/diseases/pregnancy.html [Last accessed July, 2020].
33. Merianos AL, Jandarov RA, Choi K, et al. Tobacco exposure disparities persist in US children: NHANES 1999-2014. Prev Med. 2019;123:138-42.
34. United Nations Office on Drugs and Crime. (2018). World Drug Report 2018. [online] Available from: https://www.unodc.org/wdr2018/ [Last accessed July, 2020].
35. Bloomfield MAP, Hindocha C, Green SF, et al. The neuropsychopharmacology of cannabis: a review of human imaging studies. Pharmacol Ther. 2019;195:132-61.
36. Filbey FM, Gohel S, Prashad S, et al. Differential associations of combined vs. isolated cannabis and nicotine on brain resting state networks. Brain Struct Funct. 2018;223(7):3317-26.
37. Manza P, Tomasi D, Volkow ND. Subcortical local functional hyperconnectivity in cannabis dependence. Biol Psychiatry Cogn Neurosci Neuroimaging. 2018;3(3):285-93.
38. Miller ML, Chadwick B, Dickstein DL, et al. Adolescent exposure to Δ9-tetrahydrocannabinol alters the transcriptional trajectory and dendritic architecture of prefrontal pyramidal neurons. Mol Psychiatry. 2019;24(4):588-600.
39. Filbey FM, Aslan S, Calhoun VD, et al. Long-term effects of marijuana use on the brain. Proc Natl Acad Sci U S A. 2014;111(47):16913-8.
40. Windle M, Gray JC, Lei KM, et al. Age sensitive associations of adolescent substance use with amygdalar, ventral striatum, and frontal volumes in young adulthood. Drug Alcohol Depend. 2018;186:94-101.
41. Szutorisz H, DiNieri JA, Sweet E, et al. Parental THC exposure leads to compulsive heroin-seeking and altered striatal synaptic plasticity in the subsequent generation. Neuropsychopharmacology. 2014;39(6):1315-23.
42. Han BH, Palamar JJ. Marijuana use by middle-aged and older adults in the United States, 2015-2016. Drug Alcohol Depend. 2018;191:374-81.
43. ACOG. (2015). Committee Opinion #722. Marijuana Use During Pregnancy and Lactation. [online] Available from: https://www.acog.org/Clinical-Guidance-and-Publications/Committee-Opinions/Committee-on-Obstetric-Practice/Marijuana-Use-During-Pregnancy-and-Lactation [Last accessed July, 2020].
44. Conner SN, Bedell V, Lipsey K, et al. Maternal marijuana use and adverse neonatal outcomes: a systematic review and meta-analysis. Obstet Gynecol. 2016;128(4):713-23.
45. Ko JY, Tong VT, Bombard JM, et al. Marijuana use during and after pregnancy and association of prenatal use on birth outcomes: A population-based study. Drug Alcohol Depend. 2018;187:72-8.
46. HHS.gov. U.S. Surgeon General's Advisory: Marijuana Use and the Developing Brain. [online] Available from: https://www.hhs.gov/surgeongeneral/reports-and-publications/addiction-and-substance-misuse/advisory-on-marijuana-use-and-developing-brain/index.html [Last accessed July, 2020].
47. Graf EN, Wheeler RA, Baker DA, et al. Corticosterone acts in the nucleus accumbens to enhance dopamine signaling and potentiate reinstatement of cocaine seeking. J Neurosci. 2013;33(29):11800-10.
48. Cates HM, Heller EA, Lardner CK, et al. Transcription factor E2F3a in nucleus accumbens affects cocaine action via transcription and alternative splicing. Biol Psychiatry. 2018;84(3):167-79.

49. Matsui A, Alvarez VA. Cocaine inhibition of synaptic transmission in the ventral pallidum is pathway-specific and mediated by serotonin. Cell Rep. 2018;23(13):3852-63.
50. Wright AM, Zapata A, Baumann MH, et al. Enduring loss of serotonergic control of orbitofrontal cortex function following contingent and noncontingent cocaine exposure. Cerebral Cortex. 2017;27(12):5463-76.
51. Sabrini S, Wang GY, Lin JC, et al. Methamphetamine use and cognitive function: a systematic review of neuroimaging research. Drug Alcohol Depend. 2019;194:75-87.
52. McKetin R, Leung J, Stockings E, et al. Mental health outcomes associated with of the use of amphetamines: a systematic review and meta-analysis. EClinicalMedicine. 2019;16:81-97.
53. Stuart A, Baker AL, Bowman J, et al. Protocol for a systematic review of psychological treatment for methamphetamine use: an analysis of methamphetamine use and mental health symptom outcomes. BMJ Open. 2017;7:e015383.
54. Stoner SA. Effective Treatments for Methamphetamine Use Disorder: A Review. Seattle: Alcohol and Drug Abuse Institute, University of Washington; 2018.
55. Arunogiri S, Foulds JA, McKetin R, et al. A systematic review of risk factors for methamphetamine-associated psychosis. Aust N Z J Psychiatry. 2018;52(6):514-29.
56. Chan B, Freeman M, Kondo K, et al. Pharmacotherapy for methamphetamine/amphetamine use disorder—a systematic review and meta-analysis. Addiction. 2019;114(12):2122-36.
57. Honein MA, Boyle C, Redfield RR. Public health surveillance of prenatal opioid exposure in mothers and infants. Pediatrics. 2019:143(3):e20183801.
58. Winkelman TNA, Villapiano N, Kozhimannil KB, et al. Incidence and costs of neonatal abstinence syndrome among infants with Medicaid: 2004–2014. Pediatrics. 2018;141(4):e20173520.
59. Lisonkova S, Richter LL, Ting J, et al. Neonatal abstinence syndrome and associated neonatal and maternal mortality and morbidity. Pediatrics. 2019;144(2):e20183664.
60. Cragg A, Hau JP, Woo SA, et al. Risk factors for misuse of prescribed opioids: a systematic review and meta-analysis. Ann Emerg Med. 2019;74(5):634-46.
61. Axeen S, Seabury SA, Menchine M. Emergency department contribution to the prescription opioid epidemic. Ann Emerg Med. 2018;71(6):659-67.e3.
62. Friedman BW, Ochoa LA, Naeem F, et al. Opioid use during the six months after an emergency department visit for acute pain: a prospective cohort study. Ann Emerg Med. 2020;75(5):578-86.
63. Desai RJ, Hernandez-Diaz S, Bateman BT, et al. Increase in prescription opioid use during pregnancy among Medicaid-enrolled women. Obstet Gynecol. 2014;123(5):997-1002.
64. Hand DJ, Short VL, Abatemarco DJ. Substance use, treatment, and demographic characteristics of pregnant women entering treatment for opioid use disorder differ by United States census region. J Subst Abuse Treat. 2017;76:58-63.
65. Kozhimannil KB, Graves AJ, Jarlenski M, et al. Non-medical opioid use and sources of opioids among pregnant and non-pregnant reproductive-aged women. Drug Alcohol Depend. 2017;174:201-8.
66. Patrick SW, Schumacher RE, Benneyworth BD, et al. Neonatal abstinence syndrome and associated health care expenditures: United States, 2000-2009. JAMA. 2012;307(18):1934-40.
67. Patrick SW, Davis MM, Lehman CU, et al. Increasing incidence and geographic distribution of neonatal abstinence syndrome: United States 2009 to 2012. J Perinatol. 2015;35(8):667.
68. Ko JY, Patrick SW, Tong VT, et al. Incidence of neonatal abstinence syndrome - 28 States, 1999-2013. MMWR Morb Mortal Wkly Rep. 2016;65(31):799-802.
69. Metz TD, Rovner P, Hoffman MC, et al. Maternal deaths from suicide and overdose in Colorado, 2004-2012. Obstet Gynecol. 2016;128(6):1233-40.
70. Milliren CE, Gupta M, Graham DA, et al. Hospital variation in neonatal abstinence syndrome incidence, treatment modalities, resource use, and costs across pediatric hospitals in the United States, 2013 to 2016. Hosp Pediatr. 2018;8(1):15-20.
71. Grossman MR, Berkwitt AK, Osborn RR, et al. An initiative to improve the quality of care of infants with neonatal abstinence syndrome. Pediatrics. 2017;139(6):e20163360.
72. Wachman EM, Grossman M, Schiff DM, et al. Quality improvement initiative to improve inpatient outcomes for Neonatal Abstinence Syndrome. J Perinatol. 2018;38(8):1114-22.
73. Hudak ML, Tan RC, Committee on Drugs, et al. Neonatal drug withdrawal. Pediatrics. 2012;129(2):e540-60.
74. Reddy UM, Davis JM, Ren Z, et al. Opioid Use in Pregnancy, Neonatal Abstinence Syndrome, and Childhood Outcomes: Executive Summary of a Joint Workshop by the Eunice Kennedy Shriver National Institute of Child Health and Human Development, American College of Obstetricians and Gynecologists, American Academy of Pediatrics, Society for Maternal-Fetal Medicine, Centers for Disease Control and Prevention, and the March of Dimes Foundation. Obstet Gynecol. 2017;130(1):10-28.
75. Azuine RE, Ji Y, Chang H, et al. Prenatal risk factors and perinatal and postnatal outcomes associated with maternal opioid exposure in an urban, low-income, multiethnic US population. JAMA Netw Open. 2019;2(6):e196405.
76. Committee on Obstetric Practice. Committee Opinion Number 711: Opioid Use and Opioid Use Disorder in Pregnancy. Obstet Gynecol. 2017;130(2):e81-e94.
77. Howard MB, Schiff DM, Penwill N, et al. Impact of parental presence at infants' bedside on neonatal abstinence syndrome. Hosp Pediatr. 2017;7(2):63-9.
78. Abrahams RR, Kelly SA, Payne S, et al. Rooming-in compared with standard of care for newborns of mothers using methadone or heroin. Can Fam Physician. 2007;53(10):1772-30.
79. Newman A, Davies GA, Dow K, et al. Rooming-in care for infants of opioid dependent mothers. Can Fam Physician. 2015;61(12):e555-61.
80. Bada HS, Sithisarn T, Gibson J, et al. Morphine versus clonidine for neonatal abstinence syndrome. Pediatrics. 2015;135(2):e383-91.
81. March of Dimes. (2019). Neonatal Abstinence Syndrome (NAS). [online] Available from: https://www.marchofdimes.org/complications/neonatal-abstinence-syndrome-(nas).aspx [Last accessed July, 2020].
82. CDC. (2020). About Opioid Use During Pregnancy. [online] Available from: https://www.cdc.gov/pregnancy/opioids/basics.html [Last accessed July, 2020].

83. Association of State and Territorial Health Officials. (2015). How State Health Departments Can Use the Spectrum of Prevention to Address Neonatal Abstinence Syndrome. [online] Available from: https://www.astho.org/Prevention/Rx/NAS-Framework/ [Last accessed July, 2020].
84. National Institute on Drug Abuse. (2019). New studies clarify risk factors for neonatal abstinence syndrome. [online] Available from: https://www.drugabuse.gov/news-events/nida-notes/2019/1/new-studies-clarify-risk-factors-neonatal-abstinence-syndrome [Last accessed July, 2020].
85. Miller WC, Hoffman IF, Hanscom BS, et al. A scalable, integrated intervention to engage people who inject drugs in HIV care and medication-assisted treatment (HPTN 074): a randomised, controlled phase 3 feasibility and efficacy study. Lancet. 2018;392(10149):747-59.
86. Loeliger KB, Altice FL, Ciarleglio MM, et al. All-cause mortality among people with HIV released from an integrated system of jails and prisons in Connecticut, USA, 2007-14: a retrospective observational cohort study. Lancet HIV. 2018;5(11):e617-e628.
87. Brinkley-Rubinstein L, McKenzie M, Macmadu A, et al. A randomized, open label trial of methadone continuation versus forced withdrawal in a combined US prison and jail: Findings at 12 months post-release. Drug Alcohol Depend. 2018;184:57-63.
88. Yip SW, Scheinost D, Potenza MN, et al. Connectome-based prediction of cocaine abstinence. Am J Psychiatry. 2019;176(2):156-64.
89. Rosenberg MD, Zhang S, Hsu WT, et al. Methylphenidate modulates functional network connectivity to enhance attention. J Neurosci. 2016;36(37):9547-57.
90. Ding H, Kiguchi N, Yasuda D, et al. A bifunctional nociceptin and mu opioid receptor agonist is analgesic without opioid side effects in nonhuman primates. Sci Transl Med. 2018;10(456):eaar3483.
91. National Institute on Drug Abuse. (2019). Principles of Drug Addiction Treatment: A Research-Based Guide (Third Edition). [online] Available from: https://www.drugabuse.gov/publications/principles-drug-addiction-treatment-research-based-guide-third-edition [Last accessed July, 2020].
92. American Addiction Centers. (2019). Rehab Success Rates and Statistics. [online] Available from: https://americanaddictioncenters.org/rehab-guide/success-rates-and-statistics [Last accessed July, 2020].
93. Substance Abuse and Mental Health Services Administration. (2020). SAMHSA's National Helpline. [online] Available from: https://www.samhsa.gov/find-help/national-helpline [Last accessed July, 2020].
94. Spearman CW, Dusheiko GM, Hellard M, et al. Hepatitis C. Lancet. 2019;394(10207):1451-66.

# SECTION 10

# Other Common Newborn Conditions

- Skin Disorders in the Newborn
  *Noah Craft, Zachary Max Goldstein, Ki-Young Yoo*

- Common Orthopedic Problems in the Newborn
  *Robert M Bernstein, Ronald A Roiz*

- Oxygenation, Oxygen Saturation, Retinopathy of Prematurity and Other Hyperoxia-related Damage in Newborn Infants:
  A Return to the Basics
  *Augusto Sola, Lily C Chen*

- Neonatal Gastrointestinal and Liver Disease
  *Christopher Fink*

- Nephrology in the Neonate
  *Dechu P Puliyanda, Rashmi Kirpekar*

# CHAPTER 41

# Skin Disorders in the Newborn

*Noah Craft, Zachary Max Goldstein, Ki-Young Yoo*

## ABSTRACT

Skin disorders in the newborn are many and it is important to distinguish what is benign from what warrants concern. We present an overview of both common and uncommon skin disorders that are important for clinicians to recognize. This overview is organized to group skin disorders based on how they appear to the clinician.

## MACULES (FLAT SPOTS) WITH ASSOCIATED COLOR CHANGE

### Salmon Patch (Nevus Simplex) (Fig. 1)

*What is It?*

The salmon patch represents a capillary malformation. It has different names depending on the location, which can affect prognosis. When located on the back of the neck, it is referred to as a "stork bite." When the eyelids or forehead is involved, the lesion is known as an "angel kiss." This lesion is quite common, affecting 40–60% of all newborns with no sex predilection.[1,2]

*Clinical Presentation*

On examination, nevus simplex should appear as a pink or red, blanchable flat spot. It is commonly found on the face (on the mid forehead, glabella, nose, eyelids, and/or philtrum), but can present also on the midline of the occiput or back. They are usually centrally located without a dermatomal distribution.[3]

*Diagnostic Evaluation*

The salmon patch is generally a clinical diagnosis that does not require further evaluation.[3] One exception to this rule are those that present on the sacrum (*see* "Management and Prognosis") in which imaging studies may be recommended.[4]

*Management and Prognosis*

A salmon patch on the face will usually resolve spontaneously within the first 2 years of life. On the other hand, those that present on the back of the neck ("stork bite") tend to persist.[1,2] They generally require no treatment. However, those that present on the lumbosacral area, particularly

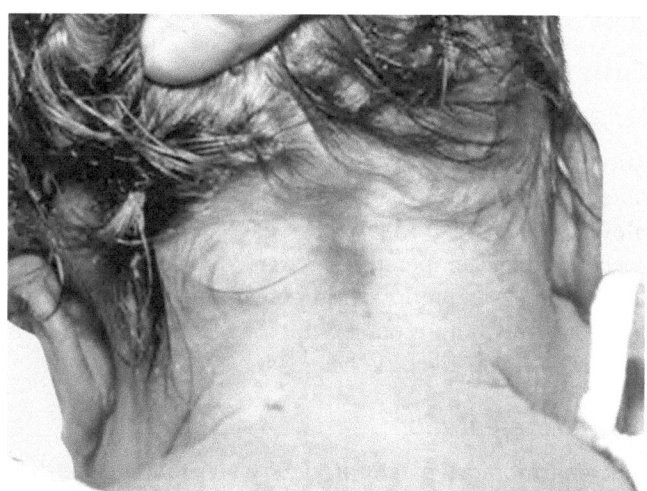

**Fig. 1:** Salmon patch *(For color version see Plate 5).*
*Source:* Image appears with permission from VisualDx (www.visualdx.com).

when associated with other skin disorders at this site, may warrant imaging studies to evaluate for spinal dysraphism.[4]

### Port-Wine Stain (Fig. 2)

*What is It?*

Similar to nevus simplex, port-wine stains (PWS) represent capillary malformations. They are typically sporadic lesions present in up to 0.2% of infants but may have an inheritance component (especially in families with multiple PWS).[1,2] Of concern are those lesions that involve the first trigeminal nerve on the face. Those infants who present with large involvement of the extremities may also require further evaluation (*see* "Management and Prognosis").

*Clinical Presentation*

Port-wine stains appear as uniform pink, red, or purple patches, and when on the face, they may present in a dermatomal distribution.[5] They can temporarily lighten during age 3–6 months, but typically darken and sometimes thicken over a lifetime.[1]

*Diagnostic Evaluation*

Similar to nevus simplex, this is a clinical diagnosis.[5]

*Management and Prognosis*

Although both nevus simplex and PWS represent capillary malformations, the latter do not improve on their own.[5] Pulsed dye laser therapy has been used for treatment, proving to be both safe and effective although multiple treatments may be needed.[6] Consideration of Sturge–Weber syndrome and ocular complications is important in patients whose PWS involves the first trigeminal nerve distribution. Patients with large involvement of the extremities should be referred for evaluation of Klippel–Trénaunay syndrome, which is a syndrome consisting of PWS, venous malformations, and limb hypertrophy.[2,7]

### Cutis Marmorata (Fig. 3)

*What is It?*

Cutis marmorata is vascular physical phenomenon that reflects the neonate's inability to properly adjust cutaneous blood flow in response to the external environment, specifically cold temperatures.[1] It may continue up to 4 weeks of age and is seen more commonly in premature infants.[8] In infants in whom it persists for longer, other conditions should be suspected (*see* "Diagnostic Evaluation").

*Clinical Presentation*

Cutis marmorata typically presents with a mottled, net-like appearance often described as having a violaceous hue. It should be blanchable and improve with warming.[8]

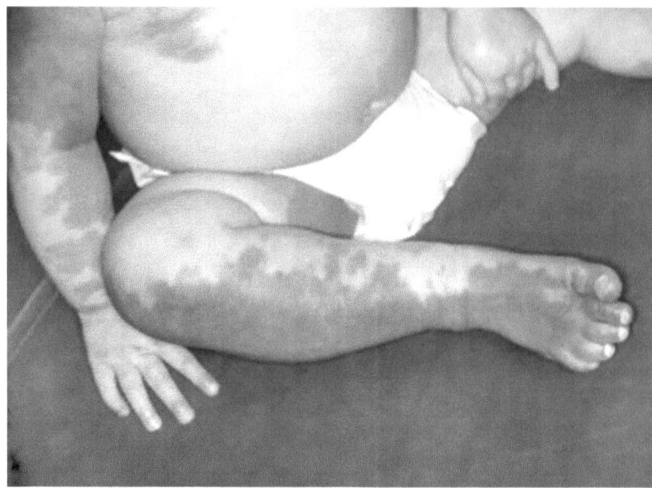

**Fig. 2:** Port-wine stain *(For color version see Plate 5).*
Source: Image appears with permission from VisualDx (www.visualdx.com).

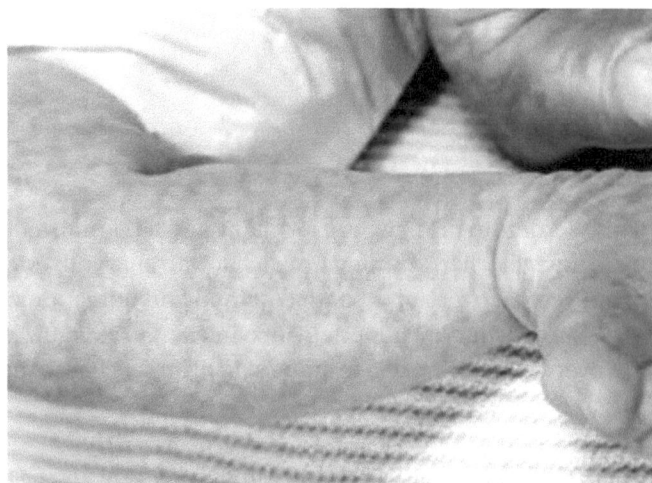

**Fig. 3:** Cutis marmorata *(For color version see Plate 5).*
Source: Image appears with permission from VisualDx (www.visualdx.com).

*Diagnostic Evaluation*

No tests are needed as it is mainly a clinical diagnosis. In those infants in whom it does not resolve, a separate cause should be suspected (e.g. hypothyroidism and cutis marmorata telangiectatica congenita).[8]

*Management and Prognosis*

No treatment is needed for this disorder.[9] In those infants in whom it does not respond to warming, one should consider cutis marmorata telangiectatica congenita (which has an asymmetric presentation sometimes associated with other findings).[8]

### Café-Au-Lait Macule (Fig. 4)

*What is It?*

As the name implies, café-au-lait macules (CALMs) are flat brown spots whose color resembles "coffee with milk".[10]

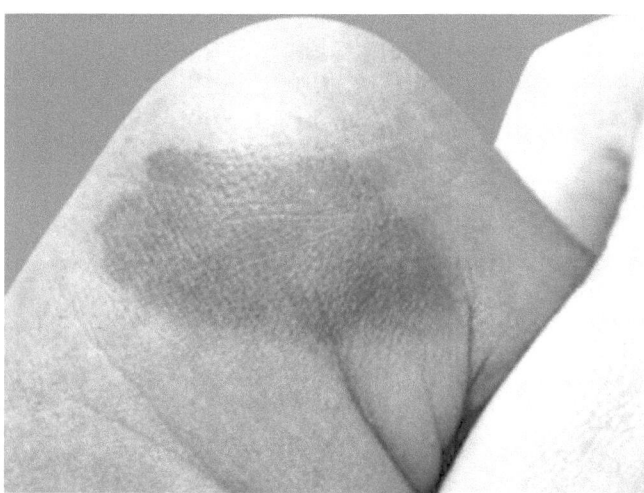

**Fig. 4:** Café-au-lait macule *(For color version see Plate 5)*.
Source: Image appears with permission from VisualDx (www.visualdx.com).

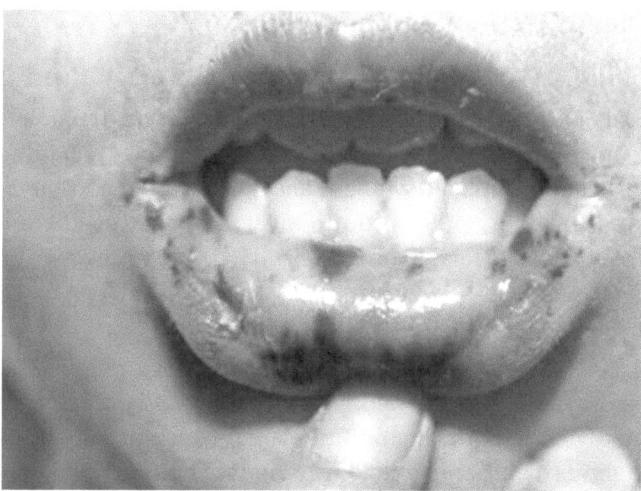

**Fig. 5:** Peutz–Jeghers syndrome *(For color version see Plate 5)*.
Source: Image appears with permission from VisualDx (www.visualdx.com).

While they are found in up to 35% of the general population, only 1% of the population have more than three CALMs.[10,11] With the exception of certain conditions (*see* "Management and Prognosis"), the etiology is unknown and attributed to increased melanogenesis.[11]

### Clinical Presentation

Café-au-lait macules have a distinct appearance presenting as light-brown, hairless spots that can vary in size and location on the body.[1,10] It is important to count the number of lesions, as having more than six may suggest neurofibromatosis (NF).[10]

### Diagnostic Evaluation

Like the other flat lesions, CALMs can generally be diagnosed based on appearance.[1] Should biopsy be performed, one would see increased epidermal pigment without melanocytic proliferation.

### Management and Prognosis

While there is no required treatment for CALMs, pigment-specific lasers can be used for cosmetic purposes.[1,11] As noted above, CALMs can be associated with systemic disorders, including NF type 1 (NF1). The presence of 6 or more CALMs measuring greater than 1.5 cm or 0.5 cm in postpubertal and prepubertal individuals, respectively, should prompt further evaluation, as this is one of the diagnostic criteria for NF1.[12]

## Lentigo (Lentigines Plural)

### What is It?

Lentigines are well-demarcated brown spots that are generally less than 5 mm in diameter and typically darker than ephelides (freckles).[13] They can develop on any surface of the skin.

### Clinical Presentation

In addition to being darker than freckles, lentigines tend to have a scattered distribution without necessarily favoring sun exposed sites.[13] They may appear early in life and increase in number over the years. When they develop in a cluster, in what appears to be a broad territory of skin, they are referred to as speckled lentiginous nevus or segmental lentiginosis.

### Diagnostic Evaluation

Certain presentations of lentiginosis should bring up the question of a genodermatosis. In Peutz–Jeghers (**Fig. 5**), lentigines appear on the oral mucosal, perinasal and periorbital skin, and acral skin. This syndrome is associated with visceral tumors and gastrointestinal polyps. Lentigines on the penis can be seen in Bannayan–Zonana syndrome, characterized by macrocephaly, lipomas, and hemangiomas. Lentigines on the nose and cheeks may be associated with mental retardation, congenital mitral valve stenosis, seizures, and other anomalies. In other syndromes, such as LEOPARD (lentigines, electrocardiogram conduction abnormalities, ocular hypertelorism, pulmonic stenosis, abnormal genitalia, retardation of growth, and sensorineural deafness) and Carney complex, extensive lentigines do not appear until childhood or puberty.[14]

### Management and Prognosis

Lentigines developing during early infancy or childhood may lighten or fade over time. When they are suspected to be associated with a genodermatosis, further evaluation may be warranted.[14]

## Nevus Depigmentosus (Fig. 6)

### What is It?

This is a light (hypopigmented) spot, as opposed to complete depigmentation seen in vitiligo. This lesion is thought to result from impaired synthesis and transfer of melanosomes, and they may present up to 3 years of age (usually no later).[1,15] They tend to be stable and fixed over time.

### Clinical Presentation

Nevus depigmentosus presents as a hypopigmented flat spot with a well-defined, possibly serrated borders. Hair may be seen growing from the area, which usually has a lighter shade compared to surrounding hairs.[1,15]

### Diagnostic Evaluation

Wood's lamp (an instrument that uses ultraviolet light with peak wavelength 365 nm) examination can be helpful in supporting the diagnosis. Unlike the chalk-white lesions seen in vitiligo under Wood's lamp examination, nevus depigmentosus will most likely present as off-white lesions without fluorescence.[15]

### Management and Prognosis

Although these lesions may enlarge in proportion with the baby's growth, the shape and number should remain stable. While there is no mandated treatment, dyes and makeups can be used for cosmetic purposes.[1,15]

## Ash Leaf Macule (Fig. 7)

### What is It?

The ash leaf macule is a hypopigmented spot that can be associated with tuberous sclerosis.[16] More than three such spots with a diameter of 5 mm or greater should raise consideration for tuberous sclerosis complex (see "Diagnostic Evaluation").[17]

### Clinical Presentation

This presents as a well-defined hypopigmented spot that resembles the lance-ovate-shape similar to ash leaves (hence the name). This is in contrast to nevus depigmentosus, which has irregular borders and typically follows the lines of Blaschko.[18]

### Diagnostic Evaluation

The presence of multiple ash leaf spots in young babies should raise the consideration of tuberous sclerosis in addition to the findings of raised, pink/brown bumps on the forehead, angiofibromas, and Shagreen patches (thickened skin resembling an orange peel).[16,18] While there are many

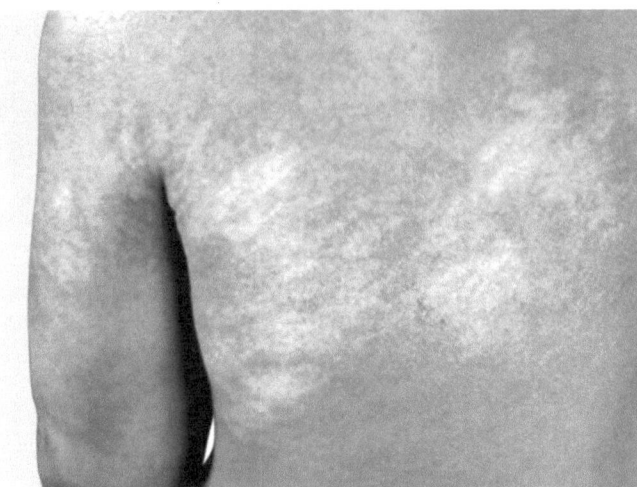

**Fig. 6:** Nevus depigmentosus *(For color version see Plate 5).*
*Source:* Image appears with permission from VisualDx (www.visualdx.com).

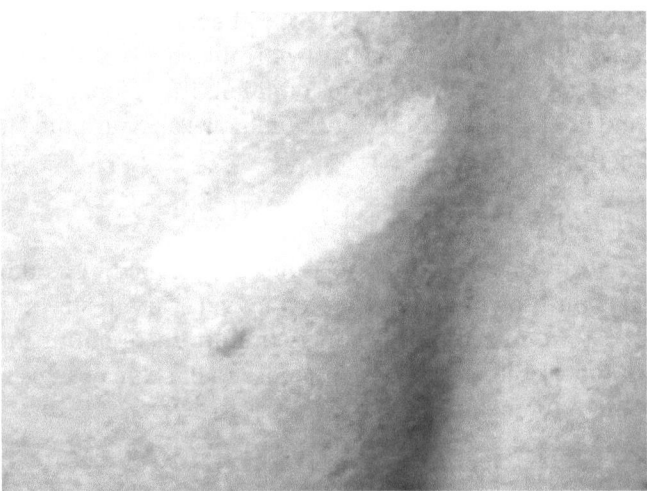

**Fig. 7:** Ash leaf macule *(For color version see Plate 6).*
*Source:* Image appears with permission from VisualDx (www.visualdx.com).

other features for diagnosing tuberous sclerosis, presence of two of these features meets the diagnostic criteria.[17]

### Management and Prognosis

While the presence of a single hypopigmented spot does not meet the criteria for tuberous sclerosis, multiple ash leaf spots associated with other clinical findings described above should prompt further evaluation.[18]

## Mongolian Spot (Blue-Gray Spot) (Fig. 8)

### What is It?

A Mongolian spot is a commonly encountered lesion in newborns with a marked difference in prevalence depending on ethnicity. One study examining 1,058 newborns reported rates as high as 9.6% in newborns of European origin, 95.5% in newborns of African origin, 81% in newborns of East

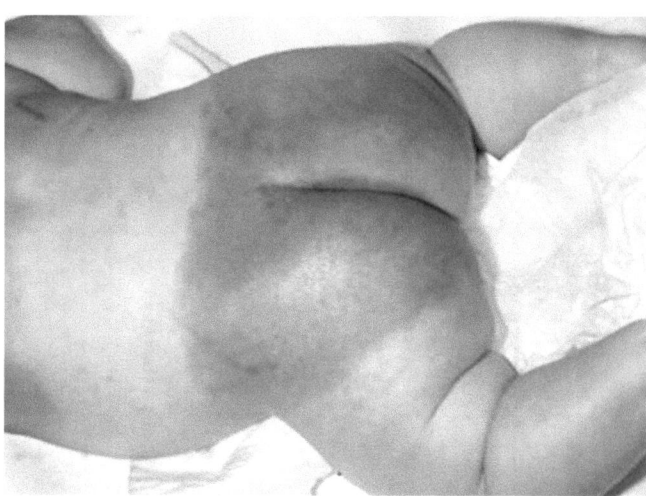

**Fig. 8:** Blue-gray spot (Mongolian spot) *(For color version see Plate 6).*
*Source:* Image appears with permission from VisualDx (www.visualdx.com).

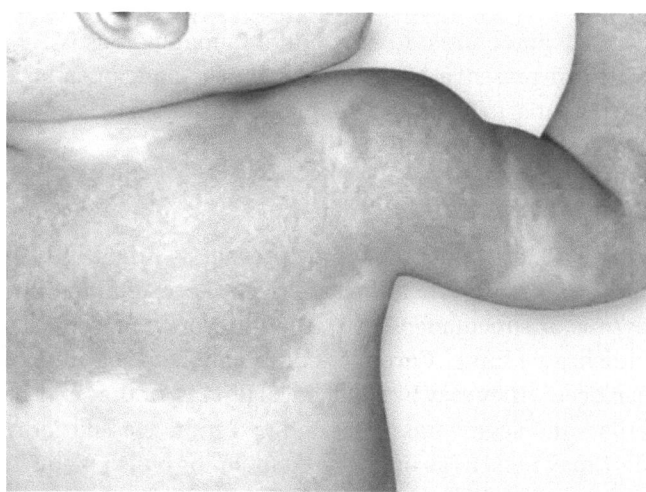

**Fig. 9:** Nevus of Ito *(For color version see Plate 6).*
*Source:* Image appears with permission from VisualDx (www.visualdx.com).

Asian origin, and 70.1% in newborns of Latin American-American Indian origin.[19] These lesions are attributed to delayed disappearance of dermal melanocytes.[9]

### Clinical Presentation

These present as blue-green or blue-gray flat spots, usually located in sacrogluteal area.[20] Similar lesions on the shoulder and periorbital regions are referred to as nevus of Ito **(Fig. 9)** and nevus of Ota, respectively.[21]

### Diagnostic Evaluation

The diagnosis is usually made clinically, but Mongolian spots can be mistaken as bruises secondary to child abuse.[9] Skin biopsy reveals scattered dendritic and melanin-laden melanocytes in the dermis with occasional melanophages.[22]

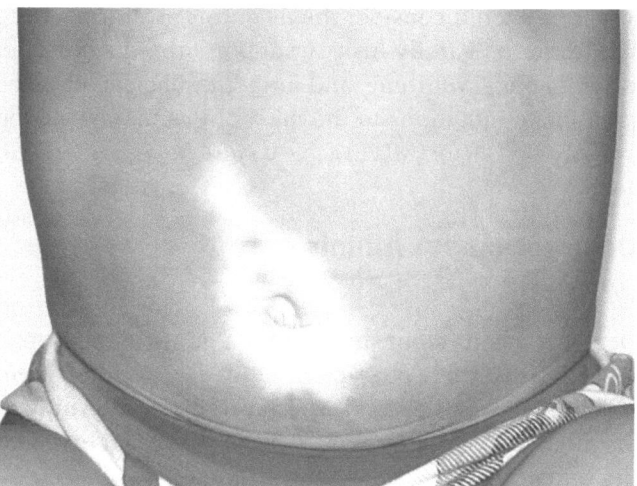

**Fig. 10:** Piebaldism *(For color version see Plate 6).*
*Source:* Image appears with permission from Dr Ki-Young Yoo.

### Management and Prognosis

Mongolian spots typically resolve spontaneously by age of 10 years; however, follow-up is warranted to rule out bruises should child abuse be suspected.[9] Of note, nevus of Ota may warrant a referral to ophthalmology for rare complication of glaucoma or ocular melanoma.[23]

## Piebaldism (Fig. 10)

### What is It?

This is an autosomal dominant condition characterized by hypopigmented or depigmented spots. It is thought to result from a failure of melanocyte migration during embryogenesis.[1] Although the light-colored spots can be seen anywhere on the body, it typically occurs on the hair and scalp (80–90%) resulting in a white forelock.[24]

### Clinical Presentation

The white forelock is a characteristic seen in a large majority of patients. The hypopigmented or depigmented patches of skin are usually present at birth. In addition to the face and forelock, other areas can be involved, such as the trunk and extremities. There may be repigmentation with the light-colored patches, as well as a rim of hyperpigmentation.[24]

### Diagnostic Evaluation

This is a clinical diagnosis.[24] Features of piebaldism can also been seen in Waardenburg syndrome, in which case further testing should be ordered (*see* "Management and Prognosis").

### Management and Prognosis

The depigmentation in piebaldism is permanent, however, patients are usually otherwise healthy.[25] If other findings are present such as facial dysmorphism, irides heterochromia (color difference of the irises), or sensorineural hearing loss, one should consider the diagnosis of Waardenburg syndrome.[1,26] Family history supports the diagnosis of Waardenburg syndrome, and further testing can be done to evaluate mutations in the microphthalmia-associated transcription factor (MITF) gene or *paired box gene 3* (*PAX3*) gene.[27]

## Oculocutaneous Albinism

### What is It?

Oculocutaneous albinism (OCA) is a group of autosomal recessive disorders characterized by decreased pigment in skin, hair, and eyes as a result of melanin synthesis disorder.[1] This disorder is classified as OCA 1–4, based on the genetic defect.

### Clinical Presentation

Patients with OCA type 1A have absence of pigment and present with snow-white hair, blue eyes, and white skin. Ocular anomalies include photophobia, nystagmus, strabismus, and decreased visual acuity. Those with OCA type 1B have some amount of pigment production and may display blond or light-brown hair, some darkening of the eye, or interestingly even have a temperature-sensitive phenotype in which cooler sites such as the acral site show pigment production. OCA types 2 and 4 display variable pigment decrease. Sometimes the disorder may not be obvious unless the pigmentation of the affected individual is compared to those of unaffected family members. Type 2 most commonly affects African-Americans, and type 4 most commonly affects the Japanese. Individuals with OCA type 3 have red hair and blue/brown eyes.[25,28]

### Diagnostic Evaluation

This is a clinical diagnosis although the hair bulb tyrosinase assay can be used to classify the type of OCA.[28] Genetic testing is available for some of the subtypes.

### Management and Prognosis

Given the defect in pigment synthesis, patients are at an increased risk for skin cancers and actinic damage.[25] A study examining skin cancer in 111 patients revealed an overall rate of 23.4% with risk increasing with age.[29] Ophthalmologic care is crucial to prevent complications such as strabismus, impaired visual acuity, nystagmus, and photophobia.[25]

## ■ PLAQUES AND NODULES (RAISED BUMPS)

### Hemangioma (Fig. 11)

### What is It?

Infantile hemangiomas (IHs) represent benign tumors composed of endothelial-like cells. IHs represent the most

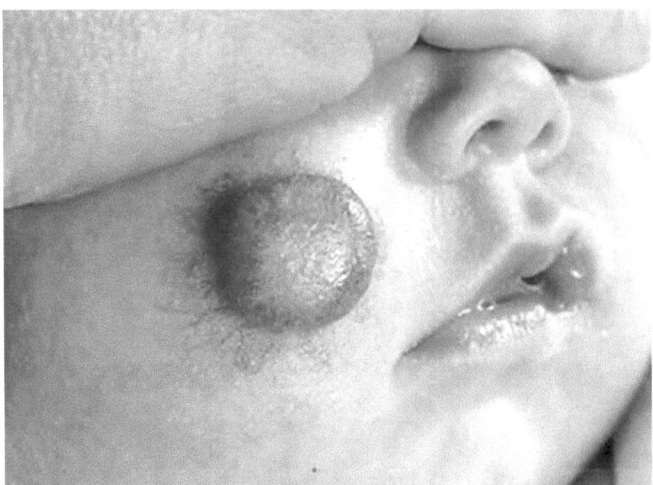

**Fig. 11:** Hemangioma, infantile *(For color version see Plate 6)*.
*Source:* Image appears with permission from VisualDx (www.visualdx.com).

common vascular tumor in healthy newborns, presenting in up to 2%.[30] They are often first seen around 3 weeks of birth, which is in contrast to congenital hemangiomas (CHs), which are present at birth. Both types of hemangiomas have the potential to involute on their own, although CHs do not proliferate after birth as can IHs.

### Clinical Presentation

When IHs are superficial, they present as bright red flat spots or bumps. When they are deep (i.e. extend into the dermis or subcutaneous fat), then they may present as a bluish/gray lump. Certainly combinations of both types can occur. They may be small, focal lesions, or they may be broad and segmental.[30] Depending on the classification, they may present as bright red papules or bluish plaques. Although multiple hemangiomas can be present (*see* "Management and Prognosis"), generally infants have a single hemangioma (75–90%) on the neck or head.

### Diagnostic Evaluation

The distinct natural growth history is helpful in the diagnosis of IHs. They tend to undergo rapid proliferation until about 5 months of age, followed by a "plateau" phase and a slow involutional phase over several years. Certain types of hemangiomas should prompt further evaluations. Segmental hemangiomas of the face can suggest PHACE syndrome (i.e. posterior fossa malformation, hemangioma, arterial lesions, cardiac and eye abnormalities), for which infants may require magnetic resonance imaging (MRI) of the brain, magnetic resonance angiography (MRA)/magnetic resonance venography (MRV) of the brain and neck, echocardiogram, and ophthalmologic evaluation.[31] Segmental hemangiomas in the perineal and lumbosacral area have been associated with the syndromes PELVIS (i.e. perineal hemangioma, external genital abnormalities, lipomyelomeningocele, vesicorenal malformation, imperforate anus, and skin tag) and SACRAL (spinal dysraphism, anogenital, cutaneous, renal and urologic anomalies, and lumbosacral hemangioma), respectively.[32,33]

### Management and Prognosis

Most hemangiomas are uncomplicated. However, a minority may have associated complications that require treatment, such as ulceration, functional impairment, and anatomic distortion or deformities. Thus, prompt referral to an expert should be sought.[30] Recently systemic propranolol has emerged as the treatment of choice for complicated IHs, surpassing the use of oral corticosteroids.[30] For small, thin IHs, topical treatment with timolol, clobetasol (a topical steroid), and pulsed dye laser have been shown to be effective.[30]

## Subcutaneous Fat Necrosis

### What is It?

Subcutaneous fat necrosis (SCN) is a benign skin disorder in which firm subcutaneous nodules result from inflammatory destruction of fat.[34,35] This usually presents during the first few days to weeks of life. It has been associated with various conditions such as perinatal trauma, asphyxia, and hypothermia. It affects healthy full-term newborns and infants.

### Clinical Presentation

Subcutaneous fat necrosis appears as nodules, usually with overlying redness of the skin, usually on the cheeks, back, buttocks, arms, and thighs.[34]

### Diagnostic Evaluation

Diagnosis can be confirmed by skin biopsy, which can show fat necrosis, needle-shaped clefts in adipocytes, and granulomatous inflammation.[34,35]

### Management and Prognosis

Reassurance is important, as SCN tends to resolve over several months. There have been reports of associated hypercalcemia, and thus monitoring by serologic testing for several months is advised.[34,35]

## Nevus Sebaceous (Fig. 12) and Epidermal Nevus (Fig. 13)

### What is It?

Epidermal nevi represent benign overgrowths of structures in the epidermis. They can be divided into two groups,

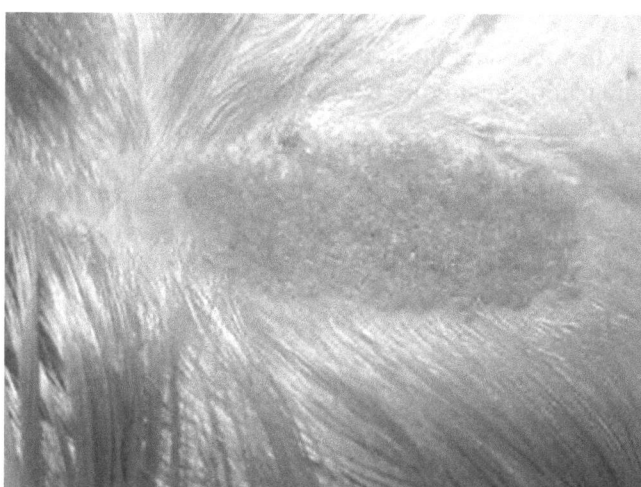

**Fig. 12:** Nevus sebaceous *(For color version see Plate 6).*
Source: Image appears with permission from VisualDx (www.visualdx.com).

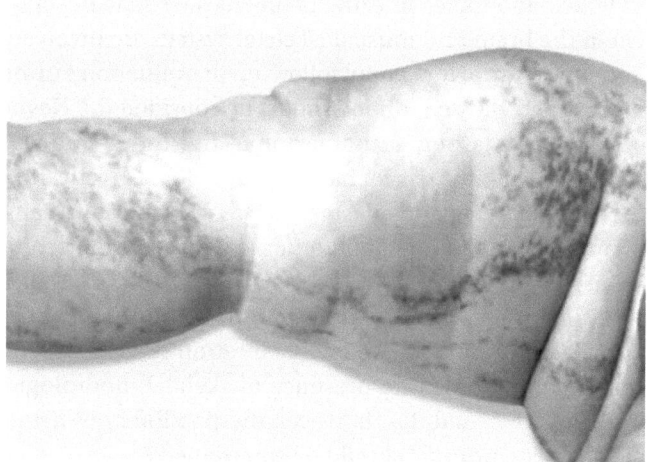

**Fig. 13:** Epidermal nevus *(For color version see Plate 7).*
Source: Image appears with permission from VisualDx (www.visualdx.com).

depending on whether they involve only keratinocytes or other epidermal cells like sebaceous glands. Keratinocytic epidermal nevi (often referred to as "epidermal nevi") are typically noticed at birth and are usually found along the lines of Blaschko. They have been reported to affect 0.1% of all newborns.[36-38] Sebaceous nevus or nevus sebaceous of Jadassohn is seen on the scalp and face, and do not appear to be influenced by ethnicity or sex.[39,40] In one study examining 4,641 newborns, the incidence of nevus sebaceous was reported to be 0.3%.[41]

### Clinical Presentation

The lesion of nevus sebaceous may be present at birth as a yellow or pink-orange linear plaque, although the lesion may not be noticed until it darkens and thickens later in life (secondary to hormonal influence).[1,40] They may develop a cobblestone appearance with time and can present with alopecia when located on the scalp. In contrast, epidermal nevi appear as thin warty plaques distributed in a linear and whorled pattern.[38] It is not uncommon for the lesions to become thicker or darker in appearance with age.

### Diagnostic Evaluation

Both epidermal nevi and nevus sebaceous can be diagnosed clinically, although a skin biopsy can confirm the diagnosis or rule out other disorders (e.g. mosaic epidermolytic ichthyosis).[37,38,40]

### Management and Prognosis

Most epidermal nevi are benign, isolated findings but can be a bothersome cosmetic issue.[1,38] Excisional surgery and carbon dioxide laser may be used but can result in scarring. In those individuals with extensive or large involvement, however, epidermal nevus syndrome should be considered, in which anomalies in extracutaneous sites may develop. Often the brain and musculoskeletal system are involved, and thus referral for careful follow-up or evaluation during infancy and early childhood should be considered.[37] Nevus sebaceous is a benign hamartoma, but there is a <1% associated lifetime risk for basal cell carcinoma arising from it.[42,43] Other benign neoplasms, such as trichoblastoma and syringocystadenoma papilliferum, have been reported to be associated with nevus sebaceous as well.[44] Watchful monitoring is a therapeutic option, but full-thickness surgical excision is also a consideration if cosmetically bothersome.[39,40] In the presence of skeletal, neurologic, and eye abnormalities, however, the possibility of nevus sebaceous syndrome should be entertained.[40]

## Congenital Melanocytic Nevus (Fig. 14)

### What is It?

Congenital melanocytic nevi (CMN) are melanocytic proliferations that usually are present at birth or develop shortly thereafter.[1] They are generally classified by size: (1) small for those less than 1.5 cm, (2) medium for those between 1.5 and 19.9 cm, and (3) large for those equal to or greater than 20 cm. Congenital nevi that cover an extensive surface area are called giant congenital nevi (**Fig. 15**) and have also been termed "garment" or "bathing trunk" nevi. Whereas CMN are present in up to 3% of newborns, only 1 in 20,000 births have large CMN.[45]

### Clinical Presentation

Congenital melanocytic nevus present as tan to dark brown, flat or elevated lesions.[1,46] The texture can vary, ranging from mildly palpable with a smooth quality to a verrucous appearance. Hair may be noted within the lesion.

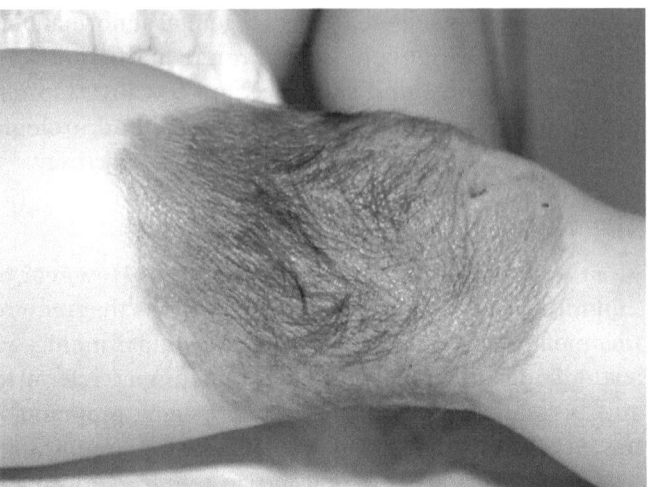

**Fig. 14:** Medium congenital nevus *(For color version see Plate 7)*.
*Source:* Image appears with permission from Dr Ki-Young Yoo.

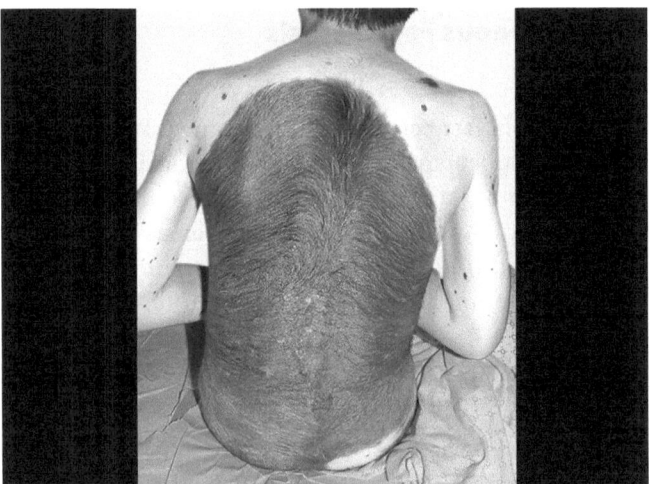

**Fig. 15:** Giant congenital nevus *(For color version see Plate 7)*.
*Source:* Image appears with permission from Dr Ki-Young Yoo.

### Diagnostic Evaluation

Congenital melanocytic nevus are viewed as a clinical diagnosis although biopsy can be pursued, if there is concern for malignancy.[46]

### Management and Prognosis

Congenital melanocytic nevus should be followed carefully. Depending on the size, there is an associated risk of malignant melanoma. Small and medium-sized CMN appears to have a lower risk than once thought, with a recent study reporting the risk of melanoma as less than 1%.[47] Large or giant CMN may be associated with 5–10% risk of melanoma, usually during the prepubertal years.[48] Large CMN may be associated with neurocutaneous melanosis, which refers to a condition in which nevus cells

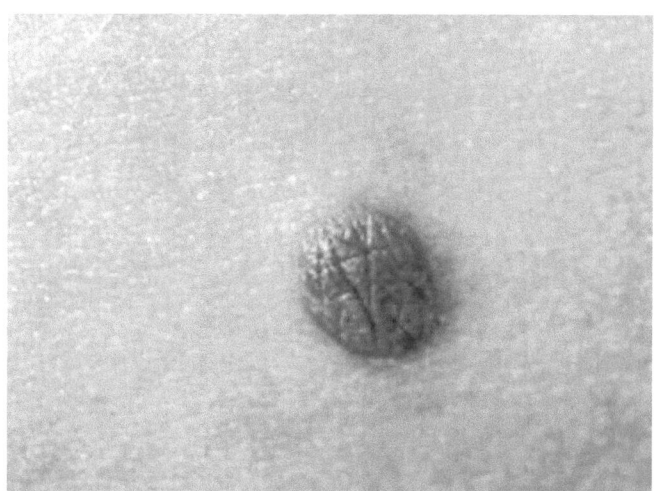

**Fig. 16:** Juvenile xanthogranuloma *(For color version see Plate 7).* Source: Image appears with permission from VisualDx (www.visualdx.com).

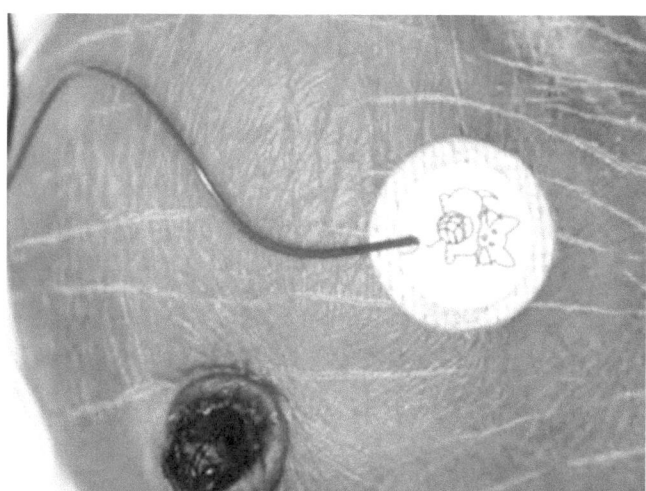

**Fig. 17:** Postmaturity desquamation *(For color version see Plate 7).* Source: Image appears with permission from VisualDx (www.visualdx.com).

proliferate in the central nervous system (CNS). This may result in neurologic symptoms. MRI may be considered for those who have large or giant CMN. While smaller lesions can generally be observed by a dermatologist, larger CMNs may need surgical removal.[46] Disfiguring scars may result from surgical removal, so careful discussion with an experienced surgeon is an important part of individualizing management strategies for patients with large or giant CMN.

## Juvenile Xanthogranuloma (Fig. 16)

### What is It?

Juvenile xanthogranulomas (JXGs) represent a benign proliferation of histiocytic cells.[49] They typically appear within the first year of life and may increase in size and number several months after.[50] Most often they present on the skin from the waist up, although 4% of all cases may present on extracutaneous sites (e.g. the eye and other internal organs).[49]

### Clinical Presentation

Juvenile xanthogranulomas typically present as bumps that can range a few millimeters to centimeters. Early lesions appear red or pink, but over time they evolve to become yellow. Typically lesions are solitary, although some children may have multiple.[50] Some lesions may even ulcerate or crust.

### Diagnostic Evaluation

The diagnosis of JXG can be made on appearance, however, skin biopsy can help confirm the diagnosis.[49]

### Management and Prognosis

Treatment may not be necessary for cutaneous JXGs, as most lesions resolve in 3–6 years.[49,50] Occasionally extracutaneous involvement may occur, which should be suspected for younger children who have multiple lesions. The eye is the most common site of extracutaneous involvement. For children with multiple lesions, the association with juvenile chronic myelogenous leukemia should also be considered, especially if the child has multiple café-au-lait spots or has a history of type 1 NF.

## PAPULOSQUAMOUS ERUPTION (BUMPS AND/OR SCALE)

### Postmaturity Desquamation (Fig. 17)

### What is It?

Postmaturity desquamation is often seen in postmaturity syndrome (approximately 2.2% of deliveries).[51] It is the result of placental insufficiency and usually occurs within the first day of birth. This is an important contrast to normal physiologic desquamation, which usually occurs between 24 hours and 36 hours.

### Clinical Presentation

Desquamation is characteristic of this disorder although other findings such as decreased subcutaneous fat, long hair and nails, or scaling of soles and palms may be present.[51]

### Diagnostic Evaluation

The diagnosis can be made on clinical grounds (as noted above, timing plays an important role).[51]

### Management and Prognosis

Both postmaturity desquamation and normal physiologic desquamation resolve on their own (usually within weeks) and thus require no treatment. Emollients can be used in dry areas.[51]

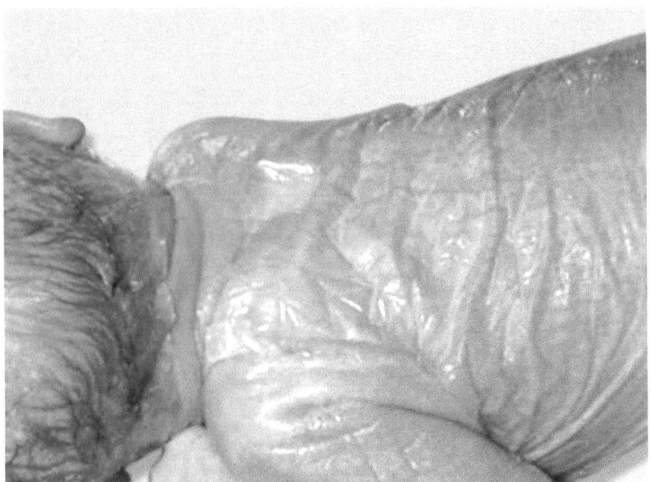

**Fig. 18:** Collodion baby *(For color version see Plate 7)*.
*Source:* Image appears with permission from VisualDx (www.visualdx.com).

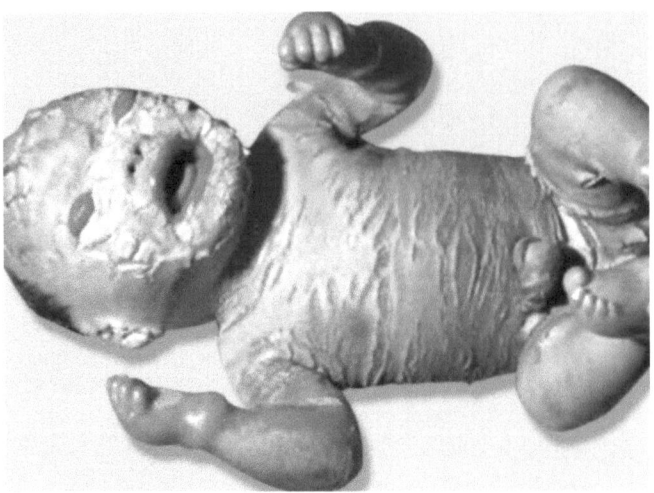

**Fig. 19:** Harlequin fetus *(For color version see Plate 8)*.
*Source:* Image appears with permission from VisualDx (www.visualdx.com).

## Collodion Baby (Fig. 18)

### What is It?

Collodion baby refers to the skin phenotype of a membrane-like covering, and it can be an early sign of several different disorders, the more common including nonbullous congenital ichthyosiform erythroderma (NICH), lamellar ichthyosis, and self-healing collodion baby.[1] While the pathogenesis of the individual disorders is beyond the scope of this chapter, all present at birth with the characteristic tight, "plastic wrapped" membrane appearance.[52]

### Clinical Presentation

In addition to the "plastic wrapped" appearance, the collodion baby may present with facial and extremity distortion along with other complications. Infants may present with ectropion (eversion of the eyelids), peripheral edema, and difficulty breathing due to the thick membrane restricting chest expansion. The membrane itself is a poor barrier, and the infant may suffer from hypernatremic dehydration.[36,53] Erosions are not uncommon and over time, skin changes may manifest, such as thick scales that can be seen in nonbullous icthyosiform erythroderma (NICH) or lamellar ichthyosis (which is usually less red than NICH and often has darker scales).[54]

### Diagnostic Evaluation

The diagnosis is made clinically. After the collodion membrane sheds, the baby's skin may be normal (self-healing collodion), or over time, the underlying ichthyosis may become more apparent. Skin biopsy is generally not helpful. Genetic testing should be pursued to further characterize the underlying ichthyosis.[52,54]

### Management and Prognosis

Acutely, the baby should be monitored carefully in the neonatal intensive care unit (NICU). Because the collodion membrane has poor barrier function, the baby should be placed in a humidified incubator, where thermal, electrolyte, fluid, and metabolic stability can be better managed. Careful surveillance for infection should also be performed.[52]

## Harlequin Ichthyosis (Fig. 19)

### What is It?

Ichthyosis is a broad term that encompasses many different disorders in which there is problem with keratinization resulting in widespread scaling of the skin.[55] Included in this group are NICH and lamellar ichthyosis (*see* above), which represent autosomal recessive congenital ichthyoses. Harlequin ichthyosis deserves special attention, as it can be associated with a high neonatal mortality rate.[1]

### Clinical Presentation

Harlequin ichthyosis has a distinct and dramatic presentation with thick, "armor-like" scales often presenting with underdeveloped appendages, ectropion, and eclabium (eversion of lips).[1] Eyelashes and eyebrows are typically absent as well.[56]

### Diagnostic Evaluation

Few other conditions resemble harlequin ichthyosis. It is considered a diagnosis of infancy, however, prenatal diagnosis involving fetal skin biopsy can be done.[56]

### Management and Prognosis

Management in the NICU is crucial upon recognition of harlequin ichthyosis, as the skin barrier is defective and

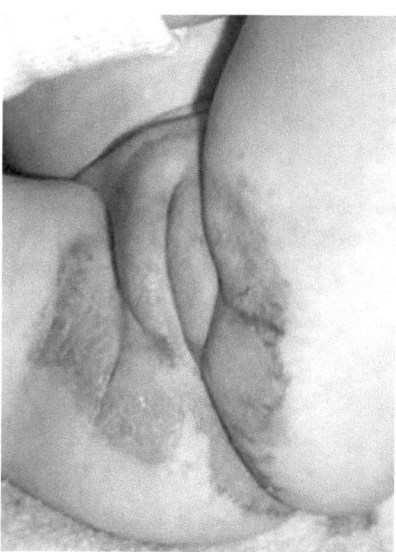

**Fig. 20:** Hereditary acrodermatitis enteropathica
*(For color version see Plate 8).*
*Source:* Image appears with permission from VisualDx (www.visualdx.com).

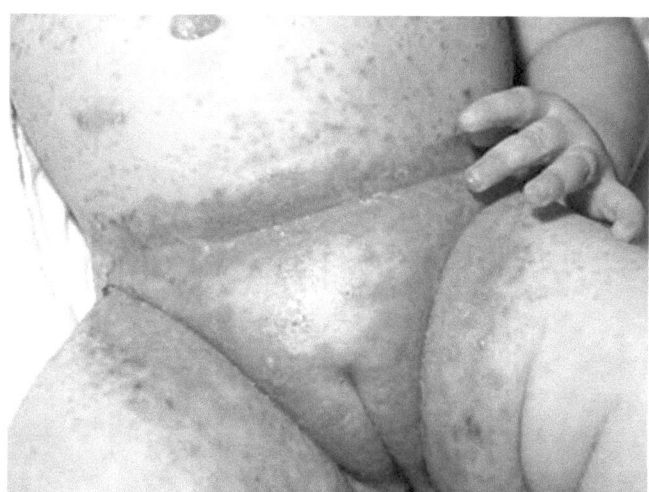

**Fig. 21:** Langerhans cell histiocytosis *(For color version see Plate 8).*
*Source:* Image appears with permission from VisualDx (www.visualdx.com).

can result in thermal, electrolyte, fluid, and metabolic instability. Many newborns with harlequin ichthyosis may die during the first few days of life. Those who survive may benefit from topical or systemic retinoid therapy, in addition to other supportive measures that may involve specialists such as surgeons and ophthalmologists.[56]

## Hereditary Acrodermatitis Enteropathica (Fig. 20)

### What is It?

This is a rare nutritional disorder inherited in an autosomal recessive fashion. As a result of poor zinc absorption, the infant develops the "classic triad" of diarrhea, dermatitis, and alopecia.[57] This usually present when the child no longer receives breast milk, but can present as early as 4–10 weeks (e.g. in infants exclusively fed formula).

### Clinical Presentation

The skin eruption may be red and scaly or blisters, and these tend to develop on acral and periorificial (mouth, nose, ears, eyes, and perineum) sites. Nail deformity is not uncommon. Infants with this disease are irritable and may show failure to thrive. Of note, acquired forms of zinc deficiency can also present with these findings. The acquired form can result from inadequate secretion of zinc in maternal milk, or those who otherwise cannot properly absorb or store zinc.[36,57]

### Diagnostic Evaluation

Low serum zinc level (50 ug/dL or lower) can be used to reaffirm the diagnosis in conjunction with the clinical picture.[36] Skin biopsy may also be a helpful tool.[57]

### Management and Prognosis

Zinc supplementation is crucial for treatment. Rapid improvement is often noted, although lifelong supplementation is needed.[57]

## Langerhans Cell Histiocytosis (Fig. 21)

### What is It?

Langerhans cell histiocytosis (LCH) is the result of the overaccumulation of dendritic histiocytes in one or more organs (e.g. skin, liver, and bone).[58] Symptoms can range depending on the site of involvement, including osteolytic lesions due to bone involvement and diabetes insipidus as a result of CNS involvement.[59] A majority of cases present before the age of 4, with younger children typically having more severe disease.[58,59] Although rare, this is an important disease to consider, especially in a child with resistant and/or atypical diaper rash.

### Clinical Presentation

The skin is involved in approximately 40% of cases and can vary in presentation from scaly red-brown bumps to small blister-like lesions.[36,58,59] The scalp, ears, and perineum may be involved, with a seborrheic dermatitis-like eruption being the classic finding. As mentioned above, diaper dermatitis with features of petechiae or oozing should include LCH in the differential. Given the potential for systemic involvement, it is important to consider other signs of organ dysfunction in addition to other constitutional findings such as fever and weight loss.

### Diagnostic Evaluation

Skin biopsy can be helpful in confirming the diagnosis, with the characteristic findings of CD1a infiltrate and S100

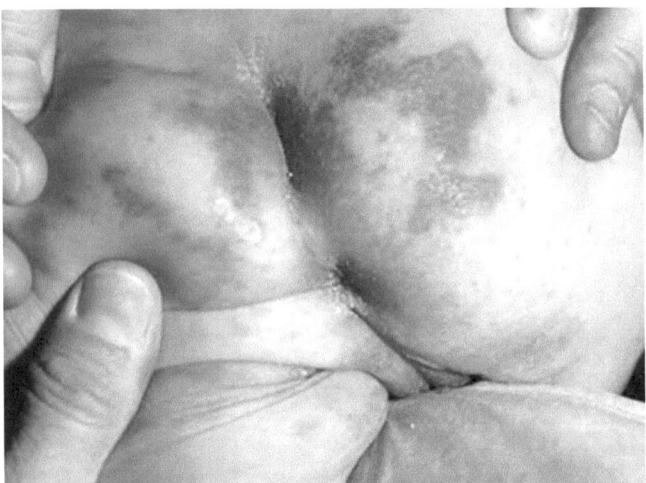

**Fig. 22:** Psoriasis *(For color version see Plate 8).*
Source: Image appears with permission from VisualDx (www.visualdx.com).

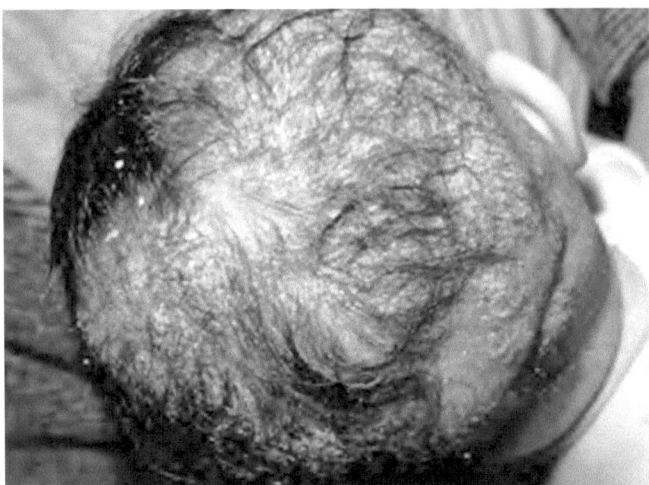

**Fig. 23:** Seborrheic dermatitis *(For color version see Plate 8).*
Source: Image appears with permission from VisualDx (www.visualdx.com).

positive histiocytic cells on immunohistochemistry. Further testing may be required, however, such as radiologic studies to determine the extent of involvement and require the care of a pediatric oncologist.[58]

### Management and Prognosis

There is an estimated 80% 3-year survival rate for patients with LCH, although prognosis is affected by age of diagnosis and organ involvement. Topical steroids, nitrogen mustard, or systemic therapy can be used for isolated skin involvement, although a multidisciplinary approach may be warranted with greater organ involvement and chemotherapy may even be indicated.[58]

## Infantile Psoriasis (Fig. 22)

### What is It?

Psoriasis is seen in approximately 2% of the pediatric population by the age of 2 years.[60] Resulting from hyperproliferation of the epidermal layer, infantile psoriasis is similar to that of the adult form in its presentation of discrete erythematous plaques. Individuals often have a strong family history and may present with nail findings such as pitting and oil spots. Infantile psoriasis is unique in that it is typically not pruritic and/or generalized.

### Clinical Presentation

As noted above, infantile psoriasis may present similarly to adult psoriasis with discrete erythematous plaques.[60] There may be less white scale, however, especially in the diaper region.

### Diagnostic Evaluation

Lesions can be treated empirically with topical steroids prior to further evaluation. Other tests such as potassium hydroxide (KOH) preparation and skin biopsy can be considered if other conditions are suspected (e.g. seborrheic dermatitis, candida).[60]

### Management and Prognosis

Topical therapy usually suffices for infantile psoriasis, with topical steroids as the mainstay of treatment.[60] Depending on the area of involvement, other treatments can be used as well (e.g. barrier creams in the diaper area).

## Seborrheic Dermatitis (Fig. 23)

### What is It?

In a newborn or infant, seborrheic dermatitis can affect many different areas. It is an inflammatory disorder believed to result from hormonal effects on sebaceous glands. It is an important diagnosis to keep in the differential for diaper dermatitis, and is often referred to as "cradle cap" when it involves the scalp.[36,61]

### Clinical Presentation

Seborrheic dermatitis of infancy presents with an erythematous base often with overlying soft white/yellow scale[61] **(Fig. 24)**. The soft white/yellow scale is helpful in making the diagnosis as other disorders such as psoriasis and atopic dermatitis can manifest in a similar pattern.

### Diagnostic Evaluation

The diagnosis of seborrheic dermatitis is typically made on clinical grounds.[61]

### Management and Prognosis

The disease itself is usually active during the first year of life, mostly during the first few months. Therapy such as mild shampoo or mineral/baby oil can be used for the

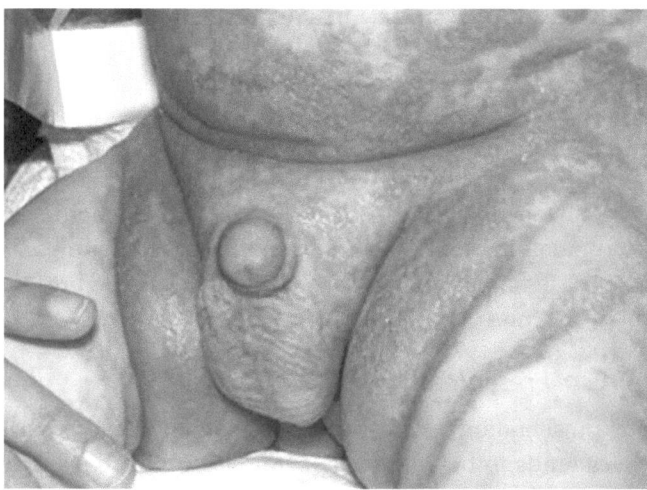

**Fig. 24:** Seborrheic dermatitis *(For color version see Plate 8).*
Source: Image appears with permission from VisualDx (www.visualdx.com).

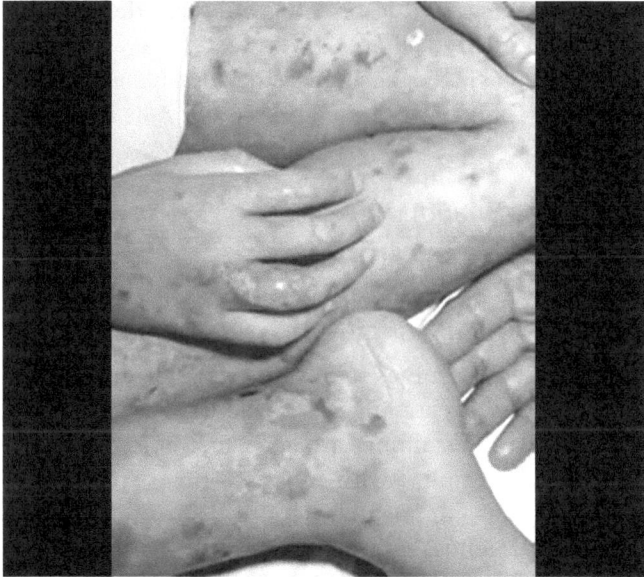

**Fig. 25:** Epidermolysis bullosa simplex *(For color version see Plate 9).*
Source: Image appears with permission from VisualDx (www.visualdx.com).

scalp, although low-potency topical steroids can be used to help with inflammation and spots on the body. Antifungal creams like ketoconazole may also help with spots on the body. The disease usually responds well to treatment after a couple of weeks, prompting other diagnoses should the spots prove to be resistant to treatment.[61]

## ■ VESICULOPUSTULAR ERUPTIONS (BLISTERS AND/OR PUSTULES)

### Epidermolysis Bullosa (Fig. 25)

#### What is It?

Epidermolysis bullosa (EB) is an inherited disorder of skin fragility, in which blisters form as a result of varying degrees of friction or trauma.[62] They are classified according to the site of skin cleavage and the mode of inheritance. The most common form is epidermolysis bullosa simplex (EBS), which is the result of intraepidermal skin separation and generally presents with blistering without residual scarring.[63] Junctional epidermolysis bullosa (JEB) is the result of separation of skin between the epidermis and dermis, more specifically within the lamina lucida, and presents as blistering with scarring. Dystrophic epidermolysis bullosa (DEB) results from skin separation in the dermis, below the basement membrane, and also manifests as blistering associated with scarring. Some subtypes of EB can present within days of birth and can carry high mortality rates.[1,64]

### Clinical Presentation

The subtypes of EB can have characteristic presentations, and each can be associated with good or poor outcomes. The details of each subtype are beyond the scope of this chapter. However, it is important to note that there can be much overlap in the neonatal period. Early in life, a newborn who may have a subtype of EB with good prognosis may present with severe, widespread blistering, making the precise diagnosis based on clinical evaluation alone difficult.[65] Many of the classic phenotypes may not appear until the child is older.[62] The severe phenotypes seen in the neonatal period may include generalized blistering erosions or ulcers. Milder phenotypes may also be apparent in the newborn period, such as localized blisters of the dorsal hands or extensor surfaces of extremities in young infants with the dominantly-inherited form of dystrophic EB.

### Diagnostic Evaluation

In order to diagnose the specific type of EB, a skin biopsy of a fresh blister is important. The skin biopsy specimen should be sent for immunofluorescent mapping or electron microscopy.[1] When doing a skin biopsy to evaluate for EB, selecting a fresh blister is very important. Family history can often be helpful as many of the EB subtypes are inherited in an autosomal dominant pattern.[62]

### Management and Prognosis

Although there is no cure for EB, several measures can be undertaken, especially in the neonatal setting, to minimize morbidity and mortality.[65] It is important to take a multidisciplinary approach to treating EB, and treatment should occur in a facility with appropriate resources to manage the complications associated with widespread skin blistering or erosions.[66] Prevention of new blisters is important and requires numerous measures such as gentle handing of the infant, generous application of lubricant, and avoiding overheating, which can make skin fragility worse.[65] Wounds require specific management with special attention to nonadherent dressings and tapes in addition to infection control measures.[66] Severe forms of EB may also require nutritional support, and extracutaneous involvement (e.g. ocular lesions) should be actively sought given that certain subtypes such as recessive dystrophic EB may require further follow up. Pain control is important throughout the process in addition to psychosocial support, which is also crucial to treatment.[65,66]

### Aplasia Cutis Congenita (Fig. 26)

*What is It?*

Aplasia cutis congenita (ACC) refers to an absence of skin in the newborn. In a majority of newborns, this presents as an isolated finding, however, it may be associated with other malformations, including trisomy 13.[67]

*Clinical Presentation*

Aplasia cutis congenita may occur on any part of the body, although it characteristically occurs on the head. One should pay attention to the "hair collar sign" (thick rim of hair around the lesion) when the lesion occurs on the scalp as it may signify CNS dysraphism. The lesion can present as an open erosion or healing scar with overlying bulla that may drain and refill.[67]

*Diagnostic Evaluation*

No specific tests are necessary although imaging may be needed in certain situations (e.g. hair collar sign).[67]

*Management and Prognosis*

The lesions of ACC have the potential to heal on their own and should receive proper wound care. Intralesional steroid injections and/or surgery may be needed in some cases, however.[67]

### Mastocytosis

*What is It?*

Mastocytosis is a disorder of mast cells in which there is an accumulation in the skin and sometimes in other organs. Most cases are evident in early childhood but can present in the newborn.[68,69]

*Clinical Presentation*

The presentation on the skin for congenital or early-onset cases tends to be—(1) mastocytomas, in which a single or multiple bumps that are skin-colored or yellow/tan develop; these usually have a "peau d'orange" (orange peel-like) surface or (2) urticaria pigmentosa, in which numerous brown or dull-red spots or bumps develop, and may be generalized all over the body with easy blistering. A helpful point in diagnosing mastocytosis is Darier's sign, in which rubbing or repeated pressure results in redness and wheal.[68,69]

*Diagnostic Evaluation*

Skin biopsy can be used to confirm the diagnosis.[68]

*Management and Prognosis*

Management involves avoiding triggers of mast cell degranulation. Treatment can be offered for symptomatic cases, and antihistamines are good first-line options.[68,69] Localized treatment with potent topical steroids for mastocytomas can also be helpful. In pediatric cases, mastocytosis tends to resolve spontaneously, often before puberty. The involvement of extracutaneous sites or hematologic malignancy is rare.

### Incontinentia Pigmenti (Fig. 27)

*What is It?*

Incontinentia pigmenti is an X-linked dominant disorder that results from mutations in nuclear factor-KB (NF-KB) essential modulator (NEMO) gene. Given this mode of inheritance, it is usually seen in females; it tends to be lethal in males. The disorder can involve the skin, teeth, CNS, and eyes. Skin involvement may be the most prominent finding in the newborn (90% have skin involvement by week 2 of life).[36,70,71]

*Clinical Presentation*

There are four stages that can be seen in the skin. The first stage involves red bumps and blisters forming along

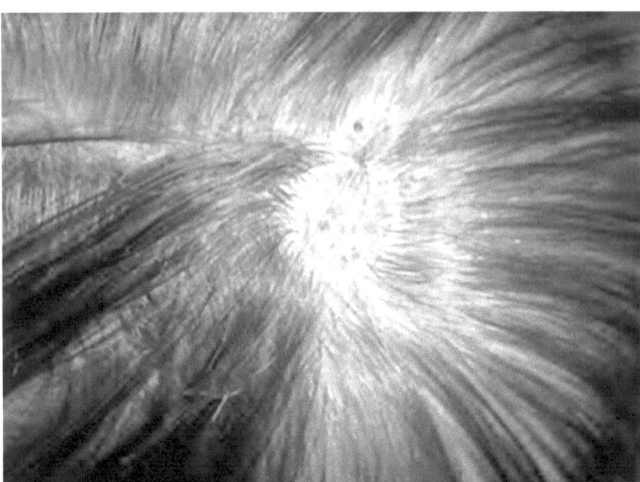

**Fig. 26:** Aplasia cutis congenita *(For color version see Plate 9).*
Source: Image appears with permission from VisualDx (www.visualdx.com).

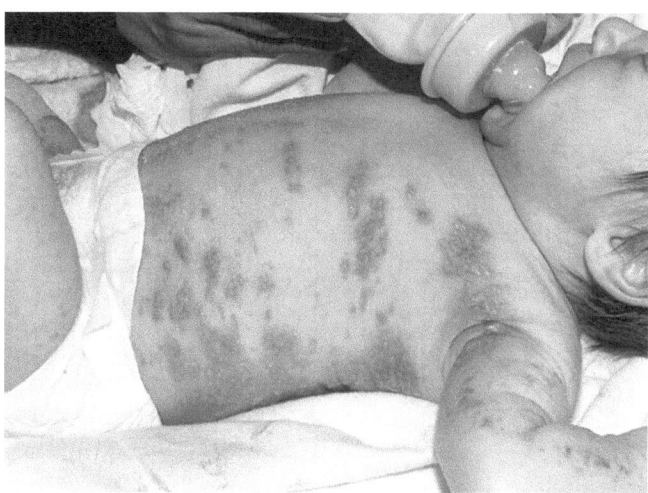

**Fig. 27:** Incontinentia pigmenti *(For color version see Plate 9).*
Source: Image appears with permission from Dr Ki-Young Yoo.

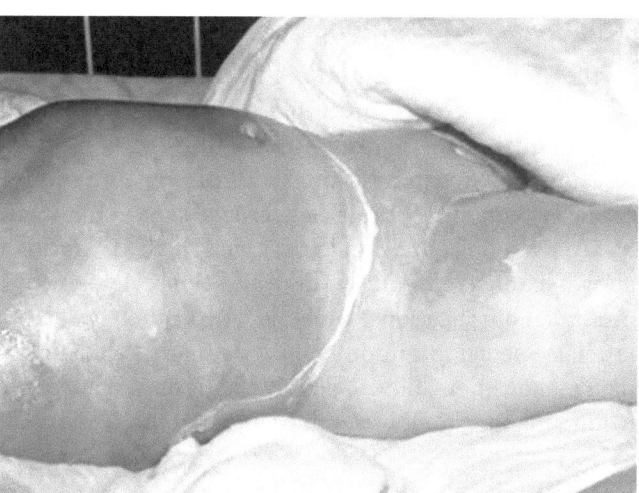

**Fig. 28:** Staphylococcal scalded skin syndrome *(For color version see Plate 9).*
Source: Image appears with permission from VisualDx (www.visualdx.com).

the lines of Blaschko, which may last for months. 70% of patients may then progress into the second stage, which is characterized by warty lesions forming in a linear or swirled pattern. 80% of patients may then experience the third stage that presents as hyperpigmentation in a "marble cake pattern," ultimately evolving into atrophic and/or hypopigmented streaks in the final stage. It is important to note that although these four stages have unique findings, they may overlap in timing.[36,70]

### Diagnostic Evaluation

Skin biopsy can be used to aid in the diagnosis. Genetic testing may also be used, with 85% of patients having a mutation in the *NEMO gene*.[70,72] It is important to also examine the mother, as the affected child's mother may have history of skin changes and tooth/hair loss at an early age, which may further suggest the diagnosis.[71]

### Management and Prognosis

Multidisciplinary management is important involving neurology, ophthalmology, and genetics. The blisters and warty changes of the earlier stages tend to involute, whereas bleaching agents can be used to assist with any pigmentary changes of the later stages.[71]

## Staphylococcal Scalded Skin Syndrome (Fig. 28)

### What is It?

Staphylococcal scalded skin syndrome (SSSS) is an important clinical diagnosis that can have fatal consequences if not treated appropriately.[73] It is a blistering skin disease that results from a toxin released by the bacteria *Staphylococcus aureus,* often secondary to a site of focal infection (e.g. the nose, eyes, umbilicus, or perineum). Infants are believed to be at increased risk due to their poor ability to excrete the toxin and lack of antitoxin antibodies.[36] Although cases in older children may be mild, neonates and infants with extensive skin blistering or peeling require hospitalization with special attention to supportive care (*see* "Management and Prognosis").[36,73]

### Clinical Presentation

The rash of SSSS classically begins with extensive erythema followed by large fragile blisters.[36,73] Infants may also present with sudden irritability and fever in addition to radial fissuring around the mouth, nose, and eyes. The eruption is often most notable in the flexural creases, and the blisters display the interesting phenomenon referred to as "Nikolsky sign" (gentle pressure causing extension of the blister). This can be further complicated by extensive shedding of the skin, which puts the child at increased risk of complications such as infection, poor temperature regulation, and fluid/electrolyte imbalances.

### Diagnostic Evaluation

Staphylococcal scalded skin syndrome can usually be diagnosed clinically, however, it is important to distinguish it from toxic epidermal necrolysis, which is an extensive blistering disorder in which the full thickness of the skin is necrosed; this disorder is usually secondary to a medication reaction and is therefore rare in newborns.[36] One useful distinction is that SSSS does not affect mucosal surfaces, although sloughed skin can be examined by frozen sections if the diagnosis remains in question.[73] Cultures from suspected sites of infection (e.g. nose and eyes) should be obtained as fluid from the blisters is generally sterile.

## Management and Prognosis

In the neonate, treatment of SSSS revolves around eliminating toxin production and supportive care. This requires intravenous penicillinase-resistance antistaphylococcal antibiotics and proper initiation of contact isolation.[36,73] The latter is crucial as SSSS outbreaks have been reported in nurseries as well as NICUs. As noted above, extensive denudation of the skin carries with it multiple complications, which is why supportive care is crucial. Special attention should be made in regards to pain management, fluid/electrolyte control, and infection/wound management including generous emollient use.

## Benign Transient Eruptions

### Erythema Toxicum Neonatorum (Fig. 29)

Erythema Toxicum Neonatorum (ETN) is a fairly common presentation in the newborn, being reported in as many as 72% of all newborns.[74] The exact cause is not known; it rarely presents in premature infants.[75] The lesions typically present after birth (within 2-4 days) and are characterized by multiple papules and pustules with an inflammatory base. The hands and feet are typically spared, which is not the case in transient neonatal pustular melanosis (TNPM). The disease typically resolves within hours, requiring no treatment, although a Wright stain can be performed to confirm the diagnosis.

### Transient Neonatal Pustular Melanosis (Fig. 30)

Similar to ETN, TNPM usually presents in term newborns, although it typically occurs in black infants.[9] The cause is unknown, and is characterized by multiple pustules that are present at birth that may rupture and leave behind

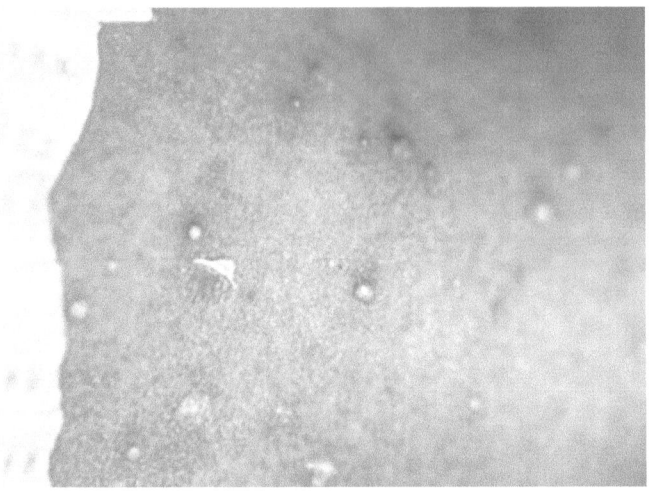

**Fig. 30:** Transient neonatal pustular dermatosis *(For color version see Plate 9).*
*Source:* Image appears with permission from VisualDx (www.visualdx.com).

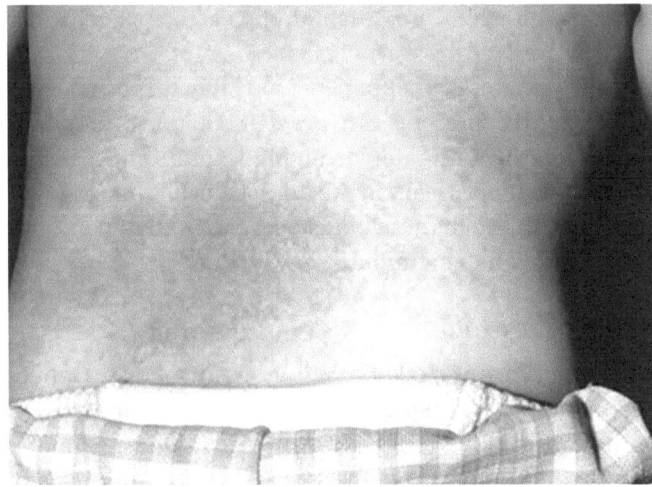

**Fig. 31:** Miliaria rubra *(For color version see Plate 10).*
*Source:* Image appears with permission from VisualDx (www.visualdx.com).

pigmented macules and/or scale.[76] TNPM, like ETN, resolves on its own and requires no therapy (although a Wright stain can be performed to confirm the diagnosis).

### Miliaria (Figs. 31 and 32)

Not to be confused with milia (keratin cysts), miliaria represent an occlusion of sweat ducts.[9] Several distinct forms may present in the newborn. This includes miliaria crystallina (which resembles "dewdrops") and miliaria rubra ("heat rash"). Like ETN, this typically does not present at birth but rather within the first week. The rash tends to involve the head and the intertriginous areas and may be associated with factors related to warming or occlusion. Wright stain may be used to confirm the diagnosis, although like ETN and TNPM, miliaria is benign and can be alleviated with cooling measures.

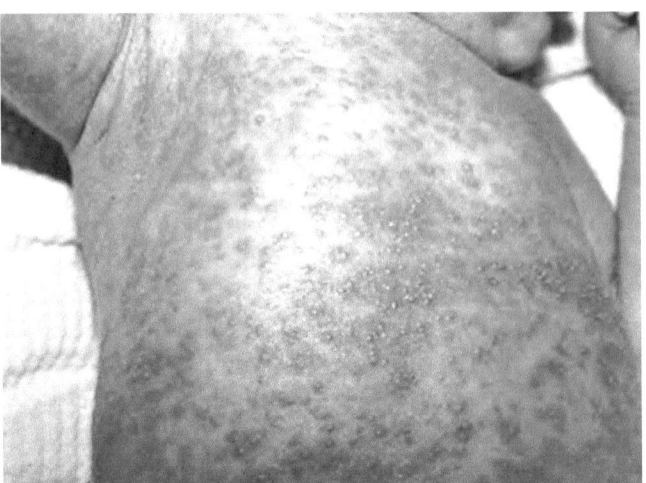

**Fig. 29:** Erythema toxicum neonatorum *(For color version see Plate 9).*
*Source:* Image appears with permission from VisualDx (www.visualdx.com).

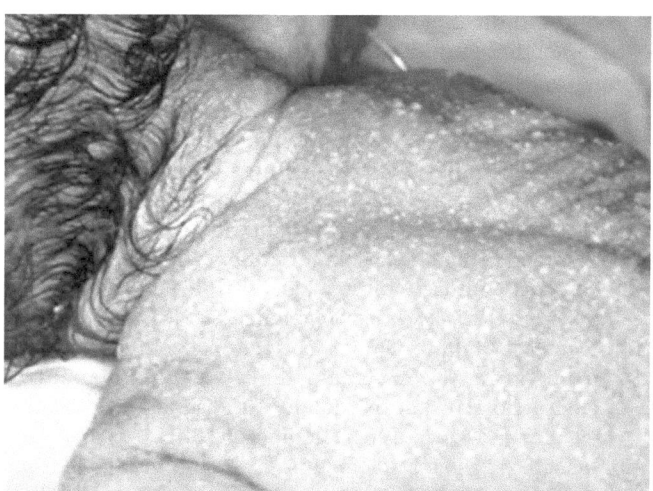

**Fig. 32:** Miliaria crystallina *(For color version see Plate 10).*
*Source:* Image appears with permission from VisualDx (www.visualdx.com).

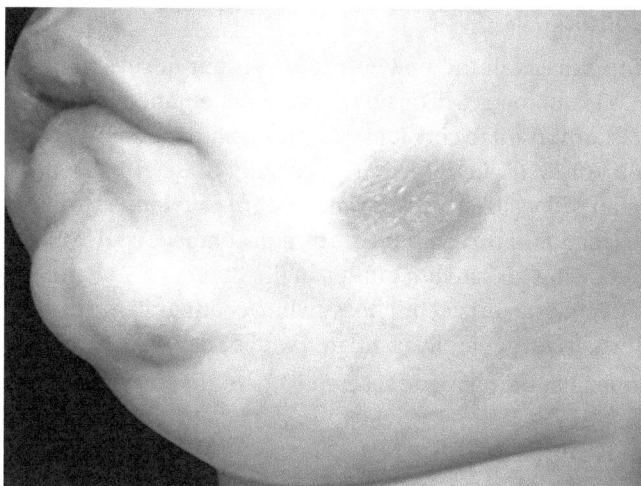

**Fig. 33:** Herpes simplex virus *(For color version see Plate 10).*
*Source:* Image appears with permission from VisualDx (www.visualdx.com).

## Miscellaneous Eruptions

### Herpes Simplex (Fig. 33) and Varicella (Fig. 34)

Unlike their adult forms, both herpes simplex virus (HSV) and *varicella-zoster virus* (VZV) can manifest in different ways in the neonate. HSV is typically acquired from close contacts and may not appear as grouped lesions as it does in adults.[77] In contrast, varicella can be contracted in utero, at birth, or by close contacts.[78] In addition, it can have severe consequences in low birth weight infants or those born before 28 weeks. Diagnosis can be confirmed in both by using several different tests (Tzanck prep, culture, and polymerase chain reaction).[77,78] Treatment may entail isolation in both conditions along with antiviral therapy. Whereas HSV usually utilizes an acyclovir regimen, treatment for VZV depends on several factors and may require both varicella-zoster immune globulin (human) and acyclovir.

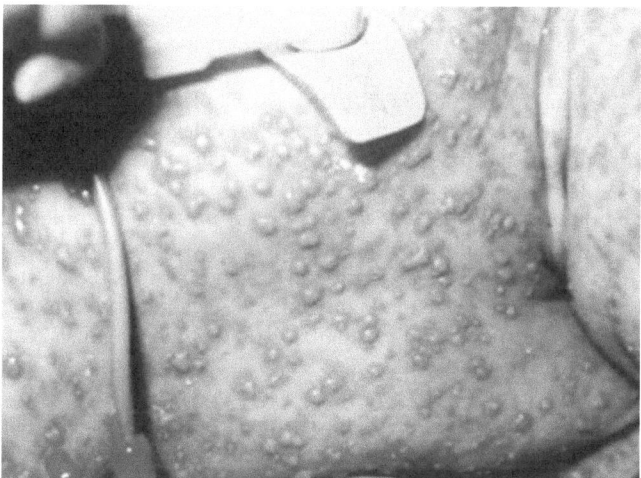

**Fig. 34:** Neonatal varicella (chickenpox) *(For color version see Plate 10).*
*Source:* Image appears with permission from VisualDx (www.visualdx.com).

### Scabies (Fig. 35)

In the infant, scabies can present as a multiple small bumps or even small blisters that can affect any site of the skin, including the face and scalp. This is in contrast to adults who usually do not have involvement of the face and scalp. Itching is the primary symptom, although young infants who cannot scratch may manifest pruritus in other ways such as head rubbing or irritability. Mineral oil scraping can be used to confirm the diagnosis, and infants older than 2 months can be treated with permethrin 5% cream (6% sulfur ointment for those younger than 2 months). Questioning family members is crucial, as similar symptoms may aid in the diagnosis and appropriate treatment of the family is needed to ensure successful resolution.[36,79,80]

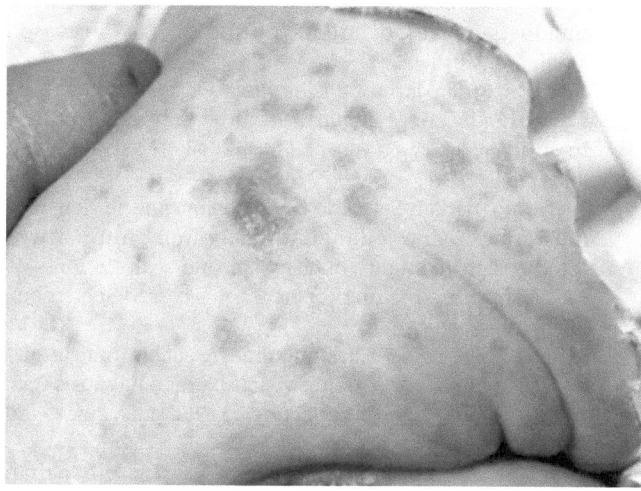

**Fig. 35:** Scabies *(For color version see Plate 10).*
*Source:* Image appears with permission from VisualDx (www.visualdx.com).

## Candidiasis

Candidiasis in the newborn can present in several ways. While our focus will be on limited mucocutaneous disease, it is important to consider widespread cutaneous infection and/or systemic infection, especially in low birth weight infants. Localized disease generally presents either as diaper dermatitis or thrush, with the former characterized by beefy red rash with satellite bumps in the diaper region and the latter characterized by cheesy white coatings in the mouth. Thrush can generally be treated with oral nystatin, whereas topical antifungals are reserved for cutaneous disease.[36, 81]

## REFERENCES

1. Eichenfield L, Frieden I, Mathes E, et al. Neonatal Dermatology, 2nd edition. Philadelphia: Saunders Elsevier; 2007.
2. UptoDate. Vascular Lesions in the Newborn. [online] Available from: http://www.uptodate.com/contents/vascular-lesions-in-the-newborn. [Last accessed September, 2019].
3. VisualDx. Salmon Patch. [online] Available from: http://www.visualdx.com/visualdx/visualdx6/getDiagnosisText.do?moduleId=23&diagnosisId=53402. [Last accessed September, 2019].
4. Juern AM, Glick ZR, Drolet BA, et al. Nevus simplex: a reconsideration of nomenclature, sites of involvement, and disease associations. J Am Acad Dermatol. 2010;63(5):805-14.
5. VisualDx. Port-Wine Stain. [online] Available from: http://www.visualdx.com/visualdx/visualdx6/getDiagnosisText.do?moduleId=10&diagnosisId=52030. [Last accessed September, 2019].
6. UptoDate. Laser and Light Therapy for Cutaneous Vascular Lesions. [online] Available from: http://www.uptodate.com/contents/laser-and-light-therapy-for-cutaneous-vascular-lesions. [Last accessed September, 2019].
7. UpToDate. Capillary Malformations (Port Wine Stains): Clinical Features, Diagnosis, and associated Syndrome. [online] Available from: www.uptodate.com/contents/capillary-malformations-port-wine-stains-clinical-features-diagnosis-and-associated-syndromes. [Last accessed September, 2019].
8. VisualDx. Cutis Marmorata. [online] Available from: http://www.visualdx.com/visualdx/visualdx6/getDiagnosisText.do?moduleId=23&diagnosisId=52641. [Last accessed September, 2019].
9. UpToDate. Benign Skin and Scalp Lesions in the Newborn and Young Infant. [online] Available from: http://www.uptodate.com/contents/benign-skin-and-scalp-lesions-in-the-newborn-and-young-infant. [Last accessed September, 2019].
10. VisualDx. Café au Lait Macule. [online] Available from: http://www.visualdx.com/visualdx/visualdx6/getDiagnosisText.do?moduleId=23&diagnosisId=53196. [Last accessed September, 2019].
11. UpToDate. Benign Pigmented Skin Lesions other than Melanocytic Nevi (Moles). [online] Available from: www.uptodate.com/contents/benign-pigmented-skin-lesions-other-than-melanocytic-nevi-moles. [Last accessed September, 2019].
12. UpToDate. Neurofibromatosis Type 1 (NF1): Pathogenesis, Clinical Features, and Diagnosis. [online] Available from: www.uptodate.com/contents/neurofibromatosis-type-1-nf1-pathogenesis-clinical-features-and-diagnosis. [Last accessed September, 2019].
13. UpToDate. Approach to the Patient with Hyperpigmentation Disorders. [online] Available from: http://www.uptodate.com/contents/approach-to-the-patient-with-hyperpigmentation-disorders. [Last accessed September, 2019].
14. VisualDx. Multiple Lentigines Syndrome. [online] Available from: http://www.visualdx.com/visualdx/visualdx6/getDiagnosisText.do?moduleId=10&diagnosisId=51984&view=text. [Last accessed September, 2019].
15. VisualDx. Nevus Depigmentosus. [online] Available from: www.visualdx.com/visualdx/visualdx6/getDiagnosisText.do?moduleId=10&diagnosisId=52028. [Last accessed Sepember, 2019].
16. UpToDate. Tuberous Sclerosis Complex: Genetics, Clinical Features, and Diagnosis. [online] Available from: www.uptodate.com/contents/tuberous-sclerosis-complex-genetics-clinical-features-and-diagnosis. [Last accessed September, 2019].
17. UpToDate. Diagnostic Criteria for Tuberous Sclerosis Complex. [online] Available from: http://www.uptodate.com/contents/image?imageKey=NEURO/66759&topicKey=PEDS%2F6175&source=outline_link&search=Tuberous+sclerosis+complex%3A+Genetics%2C+clinical+features%2C+and+diagnosis&utdPopup=true. [Last accessed September, 2019].
18. VisualDx. Tuberous Sclerosis. [online] Available from: http://www.visualdx.com/visualdx/visualdx6/getDiagnosisText.do?moduleId=10&diagnosisId=52449. [Last accessed September, 2019].
19. Jacobs AH, Walton RG. The incidence of birthmarks in the neonate. Pediatrics. 1976;58(2):218-22.
20. Cordova A. The Mongolian spot: a study of ethnic differences and a literature review. Clin Pediatr (Phila). 1981;20:714-9.
21. VisualDx. Blue-Gray Spot. [online] Available from: http://www.visualdx.com/visualdx/visualdx6/getDiagnosisText.do?moduleId=23&diagnosisId=51967. [Last accessed September, 2019].
22. Hoang MP, Mihm MC Jr. Melanocytic Lesions: A Case Based Approach, 1st edition. New York: Springer; 2014.
23. VisualDx. Nevus of Ota. [online] Available from: http://www.visualdx.com/visualdx/visualdx6/getDiagnosisText.do?moduleId=23&diagnosisId=52032&view=text. [Last accessed September, 2019].
24. VisualDx. Piebaldism. [online] Available from: http://www.visualdx.com/visualdx/visualdx6/getDiagnosisText.do?moduleId=23&diagnosisId=52159. [Last accessed September, 2019].
25. UpToDate. The Genodermatoses. [online] Available from: http://www.uptodate.com/contents/the-genodermatoses. [Last accessed September, 2019].
26. UpToDate. Hearing Impairment in Children: Etiology. [online] Available from: http://www.uptodate.com/contents/hearing-impairment-in-children-etiology. [Last accessed September, 2019].

27. VisualDx. Waardenburg Syndrome. [online] Available from: http://www.visualdx.com/visualdx/visualdx6/getDiagnosisText.do?moduleId=10&diagnosisId=52508. [Last accessed September, 2019].
28. VisualDx. Albinism. [online] Available from: http://www.visualdx.com/visualdx/visualdx6/getDiagnosisText.do?moduleId=23&diagnosisId=51077. [Last accessed September, 2019].
29. Kromberg JG, Castle D, Zwane EM, et al. Albinism and skin cancer in Southern Africa. Clin Genet. 1989;36(1):43-52.
30. VisualDx. Hemangioma, Infantile. [online] Available from: http://www.visualdx.com/visualdx/visualdx6/getDiagnosisText.do?moduleId=24&diagnosisId=51673. [Last accessed September, 2019].
31. Drolet BA, Frommelt PC, Chamlin SL, et al. Initiation and use of propranolol for infantile hemangioma: report of a consensus conference. Pediatrics. 2013;131(1):128-40.
32. Girard C, Bigorre M, Guillot B, et al. PELVIS syndrome. Arch Dermatol. 2006;142(7):884-8.
33. Stockman A, Boralevi F, Taïeb A, et al. SACRAL syndrome: spinal dysraphism, anogenital, cutaneous, renal and urologic anomalies, associated with an angioma of lumbosacral localization. Dermatology. 2007;214(1):40-5.
34. UpToDate. Skin Nodules in Newborns and Infants. [online] Available from: http://www.uptodate.com/contents/skin-nodules-in-newborns-and-infants. [Last accessed September, 2019].
35. VisualDx. Subcutaneous Fat Necrosis of the Newborn. [online] Available from: http://www.visualdx.com/visualdx/visualdx6/getDiagnosisText.do?moduleId=23&diagnosisId=52738. [Last accessed September, 2019].
36. Pallor AS, Mancini AJ. Hurwitz Clinical Pediatric Dermatology: A Textbook of Skin Disorders of Childhood and Adolescence, 4th edition. New York: Elsevier Saunders; 2011.
37. UpToDate. Epidermal Nevus and Epidermal Nevus Syndrome. [online] Available from: http://www.uptodate.com/contents/epidermal-nevus-and-epidermal-nevus-syndrome. [Last accessed September, 2019].
38. VisualDx. Epidermal Nevus. [online] Available from: http://www.visualdx.com/visualdx/visualdx6/getDiagnosisText.do?moduleId=12&diagnosisId=52045. [Last accessed September, 2019].
39. UpToDate. Nevus Sebaceous and Nevus Sebaceous Syndrome. [online] Available from: http://www.uptodate.com/contents/nevus-sebaceous-and-nevus-sebaceous-syndrome. [Last accessed September, 2019].
40. VisualDx. Nevus Sebaceus. [online] Available from: http://www.visualdx.com/visualdx/visualdx6/getDiagnosisText.do?moduleId=11&diagnosisId=52033. [Last accessed September, 2019].
41. Alper J, Holmes LB, Mihm MC Jr. Birthmarks with serious medical significance: nevocellular nevi, sebaceous nevi, and multiple cafe au lait spots. J Pediatr. 1979;95(5 Pt 1):696-700.
42. Cribier B, Scrivener Y, Grosshans E. Tumors arising in nevus sebaceous: A study of 596 cases. J Am Acad Dermatol. 2000;42(2 Pt 1):263-8.
43. Rosen H, Schmidt B, Lam HP, et al. Management of nevus sebaceous and the risk of basal cell carcinoma: an 18-year review. Pediatr Dermatol. 2009;26(6):676-81.
44. Jaqueti G, Requena L, Sánchez Yus E. Trichoblastoma is the most common neoplasm developed in nevus sebaceus of Jadassohn: a clinicopathologic study of a series of 155 cases. Am J Dermatopathol. 2000;22(2):108-18.
45. UpToDate. Congenital Melanocytic Nevi. [online] Available from: http://www.uptodate.com/contents/congenital-melanocytic-nevi. [Last accessed September, 2019].
46. VisualDx. Congenital Melanocytic Nevus. [online] Available from: http://www.visualdx.com/visualdx/visualdx6/getDiagnosisText.do?moduleId=12&diagnosisId=52631. [Last accessed September, 2019].
47. Price HN, Schaffer JV. Congenital melanocytic nevi-when to worry and how to treat: Facts and controversies. Clin Dermatol. 2010;28(3):293-302.
48. VisualDx. Congenital Nevus Giant. [online] Available from: http://www.visualdx.com/visualdx/visualdx6/getDiagnosisText.do?moduleId=24&diagnosisId=52046. [Last accessed September, 2019].
49. UpToDate. Juvenile Xanthogranuloma (JXG). [online] Available from: http://www.uptodate.com/contents/juvenile-xanthogranuloma-jxg. [Last accessed September, 2019].
50. VisualDx. Juvenile Xanthogranuloma. [online] Available from: http://www.visualdx.com/visualdx/visualdx6/getDiagnosisText.do?moduleId=12&diagnosisId=51778. [Last accessed September, 2019].
51. VisualDx. Postmaturity Desquamation. [online] Available from: http://www.visualdx.com/visualdx/visualdx6/getDiagnosisText.do?moduleId=23&diagnosisId=53655. [Last accessed September, 2019].
52. VisualDx. Collodion Baby. [online] Available from: http://www.visualdx.com/visualdx/visualdx6/getDiagnosisText.do?moduleId=23&diagnosisId=53039&view=text. [Last accessed September, 2019].
53. Buyse L, Graves C, Marks R, et al. Collodion baby dehydration: The danger of high transepidermal water loss. Br J Dermatol. 1993;129(1):86-8.
54. VisualDx. Ichthyosiform Erythroderma, Congenital Non-Bullous. [online] Available from: http://www.visualdx.com/visualdx/visualdx6/getDiagnosisText.do?moduleId=23&diagnosisId=53365&view=text. [Last accessed September, 2019].
55. UpToDate. Overview of the inherited ichthyoses. [online] Available from: http://www.uptodate.com/contents/overview-of-the-inherited-ichthyoses. [Last accessed September, 2019].
56. VisualDx. Harlequin Fetus. [online] Available from: http://www.visualdx.com/visualdx/visualdx6/getDiagnosisText.do?moduleId=23&diagnosisId=51666. [Last accessed September, 2019].
57. VisualDx. Acrodermatitis Enteropathica. [online] Available from: http://www.visualdx.com/visualdx/visualdx6/getDiagnosisText.do?moduleId=23&diagnosisId=51047&view=text. [Last accessed September, 2019].
58. VisualDx. Histiocytosis, Langerhans Cell. [online] Available from: http://www.visualdx.com/visualdx/visualdx6/getDiagnosisText.do?moduleId=23&diagnosisId=52679&view=text. [Last accessed September, 2019].
59. UpToDate. Clinical Manifestations, Pathologic Features, and Diagnosis of Langerhans Cell Histiocytosis. [online] Available from: http://www.uptodate.com/contents/clinical-manifestations-pathologic-features-and-diagnosis-of-langerhans-cell-histiocytosis. [Last accessed September, 2019].

60. VisualDx. Psoriasis, Infantile. [online] Available from: http://www.visualdx.com/visualdx/visualdx6/getDiagnosisText.do?moduleId=23&diagnosisId=53224. [Last accessed September, 2019].
61. VisualDx. Dermatitis, Seborrheic. [online] Available from: http://www.visualdx.com/visualdx/visualdx6/getDiagnosisText.do?moduleId=23&diagnosisId=51409&view=text. [Last accessed September, 2019].
62. VisualDx. Epidermolysis Bullosa Simplex. [online] Available from: http://www.visualdx.com/visualdx/visualdx6/getDiagnosisText.do?moduleId=10&diagnosisId=51504. [Last accessed September, 2019].
63. UpToDate. Epidemiology, pathogenesis, and clinical features of epidermolysis bullosa. [online] Available from: http://www.uptodate.com/contents/epidemiology-pathogenesis-and-clinical-features-of-epidermolysis-bullosa. [Last accessed September, 2019].
64. VisualDx. Junctional Epidermolysis Bullosa. [online] Available from: http://www.visualdx.com/visualdx/visualdx6/getDiagnosisText.do?moduleId=23&diagnosisId=51507&view=text. [Last accessed September, 2019].
65. Gonzalez ME. Evaluation and treatment of the newborn with epidermolysis bullosa. Semin Perinatol. 2013;37(1):32-9.
66. UpToDate. Overview of the Management of Epidermolysis Bullosa. [online] Available from: http://www.uptodate.com/contents/overview-of-the-management-of-epidermolysis-bullosa. [Last accessed September, 2019].
67. VisualDx. Aplasia Cutis Congenita. [online] Available from: http://www.visualdx.com/visualdx/visualdx6/getDiagnosisText.do?moduleId=23&diagnosisId=51132. [Last accessed September, 2019].
68. VisualDx. Urticaria Pigmentosa. [online] Available from: http://www.visualdx.com/visualdx/visualdx6/getDiagnosisText.do?moduleId=23&diagnosisId=52472&view=text. [Last accessed September, 2019].
69. VisualDx. Mastocytoma. [online] Available from: http://www.visualdx.com/visualdx/visualdx6/getDiagnosisText.do?moduleId=12&diagnosisId=51929. [Last accessed September, 2019].
70. UptoDate. Vesiculobullous and Pustular Lesions in the Newborn. [online] Available from: http://www.uptodate.com/contents/vesiculobullous-and-pustular-lesions-in-the-newborn. [Last accessed September, 2019].
71. VisualDx. Incontinentia Pigmenti. [online] Available from: http://www.visualdx.com/visualdx/visualdx6/getDiagnosisText.do?moduleId=23&diagnosisId=51767. [Last accessed September, 2019].
72. Smahi A, Courtois G, Rabia SH, et al. The NF-kappaB signalling pathway in human diseases: from incontinentia pigmenti to ectodermal dysplasias and immune-deficiency syndromes. Hum Mol Genet. 2002;11(20):2371-5.
73. VisualDx. Staphylococcal Scalded Skin Syndrome. [online] Available from: http://www.visualdx.com/visualdx/visualdx6/getDiagnosisText.do?moduleId=23&diagnosisId=52340&view=text. [Last accessed September, 2019].
74. Carr JA, Hodgman JE, Freedam RI, et al. Relationship between toxic erythema and infant maturity. Am J Dis Child. 1966;112(2):129-34.
75. VisualDx. Erythema Toxicum Neonatorum. [online] Available from: http://www.visualdx.com/visualdx/visualdx6/getDiagnosisText.do?moduleId=23&diagnosisId=51535. [Last accessed September, 2019].
76. VisualDx. Transient Neonatal Pustular Dermatosis. [online] Available from: http://www.visualdx.com/visualdx/visualdx6/getDiagnosisText.do?moduleId=23&diagnosisId=52239. [Last accessed September, 2019].
77. VisualDx. Herpes Simplex Virus. [online] Available from: http://www.visualdx.com/visualdx/visualdx6/getDiagnosisText.do?moduleId=23&diagnosisId=51694&view=text. [Last accessed September, 2019].
78. VisualDx. Varicella, Neonatal. [online] Available from: http://www.visualdx.com/visualdx/visualdx6/getDiagnosisText.do?moduleId=23&diagnosisId=53573. [Last accessed September, 2019].
79. Paller AS. Scabies in infants and small children. Semin Dermatol. 1993;12(1):3-8.
80. VisualDx. Scabies (Pediatric). [online] Available from: https://www.visualdx.com/visualdx/visualdx6/getDiagnosisText.do?moduleId=23&diagnosisId=53975&view=text. [Last accessed September, 2019].
81. VisualDx. Neonatal Candidiasis. [online] Available from: http://www.visualdx.com/visualdx/visualdx6/getDiagnosisText.do?moduleId=23&diagnosisId=53819. [Last accessed September, 2019].

# CHAPTER 42

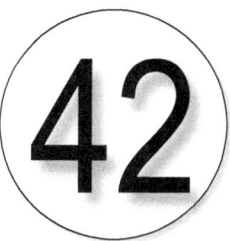

# Common Orthopedic Problems in the Newborn

*Robert M Bernstein, Ronald A Roiz*

## ABSTRACT

Common orthopedic problems in the newborn is not a comprehensive review of the orthopedic pathologies that affect the neonate, but rather an overview of the most common pathologies, particularly those seen in the neonatal intensive care unit (NICU) and their workups. The chapter reviews unique aspects of the neonate's anatomy and how to evaluate the neonate. In particular, the chapter addresses infection, common fractures, metabolic bone disease, neurologic pathologies, and finally common congenital abnormalities including hip dysplasia, club foot, VACTERL (vertebral defects, anal atresia, cardiac defects, tracheo-esophageal fistula, renal anomalies, and limb abnormalities) association, polydactyly, limb deficiencies, and hyperextension of the knee.

## INTRODUCTION

For the treating physician, neonatal patients can present some unique orthopedic problems. A neonate's musculoskeletal system grows more rapidly than it will at any other time in life. The changes that occur in the physes and joints make children in this stage susceptible to injury or disease that can significantly affect their development. In addition, the effects of prenatal care and maternal nutrition, or lack thereof (e.g. folate deficiency and its association with myelodysplasia), can result in devastating congenital abnormalities that will last the entire life of the individual. For these reasons, the neonatal period should be viewed as truly unique and may have lifelong consequences.

Pediatricians frequently state, "children are not just young adults." In fact, we should also say that "neonates are not just small children," and their orthopedic problems and treatments may be different from those of infants and children. For instance, the physeal structure is different between a neonate and an infant, resulting in different patterns of infection and fractures. Vessels cross the neonatal physis, allowing bacteria to access the joint and to easily destroy the growth plate, whereas, after a year of age, these vessels cease to cross the physis, resulting in decreased risk of growth arrest. Finally, the potential treatments and access required in the NICU by neonatal staff may affect the timing of orthopedic treatment. For instance, application of bilateral clubfoot casts makes access for heel sticks for blood draw impossible. Therefore, delaying treatment of the clubfeet would be necessary. Numerous conditions affect the neonate. in this chapter, we will focus on the conditions most commonly encountered and treated in the NICU.

## UNIQUE ASPECT OF NEONATAL BONE/JOINTS

There are a number of unique aspects that differentiate the perinatal skeleton from that of the infant. Between 24 weeks and full term, approximately 80% of calcium, phosphate, and magnesium is accrued in the skeleton.[1] Infants born prematurely have significantly decreased ossification of skeletal structures, which may increase their susceptibility to fractures and metabolic bone disease. Radiographic findings of rickets have been noted in up to 55% of infants with a birth weight of less than 1,000 g and in almost a quarter of infants weighing less than 1,500 g at birth.[2] Recent studies have also shown that adult osteoporosis may have links to fetal and neonatal bone development. Thus, attention to neonatal bone health may prevent some forms of adult metabolic bone disease.[3,4] Currently the best available screening method for low bone mineral density in preterm infants is serum total alkaline phosphatase activity and serum inorganic phosphate concentrations.[5] In addition, treatment of preterm labor with magnesium sulfate can have short-term effects on fetal/neonatal bone development.[6] Very low-birth weight infants and those treated with dexamethasone are at risk of short stature and low bone mass.[7] Finally, necrotizing enterocolitis can significantly increase bone resorption in premature infants.[8] It is clear that both prenatal and neonatal factors affect growth of the skeleton and development of bone mass and should be considered when evaluating the neonate for any abnormalities.

## EVALUATION OF THE NEONATE

An accurate history of the presentation of the neonate and any complications during delivery is essential to the diagnosis of many birth injuries. For instance, shoulder dystocia predisposes the child to clavicle fracture (sometimes a purposeful maneuver by the obstetrician) and brachial plexus injury. Moreover, breech positions are associated with congenital hip dysplasia. Many of the pathologies discussed below are associated with delivery in a neonate, with or without predisposing factors, and obtaining a detailed history of the birth can aid in ensuring an accurate diagnosis.

The clinician should assess the skin for any abnormal markings (hemangiomas, simian creases, skin dimples, and constricting bands); palpate all extremities looking for fractures, especially in the setting of a traumatic birth; check range of motion of the neck and major joints of the extremities; assess the hips for dysplasia; and examine the feet for contracture or hypermobility. Mild flexion contractures of the hips and knees that spontaneously resolve after birth are normal.

Examination of the neonate can be challenging, but a clinician can use indirect signs for evaluation of function. Eliciting the Moro reflex is an elegant way to test all extremities to look for deficits.[9-11] Pseudoparalysis and apparent pain may indicate a fracture or infection.[10] Primitive reflexes are normally present, but their absence or an asymmetry may indicate a palsy, while the persistence of a reflex beyond a certain age may indicate cerebral palsy.[9]

## INFECTION

### Osteomyelitis and Septic Arthritis

Musculoskeletal infections in the neonate can cause serious complications including damage to the physis and growth arrest, as well as joint destruction. The growth of the lower extremities is the main contributor of height in the child's development, particularly the growth plates around the knee, which contribute 60–70% of total limb growth.[10] Therefore, any damage (e.g. infection) to those growth plates can lead to early closure and significantly decrease the total length potential.

Osteomyelitis and septic arthritis in the neonate are different than in older children,[10,12] in terms of anatomy, source of infection, and presentation. As previously mentioned, in the neonate the physis has a blood supply, which is in close proximity to the joint. Bacteremia resulting from a line infection or sepsis can lead to osteomyelitis; there is usually an identifiable infection that precedes the onset of osteomyelitis.[10] Unlike adults, the neonate may not display a fever; however, hypothermia may indicate infection.[9,10,12-14] Moreover, swelling and/or pseudoparalysis is present in 95% of cases.[12,15] The hip, distal femur, proximal humerus, and proximal tibia are the most common locations for infection, but it is important to note that up to 18–40% are multifocal.[12,15] Delay in detection can result in severe physeal damage **(Fig. 1)**.

Once osteomyelitis is suspected, the workup is similar at any age. Blood cultures should be sent for testing; however, they are only positive 21–47% of the time for neonatal infections.[9,16] Cultures to send include aerobic, anaerobic, tuberculosis (TB), and fungal cultures, keeping in mind that the typical pathogen is *Staphylococcus aureus* in 72% of cases.[15] *Streptococcus* is seen in 28% of cases;[15] *Haemophilus influenzae* has also been reported.[10,12,15,17] Fungal infections can be seen around the knee of neonates who have low-birth weight or who have had a prolonged antibiotic course.[10,18] In terms of laboratory testing, WBC is typically normal or

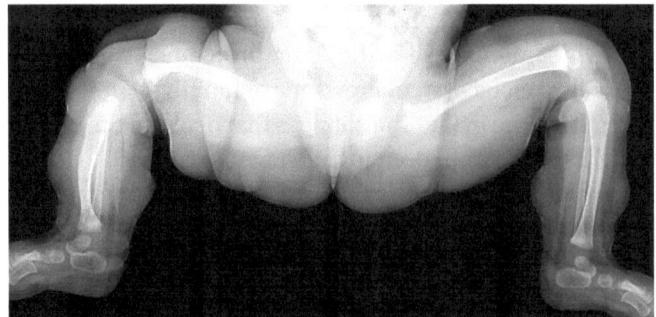

**Fig. 1:** Physeal damage in a 6-month-old following multifocal joint sepsis. Note the growth arrest and abnormalities of the right distal femur, right distal tibia, and left hip.

depressed and erythrocyte sedimentation rate (ESR) is not a reliable test for the neonatal population.[9] C-reactive protein (CRP) in combination with interleukin-6 (IL-6) is 89% sensitive for infection at initial presentation, but with only a 70% positive predictive value. However, the two tests have 90% negative predicitive value and are useful for ruling out an infection.[19] Direct aspiration with 18G needle should be part of the standard workup, and obtaining a cell count and Gram stain is important. In terms of imaging, X-ray may only show soft tissue swelling[10] but may also show rarefaction and periosteal reaction.[12] Ultrasound can be useful in revealing a subperiosteal abscess.[12] Bone scans have been reported to have a large range of sensitivities (32–87%) for detecting subclinical osteomyelitis in neonates, even though it is an effective modality in older children.[20] Magnetic resonance imaging (MRI) is a highly sensitive tool in imaging localized disease, which can be useful for aspirations or drainage, but its utility for detecting subclinical multifocal disease is not well defined, as the use of a whole-body MRI is an emerging concept.[20]

The mainstay of treatment for osteomyelitis is antibiotics, which should be started after direct aspiration and blood cultures are drawn, unless the patient is septic, in which case the patient can be treated empirically. It is important to note that direct aspiration will not alter MRI or bone scan results. Intravenous antibiotics are recommended for a minimum of 48 hours followed by oral antibiotics for up to 6 weeks.[15] Other studies have reported a shorter duration of antibiotics for older children but do not give a definite duration for the neonate.[21] Surgical drainage of any subperiosteal abscesses should be performed.[10,21] In order to prevent stiffness and deformity, an affected limb should be immobilized until the patient can move it.[10,12,15]

Septic arthritis typically presents with metaphyseal osteomyelitis with up to 76% of the patients with septic arthritis having a preceding osteomyelitis.[9] Typically there is local extension from the osteomyelitis through the thin plate into the epiphysis and then via the periosteum into the joint.[10] Similarly to osteomyelitis, septic arthritis may be multifocal and therefore all joints need to be examined. Cultures should be sent, but bear in mind that 43% of cultures are negative.[9,16] Treatment is similar to septic arthritis at any age, with surgical drainage and intravenous antibiotics. Additionally, immobilization is necessary to prevent contractures and deformity, and should be employed until the neonate can move the limb normally.[10]

### Necrotizing Fasciitis

This is a rare infection of the subcutaneous tissue and fascial planes, typically of the abdominal wall, with reported mortality of >50%.[22,23] The infection is typically associated with omphalitis, balanitis, or mammitis, but it has been described secondary to fetal monitoring, septicemia, necrotizing enterocolitis, and immunodeficiency, and rarely occurs without apparent cause.[22,23] Patients will present with swelling, erythema, and warmth surrounding an area of skin that can appear dusky.[10,22] Prompt debridement, antibiotics, and fluid resuscitation are the mainstays of treatment.[10,22,23]

### Gangrene of Newborns

Neonatal gangrene is an extremely rare occurrence with multiple predisposing conditions that lead to an arterial occlusion and localized ischemia, particularly prematurity, polycythemia, umbilical artery catheterization, and intensive care treatment for other life-threatening illnesses.[24] The patient often presents on the first day of life with marked edema, blistering, and possible cyanosis of the proximal aspect of the affected extremity. The edema will limit circulation and motion. Fasciotomies might be required to restore circulation.[12] Muscle necrosis may have already occurred and can leave the patient with weakness of the affected extremity. Allowing the necrosis to demarcate and then proceed with amputation is recommended by some authors to minimize tissue loss.[10,24] Medical measures may include antibiotics and gamma globulin.[12]

## FRACTURES

Perinatal fractures are not uncommon in neonates, with most fractures being associated with birth. Radiographs can be a useful modality for diagnosis, but some fractures can be difficult to visualize on X-ray. Ultrasound can be a useful adjunct to diagnose occult fractures, particularly those associated with the epiphysis.[9]

The clavicle is the most commonly fractured bone during birth.[9,25] The incidence ranges from 0.3% to 2.9%;[9,10,12,25] however, this fracture is commonly missed as it may be asymptomatic, and therefore underreported.[25] Predisposing factors include large birth weight, prolonged second stage of birth, instrumented delivery, shoulder dystocia, or simply a vaginal delivery.[9,25] The typical mechanism is from digital pressure applied to the clavicle while pulling on the shoulders to aid in delivery.[12] Shoulder immobilization for 7–10 days is typically sufficient to manage this fracture.[25]

Fractures of the long bones can also occur in neonates, with the most common sites for long bone fracture being the humerus and femur. Humerus fractures and other upper extremity fractures typically heal within 7–10 days of immobilization. A simple cotton stockinette is an effective way to immobilize the upper extremity, as conventional slings and immobilizers are too large for the neonatal arm.[9] Though most fractures of the humerus occur in the midshaft, epiphyseal separation of the proximal humerus can also occur; it is important to recognize this pathology, as the proximal humerus accounts for 80% of the total growth of the humerus.[10,26] Epiphyseal separations of the proximal humerus are often mistaken for shoulder dislocations, which are rare.[10] Closed reduction is indicated for large displacement; however, minor residual displacement and malalignments will correct with time.[10,27]

Midshaft femur fractures are usually evident at the time of incident by noting clinical signs of shortening and increased thigh circumference.[10,28] Femoral fractures can be sufficiently treated with a Pavlik harness;[29,30] given the efficacy of the Pavlik harness, the use of Bryant's traction should be discouraged due to the possibility of complications.[10,31] Similar to the humerus, the proximal epiphysis of the femur can separate. It can be mistaken for a hip dislocation,[10] but unlike a true congenital hip dislocation, the acetabulum will be properly formed and will appear normal on radiograph.[32] Traumatic hip dislocations have never been demonstrated.[10] Early recognition of this pathology is critical, as bony deformity can result from delayed care.[33] A history of breech position and a clinical presentation of a leg with pseudoparalysis that is abducted, flexed, and externally rotated are key indicators of long bone fracture, and an arthrogram can confirm the diagnosis.[34] Closed reduction and immobilization is typically a sufficient treatment, but internal fixation might be required if the reduction is unstable.[10,33]

## Osteomalacia/Rickets and Osteopenia of Prematurity

When a neonate presents with a fracture, the healthcare provider should consider osteopenia of prematurity and osteogenesis imperfecta. Abuse should be on the differential but rarely occurs before the age of 3 months.[10]

Osteopenia of prematurity and osteomalacia/rickets are two conditions seen in patients with a gestational age of less than 28 weeks. Osteopenia is caused by a diminished synthesis or increased absorption of bone in the setting of severe disease, medication (e.g. steroids), or lack of mechanical stimulation.[35] James et al. found that premature infants have decreased bone length and bone mineral content, which persists when they reach full term.[36] Fractures seen in these patients typically affect the ribs, but can also affect a number of other bones, and there are usually multiple fractures.[37] Previously seen rates of fracture have been diminished, as premature neonates are immobilized for shorter periods of time on mechanical ventilation.[35]

Osteomalacia, which is a deficiency of the mineralization of organic bone matrix, and rickets, which is the same deficiency but specific to the growth plate, are both caused by a lack of phosphorus.[35] Greater than six times the normal upper limit of alkaline phosphatase can be measured in neonates with osteomalacia/rickets;[36] however, an increase in alkaline phosphatase is not pathognomonic of the disease as it is also seen in liver disease and during high rates of growth.[35] Fractures associated with osteomalacia/rickets typically occur at 75 days of life.[38]

Current management of these conditions is varied amongst institutions and prevention is considered to be paramount.[39] Treatment is reliant on both adequate supply of minerals, as well as physiologic demands of the bone.[35] Screening is suggested for all neonates with gestation ≤28 weeks, any neonate requiring total parenteral nutrition for >4 weeks, or any neonate given a course of steroids or diuretics.[39] Serum calcium, serum alkaline phosphatase, and serum phosphate levels should be monitored weekly and supplementation adjusted accordingly.[39] Rigo et al. recommended supplementation of 100-160 mg/kg/day of highly bioavailable calcium salts, 60-90 mg/kg/day of phosphorus, and 800-1,000 IU of vitamin D per day.[40] Additionally, mechanical stimulation is vital, and exercise programs, like the one created by Moyer-Mileur have been shown to increase bone length, bone mineral content, and fat-free mass.[35]

## Osteogenesis Imperfecta

Another pathological entity that can present with multiple fractures is osteogenesis imperfecta. There are multiple variants of osteogenesis imperfecta, with the congenita form presenting at birth. The classic blue sclera is not present in all types, so the clinician may need to look for other signs including hypermobility of joints, skull deformity, teeth abnormality, and possibly deafness.[12] Radiographic features can be appreciated in the neonatal period, with characteristic widening and thinning of the diaphysis of long bone, ribs that are atrophic, and skull bones are Wormian at the suture line.[12] The patient can present with multiple fractures of long bones, ribs, or even the skull, so suspicion of subdural hematomas should be high; additionally, neonates with rib fractures may require respiratory support. This disease can be mistaken for child abuse because of the multiple fractures; achondroplasia is also part of the differential diagnosis given the body morphology with short limbs and an enlarged head. The treatment is primarily supportive in the perinatal setting, especially in the setting of subdural hematomas and multiple rib fractures. Further management is geared toward fracture prevention, deformity correction, and reduction of osteoporosis.[12]

## Dwarfism

Dwarfism and other skeletal dysplasias are sometimes apparent at birth. Many can be detected by ultrasound in the prenatal period.[41] Dwarfism is a condition in which a patient exhibits short stature with a standing height in adulthood below 4 ft 10 in or below the third percentile as the result of a medical or genetic condition. Dwarfism can be proportionate (as in a pituitary dwarf or primordial dwarf) or disproportionate (e.g. achondroplasia). As proportionate dwarfism does not generally require orthopedic treatment, we will focus on disproportionate conditions, many of which have significant orthopedic issues.

Determination of which portion of the limb is short, can help to determine the type of skeletal dysplasia. For instance, achondroplasia (the most common form of dwarfism which occurs sporadically as a new mutation or autosomal dominant, occurring in 1:10,000 live births) has rhizomelic (proximal) limb shortening. The trunk is normal in length. Achondroplasia affects endochondral ossification through an abnormality in the *FGFR3* gene.[42] All parts of the skeleton that form by endochondral ossification will be affected (face and occipital bones, pedicles, and long bones). Those areas that are formed by membranous ossification (the upper cranium and ribs) are not affected. Thus, children with achondroplasia are affected by frontal bossing, stenosis of the foramen magnum, and spinal stenosis. They will have splaying of the fingers, known as a trident hand. Hyperlaxity of the joints is often apparent, and kyphosis when placed in a sitting position is common but usually resolves when the child learns to stand.

Other types of dwarfism include diastrophic dysplasia (caused by mutation in the *SLC26A2* gene), spondyloepiphyseal dysplasia (caused by mutations in the *COL2A1* gene), pseudoachondroplasia (caused by a mutation in the *COMP* gene), and metatropic dysplasia (caused by a mutation in the *TRPV4* gene).[43-46] Each of these disorders has unique orthopedic problems and prognoses. Thus, once a skeletal dysplasia is considered, a geneticist should provide an immediate evaluation.

## Abuse

Abuse of the neonate is uncommon, with the peak incidence of abuse occurring at 3 months of age.[10] There are important signs of abuse which should not be missed. Shaken baby syndrome is perhaps the worst type of abuse without external signs; however, whiplash causes hemorrhaging in spinal cord, brain, and retina. If symmetrical metaphyseal fractures are found on radiograph, it may have occurred from the perichondrium being violently avulsed from the cortex[10] and is more commonly present in the abused child.[47] Though spiral fractures are common in abused children under the age of 15 months, particularly of the femur, it is also seen in the non-abused child.[47] Multiple rib fractures are indicative of abuse, but they are not necessarily located posteriorly, as it is classically taught.[47] The skull, clavicle, and spine can be affected, but obstetrical fractures affect the same bones and so it can lead to confusion.[10] Also, classically, multiple fractures in different stages of healing are found in abuse, but as multiple fractures can be found in other pathologies, other signs of neglect can be useful in determining abuse.

## ■ BRACHIOPLEXOPATHIES

Another group of injuries presenting at birth that are important to recognize are brachioplexopathies. They typically result because of obstetrical complications. The reported incidence is from 0.13 per 1,000 live births to 3.6 per 1,000 live births.[9,48-50] C5 and C6 are most commonly injured, causing an Erb's palsy[9]; C8 and T1 injuries cause Klumpke's palsy. Maternal diabetes, high birth weight, prolonged labor, and shoulder dystocia are risk factors.[50] If the entire plexus is involved, the infant may have an associated Horner's syndrome (ptosis, enopthalmos, and miosis) and should be evaluated for ipsilateral diaphragmatic paralysis.[50]

Since intervention is complicated and controversial, it is important to know the natural history. About 95% of infants will recover completely.[49] Most patients will recover by the first month,[51] with 92% recovering by 3 months.[49] Moreover, neurologic recovery within the first month will result in normal function.[51] However, if biceps function does not return by 3 months, it is unlikely to ever have normal function.[51]

The management of patients without spontaneous recovery is not well defined. While awaiting return of function, immobilization is no longer recommended; in the case there is complete paralysis of the upper limb, splinting of the wrist and hand are indicated.[12] Gentle stretching and passive exercises are recommended to prevent contractures.[12] Many authors recommend that a lack of return of biceps function is an indication for surgery. However, there is no consensus as to the appropriate timing for surgical intervention. Authors report waiting anywhere from 3 months to 12 months of age.[51] Possible surgical interventions include interpositional nerve grafts and direct neurorrhaphy. Further surgery including humeral osteotomies, and muscle release and transfer might be necessary in the cases of bony deformity, contracture, and muscle imbalance.

## ■ CONGENITAL BIRTH DEFECTS

### Congenital (Developmental) Hip Dysplasia

Congenital hip dysplasia is a prevalent, very treatable condition if monitoring is effective and timely. The incidence of frank dislocation is 1 in 1,000 births, but subluxation is as high as 10 in 1,000 births.[52] Predisposing factors include family history of congenital hip dysplasia, breech presentation, being a female or first born, having another foot deformity (e.g. metatarsus varus or clubfoot), or torticollis.[9,12] In congenital hip dysplasia, the hip dislocation will generally present at birth. Note if patient develops subluxation of the hip after normal hip examination, it might be associated with a septic arthritis. Dislocations that happen in utero are rare (<2%), and a teratologic/developmental etiology should be considered.[10]

Classically, the Ortolani maneuver reduces frank dislocations and Barlow maneuver dislocates hips, but it is important to note that teratologic hip dysplasia may be very difficult to reduce.[9,12,52] The Klisic test is a way to evaluate the relative position of the femur to the pelvis by placing a middle finger on the greater trochanter and an index finger on the anterior superior iliac spine. With normal anatomy, an imaginary line between the fingers should point toward the umbilicus. With hip dislocations, the line will point inferior to the umbilicus.[9]

Ultrasound is the imaging modality of choice, and can be effective in picking up acetabular dysplasia and mild subluxation.[9] However, it has a high rate of false positives, especially in the neonatal period (up to 1 month old);[9,53,54] some clinicians worry about losing the patient to follow-up and initiate testing early on. The use of Graf's criteria for the measurement of alpha and beta angles, and Harcke's dynamic hip ultrasonographic techniques aide in the diagnosis of congenital diaphragmatic hernia (CDH).

Many neonates that have acetabular dysplasia and mild subluxation can be managed with observation for 3-4 weeks, as they will have spontaneous resolution.[52] However, if the neonate has a persistent positive Barlow or Ortolani, then they will require intervention. The Pavlik harness is an effective treatment modality. However, the harness should not be used for more than 4 weeks, if the hip is not reduced, so as not to wear away the posterior aspect of the acetabulum.[55] The triple diaper method has been shown to be ineffective in the early period, as it does not change the natural course.[52] Results are excellent, with few complications and a success rate of 90% in children treated early on with a Pavlik harness.[52]

## Clubfoot

Clubfoot is another common problem that presents at birth, with an incidence of 1-2 per 1,000 births and a multifactorial pathogenesis; it can be treated effectively if recognized early on. Talipes equinovarus is characterized by cavus, forefoot adduction, hindfoot varus, and equines. Its presentation varies from flexible to rigid, with the latter being associated with an underlying disorder such as arthrogryposis, myelomeningocele, or Larsen syndrome.[9] There is geographic variability, an increased prevalence of 2-2.5:1 in men over women, and an increased rate of clubfoot in families with a history of clubfeet, especially if the mother is affected.[9,12,56]

The goal of treatment is the restoration of a plantigrade foot that is painless and functional for walking. Both surgical and nonsurgical methods have been used, but more recent data suggests that nonsurgical methods like the Ponseti method should be implemented initially given its high efficacy.[56] In a recent meta-analysis using the Laaveg-Ponseti grading system, the Ponseti method resulted in good-to-excellent results in 78% of patients, while patients treated with surgery only 43% had a good-to-excellent outcome.[56] Some authors argue that starting treatment early takes advantage of ligamentous laxity and gives parents a sense that the deformity is being addressed.[9] Moreover, it is recommended to start the Ponseti method in the first month of life to achieve correction in 95% of patients without the use of a posteromedial and lateral release.[57] However, a study by Dobbs et al. showed no increased risk of recurrence of clubfoot with later onset of treatment, with a mean initiation of treatment at 12 weeks (a range of 1-60 weeks), and that correction can be achieved even with a later onset of treatment.[58] Dobbs did find that noncompliance and the educational level of the parents (high-school education or less) were strong risk factors for recurrence, and in these patients, the clinician may need to provide additional education or support to the parents.[58]

## VACTERL Association

VACTERL Association refers to the collection of associated findings of congenital abnormalities of the Vertebral bodies, Anal atresia, Cardiac defects, Tracheo-Esophageal fistula, Renal anomalies and Limb abnormalities. At least three of these features need to be present for the diagnosis. This is a sporadic condition and its cause is unknown.[59]

The importance of the clinician being familiar with this association is that when a congenital abnormality is found in the neonate in one organ system such as the spine, other organ systems such as the urogenital system should be evaluated.

## Polydactyly

Polydactyly (duplication of a digit) can occur on the hand and/or foot and can be sporadic or inherited and can be associated with other abnormalities. It is generally separated into preaxial and postaxial (they are rarely central). Preaxial polydactyly is present when the duplication is on the radial (thumb) side of the hand or on the medial (big toe) side of the foot. When this occurs, it can be associated with cardiac abnormalities (Holt-Oram syndrome). When it occurs postaxially (on the ulnar side of the hand or lateral side of the foot), it is usually inherited as an autosomal dominant trait. Postaxial polydactyly can be associated with Ellis-van Creveld syndrome (chondroectodermal dysplasia).[60]

Treatment of polydactyly usually involves removal of the extra digits for cosmetic reasons. However, it is important to recognize and evaluate the patient with preaxial polydactyly for cardiac problems.

## Limb Deficiencies

Congenital limb deficiencies are relatively rare and usually sporadic. Limb deficiencies can be segregated into transverse deficiencies (such as those that occur in constriction band syndrome) and longitudinal deficiencies (such as fibular absence). Congenital constriction band syndrome (also known as amniotic band syndrome or Streeter's dysplasia) can result in intrauterine amputations of digits or even limbs[61] **(Figs. 2 and 3)**. These amputations act like traumatic or surgical transosseous amputations. As a result, terminal overgrowth can result in problems with prosthetic fitting as the child grows. In addition, there is a high rate of clubfoot associated with this condition, which tends to be more intransigent to treatment than idiopathic clubfeet. Cleft lip and palate can also be associated.

Other limb deficiencies include proximal femoral focal deficiency (PFFD), partial or complete fibular absence, tibial absence (sometimes associated with a cleft foot and is autosomal dominant), and radial club hand (radial aplasia), and thrombocytopenia with absent radius (TAR) syndrome (thrombocytopenia and absent radii). PFFD is sporadic and results in a shortened femur, often with fibular and foot involvement. Fibular absence **(Fig. 4)** is sporadic and

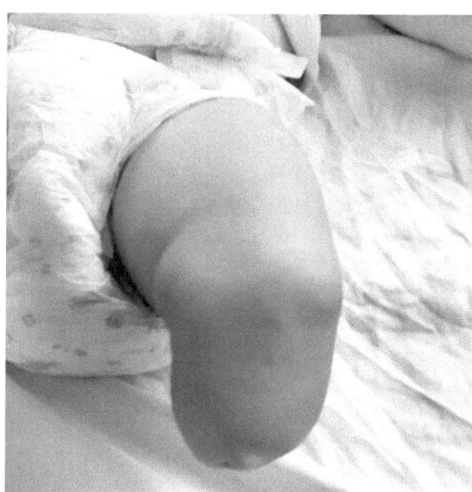

**Fig. 3:** Intrauterine transtibial amputation in the same child as the result of congenital constriction band syndrome *(For color version see Plate 11).*

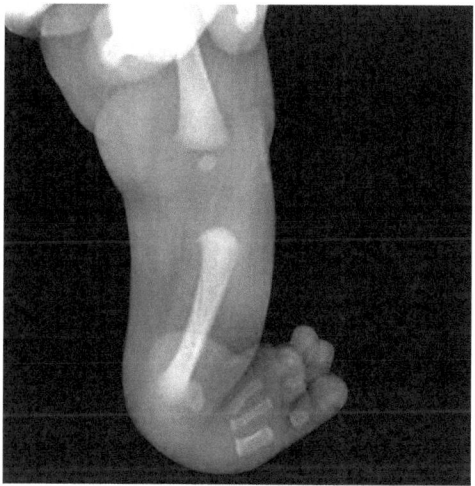

**Fig. 4:** Fibular absence in a neonate with a three rayed foot.

is often associated with a lateral foot absence and tarsal coalitions.[62] Treatment for these problems should focus on joint stability, limb alignment, and the expected leg length discrepancy at maturity.

Radial club hand can be associated with Holt-Oram syndrome and should be differentiated from TAR syndrome. One clue is presence or absence of the thumb. The thumb is always present in TAR syndrome[63] **(Fig. 5)** but absent in radial club hand. The treatment of radial club hand includes creating a new thumb out of the index finger, a procedure called "pollicization." This is generally done about a year after birth. If the diagnosis is TAR, care should be taken as the thrombocytopenia can cause life-threatening bleeding if surgery is performed. The thrombocytopenia usually resolves by 1 year of age but does not always resolve. Pancytopenia (Fanconi's anemia) can also be associated with TAR and Holt-Oram syndrome. There can also be associated knee abnormalities with both these syndromes.[64]

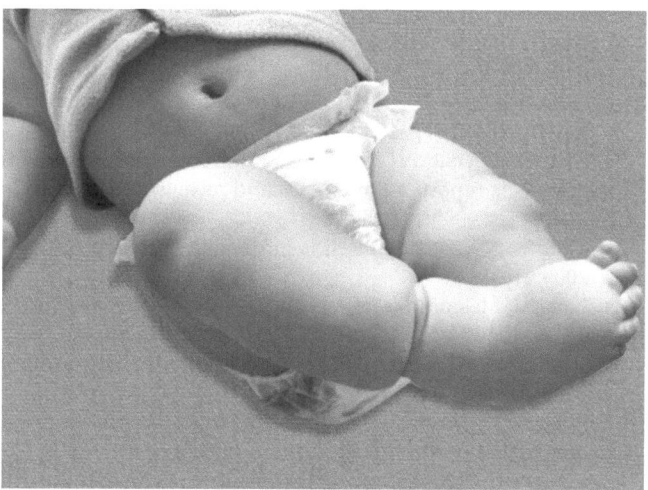

**Fig. 2:** Congenital constriction band of the distal tibia *(For color version see Plate 11).*

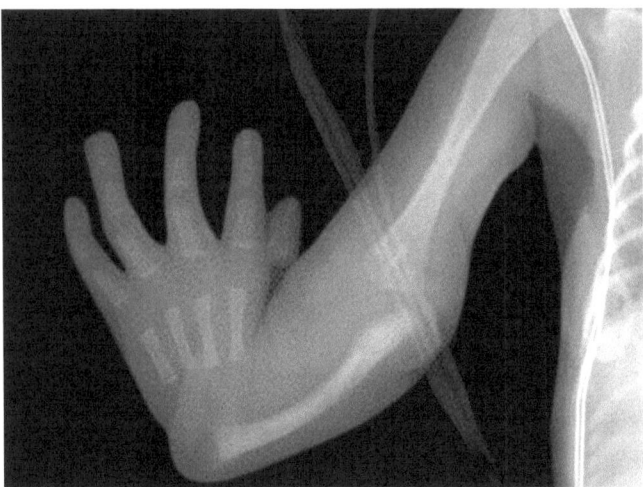

**Fig. 5:** TAR (thrombocytopenia with absent radius) syndrome in a newborn. Note the presence of the thumb.

## Hyperextension of the Knee

Congenital hyperextension (or dislocation) of the knee is perhaps one of the most surprising abnormalities that can be seen at birth. This may be associated with amyoplasia or other forms of arthrogryposis.[65] Casting is generally performed soon after birth to gradually reduce the position of the knee to 90° of flexion. Percutaneous release of the quadriceps can be performed, if the casting fails to improve the position.[66]

## ■ CONCLUSION

Orthopedic problems presenting in the neonatal period are unique and complex, involving bone injury as the result of fracture or infection, or a myriad of congenital anomalies, some of which are genetic and some of which are sporadic. Careful evaluation of functional deficits or structural deficiencies, and recognition of associated pathologies can lead to early improved outcomes.

## ■ REFERENCES

1. Demarini S. Calcium and phosphorus nutrition in preterm infants. Acta Paediatr Suppl. 2005;94(449):87-92.
2. Backström MC, Kuusela AL, Mäki R. Metabolic bone disease of prematurity. Ann Med. 1996;28(4):275-82.
3. Done SL. Fetal and neonatal bone health: update on bone growth and manifestations in health and disease. Pediatr Radiol. 2012;42(Suppl 1):S158-76.
4. Godfrey K, Walker-Bone K, Robinson S, et al. Neonatal bone mass: influence of parental birthweight, maternal smoking, body composition, and activity during pregnancy. J Bone Miner Res. 2001;16(9):1694-703.
5. Backström MC, Kouri T, Kuusela AL, et al. Bone isoenzyme of serum alkaline phosphatase and serum inorganic phosphate in metabolic bone disease of prematurity. Acta Paediatr. 2000;89(7):867-73.
6. Santi MD, Henry GW, Douglas GL. Magnesium sulfate treatment of preterm labor as a cause of abnormal neonatal bone mineralization. J Pediatr Orthop. 1994;14(2):249-53.
7. Wang D, Vandermeulen J, Atkinson SA. Early life factors predict abnormal growth and bone accretion at prepuberty in former premature infants with/without neonatal dexamethasone exposure. Pediatr Res. 2007;61(1):111-6.
8. Cakir M, Mungan I, Karahan C, et al. Necrotizing enterocolitis increases the bone resorption in premature infants. Early Hum Dev. 2006;82(6):405-9.
9. Sankar WN, Weiss J, Skaggs DL. Orthopaedic conditions in the newborn. J Am Acad Orthop Surg. 2009;17(2):112-22.
10. Hensinger RN, Jones ET. Neonatal Orthopaedics. New York; Grune & Stratton; 1981.
11. Futagi Y, Tagawa T, Otani K. Primitive reflex profiles in infants: differences based on categories of neurological abnormality. Brain Dev. 1992;14(5):294-8.
12. De Mazumder N. Neonatal Orthopaedics, 2nd edition. New Delhi: Jaypee Brothers Medical Publishers (P) Ltd.; 2013.
13. Dennison WM, MacPherson DA. Haematogenous osteitis of infancy. Arch Dis Child. 1952;27(134):375-81.
14. Skaggs DL, Flynn JM. Issues of the newborn. In: Skaggs DL, Flynn JM (Eds). Staying Out of Trouble in Pediatric Orthopaedics. Philadelphia, PA: Lippincott Williams & Wilkins; 2006. p. 135.
15. Knudsen CJ, Hoffman EB. Neonatal osteomyelitis. J Bone Joint Surg Br. 1990;72(5):846-51.
16. Deshpande SS, Taral N, Modi N, et al. Changing epidemiology of neonatal septic arthritis. Journal of orthopaedic surgery (Hong Kong). 2004;12(1):10-3.
17. Lilien LD, Yeh TF, Novak GM, et al. Early-onset Haemophilus sepsis in newborn infants: clinical, roentgenographic, and pathologic features. Pediatrics. 1978;62(3):299-303.
18. Svirsky-Fein S, Langer L, Milbauer B, et al. Neonatal osteomyelitis caused by Candida tropicalis. Report of two cases and review of the literature. J Bone Joint Surg Am. 1979;61(3):455-9.
19. Laborada G, Rego M, Jain A, et al. Diagnostic value of cytokines and C-reactive protein in the first 24 hours of neonatal sepsis. Am J Perinatol. 2003;20(8):491-501.
20. Karmazyn B. Imaging approach to acute hematogenous osteomyelitis in children: an update. Semin Ultrasound CT MR. 2010;31(2):100-6.
21. Pääkkönen M, Peltola H. Antibiotic treatment for acute haematogenous osteomyelitis of childhood: moving towards shorter courses and oral administration. Int J Antimicrob Agents. 2011;38(4):273-80.
22. Hsieh WS, Yang PH, Chao HC, et al. Neonatal necrotizing fasciitis: a report of three cases and review of the literature. Pediatrics. 1999;103(4):e53.
23. Nazir Z. Necrotizing fasciitis in neonates. Pediatr Surg Int. 2005;21(8):641-4.
24. Letts M, Blastorah B, al-Azzam S. Neonatal gangrene of the extremities. J Pediatr Orthop. 1997;17(3):397-401.
25. Uhing MR. Management of birth injuries. Clin Perinatol. 2005;32(1):19-38, v.
26. Sherk HH, Probst C. Fractures of the proximal humeral epiphysis. Orthop Clin North Am. 1975;6(2):401-13.
27. Dameron TB Jr, Reibel DB. Fractures involving the proximal humeral epiphyseal plate. J Bone Joint Surg Am. 1969;51(2):289-97.

28. Madsen ET. Fractures of the extremities in the newborn. Acta Obstet Gynecol Scand. 1955;34(1):41-74.
29. Podeszwa DA, Mooney JF 3rd, Cramer KE, et al. Comparison of Pavlik harness application and immediate spica casting for femur fractures in infants. J Pediatr Orthop. 2004;24(5):460-2.
30. Stannard JP, Christensen KP, Wilkins KE. Femur fractures in infants: a new therapeutic approach. J Pediatr Orthop. 1995;15(4):461-6.
31. Lidge RT. Complications following Bryant's traction. Arch Surg. 1960;80:557-63.
32. Wojtowycz M, Starshak RJ, Sty JR. Neonatal proximal femoral epiphysiolysis. Radiology. 1980;136(3):647-8.
33. Towbin R, Crawford AH. Neonatal traumatic proximal femoral epiphysiolysis. Pediatrics. 1979;63(3):456-9.
34. Ogden JA, Lee KE, Rudicel SA, et al. Proximal femoral epiphysiolysis in the neonate. J Pediatr Orthop. 1984;4(3):285-92.
35. Rauch F, Schoenau E. Skeletal development in premature infants: a review of bone physiology beyond nutritional aspects. Arch Dis Child Fetal Neonatal Ed. 2002;86(2):F82-5.
36. James JR, Congdon PJ, Truscott J, et al. Osteopenia of prematurity. Arch Dis Child. 1986;61(9):871-6.
37. Amir J, Katz K, Grunebaum M, et al. Fractures in premature infants. J Pediatr Orthop. 1988;8(1):41-4.
38. Dabezies EJ, Warren PD. Fractures in very low birth weight infants with rickets. Clin Orthop Relat Res. 1997;(335):233-9.
39. Harrison CM, Gibson AT. Osteopenia in preterm infants. Arch Dis Child Fetal Neonatal Ed. 2013;98(3):F272-5.
40. Rigo J, Pieltain C, Salle B, et al. Enteral calcium, phosphate and vitamin D requirements and bone mineralization in preterm infants. Acta Paediatr. 2007;96(7):969-74.
41. Hsieh FJ, Jou HJ, Ko TM, et al. Intrauterine diagnosis of short-limbed dwarfism. Taiwan Yi Xue Hui Za Zhi. 1989;88(10):1032-7.
42. Bellus GA, Hefferon TW, Ortiz de Luna RI, et al. Achondroplasia is defined by recurrent G380R mutations of FGFR3. Am J Hum Genet. 1995;56(2):368-73.
43. Krakow D, Vriens J, Camacho N, et al. Mutations in the gene encoding the calcium-permeable ion channel TRPV4 produce spondylometaphyseal dysplasia, Kozlowski type and metatropic dysplasia. Am J Hum Genet. 2009;84(3):307-15.
44. Hecht JT, Montufar-Solis D, Decker G, et al. Retention of cartilage oligomeric matrix protein (COMP) and cell death in redifferentiated pseudoachondroplasia chondrocytes. Matrix Biol. 1998;17(8-9):625-33.
45. Spranger J, Winterpacht A, Zabel B. The type II collagenopathies: a spectrum of chondrodysplasias. Eur J Pediatr. 1994;153(2):56-65.
46. Rossi A, van der Harten HJ, Beemer FA, et al. Phenotypic and genotypic overlap between atelosteogenesis type 2 and diastrophic dysplasia. Hum Genet. 1996;98(6):657-61.
47. Kemp AM, Dunstan F, Harrison S, et al. Patterns of skeletal fractures in child abuse: systematic review. BMJ. 2008;337:a1518.
48. Hardy AE. Birth injuries of the brachial-plexus: incidence and prognosis. J Bone Joint Surg Br. 1981;63-B(1):98-101.
49. Greenwald AG, Schute PC, Shiveley JL. Brachial-plexus birth palsy: a 10-year report on the incidence and prognosis. J Pediatr Orthop. 1984;4(6):689-92.
50. Piatt JH Jr. Birth injuries of the brachial plexus. Clin Perinatol. 2005;32(1):39-59, v-vi.
51. Waters PM. Comparison of the natural history, the outcome of microsurgical repair, and the outcome of operative reconstruction in brachial plexus birth palsy. J Bone Joint Surg Am. 1999;81(5):649-59.
52. Guille JT, Pizzutillo PD, MacEwen GD. Developmental dysplasia of the hip from birth to six months. J Am Acad Orthop Surg. 2000;8(4):232-42.
53. American Academy of Pediatrics. Clinical practice guideline: Early detection of developmental dysplasia of the hip. Committee on Quality Improvement, Subcommittee on Developmental Dysplasia of the Hip. American Academy of Pediatrics. Pediatrics. 2000;105(4 Pt 1):896-905.
54. Rosendahl K, Markestad T, Lie RT. Ultrasound screening for developmental dysplasia of the hip in the neonate: the effect on treatment rate and prevalence of late cases. Pediatrics. 1994;94(1):47-52.
55. Jones GT, Schoenecker PL, Dias LS. Developmental hip-dysplasia potentiated by inappropriate use of the pavlik harness. J Pediatr Orthop. 1992;12(6):722-6.
56. Lykissas MG, Crawford AH, Eismann EA, et al. Ponseti method compared with soft-tissue release for the management of clubfoot: A meta-analysis study. World J Orthop. 2013;4(3):144-53.
57. Noonan KJ, Richards BS. Nonsurgical management of idiopathic clubfoot. J Am Acad Orthop Surg. 2003;11(6):392-402.
58. Dobbs MB, Rudzki JR, Purcell DB, et al. Factors predictive of outcome after use of the Ponseti method for the treatment of idiopathic clubfeet. J Bone Joint Surg Am. 2004;86(1):22-7.
59. Solomon BD. VACTERL/VATER Association. Orphanet J Rare Dis. 2011;6:56.
60. Sasalawad SS, Hugar SM, Poonacha KS, et al. Ellis-van Creveld syndrome. BMJ Case Rep. 2013;2013. pii: bcr2013009463.
61. Koskimies E, Syvanen J, Nietosvaara Y, et al. Congenital constriction band syndrome with limb defects. J Pediatr Orthop. 2015;35(1):100-3.
62. Grogan DP, Holt GR, Ogden JA. Talocalcaneal coalition in patients who have fibular hemimelia or proximal femoral focal deficiency. A comparison of the radiographic and pathological findings. J Bone Joint Surg Am. 1994;76(9):1363-70.
63. Hall JG, Levin J, Kuhn JP, et al. Thrombocytopenia with absent radius (TAR). Medicine (Baltimore). 1969;48(6):411-39.
64. Schoenecker PL, Cohn AK, Sedgwick WG, et al. Dysplasia of the knee associated with the syndrome of thrombocytopenia and absent radius. J Bone Joint Surg Am. 1984;66(3):421-7.
65. Ko JY, Shih CH, Wenger DR. Congenital dislocation of the knee. J Pediatr Orthop. 1999;19(2):252-9.
66. Roy DR, Crawford AH. Percutaneous quadriceps recession: a technique for management of congenital hyperextension deformities of the knee in the neonate. J Pediatr Orthop. 1989;9(6):717-9.

CHAPTER

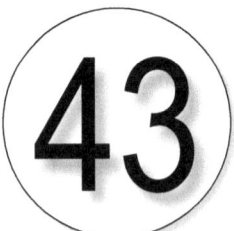

# Oxygenation, Oxygen Saturation, Retinopathy of Prematurity and Other Hyperoxia-related Damage in Newborn Infants: A Return to the Basics

*Augusto Sola, Lily C Chen*

## ABSTRACT

Oxygen is a neonatal health hazard. In caring for newborns, pediatricians, neonatologists and nurses have administered oxygen in excess for almost a century. This continues to be so all over the world and has led to significant short- and long-term morbidities, including serious incapacitating conditions such as retinopathy of prematurity (ROP) and injury to the developing brain. For the most part, these illnesses are preventable with careful and precise oxygen monitoring form the time of birth in order to guide oxygen administration and dose according to the individual newborn's needs. In this chapter we summarize salient aspects of ROP, oxidative stress, oxidant injury and physiology of oxygenation. We then discuss clinical aspects on oxygen management, oxygen in blood and saturation, focusing on proven concepts that can be useful for neonatal health care providers to avoid hyperoxemia and hyperoxia and associated induced damage.

## INTRODUCTION

Oxygen used in excess increases an infant's risk for retinopathy of prematurity (ROP) and other morbidities that can be prevented. Severe ROP is a threat to the vision and development of babies worldwide, especially where increasing numbers of premature babies are surviving. Oxygen ($O_2$) is among the most widely used drugs in newborn care, but the adverse effects of excess $O_2$ administration can be serious. Hypoxemia or hypoxia are neither deliberately induced nor accepted as normal in neonatal care; yet hyperoxemia and hyperoxia are not always carefully managed. When they occur, it is always due to the interventions of healthcare providers.

The key to any issue related to oxidative damage is prevention. Throughout the history of neonatal medicine, the administration of $O_2$ has been fraught with problems, misunderstandings, and errors.[1] Although there is ongoing debate and research regarding oxygen saturation ($SpO_2$) ranges in different phases of infant development, currently there is insufficient education about the potential damaging effects of excess $O_2$.

This chapter briefly discusses ROP and then, in more detail, how oxidative stress and oxidant injury can make $O_2$ a neonatal health hazard. We review concepts of physiology of oxygenation and $O_2$ management, including clinical aspects related to $O_2$ in blood and saturation, focusing on avoiding hyperoxemia and hyperoxia, and end with recommendations for clinical care and $SpO_2$ targeting in different neonatal conditions. The supporting bibliography for all topics presented is extensive. Due to space limitations, we have selected only some original publications and significant reviews which include extended lists of references that support all that we present in this chapter.

## RETINOPATHY OF PREMATURITY

Retinopathy of prematurity, a developmental abnormality of the retina and vitreous that occurs in premature infants, remains a leading cause of vision impairment and blindness in children around the world. Its occurrence can be decreased with improved $O_2$ management.[2-10]

In industrialized nations, ROP occurs almost exclusively in extremely low-birth weight infants. In contrast, in developing countries, ROP also occurs in larger preterm infants since the number of intensive care units for neonates has increased but often with suboptimal standards of care, causing a "third epidemic" of ROP.[11-13] An estimated 15 million preterm babies are born every year, and preterm birth rates are increasing in most countries. This increase in survival of preterm babies is associated with an increased number of infants with morbidities.

Retinopathy of prematurity and loss of vision are problems that have been frequently described in the literature in association with $O_2$ therapy. Therefore, it is imperative that measures governing $O_2$ administration improve.

The pathogenesis of ROP is unclear, complex, and multifactorial. ROP is due to abnormal angiogenesis, in which retinal blood vessels fail to grow and develop normally in infants born prematurely. The disease is associated with, and affected by, survival rates and severity of systemic disease. It is of variable severity, classified after detailed ophthalmologic funduscopic examination with indirect ophthalmoscopy. An International Classification of Retinopathy of Prematurity (ICROP) has existed for many years[14] **(Fig. 1)**, describing classic disease stages of increasing severity (stages 1–4) and dividing the eye into zones, according to which area is affected. Zone I is the most central zone, close to the optic nerve, most critical to central vision and the worst zone in which to have abnormal vessel formation. Zone II is an intermediate zone, and zone III is peripheral. The term *threshold ROP* is used when treatment is indicated. *Prethreshold* places the infant at very high risk for treatment. *Plus disease* requires at least two quadrants of dilation and tortuosity of posterior pole retinal blood vessels. The Early Treatment for Retinopathy of Prematurity (ETROP) study[15] put forth the concept that flat neovascularization in zone I should be considered stage 3, and proposed two types of ROP (I and II) to decide on the more severe cases and therapy, based on zone and on the presence or absence of plus disease.

Hyperoxemia and fluctuations in the concentration of arterial $O_2$ levels during $O_2$ therapy have been associated with increased risk for severe or threshold ROP in animals and humans. There has been improved understanding of the pathophysiology of ROP, including the role of vascular endothelial growth factor (VEG-F) and insulin-like growth factor-1 (IGF-1).[16,17] Anti-IGF-1 and anti-VEG-F may have their place in future therapy for ROP, but there is a need for more clinical studies to address safety considerations.

Oxygen therapy should be carefully adjusted (but not restricted or curtailed) to prevent alternating episodes of retinal hyperoxia and hypoxia. Investigations into the consequences of tighter $O_2$ saturation control on the development of stages 3 and 4 ROP have concluded that the severity of ROP can be reduced significantly with the use of adequate $SpO_2$ monitoring,[2,9,18-20] education of care providers, and clinical guidelines, with careful attention to $O_2$ and $SpO_2$ administration beginning at birth. These measures also are associated with improvement in other outcomes such as chronic liver disease (CLD) and other long-term outcomes.

It is impossible to know how many preterm babies become severely visually impaired or blind every year due to ROP, but it may be as many as 50,000, with the highest incidence in Asia. This number becomes even more troubling if we consider the effect on quality-adjusted life

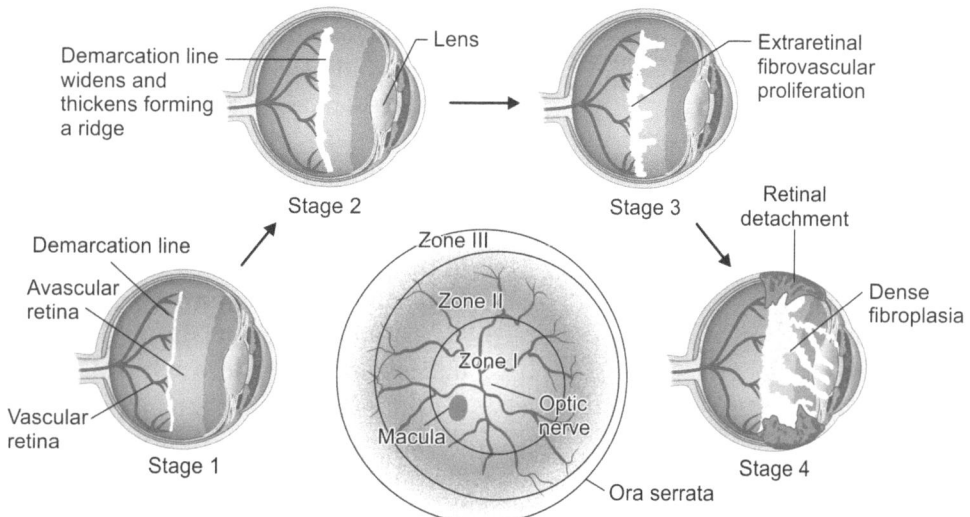

**Fig. 1:** International classification of ROP (ROP: retinopathy of prematurity).

years. Improving education together with utilizing adequate $SpO_2$ monitoring with signal extraction technology (SET), decreases ROP significantly. We can estimate that with these two changes in clinical practice, the number of infants who survive with severe ROP would decrease by at least 60%.

## SAFETY IN OXYGEN ADMINISTRATION

Oxygen is a very potent drug and is still used in unsafe ways in many situations. Various environmental stresses lead to excessive production of reactive oxygen species (ROS), causing progressive oxidative damage and ultimately cell death. The health hazards of excess $O_2$ are completely in the hands of healthcare delivery. Excess administration of $O_2$ may cause a $PaO_2$ greater than normal in a human being of any age. Judicious use of supplemental $O_2$ when a newborn infant is not hypoxemic must include eliminating the use of 100% free-flowing $O_2$ to avoid the oxidative stress and damage associated with hyperoxia.

Excess $O_2$-induced damage during the perinatal period is presented in **Box 1**. Normal birth without $O_2$ administration is associated with maternal and fetal oxidative stress with altered lipid peroxidation levels and antioxidant capacity. This is worse in cesarean sections. Unnecessary $O_2$ supplementation has been shown to be potentially dangerous for mother, fetus and placenta **(Box 2)**. Therefore, this practice should be reserved only for documented maternal hypoxia.

**Box 3** shows mechanisms of injury and undesired effects of pediatric and neonatal $O_2$ excess summarizing the impact of neonatal hyperoxia on models of pulmonary hypertension and on the master regulators of circadian rhythm among others. The combination of drugs and excess $O_2$ has been associated with potentially bad outcomes in the developing brain and eyes but anesthetic and sedative drugs could be poisonous by themselves.[4] The association of hyperoxia-induced oxidative stress and anesthetic drugs should be eluded and the practice of preoxygenation should not be utilized.

Other practices that should be eradicated are the routine usage of pure $O_2$ (i.e. inspired fraction of oxygen $FiO_2$ 1.0) in the delivery room, the use of the "hyperoxic challenge test" for differential diagnosis of heart versus lung disease and the procedure of "nitrogen washout" for a mildly to moderately symptomatic pneumothorax. These practices have inherent various potential damages and no demonstrated important benefits.

While supplemental $O_2$ need never be denied, $FiO_2$ 1.0 is almost never indicated in neonatal care. In the rare cases when it is initiated, it should be weaned as soon as possible as ROS can damage all components of the cell (proteins, lipids, and DNA). The antioxidant system has individual variability in adults but is poorly developed or markedly impaired in newborns, more so in preterm infants. Thus, oxidative damage is more serious during development.

## PHYSIOLOGY OF TISSUE OXYGENATION

The factors related to tissue oxygenation are summarized in **Box 4**. $PaO_2$ is among the least important of all the factors related to tissue oxygenation shown in the table. Furthermore, several of the involved factors described are difficult or impossible to assess in clinical care.

The alveolar gas equation is shown in **Table 1**. In room air the $FiO_2$ is 0.21 regardless of the altitude above sea level. This means that 21% of the atmospheric pressure (Patm) is $O_2$. The rest (0.79) is nitrogen. The pressure of dry gas can be easily calculated by subtracting the relative ambient

---

**BOX 1:** Risk factors for perinatal hyperoxia.

Women who undergo C-sections experience higher oxidative stress than those who give birth vaginally.
    During labor/delivery and in C-sections, unnecessary use of $O_2$ may lead to:
- Diminished fetal/maternal total antioxidant capacity, total oxidant status, and worse oxidative stress index when 40% $O_2$ is administered with spinal anesthesia instead of room air
- Higher ROS, $PaO_2$, and free $O_2$ radicals in both infants and pregnant women who receive supplemental $O_2$ during C-section with regional anesthesia

Supplemental $O_2$ should not be given for fetal resuscitation, as the benefit is unproven.

(ROS: reactive oxygen species).

---

**BOX 2:** Harmful effects of excess $O_2$ on placenta.

- Changes in $O_2$ tension and delivery may alter fetal resistance to drugs and toxins
- Tissue injury may result from harmful $O_2$ by-products after uterine hyperoxia

---

**BOX 3:** Harmful effects of hyperoxia on the infant.

- Abnormal activation of the insula, hypothalamus, and hippocampus
- Increased risk of childhood leukemia/cancer
- Cell death in the infant brain, leading to poor long-term neurodevelopmental outcomes and disabling cerebral palsy
- Changes in genes and enzymes deleterious to healthy newborn cardiopulmonary transition
- Proteome changes in the developing brain, induced by oxidative stress
- Alteration of whole-genome expression, e.g. increased risk of ROP
- Circadian rhythm disruption by altered Circadian genes
- If during anesthesia or post-surgery; reabsorption atelectasis, poor ventilation perfusion, coexisting adverse sedative agents, e.g. Midazolam and ketamine may alter risk of brain or retinal injury

(ROP: retinopathy of prematurity).

| BOX 4: Tissue oxygenation—factors to consider. | |
|---|---|
| • Cardiac output (Heart rate; stroke volume; minute volume)<br>• Peripheral vascular resistance<br>• Systemic blood flow<br>• Oxygen Delivery<br>• $PaO_2$ (mm Hg)<br>• Hb concentration (anemia) and quality (Hb F; Hb A; dyshemoglobins)<br>• Hb-$O_2$ relationship (Saturation in %)<br>• Oxygen content ($CaO_2$; in mL of $O_2$/dL)<br>• $[(SaO_2 \times Hb \times 1.34) + 0.003$ mL $O_2$/mm Hg $PaO_2]$ | • Temperature<br>• Glycemia<br>• Local $PO_2$ (4–20 mm Hg)<br>• Distance to mitochondria<br>• Microcirculation<br>• $O_2$ consumption<br>• Pulmonary vascular resistance and blood flow<br>• Hematocrit (hyperviscosity)<br>• pH<br>• $CO_2$ (local and systemic) |

| TABLE 1: Concepts and formulas derived from the alveolar gas equation. | |
|---|---|
| • Partial pressure of inspired $O_2$ ($PiO_2$)<br>• At sea level Patm is about 760–765 mm Hg. Therefore, $PiO_2$ reaching the airways and is about 150 mm Hg for dry gas<br>• Alveolar $PO_2$ ($PAO_2$)<br>• In the alveoli there is $CO_2$, at an alveolar partial pressure ($PACO_2$) of about 40 mm Hg. Therefore, "dry" $PAO_2$ in room air and at any $FiO_2$ can be derived from the formulas using the values for "dry" $PiO_2$<br>• $PaO_2$ is derived from the $PAO_2$ minus any existing shunts<br>• Normal $PaO_2$ is about 100 mm Hg at sea level in adults and 50–75 mm Hg in newborns | • $PiO_2$ in room air: Patm – $PH_2O \times 21/100$<br>• $PiO_2$ when breathing supplemental $O_2$ = $FiO_2 \times$ Patm – $PH_2O/100$<br>• $PiO_2$ in room air at sea level = 21 × Patm – $PH_2O/100$; approximately 150 mm Hg<br>• $PiO_2$ in pure $O_2$ at sea level = 100 × Patm – $PH_2O/100$; approximately 710 mm Hg<br>• $PAO_2$ = $PiO_2$ – $PACO_2$<br>• $PAO_2$ in room air at sea level = about 110 mm Hg<br>• $PAO_2$ at sea level but breathing pure $O_2$ is about 670 mm Hg<br>• With normal lungs, if a newborn is given pure $O_2$ and the $SpO_2$ is > 95%, the $PaO_2$ could be 250–400 mm Hg |

humidity or water vapor pressure ($PH_2O$) from the Patm (Patm – $PH_2O$). At sea level the pressure of dry gas is around 713 mm Hg (i.e. 760 mm Hg minus 47 mm Hg). Therefore, the partial pressure of inspired $O_2$ ($PiO_2$) in room air at sea level is 21% of 713 mm Hg, or about 150 mm Hg **(Table 1)**. When breathing 100% $O_2$ the $PiO_2$ will be approximately 710 mm Hg at sea level.

**Table 1** also shows the calculation for the alveolar partial pressure of $O_2$ ($PAO_2$) and the normal $PaO_2$ at sea level in adults and neonates.

In summary, tissue oxygenation is a complex process. It is, therefore imperative for healthcare providers not to induce hyperoxemia, with subsequent hyperoxia, oxidative stress, and oxidant injury.

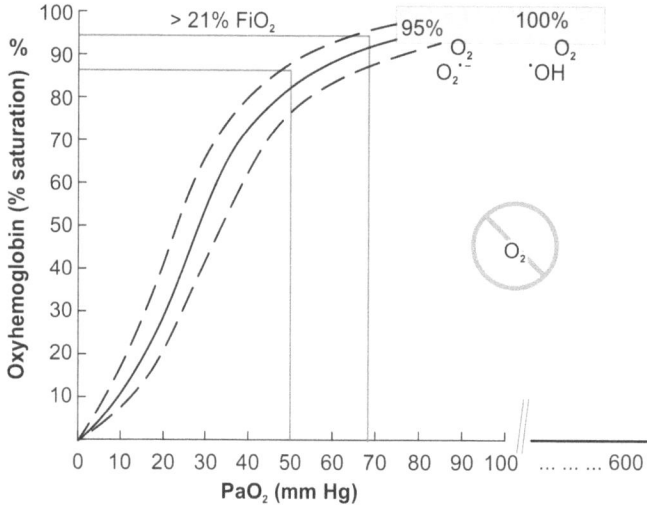

**Fig. 2:** Hb–$O_2$ relationship when breathing supplemental $O_2$. With $SpO_2$ 95–100%, $PaO_2$ could be >80 mm Hg and free dissolved $O_2$ will be circulating.
*Source:* Reprinted with permission from Augusto Sola, MD, of SIBEN.

## Assessment of Saturation in Clinical Care

The main function of hemoglobin (Hb) is to "solubilize" $O_2$ and transport it from the lungs to the tissues. The bond between $O_2$ and Hb is fascinating **(Fig. 2)**.

Oxygen saturation is expressed as percent (%); when all available Hb binding sites are completely occupied by $O_2$ molecules, the saturation is at its maximum or 100%. $SaO_2$ and Hb concentration are the key factors that determine the arterial $O_2$ content ($CaO_2$), while the contribution of $O_2$ dissolved in plasma is negligible (.003 mL $O_2$/mm Hg $PaO_2$; which is to say only 3 mL $O_2$/dL plasma when the $PaO_2$ is 100 mm Hg). With $SaO_2$ of 100% and Hb of 20 g/dL the $CaO_2$ is 26.8 mL/dL. If only 90% of the Hb binding sites were occupied with $O_2$ molecules (i.e. $SaO_2$ of 90%), $CaO_2$ would be 24.12 mL/dL. This $CaO_2$ is much higher than with 100% $SaO_2$ and Hb of 8 g/dL, where the $CaO_2$ will only be 10.72 mL/dL. As importantly, if $O_2$ is given unnecessarily, $PaO_2$ will increase but $O_2$ molecules cannot occupy any more of the Hb binding sites and they stay free in plasma, with risk for toxicity.

Situations where there may be tissue hypoxia even in the face of normal $SaO_2$ and $PaO_2$ include anemia, altered affinity of Hb for binding $O_2$ (e.g. methemoglobinemia), poor perfusion, decreased $O_2$ delivery, and altered microcirculation and related factors. On the other hand, a low $PaO_2$ in blood (hypoxemia) is not necessarily associated with inadequate tissue oxygenation (hypoxia), if there is adequate compensation by cardiac output, blood flow, and $O_2$ delivery.

The normal $SaO_2$ in room air (i.e. $FiO_2$ 0.21) is 95–100%, except during the transition from fetal to neonatal life as normal neonates may take up to 15-20 minutes after birth to reach this $SaO_2$.

As illustrated in **Figure 2**, the normal $SaO_2$ of 95-100% in room air is not recommended when breathing $FiO_2$ > 0.21. With supplemental $O_2$ and $SaO_2$ of 95-100%, the sigmoid $Hb-O_2$ relationship is "lost" and it is impossible to predict $PaO_2$ from $SaO_2$. In the example in **Figure 2**, when a newborn receives supplemental $O_2$ and the $SaO_2$ is 86-93%, the $PaO_2$ is between 50 mm Hg and 68 mm Hg. In contrast, when $SpO_2$ is 95-100%, the $PaO_2$ cannot be predicted and could be much higher than 80 mm Hg depending on the administered $FiO_2$ and the existing shunt. Free dissolved $O_2$ and ROS will then increase.

## Assessment of Oxygen in Blood

**Table 2** presents topics related to clinical assessment of $O_2$ in blood (but not in tissues). Transcutaneous $pO_2$ was continuously monitored in the past but this is not presently used for several reasons. Continuous noninvasive pulse oximeters ($SpO_2$), which are clinically used for continuous monitoring, are currently being considered as a "fifth vital sign". Pulse oximetry aids in the diagnosis of desaturation and hypoxemia but are of little or no value without the whole picture on tissue oxygenation. The functions, strengths, and limitations of $SpO_2$ monitors have been described by us[8] and others. In summary, they function by establishing the ratio between red and infrared wave lengths and displaying this as $SpO_2$. These monitors have an inherent bias (equipment error or "standard deviation"), which could be as low as 2% in some monitors but as high as 5% in others. Therefore in clinical care, it is irrelevant to argue about differences in $SpO_2$ values of 1-2%. Additionally, $SpO_2$ monitors vary by manufacturer. There are >100 published studies that demonstrate differences in $SpO_2$ monitors. The monitor with SET® has better specificity and sensitivity, less false alarms, and missed events, and functions the best during critical illness and periods of low perfusion and motion. At present, only one monitor in the market actually uses many wavelengths and not just two. In addition to $SpO_2$, this monitor measures Hb, methemoglobin and carboxyhemoglobin, and can also calculate perfusion index and plethysmographic variability index (Rainbow, Masimo Corporation, Irvine, CA).

## $SpO_2$ in Clinical Practice

In newborns in room air ($FiO_2$ 0.21) the normal $SpO_2$ is 95-100%, whether they are breathing spontaneously, on

**TABLE 2:** Clinical assessment of oxygen in blood.

| Method | Comments |
|---|---|
| $PaO_2$ measurements in arterial or venous blood | Not only do over-frequent blood samples lead to anemia/hypovolemia, but each is representative of only one point in time |
| Intermittent $SaO_2$ measurements through co-oximeters (highest standard for measuring $SaO_2$) | Using continuous wave spectrophotometers is expensive, requires blood samples, and provides intermittent monitoring only |
| Cyanosis—used to assess $O_2$ needs and fine-tune levels of $O_2$ administration | • Monitoring for bluish skin color and pale mucous membranes is problematic because the list that follows are the reasons:<br>  – Discoloration could be due to increased concentration of reduced (not saturated) Hb<br>  – People vary in their perception of color, therefore it is unreliable in diagnosis<br>  – Factors such as total Hb concentration, race, skin thickness, and illumination affect assessment<br>  – Some infants who are hypoxemic do not exhibit cyanosis<br>  – Even those infants who exhibit cyanosis may not require supplemental $O_2$ |
| Delivery room tongue color | • If the tongue is pink, the infant's $SpO_2$ is probably greater than 70%. Supplemental $O_2$ may not be required |
| Using formulas/algorithms to calculate $SaO_2$ from an arterial blood gas (based on $PaO_2$ and other factors) | • This method should not be used for clinical management of newborns<br>• Using formulas/algorithms supposes a normal adult $O_2$ dissociation curve and $O_2$ affinity, with normal 2,3 DPG, temperature, pH, $PaCO_2$, and Hb concentration. Furthermore, the assumption is made that the patient has no dyshemoglobinemia, nor fetal hemoglobin (Hb F)<br>• $SaO_2$ values calculated or transformed from a blood gas should not be compared to continuously monitored $SpO_2$ values |
| • Noninvasive pulse oximetry ($SpO_2$)<br>• Transcutaneous $PO_2$ | Please see description in chapter |

(DPG: diphosphoglycerate).

continuous positive airway pressure (CPAP), with a nasal cannula or on a respirator; the neonatal $PaO_2$ will be 50–75 mm Hg. On the other hand, when breathing supplemental $O_2$ and the $SpO_2$ is >94%, a $PaO_2$ >80 mm Hg occurs in 60% of the arterial samples.[19] Therefore, $FiO_2$ should be weaned. An adequate $SpO_2$ monitor that measures $SpO_2$ through poor perfusion and motion is necessary to more accurately adjust the amount of $O_2$ administered.

## Oxygen Practices and $SpO_2$ during Resuscitation

**Box 5** summarizes some clinical recommendations for $SpO_2$ targeting during various conditions. During resuscitation in the delivery room, most infants do not need any supplemental $O_2$.

Neonates should not be expected to have $SpO_2$ similar to that of fetuses, which is normally 60% just before birth and can decrease to as low to 30% during labor. In the transition period, $SpO_2$ increases steadily but slowly and is higher pre-ductal. Preterm infants and infants born by elective cesarean section take a bit longer to increase their $SpO_2$ to >94–95%. The right hand is always pre-ductal; if the right hand is unavailable, the left hand may be used since it is pre-ductal too in >80% of babies. The sensors should be applied according to manufacturers' specifications and Food and Drug Administration (FDA) approval. Acceptable ranges and percentiles of $SpO_2$ according to minutes after birth are summarized in **Box 5**. They are not the same for term and preterm babies and they vary according to mode of delivery and time of cord clamping. Additionally, as shown by Vento et al. in 2013, if CPAP is used in babies in room air, the increase in $SpO_2$ occurs more rapidly. It is uncertain whether this faster transition and earlier exposure to potential oxidation confers benefit or added risk.

## Clinical Recommendations for $SpO_2$ Targeting in Various Conditions

When intervention is needed in the neonatal intensive care unit (NICU) for apnea, it is better to ventilate the alveoli (breathe) and circulate, but not to give excess $O_2$ if the infant saturates adequately. With impaired alveolar ventilation and desaturation, the treatment is to ensure adequate alveolar ventilation. The risk of increasing the $FiO_2$ is induction of hyperoxemia-reperfusion after the alveolar ventilation is recovered. Additionally, if alveolar ventilation does not improve, hypoxemia will persist regardless of the

---

**BOX 5:** Suggestions for $FiO_2$ and $SpO_2$ targeting in various neonatal conditions.

*Delivery room*
$SpO_2$ increases steadily over time, reaching > 90% in about 8 minutes in term infants and a little more time in preterm infants and after cesarean sections.
   Simply stated, a term baby with pre-ductal $SpO_2$ <90% at or after 10 minutes of age should be evaluated and the underlying cause treated if necessary.

*Neonatal resuscitation*
*In term or near-term infants:* When the lungs are healthy there is no need to provide supplemental $O_2$, less so 100% $O_2$.
   Start with room air (If significant lung disease is anticipated, use higher $FiO_2$, i.e. 0.30–0.40).
*In tiny preterm infants:* Starting $FiO_2$ not well-defined yet (0.21–0.30).
   Subsequently, in both term and preterm infants adjust $FiO_2$ aiming to maintain pre-ductal $SpO_2$ within published nomograms, summarized below:
- *1 minute of age:* 10th and 90th percentiles 40%–85%
- *2 minutes of age:* 10th and 90th percentiles 46%–91%
- *3 minutes of age:* 10th and 90th percentiles 55%–92%
- *5 minutes of age:* 10th percentile 73% (90th percentile is 97%).

Decrease $FiO_2$ if $SpO_2$ >93–95%:
- *Apnea:* Ventilation with the same $FiO_2$ the infant was receiving, even if it was room air.
- *CPAP and room air ($FiO_2$ 0.21):* $SpO_2$ of 95–100% is normal with acceptable ranges of $PaO_2$. If $SpO_2$ < 94% evaluate and decide if more pressure or supplemental $FiO_2$ or both are needed.
- *Nasal cannula (high or low flow):* Similar as above. When the infant is in the hospital, it is safer to use a blender, and wean the $FiO_2$ all the way to room air if $SpO_2$ >95%. If 100% $FiO_2$ is used, the only alternative is to decrease flow if $SpO_2$ >95%, but this is more unpredictable.
- *Surgery and anesthesia:* Avoid hypoxia and hyperoxia. If $SpO_2$ 96–100%, wean $FiO_2$.
- *Suction of endotracheal tube:* Avoid hypoxia and hyperoxia. Do not "preoxygenate". If $SpO_2$ decreases do not increase $FiO_2$ abruptly or unnecessarily. Recover functional residual capacity.
- *Congenital diaphragmatic hernia and PPHN:* $SpO_2$ in the preductal territory between 91 and 96%; weaning pressures and $FiO_2$ when $SpO_2$ >96%. Avoid using 100% $O_2$ as much as possible.
- *Established BPD:* Persistent hypoxia can lead to right ventricular hypertrophy, pulmonary vasoconstriction and hypertension, cor pulmonale and bronchoconstriction. When breathing supplemental $O_2$, it may be prudent to adjust the $FiO_2$ to try maintain $SpO_2$ 91–95%, cautiously weaning the $FiO_2$ when $SpO_2$ > 95–96%.

(BPD: bronchopulmonary dysplasia; PPHN: persistent pulmonary hypertension of the newborn; CPAP: continuous positive airway pressure).

amount of $O_2$ used. The hypoxemia during endotracheal tube suctioning may be due to a diminished functional residual capacity. Higher positive end-expiratory pressure (PEEP) and/or respiratory rate (with the same $FiO_2$) during a few minutes may recover this. Preoxygenation is not a good option; it leads to hyperoxemia before suctioning and may not prevent the hypoxemia during suctioning. Hypoxemia should be promptly treated and hyperoxemia should not be induced in clinical care during neonatal resuscitation, apnea, and all other conditions listed in **Box 5**.

## Clinical Studies and $SpO_2$ Targeting for Small Preterm Infants during the First Weeks of Life

The intention to treat for $SpO_2$ in preterm infants breathing $O_2$ has been reported in the last two decades.[2,9,20-31] Despite five randomized controlled trials (RCTs),[21-25] we still do not know the optimal or perfect $SpO_2$ ranges. However, we know what $SpO_2$ values we must try to avoid. Several recent reviews summarize the salient findings and concerns of the recent RCTs that compared only two $SpO_2$ ranges as intention to treat—85-89% versus 91-95%.[7,20,26-32]

Grades of Recommendation, Assessment, Development and Evaluation (GRADE criteria) has shown that the level of confidence in some of these RCTs is only low to moderate.[32-34] There is no evidence that $SpO_2$ 91-95% is the safest range for all small preterm babies during the first weeks of life.

$SpO_2$ varies and the desired intention to treat is achieved less than 50% of the time in some infants.[35] Recently, automated $O_2$ delivery devices have been developed which have improved the proportion of time spent within the desired intention to treat.[36,37] However, they are not the final solution and are not available for routine clinical use in many countries.

## $SpO_2$ Targeting in Clinical Care

Differences in available $SpO_2$ monitors for neonates have been described as early as 2002 and only one brand was used in all RCTs. In practice, we need not be limited to target $SpO_2$ of 85-89% or 91-95%.[30] Some recommended using target ranges 90 or 91-95% based on initially reported findings of a couple of the RCTs.[21] The clinical impact was that some centers around the world changed clinical practice and increased ROP rates occurred in several of them. Many publications have suggested that prevention of severe ROP can occur without increase in mortality through improvements in clinical practice and $SpO_2$ technology.[38-41] For preterm infants in the first weeks of life, perhaps a safe $SpO_2$ intent-to-treat is between 86% and 94% in the first weeks of life when they breathe supplemental $O_2$, setting low alarms at 85% and high alarms at 95%. $SpO_2$ alarms must always be operative when a neonate is receiving supplemental $O_2$ to avoid hypoxia/hyperoxemia.

## SUMMARY

It is necessary to prevent and treat hyperoxemia as it is potentially dangerous and can damage the developing brain, alter gene expression, and be associated with childhood leukemia and cancer among other things. Cellular oxygenation, tissue hyperoxia, and hyperoxic-induced damage are complex issues. We make clinical decisions based on $SpO_2$ monitors that alert us to treatable hypoxemia but not severity of hyperoxemia. Additionally, monitor technology varies. Monitors with SET have proven optimal for newborns in many peer-reviewed publications. In the future, we need to better measure and assess tissue hypoxia, hyperoxia, and hyperoxic-induced damage. In the meantime, we must ensure sufficient $O_2$ delivery to the tissues while minimizing $O_2$ toxicity and oxidative stress. We cannot ignore the existing evidence that rates of severe ROP without increase in mortality have been associated with changes in practice including monitoring $SpO_2$ with SET technology together with educating bedside staff to decrease hyperoxemia and episodes of hypoxemia followed by hyperoxia-reperfusion from the time of birth.

Intention to maintain $SpO_2$ 91-95% may not be the safest target. The available evidence allows us to say better what we should not do rather than what we "must" do. The "magic" $SpO_2$ range for all babies at all times is not known, and it is likely that it will never be known. Therefore, any significant change in the practice of $SpO_2$ targets should be based on all available evidence and on thorough review of each center's own data. We must try to avoid tissue hypoxia, $SpO_2 \geq 95\%$ and the induction of significant fluctuations in $SpO_2$ when babies breathe supplemental $O_2$.

## CONCLUSION

Hyperoxemia is not caused by any illness or disease. Hyperoxia is caused by health care providers, does not occur in nature and evolution has not equipped the body to defend against it. It is potentially dangerous and can damage the eye and developing brain, alter gene expression, and be associated with childhood leukemia and cancer among other things. While we must always detect hypoxemia and treat its cause, at the same time we must change our clinical practices that cause hyperoxemia. We should stay away from delivering 100% $O_2$ and avoid administering any concentration of $O_2$ without having proven that the newborn is in fact in need of $O_2$. The utilization of continuous $SpO_2$ monitoring with signal extraction technology from the time of birth has proven of value to accomplish these important objectives in neonatal clinical care.

# REFERENCES

1. Silverman WA. Retrolental Fibroplasia: A Modern Parable. New York: Grune & Stratton; 2002.
2. Chow LC, Wright KW, Sola A; CSMC Oxygen Administration Study Group. Can changes in clinical practice decrease the incidence of severe retinopathy of prematurity in very low birth weight infants? Pediatrics. 2003;111(2):339-45.
3. Sola A, Rogido MR, Deulofeut R. Oxygen as a neonatal health hazard: call for détente in clinical practice. Acta Paediatr. 2007;96(6):801-12.
4. Sola A. Oxygen in neonatal anesthesia: friend or foe? Curr Opin Anaesthesiol. 2008;21(3):332-9.
5. Sola A, Saldeño YP, Favareto V. Clinical practices in neonatal oxygenation: where have we failed? What can we do? J Perinatol. 2008;28(Suppl 1):S28-34.
6. Sola A, Zuluaga C. Effects of oxygen on the development and severity of retinopathy of prematurity. J AAPOS. 2013;17(6):650-2.
7. Sola A, Golombek SG, Montes Bueno MT, et al. Safe oxygen saturation targeting and monitoring in preterm infants: can we avoid hypoxia and hyperoxia? Acta Paediatr. 2014;103(10):1009-18.
8. Sola A, Chow L, Rogido M. Pulse oximetry in neonatal care in 2005. A comprehensive state of the art review. An Pediatr (Barc). 2005;62(3):266-81.
9. Deulofeut R, Critz A, Adams-Chapman I, et al. Avoiding hyperoxia in infants < or = 1250 g is associated with improved short- and long-term outcomes. J Perinatol. 2006;26(11):700-5.
10. Bizzarro MJ, Li FY, Katz K, et al. Temporal quantification of oxygen saturation ranges: an effort to reduce hyperoxia in the neonatal intensive care unit. J Perinatol. 2014;34(1):33-8.
11. Gilbert C, Rahi J, Eckstein M, et al. Retinopathy of prematurity in middle-income countries. Lancet. 1997;350(9070):12-4.
12. Blencowe H, Lawn JE, Vazquez T, et al. Preterm-associated visual impairment and estimates of retinopathy of prematurity at regional and global levels for 2010. Pediatr Res. 2013;74(Suppl 1):35-49.
13. Gilbert C. Retinopathy of prematurity: a global perspective of the epidemics, population of babies at risk and implications for control. Early Hum Dev. 2008;84(2):77-82.
14. International Committee for the Classification of Retinopathy of Prematurity. An international classification of retinopathy of prematurity. The Arch Ophthalmol. 1984;102(8):1130-4.
15. Good WV, Hardy RJ, Dobson V, et al.; Early Treatment for Retinopathy of Prematurity Cooperative Group. The incidence and course of retinopathy of prematurity: findings from the early treatment for retinopathy of prematurity study. Pediatrics. 2005;116(1):15-23.
16. Dong L, Nian H, Shao Y, et al. PTB-associated splicing factor inhibits IGF-1-induced VEGF upregulation in a mouse model of oxygen-induced retinopathy. Cell Tissue Res. 2015;360(2):233-43.
17. VanderVeen DK, Melia M, Yang MB, et al. Anti-Vascular Endothelial Growth Factor Therapy for Primary Treatment of Type 1 Retinopathy of Prematurity: A Report by the American Academy of Ophthalmology. Ophthalmology. 2017;124(5):619-33.
18. Lim K, Wheeler KI, Gale TJ, et al. Oxygen saturation targeting in preterm infants receiving continuous positive airway pressure. J Pediatr. 2014;164(4):730-6.e1.
19. Castillo A, Sola A, Baquero H, et al. Pulse oximetry saturation levels and arterial oxygen tension values in newborns receiving oxygen therapy in the neonatal intensive care unit: is 85% to 93% an acceptable range? Pediatrics. 2008;121(5):882-9.
20. Castillo A, Deulofeut R, Critz A, et al. Prevention of retinopathy of prematurity in preterm infants through changes in clinical practice and $SpO_2$ technology. Acta Paediatr. 2011;100(2):188-92.
21. Carlo WA, Finer NN, Walsh MC, et al.; SUPPORT Study Group of the Eunice Kennedy Shriver NICHD Neonatal Research Network. Target ranges of oxygen saturation in extremely preterm infants. N Engl J Med. 2010;362(21):1959-69.
22. Vaucher YE, Peralta-Carcelen M, Finer NN, et al.; SUPPORT Study Group of the Eunice Kennedy Shriver NICHD Neonatal Research Network. Neurodevelopmental outcomes in the early CPAP and pulse oximetry trial. N Engl J Med. 2012;367(26):2495-504.
23. Stenson BJ, Tarnow-Mordi WO, Darlow BA, et al.; BOOST II United Kingdom Collaborative Group; BOOST II Australia Collaborative Group; BOOST II New Zealand Collaborative Group. Oxygen saturation and outcomes in preterm infants. N Engl J Med. 2013;368(22):2094-104.
24. Schmidt B, Whyte RK, Asztalos EV, et al.; Canadian Oxygen Trial (COT) Group. Effects of targeting higher vs lower arterial oxygen saturations on death or disability in extremely preterm infants: a randomized clinical trial. JAMA. 2013;309(20):2111-20.
25. Darlow BA, Marschner SL, Donoghoe M, et al.; Benefits of Oxygen Saturation Targeting-New Zealand (BOOST-NZ) Collaborative Group. Randomized controlled trial of oxygen saturation targets in very preterm infants: two year outcomes. J Pediatr. 2014;165:30-5.e2.
26. Sola A. Oxygen saturation in the newborn and the importance of avoiding hyperoxia-induced damage. Neoreviews. 2015;16(7):e393.
27. Whyte RK, Nelson H, Roberts RS, et al. Benefits of Oxygen Saturation Targeting Trials: Oximeter Calibration Software Revision and Infant Saturations. J Pediatr. 2017;182:382-4.
28. Schmidt B, Whyte RK, Roberts RS. Oxygen Targeting in Infants Born Extremely Preterm who Are Small for Gestational Age: A Need for Heightened Vigilance. J Pediatr. 2017;186:9-10.
29. Cummings JJ, Polin RA; AAP Committee on Fetus and Newborn. Oxygen Targeting in Extremely Low Birth Weight Infants. Pediatrics. 2016;138(2). pii: e20161576.
30. Askie LM, Darlow BA, Davis PG, et al. Effects of targeting lower versus higher arterial oxygen saturations on death or disability in preterm infants. Cochrane Database Syst Rev. 2017;4:CD011190.
31. Manja V, Saugstad OD, Lakshminrusimha S. Oxygen Saturation Targets in Preterm Infants and Outcomes at 18-24 Months: A Systematic Review. Pediatrics. 2017;139(1). pii: e20161609.
32. Lakshminrusimha S, Manja V, Mathew B, et al. Oxygen targeting in preterm infants: a physiological interpretation J Perinatol. 2015;35(1):8-15.

33. Manja V, Lakshminrusimha S, Cook DJ. Oxygen saturation target range for extremely preterm infants: a systematic review and meta-analysis. JAMA Pediatr. 2015;169(4):332-40.
34. Schmidt B, Whyte RK, Roberts RS. Trade-off between lower or higher oxygen saturations for extremely preterm infants: the first benefits of oxygen saturation targeting (BOOST) II trial reports its primary outcome. J Pediatr. 2014;165(1):6-8.
35. Schmidt B, Roberts RS, Whyte RK, et al.; Canadian Oxygen Trial Group. Impact of study oximeter masking algorithm on titration of oxygen therapy in the Canadian oxygen trial. J Pediatr. 2014;165(4):666-71.e2.
36. Claure N, Bancalari E. Role of automation in neonatal respiratory support. J Perinat Med. 2013;41(1):115-8.
37. Zapata J, Gómez JJ, Matiz Rubio A, et al. A randomized controlled trial of automated oxygen delivery algorithm in preterm neonates receiving supplemental oxygen without mechanical ventilation. Acta Paediatr. 2014;103(9):928-33.
38. Saugstad OD. Take a breath--but do not add oxygen (if not needed). Acta Paediatr. 2007;96(6):798-800.
39. Synnes A, Miller SP. Oxygen therapy for preterm neonates: The elusive optimal target. JAMA Pediatr. 2015;169(4):311-3.
40. Saugstad OD, Aune D. Optimal oxygenation of extremely low birth weight infants: a meta-analysis and systematic review of the oxygen saturation target studies. Neonatology. 2014;105(1):55-63.
41. Vento M. Oxygen supplementation in the neonatal period: changing the paradigm. Neonatology. 2014;105(4):323-31.

# CHAPTER 44

# Neonatal Gastrointestinal and Liver Disease

*Christopher Fink*

## ABSTRACT

This chapter addresses conditions such as gastroesophageal reflux disease (GERD) as they relate to respiratory health and offers a systematic approach to the differential diagnosis of newborn cholestasis and hepatitis.

## REFLUX, REGURGITATION, AND VOMITING

### Definitions and Distinctions

Gastroesophageal reflux (GER) is the effortless passage of stomach contents into the esophagus through the lower esophageal sphincter. It is a physiologic process that occurs many times per day in all humans. GER can be normal, cause disease, or be a manifestation of disease.

*Regurgitation* or "spitting up" in infants is the passage of stomach contents to the mouth. It occurs daily in ~2/3 of healthy infants and peaks at 4-6 months of age, but by 1 year, only 5% still experience daily regurgitation.[1] Infants are at increased regurgitation risk because of proportionately larger liquid intake, time spent supine, frequent meals (i.e., more time postprandial), smaller esophageal volume, increased abdominal pressure from crying and straining, and lower esophageal sphincter tone. Delayed gastric emptying also contributes, especially in children with neurological deficits.[2,3]

Vomiting (expulsion of stomach contents with force through the mouth)[4] is best diagnosed by observation. It is always pathological and requires medical attention to determine its cause **(Table 1)**. Vomiting is a reflex to many potential inputs including intestinal distention, activation of chemoreceptors, smells, and sights. Afferent pathways lead back to central integration, and thence to the efferent pathway, triggering vomiting. It may be preceded by nausea and autonomic manifestations, including cutaneous vasoconstriction, mottling, sweating, lacrimation, and salivation. The esophagus shortens and pulls the proximal stomach across the diaphragm into the thorax, which has lower pressure relative to the abdomen. Coordinated rhythmic contractions of respiratory and abdominal musculature

**TABLE 1:** Differential diagnosis of vomiting in the infant.

| Non-bilious | Bilious |
|---|---|
| • Pyloric stenosis<br>• *Metabolic:* MCAD deficiency, OTC deficiency, MELAS, acute intermittent porphyria<br>• *Central:* Bleed, trauma, subtentorial tumor, Arnold Chiari malformation<br>• *Endocrine:* Addison's disease adrenal hyperplasia<br>• *Infectious:* Pyelonephritis<br>• *Renal:* Ureteropelvic junction, uremia<br>• Pancreatitis | • *Proximal obstruction:* Duodenal atresia, annular pancreas, malrotation/volvulus, jejunal obstruction/atresia<br>• *Distal obstruction:* Ileal atresia, meconium ileus, colonic atresia, meconium plug (hypoplastic left colon syndrome), Hirschsprung disease<br>• Motility disorders including CIPO, prune belly syndrome, megacystis microcolon intestinal hypoperistalsis syndrome |

(CIPO: chronic intestinal pseudo-obstruction; MCAD: medium-chain acyl-CoA dehydrogenase deficiency; MELAS: mitochondrial encephalomyopathy, lactic acidosis, stroke-like episodes; OTC: ornithine transcarbamylase)

produce *retching*, a feature unique to vomiting. With stomach contraction, forceful expulsion of stomach contents follows.[5] In neonates, the forcefulness of vomiting contrasts with regurgitation, which is effortless. Vomiting is rarer.

## Gastroesophageal Reflux and Regurgitation

Gastroesophageal reflux, a physiologic process, is often implicated in newborn disease, including respiratory disease, perceived abdominal discomfort (excessive crying, drawing up of the legs or back-arching), apnea with bradycardia and desaturations, or brief resolved unexplained events. Refusal to feed, especially in a previously feeding infant with failure to thrive, is concerning for GERD, albeit only one cause for infant dysphagia.[6] The diagnosis is essential to protecting respiratory health, especially in infants likely to have lung disease.

### Gastroesophageal Reflux Disease and Respiratory Disease in the Newborn

Because most GER in neonates is insufficiently acidic to be detected by pH, it was not until impedance became available that the temporal relationship between apnea of prematurity and GER could be carefully examined. While both apnea of prematurity and GER are common in premature infants, they are not temporally related, a prerequisite to causality.[7] A similar lack of causal clarity exists between the bradycardia and desaturations frequently associated with apnea of prematurity. In 2008, ~25% of <1,000 g infants were discharged on GERD medications.[8] Central apnea and apnea with bradycardia and/or desaturation are not typically caused nor worsened by GER, while obstructive apnea might be.[9-11] Apnea may be precipitated by laryngeal but not pharyngeal penetration, but laryngeal penetration is unlikely during normal GER.[10] Laryngeal penetration may occur in reflux with tracheal aspiration or dysphagia associated with aspiration. A bedside or video swallow evaluation may determine that. These evaluations are done in infants with neurological deficits at risk for aspiration, and those with chronic lung disease (CLD) in whom aspiration exacerbates dyspnea.

## Diagnosis

Gastroesophageal reflux is detected by pH monitoring, or multichannel intraluminal impedance and pH monitoring (MII-pH). These detect either acid or acid and nonacid reflux, respectively. Impedance pH provides more information than pH alone **(Table 2)**. Discriminating acid from nonacid reflux is advantageous in neonates because very little reflux is acidic. Antegrade and retrograde bolus transit allows differentiation of reflux from swallowing and suggests air-swallowing versus eructation. Before

**TABLE 2:** MII-pH and pH monitoring compared.

| pH | MII-pH |
|---|---|
| • Detects acid reflux<br>• Correlates with symptoms | • Detects acid and non-acid<br>• Correlates with symptoms<br>• Characterizes reflux composition:<br>　– Acid versus non-acid<br>　– Liquid versus gas versus mixed<br>• Differentiates antegrade and retrograde transit |

(MII-pH: multichannel intraluminal impedance and pH monitoring)

either study is performed, antisecretory medications are discontinued. Proton pump inhibitors are discontinued for 7 days; $H_2$ blockers are discontinued for 3 days. Acidification of feeds with apple juice or hydrochloric acid increases sensitivity of pH monitoring.

Gastroesophageal reflux is physiological and there are few standards for how much an infant or preterm infant should reflux per day.[12,13] Determining that an infant refluxes more than arbitrary standards is less helpful than temporally correlating GER events with specific symptoms.

During pH or impedance monitoring, the infant receives bolus feeds by mouth or by nasogastric tube. Continuously fed patients or patients not being fed enterally cannot be compared to normal controls.

The upper gastrointestinal (UGI) series is an enteral contrast-enhanced fluoroscopic study used to define anatomy and exclude intestinal malrotation, pyloric stenosis, duodenal web, and esophageal disease, e.g., hiatal hernia. Reflux visualized during examination does not confirm GERD since it could be physiologic. If the infant struggles and cries, the study may be inconclusive. UGI (compared to pH impedance) has reflux detection sensitivity of 43% and negative predictive value of 24%.[14]

Esophagogastroduodenoscopy identifies mucosal lesions and some structural lesions causative or resultant of GER, but is seldom used as erosive esophagitis and eosinophilic esophagitis are unusual in infants. UGI is a less invasive means of identifying abnormal anatomy.

## Treatment

Gastroesophageal reflux may not cause but rather result in problems in the infant such as CLD, upper airway obstruction, infection, food protein allergy or intolerance, increased intra-abdominal pressure, delayed gastric emptying, or transient relaxation of the lower esophageal sphincter. Secondary GERD treatment must focus on the underlying cause.

The National Association of Pediatric Gastroenterology, Hepatology and Nutrition (NASPGHAN) clinical practice guidelines state that prior to initiating therapy for suspected GER, a study should be conducted to demonstrate the condition.[4] This may not be applicable to complicated or unstable neonatal intensive care unit (NICU) patients who might not safely tolerate probe or bolus feeds. Here, trial of pharmacologic therapy may be appropriate, provided a plan is in place to discontinue medications if improvement is not observed. Such "provocative testing" is used to resolve specific symptoms caused by GERD.

Gastroesophageal reflux treatment includes parental reassurance, counseling to avoid overfeeding, burping, and holding the infant upright after feeding. Sitting the infant upright, such as in a car seat, may increase reflux due to increased intra-abdominal pressure. Apnea and desaturation increase significantly when high-risk infants are placed in car seats; testing for desaturation, apnea, or bradycardia prior to discharge is now standard in many units.[15] Prone, followed by left lateral, are positions best for reflux, while supine and right lateral are the worst.[16] Due to risk of sudden infant death syndrome, infants should be placed supine for sleep.[17]

Treatment proceeds from least to most invasive **(Table 3)**. When regurgitation results in poor weight gain or parental distress, thickening expressed breast milk or formula may help. Rice cereal is used 1 tablespoon per 2-3 ounces milk to delay gastric emptying. It may worsen GER even while decreasing regurgitation. Recent concern that xanthan gum thickening may be associated with necrotizing enterocolitis (NEC) in preterm infants has curbed its use.[18,19] A formula change to soy or protein hydrolysate may help, if milk protein allergy is suspected. Hydrolysate formulas may speed gastric emptying time and improve GER even in infants without cow's milk protein allergy. In the absence of other symptoms such as hematochezia, improvement in GER with hydrolysate formula does not automatically lead to a diagnosis of cow's milk protein allergy. A diagnosis of cow's milk protein allergy should not be made because of improvement in GER with hydrolysate formula. Formula volume and osmolality are directly proportional to GER volume. Smaller, more frequent feeds or lower caloric density may diminish reflux.

Newborn acid production is less than in older children and adults, while greater feeding frequency (which neutralizes acid) makes it less likely to cause symptomatic GERD. Some infants respond to antisecretory medications, and their use as a provocative test is attractive versus more invasive and less available pH-impedance monitoring. Antisecretory medications may decrease volume of gastric secretions and thus be useful for infants who continue regurgitation even with transpyloric feeding.

**TABLE 3:** Gastroesophageal reflux disease and regurgitation therapies (in ascending order of invasiveness and potential harm to patient).

| Treatment | Risk | Comment |
|---|---|---|
| Reassurance | None | GER and regurgitation are physiologic processes requiring no treatment in most patients |
| Reflux precautions | None, if "back to sleep" recommendations are maintained | Observing the infant feed and subsequent symptoms assist in making sound recommendations |
| Thickening of milk | Decreased absorption of certain minerals, risk of colic and diarrhea, rare reports of intestinal obstruction, allergic reaction, and expense | Thickeners may decrease regurgitation but are unlikely to help and might worsen reflux |
| Formula change | Poor palatability resulting in decreased intake, expense | Useful if milk protein intolerance is the mechanism for GERD in a specific infant |
| Antisecretory medication | Increased respiratory and GI infections, e.g. *Clostridium difficile*. Decreased iron and calcium absorption. Abnormal GI flora. Hypergastrinemia and formation of gastric nodules and polyps | Both $H_2$ blockers and PPI are implicated in these risks. If acid suppression is started empirically, discontinue if reflux not lessened. PPI weaning is recommended |
| Prokinetics | QTc prolonged with all agents, subsequent arrhythmia documented in some. Metoclopramide commonly causes central nervous system and endocrine effects—limited use in infants. Risk of hypertrophic pyloric stenosis with erythromycin | In the USA, only metoclopramide, erythromycin, and domperidone are available |
| Transpyloric feeding | Continuous hydrolyzed feeds are necessary. Requires procedure to replace. Poor availability of small size tubes. Possible risk of intestinal perforation | A major advantage of this procedure over fundoplication is reversibility |
| Fundoplication | Morbidity, mortality, and failure rates are associated. Not practically reversible | For reflux and regurgitation in severe neurologically debilitated/consequences in those expected to worsen/never recover. Fundoplication may be life-saving in some |

(GER: gastroesophageal reflux; GERD: gastroesophageal reflux disease; GI: gastrointestinal; PPI: proton pump inhibitor)

Weaning proton pump inhibitor (PPI) over a week or more prevents rebound hypersecretory hypergastrinemia associated with immediate discontinuation. This effect should not be construed as PPI dependence for symptom relief.

Transpyloric feeding is accomplished by passage of nasojejunal (NJ) tube or, in a patient with a gastrostomy tube (G-tube), a gastrojejunal (GJ) feeding tube. GJ tubes are only available for larger infants due to perceived risk of jejunal perforation in smaller patients.[20] Transpyloric feeds must be continuous, though not necessarily around-the-clock, with the disadvantage of being tethered to a feeding pump for many hours daily. As the feeding tube bypasses the stomach, it cannot regulate the speed of delivery to the small intestine, resulting in diarrheal risk unless a hydrolyzed formula is used.

Transpyloric tubes are more cumbersome than gastric tubes. While NJ tubes are placed at bedside, GJ tubes are often placed under fluoroscopy. Frequent changes and replacements due to dislodgement increase the infant's exposure to radiation. Tube dislodgement may necessitate urgent return to a medical center if the infant's hydration depends on it.

Fundoplication is antireflux surgery. The commonly performed (Nissen) fundoplication wraps the gastric fundus around the gastroesophageal junction, tightening it and decreasing relaxation of the lower esophageal sphincter. This procedure is reserved for infants at risk of serious complications from GERD and for those not expected to improve.

While laparoscopic fundoplication is a common procedure, the level and quality of evidence supporting it is poor.[21] Benefit widely assumed in the 1980s called for inclusion of antireflux surgery for every child receiving a G-tube. Currently, children needing enteral access are not routinely offered concomitant antireflux surgery.

Preemptive Nissen fundoplication in infants with severe neurologic impairment is controversial. In 863 pediatric patients undergoing G-tube placement, presence of cerebral palsy was the only preoperative indicator predicting risk of fundoplication. Gastric emptying studies and UGI series were not predictive, even with clinical history of significant emesis.[22] In several studies, including one with age of fundoplication <1 year, neurologically impaired patients had the highest mortality rates.[23,24] Neurologically impaired patients also undergo significantly more reoperation than the neurologically normal.[21] Reasons for reoperation include wrap failure, esophageal stenosis, recurrent hiatal hernia, and the necessary pyloroplasty for delayed gastric emptying. Several studies reporting fundoplication outcomes fail to analyze neurologically impaired patients separately, despite worse outcomes.

Early studies documented high fundoplication success, but had methodological problems such as being based on parent surveys, with inadequate follow-up. Recent studies report no pediatric fundoplication benefit when performed to prevent respiratory disease, respiratory distress, and apnea.[25,26] In a study of 342 patients (45% with a well-documented neurologic disorder), hospital admissions were analyzed before and after fundoplication. Respiratory indications for admission after fundoplication did not improve and in some cases worsened.[25] Ideally, antireflux procedures should be performed only in children with well-documented GERD who have failed medical management.[25]

A study of 470 children <1.5 years of age undergoing UGI for various indications found GER in 80%.[27] Thus, objective evidence of preoperative GER as an indication to include antireflux surgery with G-tube placement would be self-fulfilling. At least one study shows no association between GER seen on UGI and ultimate need for an antireflux procedure,[22] which is unsurprising as UGI is a poor study to identify GERD.[14]

None of the prior interventions reduced risk of aspirating oral/nasopharyngeal secretions. Aspiration is considered separately from GERD and most commonly treated with anticholinergic agents such as glycopyrrolate or a tracheostomy.

# ENTERAL TUBES

## Definitions and Distinctions

Enteral tubes are used to deliver nutrition to those patients who eat insufficiently by mouth, or for decompressing/suctioning gastrointestinal content. Feeding tubes are typically smaller and softer than those used for suctioning; the latter must be stiff enough not to collapse under negative pressure. Gastrostomy and GJ tubes may be placed surgically by interventional radiology or endoscopically.

## Removing or Changing Gastrostomy Tubes

Removing or changing a tube passing through a gastrostomy requires knowledge of what holds the tube in place at the stomach. This bolster or "bumper" may be a collapsible soft disk when pulled with enough force, a balloon filled with water that must be deflated prior to pulling, or a mushroom-shaped bumper that must be straightened by pushing a separately supplied obturator while pulling the tube. Initial G-tube placement requires at least 6 weeks for the stomach to adhere firmly to the abdominal wall. After changing a tube, any question of tube placement or difficulty placing the new tube should prompt a study (usually X-ray) with a small amount of water-soluble contrast, to confirm placement and guard against feeding extraluminally. A G-tube site closes in a few hours without a tube to ensure patency. Parents and caregivers should be trained to replace a dislodged G-tube before the gastrostomy closes.

## Common Enteral Feeding Tube Problems and Solutions

### Preventing Clogging and Regaining Patency

Tube clogging is preventable by proper flushing after checking for residuals, after bolus feeds, and every 4 hours during continuous feeds, as well as after and between medications. Flush volumes may be limited by fluid restriction and it is important to be cognizant that tube length, rather than diameter, increases flush volume.

Clogged enteral tubes are not uncommon and in postoperative/unstable patients replacing the tube may be neither safe nor easy. Warm water in a small syringe (e.g. a 1-cc tuberculin syringe), infuses small volumes under high pressure. Avoid cola or other liquids, as stickiness worsens the problem. If the tube is still clogged, it is important to exclude formula or medication delivery at the time of malfunction. For formula clogs, papain (meat tenderizer) is used. For clogged medication, activated Viokase (pancreatic enzyme preparation) may be used—one crushed tablet of Viokase or 1 teaspoon of Viokase powder, one crushed non-enteric coated 324 mg sodium bicarbonate tablet or one-eighth teaspoon baking soda in 5 mL warm water. With papain or Viokase, using a small syringe, as much solution as possible is instilled into the clogged tube and left for 30–60 minutes, repeated as necessary. It is safe to push the solution through once the clog is dislodged.

A leaking gastrostomy or GJ tube leads to granulation tissue and skin breakdown. Leaking tubes are replaced. If the leak comes from around the tube, then consider—(1) if there is an internal balloon (bolster on the gastric side), check that it has not leaked or ruptured. Adding air to the balloon helps slow the leak, but this solution is temporary. For low-profile tubes, discourage stacking gauze or "2 × 2's" under the external bolster. This will dilate the tract and may lead to "buried bumper syndrome". One frequently changed 2 × 2 gauze to soak up leaked contents is acceptable; (2) too large a gastrostomy may require removing the tube for ~45 minutes to allow the gastrostomy site to partially close. Checking frequently is important to prevent complete closure. Leaking leads to bulky granulation that, when asymmetrical, will cause the tube to fit incorrectly and lead to more leaking. Attention to granulation tissue interrupts this vicious cycle. If skin is broken, the area is kept dry, or a water-repelling ointment is used to limit contact with gastric secretions. In severe cases, acid suppression may help healing. Satellite lesions may be indicative of yeast, in which case topical antifungal powder works better than ointment on wet surfaces.

Connective tissue at the gastrostomy site (i.e. granulation), is typically pink in color, looks overgrown, and is friable (bleeds easily). It can be chemically cauterized with silver nitrate applied once every several days until the tissue recedes. Steroids such as triamcinolone are also applied to discourage regrowth. Asymmetrical granulation may result from the feeding tube or extension tubing pulling to one side more than the other (remediable by alternating side of the patient the tube hangs from). Granulation should be distinguished from prolapsed gastric mucosa, through the gastrostomy, as gastric mucosa is not cauterized. Though rarely necessary, biopsy with histological examination distinguishes granulation from stomach mucosa. Usually mucosa may be pushed back into the stomach, the tube left out to allow partial gastrostomy closure, making prolapse recurrence less likely. The last option is surgical and repositioning the gastrostomy may be required (closing the problematic gastrostomy site and creating a new one).

Gastrostomy-associated cellulitis is overdiagnosed, but occurs and is treated with the same empiric agents as cellulitis in other locations. Tenderness and expanding erythema are concerning. Rarer than cellulitis is a gastrostomy-associated abscess, best localized by ultrasound.

## NEONATAL LIVER DISEASE

Neonatal cholestasis is challenging as the differential diagnosis includes common, self-limiting conditions, as well as serious and life-threatening problems. As diagnostic tests are invasive, expensive, or time-consuming, clinicians determine which patient can be observed and who needs to be subjected to study/intervention.

Although neonatal cholestasis occurs in ~1/2,500 infants, it is not uncommon in the NICU.[28] It occurs frequently with extended parenteral nutrition use, and in perioperative patients with prolonged bowel rest. Unlike older children, neonates have less mature hepatic excretory function. Cholestasis may be a presenting feature of sepsis, surgical abdomen, poor cardiac output, metabolic disease, and several other conditions.

Cholestatic jaundice is often continuous with physiologic jaundice and thus easily missed. Whenever bilirubin is measured in an infant, it is prudent to fractionate into conjugated and unconjugated (direct and indirect, respectively).

## Pathophysiology

Liver disease is categorized as *cholestatic*, the result of bile duct injury or obstruction, or *hepatitic*, the result of hepatocellular injury. Cholestasis is characterized by elevated conjugated bilirubin, often with elevations of alkaline phosphatase or gamma-glutamyl transferase (GGT). GGT is useful in premature infants because elevated alkaline phosphatase also occurs with osteopenia. Newborn GGT <28 days may be slightly increased beyond normal reference values.[29] Neonatal age explains only mild elevations, and does not explain a rising trend. GGT usually rises as biliary atresia worsens, much as in other specific causes of extrahepatic cholestasis. GGT may also be of prognostic value in cases of intrahepatic cholestasis. In spite of the broader diversity of etiologies of intrahepatic versus extrahepatic cholestasis, GGT is a sensitive though not specific predictor of poor outcome (persistent disease, death, or liver transplantation before 1 year of age) when <75 U/L or >300 U/L.[30]

Hepatitis may be present with elevated serum liver enzymes, including aspartate aminotransferase (AST), alanine aminotransferase (ALT), and lactate dehydrogenase (LDH). Of these, ALT is most specific to the liver. It is good to consider extrahepatic sources of these enzymes when liver injury does not explain their elevation. Newborn cholestasis and hepatitis are rarely perfectly distinct as cholestasis may result in hepatocellular dysfunction due to toxic effects of bile within the hepatocytes. Hepatocellular injury also results in reduced bile flow and stasis with elevated serum-conjugated bilirubin. The differential diagnosis for cholestasis and hepatitis in the newborn is thus overlapping.

## Acute Care of the Patient with End-stage Liver Disease

Definitively diagnosing cause of a newborn cholestasis is time-consuming, but supportive care must be immediate. This includes assessment of coagulation and repletion as necessary with vitamin K. Albumin and prothrombin time (PT) are indicators of liver synthetic function. Synthetic dysfunction is a late sign of liver disease, but impaired PT may also indicate vitamin K deficiency due to malabsorption of this fat-soluble vitamin, potentially dangerous for the relatively vitamin K-deficient newborn.

In very ill babies, early identification and prompt treatment of sepsis, NEC, or inborn errors of metabolism (IEM) are crucial. In those with liver disease at or soon after birth, neonatal hemochromatosis must be excluded, as this alloimmune disease is potentially treatable, if recognized early.

Less urgent but still important is the identification of patients with biliary atresia (discussed in the surgical chapter of this book) before ~2 months of age, when the success rate of the Kasai portoenterostomy declines and liver transplantation becomes inevitable.[31] Once both biliary atresia and acute life-threatening causes of cholestasis have been excluded in the cholestatic infant, the broad differential diagnosis of neonatal hepatitis and cholestasis inclusive of congenital/syndromic etiology merits consideration.

## Approach to Neonatal Liver Disease

The genetic and molecular basis of hereditary forms of cholestasis are now better understood.[28] Over the last 40 years, "neonatal hepatitis" (a descriptive reference to newborns with hepatitis or cholestasis of unknown cause) has dropped from 65% of infants with cholestasis to just 10%. Currently biliary atresia accounts for ~25–30% of those diagnosed, genetic disorders for 25%, metabolic disease for 20%, and alpha-1-antitrypsin deficiency for 10%. A German tertiary medical center found similar proportions—biliary atresia (41%), idiopathic (13%), progressive familial intrahepatic cholestasis (10%), and alpha-1-antitrypsin deficiency, Alagille syndrome, portacaval shunts, mitochondriopathy, and biliary sludge (all 2%).[32]

## History

Relevant history includes prenatal care when available and if not, the mother's pregnancy history, including HIV and hepatitis B status. Perinatal febrile illness might indicate bacterial newborn sepsis. Earlier in pregnancy, other vertically transmitted infections such as herpes simplex, cytomegalovirus (CMV), and syphilis bear exclusion. These three agents can also have neurological manifestations.[33] Miscarriage, prior neonatal demise, or family history of previous children with liver disease or chronic medical conditions is important. As IEM are often autosomal recessive, consanguinity must be excluded. Neonatal hemochromatosis is an alloimmune neonatal hepatitis that will affect most subsequent pregnancies in mothers not receiving gestational intravenous (IV) immunoglobulin therapy. Prior miscarriage may also suggest this disease. Alagille syndrome is autosomal dominant even if not previously diagnosed in other family members. Some cases are *de novo* mutations, and thus absence of family history of the syndrome does not rule it out **(Table 4)**.

## Physical Examination

Aside from jaundice, skin examination may reveal a rash consistent with congenital TORCH (Toxoplasmosis, Other agents, rubella, CMV, herpes simplex) infection or cutaneous hemangiomatoses with liver involvement. Cutaneous stigmata of liver disease, such as spider angiomata and xanthomas, are unusual in neonates, and palmar erythema may occur but often is a late finding.[34]

When palpating for the infant's liver edge with the pads of the fingertips, press gently to maintain sensitivity. A relaxed abdomen in a calm infant provides optimal

**TABLE 4:** Historical and physical clues to the newborn with liver disease.

| Clue | Points to | Comment |
|---|---|---|
| Dark urine, acholic stools | Biliary atresia, choledochal cyst, other biliary obstruction | Break up stool to verify pigment is deeper than superficial. Pigment can be deposited on stool surface by bowel wall jaundice |
| Murmur | Syndromic biliary atresia or Alagille syndrome | About 20% of biliary atresia is "syndromic" and may include cardiac defects, situs inversus, intestinal malrotation, polysplenia or asplenia. Alagille murmur often due to peripheral pulmonic stenosis |
| Nystagmus, blindness, and endocrinopathies | Panhypopituitarism | MRI brain and serum levels of pituitary hormones. Check serum calcium and phosphorus levels. |
| Fever, elevated or depressed serum white blood cells, + or − rash | Bacterial or viral sepsis or urinary tract infection | TORCH infections. *E. coli* sepsis associated with galactosemia. Cutaneous evidence of extramedullary hematopoiesis "Blueberry muffin baby" may suggest rubella, CMV, other congenital infection[39] |
| Maternal fever | Chorioamnionitis | Cholestasis associated with newborn sepsis |
| Poor feeding, poor weight gain, hypotonia, hypoglycemia, vomiting, or seizures | Inborn errors of metabolism | Newborn screening results if available. Normalize serum glucose until disorder identified |
| Previously affected or deceased newborn, history of miscarriages | Neonatal hemochromatosis, Langerhans histiocytosis, IEM | Check newborn screen |
| Delayed passage of meconium, meconium ileus, pulmonary problems | Cystic fibrosis | Review newborn screen, confirm genetic studies or sweat chloride test |
| History of umbilical arterial catheter, and umbilical venous catheter | Thrombus and hepatic abscess | Doppler liver ultrasound |
| Maternal hepatitis, IV drug use, and previous transfusion | Perinatal hepatitis infection | Infant antibodies reflect maternal serum for 3–4 months |
| IUGR, microcephaly, chorioretinitis, purpura, and multisystem organ failure | TORCH | Blueberry muffin syndrome |
| Splenomegaly | Portal hypertension, metabolic storage disease, hemolysis with splenic clearance and extramedullary hematopoiesis, malignant infiltration | Thrombocytopenia accompanies splenomegaly; is transfusion-resistant |
| Ascites | Portal hypertension, low serum oncotic pressure, low albumin due to impaired production or increased loss, e.g. protein-losing enteropathy | Paracentesis used less often in infants than adults with ascites because of rapid reaccumulation and large fluid shifts affecting vital signs and electrolytes |
| Congenital heart block, rash | Neonatal lupus erythromatosis | Mother may be asymptomatic when infant diagnosed[40] |

(CMV: cytomegalovirus; IEM: inborn errors of metabolism; MRI: magnetic resonance imaging; TORCH: toxoplasmosis, other agents, rubella, CMV, herpes simplex; IV: intravenous; IUGR: intrauterine growth retardation)

examination. Palpation starts in the pelvis and moves cephalad as the liver edge can be surprisingly low. If a low-lying edge is found, the costal margin is traced to distinguish liver from spleen. In the right midclavicular line, the normal newborn liver can be as low as 3.5 cm below the costal margin. The liver edge may be displaced by thoracic, abdominal, retroperitoneal mass, organomegaly, fluid, or pneumothorax. Chest deformity may displace the liver inferiorly. A choledochal cyst or perihepatic abscess may be mistaken for hepatomegaly. A Riedel (elongated left) lobe of the liver is a normal variant. Other normal variants exist and can usually be distinguished from pathological hepatomegaly by ultrasound. Measuring liver span instead of liver edge is a more accurate way to identify hepatomegaly. Normal newborn liver span is 4.5-5 cm. It is determined by percussing the upper edge and palpating or auscultating (scratch test) to find the lower edge. To auscultate, one listens with the stethoscope just below the xiphoid process and starts scratching from the right lower quadrant until sound enhancement is heard.[35]

Liver firmness and nodularity may indicate fibrosis. Liver ballottement indicates free fluid in the abdomen, possibly ascites.

Splenomegaly, especially with thrombocytopenia in the setting of liver disease, suggests portal hypertension. However, it can also occur during hemolysis, metabolic storage disease, or malignancy.

Abnormal bleeding from attempted IV sites and abnormal bruising may indicate advanced liver disease with synthetic impairment, but more often reflects vitamin K malabsorption with resulting deficiency. Indeed, bleeding may be the sole presenting feature of biliary atresia[36] (*see* Table 4).

## Causes of Neonatal Cholestasis

### Sepsis

Premature and small-for-gestation newborns have many reasons to be cholestatic. Cholestasis secondary to sepsis and total parenteral nutrition (TPN) is common in the NICU.

In 153 neonates with (blood culture +) sepsis, 43% developed cholestasis.[37] Onset occurred <3 days, peaked ~10th day and 15% of cases remained cholestatic >30 days from onset, with resolution by 60 days.

### Intestinal Failure-related Liver Disease

Approximately 20% of neonates receiving parenteral nutrition >2 weeks develop cholestasis.[38] In infants and children treated for >3 months with parenteral nutrition who subsequently achieved full enteral nutrition, mean time to normalization of direct bilirubin and ALT were 13 weeks and 35 weeks, respectively. Persistent ALT elevations seen in children in whom direct bilirubin has returned to normal may indicate ongoing liver injury even after parenteral nutrition withdrawal.[41] Improvement of direct bilirubin and transaminases may not occur until full enteral nutrition is achieved and parenteral nutrition withdrawn; some patients will exhibit a 1-month plateau phase.[42] A more recent study confirmed that ~2/3 of infants experience not a plateau but a rise in bilirubin that can last for weeks after parenteral nutrition is stopped.[43]

Intestinal failure-related liver disease (IFRLD) is used in place of TPN cholestasis to emphasize the multifactorial disease. The degree of hepatobiliary dysfunction after TPN is worse in infants with intrauterine growth restriction.[46] Gestational age is inversely associated with time to normalization of direct bilirubin.[41] Other factors contributing to TPN-associated cholestasis are infection (catheter-related sepsis, peritonitis, and urinary tract infection) and intestinal stasis.[47]

**TABLE 5:** Measures to improve IFRLD in infants receiving TPN.

- In advanced liver disease, critically ill, very premature, or malnourished infants, treatment includes glucose infusion
- If not, cycle the TPN (run it faster over fewer hours per day)
- Adjust trace elements
- Omegaven or other omega-3 source of intravenous lipid emulsion
- Trophic feeds—even a few milliliters per hour may help
- Long-term, restoring bowel continuity in ostomy patients
- Prevent line infections with line care and possibly ethanol locks
- Ursodeoxycholic acid[44,45]

(IFRLD: intestinal failure-related liver disease; TPN: total parenteral nutrition)

Although lipid composition (omega-3 versus omega-6 fatty acids) receives much attention for IFRLD, evidence suggests IV dextrose is important in liver toxicity.[48]

Evaluating infants with prolonged TPN or persistent cholestasis is difficult. Most infants are a few weeks old, making neonatal hemochromatosis less likely. After eliminating other life-threatening conditions such as sepsis and NEC that occur in older infants, biliary atresia needs exclusion. Infants over a few months of age with mild elevations of direct bilirubin are unlikely to have biliary atresia. Excluding syndromic biliary atresia and associated cardiac defects, the typical infant with biliary atresia is usually term without other medical problems and growing well. In an infant currently or previously maintained on parenteral nutrition for several weeks, this small risk must be weighed against the >20% chance that cholestasis has resulted from IFRLD. Given low prevalence, clinicians must maintain vigilance without administering excessive invasive and expensive tests.

Therapy for patients with IFRLD is initiation and advancement of enteral feeds (**Table 5**). In a retrospective study of infants treated with ursodeoxycholic acid (ursodiol), the onset of cholestasis was later and the duration shorter.[45] A prospective study with no control group found similar results.[49] Randomized controlled trials are needed.

### Progressive Familial Intrahepatic Cholestasis Syndromes and Defects of Bile Acid Biosynthesis

Bile acid output comprises ~40% volume of bile and is directly proportional to bile flow. It is not just volume of bile acids but their composition that affects biliary health. Certain bile acids, like cholic acid, may be trophic and choleretic to the biliary system while others, e.g. lithocholic acid, is toxic and promotes cholestasis.[50] Therefore, IEM in bile acid biosynthesis or membrane transport lead to cholestasis by either decreased total production, or by underproduction or overproduction of specific constituent bile acids. Many enzymes are necessary in the pathways leading from cholesterol to the various specific bile acids, thus many possible IEM occur. Many of these errors have been described clinically.[51] Prompt diagnosis and treatment with oral cholic acid sometimes results in histologic improvement and reduces liver transplantation.[52,53] Early identification of bile acid synthesis and transport disorders is important because safe and effective treatments exist.

Progressive familial intrahepatic cholestasis (PFIC) is a family of bile acid transporter defects. Serum bile acids are low in bile acid synthesis defect and high in PFIC. If PFIC is suspected, serum GGT can distinguish PFIC type 1 or 2, which will have low or normal GGT, from PFIC type 3, which will have high GGT. PFIC1 often has extrahepatic manifestations while PFIC2 does not. Genetic evaluation for inherited intrahepatic cholestasis syndromes can be ordered separately or simultaneously using the Jaundice Chip.[54]

Early referral is crucial for patients with worsening liver disease and for those needing liver transplantation. As liver disease progresses, cerebral edema and hepatic encephalopathy ensue, cardiopulmonary status becomes unstable, especially with secondary infections, and fluids and electrolytes become increasingly challenging. Liver failure patients require blood products, mechanical ventilation, and dialysis. Liver transplant is an option for some but for very young patients, the wait can be long. Early referral for transplantation enhances survival in these cases.

## CONCLUSION

Newborn gastrointestinal conditions are common and may be benign, or indicative of serious underlying disease. There are many emerging therapies; several centers have aerodigestive teams to address complex and chronic gastrointestinal reflux disease, which sometimes coexists with chronic or developmental lung disease, especially in premature infants.

Some infants with oral aversion may require varying durations of tube feedings. It is important to involve a pediatric gastroenterologist in the management of these babies' care. Interdisciplinary discussions with speech therapists, other therapists, and specialists, including pediatric surgeons, is often necessary to optimize outcomes.

Timely recognition and treatment of neonates with liver disease is imperative in order to fully support these patients and their families. Advances in parenteral nutrition support with minimizing exposure to phytocholesterols have resulted in less acquired liver injury from prior neonatal therapies. This has allowed infants with congenital liver disease to grow and thrive as they await organ transplant.

While previously underappreciated, pediatric gastroenterology and hepatology have become dynamic fields with exponential advances in understanding which will lead to new therapies and insights in the coming years.

## REFERENCES

1. Orenstein SR, Shalaby TM, Cohn JF. Reflux symptoms in 100 normal infants: diagnostic validity of the infant gastroesophageal reflux questionnaire. Clin Pediatr (Phila). 1996;35(12):607-14.
2. Fonkalsrud EW, Ament ME. Gastroesophageal reflux in childhood. Curr Probl Surg. 1996;33(1):1-70.
3. Stacher G, Lenglinger J, Bergmann H, et al. Gastric emptying: a contributory factor in gastro-oesophageal reflux activity? Gut. 2000;47(5):661-6.
4. Rudolph CD, Mazur LJ, Liptak GS, et al.; North American Society for Pediatric Gastroenterology and Nutrition. Guidelines for evaluation and treatment of gastroesophageal reflux in infants and children: recommendations of the North American Society for Pediatric Gastroenterology and Nutrition. J Pediatr Gastroenterol Nutr. 2001;32(Suppl 2):S1-31.
5. Behrman RE, Kliegman RM, Jenson HB. Nelson textbook of pediatrics, 17th edition. London, United Kingdom: Saunders; 2003. pp. 1-2672.
6. Burklow KA, Phelps AN, Schultz JR, et al. Classifying complex pediatric feeding disorders. J Pediatr Gastroenterol Nutr. 1998;27(2):143-7.
7. Peter CS, Sprodowski N, Bohnhorst B, et al. Gastroesophageal reflux and apnea of prematurity: no temporal relationship. Pediatrics. 2002;109(1):8-11.
8. Malcolm WF, Gantz M, Martin RJ, et al.; National Institute of Child Health and Human Development Neonatal Research Network. Use of medications for gastroesophageal reflux at discharge among extremely low birth weight infants. Pediatrics. 2008;121(1):22-7.
9. Poets CF. Gastroesophageal reflux: a critical review of its role in preterm infants. Pediatrics. 2004;113(2):e128-32.
10. Rudolph CD. Supraesophageal complications of gastroesophageal reflux in children: challenges in diagnosis and treatment. Am J Med. 2003;115(Suppl 3A):150S-6S.
11. Suys B, De Wolf D, Hauser B, et al. Bradycardia and gastroesophageal reflux in term and preterm infants: is there any relation? Journal of pediatric gastroenterology and nutrition. 1994;19(2):187-90.
12. López-Alonso M, Moya MJ, Cabo JA, et al. Twenty-four-hour esophageal impedance-pH monitoring in healthy preterm neonates: rate and characteristics of acid, weakly acidic, and weakly alkaline gastroesophageal reflux. Pediatrics. 2006;118(2):e299-308.
13. Martin RJ, Hibbs AM. Diagnosing gastroesophageal reflux in preterm infants. Pediatrics. 2006;118(2):793-4.
14. Macharia EW. Comparison of upper gastrointestinal contrast studies and pH/impedance tests for the diagnosis of childhood gastro-oesophageal reflux. Pediatr Radiol. 2012;42(8):946-51.
15. Elder DE, Russell L, Sheppard D, et al. Car seat test for preterm infants: comparison with polysomnography. Arch Dis Child Fetal Neonatal Ed. 2007;92(6):F468-72.
16. Ewer AK, James ME, Tobin JM. Prone and left lateral positioning reduce gastro-oesophageal reflux in preterm infants. Arch Dis Child Fetal Neonatal Ed. 1999;81(3):F201-5.
17. Carroll AE, Garrison MM, Christakis DA. A systematic review of nonpharmacological and nonsurgical therapies

17. for gastroesophageal reflux in infants. Arch Pediatr Adolesc Med. 2002;156(2):109-13.
18. Beal J, Silverman B, Bellant J, et al. Late onset necrotizing enterocolitis in infants following use of a xanthan gum-containing thickening agent. J Pediatr. 2012;161(2):354-6.
19. Woods CW, Oliver T, Lewis K, et al. Development of necrotizing enterocolitis in premature infants receiving thickened feeds using SimplyThick®. J Perinatol. 2012;32(2):150-2.
20. King M, Barnhart DC, O'Gorman M, et al. Effect of gastrojejunal feedings on visits and costs in children with neurologic impairment. J Pediatr Gastroenterol Nutr. 2014;58(4):518-24.
21. Martin K, Deshaies C, Emil S. Outcomes of pediatric laparoscopic fundoplication: a critical review of the literature. Can J Gastroenterol Hepatol. 2014;28(2):97-102.
22. Novotny NM, Jester AL, Ladd AP. Preoperative prediction of need for fundoplication before gastrostomy tube placement in children. J Pediatr Surg. 2009;44(1):173-7.
23. Thompson WR, Hicks BA, Guzzetta PC Jr. Laparoscopic Nissen fundoplication in the infant. J Laparoendosc Surg. 1996;6(Suppl 1):S5-7.
24. Kawahara H, Okuyama H, Kubota A, et al. Can laparoscopic antireflux surgery improve the quality of life in children with neurologic and neuromuscular handicaps? J Pediatr Surg. 2004;39(12):1761-4.
25. Lee SL, Shabatian H, Hsu JW, et al. Hospital admissions for respiratory symptoms and failure to thrive before and after Nissen fundoplication. J Pediatr Surg. 2008;43(1):59-63-5.
26. Thakkar K, Boatright RO, Gilger MA, et al. Gastroesophageal reflux and asthma in children: a systematic review. Pediatrics. 2010;125(4):e925-30.
27. Boyle JT. Gastroesophageal reflux disease in 2006. The imperfect diagnosis. Pediatr Radiol. 2006;36(Suppl 2):192-5.
28. Balistreri WF, Bezerra JA. Whatever happened to "neonatal hepatitis"? Clin Liver Dis. 2006;10(1):27-53, v.
29. Hirfanoglu IM, Unal S, Onal EE, et al. Analysis of serum γ-glutamyl transferase levels in neonatal intensive care unit patients. J Pediatr Gastroenterol Nutr. 2014;58(1):99-101.
30. Lu FT, Wu JF, Hsu HY, et al. γ-Glutamyl transpeptidase level as a screening marker among diverse etiologies of infantile intrahepatic cholestasis. J Pediatr Gastroenterol Nutr. 2014;59(6):695-701.
31. Nio M, Wada M, Sasaki H, et al. Effects of age at Kasai portoenterostomy on the surgical outcome: a review of the literature. Surg Today. 2015;45(7):813-8.
32. Hoerning A, Raub S, Dechêne A, et al. Diversity of disorders causing neonatal cholestasis - the experience of a tertiary pediatric center in Germany. Front Pediatr. 2014;2:65.
33. Bilavsky E, Schwarz M, Bar-Sever Z, et al. Hepatic involvement in congenital cytomegalovirus infection - infrequent yet significant. J Viral Hepat. 2015;22(9):763-8.
34. Greydanus DE, Feinberg AN, Patel DR, Homnick DN. The Pediatric Diagnostic Examination, 1st edition. McGraw-Hill; 2007. pp. 1-832.
35. Algranati PS. The Pediatric Patient: An Approach to History and Physical Examination. Williams & Wilkins; 1992. pp. 1-217.
36. Faverey LC, Vandenplas Y. Hemorrhagic diathesis as the presenting symptom of neonatal cholestasis. Pediatr Gastroenterol Hepatol Nutr. 2014;17(3):191-5.
37. Khalil S, Shah D, Faridi MM, et al. Prevalence and outcome of hepatobiliary dysfunction in neonatal septicaemia. J Pediatr Gastroenterol Nutr. 2012;54(2):218-22.
38. Jolin-Dahel K, Ferretti E, Montiveros C, et al. Parenteral nutrition-induced cholestasis in neonates: where does the problem lie? Gastroenterol Res Pract. 2013;2013:163632.
39. Mehta V, Balachandran C, Lonikar V. Blueberry muffin baby: a pictoral differential diagnosis. Dermatol Online J. 2008;14(2):8.
40. Singalavanija S, Limpongsanurak W, Aoongern S. Neonatal lupus erythematosus: a 20-year retrospective study. J Med Assoc Thai. 2014;97 Suppl 6:S74-82.
41. Yang CF, Lee M, Valim C, et al. Persistent alanine aminotransferase elevations in children with parenteral nutrition-associated liver disease. J Pediatr Surg. 2009;44(6):1084-8.
42. Javid PJ, Collier S, Richardson D, et al. The role of enteral nutrition in the reversal of parenteral nutrition-associated liver dysfunction in infants. J Pediatr Surg. 2005;40(6):1015-8.
43. Mangalat N, Bell C, Graves A, et al. Natural history of conjugated bilirubin trajectory in neonates following parenteral nutrition cessation. BMC Pediatr. 2014;14:298.
44. Thibault M, McMahon J, Faubert G, et al. Parenteral nutrition-associated liver disease: a retrospective study of ursodeoxycholic Acid use in neonates. J Pediatr Pharmacol Ther. 2014;19(1):42-8.
45. Simić D, Milojević I, Bogićević D, et al. Preventive effect of ursodeoxycholic acid on parenteral nutrition-associated liver disease in infants. Srp Arh Celok Lek. 2014;142(3-4):184-8.
46. Baserga MC, Sola A. Intrauterine growth restriction impacts tolerance to total parenteral nutrition in extremely low birth weight infants. J Perinatol. 2004;24(8):476-81.
47. Kubota A, Yonekura T, Hoki M, et al. Total parenteral nutrition-associated intrahepatic cholestasis in infants: 25 years' experience. J Pediatr Surg. 2000;35(7):1049-51.
48. Gupta K, Wang H, Amin SB. Parenteral nutrition-associated cholestasis in premature infants: role of macronutrients. JPEN J Parenter Enteral Nutr. 2016;40(3):335-41.
49. Al-Hathlol K, Al-Madani A, Al-Saif S, et al. Ursodeoxycholic acid therapy for intractable total parenteral nutrition-associated cholestasis in surgical very low birth weight infants. Singapore Med J. 2006;47(2):147-51.
50. Hofmann AF. Bile acids: trying to understand their chemistry and biology with the hope of helping patients. Hepatology. 2009;49(5):1403-18.
51. Setchell KD, Heubi JE, Shah S, et al. Genetic defects in bile acid conjugation cause fat-soluble vitamin deficiency. Gastroenterology. 2013;144(5):945-55.
52. Riello L, D'Antiga L, Guido M, et al. Titration of bile acid supplements in 3beta-hydroxy-Delta 5-C27-steroid dehydrogenase/isomerase deficiency. J Pediatr Gastroenterol Nutr. 2010;50(6):655-60.
53. Gonzales E, Gerhardt MF, Fabre M, et al. Oral cholic acid for hereditary defects of primary bile acid synthesis: a safe and effective long-term therapy. Gastroenterology. 2009;137(4):1310-20.
54. Liu C, Aronow BJ, Jegga AG, et al. Novel resequencing chip customized to diagnose mutations in patients with inherited syndromes of intrahepatic cholestasis. Gastroenterology. 2007;132(1):119-26.

# CHAPTER 45

# Nephrology in the Neonate

*Dechu P Puliyanda, Rashmi Kirpekar*

## ABSTRACT

Primary renal disorders in the newborn are often related to abnormal development of kidneys or urinary system or both. Our understanding of the renal development including genetic and nongenetic factors is presented in this chapter. Hypertension in the NICU is rare, detection and management of hypertension is challenging and discussed briefly. Lastly, recognition and management of AKI, including invasive and noninvasive procedures including hemo and peritoneal dialysis are described.

## INTRODUCTION

The understanding of renal disorders in the neonate is not complete without understanding normal renal physiology and function. Renal disorders can result from either congenital anomalies or prenatal and perinatal events. Advances in fetal imaging have led to increased recognition and early detection of congenital anomalies of the kidney and urinary tract (CAKUT). This chapter will cover normal renal structure and function, and congenital anomalies in the fetus and newborn. It will also address renal hypertension and provide a brief summation of modalities employed in renal replacement therapy (RRT).

## RENAL FUNCTION IN THE FETUS AND NEWBORN

The first nephrons develop following communication between the ureteric bud and the metanephric blastema. At the molecular level, this communication is a result of several transcription factors, including Wilms' tumor suppressor gene (WT1), glial-derived neurotropic factor (GDNF), hepatocyte growth factor (HGF), fibroblast growth factor 2 (FGF2), bone morphogenetic protein 7 (BMP7), the transcription factor gene *PAX2*, and Wnt signaling pathway.[1]

Urine is formed between 9 weeks and 12 weeks' gestation. However, it is the placenta that functions as the kidney and maintains normal electrolyte and acid/base balance. Urine in the fetus primarily serves to maintain the volume of amniotic fluid, which in turn promotes lung development and allows for the creation of a fluid-filled sac in which the fetus grows.

Nephrogenesis or the birth of new nephrons occurs until 36 weeks' gestation and then ceases. Premature infants are born with decreased consignment of nephrons compared to term infants. Renal function in the preterm neonate is not only immature at birth, but is also significantly delayed in achieving full capacity. This contributes to the increased risk of acute kidney injury (AKI) in preterm compared to term infants. However, preterm infants recover from transient renal injuries, as they are still developing new nephrons.

### Glomerular Function

Glomerular filtration rate (GFR) increases dramatically from fetal to neonatal life. This is a result of increased renal blood flow and other adaptive changes. Renal blood flow in the fetus is very low (2–4% of the cardiac output) compared with that of term infants (15–18%) and adult kidneys (20–25%). In general, GFR at 40 weeks of gestation is 40 ± 10 mL/min/

| TABLE 1: Glomerular filtration rate (GFR) median values in preterm infants. | | | | | |
|---|---|---|---|---|---|
| | 27 weeks | 28 weeks | 29 weeks | 30 weeks | 31 weeks |
| Day 7 | 13.4 | 16.2 | 19.1 | 21.9 | 24.8 |
| (Range) | 7.9–18.9 | 10.7–21 | 13.6–24.6 | 16.4–27.4 | 19.3–30.3 |
| Day 28 | 21 | 23.9 | 26.7 | 29.6 | 32.4 |
| (Range) | 15.5 to 26 | 18.3–29.4 | 21.1–32.2 | 24–35 | 26.9–37.9 |

1.73 m² and doubles by 8 weeks after birth. GFR median values in preterm infants are shown in **Table 1** (expressed as mL/min/1.73 m²).[2]

Serum creatinine values are used to estimate GFR. Serum creatinine in the first 48 hours of life, however, is a reflection of maternal creatinine. After 48 hours, the creatinine falls and reaches values of 0.5–0.6 by 2 weeks of life.

## Tubular Function

Tubules of the kidney play a key role in maintenance of electrolyte and acid-base balance. Their maturation follows glomerular maturation. Preterm infants are obligate "sodium wasters"; as they grow to term, the ability to reabsorb sodium increases, which is measured by the fractional excretion of sodium (FENa). The FENa in premature infants can exceed 10%; this decreases to <2% at birth. Tubular immaturity leads to inappropriate handling of an acid load, which improves at term. Premature infants also have a decreased capacity to concentrate urine. This is related to the low tonicity of the medullary interstitium. Urinary concentrating ability increases from 350 mOsm/kg at birth to 900 mOsm/kg by 30 days of life.

## STRUCTURAL DISORDERS: CONGENITAL ANOMALIES OF KIDNEYS AND URINARY TRACT MALFORMATIONS

Congenital anomalies of kidneys and urinary tract is an acronym for disorders involving the kidneys and urinary tract that share common pathogenic and genetic causes. As a group, they constitute the most common cause of chronic kidney disease (CKD) and end-stage renal disease (ESRD) in children.[3] If detected early and with supportive care, the onset of ESRD may be delayed.

The urinary system develops during the fifth week of gestation and is complete by 36 weeks. It is initiated by the coming together of the ureteric bud and metanephric mesenchyme. Several 100 genes work in concert to orchestrate the complex process of dual development of glomeruli and the urinary collecting system to form the metanephric mesenchyme and ureteric bud, respectively.

The classification of these disorders is difficult because of the heterogeneous etiology and clinical presentations. They share common features, as these defects arise mostly during nephrogenesis and can present as defects either of the kidney alone, the collecting system, or a combination of both. For example, a defect in the paired box (Pax) gene may present as an isolated renal agenesis or the dysplasia may be associated with vesicoureteral reflux.

In addition to the genetic factors, environmental factors including vitamin A exposure and maternal factors such as urinary tract infections (UTIs), diabetes, etc. have been implicated in CAKUT.

## Clinical Features of CAKUT

The abnormalities may include the kidney, the urinary system, or both. They may be sporadic or familial. While CAKUT may be isolated or part of a syndrome with extrarenal manifestations, e.g. renal coloboma syndrome due to the *PAX-2* gene, the majority of CAKUT cases are nonsyndromic.[4] **Table 2** lists clinical features of CAKUT.

## Abnormal Structure

### Renal Agenesis

Bilateral renal agenesis is generally incompatible with life.[5] It is associated with high rates of mortality and morbidity, and often is associated with the characteristic Potter sequence, with typical facial appearance, abnormal limbs with contractures, oligohydramnios, and pulmonary hypoplasia, which usually dictates survival.

Unilateral agenesis of the kidney is more common than bilateral and the most likely etiology of "single kidney" in adults. Often detected on antenatal ultrasound, it is more common in infants of diabetic mothers and in syndromes such as Poland syndrome, Fraser syndrome, branchio-oto-renal syndrome, and VACTERL (vertebral defects, anal atresia, cardiac defects, tracheo-esophageal fistula, renal anomalies, and limb abnormalities) association.[6] In females, there is a high incidence of Müllerian duct abnormalities, e.g. uterine and vaginal agenesis to duplication of the uterus and vagina, to minor uterine cavity abnormalities.

No specific causative gene defect has been identified, but this process likely begins early, during nephrogenesis. Lack of compensatory hypertrophy of the contralateral kidney suggests bilateral involvement of the "solitary

**TABLE 2:** Clinical features of congenital abnormalities of the kidney and urinary tract (CAKUT).

| Kidney | Condition | Complications | Outcome |
|---|---|---|---|
| Abnormal structure | Agenesis | Potter sequence if bilateral | Fatal if bilateral |
| | Hypoplasia | Asymptomatic | |
| | Dysplasia/cysts | Vater<br>VACTREL<br>Hnf-1b | |
| | Multicystic dysplastic kidney | Most common | Fatal if bilateral |
| | Bilateral cystic kidneys | • Autosomal recessive polycystic kidney disease (ARPKD)<br>• Autosomal dominant polycystic kidney disease (ADPKD)<br>• Glomerulocystic kidney, nephronophthisis | |
| Abnormal migration | Horseshoe kidney | Most common, tumors | |
| | Fused kidney | | |
| | Duplex | Associated duplicated collecting system | |
| Lower tract | | | |
| Obstruction | Ureteropelvic junction (UPJ), ureterovesical junction (UVJ), posterior urethral valve (PUV) | UPJ obstruction with or without renal dysplasia | Asymptomatic, UTIs, sometime renal insufficiency |
| | Hydroureter | | UTIs |
| Reflux | Retrograde flow of urine without any obstruction | Hydronephrosis, reflux nephropathy with associated renal dysplasia | UTIs, CKD |
| Duplication | Duplicated system associated with fused ectopia of the kidneys | Reflux, ectopic ureteral insertion | UTIs, incontinence |
| Bladder | Ureterocele | Associated with bilateral hydronephrosis with and without dysplasia | Urinary symptoms |
| Urethra | Posterior urethral valves | Most common obstructive lesions, CKD and ESRD | |
| | Prune belly syndrome | CKD, ESRD | |

(CKD: chronic kidney disease; UTI: urinary tract infection; ESRD: end-stage renal disease; VACTREL: vertebral defects, anal atresia, cardiac defects, tracheo-esophageal fistula, renal anomalies, and limb abnormalities).

kidney", which may be associated with hypertension, proteinuria, or decreased renal function in later years.

### Hypoplasia/Dysplasia

Although nephron number is reduced in this condition, the glomeruli are usually normal but may hypertrophy to compensate for the reduced number. They may also be associated with extrarenal manifestations involving the ears and the skeletal and cardiovascular systems. Such manifestations include renal coloboma syndrome, branchio-oto-renal syndrome, and renal hypoplasia with vesicoureteral reflux.

Renal dysplasia with cyst formations is often noted when abnormal nephrogenesis is due to urinary obstruction during development.

### Multicystic Dysplastic Kidney

Unilateral multicystic dysplastic kidney (MCDK) is the most common cystic lesion seen on prenatal ultrasound with an incidence of 1:4,000. There is compensatory hypertrophy of the contralateral kidney, with possible increased incidence of vesicoureteral reflux in the contralateral kidney. There is a slight increase in the risk of UTIs.

Diagnosis is made on renal ultrasound with thin-walled noncommunicating cysts arranged in random order. The kidney is enlarged, does not retain its shape, and renal pelvis or calyces may not be clearly visible. Ureteral atresia accompanies minimal to no function in the affected kidney. It is often confused with severe hydronephrosis.

The etiology is unknown, but likely to be multifactorial including genetic or epigenetic factors as well as exposure to viral infections, UTIs, or medications. Evidence for this includes increased incidence within family members, association with vesicoureteral reflux, and ipsilateral abnormalities of genital tracts especially in females, such as didelphys uterus or vaginal abnormalities.

Complete involution usually occurs by 2 years, but a small remnant may remain for years. Compensatory hypertrophy of the contralateral kidney is usually noted. Absence of hypertrophy may suggest underlying renal hypoplasia or dysplasia in the contralateral kidney.

There is increased risk of hypertension and proteinuria with MCDK. There is also a small risk of malignant transformation of the cysts, for which periodic monitoring is recommended.[7] Recent reports suggest that risk of malignant transformation is very rare or nonexistent.[8]

Bilateral MCDK is fatal. The abnormal development of entire renal structures results in multiple cysts, which are noncommunicating and grouped together with abnormal renal parenchyma. Bilateral MCDK is often confused with severe hydronephrosis, which may appear as a cystic mass. However, the normal reniform of the kidney is preserved, and the cysts communicate in the presence of renal function.

## Polycystic Kidneys

Bilateral renal cysts are seen in many conditions, including:
- Hereditary cystic kidney diseases, e.g. autosomal recessive polycystic kidney disease (ARPKD), and autosomal dominant polycystic kidney disease (ADPKD).
- Cystic kidneys associated with syndromes—tuberous sclerosis, Von Hippel–Lindau syndrome, Bardet-Biedl syndrome, juvenile nephronophthisis, etc.
- Cystic kidneys—isolated.

Hereditary cystic kidney diseases, the most common cystic kidney diseases, include ARPKD and ADPKD. Although both have renal and extrarenal manifestations and occur at all ages, they have significant differences, including cyst size, age of onset, and progression to ESRD.[9]

*Autosomal recessive polycystic kidney disease:* Autosomal recessive polycystic kidney disease is rare, occurring in approximately 1:20,000 individuals. Previously it was referred to as infantile polycystic kidney disease, but because of its presentation in early childhood or adolescence, it is now referred to as ARPKD. It is the most common cause of bilateral kidney enlargement in the neonatal period.

*Clinical presentation of ARPKD:* There is a wide spectrum of manifestations, with the severest forms occurring earlier in life with increased mortality and morbidity. Those who survive the immediate neonatal period usually have hypertension and feeding problems, and will develop CKDs and ESRD later in childhood and early adulthood.

In severe cases, bilateral cystic kidneys with oligohydramnios may be detected on prenatal ultrasound with accompanying pulmonary hypoplasia and Potter sequence (oligohydramnios syndrome). Mortality rate in the neonatal period can be as high as 30%, mostly secondary to respiratory failure.[10] The normal reniform of the kidney is maintained despite the enormous size of the kidney. Birth may be complicated by dystocia due to severe abdominal distension.[9]

Hypertension can occur early in the neonatal period and generally is refractory to treatment. Often, multiple antihypertensive medications may be necessary to control hypertension.

Liver abnormalities in ARPKD include hepatic fibrosis, which is present universally. In addition, bile duct dilatation and ectasia (Caroli disease) may be noted. Hepatosplenomegaly and portal hypertension are late occurrences and can lead to life-threatening bleeding.

*Autosomal recessive polycystic kidney disease pathophysiology:* The cysts in the kidneys begin at conception and originate in the collecting tubules with a normally formed nephron; hence the glomeruli are normal in structure and function. The cysts are usually small (<3 mm) and appear as enlarged and echogenic kidneys with loss of corticomedullary demarcation. The urinary concentrating mechanism is impaired.[11] Absence of dysplasia distinguishes this group from the CAKUT malformations.

*Etiology:* ARPKD is caused by mutations in the *PKHD1* gene, which is located on the short arm of chromosome 6p12. It encodes for the protein fibrocystin (also known as polyductin), which maintains tubular architecture via the primary cilia.

*Management:* There is no cure for ARPKD. Treatment involves supportive care and management of complications, which include respiratory distress from pulmonary hypoplasia and severe abdominal distension, hypertension, and liver abnormalities, especially portal hypertension and inflammation of the biliary tract.[12]

*Autosomal dominant polycystic kidney disease:* Autosomal dominant polycystic kidney disease is the most common polycystic kidney disease in the world and affects both kidneys. In this condition, the extrarenal manifestations are cysts in the liver, pancreas, and ovary, intracranial aneurysms, and mitral valve prolapse.

Family history of cystic kidney disease is a diagnostic criterion, but sporadic cases secondary to new mutations are occasionally seen. Presence of cystic kidneys on prenatal ultrasound and presence of renal cysts in a family member strongly suggest a diagnosis of ADPKD.

The genes *PKD1* and *PKD2*, located on chromosomes 16 and 4, respectively, code for the proteins polycystin-1 and -2, which reside in the ciliary apparatus of tubular cells. Polycystin-1 and -2 are involved in maintaining tubular integrity, and disruption of these proteins is one cause of cyst formation.

In neonates, large cysts may not be present and it is sometimes difficult to differentiate ADPKD from ARPKD. Presence of renal cysts in parents or other family members helps in differentiating the two conditions.[13]

### Other Heritable Cystic Kidney Diseases

Hereditary nephronophthisis is an autosomal recessive condition associated with very small cysts in both kidneys, which may not be detected on renal ultrasound. The kidneys appear hyperechogenic but usually are of normal size. Renal failure occurs in childhood. Patients usually are asymptomatic and may present with polyuria and polydipsia. Interstitial fibrosis is noted on renal biopsy. Abnormal ciliary function of the cell leads to cyst formation.

Medullary sponge kidney is an autosomal dominant condition similar to nephronophthisis, associated with bilateral cystic kidney disease. Medullary sponge kidneys appear as hyperechoic, normal-sized kidneys because the cysts are very small and arise in the collecting ducts. This condition usually manifests as kidney stone disease in adults.

## Abnormal Migration

These are abnormalities occurring during the ascent or fusion of the kidneys, which lead to the kidneys not being in the renal fossa.

Horseshoe kidney, the most common abnormality, is due to failure of ascent of the kidneys. It is associated with vesicoureteral reflux and is a common renal manifestation in Turner syndrome.

Renal ectopia, pelvic kidney, and crossed fused ectopia are abnormalities that are usually asymptomatic, but their presence means increased incidence of reflux, UTIs, renal stone disease, or increased risk of injury due to blunt abdominal trauma.

## Abnormalities of the Lower Tract

### Obstructive Lesions

*Hydronephrosis:* Fetal renal pelvis enlargement is usually seen on second trimester antenatal ultrasound. Obstruction to urine flow is the likely cause, albeit not very specific, and may encompass disorders ranging from transient physiologic dilatation to severe hydronephrosis with impaired renal function.

A grading system is used to define severity of lesions **(Figs. 1A to E)**.[14]

The Society for Fetal Urology (SFU) system, though not widely used, includes the renal parenchyma measurements as well.

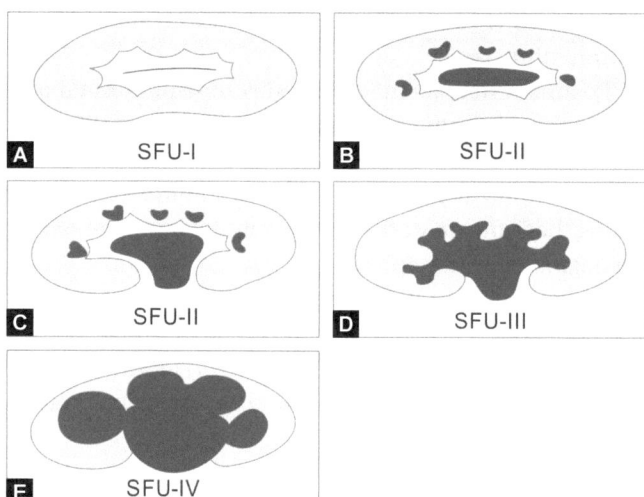

**Figs. 1A to E:** Society for Fetal Urology (SFU) grading system.

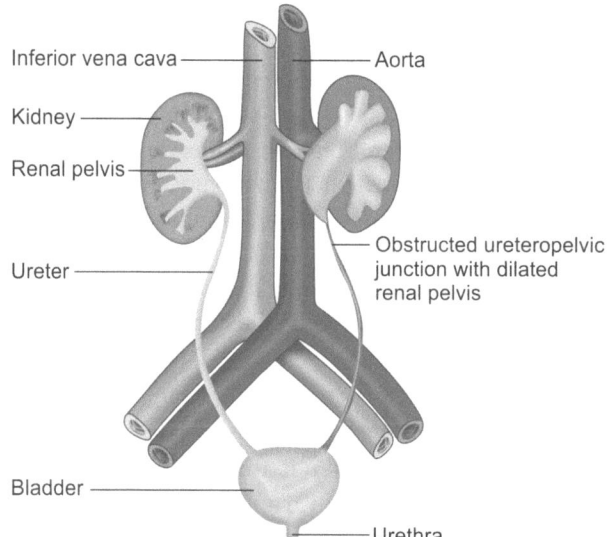

**Fig. 2:** Ureteropelvic junction obstruction.

*The Society for Fetal Urology grading system for postnatal hydronephrosis:* The grading system is based on renal ultrasonography findings of the degree of renal-pelvic and calyceal dilation and takes into account the integrity of the parenchyma. Grade 0 is normal and not represented in the figure.

| Grade | APD 2nd trimester | APD 3rd trimester |
| --- | --- | --- |
| Mild | 4 mm ≤ 7 mm | 7 ≤ 9 mm |
| Moderate | 7–10 mm | 9–15 mm |
| Severe | >10 mm | >15 mm |

(APD: anterior posterior diameter).

Ureteropelvic junction (UPJ) obstruction **(Fig. 2)** is the most common cause of unilateral hydronephrosis. Other causes include ureterovesical junction (UVJ) obstruction, vesicoureteral reflux (VUR), bladder abnormalities, and urethral obstruction. The latter is likely to cause bilateral hydronephrosis.

Postnatal management includes repeating renal and bladder ultrasounds, preferably after 48 hours of life. This is because there is relative oliguria and dehydration in the newborn in the first 48 hours of life, and ultrasound done during that time may erroneously suggest improvement in the degree of hydronephrosis.

For unilateral mild hydronephrosis, a repeat renal ultrasound by 1-2 months of age is recommended. The role of voiding cystourethrogram (VCUG) in this situation is controversial and may be deferred, if there is no ureteral dilatation.

A VCUG should be considered for bilateral hydronephrosis, hydroureter, or abnormal bladder images. UTI prophylaxis with oral antibiotics is recommended. Complete resolution of the mild hydronephrosis by 2-3 years of age occurs in most cases.

Vesicoureteral reflux is usually noted during a workup for antenatal hydronephrosis, ureteral ectopia, or multicystic kidney disease. It can occur secondary to bladder obstruction or neurogenic bladder. Reflux can be associated to reflux nephropathy with accompanying renal hypoplasia and dysplasia, but is most often diagnosed following an episode of UTI.

Reflux is graded according to the VCUG results, which are based on the international reflux study grade scheme, grades I through V **(Fig. 3)**.[15]

## Evaluation of CAKUT

A thorough family history is important to ascertain the presence of renal abnormalities in other family members. Maternal factors are important, including use of medications such as angiotensin-converting enzyme (ACE) inhibitors (captopril and enalapril) during pregnancy, presence of diabetes, UTIs, and nutritional factors such as vitamin A deficiency.

Antenatal renal ultrasound is the most common modality to detect renal tract abnormalities and other organ systems in the fetus. In addition, adequacy of amniotic fluid volume by the second trimester may suggest normal urine output. Renal size and echogenicity is also measured. A dysplastic kidney often appears enlarged and bright.

Postnatal imaging including VCUG and renal scans are discussed below.

## Management of CAKUT

Given the varied clinical presentations, the management of the CAKUT is based on appearance of the renal ultrasound and clinical presentation. Termination of pregnancy may be considered in situations where there are bilateral renal agenesis, early severe oligohydramnios, and severe pulmonary hypoplasia.

Intrauterine intervention such as vesicoamniotic shunt placement may be considered if clinical criteria are favorable, although long-term improvement in renal function is not favorable.[16]

For MCDK, periodic renal ultrasounds are performed to ascertain involution of the dysplastic kidney and compensatory hypertrophy of the contralateral kidney.

For mild unilateral hydronephrosis, periodic renal ultrasound is recommended to monitor the hydronephrosis. For worsening hydronephrosis, lasix renogram detects obstruction and function of the kidney, and surgical intervention such as pyeloplasty/nephrostomy or stent placement for improvement of obstruction may be considered. Renal function may improve by following procedures:

- Patients with CAKUT require periodic monitoring of blood pressure and urine protein excretion since renal dysfunction may not occur until adulthood.
- Genetic testing seems promising but is controversial given the phenotypic variability in expressions. Even if an abnormal gene is found, it may not be able to predict the outcome.

*Summary*: The risk of renal dysplasia or hypoplasia increases with bilateral ureteral involvement or lower urinary tract obstructions. There is also an increased risk of developing CKD or ESRD. Early intervention and treatment may delay the onset of CKD but will not reverse it.

On the other hand, unilateral lesions are typically asymptomatic. The etiology is usually not obvious but familial clustering is noted, suggesting genetic origins.

Lastly, there is an increased risk of patients developing hypertension, proteinuria, and renal dysfunction. Even in

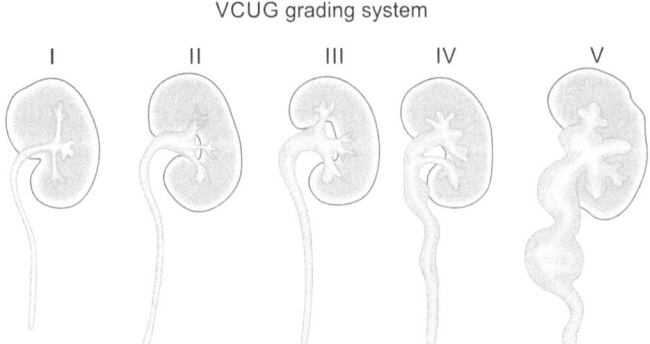

Grade I   Into nondilated ureter
Grade II  Into pelvis and calyces without dilatation
Grade III Mild-to moderate dilatation of ureter and renal pelvis
Grade IV  Moderate dilatation and/or tortuosity of ureter
Grade V   Severe dilatation and tortuosity of ureter, renal pelvis and calyces

**Fig. 3:** Voiding cystourethrogram (VCUG) grading system.

seemingly asymptomatic CAKUT, long-term follow-up is recommended.

## ACUTE KIDNEY INJURY

There is no precise definition of AKI in the neonate since the GFR tends to vary from preterm infants to term, and the serum creatinine is not a reliable measure in the first 48 hours of life. In general, the serum creatinine (>1.5 mg/dL on after 72 hours of life) and/or decrease in urine output (oliguria defined as <1 mL/kg/hr) are indicators of AKI. Keep in mind that certain types of AKI are associated with normal to increased renal output.

### Etiology of Acute Kidney Injury

Neonatal AKI is multifactorial but etiology is grouped into three broad categories:
1. *Prerenal*:
   - Hypotension secondary to hemorrhage, sepsis, or dehydration
   - Perinatal asphyxia
   - Respiratory distress syndrome
   - Congenital heart failure.
2. *Renal*:
   - Intrinsic renal disease secondary to renal hypoplasia or dysplasia
   - Bilateral renal agenesis
   - Polycystic kidney disease
   - Nephrotoxic medications, i.e. aminoglycosides, indomethacin, and maternal ACE inhibitors
   - Renal vein thrombosis
   - Renal artery occlusion.
3. *Postrenal*:
   - Bilateral UPJ obstruction or obstruction in a solitary kidney
   - Posterior urethral valve
   - Neurogenic bladder
   - Prune belly syndrome.

### Prerenal Acute Kidney Injury

Prerenal AKI results from decreased perfusion to the kidneys as a result of true volume depletion or decreased effective blood volume. True volume contraction results from hemorrhage (antepartum hemorrhage, twin-to-twin transfusion, and intraventricular bleeding), dehydration due to gastrointestinal losses, central or nephrogenic diabetes insipidus, and third space losses as seen in sepsis, capillary leak syndrome, and postoperative conditions. Decreased effective blood volume occurs when the true blood volume is normal or increased, but renal perfusion is decreased due to diseases such as congestive heart failure or severe hypoalbuminemia. Whatever is the underlying etiology, renal function returns to normal as long as the etiology is transient. If the insult is ongoing or severe, it results in an entity known as acute tubular necrosis (ATN).

*Acute tubular necrosis*: Severe vasoconstriction due to any prerenal insult results in necrosis of the tubules. This is clinically characterized by decreased renal output and a marked increase in serum creatinine. If the ongoing insult persists, ATN can evolve into microthrombi formation in the renal glomeruli, a condition referred to as cortical necrosis. While recovery from ATN results in normal renal function, cortical necrosis is associated with very high mortality—30-50% of survivors develop CKD. Overall mortality and morbidity of newborns with acute renal failure (ARF) are much worse in neonates with multi-organ failure.[17]

### Renal Acute Kidney Injury

Disorders such as renal hypoplasia, renal dysplasia, and bilateral renal agenesis are discussed under the collective term CAKUT.

*Nephrotoxic medications:* Many different drugs and agents may result in nephrotoxic ARF. Aminoglycoside use is the most common cause of nephrotoxicity and usually presents with nonoliguric ARF with a urinalysis showing minimal urinary abnormalities. Nephrotoxicity from aminoglycoside use is related to dose and duration of the antibiotic therapy, as well as the level of renal function prior to beginning medication. The etiology is thought to be secondary to injury to the proximal renal tubules. It is reversible once the offending agents have been discontinued, even though there may be a small increase in creatinine for a few days following the discontinuation.[18] Monitoring of drug levels whenever possible may prevent or decrease nephrotoxicity.

Indomethacin is a powerful afferent vasoconstrictor and therefore reduces GFR. Nephrotoxicity occurs more commonly in premature infants and in neonates with preexisting renal abnormalities. As with aminoglycosides, AKI is usually reversible after discontinuation of the drug.[19,20]

Other less common agents that can result in drug-induced AKI include amphotericin, contrast agents, and *cyclooxygenase-2* (COX-2) inhibitors.

Renal artery thrombosis and renal vein thrombosis (RVT) will result in renal failure if bilateral, or if either, occurs in a solitary kidney. RVT is much more common than renal artery thrombosis, and >80% of RVT occurs in the newborn period.[21]

The risk factors for renal vascular thrombosis are umbilical artery catheterization, birth asphyxia, being the infant of a diabetic mother, volume contraction, polycythemia, cyanotic heart disease, and coagulation abnormalities. The classic triad of RVT, consisting of gross hematuria, flank mass (unilateral or bilateral enlargement of kidneys), and thrombocytopenia, is not always seen. Instead, hypertension with or without oliguria may be the presenting feature. Laboratory tests may reveal hematuria, proteinuria, polycythemia, hemolytic anemia, thrombocytopenia, and possibly AKI. The etiology for hypercoagulability should be investigated if the common causes are excluded. A renal ultrasound may be normal or show enlarged kidneys. A renal Doppler ultrasound is the gold standard for diagnosis as it will show little or no blood flow. Therapy should be aimed at treating the cause. If the clot is large, antifibrinolytic therapy could be considered.[22]

### Postrenal Acute Kidney Injury

Postrenal AKI refers to AKI developing in kidneys that would have been normal at birth but are compromised secondary to obstruction of the flow of urine at the UPJ and UVJ, posterior urethral valve, and neurogenic bladder. These disorders are discussed in the section on CAKUT.

## Clinical Presentation and Diagnosis of AKI in Neonates

Any one or more of the following clinical findings can be seen in neonates with AKI:

- Increase in the serum creatinine after the first 48 hours of life. This is usually, but not always, associated with an increase in blood urea nitrogen (BUN).
- *Oligoanuria*—>50% of newborns void by 8 hours of age and >95% of newborns void within 24 hours.[23] Oligoanuria is, therefore defined as urine output of <1 m/min/1.73 m$^2$ in a euvolemic newborn after the first 24 hours of life.
- *Hyponatremia*—usually results from decreased urine output and can be exacerbated by an increase in sodium loss in premature neonates.
- *Hyperkalemia*—is not the most important feature of AKI in neonates. It is seen when AKI is associated with oliguria, severe metabolic acidosis, or due to disturbances of aldosterone secretion as seen in congenital adrenal hyperplasia.
- *Metabolic acidosis*—is seen secondary to H$^+$ retention from AKI. Metabolic acidosis commonly exacerbates hyperkalemia.

## Evaluation

A thorough history and physical examination, paying close attention to the etiologies and the clinical features as described above, are important first steps in the evaluation of AKI.

### Electrolyte and Renal Function Tests

Findings include abnormalities in serum creatinine, sodium, potassium, and acid base disturbances.

### Urinalysis

Urinalysis is fairly normal in neonatal AKI but can show significant abnormalities including granular, epithelial and red cell casts indicative of ATN. Glucosuria secondary to tubular immaturity is fairly common in a preterm infant and should not be considered abnormal.

*Urinary indices:* An important way for the kidneys to conserve water is to conserve sodium. Therefore, if true volume depletion is the cause of AKI and the kidneys conserve sodium to conserve water, then the urinary sodium is low, usually <20–30 mEq/L. Since sodium conservation is decreased due to tubular impairment in intrinsic renal disease, the urinary sodium is >30–40 mEq/L. Because the urine sodium can be affected by volume expanders and there is a range of urinary sodium excretion, the FENa is used. It is calculated by the formula:

$$\frac{UNa \times PCr}{PNa \times UCr}$$

UNa: Urine sodium (mEq/L); PNa: Plasma sodium (mEq/L); PCr: Plasma creatinine (mg/dL); UCr: Urine creatinine (mg/dL)

A FENa of <2% is generally indicative of prerenal AKI, whereas in the absence of diuretic therapy, >3% is indicative of intrinsic renal disease causing AKI. Since preterm infants are obligate sodium losers, FENa can be used as an indicator only in neonates >37 weeks gestational age.[24]

Urine osmolality can be used only in term infants. A low urine osmolality (<400 mOsmol/kg) is indicative of intrinsic renal disease, while high urine osmolality is indicative of prerenal AKI.

*Urinary biomarkers:* Several biomarkers are being studied in AKI neonates to facilitate early detection (before elevation of serum creatinine and oligoanuria) and management. For example, urine beta-2-microglobulin is a sensitive marker of tubular dysfunction.[25]

### Imaging

*Renal ultrasound*: Ultrasound evaluates kidney size, anatomy (number of kidneys and their location), echogenicity, and corticomedullary differentiation. Kidneys of term infants are generally 4 cm in size and have normal echogenicity and corticomedullary differentiation. Preterm infant kidneys are echogenic. Renal ultrasound is also useful in evaluating the renal parenchyma for cysts and for the presence of hydronephrosis, hydroureter, and the urinary bladder.

Voiding cystourethrogram is useful for diagnosis of vesicoureteral reflux, posterior urethral valve, bladder wall hypertrophy, and presence of ureterocele.

*Mercaptoacetyltriglycine (MAG 3) lasix renal scan:* The MAG 3 is a radionuclide tracer that has an uptake phase and an excretory phase in the kidney. A normal uptake indicates normally functioning kidneys and a normal excretion indicates the absence of obstruction. A nuclear scan to evaluate renal function is not usually done in the neonatal period as the GFR in neonates is very low, which can result in a low-uptake phase.

*Dimercaptosuccinic acid (DMSA):* Dimercaptosuccinic acid is a radionuclide tracer that only has an uptake phase in the kidney, therefore is useful in studying renal function and the presence of renal scars. This scan is very rarely performed in neonates and is reserved for evaluating function in bilateral renal agenesis and cystic dysplastic kidneys.

## Management of Acute Kidney Injury

### Fluids

A fluid bolus consisting of isotonic saline 10–20 mL/kg given over 1–2 hours is the first line of management in an oligoanuric infant with AKI without congestive heart failure. There is little indication for albumin except in hypoalbuminemic infants where third-spacing is suspected. Albumin can increase risk of infection and protein leakage into the lungs, leading to pulmonary edema.[26]

If there is no response to fluid therapy, then intrinsic renal disease is likely to cause AKI in the neonate. At this point, it is prudent to restrict fluids, attempt diuretics for fluid overload, and consider RRT if needed.

For maintenance of fluids, it is best to limit fluids to insensible and visible losses, which include urine and stool output. Infants under radiant warmers may require 25–100% more fluids; infants under phototherapy may require an extra 20 mg/kg/day.

### Dopamine

Dopamine increases systemic blood pressure and therefore may increase renal blood flow and urine output. It is restricted to neonates with heart failure and/or hypotension unresponsive to fluid repletion.

### Diuretics

*Furosemide (1–5 mg/kg/dose IV every 6 hours or furosemide drip):* Furosemide also increases urine flow to decrease intratubular obstruction and inhibits Na-K-ATPase, thus limiting oxygen consumption in already damaged tubules with a low oxygen supply.

### Hyperkalemia

It is best to remove potassium in all IV and parenteral fluids in infants with AKI unless they are hypokalemic.

The management of hyperkalemia can be achieved by a combination of the following measures:
- Albuterol (2.5 mg by nebulization)
- Sodium bicarbonate (1–2 mEq/kg IV over 5–10 minutes)
- Insulin and glucose (0.05 units/kg regular insulin with 2 mL/kg of 10% dextrose) followed by a continuous infusion of insulin (0.1 units/kg with 2–4 ml/kg/hr of 10% dextrose)
- Furosemide (1 mg/kg/dose IV 6 hourly or a furosemide drip)
- Kayexalate, a sodium-potassium exchange resin that can be given rectally (1 g/kg). Since this is an exchange resin, infants can become very hypernatremic and therefore electrolytes should be monitored. Other complications are fluid retention, constipation, and risk of perforation and intestinal necrosis.[27,28]

### Metabolic Acidosis

Treat the underlying cause. Avoid $NaHCO_3$ boluses as they can cause intraventricular hemorrhage (IVH), deterioration of cardiac function, and worsening of intracellular acidosis.

### Nutrition

It is recommended that infants are provided at least 100 kcals/kg/day of nutrition. Formula-fed infants should receive a formula low in potassium and phosphorus with low renal solute load (such formulas are commercially available). Infants receiving parenteral nutrition should receive amino acids up to maximum 1.5 g/kg/day and intralipids up to maximum 2 g/kg/day. Sodium, potassium, calcium, phosphorus, and glucose should be adjusted based on serum electrolyte concentrations.

### Hypertension

Hypertension is seen in up to 10–20% of AKI infants. Early detection and prompt treatment should be initiated.

### Renal Replacement Therapy

The purpose of acute RRT is to remove endogenous and exogenous toxins, and to maintain fluid, electrolyte and acid-base balance until renal function returns. The modalities include peritoneal dialysis, intermittent hemodialysis, and RRT used in the treatment of ARF. Recognizing the usefulness and limitations of various modalities before starting therapy is ideal.

### Indications

- Fluid overload, where fluid restriction makes it difficult to provide adequate nutrition
- Intractable hyperkalemia
- Intractable acidosis

- Hyponatremia or fluid overload in patients with congestive heart failure or pulmonary edema
- *Inborn errors of metabolism:* In maple syrup urine disease, and hyperammonemia states, the small molecules are effectively cleared by hemodialysis.[29]

## Modalities

*Peritoneal dialysis*: Although less effective in removal of fluid, this is a gentle method that can be applied continuously without need for extracorporeal blood flow, systemic heparinization, or vascular access. It can be used safely in hemodynamically unstable patients. It requires very simple equipment and can be initiated with low-volume dialysate as soon as the dialysis catheter is placed. Complications of peritonitis, inguinal or umbilical hernia, and leakage of peritoneal fluid must be kept in mind. Access to the peritoneal cavity is usually through a Tenckhoff catheter (double-cuff catheter). Dextrose-containing dialysate solutions come in 1.5%, 2.5%, and 4.25% concentrations. In older children, peritoneal dialysis is usually initiated with volumes of 15–20 mL/kg body weight while neonates usually initiate peritoneal dialysis with slightly lower volumes of 5–10 mL/kg body weight. Low-volume peritoneal dialysis will have a milder effect on the hemodynamic status of the neonate and has been shown to effectively control uremia and promote ultrafiltration.[30]

Hemodialysis results in the rapid change in the plasma electrolyte composition and a more rapid fluid removal. The need for extracorporeal blood flow, good vascular access, and systemic heparinization can be challenging and is sometimes not tolerated in unstable patients.[31,32] Maximally purified water provided by a reverse osmosis system and skilled nursing personnel are required.

*Continuous renal replacement therapy:* The use of continuous venovenous hemodiafiltration (CVVHD) is increasing in neonatal intensive care units with the advent of very small dialyzers and neonatal lines requiring minimal extracorporeal volume. Compared to peritoneal dialysis and hemodialysis, CVVHD has the advantage of removal of cytokines in sepsis, and allows for more precise volume and electrolyte changes.[33]

## Prognosis

In the neonate, the prognosis and recovery from AKI is variable and dependent upon the underlying etiology. In general, mortality is high and is seen in preterm infants and those with multi-organ failure and severe hemodynamic instability requiring RRT.[34]

Mortality is lower in neonates with non-oliguric AKI. In survivors, more than 50% are left with sequelae that include chronic renal failure, proteinuria, and hypertension; these children need to be closely monitored.

## NEONATAL HYPERTENSION

The incidence of hypertension ranges from 0.2% to 3%, and may be higher in preterm infants and those with umbilical artery catheterization.[35]

There is a paucity of good data on normative blood pressure (BP) values in the newborn. Since BP increases with age and weight gain, it makes it more difficult to have normative values. It is important to remember that BP in a neonate should be obtained while asleep or calm with a proper size neonatal cuff.

At term the mean arterial BP (MAP) is 60 mm Hg with the 50th percentile for BP being 80/50.[36]

Causes for neonatal hypertension are listed in **Box 1**.

### Clinical Presentation

Most neonates are asymptomatic but nonspecific findings include poor feeding, irritability, lethargy, and in severe cases cardiogenic shock.[37] If AKI is present, oliguria or polyuria and proteinuria may be seen.

### Evaluation

A complete history including maternal drug use and prenatal ultrasounds showing renal or urologic abnormalities are important. Physical examination should include four-extremity BP, attention to dysmorphic features and palpation of abdomen for masses.

---

**BOX 1:** Etiology of neonatal hypertension.

*Vascular:*
- Umbilical arterial catheterization
- Renal artery stenosis
- Renal vein thrombosis
- Coarctation of aorta

*Renal parenchymal disease:*
- Cystic kidney disease
- Acute tubular necrosis
- Urinary obstruction
- Congenital nephrotic syndrome

*Neurologic:*
- Increased intracranial pressure
- Pain
- Seizures

*Medications:*
- Dexamethasone
- Caffeine
- Phenylephrine
- Maternal cocaine

*Miscellaneous:*
- Congenital adrenal hyperplasia
- Bronchopulmonary hemorrhage
- Hypercalcemia
- Fluid overload

## Laboratory Testing

In addition to routine testing for a metabolic panel and urine analysis, measurement of thyroid function tests are valuable.

Renal ultrasound with Doppler should always be obtained in the evaluation of a neonate with hypertension. This will not only provide important information about the anatomy of the kidneys and rule out any congenital anomalies, but it may also assist in detecting renal venous thrombosis. In addition, an echocardiogram is useful to obtain to rule out congenital cardiac abnormalities.

In infants with persistent hypertension with inconclusive renal ultrasound and echocardiogram, an angiogram is the gold standard for making a diagnosis. CT angiogram and MR angiogram are less useful in neonates, as these will not rule out branch vessel disease.

## Management

The cause of hypertension should be investigated and treatment initiated. Treatment lies in addressing the cause of hypertension if possible. It is best to start with a short-acting agent, either IV or oral, and depending upon the need for ongoing antihypertensive therapy, proceed to use long-acting agents.

### ACE Inhibitors

Captopril (0.1–0.5 mg/kg/dose) three times daily or enalapril 0.01–0.1 mg/kg/dose twice daily are first-line agents in the treatment of neonatal hypertension. ACE inhibitors can precipitate AKI; renal function and potassium should be monitored.

*Beta-blockers:* Labetalol (0.2–3 mg/kg/hr) as a constant IV infusion can be used. Avoid use in neonates with heart failure or chronic lung disease.

### Calcium Channel Blockers

Nicardipine at 1–3 mcg/kg/min as a constant infusion can be used in severe hypertension. Amlodipine 0.1–0.3 mg/kg/dose up to a maximum of 0.6 mg/kg/day can be used orally.

### Diuretics

These are not the first-line therapy, unless there is evidence of fluid overload.

Hydrochlorothiazide 1–3 mg/kg/dose once daily or furosemide 1 mg/kg/dose every 6 hours can be used. Electrolytes should be monitored closely.

### Vasodilators

Hydralazine 0.3–1 mg/kg/dose up to a maximum of 7 mg/kg/day can be given orally three times daily. Diuretics can be used in combination with vasodilators to potentiate the effect of vasodilators alone, which can cause fluid retention.

## Outcome

Infants with hypertension should be monitored and antihypertensives carefully adjusted as blood pressure gets better or as the infant grows and needs increased doses of medications. Yearly echocardiograms to rule out left ventricular hypertrophy are necessary for infants with sustained hypertension.

# NEPHROCALCINOSIS

## Introduction

Nephrocalcinosis implies a radiological diagnosis and is defined as ultrasound evidence of bright, echogenic, usually small fleck-like spots within the medullary regions of the kidney.[38,39]

The reported prevalence is 7–41%. This wide range of occurrence could be explained by the ultrasound equipment used, some interobserver variation, and the populations studied.[40]

## Etiology of Nephrocalcinosis

Urine is a delicate balance between promoters and inhibitors of stone formation. An increase in the promoters and/or a decrease in the inhibitors results in nephrocalcinosis. Overall the cause is multifactorial **(Table 3)**.

## Detection

Nephrocalcinosis is usually an incidental finding when an abdominal ultrasound is done for other purposes.

**TABLE 3:** Promoters and inhibitors of stone formation.

| Promoters of stone formation | Inhibitors of stone formation |
|---|---|
| Dehydration | Hydration |
| Prematurity | Use of thiazides |
| Low-birth weight | Citrate |
| Severe respiratory disease | Normal GU anatomy |
| *Medications:* Furosemide, glucocorticoids, vitamin D | |
| *Genetic causes:* Hyperoxaluria and hypocitraturia, Bartter syndrome | |
| Hypercalciuria | |
| Renal tubular acidosis | |
| High calcium intake | |
| Parenteral nutrition | |
| Urinary obstruction | |

(GU: genitourinary).

Hematuria is not a common finding unless urolithiasis is present. Renal ultrasound is a very sensitive imaging modality to detect nephrocalcinosis. A CT scan is very specific; however, CT scans are not usually performed in neonates due to risk of radiation. Nephrocalcinosis on renal ultrasound appears as an increase in medullary echogenicity in the kidneys. It is important to remember that increased medullary echogenicity can be seen in other conditions like infections—especially cytomegalovirus (CMV), fungal infections of the kidney, RVT, ARF from any cause, and prominence of sinus fat, since fat is also echogenic.

A urine calcium-to-creatinine ratio is a good screening test to check for hypercalciuria. A ratio of >0.8 is considered significant (up to 7 months of age, and then >0.6 is significant up to 18 months of age).

## Management

The mainstay of management is to identify the etiology and treat it. For example, hypercalciuria is treated with the use of thiazide diuretics, while hyperoxaluria is treated initially with citrates, which combine with calcium to form urine-soluble calcium citrate.

The possible long-term consequences include hypertension and the development of urolithiasis, both of which are quite rare.

Follow-up renal ultrasound should be performed every 6 months until the disappearance of the nephrocalcinosis is confirmed.

Overall, nephrocalcinosis is associated with a very high-resolution rate and good renal outcome.

## SUMMARY

The majority of advances in fetal imaging have led to increased recognition and early detection of CAKUT. AKI in the neonatal period is another important reason for consultation with the nephrologist in the newborn period. AKI is multifactorial and resolves as the inciting event is managed. Long-term follow-up for newborns is essential to ensure that residual damage does not lead to chronic renal disease.

## CONCLUSION

Abnormalities of kidney and urinary system development or CAKUT malformations are a leading cause of chronic kidney disease in children and young adults. They may occur as isolated or in a syndrome. Early recognition is important in the management of morbidity and mortality.

Neonatal hypertension is uncommon and often secondary to an underlying cause, e.g. renovascular, BPD, PDA, etc. Early recognition and treatment can influence morbidity. Nephrocalcinosis is less common with decrease use of chronic lasix therapy but can occur in tubular disorders such as RTA, Bartters, etc.

Acute kidney injury maybe secondary to severe underlying illness such as overwhelming sepsis or severe cardiac condition often managed conservatively. Renal replacement therapy aka hemo or peritoneal dialysis are important life saving interventions, particularly for acute electrolyte and fluid management.

## REFERENCES

1. Davies JA, Fisher CE. Genes and proteins in renal development. Exp Nephrol. 2002;10(2):102-13.
2. Vieux R, Hascoet JM, Merdariu D, et al. Glomerular filtration rate reference values in very preterm infants. Pediatrics. 2010;125(5):e1186-92.
3. Schedl A. Renal abnormalities and their developmental origin. Nat Rev Genet. 2007;8(10):791-802.
4. Woolf AS. A molecular and genetic view of human renal and urinary tract malformations. Kidney Int. 2000;58(2):500-12.
5. Shapiro E. Upper urinary tract anomalies and perinatal renal tumors. Clin Perinatol. 2014;41(3):679-94.
6. Avner ED, Harmon WE, Niaudet P, Yoshikawa N (Eds). Pediatric Nephrology, 6th edition. USA: Springer; 2009. pp. 1-2063.
7. Kiyak A, Yilmaz A, Turhan P, et al. Unilateral multicystic dysplastic kidney: single-center experience. Pediatr Nephrol. 2009;24(1):99-104.
8. Hayes WN, Watson AR; Trent & Anglia MCDK Study Group. Unilateral multicystic dysplastic kidney: does initial size matter? Pediatr Nephrol. 2012;27(8):1335-40.
9. Verghese P, Miyashita Y. Neonatal polycystic kidney disease. Clin Perinatol. 2014;41(3):543-60.
10. Bergmann C. ARPKD and early manifestations of ADPKD: the original polycystic kidney disease and phenocopies. Pediatr Nephrol. 2015;30(1):15-30.
11. Torres VE, Harris PC. Mechanisms of Disease: autosomal dominant and recessive polycystic kidney diseases. Nat Clin Pract Nephrol. 2006;2(1):40-55.
12. Büscher R, Büscher AK, Weber S, et al. Clinical manifestations of autosomal recessive polycystic kidney disease (ARPKD): kidney-related and non-kidney-related phenotypes. Pediatr Nephrol. 2014;29(10):1915-25.
13. Verghese P, Kim Y. Unilateral localized cystic kidney. Pediatr Nephrol. 2011;26(5):713-6.
14. Fernbach SK, Maizels M, Conway JJ. Ultrasound grading of hydronephrosis: introduction to the system used by the Society for Fetal Urology. Pediatr Radiol. 1993;23(6):478-80.
15. Baracco R, Mattoo TK. Diagnosis and management of urinary tract infection and vesicoureteral reflux in the neonate. Clin Perinatol. 2014;41(3):633-42.
16. Morris RK, Malin GL, Khan KS, et al. Systematic review of the effectiveness of antenatal intervention for the treatment of congenital lower urinary tract obstruction. BJOG. 2010;117(4):382-90.
17. Andreoli SP. Acute renal failure. Curr Opin Pediatr. 2002;14(2):183-8.
18. Humes HD. Aminoglycoside nephrotoxicity. Kidney Int. 1988;33(4):900-11.

19. Gersony WM, Peckham GJ, Ellison RC, et al. Effects of indomethacin in premature infants with patent ductus arteriosus: results of a national collaborative study. J Pediatr. 1983;102(6):895-906.
20. Itabashi K, Ohno T, Nishida H. Indomethacin responsiveness of patent ductus arteriosus and renal abnormalities in preterm infants treated with indomethacin. J Pediatr. 2003;143(2):203-7.
21. Moudgil A. Renal venous thrombosis in neonates. Curr Pediatr Rev. 2014;10(2):101-6.
22. Payne RM, Martin TC, Bower RJ, et al. Management and follow-up of arterial thrombosis in the neonatal period. J Pediatr. 1989;114(5):853-8.
23. Clark DA. Times of first void and first stool in 500 newborns. Pediatrics. 1977;60(4):457-9.
24. Ishizaki Y, Isozaki-Fukuda Y, Kojima T, et al. Evaluation of diagnostic criteria of acute renal failure in premature infants. Acta Paediatr Jpn. 1993;35(4):311-5.
25. Piscator M. Early detection of tubular dysfunction. Kidney Int Suppl. 1991;34:S15-7.
26. Greenough A. Use and misuse of albumin infusions in neonatal care. Eur J Pediatr. 1998;157(9):699-702.
27. Gouyon JB, Guignard JP. Management of acute renal failure in newborns. Pediatr Nephrol. 2000;14(10-11):1037-44.
28. Gerstman BB, Kirkman R, Platt R. Intestinal necrosis associated with postoperative orally administered sodium polystyrene sulfonate in sorbitol. Am J Kidney Dis. 1992;20(2):159-61.
29. Puliyanda DP, Harmon WE, Peterschmitt MJ, et al. Utility of hemodialysis in maple syrup urine disease. Pediatr Nephrol. 2002;17(4):239-42.
30. Steele BT, Vigneux A, Blatz S, et al. Acute peritoneal dialysis in infants weighing less than 1500 g. J Pediatr. 1987;110(1):126-9.
31. Donckerwolcke RA, Bunchman TE. Hemodialysis in infants and small children. Pediatr Nephrol. 1994;8(1):103-6.
32. Sadowski RH, Harmon WE, Jabs K. Acute hemodialysis of infants weighing less than five kilograms. Kidney Int. 1994;45(3):903-6.
33. Goldstein SL, Currier H, Graf CD, et al. Outcome in children receiving continuous venovenous hemofiltration. Pediatrics. 2001;107(6):1309-12.
34. Stapleton FB, Jones DP, Green RS. Acute renal failure in neonates: incidence, etiology and outcome. Pediatr Nephrol. 1987;1(3):314-20.
35. Flynn JT. Hypertension in the neonatal period. Curr Opin Pediatr. 2012;24(2):197-204.
36. Dionne JM, Abitbol CL, Flynn JT. Hypertension in infancy: diagnosis, management and outcome. Pediatr Nephrol. 2012;27(1):17-32.
37. Xiao N, Tandon A, Goldstein S, et al. Cardiogenic shock as the initial presentation of neonatal systemic hypertension. J Neonatal Perinatal Med. 2013;6(3):267-72.
38. Hoppe B, Duran I, Martin A, et al. Nephrocalcinosis in preterm infants: a single center experience. Pediatr Nephrol. 2002;17(4):264-8.
39. Schell-Feith EA, Kist-van Holthe JE, van Zwieten PH, et al. Preterm neonates with nephrocalcinosis: natural course and renal function. Pediatr Nephrol. 2003;18(11):1102-8.
40. Schell-Feith EA, Kist-van Holthe JE, van der Heijden AJ. Nephrocalcinosis in preterm neonates. Pediatr Nephrol. 2010;25(2):221-30.

# Index

Page numbers followed by *b* refer to box, *f* refer to figure, *fc* refer to flowchart, and *t* refer to table.

## A

Abdomen 125
Abdominal wall defects 182
Abdominopelvic ultrasound 186
Abruptio placenta 105, 106
Absent pulmonary valve syndrome 220
Abuse 427
Accurate diagnosis 177
Acetaminophen 382
Acetyl coenzyme A 332
Acetylcholine 277
Acetylcholinesterase 155
Acquired hydrocephalus 193
Acrocyanosis 122
Actinomycetales 278
Activated clotting time 208
Acute kidney injury
   management of 459
   postrenal 458
   prerenal 457
Addiction medicine 390
Adenosine triphosphate 328, 332
Adequate prenatal folate 5
Adiposal triglycerides 332
Advanced practice
   nurse 79
   provider 65
      role of 65
   registered nurses 67
Adverse childhood event 60
African-American infants 125
Air displacement plethysmography 324
Alanine aminotransferase 446
Alcohol 392
   spectrum disorders, fetal 392
Alfentanil 382
Allantois, developmental anomalies of 187
Alport's syndrome 193
Altman's classification 185*f*
Altruists 89
Alveolar capillary dysplasia 224
Alveolar gas equation 435*t*
Alveolar-arterial oxygen gradient 206
American Academy of Pediatrics 71, 137, 146, 193, 197, 200, 328, 340, 367, 378
American Board of Internal Medicine 72
American Board of Medical Subspecialties 70
American Board of Pediatrics 70
American College of Obstetrician and Gynecologists 100, 104
American Heart Association 197
American Speech-language Association 201
Amino acids 286, 331
   essential 333, 333*t*
Ammonia 286
Amniocentesis 155, 156
Amphetamine 394
Amplatzer duct occluder II 239
Amplitude-integrated electroencephalography 268
   addition of 7
Anal atresia 423, 452, 453
Ancient egyptian depiction 136*f*
Ancillary testing 217
Anemia 322
Anesthesia, infant 191
Angiotensin-converting enzyme 456
   inhibitors 461
Animal milks 356
Anomalous left coronary artery 216
Anomalous pulmonary venous return, partial 216, 221
Anorectal malformations 180
   classification of 187*b*
Antenatal care 101
Antenatal corticosteroids 95, 96
Antenatal glucocorticoids 236
Antenatal steroid 17, 235
   therapy 246
Antepartum risk factors 113
Anthropologic evidence 137
Antibiotic 97
   exposure 279
Antiepileptic drugs 287
Antimicrobial therapy 28
Antithrombin 208
Aorta 219*f*
   coarctation of 198, 216, 218
   critical coarctation of 216
Aortic arch 216
   descending 212
   interrupted 216, 218, 220
Aortic stenosis 198, 218
Aortopulmonary collateral arteries, major 215
Aplasia cutis congenita 416, 416*f*
Apnea 166, 237
   treatment of 15
Appendectomy 184
Approach institutional funders 88
Arachidonic acid 332
   metabolism 228*f*
Arginine 370
Arrhythmia 215, 217
   managing fetal 214
Arterial blood
   gas 286
   saturation of 208
Arteriovenous malformation 217
Ash leaf macule 406, 406*f*
Aspartate aminotransferase 446
Asphyxia 27
Asymmetric crying facies 123
Atrial septal defect 217, 225
Atrioventricular canal 218
Attention deficit hyperactivity disorder 275
Audible grunting 122
Auditory neuropathy 192
Autism in toddlers 302, 310
Autism spectrum disorders 275
Automated auditory brainstem response 194, 197
Autopsy results 52

## B

Babel problem, tower of 33
Baby's medical condition, severity of 63
Bacillales 279
Bacteroidales 278
Bacteroides 278, 279
Ballard maturational assessment 121
Ballard score 121
Balloon atrial septostomy 221
Bariatric surgery 352
Basic laboratory investigations 171
Battelle developmental inventory screening tool 309
Battlefield injuries 14
Behavior disorders 275
Behavior function 390
Bench-to-bedside 266
Benzodiazepines 288
Beraprost 230
Beta-human chorionic gonadotropin 155
Bicuspid aortic valve 218
Bifidobacteria 279
Bifidobacterium 278, 279
Bilateral renal agenesis 457
Bile acid biosynthesis, defects of 448
Bile salt-stimulated lipase 334
Biochemical disorder, variety of 171
Biochemical laboratory studies 172*b*
Biochemical maternal serum screening tests 156
Birth asphyxia 24, 96, 112, 113
   prevention of 21
   severe 192

Birth attendants 26
Birth defects 160
    congenital 427
Birth trauma 123f
Blood
    culture 286
    gas monitoring 247
    pressure 460
        low diastolic 237
    stream infections 48
    transfusion 367
        number of 17
    urea nitrogen 169, 172, 350, 458
    vessels, abnormal development of 15
Blood-brain barrier 277
Bloodstream infections 365
Blue-gray spot 406, 407f
Body composition 321
    analysis 324
Body electrolytes 321
Body fluids and solids, composition of 325
Body mass index 324
Body oriented therapy 392
Bone
    morphogenetic protein 451
        receptor 2 226
    neonatal 423
Brachial plexus injury 98
Brachioplexopathy 427
Bradycardia 381
    fetal 214
Bradyrhizobiaceae 279
Brain
    development 255
        fetal and neonatal 253
    injury, risk of 275
    structure and function 5
    volumes, maturational changes in 305f
Brain-derived neuronal growth factor, release of 265
Brainstorming maps 49
Branchio-oto-renal syndrome 193
Breast
    function of 357
    milk, human 333
Breastfeeding 380
    conditions promoting 358
    contraindications of 361
    establishing full 360
Breathing pattern 122
Bronchopulmonary dysplasia 15, 223, 226, 236, 246, 437
Bubble
    continuous positive airway pressure 247
    use of 53
Buprenorphine therapy 396

## C

Café-au-lait macule 405f
CAKUT, management of 456
Calcium 286, 334, 335t
    channel blockers 461
Caloric requirements 331t
Calorie-protein-mineral content 350t, 351t
Cannabinoid 390
Caput succedaneum 123
Carbohydrate 331, 332
    disorders 168
    enteral 332
Carbon dioxide, partial pressure of 179, 246
Cardiac axis
    and size, normal fetal 212f
    fetus with varying 212f
Cardiac catheterization, indications for 221
Cardiac defects 217t, 423, 452, 453
    congenital 218t
Cardiomyopathy 170, 221
Cardiopulmonary bypass 205, 220
Cardiorespiratory disorders 203, 244
Cardiovascular management 247
Careful physical examination 162
Catheters, malposition of 50f
Centers for Disease Control 293
    and Prevention 6, 147, 192
Centers for Medicare and Medicaid Services 67
Central nervous system 127, 208, 285, 305, 339, 340, 411
    developmental 82
    injury 295, 301
Central referral hospital 25
Cephalohematoma 123
Cerebellar injury 302
Cerebral artery, anterior 266
Cerebral calcifications 194
Cerebral complications 192
Cerebral infarction 82
Cerebral palsy 112, 116, 275, 280, 300, 301, 305-308, 313
    hierarchical classification of 308fc
    surveillance of 307
Cerebral thrombosis 82
Cerebrospinal fluid 169, 286, 297
Certified nurse midwife 67
Certified registered nurse anesthetist 67
Cesarean section 17, 146, 367
CHARGE syndrome 193
Chest 124
    auscultation of 125
    reveals, palpation of 125
Chickenpox 419f
Child developmental inventory 309
Child with birth defects, evaluation of 161

Child's neonatal intensive care unit 60
Children's healthy emotional development 60
Chorioamnionitis 293
Chorionic villus sampling 155, 156
Chorioretinitis 194
Chromosomal syndrome 215
Chromosome
    abnormalities 160
        risk of 157t
    analysis 155
    microarray 155, 158, 162
Circadian rhythm 4
Circuit diagram 207f
Cirumcised penis 139f
Clarity and focus, cognitive tool for 36
Cleft lip 360
Cleft palate 360
Clinical nurse specialist 65
Clinical practice variability 237
Clostridia 278
Clostridiales 278, 279
Clostridium 278
    difficile 279
    tetani 248
    tyrobutyricum 277
Clubfoot 428
Coagulase-negative staphylococci 278
Cocaine 394
Coenzyme A 339
Collaboration facilitates continuity 51
Collodion baby 412, 412f
Colonic atresias 181
Community health workers 26, 82
Community-acquired pneumonia, improving 72
Comparative genomic hybridization 200
Complete blood
    count 147
    panel 286
Conducting funder research 87
Congenital abnormalities, clinical features of 453t
Congenital constriction band syndrome 429f
Congenital disorders, causes of 4f
Congenital malformations 141
Conotruncal defect 217
Continuous positive airway pressure 15, 25, 259, 312, 437
Continuous renal replacement therapy 460
Continuous venovenous hemodiafiltration, use of 460
Contraception 164
Cor triatriatum 227
Cord
    blood registries 7
    clamping 5
    disorder of 109

Corynebacterium 279
COVID-19 201
Cow protein formula 334
Coxsackie 285
Cranial nerves 255
Cranial ultrasonography 297, 299
Craniofacial anomalies 360
Craniofacial malformations 193
C-reactive protein 425
Creatinine 286
Critical aortic stenosis 221
Critical congenital heart disease 5, 191, 196, 200
Critical pulmonary valve stenosis 221
Crossing quality chasm 46
Cryptorchidism 126
Cutis marmorata 404, 404f
Cyanosis 215
	treatment of 15
Cyanotic heart disease 322
Cyclic adenosine monophosphate 229
Cyclic guanosine monophosphate 227
Cyclooxygenase-2 296
	inhibitors 457
Cystic kidney disease 125
Cystic periventricular leukomalacia 293, 306
Cytomegalovirus 193, 285, 446, 447, 462

**D**

Data
	collection of 33
	Modeler's design 35
	multiple sources of 47
	sources of 47
Database design, implementation of 38
Database software application report 42f
Delayed cord clamping 5, 351
Denver developmental screening tests 310
Deoxyribonucleic acid 211, 328, 339
	maternal mitochondrial 193
Depressed tone 112
Depression, long-term 265
Detect developmental abnormalities 126
Dexmedetomidine 382
Diabetes 98
Diabetic mothers, infants of 265
Diaphragmatic hernia
	anterior 182
	congenital 179, 206, 208, 212, 212f, 223, 428
Dickens' character sairey gamp 14
Dimercaptosuccinic acid 459
Diphosphoglycerate 436
Discharge planning 76, 361
Disease burden 3
Disease progression, stages of 4f
Disseminated intravascular coagulation 369

Diuretics 459, 461
Docosahexaenoic acid 332, 342
Donabedian's triad 46
Donor
	human milk 279, 346, 349, 350
	recognition 90b
Dopamine 277, 459
Double outlet right ventricle 218
Double-check methods 52
Double-outlet right ventricle 7
Down syndrome 157
Driving brain development 264
Dual diagnosis disorder 395
Ductal areteriosus 235
Ductal arterial sensitivity 237
Ductal closure, physiology of 236
Ductus arteriosus 212, 243
	closure 238
Ductus venosus 243
Duodenal atresia 180f
Duodenal obstruction 180
Duodenojejunal junction 184
Dwarfism 426
Dynasts 89
DYNC2H1 gene 163
Dysmorphology syndrome 215
Dysplasia 453
Dystrophic epidermolysis bullosa 415

**E**

Ear 123
	anatomy, cross-section of 192f
	nose, and throat 195
Early infantile epileptic encephalopathy 167, 169
Early intervention services 314
Eat, sleep, console 149
Ebstein's anomaly 220
Echocardiogram 211, 218
Echocardiography 186
Ectopia cordis 182
Education
	and training 53
	partnerships for 23
Educational curriculum for providers 23
Educational interventions 21
Educational outcomes 27
Egyptian tomb 136
Electrocardiogram 217
Electrocardiography 170
Electroencephalogram 116, 284
Electroencephalography 313
Electrolyte 327, 327t, 458
Electronic database 31
Electronic fetal heart rate monitoring 115
Electronic health record 53
Electronic medical record 50f
Electronic neonatal intensive care unit 34, 35f

Embracing maternal social and cultural context 361
Embryology 236
Emergency department 395
Emergent ororhythmic motor behaviors 258
Emerging modalities 379
Encephalopathy, moderate-to-severe 127t
Encryption 43
End preventable deaths 22
Endocannabinoid type 1 receptor 393f
Endocrine
	disorder, variety of 171
	imbalances 324
Endothelial cells 228f
Endothelial nitric oxide synthase 228f
Endothelin 226, 228f
	converting enzyme 228f
Endotracheal tube 15
End-stage renal disease 452, 453
Engorgement and milk stasis 359
Enteral feeding 367
Enteral feeds, osmolality of 350t
Enteral nutrition 347
Enteral protein 334
Enteral tubes 444
Enteric nervous system 276
Enterobacter 278, 279
Enterobacteriaceae 278
Enterobacteriales 279
Enterococci 278
Enzyme disorders 8
Epidermal growth factor 366
Epidermal nevus 409, 409f
Epidermal skin, development of 326
Epidermolysis bullosa 415
	simplex 415, 415f
Epinephrine 277, 381
Episodes, stroke-like 441
Epithelial barrier 366
Epithelial cells 356
Epoprostenol 229
Erectile dysfunction 67
Errors, types of 52
Erythema toxicum neonatorum 418, 418f
Erythrocyte sedimentation rate 425
Erythropoietin 370
	high dose 6
Escherichia 279
	coli 147, 248, 279, 294, 337, 359
	sepsis 168
Esophageal atresia 177
Esophageal perforation 248
Essential modulator gene 416
European extracorporeal life support organization 206
Extracellular fluid 325f
	electrolytes in 325
Extracorporeal life support 205
	anticipated survival with 209

contraindications to 207
mode of 207
organization 205, 206
Extracorporeal membrane oxygenation 12, 82, 179, 193, 205, 206
circuit 207
management 208
Extramedullary hematopoiesis 194
Extrauterine growth
requirements 323t
restriction 324
Extremities, congenital abnormalities of 122
Eyes 123

## F

Face 123
congenital abnormalities of 122
Facial coding system, neonatal 379
Facial dysmorphism 171
Facial expressions 379
Facilitated tucking 380
Family centered care 18, 77
Family integrated care 5, 59, 61
Fat 356
soluble 321
Fatty acid 356
essential 332
oxidation defect 167
long-chain 170
oxidation disorder 167, 168, 171
Feeding after discharge 352
Feeding difficulties 166
Feeding preterm 359
Fentanyl 382
Fetal alcohol syndrome 392
Fetal circulation 244f
Fetal echocardiogram
level 2 212t
limitations of 213
Fetal echocardiography, role of 211
Fetal growth 331t
Fetal monitoring 97
Fetal surgery 16
success of 186
Fetal ultrasound 179
Fetus
and newborn, renal function in 451
function in 153
Fibroblast growth factor 2 451
Fibular absence 429f
First-trimester diagnosis 157
Flattened facial profile 171
Fluids 325
Fluorescent in-situ hybridization 218
studies 200
Food and Drug Administration 195, 239, 288, 437
Food and Drug Association 229
Foundation of honesty 53

Foundations of Philanthropy Program 86
Four-chamber view, fetal 211f
Fractures 425
Functional residual capacity 245
Funding proposals 90
Furosemide 459

## G

Galactosemia 168, 173
Gamma-aminobutyric acid 277, 390
activation of 287
Gamma-glutamyl transferase 446
Gangrene 425
Gastric bubble 212f
Gastroesophageal reflux disease 441-443, 443t
Gastrointestinal anastomosis 181
Gastrointestinal disease 356
neonatal 441
Gastrointestinal reflux disease 449
Gastrojejunal feeding 444
Gastroschisis 182, 184
reduction 182f
Gastrostomy tube 444
Genetic counseling 156
Genetic defects 218t
Genetic hearing loss 193
Genetic tests, consideration of 162
Genital mutilation 8
Genitalia 125
female 126
male 126
Genitourinary 461
Gestational age 34, 213, 235, 245, 258, 278, 293, 296, 306, 307f, 322, 345, 347-349, 369, 377
appropriate for 321, 349
assessment 121
large for 98, 122, 244, 323, 349
small for 114, 122, 244, 311f, 323, 333, 346, 349
Gestational diabetes mellitus 98, 99
Giant congenital nevus 410f
GJB2 gene 193
GJB6 gene 195
Glial fibrillary acid protein cells 265
Glial-derived neurotropic factor 451
Glomerular filtration rate 288, 451, 452t
Gluconeogenesis disorders 168
Glucose 381
infusion rate 332
solutions 15
transporter deficiency 167
Glutamine 370
Glycine encephalopathy 173
Glycogen storage disease 168
Glycosylation, congenital disorders of 167, 168
Gomco clamp 138, 139, 139f
Gore-tex synthetic patch 180

Great arteries
dextro-transposition of 211, 215, 219
transposition of 198
Gross motor function classification score 307, 309, 312
Growth factors 356
Growth failure 322
Growth velocity 323
Guanidinoacetate methyltransferase deficiency 167
Gut motility, impaired 381
Gut-microbiota
dysbiosis 278
neonatal 278
Gut-microbiota-brain axis 276
factors affecting 276t

## H

Haemophilus influenzae 424
Hand hygiene 49fc
Haptocorrin 334
Harlequin ichthyosis 412
Head and neck 122
Head lag, absence of 127
Healthcare Delivery and Hearing Programs 196
Healthcare
education and informatics, role of 4
facilities in rural areas 82
improvement, institute for 46
infections 53
outcome, improves 46
provider, role of 131, 133
research and quality's, agency of 52
services delivery 57
systems, manner of 3
Hearing aids, conventional 195
Hearing loss
acquired 193
diagnosis of 197fc
nonmedical treatments for 196f
prevalence of 192
resources on 201t
sensorineural 192
Heart defect
congenital 211, 215, 216, 216t, 219, 219f, 220, 221
risk of 157t
Heart disease 125
congenital 5, 7, 209, 211, 223, 227, 246
Heart failure, congenital 457
Heart rate 217
fetal 115, 214
Heel stick 26
Helping babies breathe 4, 25
Hemangioma 408, 408f
congenital 408
Hemolytic disease 17
Hemorrhage
diagnosis of intraventricular 297

intracerebral 207, 311f
postpartum 17
subgaleal 123
Hepatitis C 4, 390
Hepatocyte growth factor 451
Hepatology and nutrition 442
Hepatorenal tyrosinemia 168
Hereditary acrodermatitis enteropathica 413, 413f
Hereditary hemorrhagic telangiectasia 226
Hereditary tyrosinemia 173
Heritable cystic kidney diseases 455
Herniated viscera 183
Herpes 193, 285
Herpes simplex 447
virus 141, 419, 419f
Heterogeneity, wide spectrum of 3
Heterotaxia 184
Heterotaxy syndrome 214
High reliability organizations, hallmarks of 46
High-risk infant 74, 75
High-tech data bases 33
Hindgut, developmental anomalies of 187
Hip dysplasia, congenital 427
Holocarboxylase synthetase deficiency 173
Home visitation, alternatives to 81
Homunculus 299f
Human factors, management and 31
Human immunodeficiency virus 141, 224, 390
maternal 361
Human microbiota studies, evidence from 276
Human milk 332, 346, 347, 355
advantages of 356
Banking Association 361
composition 355
studies of 356
lactation 355
oligosaccharides 332, 367
stem cells 356
Human papillomavirus 141
Human randomized trials 6
Hyaline membrane disease 13, 15, 209, 235, 245
Hydronephrosis 455
Hydroxyglutaric aciduria 171
Hygiene disorders 4
Hyperammonemia 172
Hyperbilirubinemia 98, 145, 192
screening 148
Hyperextension, congenital 430
Hyperglycemic milieu 99
Hyperinsulinism 168
hyperammonemia syndrome 171
Hyperkalemia 458, 459

Hyperoxia
harmful effects of 434b
test 200, 218
Hypertension 99, 459
etiology of neonatal 460b
neonatal 460
Hypertonia 166
Hypocalcemia 285
Hypoglycemia 145, 168, 171, 285
management of 145
neonatal 171
screening 146
Hypomagnesemia 285
Hyponatremia 458
Hypoplasia 453
Hypoplastic left heart 220
syndrome 198, 214, 216, 218, 227
Hyporeflexia 112
Hypotension 381
Hypothermia 313f
Hypotonia 166
Hypoxemic defects 198
Hypoxia, chronic 322
Hypoxic-ischemic encephalopathy 7, 112, 127, 128, 193, 284, 292, 308, 312
infants with 127

I

Idiopathic-persistent pulmonary hypertension 206
Illicit substances 5
Illness, recognition of 26
Iloprost 229
In vitro fertilization 114
Inadequate protein 322
Incontinentia pigmenti 416, 417f
Incubator baby side 13, 13f
Individual donors, funding from 89
Individual healthcare experience 5
Individual with Disabilities Education Act 314
Indocin blocks prostaglandin E2 369
Infant bonding 76
Infant development 300
Bayley scale of 295, 295f, 307
Infant fed human milk 349
Infant mental health 5
Infant respiratory distress syndrome 243, 245, 246
Infant sepsis evaluation 72
Infantile hemangiomas 408
Infantile psoriasis 414
Infection 24, 96
control 25, 29
Infectious disease, resurgence of 4
Infertility 109
Information
age of 4
management system 38, 44b

system 33
technology 44, 53
Innate immunity 366
Inpatient paediatrics, value in 71
Inspired oxygen, fraction of 246
Institutional funders, funding from 88
Insulin-like growth factor 322, 369, 433
Intelligence quotient 293, 306, 308
Interleukin 293, 368
International Business Machines Corporation 36
International Council of Nurses 68
International Lactation Consultants Association 355
Intestinal atresia, type II 181f
Intestinal epithelial cells 366
Intestinal malrotation occurs 183
Intestinal microbiota 366
Intestinal perforation 365
Intimate mother-infant connection 60
Intracardiac defects 182
Intracellular fluid 325, 325f
Intralipid 333
Intraluminal pressure 260f
Intramural course 216
Intrapartum 114
infections
recognition of 29
treatment of 29
Intrauterine fetal demise 131
Intrauterine growth
restriction 113, 194, 265, 323, 328, 340
retardation 447
velocity 349t
Intrauterine transtibial amputation 429f
Intravenous
fluids 369
immune globulin 17
initiation of 216
lipids 333
Intraventricular hemorrhage 5, 235, 275, 286, 292, 295, 296, 297, 299, 300, 459
prophylaxis 369
risk factors for 296
risk of 306
severe 381
Invasive diagnostic testing 156
Iron 336
Isolated intestinal perforation 369
Isovaleric acid, derivatives of 172
Isovaleric acidemia 173

J

Jaundice 166, 194, 360
Jejunoileal atresias 181
Jervell and Lange-Nielsen syndrome 193
Joint commission 52
Joint Commission on Infant Hearing 192
Joints, neonatal 423

Junctional epidermolysis bullosa 415
Juvenile xanthogranuloma 411, 411f

## K

Kangaroo mother care 26, 27
Kangaroo pump 15
Kaplan-Meier curve 313f
Karyotype 200
Ketamine 383
Kidney 453t
    congenital anomalies of 451
    disease, chronic 452, 453
    enlarged 125
    injury, acute 451, 457
        etiology of 457
    malformations, congenital anomalies of 452
Klebsiella 248
Klippel-Feil syndrome 193
Knee, hyperextension of 430

## L

Labor monitoring 97
Lactate dehydrogenase 446
Lactational amenorrhea method 361
Lactic acidosis 441
    congenital 167, 168
Lactobacillales 279
Lactobacillus 276, 278, 279
    species 279
Lactoferrin 334, 356
Lactoperoxidase 334
Lactose 356
Langerhans cell histiocytosis 413, 413f
Laparoscopy 188
Laryngeal nerve, superior 257
Late onset sepsis 294, 295f
    and prematurity 294
Latent errors, method of investigating 53
Left suprasternal view, high 219f
Left ventricular
    ejection fraction 224
    outflow tract 211, 212f, 216
Lethargy 166
Leukocytes 356
Levetiracetam 288
Lidocaine 288, 381
Limb
    abnormalities 423, 452, 453
    deficiencies 429
Lipopoly saccharide 368
Listeria 248
Liver disease 170, 447t
    alcoholic 391
    chronic 433
        intestinal failure-related 448
        neonatal 441, 445, 446
Liver function tests 169, 286
Local capacity, strengthening of 29
Long-term potentiation 265

Lorazepam 382
Low birth weight 295, 300, 311, 321, 326, 365
Low gestational age newborns 300, 310
Low-cost Infection Control Program 28
Lower motoneuron 257f
    pools 256f
Lower respiratory tract 356
Lumbosacral hemangioma 409
Lung disease
    cause of developmental 226
    chronic 82, 223, 247, 265, 311f, 325, 326, 328, 333, 339, 340, 442
    developmental 226
Lung rest 208
Lysosomal storage disorders 167, 168, 170, 171
Lysozyme 334

## M

Macronutrient 331
    caloric intake 331t
Magnesium 286, 334, 336t
    disorders 335t
Magnetic resonance imaging 179, 301
    functional 258, 276
Magnetic resonance spectroscopy 169
Malaria prophylaxis 24
Male circumcision
    global map of 137f
    prevalence 137
Maple syrup urine disease 167, 168
Marijuana 5
Mass spectrometry 166
Massage therapy 381
Masticatory central pattern generation 258
Mastitis 359
Mastocytosis 416
Maternal and child health 24f
Maternal and neonatal injury 109
Maternal body mass index 100
Maternal data, table of 35
Maternal disease, contribution of 98
Maternal experience 61
Maternal factors 113
Maternal health and preconception care 5
Maternal illness, chronic 132
Maternal microbiota changes 278
Maternal-fetal medicine 211
Mature milk 351t
Mean pulmonary arterial pressure 224
Meatal stenosis 140
Mechanical ventilation 25, 237, 248
Meckel-Gruber syndrome 161
Meconium aspiration 243
    syndrome 205, 243, 248
Medical community 77
Medical management, planning for 162

Medical stabilization 177
Medical suppliers 21
Medication errors 52
    bar coding for 53
Medications substances 5
Medium congenital nevus 410f
Medium-chain triglycerides 15
Melanocytic nevus, congenital 410
Membranes
    disorder of 104
    premature rupture of 104, 293
        preterm 96, 97, 104
Mental developmental index 295f, 300, 307, 311f
Mental health 4, 59
    conditions, pre-existing 63
    professionals 62
Mercaptoacetyltriglycine lasix renal scan 459
Mesenteric artery, superior 183
Metabolic acidosis 172, 237, 458, 459
    encephalopathy
        with 170
        without 168
    evidence of 113
    neonatal 172
Metabolism, inborn errors of 166, 167b, 169, 173t, 446, 447
Methadone, chronic 396
Methamphetamine 391, 394
    associated psychosis 394
Methicillin-resistant *Staphylococcus aureus* 359
Methylmalonic acid, derivatives of 172
Methylmalonic acidemia 173
Mevalonic acidemia 167
Microbe-associated molecular products 366
Microbiota 280
    colonization occur 278
    gut-brain signaling pathways 276
Microcephaly 193
Microminerals 339t, 342
Micronutrients 331, 337
Microphthalmia-associated transcription factor 408
Midazolam 382
Miliaria 418
    crystallina 419f
    rubra 418f
Milk
    ejection reflex 359
    expression, methods of 360
Millennium development goal 85, 95
Milrinone 230
Mimic intrauterine growth velocity 323t
Minimal enteral nutrition 345, 346
Minimal neural circuitry 256, 257
Minimum enteral nutrition 334
Miscarriage 131
    causes of 132

Mitochondrial disease 173
Mitochondrial disorders 168, 171, 173
Mitochondrial encephalomyopathy 441
Mitochondrial inheritance 167
Mitral stenosis 227
Mitral valve prolapse 218
Modulate brain activity 264
Molybdenum cofactor deficiency 173
Mongolian spot 406, 407f
Morbidity and mortality, neonatal 95
Morbidly adherent placenta 104, 107
Morphine 382
    6-glucuronide 382
Mother's own milk 279, 340, 346, 350, 365
Mother's unique identifier 35
Mother-infant separation 60
Müllerian duct, developmental anomalies of 187
Multicystic dysplastic kidney 453
Multidisciplinary team 77
Multifetal gestation 109
Multiple acyl-CoA dehydrogenase deficiency 168, 173
Multisensorial stimulation 381
Murmur 215, 217
Muscle tone 379
Muscular dystrophies, congenital 167
Music therapy 381
Mycoplasma spp 368

### N

Nasogastric tube 177
National Association of Neonatal Nurse Practitioners 66
National Association of Pediatric Gastroenterology 442
National Certification Testing 14
National Institute of Child Health and Human Development 260, 296, 313
    Neonatal Research Network 293, 310
National Institutes of Health 192, 248
National Perinatal Association 59, 61
Natriuretic peptide, B-type 237
Natural disease progression 4
Near-infrared spectroscopy 7, 258, 269
Necrotizing enterocolitis 183, 184, 247, 277, 295, 295f, 311f, 321, 334, 346, 356, 365, 367, 443
    incidence of 236
    mediators of 368
    pathogenesis of 366
Necrotizing fasciitis 425
Neonatal abstinence syndrome 149, 394
    incidence of 75
    treatment of 395
Neonatal care 37
Neonatal cholestasis, causes of 448
Neonatal death worldwide, causes of 293f
Neonatal distress 167

Neonatal electrocardiogram, role of 218
Neonatal encephalopathy 18, 112
    trial 313
Neonatal factors 237
Neonatal intensive care unit 7, 12, 13, 31, 43, 51, 59, 66, 75, 88, 97, 105, 147, 178, 192, 206, 214, 223, 237, 248, 256, 268, 275, 284, 321, 349, 360, 367, 377, 412, 423, 437, 443
Neonatal morbidity and mortality 17
Neonatal mortality 28
    majority of 21, 27
    worldwide, cause of 28
Neonatal opiate withdrawal syndrome 148, 149
Neonatal Pain Control Programs 378
Neonatal Research Network 260, 296, 300, 301, 313
Neonatal resuscitation 25
    comprehensive 27
    interventions for 27
Neonatal Resuscitation Program 13
Neonatal seizures, recognition of 285
Neonatal surgery, history of 16
Neonate
    exhibit 166
    function in 153
    mouth 32
Neonatology
    evidence-based 3
    special interest group 61
Nephrocalcinosis 461
    etiology of 461
Nephrology in neonate 451
Nephrotoxic medications 457
Neuroblastoma 125
Neurodevelopment function 390
Neurodevelopmental impairment 300, 301, 312
Neurodevelopmental outcome 294, 299
Neurofibromatosis 405
Neuroimaging 173, 301
Neurological dysfunction, bilirubin-induced 148
Neurological injury 117
    neonatal 112
    suspected 128
Neuronal injury and apoptosis 289
Neuroprotection and sensory stimulation 265
Neuropsychological assessment 308
Nevus depigmentosus 406, 406f
Nevus of ito 407f
Nevus sebaceous 409, 409f
Nevus simplex 403
New interventions, trial of 47
Newborn brain, monitoring 268
Newborn care
    continuum of 24f
    enhance 85

    essential 27
    home-based 86
    improve 21
    normal 119
Newborn galactosemia 361
Newborn hearing loss 191, 196
    etiology 192
    risk factors 192
Newborn hearing screening
    guidelines for 197fc
    tests 194
Newborn medicine 1, 4
Newborn pain 377
    management of 377
    scales, different 380t
Newborn physical examination 121
Newborn populations 292
Newborn screening 174
Newborn survival, improving 29
Newborn transition, normal 214
Newborn's posture 122
Nicotinamide adenine dinucleotide phosphate 339
Nicotine 393
Nitric oxide 228f, 368
    inhaled 220, 227, 248
    therapy 206
N-methyl d-aspartate 289
Non-anxious parents 60
Nonbullous congenital ichthyosiform erythroderma 412
Non-Governmental Organization 21, 86
Non-hispanic whites 391
Nonimmune hydrops 168, 171, 171b
Non-nutritive sucking 256, 258, 258f-260f, 380
    benefits of 259
    development of 266
    frequency modulation of 259f
    support 256
Nonpharmacological analgesia 380
Nonprotein nitrogen 356
Nonsteroidal anti-inflammatory drugs 235, 382
Norepinephrine 277
Normal placenta, sonographic appearance of 108f
Nose 123
Novel viral diseases 4
Nuchal translucency 155
    measurement 157t
Nucleus accumbens 394
Nucleus ambiguus 256
Nucleus tractus solitarius 256
Nulliparity 109
Nulliparous term singleton vertex 17
Nurse
    practitioner 65
        neonatal 14, 66
    role, evolution of 14

Nutrition 14, 459
  goal of 321
Nutritional breakdown 350t
Nutritional counseling 24
Nutritional deficits evaluation, specific 324
Nutritional support, stages of 345
Nutritive sucking 257f, 258, 258f, 260, 260f
  swallow central pattern generation 256, 258

## O

Obesity 109
Occipital frontal circumference measurement 322b
Oculocutaneous albinism 408
Oligoanuria 458
Omphalocele 182, 184
Ontology 33
Operative delivery 98
Opiates 394
Opioid 381, 390
  exposed newborns 395
Optimizing neonatal care 5
Oral feeds, time-to-full 268
Organic acidemias 173
Ornithine transcarbamylase 441
Orofacial sensorium 264
Orogastric tube 177, 179
Oromotor pattern generation, building blocks for 255
Orosensory entrainment therapy 259
Orphan diseases 19
Orthopedic problems, common 423
Oscillatory ventilation, high-frequency 12, 206
Osteogenesis imperfecta 426
Osteomalacia 426
Osteomyelitis 424
Osteopenia 322, 426
Ostial stenosis 216
Otoacoustic-evoked emissions 194
Ototoxic medications 192
Oxygen 432
  administration, safety in 434
  in blood
    assessment of 436
      clinical assessment of 436t
  practices 437
  saturation 432
  therapy 230
Oxygenation 432
  index 206

## P

Pain
  and addiction 375
  inducing procedures, common 378t
  management 16, 379
  neglect 377
  newborn's response to 378t
  prevention 379
Pallor and poor pulses 215
Paper-based system 31
Papulosquamous eruption 411
Paralysis 137
Parasympathetic tone 322
Parenchymal liver disease 170
Parental anxiety 76
Parental stress 59
  frequency of 59
  impact of 60
Parenteral calcium 336t
Parenteral carbohydrates 332
Parenteral nutrition 345
  total 336, 340, 345, 347, 349, 350, 366, 448
Parenteral protein 333
Pareto chart 50
Patent ductus arteriosus 199, 215, 217, 218, 224, 235, 237, 325, 369
  closure 238, 239
  diagnosis of 237
  prophylactic treatment of 239
  risk factors of 236
  risk of 247
  treatment 239
    effect of 239
    timing of 239
Paternal experience 61
Pathogenic fecal flora 355
Patient information systems, paper-based 32
Patient safety 7, 51
  and quality 5
  improving 53
Patient Safety Program 53
Peabody picture vocabulary test 299
Peak inspiratory pressure 208
Pectus excavatum 125
Pediatric autopsy, declining 7
Pediatric cardiothoracic surgeons 211
Pediatric Endocrine Society 146
Pediatric nurse practitioner 80
Pediatric surgery 188
Pelvic floor dysfunction, manage 186
Perimembranous 217
Perinatal asphyxia 6, 18, 98, 457
Perinatal factors 236
Perinatal hyperoxia, risk factors for 434b
Perinatal sentinel events 5
Perinatal substance exposure 148
Perineal fistula 187
Peripheral pulmonary stenosis 218
Peritoneal dialysis 460
Periventricular leukomalacia 82, 296, 301, 311f
Peroxisomal biogenesis disorders 171
Peroxisomal disorders 167, 173
Persistent pulmonary hypertension 82, 199, 223, 225, 243, 437
Peutz-Jeghers syndrome 405f
Pharmacological analgesia 381
Pharyngeal perforation 248
Pharyngoesophageal manometry 258
Phenytoin 288
Philanthropy, costs of 90
Phosphate 335
Phosphodiesterase, inhibitor of 5, 227, 230
Phosphorus 321, 334, 335, 335t, 336t
Phototherapy 17
Physician assistant, role of 65
Physiologic parameters 378
Physiologic stress 322
Piebaldism 407, 407f
Placenta 434b
  accreta 107, 108f
    sonographic appearance of 108f
  disorder of 105
  increta 107
  percreta 107
  previa 104, 106, 109
    complete 107f
    diagnosis of 107
    partial 107f
Placental abruption occurs 105
Placental anomalies 7
Placental pathology examinations 7
Placental previa, marginal 107f
Placentation, spectrum of 107f
Plan-do-study-act 46, 50
  cycles 50
Plasma protein A, pregnancy-associated 155
Platelet-activating factor 368
Plus disease 433
Pneumatosis intestinalis 185f
Pneumonia 248
Pneumothorax 52
Point-of-care testing in newborn screening 191
Polycystic kidney 454
  disease 457
    autosomal dominant 454
    autosomal recessive 454
Polydactyly 428
Polymerase chain reaction 194, 367
Polyunsaturated fatty acid, long-chain 332
Ponderal index 324
Pontocerebellar hypoplasia 173
Poor cognitive function 275
Poor feeding 166
Port-wine stain 404, 404f
Positive airway pressure, nasal continuous 246
Positive end-expiratory pressure 208, 238, 438

Positive pressure ventilation, nasal intermittent 246
Postextubation atelectasis 248
Posthemorrhagic hydrocephalus 297
Postmaturity desquamation 411, 411f
Postmenstrual age 256, 264, 278, 300, 365
Postmortem radiograph 7
Postnatal gut microbiota colonization 278
Postnatal hydronephrosis, grading system for 455
Post-traumatic stress disorder 61, 395
Practical nutritional critical periods 349
Precordial pulsations 237
Predominantly veillonella 278
Preeclampsia 99
Pre-extracorporeal membrane oxygenation evaluation 206
Pregestational diabetes 98
Pregnancy
    implications for 392
    loss 129
    management 164
    to community 130
Premature birth, prevention of 17
Premature born 13
Premature infant pain profile 379
Prematurity 24, 27, 95, 295
    anemia of 351
    management of 21
    osteopenia of 351
    prevention 17
Prenatal diagnosis 155, 164
Prenatal female infanticide, selective 8
Prenatal tests, common 155t
Prenatal ultrasound 186
Preterm birth risk reduction 5
Preterm infant 255, 267f, 278, 294
    brain development and injury 280
    late 305, 306
    residual treatment guidelines for 348t
Preterm neonates 302f
Previa, absence of 108f
Prevotella species 279
Primary peritoneal drainage 185
Primitive reflexes 127
Prior pregnancy termination 109
Probiotics 370
Produce admission notes 37
Profound cyanosis 215
Progressive familial intrahepatic cholestasis syndromes 448, 449
Promote ororhythmic sucking activity 264
Prophylaxis 141
Propionibacterium 279
Propionic acid, derivatives of 172
Prostacyclin 228f, 229
    receptor 228f

Prostaglandin 213, 228f, 230
    E1 214, 230
    E2 237
    synthetase inhibitors 238
Protein 321
Proteobacteria 279
Prothrombin time 446
Proton pump inhibitor 444
Providers in different settings, types of 25
Providing skilled delivery care 24
Proximal femoral focal deficiency 429
Prune belly syndrome 457
Pseudomonas 279
Psoriasis 414f
Psychomotor developmental index 295f, 300, 310
Psychosocial function 390
Pubertal menstrual cycles 357
Public health nurse 65
Public safety net system 52
Pulmonary alveolar proteinosis 224
Pulmonary artery 180, 212, 215, 216, 219f, 224, 225f, 248
    end-diastolic pressure 225, 225f
    hypertension 223, 224
    main 212
    pressure, fetal 224
Pulmonary atresia 198, 220, 221
Pulmonary blood flow 214, 215t, 219, 221
    higher 217t
Pulmonary deterioration 237
Pulmonary hypertension 223, 224, 226, 227, 248
    classification of 223, 224b
    diagnosis of 224
    with drugs and toxins 226
    with genetic disorders 226
    world symposium on 223
Pulmonary hypoplasia 224
Pulmonary insufficiency jet 225f
Pulmonary interstitial glycogenosis 224
Pulmonary lymphangiectasia 224
Pulmonary regurgitation 225
Pulmonary valve 218
Pulmonary vascular
    disease 224
    resistance 214, 224, 243
Pulmonary vein 212
    stenosis 226
Pulmonic stenosis 214
Pulse
    oximetry 200fc
        randomized trial 247
    pressure, wide 237
Pupillary light reflexes 4
Putative premotor, schematic of 257f
Pyridoxine-responsive seizures 173
Pyruvate 286
    dehydrogenase deficiency 173

## Q

Quality and safety 46
    principles of 5
Quality improvement 46
    methods in 47
    team, development of 47

## R

Ralstonia 279
Reactive oxygen species 368, 434
Recognize parental emotional distress 62
Red blood cell 340
Red cell membrane, risk of 8
Reflux 441
    high grade 141
Registered nurse 66
Regurgitation 441
    therapies 443t
Relaxation and massage 360
Release reactive oxygen species 296
Remifentanil 382
Renal acute kidney injury 457
Renal and urologic anomalies 409
Renal anomalies 423, 452, 453
Renal artery
    occlusion 457
    thrombosis 457
Renal disease, intrinsic 457
Renal failure, acute 457
Renal function tests 458
Renal replacement therapy 451, 459
Renal scars 141
Renal vein thrombosis 457
Reproduction function 390
Residual foreskin 139f
Respiratory central pattern generator 256
Respiratory compromise 112
Respiratory disease 442
Respiratory distress 215
    developed 163
Respiratory distress syndrome 97, 104, 116, 206, 235, 246, 259, 266, 457
    died of 13
    incidence of 369
Respiratory failure 206
Respiratory management 15
Respiratory support 25
Respiratory syndrome coronavirus 2, severe acute 201
Retinitis pigmentosa 168
Retinopathy of prematurity 15, 229, 236, 332, 339, 340, 432, 433f, 434
    early treatment for 433
    international classification of 433
Retractions 122
Rhesus isoimmunization disease 17
Rickets 426
Right distal
    femur 424f
    tibia 424f

Right ventricle 215, 243
Right ventricular outflow tract 219
Ritual scarring 8
Root cause analysis 53
Rubella 193, 285

## S

Sacrococcygeal teratoma 185, 186
    types of 185*f*
Safety
    culture of 47
    improvement strategy 47
    role in 53
Salmon patch 403, 403*f*
Scabies 419, 419*f*
Scalp injury 123*f*
Scimitar syndrome 227
Screening tools, developmental 309*t*
Seborrheic dermatitis 414, 414*f*, 415*f*
Secretory immunoglobulin A 356
Seizures 166, 169*t*
    etiology of neonatal 284
    neonatal 173, 284
Sensory hair cells 193*f*
Sensory nuclei 257*f*
Sensory stimulation on brain maturation, role of 268
Sepsis 145, 183, 206, 448
    diagnosis of 29
    early-onset 147, 248, 293, 294
    management of 145
    neonatal 292
    screening for 147
    treatment of 25, 29
Septic arthritis 424
Serial fetal echoes 212*f*
Serial transverse enteroplasty procedure 181
Serotonin 390
    reuptake inhibitor, selective 225
Serratia 279
Serum
    alpha-fetoprotein, maternal 182
    bilirubin, total 148
    electrolytes 286
    screening, second-trimester 157
    sodium concentration 32
Sexually transmitted
    diseases 390
    infections 137
Short bowel syndrome 181
Short-chain fatty acids 277, 370
Shunt status 300*t*
Sick children, action for 18
Signal extraction technology 434
Sildenafil 227
Silicone nipple, inside 260*f*
Singleton children, risk factors in 307*f*
Six sigma 47

Skin
    and integumentary system 122
    care, specialized 12
    disorders 403
Sleep-wake cycling 268
Smooth muscle cells 228*f*
Society for Fetal Urology 455
Society for fetal urology grading system 455*f*
Society for Maternal Fetal Medicine 100, 104
Society of Hospital Medicine 72
Sodium, fractional excretion of 452
Soft tissue injury 123*f*
Software program applications 33
Somatosensory cortex 270
Soy protein formula 334
Soybean oil 15
Sphingomonas 279
Sphingomyelin, lecithin to 15
Spinal dysraphism 409
Stanger electrocardiogram wheel 219*f*
Staphylococcal scalded skin syndrome 417, 417*f*
Staphylococcus 278, 279
    aureus 359, 417, 424
Stenosis 220
Stillbirths, rate of 28
Stone formation, inhibitors of 461*t*
Streptococcal disease, group B 294*f*
Streptococci predominate 278
Streptococcus 278, 279, 359, 424
    disease, group B 248
    group B 104, 147, 243, 285, 294
Stress, maternal 279
Stria vascularis 193*f*
Stridor 122
Structural cardiac defects 213
Structural congenital disorders 160
Structural disorders 425
Subcutaneous fat necrosis 409
Subglottic stenosis 248
Subsequent surfactant replacement therapy 17
Substance abuse and mental health services administration 148
Suck central pattern generator 255, 257*f*
Sucrose 381
Sudden infant death syndrome 106, 132
    unexpected 132
Suicide 390
Sulfite oxidase 173
    deficiency 173
Support nutritive sucking 257
Support patient care 33
Supporting implementation, focus on 21
Supravalvar mitral ring 227
Supraventricular tachycardia 214, 216
Surfactant administration 246
Surfactant positive pressure 247

Surfactant therapy 246
Surgical conditions, common 177
Surgical deliveries 7
Surgical errors 52
Surgical repair, timing of 219
Surgical site infections 54
Sustainable family-centered care 18
Swallow central pattern generator 257
Synchronized intermittent mandatory ventilation 208
Syphilis 193
    congenital 4
Systemic vascular resistance 215, 243
Systolic murmur 237

## T

T cells 356
Tachycardia 237
Tachypnea 122, 166, 215, 216
Target oxygen saturations 247
Tblinfants 36
Teamwork and communication errors 53
Telemonitoring 81
Temporal bone abnormalities 193
Teratomas 125
Tetrahydrocannabinol 390, 393
Tetralogy of Fallot 7, 198, 214, 215, 218-220
Therapeutic hypothermia 18
Thermoregulation 13, 25, 247
    importance of 13
    remains vital 13
Thoracoscopic surgery, video-assisted 238
Three-generation pedigree 162*f*
Throat 123
Thrombocytopenia 194, 429
    syndrome 430*f*
Thromboelastography 208
Thyroid stimulating hormone 340
Tissue oxygenation 435*b*
    physiology of 434
Tobacco smoke exposure 393
Tocolysis 97
Topical analgesics 381
Topiramate 289
Total anomalous pulmonary venous return 198, 207, 217, 218
Total body
    cooling 4, 6, 18
    hypothermia 313
    water 324
Toxoplasmosis 193, 285
Tracheoesophageal fistula 177, 423, 452, 453
    classification of 178*f*
Training traditional birth attendants 28
Traintrainers method 23
Transcutaneous bilirubin 148

Transcutaneous water loss, reduce 326, 326t
Transforming growth factor β 226
Transient hyperammonemia 169
Transient neonatal pustular
    dermatosis 418f
    melanosis 418
Transient tachypnea 243, 244, 246
Transport ventilators, days of 14
Treacher Collins syndrome 193
Treponema pallidum 248
Treprostinil 229
Tricuspid annular plane systolic
    excursion 225
Tricuspid atresia 198, 220
Tricuspid regurgitation 224
Tricuspid valve abnormalities 220
Trigeminal complex, mesencephalic
    nucleus of 256
Trisomy 21 syndrome 193
Truncus arteriosus 198, 217, 218
Tuberculosis 137
Tubular function 452
Tubular necrosis, acute 457
Tumor necrosis factor alpha 296, 368
Twins, kangaroo care of 18f

## U

Ultrasound 116, 207, 351
Uniform terminology 34
United Nation's Millennium
    Development 292
United Nations International Children's
    Emergency Fund 74, 82
Unmeasured anions 171
Upper esophageal sphincter 257, 257f
Urea cycle disorders 167, 173

Ureteropelvic junction 455
    obstruction 455f
Urethral injury 140
Urethrocutaneous fistula 140
Urinalysis 458
Urinary tract 453t
    congenital anomalies of 451
    infection 452, 453
        catheter-associated 53
        risk of 141
    malformations, congenital anomalies
        of 452
Useful tools 213
Usher syndrome 193

## V

VACTERL syndrome 193
Varicella 419
    neonatal 419f
Varicella-zoster virus 419
Vasa previa 109
Vascular endothelial growth factor 296
    role of 433
Vasoactive peptide 228f
Vasodilators 461
Velamentous cord insertion 109
Vena cava
    inferior 212
    left superior 218
    superior 212, 219f
Veno-venous 207
Ventral pallidum 394
Ventral swallowing group 256, 257f
Ventricle heart disease 227
Ventricular septal defect 213, 215, 217, 224
Vertebral defects 423, 452, 453

Very low birth weight 66, 75, 236, 265, 294, 312, 348, 349, 365
Vesicoureteral reflux 455
Vesiculopustular eruptions 415
Video interaction guidance 81
Vital signs 217
Vitamin 337t
    D 340
        maternal 337
Voiding cystourethrogram
    grading system 456f
    role of 456
Vomiting 166, 441
    differential diagnosis of 441t

## W

Waardenburg syndrome 193
Waste, reducing overall 46
Water balance, evaluation of 326
Weaning 208
Wechsler intelligence scale 308
Whiskey nipple 16
White matter
    abnormalities 301
        evidence of 300
    injury 295, 301, 302f, 306
Whole exome screening 162
Wilms' tumor suppressor gene 451
Wood units 224
World Health Organization 21, 74, 78, 96, 361, 392

## X

Xanthine oxidase 368

## Z

Zika virus 4, 193
Zinc 370